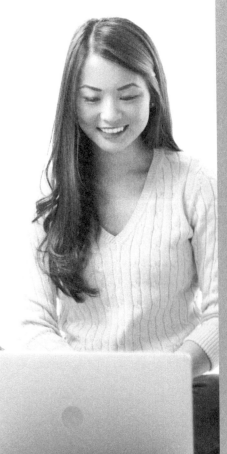

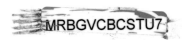

# EDELMAN *and* KUDZMA'S
# Canadian Health Promotion Throughout the Life Span

**Shannon Dames** RN, MPH, EdD
Professor/Researcher
School of Nursing
Vancouver Island University
Nanaimo, British Columbia

**Marian Luctkar-Flude** RN, PhD, CCSNE
Associate Professor
School of Nursing
Queen's University
Kingston, Ontario

**Jane Tyerman** RN, PhD, CCSNE
Assistant Professor
School of Nursing
Faculty of Health Sciences
University of Ottawa
Ottawa, Ontario

US EDITORS

**Carole Lium Edelman** MSN, GCNS-BC, CMC
Private Practice
Professional Geriatric Care Management
Westport, Connecticut

**Elizabeth Connelly Kudzma** DNSc, MPH, WHNP-BC, CNL
Professor
Director of MSN Program
School of Nursing
Curry College
Milton, Massachusetts

ELSEVIER

---

### Notices

Practitioners and researchers must always rely on their own experience and knowledge in evaluating
and using any information, methods, compounds or experiments described herein. Because of rapid
advances in the medical sciences, in particular, independent verification of diagnoses and drug dosages
should be made. To the fullest extent of the law, no responsibility is assumed by Elsevier, authors, editors
or contributors for any injury and/or damage to persons or property as a matter of products liability,
negligence or otherwise, or from any use or operation of any methods, products, instructions, or ideas
contained in the material herein.

---

**Library of Congress Control Number: 2020939702**

VP Education Content: Kevonne Holloway
Content Strategist (Acquisitions, Canada): Roberta A. Spinosa-Millman
Director, Content Development Manager: Laurie Gower
Content Development Specialist: Martina van de Velde
Publishing Services Manager: Shereen Jameel
Senior Project Manager: Umarani Natarajan
Design Direction and Cover Design: Amy Buxton

Last digit is the print number: 9 8 7 6 5 4 3 2 1

Working together
to grow libraries in
developing countries

www.elsevier.com • www.bookaid.org

To the evolving and emerging health care providers throughout Canada, may you experience health and wellness in such a way that it spills over into all that you are and do—to promote health care equity and equality for all Canadians.

**Shannon Dames, Marian Luctkar-Flude, and Jane Tyerman**


To our wonderful families, friends, students, and colleagues—that they promote health in themselves and others.

**Carole L. Edelman and Elizabeth Connelly Kudzma**

# CONTRIBUTORS

**Dr. Ellen Buck-McFadyen, RN, MScN, PhD**
Trent/Fleming School of Nursing
Trent University
Peterborough, Ontario

**Dr. Elsie Duff, BScN, RN, MEd, PhD**
Assistant Professor
College of Nursing
University of Manitoba
Winnipeg, Manitoba

**Dana S. Edge, RN, MSN, PhD**
Associate Professor (retired)
School of Nursing
Queen's University
Kingston, Ontario

**Cindy Fehr, RN, MEd, MScN, NP**
Nurse Practitioner
Family Medicine
Lorne Memorial Hospital, Swan Lake &
    Somerset Clinics
Swan Lake, Manitoba and
    CEO
Nurse Practitioner Association of Manitoba
Winnipeg, Manitoba

**Michelle Funk Borgland, RN, MScN, MHR (Palliative Care)**
Senior Lecturer
School of Nursing
Thompson Rivers University
Kamloops, British Columbia

**Bernie Garrett, RN, PGCE, PhD**
Associate Professor
School of Nursing
University of British Columbia
Vancouver, British Columbia

**Alexa Garrey, RN**
Home and Community Care
Vancouver Island Health Authority
Nanaimo, British Columbia

**Leslie Graham, RN, MN, PhD(c) CHSE, CNCC**
Professor
Faculty of Nursing
School of Health & Community Studies
Durham College
Oshawa, Ontario and
    Adjunct Professor
Faculty of Health Sciences
University of Ontario Institute of Technology
Oshawa, Ontario

**Dianne Groll, RN, PhD**
Associate Professor
Psychiatry
Queen's University
Kingston, Ontario

**Kaitlyn Hall, RN**
Healthy Babies Healthy Children Program
KFL&A Public Health
Kingston, Ontario

**Teresa Hannesson, MSN, BSN**
Professor
Bachelor of Science in Nursing
Vancouver Island University
Nanaimo, British Columbia

**Marti Harder, RN, MSN**
Professor
Bachelor of Science in Nursing
Vancouver Island University
Nanaimo, British Columbia

**Robin Humble, MPH, BSN**
Faculty Lecturer
School of Nursing
Camosun College
Victoria, British Columbia and
    Research Assistant
School of Public Health and Social Policy
University of Victoria
Victoria, British Columbia

**Emily MacLeod, BScN, MN**
Assistant Professor
School of Nursing
Cape Breton University
Sydney, Nova Scotia

**Laurie Peachey, RN, PhD**
Assistant Professor
School of Nursing
Nipissing University
North Bay, Ontario

**Maureen M. Ryan RN PhD**
Teaching Professor
School of Nursing
Faculty of Human and Social Development
University of Victoria
Victoria, British Columbia

**Bahareh Singla, RN, MN**
Congenital Cardiology Clinics
Brampton, Ontario

**Tanya Spence, BSN, MN**
Clinical Nurse Specialist
Pediatric Intensive Care Unit
Alberta Children's Hospital
Calgary, Alberta

**Collette Tattman-Melo, RN, MN-ANP, CCRN, CCN, NP(f)**
Assistant Teaching Professor
School of Nursing, Faculty of Human and
    Social Development
University of Victoria
Victoria, British Columbia and
    Nurse Practitioner
Internal Medicine
Victoria General Hospital
Victoria, British Columbia

**Sarah L. West, MSc, PhD**
Assistant Professor
Biology & Trent/Fleming School of Nursing
Trent University
Peterborough, Ontario and
    Adjunct Scientist
Translational Medicine
The Hospital for Sick Children
Toronto, Ontario

**Barbara Wilson-Keates, RN, MS, PhD**
Academic Coordinator
Faculty of Health Disciplines
Athabasca University
Athabasca, Alberta

**Erin Ziegler, PhD, NP-PHC**
Assistant Professor
Daphne Cockwell School of Nursing
Ryerson University
Toronto, Ontario

## CONTRIBUTORS TO THE US NINTH EDITION

**Lois E. Brenneman, MSN, FNP**
Family Nurse Practitioner and Adjunct
    Faculty
Fairleigh Dickinson University
Teaneck, New Jersey

**Kevin K. Chui, PT, DPT, PhD, GCS, OCS, CEEAA, FAAOMPT**
Director and Professor
School of Physical Therapy
College of Health Professions
Pacific University
Hillsboro, Oregon

**Kristi Coker, PhD, RN**
Director of Nursing for Children's Hospital
Greenville Health System
Greenville, South Carolina

**Donna DelloIacono, NP, PhD, CNL**
Nurse Practitioner
Weiner Center for Preoperative Evaluation
Brigham and Woman's Hospital
Boston, Massachusetts

**Susan Ann Denninger, PT, DPT, PCS**
Physical Therapist
Kidnetics
Greenville Health System
Greenville, South Carolina

**Christine Sorrell Dinkins, PhD**
Associate Professor of Philosophy
Wofford College
Spartanburg, South Carolina

**Susan A. Heady, PhD, RN**
Professor
Webster University
St. Louis, Missouri

**Rosanna F. Hess, BSN, MA, MSN, DNP, RN**
Research Associate
Research for Health, Inc.
Cuyahoga Falls, Ohio

**June Andrews Horowitz, PhD, RN, PMH, CNS-BC, FAAN**
Associate Dean for Graduate Programs & Research and Professor
College of Nursing
University of Massachusetts
Dartmouth, Massachusetts

**Susan Rowen James, PhD, RN**
Professor Emeritus
School of Nursing
Curry College
Milton, Massachusetts

**Debora Elizabeth Kirsch, RN, MS, CNS, PhDc**
Retired Faculty
College of Nursing
SUNY Upstate Medical University
Syracuse, New York

**Carolyn Cable Kleman, PhDc, MHA, BSN, RN**
Doctoral Candidate
Kent State University
Kent, Ohio

**Myrtle McCulloch, EdD, MS, RDN**
Assistant Professor, Nutrition
School of Nursing and Health Studies
Georgetown University
Washington, DC

**Staci McIntosh, MS, RD**
Assistant Professor
Department of Nutrition and Integrative Physiology
University of Utah
Salt Lake City, Utah

**Maureen Murphy, PhD, MSN, MEd, RN, CNM**
Professor
School of Nursing
Curry College
Milton, Massachusetts

**Anne Rath Rentfro, PhD, RN**
Professor (retired)
The University of Texas at Brownsville
Brownsville, Texas

**Susan Scott Ricci, ARNP, MSN, MEd., CNE**
Nursing Faculty
University of Central Florida
Orlando, Florida

**Ratchneewan Ross, PhD, RN, FAAN**
Cone Health Distinguished Professor
Chair, Department of Family and Community Nursing
School of Nursing
University of North Carolina at Greensboro
Greensboro, North Carolina

**Leslie Kennard Scott, PhD, APRN, PPCNP-BC, CDE, MLDE**
Associate Professor
Pediatric Nurse Practitioner BSN-DNP Programs Coordinator
College of Nursing
University of Kentucky
Lexington, Kentucky

**Jeanne M. Sorrell, PhD, RN, FAAN**
Contributing Faculty
Richard W. Riley College of Education and Leadership
Walden University
Minneapolis, Minnesota

**Frank Tudini, PT, DSc, OCS, COMT, FAAOMPT**
Professor
Sacred Heart University
Fairfield, Connecticut

**Diane Marie Welsh, DNP, RN, CNE**
Dean, School of Nursing
Regis College
Weston, Massachusetts

**Sheng-Che Yen, PT, PhD**
Assistant Professor
Department of Physical Therapy, Movement and Rehabilitation Sciences
Northeastern University
Boston, Massachusetts

# REVIEWERS

**Aliyah Dosani, RN, MPH, PhD**
Associate Professor
School of Nursing and Midwifery
Mount Royal University
Calgary, Alberta

**Nancy J. Fleming, RN, HBScN, MA(Ed)**
Professor
School of Health & Community Services
Confederation College
Thunder Bay, Ontario

**Bonnie Fournier, RN, MSc, PhD**
Associate Professor
School of Nursing
Thompson Rivers University
Kamloops, British Columbia

**Cheyenne Joseph, RN, MPH, CCHN(c)**
Senior Instructor
Faculty of Nursing
University of New Brunswick
Moncton, New Brunswick

**Denise Kall, RN, MPH, CCNE**
Professor
School of Baccalaureate Nursing
St. Lawrence College
(Laurentian University – St. Lawrence College
    Collaborative BScN Program)
Brockville, Ontario

**Anne Marie Lewis, RN, MN**
Nurse Educator
Centre for Nursing Studies (Eastern Health)
St. John's, Newfoundland

**Jo-Ann MacDonald, RN, MN, PhD**
Associate Professor
School of Nursing
University of Prince Edward Island
Charlottetown, Prince Edward Island

**Marian MacLellan, RN, MN**
Assistant Professor
Rankin School of Nursing
St. Francis Xavier University
Antigonish, Nova Scotia

**Lynn Miles, RN, PhD**
Professor of Nursing
School of Health, Nursing
Mohawk College
Hamilton, Ontario

**Laralea Stalkie, RN, MSN**
Professor and Program Coordinator
Faculty of BScN Nursing
St. Lawrence College
Kingston, Ontario

## PURPOSE OF THE BOOK

The case for promoting and protecting health, and preventing disease and injury, was established by many accomplishments in the twentieth century and has continued into the twenty-first century. Canadians and global populations are taking better care of themselves; public concerns about physical and mental fitness, good nutrition, and avoidance of health hazards, such as smoking, have become adopted in the lifestyles of global citizens. Health promotion efforts apply to all individuals, the government, health professionals, and society in general. In Canada, historically, public and private attempts to improve the health status of individuals and groups were more focused on reducing communicable diseases and health hazards; however, prevention is more than reduction of disease, and today the paradigm is shifting as we continue to recognize and prioritize the value of health promotion as a necessary and highly effective component of prevention. Concerns continue about how to deliver the best practices to improve access to and reduce costs of health services and to improve the overall quality of life for all people. Canadians increasingly recognize that the health of each individual is influenced by the health environments of all individuals worldwide.

At the helm of *Edelman and Kudzma's Canadian Health Promotion Throughout the Life Span* is the Public Health Agency of Canada (PHAC)'s 2019 mission to promote and protect the health of Canadians through leadership, partnership, innovation, and action in public health. This mission is undergirded by a respect for democracy and for people, integrity, stewardship, and excellence. The PHAC's commitment to Canadians is to promote health; prevent and control chronic disease and injury; prevent and control infection diseases; prepare for and respond to public health emergencies; serve as a central point for sharing Canada's expertise with the rest of the world; apply international research and development to Canada's public health programs; and strengthen intergovernmental collaboration on public health and facilitate national approaches to public health policy and planning.

Historically, the PHAC assessed and tracked the health of Canadians. While many factors intersect to influence health, it is recognized that the determinants of health are chief among these. They are organized into the following 12 main areas:

1. Income and social status
2. Employment and working conditions
3. Education and literacy
4. Childhood experiences
5. Physical environments
6. Social supports and coping skills
7. Healthy behaviours
8. Access to health services
9. Biology and genetic endowment
10. Gender
11. Culture
12. Race/racism

The social and economic factors included in these 12 determinants interplay and interweave with most, if not all, of the other determinants. These factors refer to an individual's social and economic capital. One's status in society is often determined by income, education, employment, race, historical trauma, and the power and influence the "group" a person identifies with in the dominant culture. Some examples of "groups" that individuals in Canada might identify with include Indigenous peoples, LGBTQ2 Canadians, Black Canadians, Asian Canadians, etc.

Even though Canada is among the healthiest countries in the developed world, we continue to grapple with significant health inequities between population groups. To attain health equity, we must continue to strive to improve access to health care services, health promotion opportunities, and contextual and cultural conditions that are more conducive to equitable health and well-being for all Canadians.

Aligning with the Public Health Agency's vision of "Healthy Canadians and communities in a healthier world" (https://www.canada.ca/en/public-health/corporate/mandate/about-agency.html), health-promotion advances require a better understanding of the environment, health risks, behaviours, and intervention measures. Outcome measures designed to assist individual and group efforts to change and improve behaviour in these areas can lead to decreases in morbidity and mortality. Professionals who undertake health-promotion strategies also need to understand the basics of health protection and disease and injury prevention. Health protection is directed at population groups of all ages and involves adherence to standards, outcomes, infectious disease control, and governmental regulation and enforcement. The focus of these activities is on reducing exposure to various sources of hazards, including those related to air, water, foods, drugs, motor vehicles, and other physical agents.

Health care providers present individuals, families, and communities with disease- and injury-prevention services, which include immunizations, screenings, health education, and counselling. To implement prevention strategies effectively, it is essential to develop activities that are targeted to and tailored for all age groups in various settings including schools, industries, the home, the health care delivery system, the larger community, and the world. Health is significantly affected by the environment in which each individual lives, works, travels, and plays. Dimensions of the environment are not only physical but also psychosocial and spiritual, including the behaviours, attitudes, and beliefs of each individual.

## APPROACH AND ORGANIZATION

This First Canadian Edition of *Edelman and Kudzma's Canadian Health Promotion Throughout the Life Span* presents health data with related theories and skills that are needed to understand and practice when providing care. Emerging from what we know about the importance of the determinants of health, this book focuses on primary prevention intervention; its three main components are: (1) health promotion, (2) specific health protection, and (3) prevention of specific diseases. Health promotion is the intervention designed to improve health, such as providing adequate nutrition, a healthy environment, and ongoing health education. Specific protection and prevention strategies, such as massive immunizations, periodic examinations, and safety features in the workplace, are the interventions used to protect against illness.

In addition to primary prevention, this book discusses secondary prevention interventions, focusing specifically on screening and education. Such programs include blood pressure, cholesterol, and diabetes screening and referral (the acute components of secondary prevention are generally not addressed in this book).

This text is presented in four parts, each forming the basis for the next.

Unit 1, *Foundations for Health Promotion,* describes the foundational concepts of promoting and protecting health, and preventing diseases and injuries, including diagnostic, therapeutic, and ethical decision-making within the Canadian health care context. Additional central concepts include cultural humility and cultural safety as they are applied to promoting the health of Canada's diverse population.

Unit 2, *Assessment for Health Promotion,* focuses on individuals, families, and communities and the factors affecting their health. The 11 functional health pattern assessments developed by Marjory Gordon (from her *Manual of Nursing Diagnosis,* 13th edition) serve as the organizing framework for assessing the health of individuals, families, and communities.

Unit 3, *Application of Health Promotion,* also uses Gordon's functional health patterns, emphasizing developmental, cultural, ethnic, and environmental variables in assessing the developing person. The intent is to address the health concerns of all Canadians regardless of gender, ethnicity, age, or sexual orientation. Although most human development theories discussed are primarily based on the research of male subjects, newer theories based on female subjects are included. The hope is to describe human development that more accurately reflects the complexity of human experiences throughout the life span.

Unit 4, *Interventions for Health Promotion,* discusses theories, methodologies, and case studies of nursing interventions, including screening, health-education counselling, stress management, and complementary and alternative strategies. The final chapter discusses changing population groups and their health needs as well as related implications for research and practice in the twenty-first century. Throughout the text, research abstracts have been added to highlight the science of nursing practice and to demonstrate to the reader the relationship among research, practice, and outcomes.

Throughout these units, the evolving health care professions and the changing health care systems, including future challenges and initiatives for health promotion, are described. Emphasis is placed on the current concerns of reducing health care costs while increasing life expectancy and improving the quality of life for all Canadians. This promotes the reader's immediate interest in thoughts about the content of the chapters.

## Key Features

- A **full-colour design,** including colour photos, is implemented throughout for better accessibility of content and visual enhancement.
- Each chapter starts with a list of **learning outcomes** to help focus the reader and emphasize the content the reader should acquire through reading the book.
- **Key Terms** including quality and safety terms are listed at the front to acquaint readers with the important terminology of the chapter.
- Each chapter's narrative begins with a **Think About It** section, the presentation of a clinical issue or scenario that relates to the topic of the chapter, followed by critical thinking questions. This promotes the reader's immediate interest in and thoughts about the chapter.
- **Research for Evidence-Informed Practice** boxes provide brief synopses on current health-promotion research studies that demonstrate the links between research, theory, and practice.
- **Diversity Awareness** boxes offer cultural perspectives on various aspects of health promotion, along with reflection questions to promote critical thinking.
- **Quality and Safety** boxes provide information regarding specific scenarios to improve health.
- **Genomics** boxes explore current genetic issues, controversies, and dilemmas with respect to health promotion, providing an opportunity for critical analysis of care issues.
- **Innovative Practice** boxes highlight inventive and resourceful projects, programs, and research studies that draw upon new ways of implementing health promotion.
- The **Case Study** highlights a real-life clinical situation relevant to the chapter topic.
- The **Care Plan** relates to the Case Study with the standardized sections of Defining Characteristics, Related Factors, Expected Outcomes, and Interventions, and details nursing issues relevant to health-promotion activities and the related interventions.
- **Review Questions** are located on the book's website to offer additional review and self-study practice.

## Features of the First Canadian Edition

- **Comprehensive inclusion** of Canadian statistics, research, references and resources, guidelines, and assessment and screening tools.
- Greater focus on connecting the research and writing with the **determinants of health.**
- A focus on **Canadian experts** speaking from a **Canadian lens.**
- **Greater emphasis placed on a societal level of health promotion** and social justice (including the Public Health Agency of Canada's Population Health Approach model; the Ottawa Charter on Health Promotion; World Health Organization and Alma-Ata Declaration; human rights; the UN Declaration on Rights of Indigenous People; the Truth and Reconciliation Commission's *Calls To Action* recommendations), weaving in the social determinants of health throughout.

- **Inclusion of Canadian cultural considerations**, as they relate to race/ethnicity, Indigenous peoples, identity, the LGBTQ2 community, family composition, and other areas, are threaded throughout all applicable chapters.
- **Fully revised "Health Defined: Health Promotion, Prevention, and Protection" chapter** reflecting the Canadian socio-environmental approach.
- **Fully revised "Diverse Populations in Canada and Health" chapter** reflecting the Canadian demographic landscape.
- **Fully revised "Ethical Issues Related to Health Promotion" chapter** covering the Canadian Nurses Association *Code of Ethics*, the Personal Information Protection Act (PIPA) and Personal Health Information Protection Act (PHIPA), Bill C-14: Medical Assistance in Dying (MAID), principles of bioethics, and more!
- **New!** Reflection Questions added to **Diversity Awareness** boxes, allowing students to reflect on their own personal cultural values while presented with cultural perspectives on various aspects of health promotion.
- **Updated art program** reflecting Canada's cultural diversity in the health care setting.
- **Expanded discussion of nursing competencies** related to health promotion.
- **Guidelines** and recommendations from **Public Health Agency of Canada**

## Evolve Resources

The expanded Evolve website for this book provides materials for both students and faculty, and is accessible at http://evolve.elsevier.com/Canada/Edelman/healthpromotion/.

### For Students
- **Review questions:** multiple choice NCLEX® examination format

### For Instructors
- **TEACH for Nurses,** including Nursing Curriculum Standards, Teaching Activities, and Case Studies
- **Image collection,** with all images from the book
- **Lecture slides,** in PowerPoint
- **Test bank,** 700 questions in NCLEX® examination format

The current trend to emphasize the developing health of individuals and population groups mandates that health care providers understand the many issues that surround individuals, families, national and world communities in social, work, and family settings, including biological, inherited, cognitive, psychological, environmental, and sociocultural factors that can put their health at risk. Most important is that they develop interventions to promote health by understanding the diverse roles these factors play in the person's beliefs and health practices, particularly in the areas of disease and injury prevention, protection, and health promotion. Achieving such effectiveness requires collaboration with other health care providers and the integration of practice and policy while developing interventions and considering the ethical issues within individual, family, and both national and world communities' responsibilities for health.

## NEXT GENERATION NCLEX

The National Council for the State Boards of Nursing (NCSBN) is a not-for-profit organization whose members include nursing regulatory bodies. In empowering and supporting nursing regulators in their mandate to protect the public, the NCSBN is involved in the development of nursing licensure examinations, such as the NCLEX-RN®. In Canada, the NCLEX-RN® was introduced in 2015 and is, as of the writing of this text, the recognized licensure exam required for practising RNs in Canada.

The NCLEX-RN® will, as of 2023, be changing in order to ensure that its item types adequately measure clinical judgement, critical thinking, and problem-solving skills on a consistent basis. The NCSBN will also be incorporating into the examination what they call the Clinical Judgement Measurement Model (CJMM), which is a framework that the NCSBN has created to measure a novice nurse's ability to apply clinical judgement in practice.

These changes to the examination come as a result of research findings which indicated that novice nurses have a much higher-than-desirable error rate with patients (i.e., errors that cause patient harm) and, upon NCSBN's investigation, the discovery that the overwhelming majority of these errors were caused by failures of clinical judgement.

Clinical judgement has been a foundation underlying nursing education for decades, based on the work of a number of nursing theorists. The theory of clinical judgement that most closely aligns to what NCSBN is basing their CJMM is the work by Christine A. Tanner.

The new version of the NCLEX-RN® is loosely being identified as the "Next-Generation NCLEX" or "NGN", and will feature the following:
- 6 key skills in the CJMM: recognizing cues, analyzing cues, prioritizing hypotheses, generating solutions, taking actions, and evaluating outcomes.
- Approved item types as of June 2020: multiple response, extended drag and drop, cloze (drop-down), enhanced hotspot (highlighting), and matrix/grid. More question types may be added.
- All new item types are accompanied by mini-case studies with comprehensive patient information—some of it relevant to the question, and some of it not.
- Case information may present a single, unchanging moment in time (a "single episode" case study) or multiple moments in time as a patient's condition changes (an "unfolding" case study).
- Single-episode case studies may be accompanied by 1-6 questions; unfolding case studies are accompanied by 6 questions.

For more information (and detail) regarding the NCLEX-RN® and changes coming to the exam, visit the NCSBNs website: https://www.ncsbn.org/11447.htm and https://ncsbn.org/Building_a_Method_for_Writing_Clinical_Judgment_It.pdf.

For further NCLEX-RN® examination preparation resources, see *Silvestri's Canadian Comprehensive Review for the NCLEX-RN Examination*, Second Edition, ISBN 9780323709385.

Prior to preparing for any nursing licensure examination, please refer to your provincial or territorial nursing regulatory body to determine which licensure examination is required in order for you to practice in your chosen jurisdiction.

# ACKNOWLEDGEMENTS

I thank Vancouver Island University for their ongoing support of my academic adventures, including the honour of joining Jane and Marian as a co-editor for the First Canadian Edition of this textbook. Thank you to the many Canadian contributors who put in countless hours to ensure the writing emerged through a Canadian lens. Thank you to my life partner, Phillip, for his unending support with our children, enabling the time and space to do this work in the cracks of life.

**–Shannon Dames**

I thank my co-editors, Jane and Shannon, for their dedication and support to complete this First Canadian Edition, and to the many contributors who stepped forward to provide their expertise. Thank you to Martina van de Velde, our Content Development Specialist, for her ongoing guidance and patience. Thank you to the Queen's University School of Nursing for supporting my nursing education scholarship endeavours. And finally, many thanks, as always, to my family for making it all worthwhile: Corey, Curt, Sarena, Cam, Kat, and Margo, and especially Richard and Brianna for holding down the fort.

**–Marian Luctkar-Flude**

A special thank you to everyone involved, especially the significant contributions of our Canadian authors. It was a special honour and privilege to work on this textbook with my amazing daughter, Kaitlyn Hall, who is a contributing author and public health nurse. I am so proud of you and our shared passion for nursing. Thank you to my wonderful husband, Glenn, and children, Kelsey and Aiden, for your unconditional support and encouragement. It was a pleasure to work with my co-editors, Marian and Shannon, both leaders in nursing education. I would also like to acknowledge the support I received from the University of Ottawa School of Nursing, which inspires excellence in nursing education and research.

**–Jane Tyerman**

We had the good fortune of receiving much assistance and support from many friends, relatives, and associates. Our colleagues read chapters, gave valuable advice and criticism, helped clarify concepts, and provided case examples.

We also acknowledge the contributions of all the authors. In developing this text, they gave the project their total commitment and support. Their professional competence aided greatly in the development of the final draft of the manuscript. The editors worked and learned from each other during the planning and development of this book; throughout the entire process, close contact prevailed. Elizabeth Kudzma, a long-standing contributor, is the co-editor of this edition. She has added much knowledge and perspective to this edition.

Many thanks to the Elsevier editorial and production team: Charlene Ketchum, Jamie Blum, Mary Pohlman, and Jeffrey Patterson. We appreciate and thank them for their ongoing help and support. It is a true pleasure working with them.

I am fortunate to have faith in the Lord, who gives courage and strength to face life's difficulties in a positive manner. My children, John and Megan Gillespie, Tom and Heather Gillespie, and Deirdre O'Brien, and my grandchildren, Ryan, Caroline, Meredith, and Colleen, bring joy to me as a mother and grandmother. Their patience and love are truly appreciated. Fredric Edelman provides much encouragement and support. Both my brother and sister in law, John and Marilyn Lium, are inspirational to me and a reminder every day that health in life is precious.

**–Carole Lium Edelman**

As a contributor from the first edition to the present, I thank Carole Edelman for inviting me to become a co-editor of this edition. The insights and clinical experiences of Curry College faculty colleagues and students are continuing sources of enrichment. Thanks also to my family, including my sister and brother (Mary and Mark), daughter Katherine, and especially to my husband, Daniel, who provided support, discussion, and insight throughout this project.

**–Elizabeth Connelly Kudzma**

# CONTENTS

1

# Health Defined: Health Promotion, Prevention, and Protection

*Dana S. Edge, RN, MSN, PhD*

Originating US chapter by *Ratchneewan Ross, RN, FAAN, PhD, Carolyn Cable Kleman, RN, MHA, PhD(c)*

## INTENDED LEARNING OUTCOMES

*After completing this chapter, the reader will be able to:*

- Analyze concepts and models of *health* as used historically and as used in this textbook.
- Discuss the history of health promotion in Canada.
- Analyze the progress made in Canada with respect to achieving the aims of the Ottawa Charter for Health Promotion.
- Differentiate between health, illness, disease, disability, and premature death.

- Compare the three levels of prevention (primary, secondary, and tertiary) with the levels of service provision available across the life span.
- Critique the role of research and evidence as well as the nurse's role in health education and research for the promotion and protection of health for individuals and populations.

## KEY TERMS

Applied research
Behavioural approach
Biomedical approach
Community-based care
Cultural safety
Disease
Ecological model of health
Empathy
Epidemiology
Ethnocentrism
Evidence-informed practice
Framework for Health Promotion in Canada
Functional health
Health
Health equity
Health inequalities
Health promotion
Health protection

Health-related quality of life (HRQL)
Illness
Interprofessional practice
Levels of prevention
Natural history of disease
Person-centred care
Ottawa Charter for Health Promotion
Population health promotion model (PHPM)
Qualitative studies
Quantitative studies
Racism
Social determinants of health
Social justice
Socioenvironmental approach
Specific protection
Strengths-based planning
Upstream thinking
Wellness

### ❓ THINK ABOUT IT

#### Use of Complementary and Alternative Therapies

One of the biggest challenges to health care providers is the blending of Western medicine and health practices with the health practices from other cultures and ethnic groups. As the demographics of Canada shift, more people use a combination of therapies in self-care and for the treatment of specific illnesses.

- What questions should the student ask to obtain information from people about their use of nontraditional therapies?
- What information should the student know about the benefits or limitations of using complementary therapies, such as acupuncture, spiritual healing, herbal remedies, or chiropractic?
- What resources should the student trust for information on the efficacy and use of herbal remedies relative to prescription medications?
- Which ideas of health would be most compatible with the use of alternative therapies?

Health is a core concept in society. This concept is modified with qualifiers such as *excellent, good, fair,* or *poor,* on the basis of a variety of factors. These factors may include age, sex, ethnicity, comparison group, current health or physical condition, past conditions, social or economic situation, geographical location, or the demands of various roles in society. In addition, there is compelling evidence that larger societal and environmental concerns determine health outcomes (Barnish, Tørnes, & Nelson-Horne, 2018; Braveman & Gottlieb, 2014). This chapter will discuss health as a concept and related concepts such as wellness, illness, and disease. In this chapter, the promotion of health for individuals, communities, and society is primarily examined from a socioenvironmental lens. Furthermore, the intersection between health promotion, disease prevention, and health protection will be explored. Some motivating factors behind the move to disease prevention and health promotion in Canada will be examined with an introduction to seminal government publications. The implementation of health promotion activities as nursing actions will also be addressed from ideal and pragmatic standpoints. Research and evidence supporting these concepts, and recommendations for further research, will be presented.

Nurses understand the pivotal role they play in promoting health and preventing disease, the important role of research in the knowledge of what is "healthy," and the central role of epidemiology (the study of health and disease in society) and public health theories in the everyday practice of nursing.

## DISEASE, ILLNESS, AND HEALTH

It is easy to think of health or wellness as the lack of disease and to consider "illness" and "disease" to be interchangeable terms. However, "health" and "disease" are not simply antonyms, and "disease" and "illness" are not synonyms. Disease literally means "without ease." Disease may be defined as the failure of a person's adaptive mechanisms to counteract stimuli and stresses adequately, resulting in functional or structural disturbances. This definition is an ecological concept of disease, which uses multiple factors to determine the cause of disease, rather than describing a single cause. This multifactorial approach increases the chances of discovering multiple points of intervention to improve health.

Illness is composed of the subjective experience of the individual and the physical manifestation of disease (Farre & Rapley, 2017). Both are social constructs within which people are in an imbalanced, unsustainable relationship with their environment and are failing in their ability to survive and create a higher quality of life. Illness can be described as a response that is characterized by a mismatch between a person's needs and the resources available to meet those needs. Additionally, illness signals to individuals and populations that the present balance is not working. Within this definition, illness has psychological, spiritual, and social components. A person can have a disease without feeling ill (e.g., asymptomatic hypertension). A person can also feel ill without having a diagnosable disease (e.g., as a result of stress). Our understanding of disease and illness within society, overlaid with our understanding of the natural history of each disease, creates a basis for promoting health.

## HEALTH AND WELLNESS

Health, as defined in this text, is a state of physical, mental, spiritual, and social functioning that realizes a person's potential and is experienced within a developmental context. Although health is, in part, an individual's responsibility, health also requires collective action to ensure a society and an environment in which people can act responsibly to support health. The culture and beliefs of people can also influence health action. This definition is consistent with the World Health Organization (WHO) definition of health as the state of complete physical, mental, and social well-being and not merely the absence of disease and infirmity (WHO, 1946), but moves beyond this definition to encompass spiritual, developmental, and environmental aspects over time. The physical aspect includes one's genetic makeup, which when combined with the other aspects, influences one's longevity. This broader definition is applicable across the life span, as well as in situations where illness may be a persistent state. For example, in this broader definition of health, a person with diabetes may be considered healthy if he or she is able to adapt to his or her illness and live a meaningful, spiritually satisfying life. A similar concept, wellness, is said to occur when one perceives their health as good, with appreciation and enjoyment. Health is considered to be part of the metaparadigm for nursing (Bender, 2018), which includes an interconnected relationship of person, health, environment, and nursing. The lack of consensus in nursing regarding a definition of health, described in a recent critical appraisal, highlights the complexity and multifaceted nature of health (Alslman, Ahmad, Hani, et al., 2017). As can be seen in the discussion thus far, health can be viewed in a variety of ways.

## HEALTH PROMOTION

The blueprint definition that most often guides health promotion in Canada is found in the 1986 document *Ottawa Charter for Health Promotion* (Hyndman & The Alder Group, 2007). The Ottawa Charter defines health promotion as "the process of enabling people to increase control over and improve their health" (WHO, 1986, p.1, para 2). More than a decade later, the WHO (1998) proposed a more expansive definition:

> Health promotion represents a comprehensive social and political process, it not only embraces actions directed at strengthening the skills and capabilities of individuals, but also action directed towards changing social, environmental and economic conditions so as to alleviate their impact on public and individual health. Health promotion is the process of enabling people to increase control over the determinants of health and thereby improve their health. (pp. 1–2)

The progression and development of health promotion approaches are outlined in the following section.

### The Evolution of Health Promotion in Canada

People involved in health promotion must consider the meaning of health for themselves and for others. Recognizing differences in the meaning of health can clarify outcomes and expectations in health promotion and enhance the quality of health care. Because health is used to describe a number of entities, including a philosophy of care (health promotion and health maintenance), a system (health care delivery system), practices (evidence-informed health practices), behaviours (personal health behaviours), and costs (health care costs), the reason that confusion continues regarding the use of the term "health" becomes clear. People's use of the term "health," and its incorporation into these various entities, has also changed over time.

Canadians who were born before 1940 have experienced the greatest changes in how health is defined. Because infectious diseases claimed the lives of many children and young adults at that time, health was viewed as the absence of disease. The physician in independent practice was the primary provider of health care services, with services provided in the private office. As the national economy expanded during and after World War II in the 1940s and 1950s, the idea of role performance became a focus in industrial research and entered the health care lexicon. This was furthered by the WHO declaration that health is "not merely the absence of disease" in 1946. Health became linked to a person's ability to fulfill a role in society. Increasingly, the physician was asked to complete physical examination forms for school, work, military, and insurance purposes, while physician practice became linked more directly to hospital-based services. It was recognized that a person might recover from a disease yet be unable to fulfill family or work roles because of residual changes from the illness episode. Concepts of disability and rehabilitation entered the health care arena. The work or school environment was viewed as a possible contributor to health, illness, disability, and death.

In this era, the biomedical approach to health promotion was predominant. Using the biomedical approach, health is defined by the absence of signs and symptoms of disease and illness is defined by the presence of signs and symptoms of disease. The target for intervention is high-risk individuals. Examples of health promotion strategies that use a biomedical approach include such activities as immunization and screening. Goals of the biomedical approach include decreased morbidity and prevalence of physiological risk factors, like high blood pressure.

From the 1940s to the present, there have been incredible changes in the provincial health care delivery systems. A result of the dreadful poverty that arose on the Prairies during the Great Depression, universal hospital insurance was initially introduced in 1947 by Saskatchewan; by 1961, universal hospital insurance was available nationally (Marchildon, 2012). Despite strong opposition from medical organizations, single-payer, universal medical care insurance was implemented in all provinces between 1962 and 1971, with the federal government agreeing to cost-share the insurance with the provinces (Marchildon, 2012; Martin, Miller, Quesnel-Vallée, et al., 2018). Universally provided health care services are commonly known as Medicare in Canada.

During the 1970s, the idea of adaptation had an important influence on the way Canadians view health. The 1974 Lalonde report ushered in a new way of thinking about health and laid the foundation to consider societal factors in the health of populations (Catford, 2014). In *A New Perspective on the Health of Canadians*, Lalonde argued:

> . . . that to improve the health of Canadians, Canada's federal health policy had to reflect the fact that illness, disease and disability were national problems that could only be successfully addressed through attention to lifestyles; the state of the environment and the organization of health care services; in addition, of course, to human biology. At the time his was a radical position aimed at revolutionizing Canadian health policy. (**Low & Thériault, 2008**, p. 201.)

Increasingly, health became linked to individuals' reactions to the environment rather than being viewed as a fixed state. Adaptation fit well with the self-help movement during the 1970s and with the progressive growth in knowledge from research of disease prevention and health promotion at the individual level using behavioural models. In the behavioural approach to health promotion, people's ability to adapt and adjust positively to social, mental, and physiological change is the measure of their health. The goal is behavioural change to improve individual lifestyles. Health is defined as the absence of disease, as well as functioning, role performance, and healthy lifestyles. Targeted messaging to high-risk groups occurs, for example to youth who are smokers. The behavioural approach draws heavily upon psychological theories that explain human behaviour and behavioural change. These theories include the theory of reasoned action by Ajzen and Fishbein (1980), theories of behaviour by Bandura (1976, 1999, 2004), the health belief model by Rosenstock (Champion & Skinner, 2008), Pender's health promotion model (Pender, Murdaugh, & Parsons, 2015), and stages of change theories by Prochaska (Prochaska, Gill, & Hall, 2004). Internet searches on each of these theories will provide numerous websites where more detailed information about them is available.

Research on self-rated health (Dávila, Polanco, & Segura, 2017; McHugh & Lawlor, 2016) and self-rated function (Shrira, Palgi, Hoffman, et al., 2018), indicates that there are multiple factors contributing to a person's perception of his or her health, sometimes referred to as functional health (Gordon, 2016) or health-related quality of life (HRQL) (Shields, Garner, & Wilkins, 2013). Multiple tools are available for measuring quality of life, including a general measure established by the (World Health Organization Quality of Life, WHOQOL-BREF (WHO 2004) and the McGill Quality of Life Questionnaire (Cohen, Mount, Bruera, et al., 1997) for use at the end of life (Quality and Safety Scenario).

By the mid-1980s, Canada became a world leader in the formulation of health promotion ideals and strategies, particularly with the unveiling of the Framework for Health Promotion in Canada (Epp, 1986) at the first WHO conference on health promotion in Ottawa. The overall goal of "achieving health for all" identifies three health challenges: reducing inequities, increasing prevention, and enhancing coping. The three health promotion mechanisms to address these challenges are self-care, mutual aid, and healthy environments. The final component of the framework consists of three implementation strategies: fostering public participation, strengthening community health services; and coordinating healthy public policy. At the end of the 1986 WHO Ottawa conference, the Ottawa Charter for Health Promotion was published with five action areas to improve the health of populations through three basic health promotion strategies: enable, mediate, and advocate (WHO, 1986). The Ottawa Charter (Fig. 1.1) has had a lasting influence on health promotion; the five action areas that continue

## ⚡ QUALITY AND SAFETY SCENARIO

### Fall Prevention in the Home

Falls in the home are a common yet preventable source of both fatal and nonfatal injuries. In 2014, Statistics Canada reported in its *Health at a Glance* section that one in three older persons aged 65 years or older were likely to fall at least once every year. Falls contributed to 73 190 hospitalizations during 2008 to 2009, based on administrative hospital data submitted to the Canadian Institute for Health Information (CIHI).

There are specific factors that contribute to fall risk, including changes to the person that are attributable to age, medication use, and environmental hazards. Nurses are in key roles to work with older persons to assess fall risks and help them gain control over this aspect of their health. The Canadian Fall Prevention Education Collaborative (CFPEC) and the Canadian Fall Prevention Curriculum (CFPC) provide resources and links to a variety of websites, programs and toolkits for fall prevention in older persons at http://canadianfallprevention.ca/resources-and-links/.

Risk factors that are attributable to the aging process include visual, hearing, and functional limitations. Although pets have proven to be beneficial for older persons by providing companionship and comfort, they can also scamper underfoot or the older person may trip over the pet because the pet is not seen or heard. Loss of night vision and depth perception can also contribute to falls when lighting is poor or when a person is moving from room to room. Older persons should be encouraged to always wear prescribed vision and hearing aids when moving about the house or apartment. Loss of upper and lower body strength can also contribute to fall risk. Lower body strength is needed to lift the legs and feet high enough to navigate stairs and changes in texture of flooring. Upper body strength allows the use of supports when a person is moving about. Watch the person manoeuvre about the living space and note the use of furniture, walls, and other objects for support.

Medications can contribute to disequilibrium. A careful review of currently used medications—both prescribed and over-the-counter medications—can help identify medications that could possibly contribute to fall risks. Environmental risks include clutter, too much furniture for the room, placement of items in typical walkways, lighting problems, needed repairs to flooring and walls, and

the need for supports such as grab bars and railings. Again, watching the person navigate through the home is helpful in recognizing potential trip hazards and areas where additional supports are needed. Adequate hydration is another consideration, especially if the person is taking medications that contribute to dehydration without regular fluid replacement, or if the temperature in the home and environment is too high.

Health outcomes for the person can be significant. Falls can cause minor injury and embarrassment, but they can also cause life-threatening injuries such as fractures and head injuries. If a fall has occurred, it is helpful to do a root cause analysis to determine those factors that contributed to the fall. Ask permission before attempting to make any alteration to the home, because items and their placement may have sentimental importance to the person. Address medication changes with the person, pharmacist, and/or primary care provider. Some medication habits may be hard for the person to change.

The nursing implications of fall risk are many and varied. Assessment skills must be practiced in a variety of settings so that the nurse is vigilant for potential hazards and individual factors that might precipitate a fall. Older persons should be routinely observed performing their daily routines to identify visual, hearing, and functional decline. Also, if a person reports a fall, that report should trigger a more extensive evaluation of that individual because falls may be indicative of future fall risk.

Falls are a frequent but preventable occurrence, especially for older persons. Falls also contribute millions of dollars each year to the cost of health care as a result of personal injury and disability. That is why fall prevention is a key feature of quality and safety education for nurses.

#### Questions
- Can you identify at least four items in your own environment that may contribute to your fall risk?
- How would you structure an interview with an older person to determine the presence of fall risks in that person's home?
- What evidence and arguments would you use to encourage an older person to modify the home environment to decrease the risk of a fall?

Source: Pearson, C., St-Amaud, J., & Geran, L. (2014). *Health at a glance: Understanding senior's risk of falling and their perception of risk*. Ottawa: Statistics Canada, Minister of Industry. Retrieved from https://www150.statcan.gc.ca/n1/pub/82-624-x/2014001/article/14010-eng.htm.

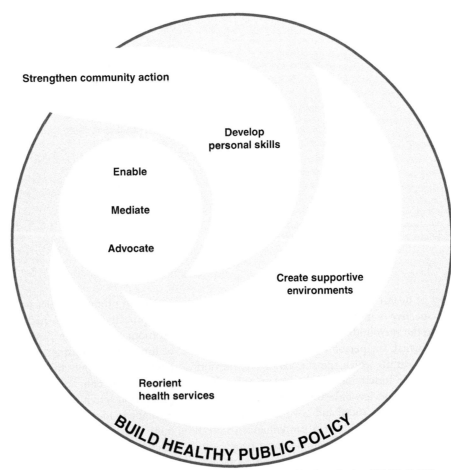

**Fig. 1.1** Health Promotion Emblem, The Ottawa Charter (From World Health Organization (WHO). [1986]. *Ottawa Charter for Health Promotion: First international conference on health promotion, 21 November 1986.* Geneva: WHO. Retrieved from www.who.int/healthpromotion/conferences/previous/ottawa/en/index4.html.)

to guide practitioners and researchers are: build healthy public policy; develop personal skills; strengthen community action; create supportive environments; and reorient health services (Vollman, 2017).

The ecological model of health emerged in the late 1980s as a comprehensive way to assess the interplay and interdependence of individuals within subsystems of the ecosystem, such as their communities, physical, and social environments (Green, Richard, & Potvin, 1996; Richard, Gauvin, & Raine, 2011). Key to the ecological model is the emphasis on the social determinants of health—those factors in society that have an influence on health and the options available to people to improve or maintain their health (Canadian Nurses Association [CNA], 2019).

The following elements form what we call the determinants of health: income and social status; social support networks; education and literacy; employment/working conditions; social environments; physical environments; healthy child development; personal health practices and coping skills; biology and genetic endowment; health services; gender; and culture (Association of Faculties of Medicine of Canada, 2018; CNA, 2019; Public Health Agency of Canada [PHAC], 2017).

Health equity means that, ideally, everyone has a fair opportunity to reach their health potential and that there is an absence of preventable or unfair differences among groups of people (WHO, 2019). When there are differences in health status between groups within society, health inequalities exist. While some disparities may be a result of biological factors, there are estimates that up to 50% of all health outcomes can be attributed to unequal distribution of social and economic factors (The Standing Senate Committee on Social Affairs, 2009). An online Canadian portal permits the examination of health inequalities in Canada using indicators from a variety of data sources, including Statistics Canada and the Canadian Institute for Health Information (CIHI). (The link to the data tool is https://health-infobase.canada.ca/health-inequalities/.)

## Current Approach in Canada to Health Promotion: Socioenvironmental

A more encompassing view of health is represented in the socioenvironmental approach to health promotion that acknowledges the interconnection between people and their physical and social environments. The approach builds upon the

| Factor | Biomedical Approach | Behavioural Approach | Socioenvironmental Approach |
|---|---|---|---|
| *Health defined as* | Biomedical, absence of disease, disability | Medical, plus functional ability, personal wellness, healthy lifestyles | Medical and behavioural, plus quality of life, social relationships |
| *Health explained by* | Pathology, physiological risk factors | Medical plus behavioural risk factors | Medical and behavioural plus psychosocial risk factors and socioenvironmental risk conditions |
| *Target for intervention* | High-risk individuals | High-risk groups | High-risk conditions |
| *Sample success criteria* | Decreased morbidity, age-standardized mortality, prevalence of physiological risk factors<br>Improved individual quality-adjusted life years (QALYs) | Improved individual lifestyles (behaviour change)<br>Adoption of healthier lifestyles earlier in "life cycle"<br>Decreased population physiological and behavioural risk factors | Improved social relationships and networks<br>Improved quality of life<br>Movement towards social equity (more equal distribution of wealth/power)<br>Movement towards environmental sustainability |

Modified from Labonte, R. (1998). Health promotion and the common good: Towards a politics of practice. *Critical Public Health, 8*(2), 107–129 (Table 1, p. 113).

ecological model of health described previously. Health from an ecological perspective is multidimensional, extending from the individual into the surrounding community, and including the context within which the person functions. It incorporates a systems approach within which the actions of one portion of the system affect the functioning of the system as a whole (Richard et al., 2011). This view of health expands on wellness by recognizing that there are social and environmental factors (i.e., social determinants of health) that can enhance or limit health and healthy behaviours. For example, most people can benefit from physical activity such as walking, and people are more likely to walk in areas where there are sidewalks or walking paths and where they feel safe. Nurses can encourage people to walk but may also need to advocate safe areas for people to walk and work with others to plan for people-friendly community development. Table 1.1 outlines the main differences in these three approaches to health promotion.

Primary care providers, including nurse practitioners and other advanced practice nurses, now attempt to involve individuals and their families in the delivery of person-centred care, and teach individuals about individual responsibilities and lifestyle choices has become an important part of their job (MOHLTC, 2015). Health care has become an interdisciplinary endeavour and is actively fostered by provincial governments, as evidenced by the establishment of family health teams in Ontario. Emphasis is being placed on the quality of a person's life as a component of health, including the reorientation of mental health services (Health Canada & PHAC, 2016), and the elimination of health inequalities (PHAC, 2018a).

The *Population Health Promotion Model* (Hamilton & Bhatti, 1996) provides an overall framework to guide health promotion by blending both health promotion and population health concepts. The three-dimensional cube reflects populations (i.e., individuals, families, communities, society), the Ottawa Charter areas for action, and the social determinants of health, with the cube based on a foundation of evidence-informed decision making and societal values (Fig. 1.2).

Health promotion goes beyond providing information. It is also proactive decision-making at all levels of society. Health promotion holds the best promise for lower cost methods of limiting the constant increase in health care costs and for empowering people to be responsible for the aspects of their lives that can enhance well-being. Based on the need for health promotion activities within the health care system, efforts must be made to identify the multiple determinants of health, determine relevant health-promotion strategies, and delineate issues relevant to social justice and access to care. The Canadian Nurses Association (CNA, 2010, p. 10) states that social justice is ". . . the fair distribution of society's benefits, responsibilities and their consequences. It focuses on the relative portion of one social group in relationship to others in society as well as on the root causes of disparities and what can be done to eliminate them." Individuals, families, and communities must be active participants in this process so that the actions taken are socially relevant, economically feasible, and supportive of changes at the individual level.

## PREVENTION

To promote health and prevent illness, disease, and disabilities, various levels of prevention are used in nursing practice. Health promotion fits as a strategy under the umbrella of primary prevention which will be expanded upon later in this section. To fully appreciate the concept of prevention, an understanding of the *natural history of disease* is helpful.

### Natural History of Disease

For many diseases, there are well-defined stages of disease progression from its inception to outcome or resolution, whether that be cure, control, disability, or death. These stages collectively are referred to as the natural history of disease (Porta, 2014); for example, we know that certain cancers (e.g., cervical) often have a long latent period from the time of pathological onset to the development of symptoms. Understanding the

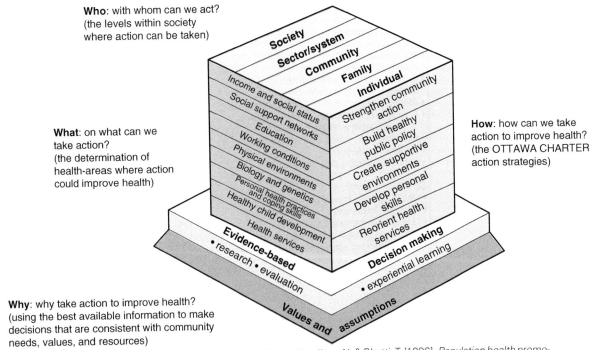

**Fig. 1.2 Population Health Promotion Model** (From Hamilton, N. & Bhatti, T. [1996]. *Population health promotion: An integrated model of population health and health promotion.* Ottawa: Health Promotion Development Division, Health Canada. Retrieved from https://www.canada.ca/en/public-health/services/health-promotion/population-health/population-health-promotion-integrated-model-population-health-health-promotion.html. ©All rights reserved. Public Health Agency of Canada. Adapted and reproduced with permission from the Minister of Health, 2019.)

typical progression of a disease assists in determining the best prevention strategies, in particular, whether screening for a disease will be beneficial.

## Levels of Prevention

Prevention, in a narrow sense, means averting the development of disease. In a broad sense, prevention consists of all measures that limit disease progression. Leavell and Clark (1965) defined three *levels of prevention*: primary, secondary, and tertiary (Fig. 1.3). Although the levels of prevention are related to the natural history of disease, they can be used to prevent disease and provide nurses with starting points for making effective, positive changes in the health status of the persons for whom they provide care.

Within the three levels of prevention, there are five steps. These steps include health promotion and specific protection (primary prevention); early diagnosis, prompt treatment, and disability limitation (secondary prevention); and restoration and rehabilitation (tertiary prevention).

Some confusion exists in the interpretation of these concepts; therefore a consistent understanding of primary, secondary, and tertiary prevention is essential. The levels of prevention operate on a continuum but may overlap in practice. The nurse must clearly understand the goals of each level to intervene effectively in keeping people healthy.

### Primary Prevention

Primary prevention refers to the timeframe *before* disease occurs (Celentano & Szklo, 2019). Primary prevention can begin as early as childhood or even prenatally and is closely linked to the determinants of health and the environment in which one lives. For example, if the social environment one grows up in discourages exercise or encourages eating high-fat foods, that environment could be targeted for primary prevention. Examples include healthy eating and activity school-based programs, reduction of sodium in the food supply, and creation of safe places to ride bikes and walk (Barekatain, Weiss, & Weintraub, 2015). Most health-promoting primary prevention directed at social determinants of health occurs at the national, provincial/territorial, and community levels and constitutes health promotion at a macro level.

Primary prevention intervention is also directed at individuals and families, and includes health promotion activities such as health education about risk factors for heart disease, and specific protection, such as immunization against hepatitis B. Its purpose is to decrease the vulnerability of the individual or population to disease or dysfunction. Health promotion interventions at the individual level encourage individuals and groups to become more aware of the means of improving health and the actions they can take at the primary preventive health level and the optimal health level. People are also taught to use appropriate primary preventive measures. However, as mentioned previously, primary prevention can also include advocating policies that promote the health of the community and electing public officials who will enact legislation that protects the health of the public.

### Secondary Prevention

Although primary prevention measures have decreased the hazards of chronic diseases such as cardiovascular disease, conditions that preclude a healthy quality of life are still prevalent.

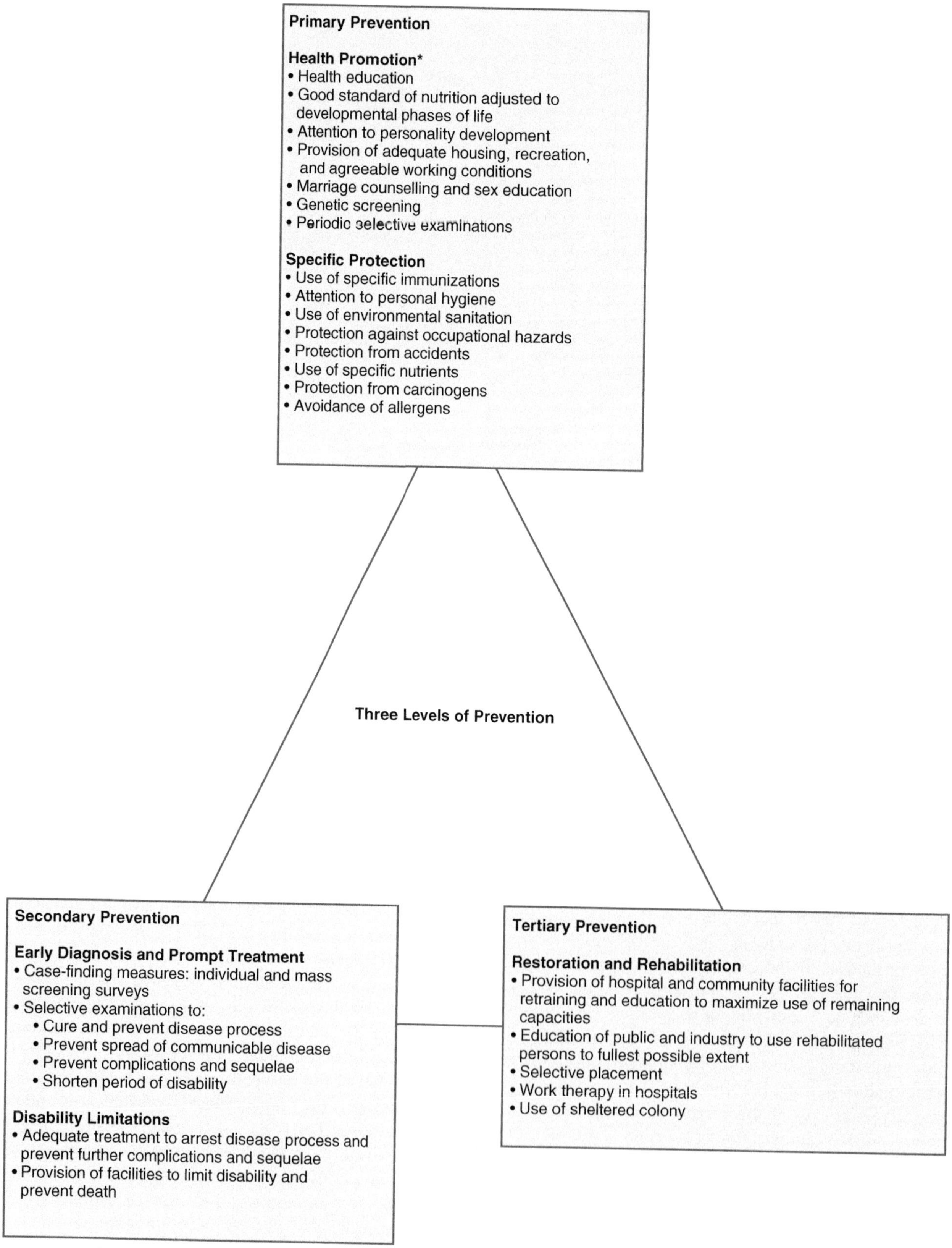

**Primary Prevention**

**Health Promotion***
- Health education
- Good standard of nutrition adjusted to developmental phases of life
- Attention to personality development
- Provision of adequate housing, recreation, and agreeable working conditions
- Marriage counselling and sex education
- Genetic screening
- Periodic selective examinations

**Specific Protection**
- Use of specific immunizations
- Attention to personal hygiene
- Use of environmental sanitation
- Protection against occupational hazards
- Protection from accidents
- Use of specific nutrients
- Protection from carcinogens
- Avoidance of allergens

**Three Levels of Prevention**

**Secondary Prevention**

**Early Diagnosis and Prompt Treatment**
- Case-finding measures: individual and mass screening surveys
- Selective examinations to:
  - Cure and prevent disease process
  - Prevent spread of communicable disease
  - Prevent complications and sequelae
  - Shorten period of disability

**Disability Limitations**
- Adequate treatment to arrest disease process and prevent further complications and sequelae
- Provision of facilities to limit disability and prevent death

**Tertiary Prevention**

**Restoration and Rehabilitation**
- Provision of hospital and community facilities for retraining and education to maximize use of remaining capacities
- Education of public and industry to use rehabilitated persons to fullest possible extent
- Selective placement
- Work therapy in hospitals
- Use of sheltered colony

Fig. 1.3 The Three Levels of Prevention (as influenced by Leavell and Clark). *The concept of Health Promotion was not part of Leavell and Clark's original theory, but was introduced in 1986 with the Ottawa Charter for Health Promotion. (Modified from Leavell, H., & Clark, A. E. [1965]. *Preventive medicine for doctors in the community.* New York: McGraw-Hill; Ali, A., & Katz, D. L. [2015]. Disease prevention and health promotion: How integrative medicine fits. *American Journal of Preventive Medicine, 49*[5], S230–S240.)

Secondary prevention ranges from providing screening activities and treating early stages of disease to limiting disability by averting or delaying the consequences of advanced disease.

Screening is secondary prevention because the principal goal is to identify individuals in an early, detectable stage of the disease process. However, screening provides an excellent opportunity to offer health teaching as a primary preventive measure. Screening activities now play an important role in the control of diseases such as heart disease, stroke, and colorectal cancer. Additionally, screening activities provide early diagnosis and treatment of nutritional, behavioural, and other related problems. Nurses play an important role in screening activities because they provide clinical expertise and educationally sound health information during the screening process.

Delayed recognition of disease results in the need to limit future disability in late secondary prevention. Limiting disability is a vital role for nursing because preventive measures are primarily therapeutic and are aimed at arresting the disease and preventing further complications. The paradox here is that health education and disease-prevention activities seem similar to those used in primary prevention, but are applied to a person or population with an existing disease. Modifications to the teaching plan must be made on the basis of the individual's current health status and ability to modify behaviour.

### Tertiary Prevention

Tertiary prevention occurs when a defect or disability is permanent and irreversible. The process involves minimizing the effects of disease and disability by surveillance and maintenance activities that are aimed at preventing complications and deterioration. Tertiary prevention focuses on rehabilitation to help people attain and retain an optimal level of functioning, regardless of their disabling condition. The objective is to return the affected individual to a useful place in society, maximize their remaining capacities, or both. The responsibility of the nurse is to ensure that persons with disabilities receive services that enable them to live and work according to the resources that are still available to them. When a person has a stroke, rehabilitating this individual to the highest level of functioning and teaching lifestyle changes to prevent future strokes are examples of tertiary prevention.

## HEALTH PROTECTION

Health protection activities focus on the reduction of threats and negative influences on health, specifically those risks over which people have no control. Ensuring safe and adequate food, water, and medical therapies for all people as well as protecting them against workplace and environmental hazards are regional, national and global objectives, and most frequently, are the responsibility of local, provincial, and federal governments (Ruger, Hammonds, Ooms, et al., 2015). At a global level, in recognition of the worldwide responsibility for social protection, a global health fund to ensure adequate protection of all the world's people concerning AIDS, tuberculosis, and malaria, was created in 2002 (The Global Fund to Fight AIDS, Tuberculosis

and Malaria, 2019). The fund partners with local people affected by the diseases, and with governments, civil society, and the private sector, to support prevention and treatment programs.

### Specific Protection

This aspect of primary prevention focuses on protecting people from injury and disease, for example, by providing immunizations and reducing exposure to occupational hazards, carcinogens, and other environmental health risks. These hazards and risks include not only protection of adults from work-related injuries (e.g., back injuries in nurses, dismemberment in machinists, exposure to chemicals used in boat repair or exposure to inhaled sawdust by carpenters), but also protection of infants and children from potential carcinogens (e.g., exposure of children to diesel emissions, damage to a fetus caused by radiation).

Primary prevention interventions are considered specific protection when they emphasize shielding or defending the body (or the public) from specific causes of injury or disease. Implementing nursing interventions that prevent a specific health problem may seem easier than promoting well-being among individuals, groups, or communities, because the variables are delineated more clearly in prevention than in promotion and the potential influences are less diverse.

## THE ACTIVE AND PASSIVE NATURE OF HEALTH PROMOTION

Health-promotion efforts, unlike those efforts directed at specific protection from certain diseases, focus on maintaining or improving the general health of individuals, families, and communities. These activities are conducted at the public level (e.g., government programs promoting adequate housing or reducing pollutants in the air), at the community level (e.g., Habitat for Humanity or community health centres), and at the personal level (e.g., voting to offer low-income housing or to elect public officials who recognize the need for public oversight). Nursing interventions are actions directed toward developing people's resources to maintain or enhance their well-being—a form of strengths-based planning. Using strengths-based nursing, the nurse focuses on what families and patients do that helps them deal with problems; through the assessment of their inner and outer strengths, this approach promotes health and facilitates healing (Gottlieb, 2014; Gottlieb & Gottlieb, 2017).

Strategies of health promotion that involve the individual may be either passive or active. Passive strategies involve the individual as an inactive participant or recipient. Examples of passive strategies include public health efforts to maintain clean water and sanitary sewage systems to decrease infectious diseases and improve health, and efforts to add vitamin D to all milk to ensure that children will not be at high risk of rickets when living in areas where sunlight is scarce. These passive strategies must be used to promote the health of the public when individual participation might be low but the benefit to society is high.

Active strategies depend on the individual becoming personally involved in adopting a proposed program of health promotion (lifestyle change). Two examples of lifestyle change are performing daily exercise as part of a physical fitness plan and adopting a stress-management program as part of daily living. A combination of active and passive strategies is best for making an individual or society healthier. This book is concerned with the nurse's role in using these strategies with individuals and families, and in fostering better community health and public health policy across the life span.

## THE ROLE OF THE PUBLIC HEALTH AGENCY OF CANADA IN HEALTH PROMOTION, PREVENTION, AND PROTECTION

Public health has always had the prevention of disease in society as its focus. However, during the past 30 years, the promotion of health with a focus to address the social determinants of health moved to the forefront within public health, becoming a driving force in health care reform.

The aim of the Public Health Agency of Canada (PHAC) is "to promote and protect the health of Canadians through leadership, partnership, innovation and action in public health" (PHAC, 2017). Among the agency's recent plans (PHAC, 2017), there are three programs: public health infrastructure; health promotion and disease prevention; and health security. The planned results for the health promotion and disease prevention program include six targets to address:

- Infectious diseases and immunization
- Healthy living and injury prevention
- Mental health promotion and suicide prevention
- Older people and aging
- Vulnerable children and families
- Innovation and experimentation

These six areas established the current federal focus for health promotion and disease prevention efforts to occur. Research in a variety of areas has clearly indicated that health disparities are directly and indirectly linked to longevity and quality-of-life issues (Marmot, 2017; PHAC, 2018a). For example, the life expectancy among Canadians living in the lowest income neighbourhoods in 2010 to 2011 was 4.1 years lower at 79.1 years than Canadians living in the highest income neighbourhoods (PHAC, 2018a). An even stronger disparity was found in areas where there was a high concentration of Indigenous peoples; for example, the life expectancy at birth in areas with high concentrations of Inuit was 12 years lower than in areas of low concentration. Adequate housing to eliminate these health inequalities that lead to poor health in Indigenous communities is one strategy being taken by the federal government (Government of Canada, 2019; National Collaborating Centre for Aboriginal Health, 2018). Much work is required to address existing disparities in health among First Nations, Inuit, and Métis people of Canada, not only from governments, but also from Canadian health care providers. The glaring inequalities among Indigenous Canadians compared to non-Indigenous Canadians include the following: high infant mortality rate; increased prevalence of diabetes; increased overall suicide rate; shortened life expectancy; and heavy infectious disease burden (HealthCareCAN, 2016). In a recent study, higher self-reported educational and income levels were deemed to be protective determinants of health for off-reserve First Nations and Métis peoples, which have wide-ranging implications for health promotion (Bethune, Absher, Obiagwu, et al., 2018). Recommendations for health care providers to address health inequalities among Indigenous people from the Truth and Reconciliation Commission of Canada can be found at http://www.healthcarecan.ca/what-we-do/health-policy/indigenous-healthcare/ (Diversity Awareness).

### 🌐 DIVERSITY AWARENESS

#### Influence of Personal Cultural Values on Health Care Delivery

Culture influences every aspect of human life, including beliefs, values, and customs regarding lifestyle and health care. As health care providers, nurses need to be aware of their own beliefs, values, and customs and how these ideas translate into behaviour. It is easy to assume that an individual's own perspective is correct and shared by others. This is especially true when one is working with other health care providers who share the same culture. This concept is referred to as ethnocentrism and can lead to a devaluing of the beliefs, values, and customs of others, known as racism. Although it is impossible for any person to ignore the cultural influences on their lives, nurses and other health care providers have a special obligation to be aware of their own social and cultural biases. Our focus as nurses must be on the cultural influences in the daily lives of individuals through the development of cultural safety and cultural humility. The ability to view other people's situations from their perspective is known as empathy. Diversity awareness will continue to challenge providers to lifelong learning about the people for whom they provide care as the ethnic mix in society changes.

Interviews were conducted with 28 immigrant women who were mothers of children with developmental disabilities in a recent qualitative study in Toronto (Khanlou, Mustafa, Vazquez, et al., 2017). The womens' regions of origin included Asia, Europe, Latin America, and the Caribbean. The authors found that the challenges associated with mothering a child with a disability were amplified and women were at increased risk of social exclusion from social services and society. They concluded that migration status, gender, and disability intersected together to affect the immigrant mothers' health.

**Reflective Questions**
- What actions can an individual undertake to develop an environment that promotes cultural safety?
- How would you engage with immigrant mothers to show cultural humility?
- Consider your own personal assumptions and biases. How might they influence the nursing care that you provide to diverse patient populations?

Source: Khanlou, N., Mustafa, N., Vazquez, L. M., et al. (2017). Mothering children with developmental disabilities: A critical perspective on health promotion. *Health Care for Women International, 38*(6), 613–634. https://doi.org/10.1080/07399332.2017.1296841.

At the federal level, the Government of Canada has committed to providing leadership in health promotion and disease prevention by improving immunization coverage, reducing tuberculosis rates among Indigenous peoples, monitoring risks related to overweight/obesity and sedentary behaviour, and working to test innovative interventions on making healthy choices, to name a few (PHAC, 2017). Health services are the responsibility of provincial governments, with each province and territory developing their own set of targets to prevent disease and promote health. A recent example of a coordinated federal/provincial health policy document is a common vision released in 2018 on reducing sedentary lifestyles called *Let's Get Moving* (PHAC, 2018b). Within this document, all government, organizations, and leaders are called upon to get Canadians to move more and sit less. One specific foundational message is "to encourage and enable Canadians of all ages in their efforts to be more physically active in all aspects of their daily living, and at all stages of their lives" (PHAC, 2018b, p. 23).

Physical activity can contribute to the maintenance or improvement in mobility, which improves the quality of life and prevents disability. It is something in which most people can participate. It enhances positive mental health through stress reduction and physical fitness, which contribute to the development of healthy behaviours. However, it takes awareness of larger socioenvironmental and social justice issues to address the need for social and physical environments that support physical activity across the life span. Access to health care to obtain a complete physical examination before starting to exercise and the quality of the work or neighbourhood environment available for exercise can contribute to success or failure of this objective (Innovative Practice).

Additionally, current knowledge of physical activity and specific populations was considered when the *Let's Get Moving* document was being created. Older Canadians, low-income populations, children, and people with disabilities are more likely to exceed the sedentary behaviour limits in the guideline than adults with moderate-to-high incomes (PHAC, 2018b). The reasons for the low activity levels amongst these vulnerable groups are diffuse, but relate back to the social determinants of health. These health disparities can influence the number of people in these groups who develop high cholesterol levels or high blood pressure, which further increases their risk of heart disease and stroke. The document addresses the need for beginning exercise activities at an early age and encouraging young adults to be actively engaged in exercise. Most importantly, the approach emphasizes personal responsibility but includes society's role in addressing the social and physical environments within which those choices are made. Organizations and governments are challenged to improve Canadians' activity levels by addressing a) cultural norms; b) spaces and places; c) public engagement; d) partnerships; e) leadership capacity building; and f) progress through accountability (PHAC, 2018b). Echoing the *Let's Get Moving* report, the Canadian Public Health Association released a position statement and developed an interactive toolbox for improving access to unstructured play for Canadian children (CPHA, 2019) (see https://www.cpha.ca/unstructured-play).

## INNOVATIVE PRACTICE
### *Process for Assessing, Evaluating, and Guiding Individuals Regarding Physical Activity*

Inactivity and sedentary behaviours are major concerns in public health because they contribute to other health problems such as high cholesterol level, high blood pressure, diabetes mellitus, heart disease, functional limitations, and disability. As part of the *Let's Get Moving* initiative, nurses have an important role to play in health education related to increasing movement and activity. More complete information about the *Canadian 24-hour Movement Guidelines* can be obtained from the Canadian Society for Exercise Physiology at https://csep-guidelines.ca.

Applying the socioenvironmental approach, the nurse recognizes how the built environment (i.e., dwellings, neighbourhood, community) directly affects a person's ability to easily participate in physical activities. Such an assessment identifies potential challenges and barriers that may make it difficult for an individual to carry out health education instructions. In addition, an individual's inability to afford exercise equipment or clothing may be an important impediment, causing some individuals or families to dismiss health education advice.

#### Make the Most of the Individual's Visit and Set an Effective Tone for Communication

Nurses ask individuals about their exercise history, weight-related health risks, and desire to become more active. The approaches used need to be respectful of a person's lifestyle, habits, housing, neighbourhood, and cultural influences. During history gathering, questions that explore social supports, accessible sidewalks and pathways, locations of local gyms, availability of community-run programs, and the individual's perception of challenges (such as time and finances) will aid in a mutual dialogue with the individual regarding a suitable, realistic plan. Discussions need to be nonjudgmental and goal directed.

#### Assess the Individual's Motivation/Readiness to Exercise

Nurses explain the role of activity in keeping people healthy. Individuals need to understand the various methods of data collection and measurement of height and weight, as well as waist circumference, risk factors, and comorbidities to get a full picture of their state of health. Nurses develop skill in determining readiness and motivation to exercise and remain active in their patients. Also key in the assessment of readiness to exercise is whether there are external barriers that require creative solutions from the nurse or others to facilitate the proposed exercise.

#### Build a Partnership With an Individual

Nurses work with individuals to determine what each person is willing to do to achieve a balanced activity level. This approach includes knowing the best practices to promote activity and exercise. If weight loss is a person's motivating factor for exercising, then use recommended diets that restrict caloric intake, set activity goals with your patients, encourage the person to keep a weekly food and activity diary, and provide information on diet and activity. Be sure to record individual goals and the treatment plan, including a health education plan. Nurses are knowledgeable about current exercise and weight treatment options and their success. Holistic approaches are needed because activity and food behaviours are influenced by many factors. Listen to individuals' stories about exercise and its role in their lives. Recommendations and therapies should fit the individual's goals and lead to lifestyle change. Finally, the identification of the lack of accessible sports facilities, walking paths, or safe neighbourhoods is the first step in alerting community health nurses, city planners, and elected officials to make changes to build healthy communities that facilitate physical activity.

## Legislative Changes Affecting Health

Responsibility for the delivery of health services in Canada rests with the provinces. Changes to public policy that have direct and indirect effects on the health of provincial residents are made through legislation and regulations. The federal government is responsible for setting national standards and developing national strategies related to health and safety. Nursing organizations often present briefs and lobby governments when it comes to health policy decisions, as do individual nurses.

The following is an example of how legislative action can influence health. Researchers, examined mortality rates from unintentional injuries in Canadian children between 1950 and 2009, and compared them against the introduction of national population-level injury prevention programs; they reported a strong association between the implementation of legislative changes and safety campaigns and a significant decline in childhood fatalities (Richmond, D'Cruz, Lokku, et al., 2016). Examples of legislation identified from the study that made a dramatic difference in childhood burn, choking, and motor vehicle collision fatalities were as follows: a) *Hazardous Products Act*—Flammability Regulations, 1971; b) *Hazardous Products Act*—Crib Regulations, 1985; and c) mandatory seat belt laws, 1976–1977. Many other forms of legislation and regulations are in place to protect the public. Ongoing societal changes require the continual evolution of new legislation, regulations, and policies.

## THE NURSE'S ROLE

Evolving demands are placed on the nurse and the nursing profession as a result of changes in society. Emphasis is shifting from acute, hospital-based care to preventive, community-based care, which is provided in nontraditional health care settings in the community. This demand for community-based services, with the home as a major community setting for care, is closely related to the changing demographics of Canada. While the home and community become the existing sites for care, nurses must assume more blended roles, with a knowledge base that prepares them to practice across settings using evidence-informed practice. Within these roles, nurses assume a more active involvement in the prevention of disease and the promotion of health. Nurses can be more independent in their practice and place a greater emphasis on promoting and maximizing health, and more than ever nurses are accountable morally, ethically, and legally for their professional behaviour.

### Nursing Roles in Health Promotion, Prevention, and Protection

Although nurses often work with people on a one-to-one basis, they seldom work in isolation. Within today's health care system, nurses collaborate with other nurses, physicians, social workers, nutritionists, psychologists, therapists, individuals, and community groups. In this interprofessional practice, nurses play a variety of roles.

### Advocate

As advocates nurses help individuals obtain what they are entitled to receive through the health care system, try to make the system more responsive to individual and community needs, and help people develop the skills to advocate for themselves. In the role of an advocate, the nurse strives to ensure that all persons receive high-quality, appropriate, safe, and cost-effective care. The nurse may spend a great deal of time identifying and coordinating resources for complex cases. As an advocate, the nurse uses social justice principles to guide assessment and decision making (CNA, 2010).

### Care Coordinator

The nurse acts as a care coordinator to prevent duplication of services, maintain quality and safety, and reduce costs. Information gathered from reliable data sources enables the care coordinator to help individuals avoid care that is unproven, ineffective, or unsafe. Reliable sources of information on best practices, evidence-informed practices, and standard protocols are available from Internet sites sponsored by the federal government (e.g., http://cbpp-pcpe.phac-aspc.gc.ca), nursing organizations (e.g., https://rnao.ca/bpg), and specialty organizations (e.g., https://www.heartandstroke.ca/what-we-do/for-professionals; https://guidelines.diabetes.ca/cpg). Successful care management depends on a collaborative relationship among the care coordinator, other nurses and physicians, the individual and his or her family, community organizations, and other care providers who work with the person. The wishes of the individual and the family need to be clear to the care coordinator as part of person-centred care provision. Facilitating communication among parties is one of the care coordinator's most important functions.

### Consultant/Collaborator

Nurses may provide knowledge about health promotion and disease prevention to individuals and groups as a consultant. Some nurses have specialized areas of expertise or advanced practice, such as in gerontology, women's health, or community/public health, and they are equipped to provide information as consultants in these areas of specialization (CNA, 2015). A gerontological nurse practitioner might be on a community planning board offering advice about what types of health-promotion activities should be considered in planning a new older person housing development. All nurses need to develop consultation and collaboration skills that can be integrated into practice and allow the individual nurse to take advantage of opportunities to provide support on an individual level or for future development at the organizational level (Norwood, 2003).

### Clinician

The core role of the nurse is the delivery of direct services such as health education, influenza vaccinations, and counselling in health promotion. Visible, direct delivery of nursing care is the foundation for the public image of nursing. The public demands that nurses be knowledgeable and competent in their delivery of services. This role is clearly expressed in the *Framework for the Practice of Registered Nurses in Canada* (CNA, 2015) and in the *CNA Code of Ethics for Registered Nurses* (CNA, 2017).

### Educator

Support for health practices in Canada are derived from the *Canada Health Act* (1984) and from societal values that consider health components such as good nutrition, industrial and highway safety, immunization, and specific medication therapy within the grasp of the total population. Even with its rich resources, society falls far short of attaining the goal of maximal health for all. The problem is not a lack of knowledge, but rather the lack of application; therefore it is incumbent on nurses to be excellent health educators. To teach effectively, the nurse must know essential facts about how people learn and the teaching–learning process (see Chapter 20).

In addition to their storehouse of scientific knowledge, nurses who are committed to their teaching role know that individuals are unique in their response to efforts to change their behaviour. This is especially true for nurses working with individuals and groups of a different ethnic or cultural background than their own (Ziabakhsh, Peterson, Prodan-Bhalla, et al., 2016). Teaching may range from a chance remark by the nurse, based on a perception of desirable individual behaviour, to structurally planned teaching according to individual needs. Selection of the methods most likely to succeed involves the establishment of teacher–learner goals. Health promotion and protection rely heavily on the individual's ability to use appropriate knowledge. Health education is one of the primary prevention techniques available to avoid the major causes of disability and death today and is a critical role for nurses.

### Facilitator of Healing

The role of facilitator of healing requires the nurse to help individuals integrate and balance the various parts of their lives (Rosa, Estes, & Watson, 2017). Healing resides in the ability to glimpse or intuit the "interior" of an individual, to sense and identify what is important to that other person, and to incorporate the specific insight into a care plan that helps that person develop his or her own capacity to heal. It requires a mindful blending of science and subjectivity (Benner, Sutphen, Leonard, et al., 2010). Nurses have a special ability to help people heal. The art of nursing is the extraordinary ability to manage a broad array of information to create something meaningful, sensible, and whole (see Chapter 24).

### Scholar/Researcher

In today's health care environment, nurses are constantly striving to understand and interpret research findings that will enhance the quality and value of individual care. To provide optimal health care, nurses need to use evidence-informed findings as their foundation for clinical decision-making. When nurses or other clinicians use research findings and the best evidence possible to make decisions, the outcome is termed evidence-informed practice. Evidence-informed practice is defined as the conscientious, explicit, and judicious use of current best evidence in making decisions about the care of individuals. The practice of evidence-informed nursing decision making means integrating individual clinical expertise with the best available external clinical evidence from systematic research (CNA, 2018).

Evidence-informed practice involves searching for the best evidence with which to answer clinical research questions. Research evidence can be gathered from quantitative studies that describe situations, correlate different variables related to care, or test causal relationships between variables related to care. Such studies become incorporated into screening and treatment standards such as those from the Canadian Task Force on Preventive Health Care (2018). Research evidence can also be gathered from qualitative studies that describe phenomena or define the historical nature, cultural relevance, or philosophical basis of aspects of nursing care. Applied research is done to directly affect clinical practice (Polit & Beck, 2017). Nursing organizations stress the use of the best evidence available to answer clinical questions and explore the next best evidence when appropriate (CNA, 2018). The next best evidence may include the individual clinical judgement that nurses acquire through clinical experience and clinical practice and other qualitative approaches to research.

Nurses need to recognize that research is important as a basis for their practice and that they need to participate in the research process. For example, nurses in Canadian long-term care facilities widely use the minimum data set (MDS) assessment tools, such as the Resident Assessment Instrument (RAI-MDS) to collect extensive data on the cognitive and physical functioning of individuals (Armstrong, Daly, & Choiniere, 2016; CIHI, 2019). These data are used as part of the quality improvement process to indicate areas for improvement in care, thereby contributing to nursing protocols.

Chapters 10 to 18 contain specific health-promotion research studies. Time should be taken to review these studies and explore the relationship between behaviour and disease, to identify which population groups are at risk, and to discover what types of health-promotion programs work and why they work. Through knowledge of research, nurses can strengthen their confidence in making daily decisions about quality care (Research for Evidence-Informed Practice).

## IMPROVING PROSPECTS FOR HEALTH

### Population Effects

Cultural and socioeconomic changes within the population unequivocally influence lay concepts of health and health promotion. Currently there are areas of Canada where Indigenous peoples outnumber any other population group. By 2036, among working-age (15 to 64 years) Canadians, between 35% to 40%, are projected to belong to a visible minority group (Morency, Malenfant, & MacIsaac, 2017). Taken together as a portent for future health-promotion strategies, these predictions about the population indicate that current knowledge of, and approaches to health promotion, may not meet the needs of the future Canadian population (see Chapter 2).

In addition to changes in the ethnic distribution within the population, the projected changes in age distribution will affect health-promotion practice. Considerable growth is expected in the proportion of the population that is aged 25 years or older. For example, it is projected that by 2063 the number of older people will more than double and potentially comprise between 24% and 28% of the overall Canadian population (Bohnert, Chagnon, & Dion, 2015). Although there was a drop in births after 1960, this decrease has been offset by an increase in immigration. Analysis of these population trends and projections helps health care providers determine changing needs. Additionally, analysis of the social and economic environment is necessary for the development of social policy concerning health.

## RESEARCH FOR EVIDENCE-INFORMED PRACTICE

### *Preventing Functional Decline in Hospitalized Older Persons*

The ability to function independently is important throughout life, but especially as one ages. Although some loss of independence in physical functioning may be expected over time, hospitalization should not contribute to physical function loss. Current practice in most hospitals is to limit a person's mobility and independence in activities of daily living. At times these limitations are imposed to prevent falls or other events for the benefit of the individual. But at other times limitations are imposed for the convenience of the staff or to decrease the risk of liability (Lafrenière, Folch, Bédard, et al., 2017).

Older persons are at risk of losing their functional abilities if the hospitalization-imposed limitations interfere with their normal level of activity. In addition, pre-existing, multiple comorbidities predispose Canadian older persons to functional decline (St. John, Tyas, Menec, et al., 2019). A prolonged hospitalization and rehabilitation period can lead to deconditioning, where the person loses muscle mass, strength, and range of motion as a result of a decrease in his or her activity. Research has demonstrated that such declines can further limit the activities of daily living for these older persons (Zisberg, Shadmi, Gur-Yasish, et al., 2015).

Evidence is now available to improve the quality of hospital and long-term care of older persons. Actions include establishing functional baseline data through geriatric assessments at the time of admission and at other set times during the stay; using protocols to improve self-care, nutrition, sleep quality, and cognition; minimizing the adverse events that may further influence loss of physical function; and improving the hospital environment to better serve older persons (Lafrenière et al., 2017; Mudge, Banks, Barrett, et al., 2017). It is still the nurse caring for the individual person who is most likely to see the need for applying this evidence to improve the care of the hospitalized older person.

Sources: Lafrenière, S., Folch, N., Bédard, L., et al. (2017). Strategies used by older patients to prevent functional decline during hospitalization. *Clinical Nursing Research, 26*(1), 6–26. https://doi.org/10.1177/1054773815601392; Mudge, A. M., Banks, M. D., Barnett, A. G., et al. (2017). CHERISH (Collaboration for Hospitalised Elders Reducing the Impact of Stays in Hospital): Protocol for a multi-site improvement program to reduce geriatric syndromes in older inpatients. *BMC Geriatrics, 17* (11), online 1–9. https://doi.org/10.1186/s12877-016-0399-7; St. John, P., Tyas, S. L., Menec, et al. (2019). Multimorbidity predicts functional decline in community-dwelling older adults. *Canadian Family Physician, 65*(2), e56–e63; Zisberg, A., Shadmi, E., Gur-Yaish, N., et al. (2015). Hospital-associated functional decline: The role of hospitalization processes beyond individual risk factors. *Journal of the American Geriatrics Society, 63*, 55–62. https://doi.org/10.1111/jgs.13193.

## SHIFTING PROBLEMS

The provision of personal health services must be influenced by current information regarding environmental health. Environmental pollution is a complex and increasingly hazardous problem. Diseases related to industry and technology, including asthma and trauma, have become important threats to health.

The physical and psychological stresses of a rapidly changing and fast-paced society present daily problems, such as psychosocial and spiritual poor health habits. Posttraumatic stress disorder is becoming a more common diagnosis. Obesity, partly attributed to a lack of exercise and increasing food portion size, is a growing health issue. The ingestion of potentially toxic, non-nutritious, high-fat foods is another contributing factor (see Chapter 21). The abuse of tobacco, medications, and alcohol also negatively affects health.

The emphasis on treating disease through the application of complex technology not only is costly but also contributes minimally to the improvement of health. An orientation toward illness clearly focuses on the effects rather than the causes of disease.

A substantial change in wellness patterns is occurring. Infectious and acute diseases were the major causes of death in the early part of the twentieth century, whereas persistent conditions, heart disease, cerebrovascular accident (stroke), and cancer are the major causes today. An emphasis on the diagnosis and treatment of disease, which were highly successful in the past, is not the answer for today's needs, which are closely related to and affected by the individual's biochemical functioning, genetics, environment, and personal choices (Genomics).

## GENOMICS

Genetic research is primarily concerned with discovering, detecting, and treating illnesses related to specific abnormal genetic sequences (Canadian Institutes of Health Research [CIHR], 2019). Genomics, as a research focus, involves the study of all human genes, which are collectively called the human genome. The study and practice of genomics is concerned with how genes express themselves and how they interact with each other and the environment to encourage or discourage disease (Molster, Bowman, Bilkey, et al., 2018). Genomic interests range from an individual level to a population-based level similar to health-promoting activities. Genomics at an individual level is concerned with an individual's risks related to that person's genomic profile and environmental stimuli. At the population level, genomics is concerned with large-scale patterns of genomic risk and how that plays out in the public arena. Therefore population-based public health genomics is involved with policy development, prioritizing useful genomic information, and ensuring that genomic information is discovered and used ethically and responsibly (Molster et al., 2018).

Lifestyle, environment, and genetics and the interaction between the three are determining factors of disease. Currently the focus of much intervention is on the lifestyle and environmental contributors to disease. Because we are just beginning to look at the genomic components of disease and how they interact with lifestyle and environment, the current scientific discussion revolves around the ethical implications of private and public genomic interventions. Current debate surrounding population genomics focuses on the public's "right not to know" (Allen, Senecal, & Avard, 2014). Genomic information can be used to formulate public health information and initiatives. There are potential social justice ramifications in sharing large-scale genomic information which may accentuate discrimination and worsen stigma. If the information is too complex or difficult to comprehend, it may demotivate people from making needed positive changes. For example, if there is a health behaviour that is linked to a particular genomic profile, knowing that could help those who do not have the genomic profile become motivated to change their behaviour, whereas people with the genetic profile might become demotivated to change their behaviour. Because it is a combination of factors that cause disease, just because a person has the genetic profile does not mean it is an absolute that the person will get the disease, so sharing this information incautiously may be a disservice to public health as opposed to a service. Careful consideration of the risks and benefits of sharing public genomic-related information is essential.

Sources: Allen, C., Senecal, K., & Avard, D. (2014). Defining the scope of public engagement: Examining the "right not to know" in public health genomics. *Public Health Genomics, 42*(1), 11–18; Molster, C. M., Bowman, F. L., Bilkey, G. A., et al. (2018). The evolution of public health genomics: Exploring its past, present, and future. *Frontiers in Public Health, 6*, 247. https://doi.org/10.3389/fpubh.2018.00247.

## MOVING TOWARD SOLUTIONS

Approximately one in eight Canadians face food insecurity and one in five struggle with housing affordability (Canada Without Poverty, 2019). Solutions are neither simple nor easy, but more sustainable solutions are found when framing issues using the population health promotion model (PHPM) discussed earlier. The PHPM assists in identifying the socioenvironmental "who, what, how, and why" of a health promotion activity. Specifically, one must determine at which level of society to take action (the "who" of the PHPM), the social determinants of health to act upon (the "what"), the appropriate Ottawa Charter action area (the "how"), and the best available evidence to make decisions (the "why"). Using the model results in a more encompassing view of a problem and leads to better solutions. Such an approach promotes upstream thinking that focuses on strategies to address economic and social factors by removing barriers and improving supports to allow people to reach their full potential (National Collaborating Centre for Determinants of Health, 2019). Solutions can be focused in two main directions: with individuals and families, or at community and governmental levels of involvement. The first direction concentrates on actions of the individual, especially actions related to lifestyle choices across the life span. The learning and the inherent changes that are involved require the adoption of a new set of skills by people who will need the assistance of nurses to make those changes.

Motivational factors play a large role in influencing attitudinal change. Health promotion programs and health education are only part of the answer. Financial incentives for prevention may be another motivating factor, and health advocacy by professionals in the health field is critical. Additionally, private and public action at all levels is needed to reduce social and environmental health hazards. Toxic agents in the environment such as particles from diesel emissions, and social conditions such as overcrowding, can present health hazards such as the spread of tuberculosis and others that may not be detected for years; therefore it is necessary for individuals and the government to play a role.

Legislation and financing that relate to primary prevention are discussed in Chapter 3. Government activity, in the form of legislation, is currently increasing in this area. For example, increasing the activity time in schools, mandating seat belt use, and implementing taxes on gasoline use to combat climate change, are specific areas for governmental intervention. Health ecology and planning are important areas for government involvement in the future. The redirection of the existing health care delivery system, putting more emphasis on primary prevention, is probably the most difficult and the most far-reaching goal; yet an emphasis on upstream thinking to the address the social determinants of health is necessary to truly improve the health of Canadians.

## CASE STUDY

### Health Assessment: Antonio (Tony) and Family

Tony's large brick home is located in Hamilton, Ontario, a few miles away from the small bungalow where his parents, Enzo and Maria, raised their family after emigrating from Italy. His parents, two older brothers, and Antonio (who was 1 year old at the time) arrived in Canada in 1963.

Tony was raised knowing the odds that unless he went to university or community college, he would likely follow his father and brothers' footsteps and work in one of the local steel mills. As his mother often reminded him, Antonio had to do better than others in school so he would not be restricted to working in the mills. Tony was intent on helping at home and building something better for his future. He graduated from high school and was awarded a scholarship to a prominent Ontario university, and eventually earned a Master of Business Administration degree. He married Sharon, his long-time girlfriend, and the two planned their future.

With a good job in a large local sales firm, Tony built his house and started a family. He moved from being a salesman to being a division head and often travelled to regional meetings, sometimes accompanied by Sharon and their three children. Tony's dream of sharing his success with his family included saving part of his earnings for his children's postsecondary education and spending money on his parents.

This new way of life meant Tony had little time for relaxation and frequently had to attend business luncheons and career-promoting social events. Tony kept late hours and worked long weekends. Good food, drinks, and cigarettes helped Tony relax before and after important business and social encounters; these softened the edges of hard bargaining and were status symbols.

Not surprisingly, Tony gained weight. He had a persistent cough, which was probably a result of the smoking habit that developed during the early years of his career. Tony's health care provider said his blood pressure and serum lipid levels were both higher than normal and that he had chronic bronchitis. The health care provider urged Tony to take the actions that Tony already recognized: reduce smoking, drinking, and intake of saturated fats and calories; get more exercise; and find ways to relax. However, Tony's life was too busy for exercise. He had to work harder because he was promoted in his company, but he also had to appear relaxed, which was an essential characteristic for a prospective vice president. To meet these goals, Tony tended to drink and smoke more. He also refused to take medication for problems he could not see. Without the outward signs of disease, Tony believed he was out of shape but generally healthy. Then Sharon noted that his chance for a job promotion might actually improve if he lost some weight; therefore Tony registered for a physical fitness program for executives that he could attend on Saturday mornings and before work during the week. At his first workout, the classic sharp pain gripped his chest and Tony had a massive heart attack.

Weeks later, Tony was convalescing at home after being released from the hospital's coronary care unit. He was lucky to survive the heart attack and he was also fortunate to have 80% of his earnings protected by the company's disability pension.

However, Tony's dreams of promotion in the company were shattered. For many months he could go to the office only two or three times a week at most, simply to deal with routine matters. He could not travel, for business or otherwise, for a long time. He was also skeptical about his cardiac rehabilitation program because his heart attack happened during exercise.

#### Reflective Questions

- What are the socioenvironmental factors that contributed to Tony's situation?
- How would you use the population health promotion model to intervene?
- As a nurse, how would you explain to Tony that his heart attack was not caused by his exercise?
- How might a family approach to diet and exercise, and a re-examination of life goals work with this family, given its structure and background?
- Are there negative behaviours in your life that are influenced by larger societal values?

# TYING IT ALL TOGETHER USING THE NURSING PROCESS

## Problem Identification

How many problems are present in Tony's situation? The answer depends on who is asked the question and his or her position in relation to Tony. Each point of view focuses on different aspects of Tony's life. His health care provider, using a biomedical approach, might say that Tony has coronary heart disease with an acute myocardial infarction, hypertension, hyperlipidemia, chronic bronchitis, and obesity. But Tony's problems also represent workplace and societal stressors that led to unhealthy behaviours. His nurse can add that he has paid little attention to his lifestyle, even after changes were recommended. Humans are creatures of habit, and Tony continues to overeat, drink too much, smoke, not exercise, and live a stressful life. Tony's employer sees a man who has potential but who is now too disabled to take on new responsibilities and perhaps unable to continue performing his previous duties. Tony's children might feel helpless and concerned about his reduced vitality. His wife, Sharon, knows that their plans for travel and enjoyment, might suffer. The human resource personnel who manage Tony's disability and pension programs would say that he has an expensive disease, and the provincial health planner would point out that Tony's problem is only one of a growing number of disabling illnesses that result from preventable causes.

To Tony, his health problems are multidimensional. His initial fear of dying, pain, dependence, and frustration decreased as he began to feel better, but Tony is haunted by his realization that he might never be able to achieve his dreams for himself and his family. Although theoretically in his prime, Tony suddenly sees himself as far older than his years, both in body and in social achievement. He believes he has reached his limit and that he will never again have the freedom to choose his future. He and his family needed to evaluate their situation and make alternative plans based on strengths planning. A care plan has been developed based on the situation of Tony and his family. (See the Care Plan at the end of this chapter.)

## Planning Interventions

Rather than emphasizing the persistent health issues and related problems, the nurse can begin with the PHPM to identify the focus of intervention; in this situation, Tony, his family, and his community. What to take action on would consider Tony's income and social status; social support network; education; culture; working conditions; physical environments; biology and genetics; and his personal health practices and coping skills. The appropriate Ottawa Charter action strategies (i.e., the how) to contemplate are: creating supportive environments; developing personal skills; and building healthy public policy. The nurse employs strength-based planning to help focus the family members and their providers on the building blocks for their future by identifying the assets or strengths of the individual, the family, and the community, and applying those assets to improve or maintain the current level of functioning.

Tony's health care providers can begin with the fact that Tony survived his first myocardial infarction. The coronary damage resulting from this event becomes the baseline for determining future change in the lives of Tony and his family. Earlier, Tony's health care provider had taken a broader time perspective when he advised Tony to reduce his cigarette smoking, which was contributing to both his bronchitis and his hypertension, and to change his high-fat diet and sedentary habits, which contributed to his weight problem and his high blood pressure. These lifestyle changes now become tools for Tony's recovery and for change within his family. His cardiac event also becomes a risk factor for heart disease in the lives of his children.

Looking at the immediate future, Tony's employer saw the effect of the event on Tony's position within the company. Tony would have a long recovery that could be successful if he continued with his cardiac rehabilitation program. Strengths planning at this level means examining how to move Tony back into his work role without further jeopardizing his health. Tony and Sharon also need to examine if he could continue in this position, given its potential effect on his health.

Tony and his family used a broader perspective than the medical personnel or the corporation. They knew that to achieve the family's economic goals and still spend time together they had to make decisions that would ultimately affect Tony's health for the positive. Similar to many Canadians, they had been willing to live with Tony's job pressures and stressful lifestyle. However, they also recognized that the strength of their family, their ability to work together to achieve goals, and their faith were assets that could be used for support.

Tony's social network of friends, relatives, and church members became an additional asset. They helped the family through the difficult initial weeks at home by delivering meals, taking care of the yard work and laundry, and providing companionship so Sharon could shop and have time alone. As Tony recovered, they would provide support for the social and lifestyle changes that Tony and his family needed to make.

The nurse-led cardiovascular rehabilitation group played a vital role in Tony's recovery. As the health care provider continued to monitor Tony's cardiac status, the nurse began the long process of working with Tony to modify his habits and to acknowledge his accomplishments. He had stopped smoking while in the hospital, but with more free time than usual, he was craving to smoke again. Using a strength-based planning approach, the nurse identified the changes that Tony needed to make to decrease the risk of a second heart attack. A plan was developed to help Tony begin to take control of his life through behaviour changes. These changes included relaxation techniques, diet modification, smoking cessation, and mild chair exercises. The support of the family was enlisted to reinforce the changes Tony was willing to make, because social support and environmental changes are shown to enhance personal decision making. His employer was contacted and agreed to a plan enabling Tony to work from home using a computer while the workplace became smoke-free. Tony became an asset to the workplace, serving as a spokesperson for the benefits of lifestyle change. He was enlisted to talk with other employees about stress management, exercise, weight reduction, and smoking cessation based on his personal experiences.

Health planners and public health officials used the broadest perspective in strength-based planning by viewing Tony as an example of a person whose potential shifted as a result of a preventable, disabling illness. The planners looked to public and private community patterns and policies that increase healthful habits and living conditions. Work schedules and work load; stress and safety in work environments; programs for increased jobs and wages; availability of public transportation systems, recreational facilities, and economically accessible housing; and regulation of health-damaging drugs such as alcohol and nicotine were all taken into consideration (Brawley, 2017; Whitsel, 2017). The strength-based planning approach emphasized the positive actions that could be made at the personal, employment, community, and societal levels to minimize the effects of Tony's illness and related diseases, thereby addressing all levels of the socioenvironmental approach to health promotion.

## What Was the Actual Cause of Tony's Problem?

It is not possible to separate one cause from another because heart disease is a multifactorial disease. In Tony's case the sources of illness were found in the many interrelationships in his life. The medical label of "heart disease" is actually a symptom of much bigger issues for Tony, such as societal pressure to accumulate wealth and status, long working hours without much appreciation or reward, and pressure to be a good provider for his family. Attempting to treat or change each factor as a separate entity can have only a limited effect on the improvement of overall health. Tony's health problems were numerous. In addition to a poor diet, weight gain, lack of exercise, and smoking, his hyperlipidemia, an adaptive biological response to the pressures in his life, further debilitated him. It eventually led to clogged coronary vessels, and his responses became maladaptive. His hypertension, resulting from his diet and time-constrained lifestyle, complicated by the buildup of plaque secondary to hyperlipidemia, was also a biological attempt to adjust to a situation that contributed to an imbalance between his personal resources and the demands of his family and the economic world. Tony's smoking was a psychosocial means to help him relieve some of the emotional pressures. Cigarette use by persons who have hypertension or high serum cholesterol levels multiplies their risk of coronary heart disease (Chan, Pang, Hooper, et al., 2015). It may have served this short-term purpose, but only at a silently rising cost to his health.

## Evaluation of the Situation

The health status of an individual or population depends on a sustainable balance of the complex responses between physiological, psychological, and social and environmental factors. Health was initially conceived as a biological state, with genetic endowment as the starting point. However, health involves psychological and social aspects and is interpreted within the context of the immediate environment.

The interconnections between biophysical, behavioural, and environmental causes and consequences did not end with Tony's heart attack. His heart attack was only the most dramatic sign that health-damaging responses outweighed health-promoting ones. The "tip of the iceberg" analogy is frequently used to illustrate the importance of identifying individuals with subclinical symptoms. High blood lipid levels, high blood pressure, obesity, smoking, and persistent worrying were no less important than the infarction in shaping the status of Tony's health. Repairing the damage to Tony's heart without changing his lifestyle, habits, and work environment would only buy a brief amount of time before further damage would occur.

The infarction and resulting disability also permanently reshaped Tony's environment. After a few months of working full-time, Tony realized that he needed to find a less stressful job. He recognized that his sales administration skills were an asset and began interviewing in the nonprofit sector. Ultimately, he landed a job at half his previous salary, but with excellent benefits and a flexible work environment. Tony found that his contacts in both the corporate and the nonprofit sectors increased his value to his new employer. Tony's entire life, internal and external, had changed. He had learned to adapt to his health problems and had developed a more holistic approach to health and life.

Tony's situation illustrates how causes and effects in life and health tend to merge into constant, inseparable interconnections between individuals and their worlds. A person's health status is a reflection of a web of relationships that characterize that person's life. Health is not an achievement or a prize, but a high-quality interaction between a person's inner and outer worlds that provides the capacity to respond to the demands of the biological, behavioural, and environmental systems of these worlds.

## ◎ CARE PLAN

### *Health Assessment: Antonio (Tony) and Family*

**Nursing Issue**

Potential for improvement in coping after myocardial infarction, given existing family and community supports.

**Defining Strengths**
- Wife and children cohesive and attentive to needs
- Extensive, supportive network of friends, extended Italian community, and church members
- Educational background is a strength for understanding long-term complications
- Financially stable for the short term
- Access to a nurse-led cardiovascular rehabilitation program
- Early success in smoking cessation while in hospital, setting the stage for further lifestyle changes
- Employer willing to make concessions to allow working from home
- Reassessment of work abilities 2 months after infarction

**Expected Outcomes**
- The person will develop realistic expectations of capabilities on the basis of rehabilitation potential.
- The nurse and person will set mutually agreeable milestones for resuming functions.
- The person will develop a revitalized sense of self.
- The person and family will use available resources to examine social and role shifts that affect the family.
- The person and spouse will express to each other their hopes and fears about the future.

**Interventions**
- Listen to the concerns of the person and spouse regarding job, social, family, and medical concerns.
- Counsel the individual and spouse about realistic goals and expectations of cardiac rehabilitation.
- Assist the individual in setting realistic and reachable short-term goals.
- Assist the individual in developing more effective problem-solving skills.
- Provide support and positive feedback as short-term goals are met.
- Explore available community services that match the goals of the family.
- Facilitate family access to needed services through advocacy and supportive guidance.
- Supervise and teach about the use of prescribed and other medications.
- Coordinate communications between providers, employers, and other organizations to meet coping needs of the individual and his or her family.

# SUMMARY

The ways individuals define health and health problems are important because definitions influence attempts to improve health and care delivery. In the case study, Tony's health was affected by obvious, immediate, and personal factors such as his diet and employment pressures. Nevertheless, his problems had their roots in the social and economic conditions of his parents; in his own early history of education and work; and in his and his family's hopes and aspirations. His health care provider defined Tony's problem in immediate biomedical terms. Community health nurses, who saw Tony's problem on a longer term population basis, sought policy solutions to the problem of preventing cardiovascular disease.

The view taken in this text is that a broad and longer term perspective of health is the best guide to promoting health more effectively, even as nurses deal with individual problems on a daily basis. Health is a sustainable balance between internal and external forces. Health allows people to move through life free from the constraints of illness and promotes healing.

Illness represents an imbalance that human choices (intertwined social, political, spiritual, professional, and personal choices) create. In Canada, communities still have time to reduce the onslaught of chronic disability and shift the direction, slow the pace, and humanize the scope of economic and social life.

Shifting directions in today's health care patterns may be possible only when nurses and other health professionals do what is expected of them as leaders in the care of health: to work with others through open processes; to provide leadership in finding the vision and the path; and to inform, educate, and re-educate themselves, their colleagues, the media, and the general public using research findings and evidence-informed practice methods.

The responsibility of nurses as health professionals today is to see the health problem in new ways and help others to do the same. Responsibility means developing new roles and examining the problem through others' viewpoints, including those of individuals, the public, other professionals, and other nations. Responsibility also means evaluating the social and individual consequences, the long-term and short-term effects, and the public and private interests that are involved when one is deciding on the set of tools to use in the care of health.

**Evolve Chapter Features**

http://evolve.elsevier.com/Canada/Edelman/healthpromotion/
- Review Questions

# REFERENCES

Ajzen, A., & Fishbein, M. (1980). *Understanding attitudes and predicting social behavior.* Upper Saddle River, NJ: Prentice Hall. [Seminal Reference].

Allen, C., Senecal, K., & Avard, D. (2014). Defining the scope of public engagement: examining the "right not to know" in public health genomics. *Public Health Genomics, 42*(1), 11–18. https://doi.org/10.1111/jlme.12114.

Alslman, E. T., Ahmad, M. M. M., Hani, M. A. B., et al. (2017). Health: A developing concept in nursing. *International Journal of Nursing Knowledge, 28*(2), 64–69.

Armstrong, H., Daly, T. J., & Choiniere, J. A. (2016). Policies and practices: The case of RAI-MDS in Canadian long-term care homes. *Journal of Canadian Studies, 50*(2), 348–367. https://doi.org/10.3138/jcs.50.2.348.

Association of Faculties of Medicine of Canada. (2018). *AFMC primer on population health* (2nd ed.). Retrieved from https://phprimer.afmc.ca/en/.

Bandura, A. (1976). *Social learning theory.* Upper Saddle River, NJ: Prentice Hall. [Seminal Reference].

Bandura, A. (1999). *Self-efficacy: The exercise of control.* New York: W.H. Freeman. [Seminal Reference].

Bandura, A. (2004). Health promotion by social cognitive means. *Health Education Behavior, 31*(2), 143–164 [Seminal Reference].

Barekatain, A., Weiss, S., & Weintraub, S. (2015). Value of primordial and primary prevention for cardiovascular diseases: A global perspective. In J. Andrade, F. Pinto, & D. Arnett (Eds.), *Prevention of cardiovascular diseases* (pp. 21–28). New York: Springer.

Barnish, M., Tørnes, M., & Nelson-Horne, B. (2018). How much evidence is there that political factors are related to population health outcomes? An internationally comparative systematic review. *BMJ Open, 8*:e020886. https://doi.org/10.1136/bmjopen-2017-020886.

Bender, M. (2018). Reconceptualizing the nursing metaparadigm: Articulating the philosophical ontology of the nursing discipline that orients inquiry and practice. *Nursing Inquiry, 25*(3). https://doi.org/10.1111/nin.12243.

Benner, P., Sutphen, P., Leonard, V., et al. (2010). *Educating nurses: A call for radical transformation.* San Francisco: Jossey-Bass. [Seminal Reference].

Bethune, R., Absher, N., Obiagwu, M., et al. (2018). Social determinants of self-reported health for Canada's indigenous peoples: A public health approach. *Public Health, online,* 1–9. https://doi.org/10.1016/j.puhe.2018.03.007.

Bohnert, N., Chagnon, J., & Dion, P. (2015). *Population projections for Canada (2013 to 2063), provinces and territories (2013 to 2038). Catalogue no. 91-520-X.* Ottawa: Statistics Canada. Retrieved from https://www150.statcan.gc.ca/n1/pub/91-520-x/91-520-x2014001-eng.htm.

Braveman, P., & Gottlieb, L. (2014). The social determinants of health: It's time to consider the causes. *Public Health Reports, 129*(Suppl. 2), 19–31. https://doi.org/10.1177/00333549141291S206.

Brawley, O. W. (2017). The role of government and regulation in cancer prevention. *The Lancet Oncology, 18,* e483–e493. https://doi.org/10.1016/S1470-2045(17)30374-1.

Canadian Institute for Health Information [CIHI]. (2019). *Continuing care metadata.* Ottawa: CIHI. Retrieved from https://www.cihi.ca/en/continuing-care-metadata.

Canadian Institutes of Health Research [CIHR]. (2019). *Institute of genetics.* Ottawa: CIHR. Retrieved from http://www.cihr-irsc.gc.ca/e/13147.html.

Canadian Nurses Association (CNA). (2019). *Social determinants of health.* Ottawa: CNA. Retrieved from https://www.cna-aiic.ca/en/nursing-practice/evidence-based-practice/social-determinants-of-health.

Canadian Nurses Association (CNA). (2018). *Position statement. Evidence-informed decision-making and nursing practice*. Ottawa: CNA. Retrieved from https://www.cna-aiic.ca/-/media/cna/page-content/pdf-en/evidence-informed-decision-making-and-nursing-practice-position-statement_dec-2018.pdf.

Canadian Nurses Association (CNA). (2017). *CNA code of ethics for registered nurses*. Ottawa: CNA. Retrieved from https://www.cna-aiic.ca/en/nursing-practice/nursing-ethics.

Canadian Nurses Association (CNA). (2015). *Framework for the practice of registered nurses in Canada*. Ottawa: CNA. Retrieved from https://www.cna-aiic.ca/en/nursing-practice/the-practice-of-nursing.

Canadian Nurses Association (CNA). (2010). *Social justice . . . a means to an end, an end in itself* (2nd ed.). Ottawa: Author. Retrieved from https://www.cna-aiic.ca/-/media/cna/page-content/pdf-fr/social_justice_2010_e.pdf.

Canadian Public Health Association (CPHA). (2019). *Projects unstructured play*. Ottawa: Author. Retrieved from https://www.cpha.ca/unstructured-play.

Canadian Task Force on Preventive Health Care. (2018). *Published guidelines*. Ottawa: CTFPC. Retrieved from https://canadiantaskforce.ca/guidelines/published-guidelines/.

Canada Without Poverty. (2019). *Just the facts*. Ottawa: Author. Retrieved from http://www.cwp-csp.ca/poverty/just-the-facts/.

Catford, J. (2014). Turn, turn, turn: time to reorient health services. *Health Promotion International, 29*(1), 1–3.

Celentano, D. D., & Szklo, M. (Eds.). (2019). *Gordis epidemiology* (6th ed.) Philadelphia: Elsevier.

Champion, V. L., & Skinner, C. S. (2008). The health belief model. In K. Glanz, B. Rimer, & K. Viswanath (Eds.), *Health behavior and health education: Theory, research and practice* (4th ed.). San Francisco: Jossey-Bass. [Seminal Reference].

Chan, D. C., Pang, J., Hooper, A. J., et al. (2015). Elevated lipoprotein(a), hypertension and renal insufficiency as predictors of coronary artery disease in patients with genetically confirmed heterozygous familial hypercholesterolemia. *International Journal of Cardiology, 201*, 633–638. https://doi.org/10.1016/j.ijcard.2015.08.146.

Cohen, S. R., Mount, B. M., Bruera, E., et al. (1997). Validity of the McGill Quality of Life Questionnaire in the palliative care setting. A multi-center Canadian study demonstrating the importance of the existential domain. *Palliative Medicine, 11*(1), 3–20 [Seminal Reference].

Dávila, M. G., Polanco, V. P., & Segura, L. (2017). Income deprivation and self-rated health. *American Journal of Public Health, 107*(11), 1688. https://doi.org/10.2105/APHA2017.304086.

Epp, J. (1986). Achieving health for all: A framework for health promotion. Ottawa, ON: Health and Welfare Canada. Retrieved from Health Canada website: http://www.hc-sc.gc.ca/hcs-sss/pubs/system-regime/1986-frame-plan-promotion/index-eng.php. [Seminal Reference]

Farre, A., & Rapley, T. (2017). The new old (and old new) medical model: Four decades navigating the biomedical and psychosocial understandings of health and illness. *Healthcare, 5*, 88. https://doi.org/10.3390/healthcare5040088.

Gordon, M. (2016). *Manual of nursing diagnosis* (13th ed.). Sudbury, MA: Jones & Bartlett.

Gottlieb, L. N. (2014). CE: Strengths-based nursing. *American Journal of Nursing, 114*(8), 24–32. https://doi.org/10.1097/01.NAJ.0000453039.70629.e2.

Gottlieb, L. N., & Gottlieb, B. (2017). Strengths-based nursing: a process for implementing a philosophy into practice. *Journal of Family Nursing, 23*(3), 319–340. https://doi.org/10.1177/1074840717717731.

Government of Canada. (2019). *Indigenous homes innovation initiative*. Ottawa: Author. Retrieved from https://impact.canada.ca/en/challenges/indigenous-homes.

Green, L. W., Richard, L., & Potvin, L. (1996). Ecological foundations of health promotion. *American Journal of Health Promotion, 10*(4), 280–281 [Seminal Reference].

Hamilton, N. & Bhatti, T. (1996). *Population health promotion: An integrated model of population health and health promotion*. Ottawa: Health Promotion Development Division, Health Canada. Retrieved from https://www.canada.ca/en/public-health/services/health-promotion/population-health/population-health-promotion-integrated-model-population-health-health-promotion.html.

Health Canada & the Public Health Agency of Canada (PHAC). (2016). *Evaluation of mental health and mental illness activities of Health Canada and the Public Health Agency of Canada 2010–2011 to 2014–2015*. Ottawa: Health Canada, PHAC. Retrieved from https://www.canada.ca/en/health-canada/corporate/transparency/corporate-management-reporting/evaluation/2010-2011-2014-2015-mental-health-mental-illness-activities-health-canada-public-health-agency-canada.html.

HealthCareCAN. (2016). *Issue brief: The Truth and Reconciliation Commission of Canada: Health-related recommendations*. Ottawa: Author. Retrieved from http://www.healthcarecan.ca/wp-content/themes/camyno/assets/document/IssueBriefs/2016/EN/TRCC_EN.pdf.

Hyndman, B., & The Alder Group. (2007). *Towards the development of competencies for health promotors in Canada: A discussion paper*. Ottawa: Health Promotion Canada. Retrieved from https://www.healthpromotioncanada.ca/resources/publications/.

Khanlou, N., Mustafa, N., Vazquez, L. M., et al. (2017). Mothering children with developmental disabilities: A critical perspective on health promotion. *Health Care for Women International, 38*(6), 613–634. https://doi.org/10.1080/07399332.2017.1296841.

Lafrenière, S., Folch, N., Bédard, L., et al. (2017). Strategies used by older patients to prevent functional decline during hospitalization. *Clinical Nursing Research, 26*(1), 6–26. https://doi.org/10.1177/1054773815601392.

Leavell, H., & Clark, A. E. (1965). *Preventive medicine for the doctor in his community*. New York: McGraw-Hill. [Seminal Reference].

Low, J., & Thériault, L. (2008). Heath promotion policy in Canada: Lessons forgotten, lessons still to learn. *Health Promotion International, 23*(2), 200–206. https://doi.org/10.1093/heapro/dan002.

Marchildon, G. P. (2012). *Making medicare: new perspectives on the history of medicare in Canada*. Toronto [Ont.]: University of Toronto Press. https://doi.org/10.3138/j.ctt2tv25c.

Marmot, M. (2017). Social justice, epidemiology and health. *European Journal of Epidemiology, 32*, 537–546. https://doi.org/10.1007/s10654-017-0286-3.

Martin, D., Miller, A. P., Quesnel-Vallée, A., et al. (2018). Canada's universal health-care system: Achieving its potential. *Lancet, 391*, 1718–1735. https://doi.org/10.1016/S0140-6736(18)30181-8.

McHugh, J. E., & Lawlor, B. A. (2016). Executive functioning independently predicts self-rated health and improvement in self-rated health over time among community-dwelling older adults. *Aging & Mental Health, 20*(4), 415–422. https://doi.org/10.1080/13607863.2015.1018866.

MOHLTC. (2015). Patients first: A proposal to strengthen patient-centered health care in Ontario. Retrieved from http://www.health.gov.on.ca/en/news/bulletin/2015/docs/discussion_paper_20151217.pdf

Molster, C. M., Bowman, F. L., Bilkey, G. A., et al. (2018). The evolution of public health genomics: Exploring its past, present, and future. *Frontiers in Public Health, 6*, 247. https://doi.org/10.3389/fpubh.2018.00247.

Morency, J. D., Malenfant, E. C., & MacIssac, S. (2017). *Immigration and diversity: Population projections for Canada and its regions, 2011 to 2036.* (Catalogue no. 91-551-X.) Ottawa: Statistics Canada. Retrieved from https://www150.statcan.gc.ca/n1/pub/91-551-x/91-551-x2017001-eng.htm.

Mudge, A. M., Banks, M. D., Barnett, A. G., et al. (2017). CHERISH (Collaboration for Hospitalised Elders Reducing the Impact of Stays in Hospital): Protocol for a multi-site improvement program to reduce geriatric syndromes in older inpatients. *BMC Geriatrics, 17*(11), online 1–9. https://doi.org/10.1186/s12877-016-0399-7.

National Collaborating Centre for Aboriginal Health. (2018). *The built environment: Understanding how physical environments influence the health and well-being of First Nations peoples living on-reserve.* Prince George, BC: NCCAH. Retrieved from https://www.nccah-ccnsa.ca/495/The_built_environment__Understanding_how_physical_environments_influence_the_health_and_well-being_of_First_Nations_peoples_living_on-reserve_.nccah?id=236.

National Collaborating Centre for Determinants of Health. (2019). *Upstream/downstream.* Antigonish, NS: Author. Retrieved from http://nccdh.ca/glossary/entry/upstream-downstream.

Norwood, S. (2003). *Nursing consultation: A framework for working with communities* (2nd ed.). Upper Saddle River, NJ: Prentice Hall. [Seminal Reference].

Pender, N. J., Murdaugh, C. L., & Parsons, M. A. (2015). *Health promotion in nursing practice* (6th ed.). Upper Saddle River, NJ: Prentice Hall.

Polit, D. F., & Beck, C. T. (2017). *Nursing research: Generating and assessing evidence for nursing practice* (10th ed.). Philadelphia: Wolters Kluwer.

Porta, M. (2014). *Dictionary of epidemiology* (5th ed.). Oxford: Oxford University Press.

Prochaska, J., Gill, P., & Hall, S. (2004). Treatment of tobacco use in an inpatient psychiatric setting. *Psychiatric Services, 55,* 1265–1270 [Seminal Reference].

Public Health Agency of Canada (PHAC). (2017). *What determines health?* Ottawa: Author. Retrieved from http://www.phac-aspc.gc.ca/ph-sp/determinants/index-eng.php#determinants.

Public Health Agency of Canada (PHAC). (2018a). *Key health inequities in Canada: A national portrait.* Ottawa: PHAC. Retrieved from https://www.canada.ca/en/public-health/services/publications/science-research-data/key-health-inequalities-canada-national-portrait-executive-summary.html.

Public Health Agency of Canada (PHAC). (2018b). *A common vision for increasing physical activity and reducing sedentary living in Canada: Let's get moving.* Ottawa: PHAC. Retrieved from https://www.canada.ca/en/public-health/services/publications/healthy-living/lets-get-moving.html.

Richard, L., Gauvin, L., & Raine, K. (2011). Ecological models revisited: Their uses and evolution in health promotion over two decades. *Annual Review of Public Health, 32,* 307–326 [Seminal Reference].

Richmond, S. A., D'Cruz, J., Lokku, A., et al. (2016). Trends in unintentional injury mortality in Canadian children 1950–2009 and association with selected population-level interventions. *Canadian Journal of Public Health, 107*(4–5), e431–3437. https://doi.org/10.17269/CJPH.107.5315.

Rosa, W., Estes, T., & Watson, J. (2017). Caring science conscious dying: an emerging metaparadigm. *Nursing Science Quarterly, 30*(1), 58–64. https://doi.org/10.1177/0894318416680538.

Ruger, J. P., Hammonds, R., Ooms, G., et al. (2015). From conceptual pluralism to practical agreement on policy: Global responsibility for global health. *BMC International Health and Human Rights, 15*(30). https://doi.org/10.1186/s12914-015-0065-8.

Shields, M., Garner, R. E., & Wilkins, K. (2013). Dynamics of smoking cessations and health-related quality of life among Canadians. *Health Reports* (no. 82-003-X). Ottawa: Statistics Canada. Retrieved from https://www150.statcan.gc.ca/n1/pub/82-003-x/2013002/article/11769-eng.htm.

Shrira, A., Palgi, Y., Hoffman, Y., et al. (2018). Subjective age as a moderator in the reciprocal effects between posttraumatic stress disorder symptoms and self-rated physical functioning. *Frontiers in Psychology, 9,* 1746. https://doi.org/10.3389/fpsyg.2018.01746.

St. John, P., Tyas, S. L., Menec, V., et al. (2019). Multimorbidity predicts functional decline in community-dwelling older adults. *Canadian Family Physician, 65*(2), e56–e63. Retrieved from http://www.cfp.ca/content/65/2/e56.

The Global Fund to Fight AIDS, Tuberculosis and Malaria. (2019). *Global fund overview.* Geneva, Switzerland. Retrieved from https://www.theglobalfund.org/en/overview/.

The Standing Senate Committee on Social Affairs, Science and Technology; the Honourable Wilbert Joseph Keon, Chair, and the Honourable Lucie Pepin, Deputy Chair. (2009). *A healthy productive Canada: a determinant of health approach. Final report of the Senate Subcommittee on Population Health.* Retrieved from https://sencanada.ca/content/sen/Committee/402/popu/rep/rephealth1jun09-e.pdf.

Vollman, A. R. (2017). Population health promotion: Essentials and essence of practice. In A. R. Vollman, E. T. Anderson, & J. McFarlane (Eds.), *Canadian Community as Partner: Theory & Multidisciplinary Practice* (4th ed.) (pp. 3–6). Philadelphia: Wolters Kluwer.

Whitsel, L. P. (2017). Government's role in promoting healthy living. *Progress in Cardiovascular Diseases, 59,* 492–497. https://doi.org/10.1016/j.pcad.2017.01.003.

World Health Organization (WHO). (2019). *Health equity.* Geneva: Author. Retrieved from https://www.who.int/topics/health_equity/en/.

World Health Organization (WHO). (2004). *The World Health Organization Quality of Life (WHOQOL)-BREF.* Geneva: Author. Retrieved from http://www.who.int/substance_abuse/research_tools/en/english_whoqol.pdf.

World Health Organization (WHO). (1998). *Health promotion glossary.* Geneva: Author. Retrieved from https://www.who.int/healthpromotion/about/HPR%20Glossary%201998.pdf?ua=1.

World Health Organization (WHO). (1986). *Ottawa Charter for Health Promotion: First international conference on health promotion,* 21 November 1986. Geneva: Author. Retrieved from https://www.who.int/healthpromotion/conferences/previous/ottawa/en/index4.html.

World Health Organization (WHO). (1946). *Preamble to the Constitution of the World Health Organization as adopted by the International Health Conference,* New York, 19–22 June 1946. Geneva: Author. Retrieved from https://www.who.int/about/who-we-are/constitution.

World Health Organization (WHO). (2004). *The World Health Organization Quality of Life (WHOQOL)-BREF.* Geneva: Author. Retrieved from http://www.who.int/substance_abuse/research_tools/en/english_whoqol.pdf.

Ziabakhsh, S., Pederson, A., Prodan-Bhalla, N., et al. (2016). Women-centered and culturally responsive heart health promotion among Indigenous women in Canada. *Health Promotion Practice, 17*(6), 814–826. https://doi.org/10.1177/1524839916633238.

Zisberg, A., Shadmi, E., Gur-Yaish, N., et al. (2015). Hospital-associated functional decline: the role of hospitalization processes beyond individual risk factors. *Journal of the American Geriatrics Society, 63,* 55–62. https://doi.org/10.1111/jgs.13193.

# 2

# Diverse Populations and Health

*Marian Luctkar-Flude, RN, PhD, CCSNE*

## INTENDED LEARNING OUTCOMES

*After completing this chapter, the reader will be able to:*

- Differentiate among ethnicity, ethnic group, and minority group.
- Differentiate among culture, values, and values orientation.
- Differentiate between cultural competency and cultural humility.
- Describe demographic data relative to diverse populations.

- Describe health concerns and issues of the following diverse populations in Canada: Indigenous persons, LGBTQ2 persons, immigrants and refugees, and homeless persons.
- Discuss selected cultural factors that may have an impact on the health and well-being of diverse populations.
- Explain strategies for health care providers to meet the needs of diverse populations.
- Describe initiatives to address the health care concerns of diverse populations.

## KEY TERMS

Complementary and alternative medicine (CAM)
Cultural competency
Cultural humility
Cultural nursing assessment
Cultural pluralism
Cultural safety
Culture
Ethnicity
Ethnocentric perspective
Female genital cutting (FGC)
Gender diversity

Gender equity
Harm reduction
Health equity
Health inequalities
Health inequity
Hidden homelessness
Homelessness
*Indian Act*
Indian status
Integrative health care
Intersectional perspective
Marginalization

Minority group
Multiculturalism
Non-status individuals
Pan-Canadian Health Inequalities Reporting Initiative
United Nations (UN) 2030 Agenda for Sustainable Development
Value orientations
Values
Visible minority

## HEALTH INEQUALITIES AND HEALTH EQUITY

Canadians are among the healthiest people in the world; however, many magnitudes of inequality, particularly in health, exist within Canada and around the world, and in some cases these inequities are growing (Raphael, 2017; Tjepkema, Wilkins, & Long, 2013). Health inequalities refer to the differences in health status between different groups in society, which can be due to biological factors, individual choices, or chance; however, many health inequalities can be attributed to the unequal and unjust distribution of social and economic factors such as income and education, and exposure to social and environmental conditions that influence health (PHAC, 2018). There has been a growing awareness globally of the conditions that affect health and the opportunity for health, such as poverty, lack of educational opportunities, and ethnic and gender discrimination. Canada,

along with 192 other countries, has committed to the United Nations (UN) 2030 Agenda for Sustainable Development, which includes goals for ending poverty and food insecurity, providing inclusive and equitable quality education at all levels, achieving gender equality, and promoting health and well-being through universal health coverage and access to quality health care for all (UN, 2015).

In Canada, efforts to address health inequalities involve first identifying and describing the magnitude and distribution of key health inequalities to inform policy and program decision making (Canadian Institute for Health Information [CIHI], 2018). Findings from the Pan-Canadian Health Inequalities Reporting Initiative revealed significant health inequalities among Indigenous people, sexual and racial minorities, immigrants and people with functional limitations, as well as a range of inequalities related to socioeconomic status (Public Health

## 🔮 THINK ABOUT IT

### *Harm Reduction for Problematic Substance Use in Canada*

- Drug-use practices, such as reuse and sharing of injection and smoking equipment, can lead to transmission of human immunodeficiency virus (HIV), hepatitis C virus (HCV), and other harms, such as overdose, which are pressing issues affecting many communities across Canada. Traditional approaches to substance use problems focused on abstinence and rehabilitation through residential and outpatient programs. Access to health care services is often a major barrier for certain marginalized people, such as those who use drugs and those who are homeless.

- A newer compassionate and science-based approach to address problematic substance use is that of **harm reduction**, which aims to assist people who use legal and illegal drugs to live safer and healthier lives. Harm reduction is one of the five pillars of the Canadian Drugs and Substances Strategy, which supports measures to reduce the harmful health, social and economic consequences of substance use on individuals, families and communities.

- This approach acknowledges that people use drugs for many reasons, and that not everyone is willing or able to enter treatment at all times. Rather than condemn or condone, harm-reduction practitioners seek to work collaboratively with the individual to reduce risks, improve health, and connect people with other key health and social services until they are ready and able to seek treatment.

Harm-reduction programs such as needle and syringe programs are both effective and cost-effective measures to reduce equipment reuse and reduce HIV incidence and prevalence. Various program service models provide opportunities for prevention education related to risks of disease transmission and overdose, and a wide array of formal and informal health and social services.

Best practice recommendations have been developed for Canadian harm reduction programs that summarize best practices about distribution of needles, syringes, and other injection equipment, handling and disposal of used drug-use equipment, safer drug-use education on crack cocaine smoking, opioid overdose prevention, and naloxone distribution. Additional recommendations focus on service models, referrals to services, and emerging areas of practice. Elements of harm reduction programs such as safe injection and consumption sites remain controversial, and as a result, policies, funding, and support vary considerably at the provincial and territorial level across Canada, despite the growing body of research evidence regarding the effectiveness of this approach. Something to think about!

Sources: Canadian Drug Policy Coalition. (2019). *Harm reduction.* Retrieved from http://drugpolicy.ca/issues/harm-reduction/; Government of Canada. (2018). *Harm reduction: Canadian drugs and substances strategy.* Retrieved from https://www.canada.ca/en/health-canada/services/substance-use/canadian-drugs-substances-strategy/harm-reduction.html; Hyshka, E., Anderson-Baron, J., Karekezi, K., et al., (2017). Harm reduction in name, but not substance: A comparative analysis of current Canadian provincial and territorial policy frameworks. *Harm Reduction Journal, 14,* 50; Working Group on Best Practice for Harm Reduction Programs in Canada. (2013/2015). *Best practice recommendations for Canadian harm reduction programs.* Retrieved from https://www.catie.ca/en/programming/best-practices-harm-reduction.

Agency of Canada [PHAC], 2018). Lower income status has been linked to poorer health outcomes, including higher mortality rates in Canada (Raphael, 2016; Tjepkema et al., 2013).

Health equity is the accomplishment of the highest level of health for all people. Health inequity refers to the unjust differences in health between persons of different social groups, and it is evaluated indirectly through monitoring of health inequalities that can be measured. Many health inequities are the result of an unfair distribution of the underlying social determinants of health (SDOH), such as access to educational and employment opportunities, and reflect forms of structural and individual discrimination and prejudice (Browne & Varcoe, 2019). Health equity is one aspect of social justice that is focused on fair distribution and access to health services to all members of society (Fig. 2.1). Attaining health equity requires valuing everyone equally with focused and ongoing societal efforts to deal with preventable inequalities, historical and contemporary injustices, and the elimination of health and health care inequities. Although the diversity of the Canadian population is one of its best assets, one of the greatest challenges is reducing the disparity in health status of Canada's vulnerable populations, including Indigenous persons, immigrants, refugees, homeless persons, and gender-diverse persons.

Efforts to eliminate inequalities and achieve health equity have focused primarily on diseases or illnesses and on health care services. However, the absence of disease does not automatically equate to good health. An individual's ability to achieve good health could be affected because of race or ethnicity, gender, sexual identity, age, disability, socioeconomic status, and geographical location (Box 2.1). Three principles of action to lessen the

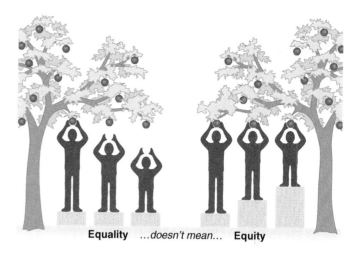

**Equality**   *...doesn't mean...*   **Equity**

Fig. 2.1 Creating Better Health for All: Health Equity

impact of SDOH and promote health equity are (1) improving the conditions of daily life; (2) addressing the inequitable distribution of power, money, and resources at global, national, and regional levels; and (3) raising public awareness of SDOH, measuring the problem, and evaluating access (WHO, 2013). Box 2.2 outlines specific recommendations for measuring health inequalities and promoting health equity within the Canadian context. In addition to SDOH, it is important to consider the degree of social cohesion and social capital present in communities and cities, as a strong sense of community belonging is closely linked to better health outcomes (Snyder, Cheff, & Roche, 2016). Fostering social cohesion means creating resilient societies where people live

## BOX 2.1   Measuring Health Inequality: Defining Stratifiers for Measuring Health Inequality

Issue: Approaches used to measure inequalities in health and health care vary and could be strengthened by the development and use of common standards.

Purpose: To identify differences in healthy equity that can be acted on and used to measure progress toward achieving health.

Strategy: CIHI held a pan-Canadian dialogue on March 22, 2016, to advance the measurement of equity in health care, with a total of 37 participants attending from 12 provinces and territories, representing ministries of health, quality councils, health regions, academia, practitioners, national organizations, and the federal government.

*Core stratifiers as highest priority for measuring equity in health care.* Age, sex, geographic location, income, education, aboriginal identity, and ethnicity.

*Additional stratifiers requiring further consideration.* Housing, disability, language, health insurance, immigrant status, sexual orientation, and gender identity.

*Low-rated stratifiers eliminated from core set.* Household status, country of birth, occupation, employment, wealth, and religion.

Sources: Canadian Institute for Health Information (CIHI). (2016). *Pan-Canadian dialogue to advance the measurement of equity in health care: Proceedings report.* Ottawa: Author; Canadian Institute for Health Information (CIHI). (2018). *In pursuit of health equity: Defining stratifiers for measuring health inequality—A focus on age, sex, gender, income, education and geographic location.* Ottawa: Author.

## BOX 2.2   Promoting Health Equity in Canada

The Public Health Agency of Canada (PHAC, 2018), in collaboration with the Pan-Canadian Public Health Network, published a report that documented Canada's health inequalities and described differences in health outcomes, daily living conditions, and structural conditions that support health among various populations. The report is supported by an online interactive database, the *Health Inequalities Data Tool*, which maps health inequalities according to the following indicators of health status and health determinants:

| Health Status | Health Determinants |
| --- | --- |
| Mortality and life expectancy | Health behaviours |
| Morbidity and disability | Physical and social environment |
| Mental illness and suicide | Working conditions |
| Physical and mental health | Health care |
| Self-assessed disease/health condition | Social protection |
| | Social inequities |
| | Early childhood development |

The report also outlines *key principles for action* and promising practices that can be adapted to advance health equity within the Canadian context:

1. Adopt a human rights approach to action on the social determinants of health and health equity.
2. Intervene across the life course with evidence-informed policies and culturally safe health and social services.
3. Intervene on both proximal (downstream) and distal (upstream) determinants of health and health equity.
4. Deploy a combination of targeted interventions and universal policies/interventions.
5. Address both material contexts (living, working, and environmental conditions) and sociocultural processes of power, privilege, and exclusion (how social inequalities are maintained across the life course and across generations).
6. Implement a "Health in All Policies" approach.
7. Carry out ongoing monitoring and evaluation.

Sources: Government of Canada. (2018). *Health Inequities Data Tool.* Ottawa: Public Health Agency of Canada; Public Health Agency of Canada (PHAC). (2018). *Key health inequalities in Canada: A national portrait.* Ottawa: Author.

together with all their differences, while developing well-being, a sense of belonging, and providing equal rights and opportunities for all (Fonseca, Lukosch, & Brazier, 2018).

The distribution of SDOH across a population is largely the result of public policies at various levels of government; thus, efforts to achieve health equity require understanding and support from the public. Overall, research suggests that Canadians perceive personal behaviour as being more important than the SDOH for determining the health of individuals, and that Canadians show relatively better understanding of the impact of income inequality and poverty on health compared with other determinants (Snyder et al., 2016).One study conducted in Ontario has demonstrated public support for targeted health equity interventions, but also that attributions of inequities (e.g., the plight of the poor versus privilege of the rich) and political affiliation are important predictors of support (Kirst, Shankardass, Singhal, et al., 2017). Implementation of health-promoting public policies that support the SDOH will require educating and engaging the public to demand changes to existing economic and political structures that currently benefit the wealthy and powerful (Raphael, 2017).

The Canadian Nurses Association (CNA) *Position Statement on Global Health and Equity* asserts that "Canadian health professionals, including registered nurses, have the right and responsibility to be cognizant and raise awareness of the root causes of inequity in global health and to participate in finding solutions" (CNA, 2009, p. 1). Health care providers can influence the health of Canadians at the patient, practice, and community levels by using a growing number of clinical decision aids, practice guidelines, and other tools available to help them address the social determinants in their day-to-day clinical practice, and by (1) asking patients about social challenges, (2) helping them access benefits and support services, (3) providing culturally safe and accessible services, and (4) partnering with local organizations and public health to get involved in health care planning and advocacy (Andermann, 2016).

## POPULATION MOSAIC OF CANADA

Indigenous people in Canada—the First Nations, Métis, and Inuit—and successive waves of immigrants and their Canadian-born descendants, have contributed to the ethnocultural diversity of the country (Statistics Canada, 2016a). Other types of diversity include religious, linguistic, sexual diversity, and ranges of ability and disability (Bourque, Bearskin, & Jakubec, 2017). Canada's multicultural society has been held up globally as a model for the integration of people from diverse ethnic backgrounds, and Canada was the first country to introduce an official multiculturalism policy (Jedwab, 2014). Multiculturalism consists of the ideas and ideals related to respect for and celebration of our cultural diversity, as well as formal initiatives at federal, provincial, and municipal levels to operationalize them (Brousseau & Dewing, 2018). Cultural pluralism refers to diverse groups within a larger society maintaining their unique cultural identities, while living together harmoniously with their values and practices accepted provided that they are consistent with human rights and freedoms guaranteed by the laws of the wider society (UNESCO, 2001). Canadian pride and support for multiculturalism has fostered high levels of immigration and its resulting cultural and economic benefits (Jedwab, 2014). Canada has grown from a commitment to diversity, inclusiveness, and pluralism; however, intolerance does exist here and threatens movement toward an ever-more inclusive, fair, and just society for all Canadians (Johnston, 2017). In addition, the diversity represented in the population mosaic of Canada presents challenges to the equitable delivery of health care and health promotion that must be considered.

## Population Statistics and Demographic Trends

Canada's population was estimated to be over 37 million in 2018, an increase of over half a million people from the previous year (Statistics Canada, 2018a). The majority of Canadians (86.4%) live in one of four provinces: Ontario (38.6%), Quebec (22.6%), British Columbia (13.5%), and Alberta (11.6%). Most (83.2%) live in an urban area, with nearly half (47%) living in one of Canada's six largest cities: Toronto, Montreal, Vancouver, Calgary, Ottawa-Gatineau, and Edmonton.

Over much of Canada's history, population growth has occurred as a result of natural increase, the change in size of a population due to the difference between the number of births and deaths in a given period (Statistics Canada, 2017a). However, over time, migratory increase has played an expanding role and now accounts for about two-thirds of Canada's population growth. International migration accounted for 79.6% of population growth in 2017/2018, the highest proportion in Canada's history, and attributable to an upward trend since the early 1990s (Statistics Canada, 2018a). The high international migratory increase represents a high number of permanent immigrants, as well as an increase in non-permanent residents, including asylum seekers and work and study permit holders.

Population growth has increased in many provinces, including Ontario (+1.8%) and Quebec (+1.1%), which saw the strongest population growth in nearly 30 years, and Alberta (+1.5%), which has seen a resurgence in population growth after 4 years of slowdown. With the exception of Newfoundland and Labrador, the Atlantic provinces have seen the highest levels of population growth since the 1980s: Prince Edward Island (+1/8%), Nova Scotia (+1.0%), and New Brunswick (+0.5%).

The proportion of females and males in the Canadian population has fluctuated over time. Historically, females comprised less than half of the population; however, over the past 40 years women and girls have accounted for just over half as a result of increases in life expectancy that have favoured females over males (Government of Canada, 2019a). Larger numbers of women can be seen in the older years compared to men, particularly at the oldest ages.

A key demographic trend in Canada is aging of the population, which is driven by increased life expectancy and lower birth rates, as well as aging of the baby boom generation who were born after the Second World War (1946–1965) and make up a significant proportion of the population (Statistics Canada, 2018a). In 2018, approximately 17% of Canadians were aged 65 years and older compared with 14% in 2011, and it is projected that by 2024, one in five will be aged 65 and older. The median age of Canadians is 40.8 years, with the youngest populations in the Prairie provinces and the territories, and the oldest populations in the Atlantic provinces. Nunavut has the youngest population (median age 26.1 years), and Newfoundland and Labrador the oldest (median 46.5 years). The median age is higher for women (41.8 years) than men (39.7 years) as women have a longer life expectancy than men (Statistics Canada, 2019a).

The aging of the population has implications for the health care system as older persons tend to be more susceptible to illness, including chronic diseases, and as a result consume higher proportions of health care resources than younger persons (Jackson, Clemens, & Palacios, 2017). The share of health care expenditure accounted for by Canadians aged 65 years and older rose from 44.3% in 2005 to 46.0% in 2015 (CIHI, 2017). Thus health promotion strategies for the older person (see Chapter 18) are particularly important to enable healthy aging and quality of life and to reduce burden on the health care system.

## Immigration in Canada

According to 2016 Census data, 76.6% of Canadians were Canadian-born, 21.9% were immigrants, and 1.5% were non-permanent residents (Statistics Canada, 2016b). In addition, 6.2% reported "Aboriginal ancestry," which refers to the Indigenous people, the original inhabitants of the land. In Canada, Indigenous people include the First Nations, Métis, and Inuit. Prior to colonization and formation of Canada there were an estimated 500,000 Indigenous people, a number that was significantly reduced by contact with French and British explorers, missionaries, and settlers (beginning in the sixteenth century) who brought infectious diseases such as influenza, smallpox, and tuberculosis to which the Indigenous inhabitants had no immunity (Bourque, Bearskin, & Jakubec, 2017). Also, successive waves of European immigrants displaced Indigenous people from their land to set up colonies.

Following Confederation, the majority of immigrants (84%) arrived from the British Isles, with only 11% from the United States, 4% from Germany, and less than 1% from France (Statistics Canada, 2018b). In the late 1800s and early 1900s new groups of immigrants arrived from Eastern Europe (Russia, Poland, and Ukraine), Western Europe, and Scandinavia. From the 1950s to the 1970s a significant number also arrived from Western Europe (Germany, the Netherlands) and Southern Europe (Italy, Greece, Portugal, and Yugoslavia), and in the 1980s and 1990s more immigrants arrived from Eastern Europe, including those from the Russian Federation and former Soviet republics, Poland and Romania.

Increasing diversity in the source countries for immigration was seen from the 1960s and onwards when the number of immigrants from Asia (China, Japan, Vietnam, Cambodia, India, and Philippines), and the Caribbean (Bermuda, Jamaica, Haiti, and

Trinidad and Tobago) began to grow. Asia, including the Middle East, is now the main origin of immigrants to Canada, while the proportion from Africa is growing (Statistics Canada, 2018b).

As a result of processes of self-selection and Canada's point system for selection, the majority of contemporary immigrants are healthy upon arrival in Canada, and tend to be healthier than the native-born population (Vang, Sigouin, Flenon, et al., 2017). However, it is also known that immigrants' health advantage may disappear and, in some cases, become worse with longer duration of residence in a new country.

## ETHNICITY, ETHNIC GROUPS, AND MINORITY GROUPS

Ethnicity is a complex and evolving concept that is not synonymous with either race or culture. Ethnicity may be defined as:

> a dynamic set of historically derived and institutionalized ideas and practices that allows people to identify or to be identified with groupings of people on the basis of presumed (and usually claimed) commonalities including language, history, nation or region of origin, customs, ways of being, religion, names, physical appearance, and/or genealogy or ancestry; can be a source of meaning, action, and identity; and confers a sense of belonging, pride, and motivation (Markus, 2008, p. 654).

More than 200 ethnic origins were reported in the 2011 Canadian National Household Survey (NHS), and over 13 different ethnic origins had achieved populations of over 1 million persons (Statistics Canada, 2019b). An individual may identify with one or more ethnic groups or population groups based on heritage or other commonalities; however, many people living in Canada self-identify as "Canadian," whether or not they were born in Canada.

In the United States, the term "race" continues to be used interchangeably with the term "ethnicity" to categorize people based on common ancestry and physical characteristics. In Canada, the term race is no longer used, because "racialization" is closely linked to *discrimination*, the systemic inequitable treatment of individuals or groups based on stratified classifications (Browne & Varcoe, 2019). Race is associated with power and indexes the history or ongoing imposition of one group's authority above another, whereas ethnicity focuses on differences in meanings, values, and ways of living (practices) (Markus, 2008).

A minority group is not, as the term implies, a group existing in proportionately smaller numbers than other groups, but is a group associated with marginalized status, most often related to ethnicity, religion, gender, or sexual orientation (Srivastava, 2007). Marginalization is a social process in which groups and individuals are pushed to the edges of society where they are excluded from the mainstream political, social, and economic life. For example, a single teenage mother's experiences of stigma and discrimination often lead them to drop out of school, which limits their future opportunities. Marginalized groups, often referred to as *vulnerable populations*, have less power, are more likely to live in poverty, and are at risk for discrimination and stigma that may impact their health and access to health care (Government of Canada, 2017; Srivastava, 2007). In Canada, vulnerable populations include Indigenous people, LGBTQ2 persons, the homeless, incarcerated people and their families, older persons, persons with physical or mental health disorders, immigrants, refugees, and visible minorities.

Another classification term that continues to be used officially in Canada is that of visible minority, which refers to "persons, other than Aboriginal peoples, who are non-Caucasian in race or non-white in colour" and consist mainly of the following groups: South Asian, Chinese, Black, Filipino, Latin American, Arab, Southeast Asian, West Asian, Korean, and Japanese (Statistics Canada, 2015). This practice is a form of scientific racism. Categorizing individuals and groups of people as visible minorities can also be perceived as being demeaning and contributing to racialization. However, health inequities are often reported based on self-identified skin colour. For example, in one study, Canadians who identified as "Black" reported the worst overall self-rated health, whereas "White" respondents reported the best self-rated health, a disparity that was attributable to differences in income (Veenstra & Abel, 2019). In the same study, Canadians who self-identified as both Black and White fell between Black and White Canadians in terms of self-rated overall health, but reported the worst self-rated mental health of the three populations.

Diversity goes beyond skin color and nationality. Attributes of visible diversity include age, gender, and physical appearance; attributes of invisible diversity include religion, sexual orientation, illness, occupation, and other characteristics that are not readily apparent. However, people who are visibly diverse have a higher risk of experiencing racialization, discrimination, and marginalization within society and the health care system (Srivastava, 2007). Nurses and other health care providers must be aware of the categories and assumptions assigned to individuals and groups of people, whether conscious or unconscious, to avoid the harmful effects of racialization and to provide culturally safe care.

## CULTURE, VALUES, AND VALUE ORIENTATION

Ethnicity is evidenced in customs that reflect the socialization and cultural patterns of the group. Culture is a dynamic and evolving concept that refers to the common values and ways of thinking and acting of a group of people that differ from those of another group (Srivastava, 2007).

Values are beliefs about the worth of something and serve as standards that influence behaviour and thinking. Cultural values "are unique, individual expressions of a particular culture that have been accepted as appropriate over time. They guide actions and decision-making that facilitate self-worth and self-esteem" (Giger, 2013). Cultural values are integral to the manner in which individuals will employ health behaviours, maintain their health, how they will seek care for themselves and others, and where they are likely to go to receive care (Boyle, 2016).

Value orientations, learned and shared through the socialization process, reflect the personality type of a particular society. The dominant value orientations are shared by the majority of the group. Kluckhohn's model (Kluckhohn, 1953) of value orientations incorporates themes regarding basic human nature, the relationship of human beings to nature, human beings' time orientation, valued personality type, and relationships between human beings.

Ethnic groups have their unique beliefs and attitudes about health and health care services (Diversity Awareness). Incongruent beliefs and attitudes about health and health care services among ethnic groups versus the rest of the population, particularly health care providers, are major barriers in improving the health status of ethnic group members. Health care providers need to become responsive to the cultural values of different peoples and to realize how this cultural understanding could augment effective and humanistic care delivery. Knowledge and culturally competent practices are essential for nurses to function effectively in rapidly changing multicultural societies to provide quality and safe care to all.

## DIVERSITY AWARENESS

### Female Genital Cutting: Taboo or Tradition?

Some practices of individuals or groups are deeply rooted in beliefs connected to culture. These practices are considered unhealthy and/or unsafe in other cultures who do not share the same beliefs. This is the case for female genital cutting (FGC), also referred to as female circumcision or female genital mutilation (FGM). The term FGC is the preferred term, as it is considered medically correct and culturally sensitive (Perron, Senikas, Burnett, et al., 2013).

What is the likelihood of health care providers having an encounter with circumcised women? It is probably high because more than 200 million girls and women alive today have undergone FGC "although the incidence of FGC in women is worldwide, rough estimates range from 114–130 million women" (Little, 2003). The increasing migration of circumcised women to Canada increases the probability of these women's presence in health care settings. In countries that legally prohibit FGC, parents often feign a holiday or vacation to the native country, where they have the young daughter circumcised.

FGC has unknown origins. However, it is believed that the practice can be traced "in Africa as far back as the fifth century BC and has taken place in ancient Egypt, ancient Rome, Arabia, and Tsarist Russia" (Little, 2003). There are four types of FGC:

- *Type 1*, also known as clitoridectomy, is the excision of the clitoral prepuce and may also involve the excision of all or part of the clitoris.
- *Type 2* is the excision of the clitoris and may also involve the excision of all or part of the labia minora.
- *Type 3*, also known as infibulation, involves excision of part or all of the external genitalia and the stitching or narrowing of the vaginal opening.
- *Type 4* refers to all other genital procedures (Momoh, 2004).

It is a myth that FGC is advocated by specific individuals in cultures or societies that advocate and support this practice. Leval, Widmar, Tishelman, et al. (2004) analyzed the ways Swedish midwives discussed sexuality in circumcised African women. Their encounters with spouses in maternity wards dispelled the myth that men are the power holders. They were described as "always tender, caring, power shares, or even subordinates in the relationship." Support for this myth buster is seen in societies where adult women advocate and support the practice as an affirmation of their roles and high regard for their bodies (Little, 2003). Parents of young girls support the practice as an assurance of economic security for their daughters (Gruenbaum, 2005). In some societies, powerful women leaders who are feared and respected promote this practice (Little, 2003).

There are many explanations for FGC. Gruenbaum (2005) offers a comprehensive discussion of these. Her analysis to approaches for proposed changes in the practice or its elimination through the passage of laws is extremely enlightening and provides a deep understanding of the complexities of FGC. There are cultural reasons for this practice, including providing health benefits, preserving virginity before marriage, serving as a rite of passage, and providing economic security for women as well as for the people performing such acts (Berg & Denison, 2012; Gruenbaum, 2005; Little, 2003). Cultural beliefs about sexuality and sexual responses are also a factor (Leval et al., 2004).

FGC has many complications. The immediate ones include hemorrhage, infections, abscesses, and urinary difficulties such as retention and straining. Long-term complications include difficulty voiding, urinary and reproductive tract infections, and incontinence. Other complications are infertility, painful intercourse, keloids, introital and vaginal stenosis, dermoid cysts, and pain. For the circumcised woman during labour, there is obstructed labour, fetal distress, perineal tears, perineal wound infection, and postpartum hemorrhage and sepsis. Obermeyer (2005) contends that complications or consequences of FGC are poorly documented because of many methodological issues, including the quality of the data collected. Valid research on female circumcision is a fertile ground. Obermeyer's (2005) review of studies on FGC is an excellent resource for interested researchers.

What are the care implications for nurses? Midwives and nurses whose area of practice is women's health are more likely to have experiences with circumcised women. "It is essential that midwives recognize the cultural complexities of FGM and show sensitivity when caring and supporting women with FGC during pregnancy, labour, and the postnatal period" (Momoh, 2004). Identification can start by asking questions such as the following: "Have you been closed?" "Did you have the cut or operation as a child?" Referrals to a specialist would facilitate discussion of legal issues and possible reversal of the procedure (infibulation). Procedures to reverse infibulation during labour might be performed. Other invasive procedures need to be avoided to eliminate possible sources of pain and stress.

Following delivery, before reinfibulation or restitching is done, the health care provider needs to consider the laws governing the practice of FGC. The mother and the baby, if female, are cared for with a view toward the future of the baby.

The information presented is but a very small representation of the continuing interests and work of people from diverse backgrounds. One powerful statement made by these scientists and caregivers is that whatever is done to eliminate FGC, "the cultural integrity of the people" (Little, 2003) must be preserved. Readers are strongly urged to read the cited references for a fuller understanding of FGC.

#### Reflective Questions

- How does a nurse practice cultural humility when cultural practices have negative consequences for the health and well-being of a patient in their care?
- What are the ethics of Western cultures forcing their ideals upon other cultures that have traditions perceived as harmful and unnecessary?

Sources: Berg, R. C., & Denison, E. (2012). *International initiative for impact evaluation: Interventions to reduce the prevalence of female genital mutilation/cutting in African countries*. Retrieved from http://www.ieimpact.org/admin/pdfs_synthetic/011%20protocol.pdf; Gruenbaum, E. (2005). Socio-cultural dynamics of female genital cutting: Research, findings, gaps, and directions. *Culture Health Sexuality, 7*(5), 420–441; Leval, A., Widmar, C., Tishelman, C., et al. (2004). The encounters that rupture the myth: Contradictions in midwives' descriptions and explanations of circumcised women's sexuality. *Health Care for Women International, 25*, 743–760; Little, C. M. (2003). Female genital circumcision: Medical and cultural considerations. *Journal of Cultural Diversity, 10*(1), 30–34; Momoh, C. (2004). Attitudes to female genital mutilation. *British Journal of Midwifery, 12*(10), 631–638; Obermeyer, C. M. (2005). The consequences of female circumcision for health and sexuality: An update on the evidence. *Culture Health Sexuality, 7*(5), 443–461; Perron, L., Senikas, V., Burnett, M., et al. (2013). Clinical practice guidelines: Female genital cutting. *Journal of Obstetrics and Gynaecology Canada, 35*(11), 1028–1045.

# CULTURAL COMPETENCY AND CULTURAL HUMILITY

Culture may have an impact on people's health, healing, wellness belief systems, perceived causes of illness and disease, behaviours of seeking health care, and attitudes toward health care providers. Culture may also influence the delivery of health care services by the providers, who use their own limited set of values to view the world.

Every culture has diverse illustrative models of illness and belief systems regarding health and healing. These models and wellness belief systems include views about the pathophysiology of diseases, the cause and the onset of symptoms, the natural history of illnesses, and the appropriate treatments for various health issues.

Cultural competency is one of the major elements in eliminating health inequities; it starts with an honest desire to disregard personal biases and to treat every person with respect. Cultural competence is a broad concept used to describe a compilation of knowledge, attitudes, and skills necessary to interact effectively with individuals and groups of the same and different cultures (Clipsham, Hampson, Powell, et al., 2011). Health care providers and persons seeking care bring their individual cultures and health beliefs and values to the health care experience. Hence, understanding the cultural underpinning of care is a challenging task because of the complexity and interaction between the person seeking care and the health care provider's cultural beliefs (Salman, McCabe, Easter, et al., 2007). In addition, providing health care services that are respectful of and responsive to diverse individuals' health beliefs, practices, and cultural needs is believed to contribute to fewer negative health outcomes.

Cultural humility has been described as a lifelong process of self-reflection and critique that encompasses the recognition of power imbalances and the development of mutually beneficial partnerships between patient and provider (Foronda, Baptiste, Reinholdt, et al., 2016, p. 213). Cultural humility incorporates reflexivity by practitioners of both their own actions with patients as well as on power and bias within the health care system and offers a dynamic practice that is grounded in health equity that promotes culturally safe care environments (Carroll, 2018). Cultural humility when viewed from an intersectional perspective recognizes that all experiences of identity are unique and may involve multiple overlapping oppressions; thus, it essential that nurses avoid language that makes superficial assumptions or seeks to define individuals by a single identity (Carroll, 2018; YWCA, 2017). Practising cultural humility places the health care provider in the role of learner as opposed to the authority in their relationship with patients, who are the experts about their own cultural experiences (Ortega & Coulborn Faller, 2011).

Cultural safety extends beyond cultural awareness and acknowledgement of difference to an understanding of the limitations of cultural competence which is focused on the knowledge, skills, and attitudes of the health care practitioner (Aboriginal Nurses' Association of Canada [ANAC], 2009). Whereas cultural humility is a process, cultural safety is an outcome based on respectful engagement that results in people feeling safe when receiving health care ([First Nations Health Authority FNHA], 2019). Cultural safety is action-oriented, and allows unequal power relations to be exposed and managed (ANAC, 2009). Providing cultural safety is historically grounded in the decolonization of health care spaces for Indigenous people (FNHA, 2019), but also applies to other population groups facing discrimination, such as gender-diverse persons (Carroll, 2018) and ethnically diverse groups. Cultural safety means that the environment is a physical, emotionally, socially, and spiritually safe space, which can improve both the quality of health care services and access to care (FNHA, 2019).

It is very important for health care providers to be aware of how persons interpret their health issues or illnesses and to be capable of providing culturally safe care. Simply recognizing and accepting cultural diversity is insufficient to attain cultural competency in health care. Culturally competent health care providers should be able to consistently and thoroughly recognize and understand the differences in their culture and the culture of others; to respect others' values, beliefs, and expectations; to understand the disease-specific epidemiology and treatment efficacy of different population groups; and to adjust the approach of delivering care to meet each person's needs and expectations (Management Sciences for Health, n.d.). Cultural competency and safety is usually reflected in a health care provider's attitude and communication style.

Douglas, Rosenkoetter, Pacquiao, and colleagues (2014) discuss universally applicable guidelines for achieving culturally safe care. Their guidelines include knowledge of culture; education and training in culturally competent care; critical reflection; cross-cultural communication; culturally competent practice; cultural competence in health care systems and organizations; patient advocacy and empowerment; a multicultural workforce; cross-cultural leadership; and evidence-informed practice and research. For each guideline they discuss strategies and provide implementation examples for caregivers and health care organizations' leaders/managers.

Truong, Paradies, and Priest (2014) conducted a systematic review of reviews on the effectiveness of interventions to improve cultural competence in health care. Nineteen reviews were included that examined a variety of health care contexts (i.e., a variety of minority populations, diseases, health care settings and providers, and interventions). In this systematic review, three main types of outcomes were reported: patient-related outcomes, provider-related outcomes, and health service access and utilization outcomes. Most of the reviews reported moderate-level evidence for improvements in provider-related outcomes and health service access and utilization outcomes. Some, but weaker, evidence was reported for patient-related outcomes. Unfortunately, many of the self-reported measures, such as patient- and provider-related outcomes, used tools that were not validated.

Recently, researchers have established and tested the Cultural Competence Health Practitioner Assessment (CCHPA-67), which purports to determine levels of cultural and linguistic competence (Harris-Haywood, Goode, Smith, et al., 2014). The 67-item questionnaire has three domains—knowledge, adapting practice, and promoting health—and has sound clinometric properties, including reliability and validity. CCHPA-67 can be used to examine the effectiveness of interventions to increase cultural and linguistic competence of health care practitioners and the association between their level of competence and health care outcomes.

## TRADITIONAL AND COMPLEMENTARY AND ALTERNATIVE MEDICINES

The traditional healing practices of several great societies developed in relative isolation from conventional Western medicine (Carr, n.d.). Within its cultural traditions, each group has a healing system that incorporates the beliefs and practices deemed essential in maintaining and restoring health. A traditional healing system embodies the beliefs, values, and treatment approaches of a particular cultural group that are products of cultural development. Conventional medicine or biomedicine, despite claims of scientific objectivity, reflects the dominant philosophical belief system of Western society (Ning, 2013).

The choice of a health care system differs among cultural population groups and among individuals within the same group. An individual's preference is motivated by their familiarity with the traditional healer, who usually speaks the same language and is knowledgeable about the beliefs, customs, and traditions of the cultural group. Easy access and the individual's ability to pay for the healer's services are real advantages when compared with the difficulty of getting appointments, the long waits, and the unfamiliar institutional settings in the professional care system. Despite ongoing developments in treatments provided by professional care systems, many traditional medicines and healing practices maintain their popularity today. When these healing practices are not effective, the individual may, as a last resort, turn to the professional care system. Through a culturally sensitive assessment process, nurses can determine which specific traditional medicines individuals are using and whether their continued use would interfere with the prescribed medical regimen. Nurses must avoid an ethnocentric perspective when working with ethnic groups. An ethnocentric perspective, which views other ways as inferior, unnatural, or even barbaric, can serve as a major obstacle in establishing and maintaining good working relationships with patients and their families. Similarly, nurses must avoid stereotyping individuals, as not all people from the same cultural group will hold the same views.

The World Health Organization (WHO) published the *WHO Traditional Medicine Strategy 2014–2023* to support member states in promoting the safe and effective use of TM to contribute to the health and wellness of the population (WHO, 2013). In some countries, TM or non-conventional medicine may be referred to as complementary medicine (CM) or complementary and alternative medicine (CAM). Traditional and complementary medicine (T&CM) is an important and often undervalued part of modern health care around the world and the demand for its services is increasing (WHO, 2013). Traditional and complementary therapies include massage therapy, acupuncture, naturopathy, and traditional Chinese medicine, as well as the traditional medicines of the Indigenous peoples of Canada.

Thus, it is imperative that nurses have a general understanding of these practices and their potential benefits and harms, and assess for their use when encountering patients in all clinical settings in order to provide holistic, patient-centred care. Within Western societies, including Canada, there is a growing trend towards integrative health care, which is rooted in the belief that individuals should have the ability to make informed choices about their health care options, and the emphasis is on wellness, and holistic, personalized care (Kania-Richmond & Metcalfe, 2017). More information about CAM therapies can be found in Chapter 24.

## INDIGENOUS PEOPLE

In Canada there are three distinct groups of Indigenous people with unique histories and cultures: the First Nations, Métis, and Inuit (Fig. 2.2). The arrival of European traders and settlers beginning in the 1600s disrupted Indigenous communities through discriminatory policies and practices that restricted their self-determination and impacted their health. The original Indian Act was created in 1876 to assimilate First Nations people (referred to as Indians) into the dominant Canadian culture and to control their lands. Indigenous communities were moved from their traditional lands to live on *reserves*, where the resources were often inferior and insufficient to support traditional ways of life. Between 1883 and 1996 approximately 150,000 First Nations, Métis, and Inuit children were removed from their families and communities and forced to attend federal residential schools, where they were required to abandon their cultural traditions and languages, and were exposed to physical, emotional, and sexual abuse (Canadian Geographic, 2018a). The *Indian Act* also specifies a person's eligibility for Indian status. Status Indians or Registered Indians have certain rights and benefits that are not available to non-status Indians, Inuit, Métis, or other Canadians, such as on-reserve housing, education, and exemptions from certain taxes (Government of Canada, 2018a).

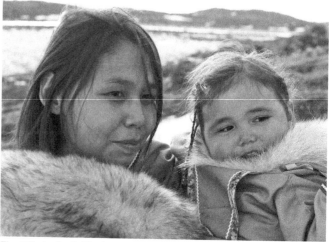

**Fig. 2.2  An Inuit Mother and Her Child** (iStockphoto/RyersonClark.)

In the 2016 Census, there were 1,673,785 Canadians who reported Indigenous heritage, which represents 4.9% of the total population (Statistics Canada, 2018c). The populations of First Nations, Métis, and Inuit are growing more rapidly than the rest of the population in Canada, as a result of increased life expectancy, relatively high birth rates, and increases in self-reported identification. The Indigenous population is, on average, nearly a decade younger than the rest of the Canadian population, reflecting the lower life expectancy among First Nations, Métis, and Inuit men and women. There were over 70 Indigenous languages reported on the 2016 Census, with the most widely spoken being Cree, Inuktitut, and Ojibway (Statistics Canada, 2018c).

## First Nations

"First Nations" is a term that describes the Indigenous people of Canada who are not Inuit or Métis, and who are typically status Indians registered with a particular home reserve, band, or community. The term "First Nations" is preferred to the historical term "Indian", which persists as a legal term in Canada, as a symbol of their status as a founding nation of Canada along with the English and French (Gadacz & Parrott, 2015). The First Nations represent a collection of more than 600 bands across the country, each with their own unique cultural heritage. In 2016 there were 744,855 First Nations people with registered or Treaty Indian status, accounting for just over 76% of the First Nations population, with 44% living on reserves (Statistics Canada, 2017b). Over half of First Nations people live in the four western provinces, and almost a quarter live in Ontario.

## Métis

The Métis are a distinct Indigenous group in Canada descended from First Nations women and European fur traders and settlers dating back to the 1700s (Canadian Geographic, 2018b). Historically, Métis communities were found in western Canada, northwest Ontario, and the Northwest Territories. In 2016 there were 587,545 Métis in Canada, with the largest proportion, one-fifth of the total Métis population, living in Ontario (Statistics Canada, 2017b); however, the only recognized Métis land base in Canada is the Alberta Métis Settlements located in Northern Alberta (Canadian Geographic, 2018b). Métis are also the most likely of the three Indigenous groups to live in urban areas, including large cities or metropolitan areas. The official language of the Métis Nation is Michif; however, the Métis speak other languages, including French Michif, a mixture of Canadian French and Algonquin linguistic features (Canadian Geographic, 2018b). As a result of their dual ancestral heritage, the Métis perspective on health draws on both Indigenous and Western knowledge and "ways of knowing" (PHAC, 2018).

## Inuit

The Inuit are the original people of the North American Arctic from Alaska to Newfoundland and Labrador. This region, known as the Inuit Nunangat is composed of four regions: the Inuvialuit Settlement Region (northern Northwest Territories), Nunavut, Nunavik (northern Quebec), and Nunatsiavut (Northern Labrador) (Canadian Geographic, 2018c). The majority of Inuit live in Nunavut, which was proclaimed to be a territory in 1993. In 2016, there were 65,025 Inuit living in Canada, with almost three-quarters of those living in the Inuit Nunangat (Statistics Canada, 2017b). More than one third of the 53 communities in Inuit Nunangat have populations of under 500 people, most of which can only be reached by air year-round and by air and sea during the summer months (Canadian Geographic, 2018c). The Inuit language is Inuktut; however, each region has its own dialect.

## Health Issues of Indigenous Populations

Whereas First Nations, Inuit, and Métis peoples in Canada have unique histories and cultural practices and beliefs, they have held similar holistic views of health as a balance between the spiritual, emotional, mental, and physical dimensions. European colonization disrupted many structural determinants of health such as self-determination, intermediate determinants such as community infrastructure and resources, and proximal determinants such as physical environment and social supports (PHAC, 2018). The creation of federal reserves displaced First Nations people from their connection to the land, their lifestyles, and sources of economic livelihoods, which in conjunction with the remote and/or rural locations of many communities has impeded access to education, employment and health care services (PHAC, 2018). Many of the health problems of Indigenous populations in Canada can be linked directly to their social and economic living conditions, which predispose them to illnesses and health problems that afflict the poor. In addition, cultural barriers, geographical and social isolation, low income, and systemic racism are factors that prevent Indigenous persons from receiving quality medical care.

Life expectancy and infant mortality rates are key indicators of overall health status. Life expectancy at birth in Canada is lower in regions with high concentrations of people who identify as Indigenous: 12 years lower in areas with a high concentration of Inuit; 11.2 years lower in areas with a high concentration of First Nations; and 6.9 years lower in regions with a high concentration of Métis (PHAC, 2018). Similarly, infant mortality rates are much higher in regions with a high concentration of Indigenous people than those living in areas with a low concentration of Indigenous people: 3.9 times higher in areas with a high concentration of Inuit; 2.3 times higher in areas with a high concentration of First Nations people; and 1.9 times higher in areas with a high concentration of Métis people (PHAC, 2018). Differences between Indigenous and non-Indigenous infant mortality rates are greatest in the post-neonatal period, and rates of key risk factors, such as preterm birth and low birthweight, are also substantially higher among Indigenous peoples (PHAC, 2018).

Unintentional injury is the leading cause of death among Canadian children and young adults and the fifth leading cause of death for all ages, and individuals living in areas with a high concentration of First Nations, Inuit, and Métis people had, respectively, 3.5, 3.2, and 2.7 times the rate of unintentional injury mortality as those living in areas with a low concentration of First Nations, Inuit, and Métis people (PHAC, 2018). There is a clear socioeconomic gradient for suicide, with suicide rates increasing as income and education levels decrease. In areas where many people identify as Inuit, First Nations, and Métis, suicide rates are, respectively, 6.5, 3.7, and 2.7 times higher than areas with a low concentration of people who identify as Indigenous; suicide rates are particularly high among Inuit males (118.2 per 100,000) (PHAC, 2018). Self-rated mental health is a subjective measure of overall mental health status, and prevalence of low self-rated mental health among First Nations living off reserve and Métis is 1.9 and 1.5 times, respectively, than that of non-Indigenous people (PHAC, 2018). Mental health services often are not available or may not be culturally appropriate for persons who identify as Indigenous.

Indigenous people have higher rates of many chronic health conditions. Arthritis is one of the most common conditions affecting Canadians, resulting in considerable economic burden. Smoking and obesity are risk factors for arthritis that are associated with social determinants of health, such as income and education; thus higher rates of arthritis are found in regions with high levels of these risk factors. The prevalence of both arthritis and asthma is 1.6 times that of non-Indigenous adults for both First Nations and Métis populations (PHAC, 2018). Similarly, the prevalence of diabetes among First Nations adults living off reserve and Métis adults is 1.9 and 1.5 times, respectively, that of non-Indigenous adults (PHAC, 2018). Indigenous Canadians are among the highest-risk populations for diabetes and diabetes-related complications, and have poor success at achieving management targets (Crowshoe, Dannenbaum, Green, et al., 2018). Dietary and lifestyle changes related to colonization have contributed to high obesity rates and prevalence of diabetes among First Nations people in Canada.

Inequities of the past that result from colonialism continue to influence the health status of First Nations, Inuit, and Métis people in Canada. The Truth and Reconciliation Commission of Canada (TRC) documented the attempted indoctrination of Indigenous people into the dominant culture through the residential school system and its effect on the health and well-being of the survivors and their families (TRC, 2015). This intergenerational trauma has contributed to the persisting disparities in health outcomes between Indigenous and non-Indigenous Canadians. In 2015, the TRC released its final report, which outlined 94 calls for action, including a call for "the federal government, in consultation with Aboriginal peoples, to establish measurable goals to identify and close the gaps in health outcomes between "Aboriginal and non-Aboriginal communities" (TRC, 2015, p. 161).

## IMMIGRANTS AND REFUGEES

In 2016, there were over 7.5 million immigrants living in Canada with origins in over 200 countries (Statistics Canada, 2019b). The main countries of origin of immigrant residents of Canada in 2016 included: India (668,565), China (649,260), Philippines (588,305), United Kingdom (499,120), United States (253,715), Italy (236,635), Hong Kong (208,935), Pakistan (202,255), Vietnam (169,250), Iran (154,420), Poland (146,470), Germany (145,840), Portugal (139,450), Jamaica,

(138,345), Sri Lanka (131, 995), South Korea (123,305), and France (105,570) (Statistics Canada, 2019b). In recent years, war in the Middle East has resulted in a wave of Syrian refugees to Canada, with the majority of those receiving government assistance and the remainder being privately sponsored by non-governmental organizations, groups, or individuals (Houle, 2019). Syrian refugees accounted for more than 60% of refugees who resettled into Canada between January 1, 2015, and May 10, 2016, followed by refugees from Iraq, Afghanistan, Eritrea, and the Democratic Republic of the Congo. Syrian refugees are younger than refugees from other countries, and most (85%) are couples with children; the majority did not know English or French at the time of the 2016 census, and government-sponsored Syrian refugees had lower employment rates than privately sponsored refugees and refugees from other countries (Houle, 2019).

There are almost 500,000 people living in Canada without status (i.e., individuals who are not authorized to enter or remain legally in Canada, often referred to as non-status or undocumented) (Aery & Cheff, 2018). The majority of non-status individuals arrived legally in Canada as temporary residents, including temporary workers, refugee claimants, and international students. Non-status individuals have limited or no access to public services, which can negatively impact their health and well-being. The Canadian cities of Toronto, Hamilton, Vancouver, and Montreal have joined the Sanctuary City movement, and more including Edmonton, Calgary, Ottawa, Regina, Saskatoon, and Winnipeg are considering becoming sanctuary cities, committed to providing services to all residents regardless of their immigration status. Sanctuary cities promote health equity through policies and programs that improve access to health care, employment and income, housing, education, food security, sense of belonging and neighbourhoods (Aery & Cheff, 2018).

## Health Care Issues for Immigrants and Refugees

Research has demonstrated a "healthy immigrant" effect for both physical and mental health compared with Canadian-born residents; however, this health advantage generally deteriorates during the first 2 years of living in Canada, particularly among female and non-European immigrants (Kim, Carrasco, Muntaner, et al., 2013). In addition, this immigrant health advantage varies across the lifespan, with the strongest effect during adulthood, and less effect during childhood, adolescence, and older age (Vang et al., 2017). People living in areas with a high concentration of Canadian-born residents had a lower life expectancy of 81.0 years compared with regions with a high concentration of immigrant residents, at 83.9 years. Health-adjusted life expectancy (HALE) at age 18 showed a similar pattern, with immigrants living 3.4 years longer in good health than non-immigrants (PHAC, 2018).

Among people living in areas with a low proportion of immigrant residents, the rate of unintentional injury mortality was 1.5 times the rate among people living in areas with a high proportion of immigrant residents (PHAC, 2018). Suicide rates were also 42.4% lower in areas with a high concentration of immigrant residents compared with areas with a low concentration of immigrant residents (PHAC, 2018). Compared with 5.8% of White Canadians, 7.1% of East/Southeast Asians and 4.2% of South Asians report low self-rated mental health (PHAC, 2018). Rates of chronic health conditions are typically lower among recent immigrants; for example, the prevalence of asthma is half that among non-immigrants (PHAC, 2018).

Immigrants and refugees may have unique health problems, and may experience cultural, economic, geographic, and language barriers accessing the Canadian health care system and social services (Ahmed, Shommu, Rumana, et al., 2015), particularly those from low- to middle-income or developing countries (Pottie, Greenaway, Feightner, et al., 2011). Forced migration, low income and limited proficiency in either English or French increase their risk for health care decline. The Canadian Collaboration for Immigrant and Refugee Health has developed evidence-informed clinical guidelines for assessment and preventative care for immigrants and refugees related to infectious diseases, mental health, chronic, and non-communicable diseases, and women's health (Pottie et al., 2011).

Some immigrants and refugees may be fearful or untrusting of Western medicine, and may continue to practice traditional healing methods from their countries of origin. For example, Asian traditional medicine uses a wide variety of herbs for healing purposes, including roots, leaves, seeds, tree bark, and parts of flowers. Some aspects of Asian traditional medicine have gained popularity within the professional care system. In general, the use or nonuse of healing traditions seems to be consistent with how closely Asians identify with their heritage (Tashiro, 2006). Of these, the best known is acupuncture. Similar alternative treatment modalities that are slowly gaining wide acceptance include meditation, therapeutic touch, massage, biofeedback, imagery, relaxation, and bipolarity. Research for Evidence-Informed Practice discusses the use of CAM in Canada.

## RESEARCH FOR EVIDENCE-INFORMED PRACTICE

### Use of Complementary and Alternative Medicine in Canada

The National Center for Complementary and Alternative Medicine (2011) defines complementary and alternative medicine (CAM) as a set of varied medical and health care practices, systems, and products that are not usually considered part of conventional medicine practiced by medical doctors, registered nurses, and nurse practitioners or allied health care providers such as physiotherapists and psychologists. Conventional medicine is also called Western or allopathic medicine. Acupuncture, biofeedback, neurofeedback, relaxation, music therapy, massage, art, music, and dance therapy are some examples of CAM. Western medicine, supported by improved knowledge and advances in technology, has been successful in addressing numerous illnesses. However, there remains a cadre of chronic illnesses and conditions that do not respond well to allopathic treatment. People who do not experience relief from chronic conditions often resort to CAM. However, the boundaries between CAM and conventional medicine are not fixed, and several CAM practices (e.g., acupuncture and music therapy) have been becoming more widely accepted.

## HOMELESS POPULATIONS

The Canadian Observatory on Homelessness (COH) defines homelessness as "the situation of an individual, family or community without stable, permanent, appropriate housing, or the immediate prospect, means and ability of acquiring it" (COH, 2012). In Canada, "homelessness emerged as a problem as a result of a large disinvestment in affordable housing, structural shifts in the economy (resulting in, for example, a rapid decline in full-time, permanent, well-paying jobs) and reduced spending on a range of social and health supports in communities all across the country" (Gaetz, Dej, Richter, et al., 2016, p. 12). Homelessness is a complex social and economic problem that continues to persist and grow. Many services and programs have been developed to address the issue, yet homelessness remains a significant problem. Homelessness encompasses a range of living situations (COH, 2012):

1. *Unsheltered:* those who are absolutely homeless and living on the streets (Fig. 2.3).
2. *Emergency sheltered:* those who are staying in overnight shelters for people who are homeless.
3. *Provisionally accommodated:* those who are staying in temporary accommodations.
4. *At risk of homelessness:* those who are not homeless, but whose current economic and/or housing situation is precarious or does not meet public health and safety standards.

It is difficult to know the exact numbers of homeless individuals as the boundary between being and not being homeless is quite fluid, and without a fixed address, individuals are unable to respond to Census Counts. Several Canadian communities use "point-in-time counts" to determine how many people are homeless on a specific day by counting the numbers of people in emergency shelters, women's shelters, unsheltered locations (e.g., parks, sidewalk, abandoned buildings), and fixed-term transitional housing (Gaetz et al., 2016). In 2016, the first nationwide point-in-time count estimated 133,000 people across Canada experienced homelessness at an emergency shelter, including women, children, families, older persons, veterans, and people with disabilities (Government of Canada, 2019a). Risk factors for homelessness include mental health and substance-use issues, marital breakdown and abusive relationships, transitions out of institutionalized care, inadequate income, cost of housing, and economic factors (Echenberg & Jensen, 2012).

The subpopulation of homeless Canadian Forces Veterans, and their differing needs, is gaining increasing recognition across Canada. There are limited data on the number of homeless veterans in Canada, but it is estimated to be relatively small (Veteran's Affairs Canada, 2019). A baseline estimate is that 2,250 veterans use emergency homeless shelters each year in Canada, representing about 2.7% of shelter users (Segaert & Bauer, 2015). Major issues that lead to homelessness among Canadian Forces veterans include mental health problems, substance use, and difficulty transitioning from military to civilian life (Ray & Forchuk, 2011).

Nearly 1 in 10 Canadians have experienced hidden homelessness, defined as ever having to live temporarily with family,

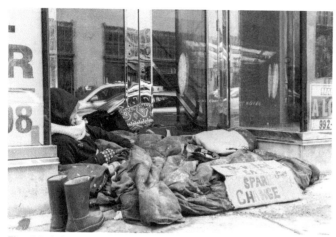

Fig. 2.3 A homeless woman in Montreal asks passersby for money, while covered in blankets to stay warm. (iStockphoto/Josie Desmarais.)

friends, or in their care because they had nowhere else to live (Rodrigue, 2016). While most experienced hidden homelessness for less than 1 year, 18% were homeless for a period longer than 1 year. Persons who reported an Indigenous identity were more than twice as likely (18%) to have experienced hidden homelessness than non-Indigenous persons (8%), whereas immigrants (6%) and individuals belonging to a visible minority group (4%) were less likely than non-immigrants (9%) or non-visible minority persons (9%) to have experienced hidden homelessness (Rodrigue, 2016).

## Health Issues of Homeless Populations

Homelessness and health care are closely interlinked. Poor health is both an effect and a cause of homelessness; however, homeless populations are likely underrepresented in the published literature (Public Health Ontario, 2019). Homelessness is associated with various behavioural, social, and environmental risks that expose individuals to many diseases. People who experience homelessness usually have complex health problems. The lives of homeless persons and families are constant battles for daily survival. Homeless persons experience exposure to extremes in temperatures, unsanitary living conditions, crowded shelters, poor nutrition, and unsafe situations, wherever they live. They experience the same situations relative to health care: poor access and inadequate resources to travel to health facilities; difficulty obtaining medications; and difficulty adhering to medication recommendations such as dietary restrictions.

As a result of poor living conditions and limited access to health care, homeless people are at a higher risk of being exposed to disease, violence, unsanitary conditions, malnutrition, stress, and addictive substances. A literature review conducted by Public Health Ontario (2019) identified the following specific outcomes associated with homelessness: infectious diseases, mental health issues, cognitive issues, nutrition deficiencies, foot issues, and chronic diseases and injuries. Homeless persons often experience co-occurring and debilitating physical, psychological, and social conditions, including disproportionate rates of infectious diseases such as tuberculosis, human

immunodeficiency virus (HIV), and hepatitis. Higher sexually transmitted infection (STI) prevalence was associated with substance use, intimate partner violence, history of incarceration, and severity of homelessness (Williams & Bryant, 2018). The review also demonstrated that homeless persons experience mental health issues at higher rates than the general population, including impaired cognitive performance among homeless youth and behavioural disorders among homeless children. While chronic illnesses such as diabetes and hypertension were prevalent among homeless persons, rates were similar to those of the general population; however, injuries such as traumatic brain injuries were found at higher rates than among non-homeless persons.

HIV/AIDS (acquired immunodeficiency syndrome) and homelessness are intricately associated. The conditions of homelessness may increase an individual's risk of becoming infected with HIV. Having substance abuse disorders and sharing or reusing needles to intravenously inject drugs greatly increases homeless peoples' risks of being infected with HIV. The homeless environment (such as limited privacy and communal sleeping and bathing at shelters) is not conducive to stable sexual relationships and makes it more likely for the homeless person to engage in risky sexual behaviours, thereby increasing the likelihood of contracting HIV. Mental health problems in homeless people also influence behaviours that could affect the progression of HIV/AIDS. Limited access to medical care prevents homeless people from receiving adequate HIV/AIDS treatment as well as education concerning HIV/AIDS prevention and risk reduction. To provide comprehensive services such as health education, HIV testing, case management, and mental health services, basic health care is needed for homeless people with HIV/AIDS.

The homeless condition may also make adherence to HIV treatment regimens challenging for homeless patients and their caregivers. In a study of HIV-infected drug users, homelessness and frequent heroin use were negatively associated with antiretroviral therapy adherence (Palepu, Milloy, Kerr, et al., 2011). In addition, methadone maintenance was positively associated with antiretroviral therapy adherences, which speaks of the importance of improving housing status and methadone maintenance to increase survival in this population. Research has demonstrated positive associations between increased housing stability and improved health outcomes among persons with HIV/AIDS in Canada (PHAC, 2013). Thus, strategies for reducing homelessness among those at risk for or living with HIV/AIDs are needed.

Stress, depression, and other mental health problems are also common in homeless people. People who are homeless experience extreme stress on a daily basis. Multiple stresses of living in shelters and on the streets, physical problems, lack of resources, psychosocial issues such as shame and stigma, and feelings of hopelessness and despair often tax the homeless person's ability to cope. Gambling problems are risk factors for homelessness, and the homeless are also more likely to have gambling problems, with 35% of men using Toronto shelter services reporting serious or severe gambling at some point in their lives; however, gambling problems are often overlooked because of competing mental health and substance use issues (Matheson, Devotta, Wendaferew, et al., 2014).

Multiple systematic reviews have demonstrated that over half of people experiencing homelessness have mental health issues, including alcohol and drug use, personality disorders, anxiety disorders, affective disorders, depression, and psychotic illness. Homeless people are also more likely to have cognitive impairment (Depp, Vella, Orff, et al., 2015), which further complicates their mental health.

The prevalence of substance abuse among homeless people is much higher than that among the general population and is both a leading cause and a consequence of the continuance of homelessness among individuals. Substance use also often arises after individuals become homeless, as they attempt to obtain temporary relief from their problems and eventually rely on drugs and alcohol to cope with their daily struggles; however, substance use only worsens their problems and makes it more difficult for them to escape their homeless status. Substance use often co-occurs with mental health problems among homeless people (Polcin, 2015). Drug use contributes to the poor health and increased mortality risk observed among homeless persons (Grinman, Chiu, Redelmeier, et al., 2010).

## Strategies to Address Homelessness

Homelessness has long been recognized as a multidimensional problem of modern-day society. The homeless situation is a problem not only of individuals but also of families, communities, and societies. This problem needs to be addressed as a dynamic and not a static phenomenon, because as societies continue to change and evolve, there will always be those who are excluded and suffer consequences. These are the risks that must be actively anticipated so that strategic planning can forestall any devastating and long-lasting effects.

Communities across the country have developed their own strategies to address homelessness. Adamo, Klodawsky, Aubry, et al. (2016), reporting on a study of 10-year housing and homelessness plans in four major Canadian cities (Calgary, Vancouver, Toronto, and Ottawa), noted that the cities had made progress in advancing program and system-level initiatives, with a stabilization in the growth of homelessness within their jurisdictions; however, none of the cities have achieved sustained reductions in the number of homeless individuals and families, and in some cities, homelessness is growing among subpopulations such as families, youth, and older persons. The study also highlighted that the 10-year plans are severely underfunded, that municipalities have limited authority over the key drivers of homelessness and precarious housing in Canada, and that cities require a comprehensive and well-integrated national plan.

*Reaching Home: Canada's Homelessness Strategy* is a new community-based program that is aimed at preventing and reducing homelessness across Canada that provides funding to urban, rural, remote, and Indigenous communities (Government of Canada, 2019a). Participating communities will work toward reducing chronic homelessness by 50% over the next 10 years. Reaching Home is part of Canada's first-ever National Housing Strategy, a 10-year, $40-billion plan to provide housing that is sustainable, accessible, mixed-income, and mixed-use (Government of Canada, 2018b).

Resolving health problems and resolving homelessness are dependently interrelated. Many health problems are highly prevalent in people experiencing homelessness. Health conditions such as diabetes, HIV/AIDS, addiction, and mental illness require ongoing treatment. If people do not have a stable place to stay, treating their health conditions and finding time for healing and recovery from health problems are almost impossible.

There is a greater degree of optimism today in dealing with the problems of homelessness. Individuals and communities are showing concern through increased involvement. Homelessness is everyone's problem, and people can ultimately affect the establishment of priorities to facilitate an improved quality of life. Increasing awareness and knowledge of the current status of homeless people will aid in understanding the problem and its ramifications.

Health care providers play a significant role in helping homeless persons. It is important for them to be capable of meeting the complex health needs of homeless people. Creative care planning is necessary for the homeless patient because standards of care may not be suitable for an individual who experiences homelessness and does not have a home where the basic requirements for self-care and recovery are available (Billings & Kowalski, 2008). Community health practitioners are also at the forefront of advocacy for the homeless as they work to effect changes and develop strategies to deal with the problems associated with the health status of homeless people. Key recommendations to address homelessness include (1) prevention through mechanisms to stop or reduce risk of homelessness, (2) provision of emergency services such as shelters and day programs, and (3) moving people into housing with necessary supports as rapidly as possible (Gaetz et al., 2016).

The Homeless Health Research Network (HHRN) is a group of researchers and health care providers who are working on developing a set of evidence-informed guidelines on how to address the health and social needs of homeless and vulnerably housed populations in Canada (Cochrane Methods: Equity, 2018). The group have identified the top four issues to prioritize: (1) facilitating access to housing, (2) mental health and addiction care, (3) care coordination/case management, and (4) facilitating access to income. Additionally, the HHRN list in their guidelines the following groups as being the top four homeless populations to prioritize: (1) Indigenous peoples, (2) women, (3) youth, and (4) people with disabilities.

# GENDER AND SEXUAL DIVERSE POPULATIONS

Gender diversity is an umbrella term used to describe a diversity of gender identities or expressions beyond masculine and feminine. These may include lesbian, gay, binary, transgender, queer, intersex, and two spirit (LGBTQ2). Nurses and health care providers do not need to know about every gender identity possible, but must acknowledge that there are many ways to identify outside of the male/female binary, and must respect those who are gender diverse and their life choices. This includes using the correct names and pronouns for gender-diverse people, and using gender neutral language.

The term "gender and sexual diversity" is considered to be more inclusive than "LGBT" because it does not specify any gender identity or sexual orientation whatsoever (Government of Canada, 2019b). The term "gender and sexual minorities" includes all people whose gender identity or sexual orientation differs from the majority of the surrounding society. The concept of *gender equality* maintains that "all human beings, regardless of their gender, are free to develop their personal abilities and make choices without the limitations set by stereotypes, rigid gender roles and prejudices, and that the different behaviours, aspirations and needs of people of all genders are considered, valued and favoured equally" (Government of Canada, 2019b). Gender equity refers to the fair treatment of all genders according to their respective needs and acknowledges that this treatment can be different but must be equivalent in terms of rights, benefits, obligations, and opportunities (Government of Canada, 2019b).

## Health Issues of Gender-Diverse Populations

There is growing evidence of inequalities faced by LGBTQ2 communities in Canada and internationally (Haas, Rodgers, & Herman, 2014); however, there is a lack of national-level data on suicide rates among LGBT people. A meta-analysis of 25 international population-based studies showed that suicide attempts among gay and bisexual men are four times more frequent than among heterosexual men, and that suicide attempts among lesbian and bisexual women are two times more frequent than among heterosexual women (King, Semlyen, Tai, et al., 2008). A study of 350 LGBTQ2 youth in Canada, the United States, and New Zealand found that over 4 out of 10 had considered suicide, and 1 in 3 had attempted suicide. Among the latter, 65% of male youth and 45% of female youth considered their attempt to be related to their sexual orientation (D'Augelli, Hershberger, & Pilkington, 2001). The prevalence of low self-rated mental health among bisexual or gay/lesbian adults is 3.1 and 1.7 times, respectively, that of heterosexual adults (PHAC, 2018).

Homelessness among youth who identify as LGBTQ2 is prevalent and poses significant risks to their physical and psychosocial well-being as they are confronted with stigma, discrimination, and exclusion (McCann & Brown, 2019). Challenges faced by LGBTQ2 homeless youth include finding shelter, getting an education, getting a job, and accessing health care and social services, and, for some, violence and abuse, mental health issues, and substance use; sexual risks complicate matters even further (McCann & Brown, 2019).

Rates of some chronic health conditions are higher among gender-diverse populations: for example, the prevalence of asthma is 1.8 times higher among lesbian women than heterosexual woman, and 1.7 times higher among bisexual adults than heterosexual adults (PHAC, 2018). The underestimation of the prevalence of the transgender population contributes to systemic discrimination and underfunding of health care services (Carroll, 2018).

# NURSING'S RESPONSE TO DIVERSE POPULATIONS AND HEALTH

The *Code of Ethics for Registered Nurses* of the Canadian Nurses Association (CNA) explicitly states the profession's commitment to individually and collectively advocate for and work toward eliminating social inequities (CNA, 2017). Additionally, the CNA describes several ethical responsibilities of nurses interacting with persons seeking care. Two responsibilities that are relevant to working with Canada's diverse populations are the following:

1. "Nurses do not discriminate on the basis of a person's race, ethnicity, culture, political and spiritual beliefs, social or marital status, gender, gender identity, gender expression, sexual orientation, age, health status, place of origin, lifestyle, mental or physical ability, socio-economic status, or any other attribute" (CNA, 2017, p. 15).
2. "Nurses respect the special history and interests of Indigenous Peoples as articulated in the Truth and Reconciliation Commission of Canada's (TRC, 2015) *Calls to Action*.

Nurses have responsibilities to be aware of specific health needs and respond to illness in all populations. Nurses continue to make many positive moves toward understanding culturally diverse populations. (See the Case Study and Care Plan regarding Mr. and Mrs. Arahan, an older adult immigrant couple, at the end of this chapter, which propose nursing interventions to ensure their quality of life in their later years.) Nurses' awareness and understanding of transcultural issues have been facilitated by the works of leaders such as Leininger, Giger, Davidhizar, Andrews, and Boyle, to name just a few. In addition, wide dissemination of research findings has been made possible through the *Journal of Transcultural Nursing* and through annual conferences and other sponsored workshops. Additionally, nurses with advanced preparation have committed their time and energy to developing approaches and models for transcultural nursing.

A major limitation of transcultural nursing models and theories is their lack of acknowledgement of power relationships, and their implicit cultural essentialism or attribution of fixed characteristics to different ethnic groups (Mulholland, 1995). The power relationship between the health care provider and patient is important to providing culturally safe care, and stereotyping cultural groups diminishes the identity of the individual and their unique circumstances. A cultural nursing assessment is a systematic way of identifying individual beliefs and values while considering their history and their current social and physical environments (Bourque, Bearskin, & Jakubec, 2017). Giger and Davidhizar's (2012) Transcultural Assessment Model considers the following factors—culturally unique individual, communication, space, social organization, and biological variations—and incorporates these data into the nursing care plan. A spiritual assessment identifies spiritual beliefs and practices and implications for health (Innovative Practice). Using this approach nurses can develop the culturally sensitive attitudes and skills that support culturally safe care. Several nursing journals focus on cultural diversity, such as the *Journal of Cultural Diversity* and the *Journal of Multicultural Nursing and Health*. These journals and a variety of other publications are constantly increasing health care providers' knowledge of health-related cultural issues.

## INNOVATIVE PRACTICE

### Spiritual Practices and Health

Spirituality and its relationship with health outcomes have been the focus of considerable interest in recent years (Como, 2007). Spirituality can mean many different things to different people, ranging from traditional institutional religion to occult practices (Fisher, 2011). Spirituality can be defined as an individual's sense of peace, purpose, and connection to others as well as the person's beliefs about the meaning of life. Spirituality is not necessarily tied to any particular religion, but religion is one way that people may express their spirituality. Individuals express their spirituality through (1) beliefs and values about life, death, suffering, and meaning; (2) traditions and practices such as prayer, meditation, religious practices, and commitment to a way of living; and (3) sacred awareness and experience of a sacred relationship, transcendence, Divine love, interconnectedness, or wholeness (Manitoba's Spiritual Health Care Partners, 2017).

Spirituality plays an important role in the lives of many Canadians. In the report called Canadians on Religion, Faith and Spirituality, participants disclosed their top reasons for being religious or spiritual, including having a set of values to follow (30%), bringing positivity into their lives (30%), providing a sense of hope (29%), and helping to cope with stress (23%) (Ipsos, 2017). According to a study by the Angus Reid Institute (2017), most Canadians have considerable personal faith and believe in the existence of God, although they might not view the word "religion" favourably; Canadians fit into four major groups: religiously devout (21%); privately faithful (30%); spiritually uncertain (30%); and non-believers (19%). The study also found that, in general, highly religious people are happier and more engaged with their communities. Faith-based communities also provide support and comfort for new Canadians; notably, sometimes the community they find support within is not associated with their own religion (Angus Reid Institute, 2018).

Spirituality and spiritual care play an important role in health and health care. Spiritual health is a fundamental dimension of overall health and well-being that permeates all other dimensions of health (physical, mental, emotional, social, and vocational) (Fisher, 2011). The CNA (2010) recognizes that spirituality is an integral dimension of health, spiritual beliefs are diverse, and that registered nurses are expected to respect this diversity, support spiritual preferences, and

attend to the spiritual needs of individuals. Considerable evidence has shown spiritual practices to be an important and effective coping strategy and a common approach to dealing with health problems, particularly chronic diseases such as cardiovascular disease and cancer (Como, 2007). Spiritual practices are likely to improve coping skills and social support, promote feelings of optimism and hope, encourage healthy behaviour, decrease feelings of depression and anxiety, and support a sense of relaxation. Many studies have found that spiritual or religious beliefs and practices help patients with cancer as well as their caregivers to cope with the disease. Studies also suggest that many patients would like health care providers to consider spirituality as a factor in their health care (Bremault-Phillips, Olson, Brett-MacLean, et al., 2015).

Holistic nursing care requires exploring the spiritual self and spiritual healing for self and others (Jaberi, Momennasab, Yektatalab, et al., 2017). Addressing spirituality at critical times in life (such as during serious illness or at the end of life) has been noted to reduce spiritual pain and distress (Bremault-Phillips et al., 2015). A spiritual assessment may help nurses and other health care providers understand how religious or spiritual beliefs will affect the way a patient copes with diseases and health problems. Few tools for assessing spiritual history and/or spiritual practices have been developed to help health care providers consider patients' spiritual needs and/or plan appropriate spiritual interventions for their patients. A spiritual practices checklist (Quinn-Griffin, Salman, Lee, et al., 2008) was developed to identify the religious or spiritual interventions used and the frequency of use of religious or spiritual interventions. The 12 items of the checklist include the most commonly used spiritual practices (e.g., prayer) and CAM interventions (e.g., meditation, yoga). The FICA Spiritual History Tool comprises questions that help to identify the presence of Faith, belief or meaning in a patient's life; the Importance of spirituality in a patient's life and health care decision-making; their spiritual Community; and interventions that may help to Address the patient's spiritual needs (Bremault-Phillips et al., 2015). Guidelines for providing spiritual care have been published by the Canadian Hospice Palliative Care Association (2013) and Manitoba's Spiritual Health Care Partners (2017).

Sources: Angus Reid Institute. (2017). A spectrum of spirituality: Canadians keep the faith to varying degrees, but few reject it entirely. Retrieved from http://angusreid.org/religion-in-canada-150/; Angus Reid Institute. (2018). Faith and immigration: New Canadians rely on religious communities for material and spiritual support. Retrieved from http://angusreid.org/faith-canada-immigration/; Bremault-Phillips, S., Olson, J., Brett-MacLean, P., Oneschuk, D., Sinclair, S., Magnus, R., Puchalski, C. M., et al. (2015). Integrating spirituality as a key component of patient care. Religions, 6, 476–498. https://doi.org/10.3390/rel6020476; Canadian Hospice Palliative Care Association. (2013). How spiritual care practitioners provide care in Canadian hospice palliative care settings: Recommended advanced practice guidelines and commentary. Retrieved from https://www.chpca.net/media/319456/chpca_spiritual_advisors_--recommended_practice_guidelines_--_31october_2013.pdf; Canadian Nurses Association. (2010). CNA Position Statement: Spirituality, health and nursing practice. Retrieved from https://www.cna-aiic.ca/-/media/cna/page-content/pdf-en/ps111_spirituality_2010_e.pdf?la=en&hash=0F2E61A2C3E07A08291F88506C523D485DC49BE7; Como, J. M. (2007). Spiritual practice: A literature review related to spiritual health and health outcomes. Holistic Nursing Practice, 21(5), 224–236; Fisher, J. (2011). The Four Domains Model: Connecting spirituality, health and well-being. Religions, 2, 17–28. https://doi.org/10.3390/rel2010017. Quinn-Griffin, M., Salman, A., Lee, Y., & Fitzpatrick, J. J. et al., (2008). A beginning look at the spiritual practices of older adults. Journal of Christian Nursing, 25(2), 100–102; Ipsos. (2017). Canadians on religion, faith and spirituality. In Jaberi, A., Momennasab, M., Yektatalab, S., Ebadi, A., & Cheraghi, M. A. et al. (2017). Spiritual health: A concept analysis. Journal of Religious Health. https://doi.org/10.1007/s10943-017-0379-z; Manitoba's Spiritual Health Care Partners. (2017). Core competencies for spiritual health care practitioners. Retrieved from https://www.gov.mb.ca/health/mh/spiritualhealth/core.html.

Nursing organizations such as the Canadian Nurses Association (CNA, 2010), the Canadian Association of Schools of Nursing (CASN, 2009, 2013), and the Registered Nurse's Association of Ontario (RNAO, 2007) publish culturally relevant materials to guide students, clinicians, and educators, with a particular focus on First Nations, Métis, and Inuit Peoples. Additionally, there is a cadre of nurses whose research on the cultural practices and beliefs of individuals and families gives nurses and other health care providers a sound base for improving practice and designing cost-effective and humanistic health care strategies. The quest to deliver culturally competent care has provided the impetus for a nursing faculty to require courses in the nursing curriculum to facilitate awareness and understanding of cultural diversity. Rowan and colleagues (2013) examined the integration of cultural competence and cultural safety into Canadian schools of nursing, identified facilitating factors, and provided theoretical and practical implications for initiation and improvement of integration strategies.

The most commonly identified environmental influence was on the need to meet competency requirements written by nursing regulatory bodies and professional organizations. Study findings suggested that few schools had developed indicators to measure whether students had learned the concepts of cultural competence and cultural safety. Results of another Canadian study that examined nurses perceptions of critical cultural competence suggest that Canadian-born nurses who share a similar culture and language as their patients scored higher perceptions of cultural competence than those who were born in different countries, demonstrating the need for ongoing education in cultural competence, particularly in health care organizations with multicultural workforces or patient populations (Almutairi, Adlan, & Nasim, 2017). It is essential for Canadian nurses to plan culturally tailored and competent care to mitigate health inequities and provide effective care in our rapidly changing multicultural societies, thereby delivering quality and safe care to all (Quality and Safety Scenario).

## QUALITY AND SAFETY SCENARIO

### Immigrants and Health Care Providers

Mr. Jade and Madam Nora have four children: Nirman (6 months), Julia (18 months), Hady (4 years), and Jamella (6 years). Mr. Jade is an economist who immigrated to Canada from Iraq 4 years ago. The family has come to the well-baby clinic because Madam Nora has been concerned about Nirman; Nirman's skin appears paler than that of her siblings, and she is also not gaining weight. Mr. Jade gave a brief health history of Nirman's situation because his wife cannot express herself in English. "My wife believes that Nirman is not growing like the rest of our children. She breastfeeds her every 2 hours, but she is not eating." My wife is "upset that Nirman is not becoming bigger." The vital signs are as follows: pulse, 125 beats per minute; respirations, 22 breaths per minute; blood pressure, 100/70 mm Hg; and rectal temperature, 37.4°C. Nirman's weight is 4.54 kg and her length is 55.88 cm. Nirman appears pale. Madam Nora, aged 28 years, is wearing a headscarf covering her hair and a long dress. When Mr. Jade and Madam Nora are left alone, nurses can hear them arguing and raising their voices in a foreign language (Arabic), and Madam Nora appeared very upset. The medical history revealed a term baby female born by normal vaginal delivery with a normal birth weight. No history of vomiting, diarrhea, or fever was reported. Pallor and jaundice were noted on physical examination. The family history revealed that both Mr. Jade and Madam Nora came from the same village and are Muslim and second-degree cousins. No genetic studies have been performed for the family members. Nirman's initial diagnosis is hemolytic anemia.

Nurses should consider the unique cultural background and family dynamics and functioning while providing care to this immigrant family to ensure safe and quality care. The family has an ineffective communication pattern and an inability to navigate through the complexity of the health care system. Madam Nora needs to communicate with health care providers through her husband, who, in turn, is not familiar with medical terminology. The fact that no genetic testing was performed among family members may be attributed to the unfamiliarity and complexity of the health care system in Canada as compared with the health services in their native country. It is important for nurses to have culturally competent skills and to identify cultural beliefs that may impact how immigrant patients may communicate with them. Hence, effective approaches may be implemented to provide safe and quality care for this population and to mitigate health inequities.

Discussion of specific health care problems and nursing care always includes cultural aspects. In the clinical setting, health care workers, through staff development and in-service programs, are provided with opportunities to learn and develop cultural humility and culturally sensitive care approaches.

## CASE STUDY

### An Older Immigrant Couple: Mr. and Mrs. Arahan

Mr. and Mrs. Arahan, an older couple in their 70s, have been living with their oldest daughter, her husband of 15 years, and their two children, aged 12 and 14 years. They all live in a middle-income neighbourhood in a suburb of a metropolitan city. Mr. and Mrs. Arahan are both university educated and worked full time while they were in their native country. In addition, Mr. Arahan, the only offspring of wealthy parents, inherited a substantial amount of money and real estate. Their daughter came to Canada as a registered nurse and met her husband, a pharmaceutical company representative. The older couple moved to Canada when their daughter became a Canadian citizen and petitioned for them as immigrants. Because the couple were facing retirement, they welcomed the opportunity to come to Canada.

The Arahans found life in Canada different from that in their home country, but their adjustment was not as difficult because both were healthy and spoke English fluently. Most of their time was spent taking care of their two grandchildren and the house. As the grandchildren grew older, the older couple found that they had more spare time. The daughter and her husband advanced in their careers and spent a great deal more time at their jobs. There were few family dinners during the week. On weekends, the daughter, her husband, and their children socialized with their own friends. The couple began to feel isolated and longed for a more active life.

Mr. and Mrs. Arahan began to think that perhaps they should return to their home country, where they still had relatives and friends. However, political and economic issues would have made it difficult for them to live there. Besides, they had become accustomed to the way of life in Canada with all the modern conveniences and abundance of goods that were difficult to obtain in their country. However, they also became concerned that they might not be able to tolerate the winter months and that minor health problems might worsen as they aged. They wondered who would take care of them if they became very frail and where they would live, knowing that their daughter had saved money only for their grandchildren's college education. They expressed their sentiments to their daughter, who became very concerned about how her parents were feeling.

This older couple had been attending church on a regular basis but had never been active in other church-related activities. The church bulletin announced the establishment of parish nursing with two retired registered nurses as volunteers. The couple attended the first opening of the parish clinic. Here, they met one of the registered nurses, who had a short discussion with them about the services offered. The registered nurse had spent a great deal of her working years as a community health nurse. She informed Mr. and Mrs. Arahan of her availability to help them resolve any health-related issues.

Reflective Questions:
- What strategies could be suggested for this older adult couple to enhance their quality of life?
- What community resources can they use?
- What can the daughter and her family do to address the feelings of isolation of the older couple?
- What health-promotion activities can ensure a healthy lifestyle for them?

## CARE PLAN

### An Older Immigrant Couple: Mr. and Mrs. Arahan

**Nursing Issue**
Risk of continued feelings of isolation

*Defining Characteristics*
- The couple no longer have a great deal of caretaking responsibilities.
- The daughter and her husband spend a great deal of time on their careers.
- Family dinners are seldom.
- The daughter and her family socialize with their own friends.
- The older couple is thinking of returning to their native country.
- The couple is concerned about life in Canada with harsh winters and their minor health problems.
- The couple is concerned about their advancing years and future living arrangements.

*Related Factors*
- Transition from the native country to Canada.
- Differing religious, ethnic, and cultural backgrounds between the native country and Canada influence care decisions.
- Differing roles in family structures between the native country and Canada.
- Conflicting roles between the two generations.
- Limited opportunities for social support and assimilation for older immigrants.
- Health and health care needs, multiple and complex, for the elder population.

*Expected Outcomes*
The Arahans will:
- Join an older person centre for socialization and other activities.

- Volunteer at a nearby hospital or school several mornings or afternoons per week.
- Work with their daughter and her family to plan at least one family meal per week.
- Pursue some neglected hobbies.
- Get involved in a church group or in a civic organization.
- Begin a discussion on future alternative living arrangements.
- Make periodic visits to the native country to see relatives and friends.

*Interventions*
- Encourage the couple to have open discussions about their concerns with their daughter and her family.
- Support them in their choice of meaningful activities such as joining the older person centre and volunteering.
- Provide information on resources for future living arrangements in Canada.
- Develop a plan for health monitoring on a regular basis.
- Provide a list of organizations that address issues and concerns of older adults
- Utilize their experience and expertise (if any) in managing the parish nursing clinic.
- Initiate an older support group in the parish with the Arahans as the first members.

The Arahans' situation is a very common one in most immigrant groups. The interventions outlined would need to consider the cultural traditions, personal preferences, health status, motivation level, physical ability, and resources of the couple to ensure positive outcomes and goal achievement.

## SUMMARY

This century will continue to be a time of great challenges as the population of Canada continues to be a nation of diverse peoples. The nation and its people have repeatedly overcome devastations by both nature and humankind itself. As citizens, diverse populations share similar concerns about life, including health, an acceptable standard of living, and quality of life. An array of cultural, economic, educational, social, and political barriers are being eroded at the local, national, and global levels to ensure the health and well-being of the people of Canada. The government, public and private industries, health care professions, and all individuals can work together to reduce health inequities and ensure a healthy nation for future generations.

**Evolve Chapter Features**

http://evolve.elsevier.com/Canada/Edelman/healthpromotion/
- Review Questions

## REFERENCES

Aboriginal Nurses Association of Canada [ANAC]. (2009). *Cultural competence and cultural safety in nursing education: A framework for First Nations, Inuit and Métis Nursing.* [Seminal Reference] https://www.cna-aiic.ca/~/media/cna/page-content/pdf-en/first_nations_framework_e.pdf.

Adamo, A., Klodawsky, F., Aubry, T., et al. (2016). *Ending homelessness in Canada: A study of 10-year plans in 4 Canadian cities.* Retrieved from https://homelesshub.ca/sites/default/files/attachments/Ending%20Homelessness%20in%20Canada_October%202016.pdf.

Aery, A., & Cheff, R. (2018). *Sanctuary city: Opportunities for health equity.* Toronto, ON: Wellesley Institute.

Ahmed, S., Shommu, N. S., Rumana, N., et al. (2016). Barriers to access to primary health care by immigrant populations in Canada: A literature review. *Journal of Immigrant and Minority Health,* 18(6), 1522–1540.

Almutairi, A. F., Adlan, A. A., & Nasim, M. (2017). Perceptions of cultural competence of registered nurses in Canada. *BMC Nursing,* 16, 47. https://doi.org/10.1186/s12912-017-0242-2.

Andermann, A. (2016). Taking action on the social determinants of health in clinical practice: A framework for health professionals. *Canadian Medical Association Journal,* 188(17–18), E474–E483. https://doi.org/10.1503/cmaj.160177.

Angus Reid Institute. (2017). *A spectrum of spirituality: Canadians keep the faith to varying degrees, but few reject it entirely.* Retrieved from http://angusreid.org/religion-in-canada-150/.

Angus Reid Institute. (2018). *Faith and immigration: New Canadians rely on religious communities for material and spiritual support.* Retrieved from http://angusreid.org/faith-canada-immigration/.

Berg, R. C., & Denison, E. (2012). *International initiative for impact evaluation: Interventions to reduce the prevalence of female genital mutilation/cutting in African countries.* Retrieved from http://www.ieimpact.org/admin/pdfs synthetic/011%20protocol.pdf.

Billings, D. M., & Kowalski, K. (2008). Teaching tips. Increasing competency in the care of homeless patients. *Journal of Continuing Education in Nursing, 39*(4), 153–154.

Bourque Bearskin, R. L., & Jakubec, S. L. (2017). Diversity and relational practice in community health nursing. In M. Stanhope, J. Lancaster, S. L. Jakubec, et al. (Eds.), *Community health nursing in Canada* (3rd ed.) (pp. 173–207). Toronto: Elsevier Canada.

Boyle, J. S. (2016). Culture, family, and community. In M. M. Andrews, & J. S. Boyle (Eds.), *Transcultural concepts in nursing care* (7th ed.) (pp. 317–358). Philadelphia: Lippincott Williams & Wilkins.

Bremault-Phillips, S., Olson, J., Brett-MacLean, P., et al. (2015). Integrating spirituality as a key component of patient care. *Religions, 6,* 476–498. https://doi.org/10.3390/rel6020476.

Brousseau, L., & Dewing, M. (2018). *Background paper: Canadian multiculturalism.* Publication No. 2009-20-E. Ottawa: Library of Parliament.

Browne, A. J., & Varcoe, C. (2019). Cultural and social considerations in health assessment. In C. Jarvis, A. J. Browne, J. Macdonald-Jenkins, et al. (Eds.), *Physical examination and health assessment* (3rd Canadian ed.) (pp. 28–45). Toronto: Elsevier Canada.

Canadian Association of Schools of Nursing (CASN). (2009). *Cultural competence and cultural safety in nursing education: A framework for First Nations, Inuit and Metis Nursing.* Retrieved from https://www.cna-aiic.ca/~/media/cna/page-content/pdf-en/first nations framework_e.pdf.

Canadian Association of Schools of Nursing (CASN). (2013). *Educating nurses to address socio-cultural, historical, and contextual determinants of health among Aboriginal peoples.* Retrieved from https://casn.ca/wp-content/uploads/2014/12/ENAHHRIKnowledgeProductFINAL.pdf.

Canadian Geographic. (2018a). *Indigenous peoples atlas of Canada.* Ottawa: Royal Canadian Geographical Society.

Canadian Geographic. (2018b). *Indigenous peoples atlas of Canada: Metis.* Ottawa: Royal Canadian Geographical Society.

Canadian Geographic. (2018c). *Indigenous peoples atlas of Canada: Inuit.* Ottawa: Royal Canadian Geographical Society.

Canadian Hospice Palliative Care Association. (2013). *How spiritual care practitioners provide care in Canadian hospice palliative care settings: Recommended advanced practice guidelines and commentary.* Retrieved from https://www.chpca.net/media/319456/chpca_spiritual_advisors_--recommended_practice_guidelines_--_31october_2013.pdf.

Canadian Institute for Health Information (CIHI). (2017). *Has the share of health spending on seniors changed?* Retrieved from https://www.cihi.ca/en/has-the-share-of-health-spending-on-seniors-changed-2017.

Canadian Institute for Health Information (CIHI). (2018). *In pursuit of health equity: Defining stratifiers for measuring health inequality: A focus on age, sex, gender, income, education and geographic location.* Ottawa: Author.

Canadian Nurses Association (CNA). (2009). *CNA position statement: Global health and equity.* Ottawa: Author.

Canadian Nurses Association (CNA). (2010). *CNA Position Statement: Spirituality, health and nursing practice.* Ottawa: Author. Retrieved from https://www.cna-aiic.ca/-/media/cna/page-content/pdf-en/ps111_spirituality_2010_e.pdf?la=en&hash=0F2E61A2C3E07A08291F88506C523D485DC49BE7.

Canadian Nurses Association (CNA). (2017). *2017 Edition: Code of ethics for registered nurses.* Ottawa: Author.

Canadian Observatory on Homelessness (COH). (2012). *Canadian definition of homelessness.* Toronto: Canadian Observatory on Homelessness Press. Retrieved from https://www.homelesshub.ca/resource/canadian-definition-homelessness.

Carr, I. (n.d.). *Folk healing, alternative, and parallel medicines.* Retrieved from http://medheritage.lib.umanitoba.ca/?page id=428.

Carroll, J. M. (2018). *Cultural humility and transgender clients: A study examining the relationship between critical reflection and attitudes of nurse practitioners.* Kingston, ON: Queen's University.

Clipsham, J., Hampson, E., Powell, L., et al. (2011). *A positive space is a healthy place: Making your community health centre, public health unit or community agency inclusive to those of all sexual orientations and gender identities.* Retrieved from https://opha.on.ca/getmedia/125e32e7-f9cb-48ed-89cb-9d954d76537b/SexualHealthPaper-Mar11.pdf.aspx?ext=.pdf.

Cochrane Methods: Equity. (2018). *Homeless health guidelines.* Retrieved from https://methods.cochrane.org/equity/projects/homeless-health-guidelines.

Como, J. M. (2007). Spiritual practice: A literature review related to spiritual health and health outcomes. *Holistic Nursing Practice, 21*(5), 224–236. [Seminal Reference].

Crowshoe, L., Dannenbaum, D., Green, M., et al. (2018). Type 2 diabetes and Indigenous peoples. *Canadian Journal of Diabetes, 42,* S296–S306. https://doi.org/10.1016/j.jcjd.2017.10.022.

D'Augelli, A. R., Hershberger, S. L., & Pilkington, N. W. (2001). Suicidality patterns and sexual orientation-related factors among lesbian, gay, and bisexual youths. *Suicide and Life-Threatening Behavior, 31*(3), 250–265. [Seminal Reference].

Depp, C. A., Vella, L., Orff, H. J., et al. (2015). A quantitative review of cognitive functioning in homeless adults. *Journal of Nervous and Mental Disease, 203*(2), 126–131.

Douglas, M. K., Rosenkoetter, M., Pacquiao, D. F., et al. (2014). Guidelines for implementing culturally competent nursing care. *Journal of Transcultural Nursing,* 1–13.

Echenberg, H., & Jensen, H. (2012). *Risk factors for homelessness.* Ottawa: Library of Parliament. Retrieved from http://publications.gc.ca/collections/collection_2016/bdp-lop/bp/YM32-2-2009-51-eng.pdf.

First Nations Health Authority [FNHA]. (2019). *Cultural humility.* Retrieved from http://www.fnha.ca/wellness/cultural-humility.

Fisher, J. (2011). The Four Domains Model: Connecting spirituality, health and well-being. *Religions, 2,* 17–28. https://doi.org/10.3390/rel2010017.

Fonseca, X., Lukosch, S., & Brazier, F. (2018). Social cohesion revisited: A new definition and how to characterize it. *Innovation: The European Journal of Social Science Research.* https://doi.org/10.1080/13511610.2018.1497480.

Foronda, C. L., Baptiste, D., Reinholdt, M. M., et al. (2016). Cultural humility: A concept analysis. *Journal of Transcultural Nursing, 27*(3), 210–217. https://doi.org/10.1177/1043659615592677.

Gadacz, R. R., & Parrott, Z. (2015). *First Nations.* Retrieved from https://www.thecanadianencyclopedia.ca/en/article/first-nations.

Gaetz, S., Dej, E., Richter, T., et al. (2016). *The state of homelessness in Canada 2016.* Toronto: Canadian Observatory on Homelessness Press. Retrieved from https://www.homelesshub.ca/sites/default/files/attachments/SOHC16_final_20Oct2016.pdf.

Giger, J. N. (2013). Introduction. In J. Giger (Ed.), *Transcultural nursing: Assessment and interventions* (6th ed.) (pp. 2–18). St. Louis: Elsevier.

Giger, J. N., & Davidhizar, R. E. (2012). *Transcultural nursing: Assessment and intervention* (6th ed.). St. Louis: Mosby Elsevier.

Government of Canada. (2017). *Inclusion of marginalized people.* Retrieved from https://international.gc.ca/world-monde/issues_development-enjeux_developpement/human_rights-droits_homme/inclusion.aspx?lang=eng.

Government of Canada. (2018a). *What is Indian status?* Retrieved from https://www.aadnc-aandc.gc.ca/eng/1100100032463/1100100032464.

Government of Canada. (2018b). *Reaching home: Canada's homelessness strategy.* Retrieved from https://www.canada.ca/en/

employment-social-development/news/2018/06/reaching-home-canadas-homelessness-strategy.html.

Government of Canada. (2019a). *Description of reaching home: Canada's homelessness strategy*. Retrieved from https://www.canada.ca/en/employment-social-development/programs/homelessness.html.

Government of Canada. (2019b). *Gender and sexual diversity glossary*. Retrieved from https://www.btb.termiumplus.gc.ca/publications/diversite-diversity-eng.html.

Grinman, M. N., Chiu, S., Redelmeier, D. A., et al. (2010). Drug problems among homeless individuals in Toronto: Canada: Prevalence, drugs of choice, and relation to health status. *BMC Public Health, 10*, 94. https://doi.org/10.1186/1471-2458-10-94.

Gruenbaum, E. (2005). Socio-cultural dynamics of female genital cutting: Research, findings, gaps, and directions. *Culture Health Sexuality, 7*(5), 420–441.

Haas, A. P., Rodgers, P. L., & Herman, J. L. (2014). *Suicide attempts among transgender and gender non-conforming adults*. Retrieved from https://queeramnesty.ch/docs/AFSP-Williams-Suicide-ReportFinal.pdf.

Harris-Haywood, S. H., Goode, T., Smith, K., et al. (2014). Psychometric evaluation of a cultural competency assessment instrument for health professionals. *Medical Care, 52*(2), e7–e15.

Houle, R. (2019). *Results from the 2016 Census: Syrian refugees who resettled in Canada in 2015 and 2016*. Ottawa: Statistics Canada. Retrieved from https://www150.statcan.gc.ca/n1/en/pub/75-006-x/2019001/article/00001-eng.pdf?st=oDG_fS7M.

Ipsos. (2017). *Canadians on religion, faith and spirituality*. Retrieved from https://www15 0.statcan.gc.ca/n1/en/pub/75-006-x/2019001/article/00001-eng.pdf?st=oDG_fS7M.

Jaberi, A., Momennasab, M., Yektatalab, S., et al. (2017). Spiritual health: A concept analysis. *Journal of Religious Health*. https://doi.org/10.1007/s10943-017-0379-z.

Jackson, T., Clemens, J., & Palacios, M. (2017). *Canada's aging population and implications for government finances*. Retrieved from https://www.fraserinstitute.org/sites/default/files/canadas-aging-population-and-implications-for-government-finances.pdf.

Jedwab, J. (2014). *The multiculturalism question: Debating identity in 21st-century Canada*. Kingston, ON: Queen's University School of Policy Studies.

Johnston, D. (2017). *Pluralism is a path to lasting peace and prosperity*. Retrieved from https://www.theglobeandmail.com/opinion/pluralism-is-a-path-to-lasting-peace-and-prosperity/article36422623/.

Kania-Richmond, A., & Metcalfe, A. (2017). Integrative health care: What are the relevant health outcomes from a practice perspective? A survey. *BMC Complementary and Alternative Medicine, 17*, 548. https://doi.org/10.1186/s12906-017-2041-4.

Kim, I. H., Carrasco, C., Muntaner, C., et al. (2013). Ethnicity and postmigration health trajectory in new immigrants to Canada. *American Journal of Public Health, 103*(4), e96–e104. https://doi.org/10.2105/AJPH.2012.301185.

King, M., Semlyen, J., Tai, S. S., et al. (2008). A systematic review of mental disorder, suicide, and deliberate self harm in lesbian, gay and bisexual people. *BMC Psychiatry, 8*(1), 70.

Kirst, M., Shankardass, K., Singhal, S., et al. (2017). Addressing health inequities in Ontario, Canada: what solutions do the public support? *BMC Public Health, 17*, 7. https://doi.org/10.1186/s12889-016-3932-x.

Kluckhohn, C. (1953). Dominant and variant value orientations. In C. Kluckhohn, H. A. Murray, & D. A. Schneider (Eds.), *Personality in nature, society, and culture* (2nd ed.). New York: Alfred A. Knopf. [Seminal Reference].

Leval, A., Widmar, C., Tishelman, C., et al. (2004). The encounters that rupture the myth: Contradictions in midwives' descriptions and explanations of circumcised women's sexuality. *Health Care for Women International, 25*, 743–760.

Little, C. M. (2003). Female genital circumcision: Medical and cultural considerations. *Journal of Cultural Diversity, 10*(1), 30–34.

Management Sciences for Health. (n.d.). *The providers guide to quality and culture: Health disparities*. Retrieved from http://erc.msh.org/mainpage.cfm?file=7.1.0.htm&module=provider&language=English.

Manitoba's Spiritual Health Care Partners. (2017). *Core competencies for spiritual health care practitioners*. Retrieved from https://www.gov.mb.ca/health/mh/spiritualhealth/core.html.

Markus, H. R. (2008). Pride, prejudice, and ambivalence: Toward a unified theory of race and ethnicity. *American Psychologist, 63*, 651–670. [Seminal Reference].

Matheson, F. I., Devotta, K., Wendaferew, A., et al. (2014). Prevalence of gambling problems among the clients of a Toronto homeless shelter. *Journal of Gambling Studies, 30*, 537–546. https://doi.org/10.1007/s10899-014-9452-7.

McCann, E., & Brown, M. (2019). Homelessness among youth who identify as LGBTQ+: A systematic review. *Journal of Clinical Nursing, 28*, 2061–2072. https://doi.org/10.1111/jocn.14818.

Momoh, C. (2004). Attitudes to female genital mutilation. *British Journal of Midwifery, 12*(10), 631–638.

Mulholland, J. (1995). Nursing, humanism and transcultural theory: The "bracketing-out" of reality. *Journal of Advanced Nursing, 22*, 442–449. [Seminal Reference].

National Center for Complementary and Alternative Medicine. (2011). What is complementary and alternative medicine? Retrieved from http://nccam.hih.hov/health/whatiscam#defininigcam.

Ning, A. M. (2013). How 'alternative' is CAM? Rethinking conventional dichotomies between biomedicine and complementary/alternative medicine. *Health: An Interdisciplinary Journal for the Social Study of Health, Illness and Medicine, 17*(2), 135–158. https://doi.org/10.1177/1363459312447252.

Obermeyer, C. M. (2005). The consequences of female circumcision for health and sexuality: An update on the evidence. *Culture Health Sexuality, 7*(5), 443–461.

Ortega, R. M., & Coulborn Faller, K. (2011). Training child welfare workers from an intersectional cultural humility perspective: A paradigm shift. *Child Welfare, 90*(5), 27–49.

Palepu, A., Milloy, M. J., Kerr, T., et al. (2011). Homelessness and adherence to antiretroviral therapy among a cohort of HIV-infected injection drug users. *Journal of Urban Health, 88*(3), 545–555.

Perron, L., Senikas, V., Burnett, M., et al. (2013). Clinical practice guidelines: Female genital cutting. *Journal of Obstetrics and Gynaecology Canada, 35*(11), 1028–1045.

Polcin, D. L. (2015). Co-occurring substance abuse and mental health problems among homeless persons: Suggestions for research and practice. *Journal of Social Distress and the Homeless, 25*(1), 1–10.

Pottie, K., Greenaway, C., Feightner, J., et al., coauthors of the Canadian Collaboration for Immigrant and Refugee Health. (2011). Evidence-based clinical guidelines for immigrants and refugees. *Canadian Medical Association Journal, 183*(12), E824–E925.

Public Health Agency of Canada (PHAC). (2013). *Population-specific HIV/AIDS status report: People living with HIV/AIDS*. Ottawa: Author. Retrieved from http://publications.gc.ca/site/eng/438877/publication.html.

Public Health Agency of Canada (PHAC). (2018). *Key health inequities in canada: a national portrait*. Ottawa: Author.

Public Health Ontario. (2019). *Homelessness and health outcomes: What are the associations?* Retrieved from https://www.publichealthontario.ca/-/media/documents/eb-homelessness-health.pdf?la=en.

Quinn-Griffin, M., Salman, A., Lee, Y., et al. (2008). A beginning look at the spiritual practices of older adults. *Journal of Christian Nursing, 25*(2), 100–102.

Raphael, D. (Ed.). (2016). *Social determinants of health: Canadian perspectives* (3rd ed.) Toronto: Canadian Scholars Press.

Raphael, D. (2017). Implications of inequities in health for health promotion practice. In I. Rootman, A. Pederson, K. L. Frolich, et al. (Eds.), *Health promotion in Canada: New perspectives on theory, practice, policy, and research* (4th ed.) (pp. 146–166). Toronto: Canadian Scholars Press.

Ray, S. L., & Forchuk, C. (2011). *The experience of homelessness among Canadian Forces and Allied Forces veterans.* Retrieved from https://www.homelesshub.ca/resource/experience-homelessness-among-canadian-forces-and-allied-forces-veterans.

Registered Nurse's Association of Ontario (RNAO). (2007). *Embracing cultural diversity in health care: Developing cultural competence.* Retrieved from Toronto: Author. [Seminal Reference] https://rnao.ca/sites/rnao-ca/files/Embracing_Cultural_Diversity_in_Health_Care_-_Developing_Cultural_Competence.pdf.

Rodrigue, S. (2016). *Insights on Canadian society: Hidden homelessness in Canada* Retrieved from. https://www150.statcan.gc.ca/n1/pub/75-006-x/2016001/article/14678-eng.html.

Rowan, M. S., Rukholm, E., Bourque Bearskin, L., et al. (2013). Cultural competence and cultural safety in Canadian schools of nursing: A mixed methods study. *International Journal of Nursing Education & Scholarship, 10*, ii. https://doi.org/10.1515/ijnes-2012-0043.

Salman, A., McCabe, E., Easter, T., et al. (2007). Cultural competence among staff nurses who participated in a family-centered geriatric care program. *Journal of Nurses Staff Development, 23*(3), 103–111.

Segaert, A., & Bauer, A. (2015). *The extent and nature of veteran homelessness in Canada. Employment and Social Development Canada.* Retrieved from https://www.canada.ca/en/employment-social-development/programs/homelessness/publications-bulletins/veterans-report.html.

Snyder, J., Cheff, R., & Roche, B. (2016). *Perceptions of the social determinants of health across Canada: An examination of the literature.* Toronto: Wellesley Institute.

Srivastava, R. (Ed.). (2007). *The healthcare professional's guide to clinical cultural competence.* Toronto: Elsevier Canada. [Seminal Reference].

Statistics Canada. (2015). *Visible minority of person.* Retrieved from http://www23.statcan.gc.ca/imdb/p3Var.pl?Function=DECI&Id=257515.

Statistics Canada. (2016a). *Census in brief: Ethnic and cultural origins of Canadians: Portrait of a rich heritage.* Retrieved from https://www12.statcan.gc.ca/census-recensement/2016/as-sa/98-200-x/2016016/98-200-x2016016-eng.cfm.

Statistics Canada. (2016b). *Census program.* Retrieved from https://www12.statcan.gc.ca/census-recensement/index-eng.cfm.

Statistics Canada. (2017a). *Population growth: Migratory increase overtakes natural increase.* Retrieved from https://www150.statcan.gc.ca/n1/pub/11-630-x/11-630-x2014001-eng.htm.

Statistics Canada. (2017b). *Aboriginal peoples in Canada: Key results from the 2016 census.* Retrieved from https://www150.statcan.gc.ca/n1/en/daily-quotidien/171025/dq171025a-eng.pdf?st=vqkFcoMr.

Statistics Canada. (2018a). *Population estimates: Key indicators.* Retrieved from https://www150.statcan.gc.ca/n1/en/subjects/population_and_demography/population_estimates.

Statistics Canada. (2018b). *150 years of immigration in Canada.* Retrieved from https://www150.statcan.gc.ca/n1/pub/11-630-x/11-630-x2016006-eng.htm.

Statistics Canada. (2018c). *First Nations people, Métis and Inuit in Canada: Diverse and growing populations.* Retrieved from https://www150.statcan.gc.ca/n1/pub/89-659-x/89-659-x2018001-eng.htm.

Statistics Canada. (2019a). *Annual demographic estimates: Canada, provinces and territories, 2018.* Retrieved from https://www150.statcan.gc.ca/n1/pub/91-215-x/91-215-x2018002-eng.htm.

Statistics Canada. (2019b). *Immigration and ethnocultural diversity in Canada.* Retrieved from https://www12.statcan.gc.ca/nhs-enm/2011/as-sa/99-010-x/99-010-x2011001-eng.cfm.

Tashiro, C. J. (2006). Identity and health in the narratives of older mixed ancestry Asian Americans. *Journal of Cultural Diversity, 13*(1), 41–49.

Tjepkema, M., Wilkins, R., & Long, A. (2013). Cause-specific mortality by income adequacy in Canada: A 16-year follow-up study. *Health Reports, 24*(7), 14–22 (Cat. no. 82-003-X). Ottawa: Statistics Canada.

Truong, M., Paradies, Y., & Priest, N. (2014). Interventions to improve cultural competency in healthcare: A systematic review of reviews. *BMC Health Services Research, 14*(99), 1–17.

Truth and Reconciliation Commission of Canada (TRC). (2015). *Honouring the truth, reconciling for the future: Summary of the final report of the Truth and Reconciliation Commission of Canada.* Retrieved from http://nctr.ca/assets/reports/Final%20Reports/Executive_Summary_English_Web.pdf.

United Nations. (2015). *Transforming our world: The 2030 agenda for sustainable development.* Retrieved from https://sustainabledevelopment.un.org/post2015/transformingourworld.

United Nations Educational, Scientific and Cultural Organization (UNESCO). (2001). *Universal Declaration on Cultural Diversity.* Retrieved from https://unesdoc.unesco.org/ark:/48223/pf0000127160.page=10.

Vang, Z. M., Sigouin, J., Flenon, A., et al. (2017). Are immigrants healthier than native-born Canadians? A systematic review of the healthy immigrant effect in Canada. *Ethnicity and Health, 22*(3), 209–241. https://doi.org/10.1080/13557858.2016.1246518.

Veenstra, G., & Abel, T. (2019). Capital interplays and social inequalities in health. *Scandinavian Journal of Public Health, 47*(6), 631–634. https://doi.org/10.1177/1403494818824436.

Veteran's Affairs Canada. (2019). *VAC support for homeless veterans.* Retrieved from https://www.veterans.gc.ca/eng/services/health/homeless/activities.

Williams, S. P., & Bryant, K. L. (2018). Sexually transmitted infection prevalence among homeless adults in the U.S.: A systematic literature review. *Sexually Transmitted Diseases, 45*(7), 494–504. https://doi.org/10.1097/OLQ.0000000000000780.

World Health Organization (WHO). (2013). *Handbook on health inequality monitoring with a special focus on low- and middle-income countries.* Retrieved from http://www.searo.who.int/entity/health_promotion/9789241548632.pdf?ua=1.

YWCA. (2017). *YW Boston Blog: What is intersectionality, and what does it have to do with me?* Retrieved from https://www.ywboston.org/2017/03/what-is-intersectionality-and-what-does-it-have-to-do-with-me/.At dolore nist, quis id unto occusae cum

# 3

# Health Policy and the Delivery System

*Cindy Fehr, RN, MEd, MScN, FNP* and *Elsie Duff, RN, MEd, PhD*

Originating US chapter by *Debora Elizabeth Kirsch, RN, MS, CNS*

## INTENDED LEARNING OUTCOMES

*After completing this chapter, the reader will be able to:*

- Examine key developments in the history of health care that influenced the philosophical basis of Canadian health care and separated preventive measures from curative measures.
- Differentiate between private and public sector functions and responsibilities in the delivery of health care.
- Describe the mechanisms by which health care in Canada is financed in both the private sector and the public sectors.

- Analyze the influence of health legislation on the health care delivery system.
- Differentiate between the purposes, benefits, and limitations of Canada's government-sponsored health care programs (medicare) in achieving health equity.
- Compare and contrast the health care delivery systems of Canada and the United States.
- Discuss the major provisions of the *Canada Health Act* of 1985 and its impact on improving population health.

## KEY TERMS

Advanced practice nurses (APNs)
Advocate
Ambulatory care
Concierge care
Fee–for-service

Hospitalist
Medicare
Nursing centres
Nurse practitioner (NP)
Third party payor

 **THINK ABOUT IT**

### The Canada Health Act

Saskatchewan introduced a universal, provincial medical insurance plan to provide doctors' services to all its residents in 1962. The federal government passed the Medical Care Act in 1966, which offered to reimburse, or cost-share, one-half of provincial and territorial costs for medical services provided by a doctor outside hospitals. Within 6 years, all of the provinces and territories had universal physician services insurance plans.

More recently, the *Canada Health Act* (1985) and subsequent health accord renewals ignited the national conversation on the role of government in health care. Within the many provisions of the law, a federal government mandate requires all Canadian citizens to have reasonable access to medicare health insurance coverage (Government of Canada, 2016). Medicare is a term used to refer to Canada's publicly funded health care system by 13 provincial and territorial health care insurance plans. Although health insurance coverage is an essential element in promoting the health of an individual, questions remain on how best to serve the health care needs of all Canadians.

- What might solve the problems of access to affordable quality health care for all citizens?
- With a major proportion of the population mandated to have basic health insurance, can the overall health of the population be improved?
- How might Canada curtail rising health care costs while maintaining quality and safety?

The health care delivery system in Canada is a complex, multi-layered federal-to-jurisdictional entity that has the capacity to provide medicare without residents having to pay out of pocket. Canada's publicly funded system is distinct from any other health care delivery system in the world, employing almost 1.7 million people in 2012, to serve more than 34 million people. Of all the health care occupations, the Canadian Institute of Health Information (CIHI, 2019a) reports that registered nurses (RNs) constitute the largest number of professionals (48%); the average median salary for RNs (general duty) is $72,933 and $97,495 for nurse practitioners (NPs) (Canadian Federation of Nurses Unions [CFNU], 2018).

The demand for nursing resources to support continuing care for Canadian older people is expected to grow 3.4% annually through 2035. Annual nursing supply statistics indicate only 0.8% increase per year, resulting in a drastic shortfall of regulated nursing supply (Conference Board of Canada, 2017). Estimated to make up 25% of the population by midcentury, older people constitute the largest consumers of health care; averaging $11,625 per year compared with those aged 15–64 years, costing $2664 annually (Jackson, Clemens, & Palacios, 2017). Hospitals and physicians are funded under the *Canada Health Act (CHA)* and are the largest health care expenditures. The rising cost of other related expenditures, such as medications and other professionals not financed by the publicly funded *CHA,* is a growing burden to working Canadian families and employers.

The Canadian health care system is costly, with rising costs of health care consuming a growing percentage of the nation's gross domestic product (GDP), and currently up to 43% of provincial GDP (Barua, Palaocios, & Emes, 2017; Sutherland, Repin, Crump, et al., 2012). The CIHI reported in 2018 that national health expenditures consumed 11.3% of the nation's GDP (i.e., more than $253.5 billion), which equates to $6839 per person, among the highest dollar amount per capita of all industrialized countries (CIHI, 2019b; Fig. 3.1).

Health care is the largest component of jurisdictional budgets and has been rising at an unsustainable pace of 116.4% since 2001 (Barua et al., 2017). Despite the vast economic resources devoted to financing the health care system, unequal access to care exists, especially among vulnerable populations. Although the availability and provision of publicly funded health insurance is an important factor in health equity, vulnerable populations face additional obstacles, leading to health inequalities across the nation (Box 3.1). Health inequities (a particular type of health difference that is closely linked with social, economic, and/or environmental disadvantage) adversely affect groups of individuals, especially vulnerable populations.

To improve the health of the population, federal and provincial/territorial governments enact health care reform policies and legislation. Canadian health care reform has been, and continues to be, a dynamic process that is responsive to federal and provincial/territorial health care analysis reports, consisting of incremental steps mainly targeted at the poor and older person(s) populations to improve health (medicare). Common criticisms of the Canadian health care system include the increasing wait times for specialist consults, diagnostic, and

---

### BOX 3.1    Determinants of Health

The main determinants of health include the following:
- Income and social status
- Employment and working conditions
- Education and literacy
- Childhood experiences
- Physical environments
- Social supports and coping skills
- Healthy behaviours
- Access to health services
- Biology and genetic endowment
- Gender
- Culture
- Race/racism

Source: Public Health Agency of Canada. (2018). *Social determinants of health and health inequalities.* Retrieved from https://www.canada.ca/en/public-health/services/health-promotion/population-health/what-determines-health.html.

---

## How much will we spend on health in 2019?

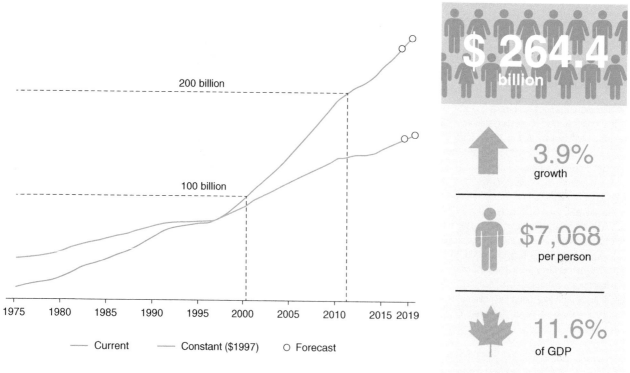

**Fig. 3.1** National Health Expenditure Trends, 1975 to 2019 (Canadian Institute for Health Information. (2019). *National Health Expenditure Trends, 1975 to 2019.* Ottawa: CIHI. Retrieved from https://www.cihi.ca/sites/default/files/docume/nhex-trends-narrative-report-2019-en-web.pdf.)

surgical procedures (Barua, 2017), and the high cost of services for only modest returns (Barua & Jacques, 2018). Despite the assumption that universal publicly funded health care equates to free health care, Canadians still report cost as a barrier to accessing health care services (Barua & Jacques, 2018).

Health care reform has been challenging. For example, through cost cuts and streamlining decision-making responsibility, several provinces (e.g., Alberta, Saskatchewan, Manitoba, Ontario) have attempted to collapse multiple health regions into fewer regions or single health authorities responsible for planning, implementing, and evaluating health care programs and services. While this structure is favoured by economists, others question the ability of this structure to make relevant decisions for the vast range of health care recipients, including those living rurally or at the margins of society, far away from where the decision makers are located.

Every Canadian citizen has the same basic primary health insurance coverage that is provided by the national health care plan or other federal health funding through the Canadian Armed Forces, First Nations and Inuit, Immigration and Refugee Board, Veterans Affairs, Royal Canadian Mounted Police, and federal correctional institutions. Each Canadian citizen or permanent resident applies for a provincial health card, and once it has been issued the card is utilized to access health care (Government of Canada, 2017a). The Canadian publicly funded health care program, called medicare, is a group of 13 provincial/territorial health insurance plans that provide health coverage to all Canadian citizens, regardless of medical history, personal income, or job status.

The *CHA*, legislated at the federal level (Government of Canada, 2017d), determines what services must be provided, similar to the Medicaid program in the United States. All provincial/territorial socialized health insurance plans cover essential health benefits, as identified in the *CHA* and established eligibility criteria, but each provincial/territorial plan is different, with some also opting to cover additional services (e.g., chiropractor visits, eye exams for specific populations; Manitoba Health, 2017). Essential health benefits include ambulatory patient services; emergency services; hospitalization and associated care; maternity, newborn, and well-child care; mental health and substance abuse services; prescription medications for those with low income (Pharmacare); laboratory services; preventive and wellness services and chronic disease management; and preventive care. Some provinces/territories also have reproductive health benefits (e.g., birth control, medical and surgical abortion) for the economically disadvantaged (Government of Canada, 2017b). Adult vision and dental care coverage are not required in the mandated essential packages, although some provinces/territories offer these benefits for specific population groups. For example, in Manitoba, individuals who have diabetes mellitus are funded for an annual dilated eye exam; discounts exist for older people's eye exam fees; residents are eligible for seven chiropractor visits annually; and pharmacists can provide specific immunizations. Most provinces/territories cover point-of-care pharmacist-provided assessments and administration of vaccines, smoking-cessation services, episodic conditions, and pain management.

Because the government is the primary payer (70%) for health care costs, Canada's health care system is referred to as a single-payer arrangement (Department of Finance Canada, 2011). Canadians pay for health care through a variety of federal and provincial taxes, just as US residents pay for Social Security and Medicare through their payroll taxes. The federal government appropriates funds to the provinces/territories by way of Canada Health Transfer (CHT) payments through cash and tax transfers. Some provinces/territories gain additional funds through health premiums, lottery proceeds, sales tax, and user fees. Some employers also offer private insurance plans to supplement services not covered by the Canadian health care plan, such as corrective lenses, medications, and home care.

At one time, the Canadian system was seen as being an ideal model that the United States and other countries should adopt; however, increasing health care costs, access issues, delays in treatment, and workforce shortages have caused political controversy and debate in Canada and abroad. A major shortage of physicians and nurses in Canada is in part due to lower reimbursement rates by the public health system and thus lower salaries, which results in some health care providers leaving Canada to practise in other countries such as the United States. Over the years, the federal government has decreased contributions to the provinces/territories because of large federal budget deficits and limited fee increases to physicians for services. Regionalization of hospitals has further resulted in issues with accessing care for those who live outside of major cities. Expansion of the Canadian system to offer better access to home care and community-based services is also an emerging issue (Health Canada, 2016).

As technology has advanced, system capacity and criticism has occurred related to queuing. *Queuing* refers to a system where a person is placed on a wait list or lineup before receiving certain types of care (e.g., emergency department care), medical tests, or surgery, allowing a person who is in need of more immediate care to receive priority attention (Rowe, 2016). If care needs are determined to be not life threatening, persons may need to wait for months to access such services as magnetic resonance imaging scans, heart bypass surgery, cataract removal, or hip replacement procedures. This ensures that persons in urgent need of the procedures are triaged higher on the list rather than services being based on a first-come-first-served basis. Although all citizens receive the same level of public health care, supplemental private insurance allows for a two-tiered system that favours Canadians with private health insurance or other financial resources to receive expedited care through private diagnostic companies or surgical centres.

Private insurance plans are designed to supplement jurisdictional essential services, but often have deductibles, co-payments, and other out-of-pocket costs for covered services; many employers offer coverage as part of an employee benefits package (Government of Canada, 2017a). Canadians who are covered by private health insurance typically have 80% of their costs covered at private clinics. The process for applying to join a plan can be challenging for many individuals, especially for those who have low literacy levels or limited health literacy. Despite supplemental private health insurance coverage for individuals, issues for the newly insured include paying for monthly premiums (if applicable), knowing how to access plan benefits effectively, finding an insured provider, navigating the health care system, and paying additional out-of-pocket expenses for deductibles and co-pays. Nurses play a key role in advocating for individuals and families to overcome these barriers.

Higher income Canadians can also pay out-of-pocket for care received at private clinics, which typically offer services with reduced wait times. For example, obtaining a magnetic resonance imaging scan at a hospital may require a waiting period of months, whereas a private diagnostic clinic could offer the scan within days to weeks. Canadians who have supplemental private health insurance or higher incomes, therefore, have access to more expedited care options (Health Canada, 2016). If a person can pay out-of-pocket, he or she may also elect to travel elsewhere (e.g., to the United States or Germany) to receive expedited health care services. Medical expenses not funded by the *CHA* (e.g., medical cannabis, some prescription medications, nursing services, home care supplies) may be eligible as a federal Revenue Canada expense on annual tax returns.

The health status of our nation compared with the United States, an examination of historical influences in the delivery of health care, a description of the structure and mechanisms to deliver public (medicare), and private health care in Canada and the United States, the financing of the health care system, and key federal legislation with emphasis on the *CHA* and provincial/territorial health accords, are addressed in this chapter. The greatest savings in health care expenditures could be realized if individuals engage in consistent health-promotion and disease-prevention practices to avoid costly consequences of acute and chronic disease. Health care transformation in Canada includes resources and incentives for services designed to promote health screenings and other preventative measures, hoping that savings will be realized from early detection, decreasing hospital admissions, and unnecessary hospital readmissions. For example, in British Columbia, family physicians' supplementary incentive payments are aimed at improving patient care for chronic disease management, complex care planning and management, mental health, palliative care, or residential care. Nurses must be knowledgeable about resources to help individuals and families navigate the health care system, and be politically active in influencing health policy as an advocate of social justice for individuals and families.

## THE HEALTH OF THE NATION

The Minster of Health portfolio is supported by the Canadian Food Inspection Agency, the Canadian Institutes of Health Research, Health Canada, the Patented Medicine Prices Review Board, and the Public Health Agency of Canada. The *CHA Annual Report* is prepared by Health Canada each year to report on the pan-Canadian administration, operation, and adherence of the CHA (Government of Canada, 2019a). To track the variety of measurable health indicators, the government relies on key reports from the Public Health Agency of Canada (PHAC), typically following census years, for example: the CIHI annual reports and data releases; other government-contracted reports with specific foci; and international reports such as those from the Organisation for Economic Co-operation and Development (OECD). These reports serve several key functions, but their

main goal is to inform policymakers and the federal/provincial/territorial governments of the trends in the nation's health and system performance in order to guide the development of sound health policy and allocation of resources to maintain and improve the health of Canadians.

The 2016 PHAC report provided data on composite indicators to speak more broadly to overall population health, social influencers of health, and health system success (PHAC, 2016a). Over the years, Health Canada has invested substantial funding for public health programs, research, provision of health care, and initiatives to support consumer education. Emerging trends indicate success in the reduction of morbidity and mortality for many diseases, control of widespread infectious diseases through widespread vaccination programs, improvement in motor vehicle safety, smoking cessation measures, and reduction of cardiovascular-related deaths. Life expectancy has increased for both men and women, and maternal and infant mortality rates on average are declining in many geographical locations, but remain poorer for Indigenous Canadians and those living at the lowest income levels (PHAC, 2016b; PHAC, 2017a). Cancer, heart disease, and cerebrovascular disease remain the top three causes of death for Canadians (Statistics Canada, 2019b).

Education regarding a healthy lifestyle, controlling hypertension, smoking cessation, using cholesterol-lowering medications, and participating in routine screening has contributed to better health for many Canadians, but concern about sedentary lifestyle, rising obesity trends, and chronic disease is noted. Recent smoking cessation interventions are demonstrating some effectiveness as the percentage of individuals who smoke dropped to 13% in 2015, compared with almost 20% of the population smoking in 2005 and 50% in 1965, although the use of cannabis is increasing among the younger Canadian population (Reid, Hammond, Rynard, et al., 2017). The percentage of adults and children who meet recommendations for daily physical activity has not significantly changed from 2011 (Colley, 2017; Statistics Canada, 2019c), likely contributing to increased rates of obesity from 22.9% in 2004 to 28.2% in 2014/2015 (PHAC, 2017b). The prevalence of childhood obesity is a growing concern—in 1978/79, 23% of children were considered overweight or obese, whereas in 2012/13 this had increased to 31.4% (Rao, Kropac, Do, et al., 2016). As obesity trends often continue into adulthood, these children are at greater risk of developing diabetes, hypertension, and cardiovascular disease earlier in life and developing the sequelae of chronic disease in adulthood.

Alarmingly, suicide and drug poisoning death rates have increased in recent years, especially among Canada's northern residents, Indigenous population, and LGBTQ2 community (MacDonald, 2016; House of Commons, 2016). Suicide is the second leading cause of death among children, youth, and young adults. Canada's opioid epidemic has also exploded, accounting for more than 9000 accidental opioid-related deaths between 2016 and 2018, crossing all sociodemographic and socioeconomic groups, among both chronic and occasional substance users (Government of Canada, 2018a; Special Advisory Committee on the Epidemic of Opioid Overdoses, 2018).

Improvements in the nation's health have not been uniform, because factors affecting health equity include an individual's income, race, sex, ethnicity, education level, and geographical location. In summary, the most effective intervention to decrease the growing cost of health care is to keep Canadians healthy—preventing chronic diseases such as diabetes and heart disease with healthy eating, routine exercise patterns, and following recommended preventative measures with routine health screenings and early intervention, if problems arise (PHAC, 2016a).

## The Pan-Canadian Healthy Living Strategy

In 2005, Canadian federal, provincial/territorial Ministers of Health endorsed a shared vision to focus on health promotion and the prevention of disease, disability, and injury as outlined in *The Integrated Pan-Canadian Healthy Living Strategy*. The goal was to collaboratively improve resources and education for Canadians to improve their overall health, so as to reduce the prevalence of chronic life-limiting diseases that share common modifiable risk factors (e.g., poor lifestyle, diet, and tobacco exposure) and disadvantaging social determinants of health. The initial progress report in 2008 noted a lack of advancement in meeting targets but faulted poor data collection rather than the actual progress of initiatives toward improving physical activity, healthy eating, and healthy weights. In 2010, the pan-Canadian health living strategy was revisited and strengthened, resulting in *The Strengthened Pan-Canadian Healthy Living Strategy Framework* (PHAC, 2010). This framework added a population health approach and intersectoral coordinated collaboration to broaden the influence and impact on a healthy Canada, including priorities of promoting healthy weights, mental health, and injury prevention (Secretariat for the Intersectoral Health Living Network, 2005).

While it takes several decades to measure the multigenerational impact of a healthier diet and lifestyle, the Pan-Canadian Public Health Network released progress reports in 2013, 2015, and 2017 to update the federal and provincial/territorial initiatives and programs focused on improving wellness through healthy nutrition, increased physical activity, healthy environments, and weight reduction (Pan-Canadian Public Health Network, 2016). Data clearly shows that there still exists disproportionate increased weight distribution among those with the lowest incomes, lowest educational attainment, or Indigenous ethnicity. One might also wonder how rural and remote residence influences access to the healthy environment and food sources that are important for healthy weight attainment.

In 2018, the PHAC released *A Common Vision for Increasing Physical Activity and Reducing Sedentary Living in Canada: Let's Get Moving* to address the issue of sedentary lifestyle on health outcomes (PHAC, 2018c). In 2019, with the goal of improving access to and consumption of healthy nutritious food, Health Canada released the new *Canada's Dietary Guidelines* (previously known as Canada's Food Guide) with updated, mobile-friendly web access (Health Canada, 2019). Implementation uptake and impact has yet to be published, but the hope is a renewed food guide that reflects current research will improve the health of Canadians for generations to come. It is anticipated that if Canadians integrate healthy food choices along with increased physical activity into their lives, the overall rate of obesity and chronic disease will decrease, and thus the cost of long-term health care expenses will improve.

The first mental health strategy report for Canada was released in 2012 by the Mental Health Commission of Canada (MHCC, 2012), with 26 priorities including mental health promotion across the lifespan, fostering recovery and well-being for those living with mental illness, providing access to appropriate services, reducing risk factor disparities, acknowledging unique circumstances and needs for Indigenous Canadians, and mobilizing leadership collaboration. Resulting from seemingly poor uptake and actioning, the MHCC (2016) undertook extensive consultations and roundtables to better understand mental health in Canada, including the barriers and facilitators to optimize mental health for all. The resulting report *Advancing the Mental Health Strategy for Canada: A Framework for Action (2017–2022)* has the overarching goal to accelerate the uptake of the 2012 mental health strategy, and outlines four key pillars (leadership and funding; promotion and prevention; access and services; and data and research), each with respective objectives.

Canada's injury and prevention task force was established in 2008 and released *Injury Prevention in Canada: An Action Plan (2011–2020)* with three priority areas: 1) preventing falls among older people; 2) preventing sports and recreation related falls; and 3) surveillance of fall-related injuries. Unfortunately, implementation response was delayed due to operational challenges and by 2011 the task force was disbanded and the report was shelved due to difficulties with implementing such broad-scoping recommendations. While the original task force may have collapsed, a few provinces, including Manitoba Health (2015), Alberta Health Services (2019), Ontario (Ontario Ministry of Health and Long-Term Care, 2018), and Nova Scotia Health (2009), and population-focused advocacy groups (Canadian Paediatric Society, 2019; Parachute Canada, n.d.; National Defence & Canadian Armed Forces, 2012) have continued in injury prevention faithfulness and published their own jurisdictional reports, recommendation plans, programs, and online support (Yanchar, Warda, Fuselli, et al., 2012).

Health inequalities adversely affect groups of people who have systematically experienced greater obstacles to health on the basis of their race, colour, or national origin; ethnic group; religion; socioeconomic status; gender; age; mental health; cognitive, sensory, or physical or other disability; sexual orientation or gender identity; geographical location; access to social resources; or other characteristics historically linked to discrimination or exclusion (PHAC, 2018d). Individuals and groups at risk of health inequity are considered vulnerable populations; disadvantaged by sociopolitical and economic constraints that limit their access to necessary social determinants of health (e.g., employment and income security, education and literacy opportunities, housing and food security, sociocultural inclusion, health services access) (PHAC & Pan-Canadian Public Health Network, 2018). See Box 3.1 for a list of Canada's social determinants of health that health care providers should consider, in addition to physical and mental contributors of health and wellness (PHAC, 2018a).

Public health nursing practice promotes and preserves the health of populations, looking at the community as a whole and its effect on the health of individuals, families, and groups. Community health nursing practice promotes, preserves, and maintains the health of populations through care provided to individuals, families, and groups, and studies the effect of their health status on that of the community as a whole (Stanhope & Lancaster, 2012). A healthy thriving community is a community that is safe and inclusive and promotes a high quality of life and well-being, which can be measured by social networks, physical assets, economic opportunity, human development, and local institutions that sustain respect and support each of the dimensions (Community Health and Empowerment Through Education and Research, 2015).

Successful population health requires effective public health infrastructure for planning, delivering, and evaluating public health. Key components of effective public health programming must be responsive in their ability to prepare for and react to national and global emergencies that result from both health and environmental crises, while also focusing on population health improvements by reducing health inequalities. This requires a well-trained, cooperative, and responsive health and social workforce; effective information and communication systems; and population access to health and social resources (Mowat & Butler-Jones, 2007). One of the main goals of the PHAC is to build a progressive, resilient, and sustainable health and social workforce, resource tools, and infrastructure. With the goal of improving public health in Canada, the federal and provincial/territorial governments established the Pan-Canadian Public Health Network in 2005 as a system for intergovernmental collaboration with experts from academia, research, nongovernmental agencies, and clinical practice. This network supports partnerships and information sharing to influence government policy; supports collaborative public health projects and programs; and educates Canadians regarding specific public health topics such as healthy weights, active outdoor play, antimicrobial stewardship, and improving immunization engagement.

## Health Indicators of a Nation

The health status of the population of one nation compared with another uses death indicators as standard measures. Although mortality-based indicators do not directly measure the health status of the living population, the data indirectly reflect the general health of a nation and are more readily available through government and world agencies. Table 3.1, International Comparisons of Core Health Indicators, compares the average life expectancy by gender and infant mortality rates of populations in select countries. According to the OECD (OECD, 2018b), the life expectancy on average (both sexes combined) in Canada for 2015 was 81.9 years compared with 82.3 years in Sweden and 78.7 years in the United States. The life expectancy in Mexico was significantly lower at 75.0 years. In 1961, life expectancy in Canada was 68.4 years (OECD, 2018b), so much progress has been made in improving the health of the country. Overall, life expectancy rates have risen sharply in the past 60 years in Canada and other industrialized countries, but in stark comparison, life expectancy in developing or poorer countries lags. For example, India, a country with low levels of health care provisions, life expectancy today is on average 66.9 years (World Health Rankings, 2018; Table 3.2). Compared with Canada, this gap is almost 13 years, and lower than the life expectancies reported for Canadians in 1961.

Infant mortality rates (Table 3.3) are one of the most important indicators of the health of a nation because they are associated with factors such as maternal health and access to health care. The Canadian infant mortality rate (number of deaths in the first year of life) estimated in 2014 was reported as 4.7 (number of deaths of infants in the first year of life per 1000 live births), a dramatic improvement from 27.3 reported in 1960 but higher than mortality rates in other developed nations (OECD, 2018a). Mexico has an infant mortality rate of slightly more than 12, which is lower than that of other poor nations such as India, which has an infant mortality rate of more than 37.9. The rationale for why Canada ranks less favourably in this health indicator than other industrialized nations is attributed to a number of factors. According to a working paper from the National Bureau of Economic Research (Chen, Oster, & Williams, 2014), there is a lack of comparable

| TABLE 3.1 | International Comparisons of Core Health Indicator Estimates for 2014–2016 | | | | | | | |
|---|---|---|---|---|---|---|---|---|
| | Afghanistan (A), South Africa (SA), and India | Canada | France | Germany | Mexico | Sweden | United Kingdom | United States |
| Life expectancy at birth: males (years) | A: 60.5 SA: 55.50 India 66.9 | 79.80 | 79.20 | 78.60 | 72.90 | 80.60 | 79.40 | 76.10 |
| Life expectancy at birth: females (years) | A: 62.0 SA 59.50 India 69.90 | 83.90 | 85.50 | 83.50 | 77.90 | 84.10 | 83.00 | 81.10 |
| Life expectancy at birth: both sexes (years) | A 61.3 SA 55.50 India 66.90 | 79.80 | 72.20 | 79.60 | 72.90 | 80.60 | 79.40 | 76.10 |
| Infant deaths per 1000 live births | A 66.0 SA 33.6 India 37.9 | 4.7 | 3.7 | 3.4 | 12.1 | 2.5 | 3.8 | 5.9 |

Data from the Organisation for Economic Co-operation and Development. (2018). *Infant mortality rates*. Retrieved from http://data.oecd.org/healthstat/infant-mortality-rates.htm.

microdata sets across countries, which may account for about 40% of the difference in infant mortality rates between comparable countries because of the variability in the reporting of births near the threshold of fetal viability, so there are differences in how and what data are collected and used. This is also a factor in comparing neonatal mortality rates (infant deaths within the first 28 days of life) as countries may differ in reporting data based on gestational age and birth weight and survival (PHAC, 2017a).

In Canada, congenital malformations and disorders related to short gestation and low birth weight, were the two top reasons for infant deaths in 2016 (Statistics Canada, 2019a). Despite data collection and reporting variations, Canada overall has large disparities in health status by geographical areas, race, ethnicity groups, social class, and education levels. For example, infant mortality rates among Indigenous peoples in Canada's (First Nations, Inuit, and Métis) babies were more than twice those of non-Indigenous Canadians (Conference Board of Canada, 2019; Sheppard, Shapiro, Bushnik, et al., 2017). A number of characteristics correlate with maternal, fetal, and infant health/death rates, including: maternal race and ethnicity, and education level; economic and geographic residence; perinatal alcohol and smoking exposure; maternal age

at conception; excess prepregnancy weight; folic acid fortified food security; and health service access, including fertility and neonatal technology care (PHAC & Pan-Canadian Public Health Network, 2018; PHAC, 2008; PHAC, 2017a). Large differences in infant death rates are readily apparent in Canada. The highest rates of infant death in Canada are among the Inuit population, at a rate almost four times greater than the general population; Indigenous people experience more than twice the rate of infant death as the general population. Geographical variations also exist within Canada, with the highest rate of neonatal mortality (0–27 days) reported (per 1,000) in Nunavut at 7.6, Northwest Territories at 5.6, and Manitoba at 4.6 (compared with the national average of 3.7). Likewise, infant mortality rates reported in Nunavut at 14, Northwest Territories at 8.7, Saskatchewan at 6.6 (compared with the national average of 5.0), and the lowest infant death rates being reported in Nova Scotia at 3.6, Prince Edward Island at 3.0, and British Columbia at 4.0 (compared with the national average of 5.0; PHAC, 2017a). In summary, decreasing the country's infant mortality rates will continue to require community advocacy and interventions aimed at improving social determinants of health while providing targeted interventions for specific racial groups, geographical areas, and perinatal exposures.

## Historical Role of Women in Health Promotion

Nurses have a long tradition of involvement in health promotion. Augustine nuns first arrived in Quebec in 1639 for medical mission, providing holistic care to patients and introducing the nursing apprenticeship model to North America. During the early nineteenth century, denominational nurses (e.g., Catholic, Anglican, Mennonite) provided health care to frontier settlers across Canada (Canadian Museum of History Online Collection, n.d.).

**TABLE 3.2  International Comparison of Life Expectancy Rates at Birth (in Years) Over Time for 1990, 2000, and 2015**

| Location | Period | Male | Female | Both Sexes |
|---|---|---|---|---|
| Australia | 2015 | 80.4 | 84.5 | 82.5 |
| | 2000 | 76.6 | 82 | 79.3 |
| | 1990 | 73.9 | 80.1 | 77 |
| Canada | 2015 | 79.8 | 83.9 | 81.9 |
| | 2000 | 76.3 | 81.6 | 79 |
| | 1990 | 73.9 | 80.5 | 77.2 |
| China | 2015 | 74.5 | 77.5 | 76 |
| | 2000 | 70.1 | 73.5 | 71.8 |
| | 1990 | 67.4 | 70.7 | 69.1 |
| Denmark | 2015 | 78.8 | 82.7 | 80.8 |
| | 2000 | 74.5 | 79.2 | 76.9 |
| | 1990 | 72 | 77.8 | 74.9 |
| France | 2015 | 79.2 | 85.5 | 82.2 |
| | 2000 | 75.4 | 83 | 79.2 |
| | 1990 | 72.8 | 81.2 | 77 |
| India | 2015 | 66.9 | 69.9 | 68.4 |
| | 2000 | 61.8 | 63.5 | 62.7 |
| | 1990 | 57.6 | 58.3 | 58 |
| Mexico | 2015 | 72.3 | 77.7 | 75 |
| | 2000 | 70.5 | 76.1 | 73.3 |
| | 1990 | 67 | 74 | 70.5 |
| United Kingdom | 2015 | 79.2 | 82.8 | 81 |
| | 2000 | 75.5 | 80.3 | 77.9 |
| | 1990 | 72.9 | 78.5 | 75.7 |
| United States | 2015 | 76.3 | 81.1 | 78.7 |
| | 2000 | 74.1 | 79.3 | 76.7 |
| | 1990 | 71.8 | 78.8 | 75.3 |

Data from the Organisation for Economic Co-operation and Development. (2018). *Life expectancy at birth*. Retrieved from http://data.oecd.org/healthstat/life-expectancy-at-birth.htm.

**TABLE 3.3  International Comparison of Infant Rates Over Time for 1960 and 2018**

| Location | Period | Deaths per 1000 Live Births |
|---|---|---|
| Australia | 2018 | 3 |
| | 1960 | 20 |
| Canada | 2018 | 4 |
| | 1960 | 28 |
| China | 2018 | 7 |
| | 1960 | 8 |
| Denmark | 2018 | 4 |
| | 2000 | 21 |
| France | 2018 | 3 |
| | 1960 | 24 |
| India | 2018 | 30 |
| | 1960 | 161 |
| Mexico | 2018 | 11 |
| | 1960 | 103 |
| United Kingdom | 2018 | 4 |
| | 1960 | 23 |
| United States | 2018 | 6 |
| | 1960 | 26 |

Data from The World Bank. (2019). *Mortality rate, infant (per1000 live births)*. Retrieved from https://data.worldbank.org/indicator/sp.dyn.imrt.in.

By the late nineteenth century, hospital nursing was more common, and it was also at this time that Florence Nightingale, the founder of modern nursing, began her good work for health promotion. In 1854 during the Crimean War, while caring for wounded soldiers in a British camp outside Constantinople, Turkey, she fought for hospital reform by crusading for nutritious food, cleanliness, and sanitation. She provided leadership for a group of nurses and comfort to the soldiers. Her careful recordings of care outcomes quantified needed reform in health promotion (University of Alabama at Birmingham, 2016). Within Canada, the *Victorian Order of Nurses (VON)* was started in 1897 by Lady Aberdeen, wife of the Governor General of Canada, to provide home and maternity care. The early twentieth century then saw the establishment of nursing programs with a focus on disease prevention, public health education, and maternal child care. By the 1920s, public health nursing turned its focus to outlying Indigenous communities and remote settlers through *The Canadian Red Cross* outpost nursing stations (Canadian Museum of History Online Collection, n.d.). These pioneers and others set the stage for nurses' unique role in health promotion. Jumping forward to 1986, health promotion became a guiding principle behind public health advancements, with an emphasis on key determinants of health following a significant federal report, *Achieving Health for All: A Framework for Health Promotion* by Jake Epp, then Minister of National Health and Welfare. It was also in 1986 that Canada hosted the first International Conference on Health Promotion (Canadian Public Health Association, n.d.-a; Rutty, Sullivan, Last, et al., 2010).

## A SAFER SYSTEM

The health care delivery system in Canada is experiencing significant changes, sparked by health care reform and recommendations from commissioned reports, along with a variety of organizations and advisory groups involved in forming health policy. Several reports have been instrumental in advising on the need to revise health policy in order to change the structure of health care delivery for provision of safer care. The Canadian Patient Safety Institute (CPSI), established by Health Canada in 2003, works with health care organizations, providers, and government to improve patient safety and quality. The *Building a Safer System* report in 2002 was instrumental in the development of CPSI for creating a safer health care system (Hassen, Hoffman, Gebran, et al., 2006). Today, a number of governments and organizations are involved in safety and quality of health care, for example, British Columbia Patient Safety and Quality Council, Health Quality Council of Alberta, Saskatchewan Health Quality Council, Manitoba Institute for Patient Safety, Health Quality Ontario, Québec Health and Welfare Commissioner, and the New Brunswick Health Council.

Several Canadian studies and reports have noted the connection between inadequate nursing staffing levels, stressed work environments, increased nursing care interruptions, poor system integration and coordination with poor patient outcomes, adverse events, increased length of stay, and readmission rates (Berry & Curry, 2012; MacPhee, Dahinten, & Havaei, 2017; Purdy, 2011). Countless other international reports also reinforce the highlighted issues and system needs identified within these Canadian studies. The overall conclusion from research on nursing-related patient outcomes is that overstretched staffing levels, combined with an increased complexity of patient conditions and stressful work environment, directly and indirectly relate to an increased frequency of adverse patient events, poor overall patient outcomes, and increasing health resource costs.

Similar to Canadian studies, the Institute of Medicine researchers in the United States found that nurse staffing ratios, fewer nurses, mandatory overtime, inadequate continuing education, and lack of nurse involvement in decisions about client care create an environment that contributes to error making. In Canada, medication incidents are a leading cause of preventable patient injury. To help combat the incidence of patient injury, the CPSI (CPSI, 2016) has advocated for improvement measures to reduce medication incidents, which are not only common but also costly to the nation (Health Canada, 2011a). It is recognized that prevention of medication incidents is a shared responsibility among government, industry, patient safety organizations, organization leadership, health care team members, and patients/consumers. Using a comprehensive approach to decreasing the prevalence of medication errors requires changes in the health care system through standardized procedures, education, and creating a non-shaming reporting culture such that errors are identified so that strategies to minimize future incidents can be developed. Health Canada, along with the CIHI and CPSI, work collaboratively to coordinate patient safety initiatives and the Canadian Medication Incident Reporting and Prevention System, a national program for collecting, analyzing, and educating about medication incidents.

The Institute of Medicine (IOM) has made recommendations in other areas promoting safety and wellness within the health care system. For example, in 2014 an IOM report, *Dying in America, Improving Quality and Honoring Individual Preferences Near the End of Life* (IOM, 2014) provided direction on improving end-of-life care for this vulnerable population. Similarly, in Canada, several reports have guided policy and legislative changes, both federally and provincially, to support end-of-life care provision and a choice about where and when to die. Carstairs (2010) highlighted the fact that 90% of those who die could benefit from palliative care, yet very few were receiving such services. This report led to a revamping of palliative and end-of-life care policy and eventually to Medical Assistance in Dying legislation (Dying with Dignity Canada, 2019).

The IOM, now called the Health and Medicine Division (HMD) has been productive in releasing hundreds of reports and workshop summaries of pressing concerns related to health and the health care system. Despite their American focus, Canadian nurses and other health care providers can glean transferable insights from these reports. New reports are generated each month by the HMD and can be found on the National Academy of Science website (see http://nationalacademics.org). Current topic areas include public health, biomedical and health research, quality and safety, diseases, health services, coverage, access, and select populations and health inequities Other subject areas include food and nutrition, health care workforce, global health, veterans' health, mental health, education, aging, and women's health.

To provide safe, evidence-informed care, nurses have a regulated and ethical responsibility to be lifelong learners to stay abreast of new scientific findings and advocate health care policy changes that improve the health of the communities in which they practice and extend to the greater global population. Although health care is often equated with medical care, which focuses on the treatment of illness, this chapter presents the evolution and ongoing development of a broader concept of health based on the definition given in Chapter 1.

# GLOBAL HEALTH

The overriding objective of the World Health Organization (WHO) is to influence health opportunities and outcomes for all people so that they can attain the highest possible level of health. The WHO recognizes the importance of families and health promotion, and has contributed to the family health policies of many nations by shaping global awareness for health promotion. The current agenda of WHO involves the following six goals: promoting development; fostering health security; strengthening health systems; harnessing research, information, and evidence; enhancing partnerships; and improving performance (WHO, n.d.-a). Internationally, shrinking health care budgets have resulted in a variable level of achievement of these goals. In developing nations, such as those in Latin America and Africa, huge inequities in health care persist.

## Historical Perspectives

The complexities of the Canadian health care system necessitate an understanding of the system as a whole before one can focus on the intermingled causative factors that have created a fragmented system of health care delivery. The relevance of the divergence between preventive and curative measures is apparent when the organization and financing of the delivery system are examined. Canada has established a system that uses two basic divisions of society to provide service: the public sector and the private sector, which are discussed in further detail throughout this chapter.

# HISTORY OF HEALTH CARE

## Early Influences

Indigenous peoples inhabited North America prior to European immigration. Historical records of early civilizations (Egyptian, Indian, Chinese, Aztec, and Greek) show that ancient peoples were concerned with disease and practised various methods of treatment. The earliest views of health can be seen as holistic in the sense that they emerged from an integrated worldview. Primitive peoples understood illness in mystical terms: sickness and cure theories were tied to the cosmic view of life, with natural and supernatural forces often inseparable. Most religions include a person's hygiene as part of their practice. For thousands of years, epidemics were viewed as divine judgements on human wickedness, with a gradual awareness that pestilence (any epidemic disease with a high death rate) has natural causes such as climate and other aspects of the physical environment. During the Middle Ages, infectious diseases in epidemic proportions (leprosy, bubonic plague, smallpox, and tuberculosis [TB]) were the leading causes of death. Clearly, health was viewed in terms of survival and absence of disease.

## Industrial Influences

The population of the Western world began to increase during the 1600s, when North America was first being explored (Rutty et al., 2010). The New World had many things to offer explorers. An adequate food supply made it possible for the population to live longer, and advances in transportation made distribution of food supplies and other goods and services possible. Manufacturing advances during the eighteenth century, through the invention of the flush toilet and cast iron pipe, made sanitary engineering possible, saving many lives by preventing diseases such as typhoid, paratyphoid, and gastroenteritis.

## Socioeconomic Influences

Although the Elizabethan poor laws (1601) in England provided a system of relief for the poor, which included infants, sick, and older people, and laborers in the workhouses, a harsher philosophy in North America regarded pauperism among able-bodied workers as a moral failing. If the worker did not earn a subsistence-level income, the attitude toward that worker was suspicious and punitive. According to this view, people are held directly accountable for their state in life, and health maintenance is the responsibility of the individual. The far-reaching implications of this ethic can be seen today in the organization, financing, and delivery of health services in the United States. While early beliefs in Canada mirrored those of the United States, the introduction of the *Hospital Insurance and Diagnostic Act* of 1957 started a revolution of socialized health care and what Canadians today proudly protect as a publicly funded health care system.

## Public Health Influences

In Canada, vessels with European immigrants arrived at the Port of Quebec; the large number of sick passengers arriving among those immigrants led to the establishment of a quarantine act in 1721, which was revised to the *Quarantine Act of Lower Canada* in 1795. This law served as a template used by British North America colonial governments to prevent the spread of infectious disease (Rutty et al., 2010).

Edwin Chadwick (1800–90) is known as the father of British and American public health. Chadwick established the English Board of Health, which emphasized environmental sanitation but excluded physicians outside times of crisis. Additionally, Chadwick was Secretary of the Poor Law Commission, which strove to improve the health of the masses for economic reasons. Chadwick's rationale was that disease among the poor was a major factor in their inability to support themselves. Therefore governmental health and welfare policies have been joined in England since the nineteenth century.

Today, public health advancements such as drinking water fluoridation, infectious disease control for diseases such as West Nile virus, motor vehicle safety education, tobacco cessation programs, occupational safety initiatives, and immigrant health programs, have improved the health of Canadians across several decades (CPHA, n.d.-b).

## Scientific Influences

Until the twentieth century, epidemics of infectious disease (plague, cholera, typhoid, smallpox, and influenza) were the most critical health problems and major causes of death and disability for Canadians. Scientific advances during the nineteenth century by Louis Pasteur (germ theory), Robert Koch (origin of bacterial infection), Joseph Lister (antisepsis), and Paul Ehrlich (chemotherapy), expanded public health from its earlier concentration on sanitation to control of communicable diseases through a broad biological base. Public health became an important force in decreasing death rates and increasing life expectancy through the application of bacteriology. International environmental conditions were improved by the development of systems that safeguard water, milk, and food supplies; promote sanitary sewage disposal; and monitor the quality of urban housing.

Between 1936 and 1954 the discovery and use of sulfonamides and other antibiotics to treat bacterial infections reduced the death rate to its lowest point in history, with deaths caused by primary infections reduced to 4%, as compared with 33% only 50 years earlier (in 1886). The death rate did not change significantly between 1954 and the mid-1960s. Another decline in the death rate began after the mid-1960s and has continued (with the exception of a slight increase in 1995) with the control of many infectious diseases (Arias & Smith, 2003). As the life expectancy of the population increases, chronic diseases and comorbidities increase as well. Data from 2016 revealed that cancer, heart disease, cerebrovascular disease, accidents, chronic lower respiratory disease, diabetes mellitus, Alzheimer's disease, influenza and pneumonia, suicide, and chronic liver disease and cirrhosis, in descending order, are the top 10 leading causes of total death in Canada (Statistics Canada, 2019b).

Despite the progress in conquering infectious diseases, in vulnerable populations infections are once again among the top leading contributors to death. Some infectious diseases are difficult to eradicate from the population (e.g., TB). The most effective strategy for eliminating TB is to monitor those infected to ensure completion of treatment is by direct observed therapy, which requires the monitoring of a person's medication adherence for first-line medications for 8 weeks and continuation of treatment for 4 to 7 months. Individuals who do not finish the prescribed medication regimen correctly are at risk of developing resistance to one or more first-line medications. Treatment of medication-resistant TB becomes more complicated and costly, and medication-resistant TB is difficult to eradicate. Resources are needed at local public health departments to provide monitoring and follow-up in this typically elusive TB-infected population.

Globally, TB is the most common infectious disease and one of the world's deadliest diseases, with one third of the world's population being infected. Major efforts have been put in place for TB prevention, screening, diagnosis, and treatment. The WHO estimates that 43 million lives were saved between 2000 and 2014 with targeted measures. Despite this progress, in 2014, 1.5 million people (1.1 million HIV-positive and 0.4 million HIV-negative) died of TB. This includes 140,000 children. TB is the leading cause of death in individuals with HIV. Targeted interventions have been distributed over wide regions of high disease–burdened countries

because the risk of infection of the population is more widespread. Regions in Africa, for example, have 28% of the world's cases, with 281 cases for every 100,000 people. Indonesia was estimated to have 1 million new cases in 2014. The WHO reported that in 2013, 9 million people around the world became ill with TB. New strains of medication-resistant TB are now emerging that are resistant not only to isoniazid and rifampin, which are the most effective first-line TB treatment medications, but also to second-line anti-TB medications. TB remains an urgent public health problem, with more than 80% of the cases identified in 22 high-burden countries. Global interventions to reduce TB include targeted population- and age-specific interventions such as administration of the bacille Calmette-Guérin (BCG) vaccine to infants and small children in countries where TB is more common. The vaccine is given only if the child has negative TB skin test findings and cannot be separated from adults who are untreated or ineffectively treated for TB (CDC, 2015; WHO, 2015).

An effective, comprehensive public health system is imperative to enable Canada to respond to local, national, and global concerns. As new diseases emerge, older diseases re-emerge (sometimes in medication-resistant forms), and natural and man-made disasters occur, a functioning public health system is warranted. While TB is still problematic in Canada, other preventable childhood diseases are also re-emerging as concerning outbreaks in under- and nonimmunized populations. In part, this is due to a globalized citizenship, where travel is abundant, including travel to countries where measles and rubella are at epidemic proportions. In 2019 Canada, had already seen 81 cases of measles, up from 29 in 2018 (Government of Canada, 2019b). According to the 2015 childhood National Immunization Coverage Survey (cNICS) conducted by the PHAC and Statistics Canada, the majority of Canadian children were vaccinated before their second birthday, but unfortunately this rate of immunization is decreasing year after year (Government of Canada, 2018b). While vaccination rates of 77–89% are commendable, these numbers continue to fall short of the Canadian target of 95% childhood vaccination coverage, and 80% for seasonal influenza immunization by 2025 (Government of Canada, 2019c).

## Special Population Influences

An important goal of health policy is to achieve health equity, eliminate disparities, and improve the health of all groups. Vulnerable populations, especially those living in poverty, are at great risk of experiencing health inequalities (CIHI, 2018; CIHI, 2015; PHAC, 2018b). For many of these disadvantaged people, the issues of preventing disease and promoting good health are often secondary to the problems associated with everyday survival. Determinants of health in a population are related strongly to socioeconomic status and education level, with populations in the lower strata having worse outcomes. However, individual lifestyle behaviours, including dietary choices, level of physical activity, use of alcohol and tobacco, substance abuse, and risky sexual behaviour, play a significant role in the health status of an individual. Access to health care for prevention, early detection, and treatment is paramount in diminishing health inequities but programs promoting positive individual lifestyle behaviours are also needed (Diversity Awareness).

## DIVERSITY AWARENESS

### Health Inequities Among Indigenous People in Canada

As a nation, health equity does not exist, especially among racial and ethnic populations, including Indigenous peoples in Canada. Health inequities are differences in health outcomes that are closely linked with social, economic, and environmental disadvantage, which are often driven by the social conditions in which individuals live, learn, work, and play. Marked differences in social determinants, such as poverty, low socioeconomic status, and lack of access to care, exist along racial and ethnic lines, leading to poor health outcomes. The burden attributable to socioeconomic health inequalities is estimated to be at least $6.2 billion annually, with Canada's lowest income group representing 60% ($3.7 billion) of health care costs. Many Indigenous people experience poorer physical environmental conditions compared to non-Indigenous Canadians, including such conditions as overcrowding; inadequate sanitation; mouldy houses; and contaminated soil, air, and water sources, which can negatively impact physical and psychosocial wellness. The major dimensions of health inequities for Indigenous people in Canada include:

- An overrepresentation among Canadians who have inadequate access to health care
- Generally poorer health, related to maternal, fetal, and infant health; child health; communicable and noncommunicable conditions; mental health; violence, abuse, and injury; and environmental health conditions, largely related to poorer social determinants of health compared to non-Indigenous Canadians
- Higher rates of obesity, tobacco use, and inadequate healthy food security that contribute to the onset of diabetes, hypertension, and cardiovascular disease (PHAC, 2016a)

Diminishing degrees of community and cultural engagement, along with limited access to culturally connected care, further disadvantage Indigenous people, resulting in greater rates of substance use and suicide.

As the demographics of Canada continue to become more diverse, and the population of Indigenous people grows, nurses must continue to cultivate cultural safety as one strategy for eliminating racial and ethnic disparities.

Diversity in the workforce is a key element of patient-centred care. Efforts to match the ethnic and racial composition of the health care workforce with the Canadian population will contribute to addressing cultural safety and health inequities. Providers who speak a second language will also be needed. Shortages of primary care providers in underserved areas significantly affect the health of ethnic and racial minorities. The primary care nurse practitioner is ideally suited to care for underserved populations in urban and rural areas. A capable and qualified workforce, sustainable pan-Canadian public health funding, and public health agencies capable of assessing and responding to public health needs, including emergency situations, are necessary for an effective public health infrastructure. Nurses can play key roles as leaders, educators, and providers of care in their communities to meet the needs of vulnerable populations and close the health disparity gap.

Sources: National Collaborating Centre for Aboriginal Health (NCCAH). (2012). *The state of knowledge of aboriginal health: A review of aboriginal public health in Canada.* Retrieved from https://www.ccnsa-nccah.ca/docs/context/RPT-StateKnowledgeReview-EN.pdf; Government of Canada. (2014). *A statistical profile on the health of First Nations in Canada: Determinants of health, 2006 to 2010.* Ottawa: Author. Retrieved from http://publications.gc.ca/collections/collection_2014/sc-hc/H34-193-1-2014-eng.pdf; Public Health Agency of Canada. (2018). *A common vision for increasing physical activity and reducing sedentary living in Canada: Let's get moving.* Ottawa: Author. Retrieved from https://www.canada.ca/en/public-health/services/publications/healthy-living/lets-get-moving.html#ex.

## Political and Economic Influences

Political and economic considerations influence the health care system, and politics determines the decision makers who will negotiate a desired outcome. Economics defines the resources that are distributed and the manner in which they are distributed. Canada's publicly funded health care is primarily financed through federal and provincial/territorial personal and corporate taxation, but additional financial support is derived through other tax revenues (e.g., provincial/territorial sales and liquor/cannabis taxation and lottery proceeds). Some provinces (e.g., Alberta, British Columbia, Ontario) also charge residents health premiums to supplement provincial health care costs.

The effect of economics and politics on the delivery of health care is illustrated by the situation in Canada during which medicare was established. Prior to the Second World War, health care was privately funded and provided. The first stage of medicare began in Saskatchewan with the introduction of a universal hospital care plan, and was then quickly followed by Alberta and Ontario enacting similar arrangements. Federal engagement began with the *Hospital Insurance and Diagnostic Act* of 1957 in which federal and provincial governments entered into an agreement to cover costs of acute hospital care and laboratory and diagnostic services. The second phase of medicare came in 1966 with the passing of the *Medical Care Act*, which established 50/50 cost sharing between the federal and provincial/territorial governments to extend health insurance to cover physician services (Dunlop, 2015). Since that time, there has been decreasing federal contribution to provincial and territorial health resource costs. Reflexively, provincial/territorial governments have seen increasing economic resources being directed toward health care, often being the greatest component of annual provincial budgets.

As stated previously, the majority of Canadian health care is publicly financed, but nearly all is privately delivered, (e.g., hospitals run by nonprofit private societies or corporations; fee-for-service private practice practitioners, privately owned residential care facilities). There are numerous medically sanctioned therapies (e.g., prescription medications, physiotherapy, orthotic devices, etc.) that are either paid for out-of-pocket by patients themselves, or through supplementary insurance packages that individuals/employers pay for. Approximately half of all prescriptions are paid privately, either by third-party insurance coverage or by patients themselves. More recently, increased numbers of privately owned clinics have been offering medical and surgical services (e.g., diagnostic tests, physiotherapy rehabilitation, and minor surgeries), paid directly by the patient and/or through third-party insurance programs.

The high-profile legal battle between private surgeon Dr. Brian Day and British Columbia's provincial government is based on a constitutional challenge of the province's restrictions on access to private health care and penalizing physicians who are trying to open up access to services by offering the option of private pay. It is argued that this contradicts the basic principles of medicare and equitable access to publicly funded services. Day argues that there already exists a two-tiered system where certain groups of patients get priority access, including patients who are covered by workers' compensation or provincial motor insurance, RCMP officers, military personnel, and federal prisoners.

## Split Between Preventive and Curative Measures

The link between environmental health and personal medical care developed when sanitarians (people who work to maintain a clean environment) realized that their efforts alone were not sufficient to prevent and cure the diseases of the population as a whole; improvement of personal health was also necessary. Early preventive services directed toward individuals originated in medical practice rather than public health, but were limited to socialized medicine (caring for individuals through organized programs). Delivery of preventive services developed separately from clinical medicine and became associated with public health. Most physicians, educated in hospitals, were interested in individuals for whom prevention had failed and whose illnesses brought them to the hospital ward.

Despite the separation of preventive and treatment services, the benefits of prevention were eventually incorporated into clinical medicine for individuals. Preventive and early detection measures became a part of pediatrics and obstetrics during the early part of the twentieth century, when vaccines and vaginal cytology examinations became available and accepted. Later in the twentieth century, internal medicine incorporated early detection of diseases such as diabetes, glaucoma, obesity, and hypertension. A shift to preventive medicine for the individual occurred, but separate educational programs for public health and medicine still divided these areas. Not until the 1960s did the emphasis begin to turn from individual to societal values (Freyman, 1980; Rutty et al., 2010).

This new emphasis on societal values parallels another evolution in the role of health in society. Greater governmental involvement in financing the health care delivery system has improved access to health care for many populations. Technological developments such as computerized medical records, should improve access to care through better communication with laboratories, primary care offices, hospitals, and care delivery agencies.

## ORGANIZATION OF THE DELIVERY SYSTEM

The structure and financing of the Canadian health care delivery system is a multifaceted network with complex interrelationships involving providers, consumers, and settings, with both the public sector and the private sector financing and providing services. The Canadian system primarily publicly funded coverage is for hospital and physician services, yet, also includes a combination of public and private delivery of services. The public sector includes voluntary and nonprofit agencies, along with official or governmental agencies. Health Canada is the principal federal regulatory agency whose goal is to enhance and protect the health and well-being of all Canadians by ensuring effective health and human services, safeguarding health devices, natural health products and pharmaceutical provisions and fostering advances in medicine, public health, and social services (Health Canada, 2011b). Delivery of services is organized

on three levels: local, provincial/territorial, and national. Each of the three levels consists of provincially/federally funded or voluntary public agencies combined with private practice providers. The nurse is often the professional who assists the health consumer to navigate throughout the complex health care delivery system; therefore a basic understanding of the system's organization is essential.

## Private Sector
### Independent Practice

While physicians are often self-employed or contractors paid through a fee-for-service remuneration model, services rendered are primarily funded through public funds. Many other health care providers, such as nurses and NPs, are traditionally health system employees who are paid a publicly funded salary, but many also work within independent, private practice settings. Other health service providers (e.g., physiotherapists, psychologists, dentists) are primarily private practice operators who bill the patient or third party insurer directly. Although health care traditionally has been disease oriented, the current emphasis on primary care and health promotion necessitates a much broader perspective. Primary health care involves continual and comprehensive care that includes efforts to keep people as healthy as possible and to prevent disease.

While not traditionally thought to exist in Canada's socialized medical system, private care options are found across numerous settings, from inpatient (private surgical services or extended care facility) to outpatient (ambulatory and community) settings. Outpatient care is defined as any health care services that are not provided on the basis of an overnight stay in which room and board costs are incurred. Ambulatory care settings include two major categories: care provided by owners and providers, and care provided in service settings (Box 3.2). These categories overlap because many providers practice in

---

**BOX 3.2 Types of Ambulatory Care Settings**

- *Owner provider:* surgical and diagnostic centres, private practice health and medical providers, home care organizations, insurance agencies
- *Service settings:* hospital or community care-based clinics/centres, solo or group medical practices, concierge and mobile/home visit practices, ambulatory surgery and diagnostic procedure centres, telehealth and online service environments, retail clinics, university and community hospital clinics, military and Veterans Affairs health centres, NP-managed clinics, colleges/universities and educational institutions, free-standing community facilities, walk-in clinics (some clinics offer free health services for uninsured refugees and new immigrants) (Canadian Centre for Refugee & Immigrant Health Care, n.d.), urgent care centres, outpatient surgery centres, cancer care centres, dialysis centres, neighbourhood and community health centres, diagnostic and mobile imaging centres, occupational health centres, women's health clinics, wound care centres, fitness-wellness centres, health department clinics, nursing centres

Source: Aliber, J. (2016). Eight ambulatory models of care: Outpatient environments come in all shapes and sizes and should be designed accordingly. *Health Facilities Management.* Retrieved from https://www.hfmmagazine.com/articles/1852-eight-ambulatory-models-of-care; Canadian Centre for Refugee & Immigrant Health Care. (n.d.). *18 years of healthcare for Canada's medically uninsured.* Retrieved from https://www.healthequity.ca/.

their own offices and contract with publicly funded care organizations or bill to third-party insurance companies that employees have additional health service coverage through.

Nurse-managed health centres, initially established as northern nursing stations, and now often situated in medically underserved rural and urban areas, primarily serve vulnerable populations in the provision of primary care to individuals and families. Nursing centres (ambulatory care centres, family practice nursing centres, community nursing centres, and birthing centres) have provided high-quality nursing care from NPs, and other advanced practice nurses (APNs). A number of nursing centres are academic nursing centres, established to provide nursing services to communities, learning experiences for students, and settings for faculty practice and research. The key components of a community nursing centre include the following: a nursing staff that is accountable and responsible for care and professional practice, and nurses as the primary providers of care. Using a multidisciplinary collaboration framework, nurses have the opportunity to provide comprehensive primary care services, including a focus on wellness and health promotion, public health programs, and targeted interventions for populations with special needs (Health Canada, 2006).

APNs, an umbrella term for master's or doctoral prepared nurses who practice in the roles of NPs, clinical nurse specialists, or nurse anaesthetists, are well suited to provide cost-effective, quality care to individuals and their families and to serve economically disadvantaged and vulnerable populations. APNs not only have specialized clinical knowledge and skills at the master's or doctoral level, but also have pursued an advanced curriculum that includes research and theoretical foundations to determine best practices, evaluate health policy issues, and understand the intricacies of the health care system and financial management. NPs play a key role within the health care system, caring for vulnerable populations in rural areas and inner cities within primary, acute, and long-term care settings.

### Concierge Medical Practices (Retainer Medicine)

Concierge care is a newer model that is popping up across Canada (e.g., in British Columbia, Alberta, Ontario), in which private practice physicians and NPs provide comprehensive health-related services in exchange for a monthly or annual membership fee paid by individuals or corporate organizations (Doherty, 2015; Keehn, 2015; McKeon, 2014; Reid, 2017). This direct patient contracting practice, while purported primarily to provide prevention and wellness-focused care and to help divert pressure from emergency department services with after-hours care, is instigating controversial questioning about how providing this type of service may contravene the expectations of the CHA. However, a rapidly emerging service is the on-demand online virtual health care offered to employees through third-party health insurance companies (e.g., Akira, Wello, and others). The debate is complex, given that only physician and hospital services are specifically named in the CHA, whereas complementary services provided by NPs are seemingly exempt. This healthy employee-focused care model is meeting the needs of a particular niche of companies and individuals who want to

focus on maintaining or improving health rather than relying on traditional illness-focused care models that are driven by fee-for-service billing pressures (Graff Mcrae, 2017).

### Third-Party Private Health Insurance Plans

Third-party private health insurance plans in Canada were designed to help individuals afford services that are not covered under the CHA (e.g., prescription medications, home care, long-term care, vision prescriptions, dental care). Premium costs vary among plan types, some with higher or lower deductibles and eligibility for health savings accounts (HSAs). A growing number of employers are offering group health insurance as an employee benefit, and these plans usually have a set annual out-of-pocket limit. Attached to these plans, an employer can offer HSAs or savings options. Typically, an employer will make quarterly or annual deposits into the individual's health savings account; individuals can withdraw money from the account at any time for health-related expenditures in addition to those covered by their standard health and dental coverage. Some plans allow preventive and care services offered by complementary care providers (e.g., chiropractors, naturopaths, podiatrists, psychologists, physiotherapists, dietitians, sports therapists, and others).

## Public Sector

The public sector contains federal and jurisdictional government agencies operating at the local, provincial/territorial, federal, and international levels. Before 1900, public health was concerned with problems related to environmental risks and infectious diseases. After the 1900s the public health agenda expanded to address the needs of children and mothers (Rutty et al., 2010). By midcentury, treating chronic disease had also been added to the agenda. As the century progressed, public health issues came to include substance abuse, mental illness, teenage pregnancy, long-term care, epidemics of violence and/or HIV/AIDS, and most recently bioterrorism and disaster preparedness (Nies & McEwen, 2014).

### The Hospitalist Movement

While the impetus for hospitalist programs in the United States was to control hospital costs without compromising quality or satisfaction with client care, the Canadian impetus for this movement was a severe shortage of family physicians who could provide hospital services. Hospitalists are physicians or NPs whose professional focus is managing the comprehensive care of the hospitalized individual, providing direct inpatient primary, critical, and consultative care 24 hours a day, often in a multidisciplinary care team. Hospitalists engage in clinical care, teaching, research, and leadership in the field of hospital medicine, and in meeting the needs of hospitalized patients with acute and chronic complex diseases. Hospitalists enhance the quality and safety of care of a patient within the hospital setting and the safe transitioning of care from the acute care hospital setting to post-acute care facilities or home (Henkel, 2013; Yousefi & Wilton, 2011). Studies have found that hospitals with a hospitalist model program have improved both the quality and the safety of care, with reduced lengths of stay, readmission rates, mortality rates, and complication rates, and with efficient use of hospital and health care resources (Khare, 2017; Yousefi & Chong, 2013).

### Salary or Fee-for-Service Tariff Code

Provinces/territories fund physician services either in negotiating an annual salary or through direct billing using a fee schedule and tariff code billing. The fee schedule is negotiated between physicians and the province/territory health department, and thus differs between provinces/territories. Ultimately, this funding falls under the health transfer agreement with the federal government. Nurses typically fall within a salaried unionized position within the health authority or other government agencies.

### Source of Power

The Canadian Constitution is a collection of statutes and orders that outline the structure and powers of Canadian government and legislatures. The *British North America Act* (Constitution of 1867) established the Dominion of Canada (Federation of Canada) and focuses on the governing structure (Senate and House of Commons), the role of British monarchy, and the provincial/territorial and federal divisions of power, with greater power and authority given to the federal government. Assigned responsibility to the federal government includes a multitude of responsibilities such as citizenship, Indigenous affairs, national defence, and penitentiaries. Similarly, provincial governments were delegated responsibility for hospitals, prisons, and schools. Within the Act, joint responsibility focuses on immigration and agriculture. The *Constitution Act* of 1982 (Canadian Charter of Rights and Freedoms) outlines Canadian citizen civil rights and how constitutional laws in Canada can be amended.

Government decision making is similar across federal and provincial/territorial governments. Within the federal government, the reigning party (Liberal, Conservative, New Democrat, Green, etc.) is citizen elected with an appointed leader who takes on the office of Prime Minister. He or she then appoints their designated department leads, including Health Minister. A dedicated civil servant staff with the lead Deputy Minister are responsible for daily running of the department, meeting with stakeholders, and developing/reviewing health policy that filters up for final approval by the Health Minister. Once approved, the ministry staff then create implementation and evaluation plans.

The federal focus of policy and decision making is for pan-Canadian influence and health strategies (e.g., pan-Canadian mental health plan) and associated financial support via the CHT payments and added financial allotments for focused health strategies (e.g., new mental health and home care programming) that are compliant with federal strategic goals. To support policy development, review, and adaptation, the federal government has created and funded eight advisory organizations (Box 3.3) and commissioned numerous review committees that are focused on health system transformation needs and specific pan-Canadian concerns. Stakeholder groups also regularly meet with ministry representatives and independently create and submit reports to influence government policy.

---

> ## BOX 3.3   Health Canada Support Organizations and Agencies
>
> Over the past three decades, the federal government has established and funded eight not-for-profit pan-Canadian organizations tasked with providing advisory and education roles, at arm's length to the government, by providing recommendations for policy and structure changes within the Canadian health care system:
>
> - *Canadian Centre on Substance Use and Addiction (CCSA)*. Created in 1998 to educate and create partnerships related to substance use and misuse.
> - *Canadian Agency for Drugs and Technologies (CADTH)*. Created in 1989 to advise government on clinical value and cost-effective adoption of medications and other technologies.
> - *Canadian Institute for Health Information (CIHI)*. Created in 1994 to collect, analyze, and report on various health data.
> - *Canadian Foundation for Healthcare Improvement (CFHI)*. Created in 1996 to help accelerate health care innovations through partnerships.
> - *Canada Health Infoway*. Created in 2001 to advise on needed investments for e-health infrastructure.
> - *Canadian Patient Safety Institute (CPSI)*. Created in 2003 to build a culture of patient safety.
> - *Canadian Partnership Against Cancer (CPAC)*. Created in 2006 to accelerate action on cancer control by working with various stakeholders, including provincial/territorial cancer agencies.
> - *Mental Health Commission of Canada (MHCC)*. Created in 2007 to develop a national strategy for mental health and to help reduce stigma associated with mental illness.
>
> Likewise, external advisory bodies, with government appointed members, have also been established to advise government on a wide range of specific topic areas. Examples include:
>
> - Advisory Council on the Implementation of National Pharmacare
> - Advisory Council on Traditional Chinese Medicine
> - Expert Advisory Group on Marketing of Opioids
> - External Review of the Federally Funded Pan-Canadian Health Organizations
> - Ministerial Advisory Council on Mental Health
> - Paediatric Expert Advisory Committee
> - Scientific Advisory Committee on Health Products for Women
> - Scientific Advisory Panel on Cannabis
> - Scientific Advisory Panel on Pharmaceutical Sciences and Clinical Pharmacology

Sources: Health Canada. (2017). *Review of federally-funded pan-Canadian health organizations*. Retrieved from https://www.canada.ca/en/health-canada/programs/external-advisory-body-pan-canadian-health-organizations/terms-of-reference.html; Health Canada. (2019). *External advisory bodies*. Retrieved from https://www.canada.ca/en/health-canada/corporate/about-health-canada/public-engagement/external-advisory-bodies.html.

Similar to the federal structure, the provincial/territorial governments have elected parties to lead provincial parliament, with a Premier as party head, appointed Minister of Health, and employed civil servants who meet with stakeholders and are responsible for the bulk of policy and program development, implementation, and evaluation. At least once annually the provincial/territorial health ministers (and support team) meet with the federal Minister of Health and his/her support team to review annual CHT payments and pan-Canadian concerns (e.g., the opioid crisis) with associated financial support requests.

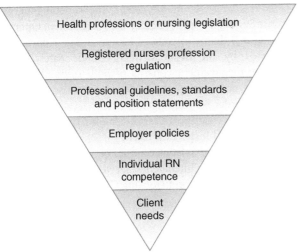

**Fig. 3.2 Scope of Practice Factors** (Canadian Nurses Association. [2015]. *Framework for the practice of registered nurses in Canada* [2nd ed., p. 14, Fig. 3]. Ottawa: Author. Retrieved from https://www.cna-aiic.ca/~/media/cna/page-content/pdf-en/framework-for-the-pracice-of-registered-nurses-in-canada.pdf).)

Since 2014–15, the federal to provincial cash allocation procedure has been on an equal per capita cash basis across provinces/territories, whereas previously there was an equalizing adjustment when the federal government reduced its basic tax rate by a specific percentage and the provinces then took up the remaining costs. CHT was agreed on as a minimum 3% annual increase, but over the past several years has been growing closer to 6% per annum, equating to approximately $38 billion annual CHT payments for provincial/territorial health funding support (Di Matteo, 2019).

The national Senate was created out of the *British North America Act* to ensure sober thought and equal jurisdictional voice into parliamentary decision making (Foot, 2019). It is comprised of 105 members, each appointed by the Governor General on advice from the Prime Minister. The main function of Senate is to review and give recommendations on national issues that influence policy while ensuring equal input from all jurisdictions.

### Nursing's Role in Leading Change

Nurses contribute to patient wellness and health care system optimization through their multidimensional leadership roles across a wide range of practice settings, including clinical, education, administration, research, and policy (Fig. 3.2). While many nurses choose formalized leadership roles with education, administration, policy, and clinical practice (advanced nursing practice roles), all nurses are called to engage in informal leadership with patients and as members of collaborative practice teams. Nurses use leadership skills every day by:

- Engaging critical thinking for decision making based on person-centred care and empirical evidence
- Practising to their full and legal scope and competence
- Pioneering new realms of practice that may push boundaries and overlapping scopes in a respectful manner
- Asking important questions to shift policy and encourage new areas of research
- Helping patients ensure continuity and coordinated care

- Delegating appropriately to other care team members
- Helping to develop innovative service delivery models
- Supporting health system sustainability by identifying gaps within current health care system and recommending needs based on their unique frontline care knowledge
- Supporting population health by helping identify and address social determinants of health
- Advocating for expansion of socialized health care coverage and modernization of the *CHA* to include a national Pharmacare program, improved palliative care, and enhanced home and community services
- Mentoring students and new graduates
- Participating on focused clinical teams to develop population-specific guidelines and practice supports (CNA, 2015, 2009; RNAO, 2013), such as Choosing Wisely diagnostic and treatment guidelines (Box 3.4).

### Official Agencies

Official agencies are tax supported and therefore accountable to the citizens through elected or appointed officials or boards. The purpose and duties of official agencies are prescribed or mandated by law. This discussion is from the perspective of the individual gaining knowledge of or access to the health care system.

*Local level.* The health department of a town, city, municipality, or health authority is the local health unit and is usually the first line of access and health responsibility for the population that it serves. The regional health authority board members are accountable to the minister of health, and generally the regional chief executive officer is appointed by the Minster of Health. The local regional health authority's role and functions centre on providing direct services to the public and depend on the jurisdictional mandate and community resources.

*Jurisdictional (provincial/territorial) level.* The Minister of Health is appointed by the elected governing party. Health services are organized by each jurisdiction, with wide

---

**BOX 3.5   Health Canada's Portfolio**

*Overarching Goals.* Maintaining and improving the health of Canadians. This is supported by the Health Portfolio which comprises:

- Health Canada
- Public Health Agency of Canada (PHAC)
- Canadian Institutes of Health Research (CIHR)
- Patented Medicine Prices Review Board
- Canadian Food Inspection Agency (CFIA)

The Health Portfolio consists of approximately 12,000 full-time equivalent employees and an annual budget of over $3.8 billion.

Source: Government of Canada. (2017). *Health portfolio.* Retrieved from https://www.canada.ca/en/health-canada/corporate/health-portfolio.html.

---

variation from one province/territory to another. The deputy minister is responsible for various units within the health portfolio, for example, administration and finance, workforce, regional services, public health, or primary care. One agency, the department/ministry of health, performs the primary responsibilities in policy, planning, and coordination of programs and services for regional health authorities.

*Federal level.* The Minister of Health is appointed by the federally elected government, who is responsible for the publicly funded national medicare plan. The federal government assumes overall responsibility for the funding of health care insurance plans and reasonable access to hospital and physician services. Health care services are shared between provincial/territorial governments and the federal government. The federal government provides health care services to specific populations including First Nations people living on reserve, Inuit people, serving members of the Canadian Armed Forces, eligible veterans, inmates in federal penitentiaries, and some groups of refugee claimants.

Health Canada, the main federal body concerned with the health of the nation, consists of a number of separate operating agencies (Box 3.5). Under each of the federal health service agencies listed there are numerous other departments.

*Federal nursing policy.* Nursing policy at the federal level consists of representation to Health Canada by the Principal Nursing Advisory Task Force (PNATF) to support the Federal/Provincial/Territorial (F/P/T) Committee on Health Workforce (CHW) and the Conference of Deputy Ministers of Health. The PNATF consists of chief nursing officers for each Canadian province/territory, Correctional Service Canada, the Department of National Defense, First Nations Inuit Health, the Public Health Agency of Canada, the Strategic Policy Branch, and Veterans Affairs Canada, to provide advice on policy, programs, and initiatives in support of effective and optimal utilization of nursing knowledge, skills, and expertise. PNATF is working on a new vision for the "Family of Nursing" in Canada (Licensed Practical Nurses [LPNs], Registered Psychiatric Nurses [RPNs], RNs, and NPs); the goal is to provide a pan-Canadian harmonization of regulation, education, and optimized scopes of practice. In some provinces/territories (e.g., Nova Scotia), the legislation has passed to merge all classification of nurses where the plan is that portability for health human resource planning will improve while simultaneously enhancing health care access for all Canadians.

*Federal emergency management.* The Federal Emergency Response System is coordinated by the Government Operations Centre (GOC) that is operated 24 hours a day, 7 days a week, coordinated by the department of Public Safety Canada. Emergency management consists of both responding to and preventing events by a number of federal departments:

- Canada Border Services Agency
- Canadian Air Transport Security Authority
- Canadian Food Inspection Agency
- Canadian Nuclear Safety Commission
- Canadian Security Intelligence Service
- Canadian Mortgage and Housing Corporation
- Environment Canada
- Global Affairs Canada
- Health Canada
- Indian and Northern Affairs Canada
- Industry Canada
- National Defence
- Natural Resources Canada
- Public Health Agency of Canada
- Privy Council Office
- Royal Canadian Mounted Police
- Transport Canada

Public Safety Canada addresses avalanches, earthquakes, floods, hurricanes, landslides, severe storms, storm surges, tornadoes, tsunamis, wildfires, bomb threats, chemical releases, nuclear emergencies, pandemic influenza, power outages, and suspicious packages. The role of the GOC is to provide an integrated federal response to emergencies of national interest to manage the federal emergency response plan. The GOC role also is to harmonize a jurisdictional, nongovernmental and private sector response to emergencies.

*Military health care at the federal level.* Canadian Armed Forces members' health care falls under the jurisdiction of the *National Defence Act*, that is, military members are excluded from the *CHA*. The Department of National Defence and the Canadian Forces provide medical and dental care to military personnel, excluding families which are covered by provincial/territorial plans. Health care is provided by regular force, reserve, and public (civilian) professionals that include nurses. Military health care services are tailored to meet the operational requirements and member needs.

Veterans Affairs Canada is made up of four branches (Service Delivery, Strategic Policy & Commemoration, Chief Financial Officer and Corporate Services, and Strategic Oversight and Communications) and three divisions (Audit and Evaluation, Bureau of Pensions Advocates, and Human Resources). The Service Delivery Branch delivers benefits and services to support Canadian Forces veterans.

*First Nations people living on reserves and Inuit people.* The federal government provides primary and supplementary services to First Nations people living on reserves, and to Inuit people. The direct services to First Nations people and the Inuit includes primary care and emergency services on remote and isolated reserves where no provincial or territorial services are readily available; community-based health programs both on reserves and in Inuit communities; and a non-insured health benefits program (medication, dental, and ancillary health services) for First Nations and Inuit people no matter where they live in Canada. In general, these services are provided at nursing stations, health centres, in-patient treatment centres, and through community health promotion programs. Increasingly, both orders of government and Indigenous organizations are working together to integrate the delivery of these services with the provincial and territorial systems (Health Canada, 2018).

*Federal penitentiaries.* Federal corrections facilities are funded by Corrections Canada. The *Corrections and Conditional Release Act (CCRA)*, Section 86(1,2), requires that inmates be provided with professionally accepted standards for essential health care and reasonable access to nonessential mental health care. The *CCRA* sets out the principle that corrections policies, programs and practices for successful rehabilitation and reintegration into the community (Correctional Service Canada, 2015).

*Refugee claimants.* Refugees coming to Canada are funded for health care under the Interim Federal Health Program (IFHP) medical services. Immigration medical exams and follow-up treatment of health conditions that would make someone inadmissible to Canada are listed in the *Immigration and Refugee Protection Act*; vaccinations, outbreak management and control, and medical support needed for safe travel are funded under this program. Additionally, there is temporary coverage of health care benefits to groups who are not eligible for provincial or territorial (PT) health insurance. The IFHP does not cover or coordinate the cost of health care services that may be claimed under a public or private health insurance plan. Similar to the health transfer funding, the IFHP covers in-patient and out-patient hospital services, services from medical doctors, RNs, and other health care providers licensed in Canada, including pre- and postnatal care, and laboratory, diagnostic and ambulance services. *Supplemental coverage* (similar to social assistance recipients by provincial and territorial governments) includes limited vision and urgent dental care, home care and long-term care, services from allied health care practitioners including clinical psychologists, psychotherapists, counselling therapists, occupational therapists, speech language therapists, physiotherapists, assistive devices, medical supplies and equipment (orthopedic and prosthetic equipment, mobility aids, hearing aids, diabetic supplies, incontinence supplies, and oxygen equipment), prescription medications, and other products listed on provincial/territorial public medication plan formularies (Immigration & Citizenship Canada, 2019).

*Living with a disability.* The Canadian Charter of Rights and Freedoms and the Canadian *Human Right Act* of 1977 require employers and health care providers to comply with protecting people with disabilities from discrimination. Other legislation that applies to disability discrimination includes the Accessible Transportation Code, *Employment Equity Act*, Policy on the Duty to Accommodate Persons with Disabilities in the Federal Public Service, *Canada Elections Act, Criminal Code,* and *Canada Evidence Act* (Section 6). An example of removing barriers for accommodation is to install wheelchair lifts in shuttle bus systems.

*Medical assistance in dying.* In 2016, the Parliament of Canada passed legislation (Bill C-14) to allow Medical Assistance in Dying (MAiD) for eligible Canadian adults. The law is inclusive of NPs who can provide medical assistance in dying under the rules set out in the *Criminal Code*. The *Criminal Code* was changed to address the Supreme Court of Canada ruling to satisfy the Canadian Charter of Rights and Freedoms. The amended law sets the rules to support access for patients who are seeking medical assistance in dying within Canada.

*Protection of personal information.* Personal information refers to material that can identify an individual, including ethnic origin, religion, marital status, age, sexual orientation, medical or dental history, education or employment history, financial information, genetic information, or any individualized numbers specific to that individual such as driver's license, health number, or social insurance number.

There are two federal privacy laws in Canada, the *Privacy Act* (1985) and the *Personal Information Protection and Electronic Documents Act* (PIPEDA) (Office of the Privacy Commissioner of Canada, 2018). The *Privacy Act* specifically pertains to ensuring the privacy of personal information collected and held by government and its affiliates, along with an individual's access to this information (Department of Justice, 1985). *PIPEDA* pertains to the private sector organizations in how they collect, store, share, and disclose personal information to others and to the individual the information relates to (Government of Canada, 2000). Each province and territory may also have its own regulations surrounding the protection of personal information. British Columbia also has legislated that residents' health information must not be stored in the United States, even if encrypted; all other provinces and territories do not have this specific requirement but the Office of the Privacy Commissioner of Canada is reviewing transborder dataflows (Government of Canada, 2008; Office of the Privacy Commissioner of Canada, 2019).

*International level.* The WHO, the United Nations' specialized agency for health, was established in 1948. The WHO comprises members from more than 190 countries, and its core functions include giving worldwide guidance in the field of health; setting global standards for health; cooperating with governments in strengthening national health programs; and developing and transferring appropriate technology, information, and standards. The following is the six-point agenda of the WHO: promoting development; fostering health security; strengthening health systems; harnessing research, information, and evidence; enhancing partnerships; and improving performance. In September 2015, a global plan of action for the next 15 years was developed with 17 Sustainable Development Goals and 169 targets. The new goals build upon what was not completed in the previous 15-year goals and seeks to meet the needs of the world's most disadvantaged people (women, children, poor), with the remaining overarching health goal of ensuring healthy lives and promoting well-being for all ages. Emerging challenges were recognized, such as noncommunicable diseases (diabetes and heart disease) and changing social and environmental factors, such as sanitation, pollution, urbanization, and climate change (WHO, n.d.-b).

## Voluntary Agencies

The voluntary (not-for-profit) health movement, which began in 1882, stems from the goodwill and humanitarian concerns that are part of the nongovernmental, free enterprise heritage of the people of the United States and Canada. Nonprofit entities that maintain a tax-free status are often powerful forces in the health field, voluntary agencies, foundations, and professional associations. The tax-free status of these organizations is challenged at times on the basis of charge that some of them serve only a limited population. Voluntary agencies are influential in promoting health affairs and research agendas at the national policy level and often have significant influence on health legislation. Their prominent role was demonstrated by the Cancer Society's early mass media announcements about the health hazards of smoking. An example of another voluntary agency is the Alzheimer Society of Canada, which has local chapters that provide resources for families, including publications, services, respite for the caregiver, and support groups for individuals and families. Many not-for-profit agencies exist in Canada, including ladies' auxiliaries, hospital foundations, and local community foundations that fund capital equipment, housing, or research.

Philanthropic foundations provide valuable stimulation to the health field and operate under fewer constraints than do other sources in supporting research or training projects. Nurses interested in research or advanced clinical study that relates to the special interests of voluntary agencies or foundations may apply for grant monies available to support their work. For example, the St. Amant Center was founded in 1931 by the Grey Nuns to improve health care for patients with TB. Today, the centre is dedicated to meeting the needs of persons with developmental disabilities funding many research projects in addition to a joint appointed Faculty of Nursing research chair position.

Professional associations, organized at the national level with provincial/territorial and local branches, are powerful political forces. Nurses can support their professional organizations in influencing the direction of health policy through membership and active participation to advanced health policy, research, or legislation.

*VON Canada.* The Victorian Order of Nurses (VON) has been a nonprofit pioneer of home care for over 120 years. In the 1890s, the National Council of Women passed a resolution which founded the VON with the first order of business to provide nursing services and establish cottage hospitals in isolated areas. In 1897, Charlotte Macleod, a Canadian who had studied with the legendary Florence Nightingale, was recruited by Dr. Alfred Worcester, a Harvard professor and founder of the Waltham Training School for Nurses in Massachusetts to set up the VON Canada. Today, the VON delivers 75 different health program and services, for example acute pediatric care, adult day programs, Alzheimer's programs, bereavement services, breastfeeding consultation, caregiver support, case management. and more (VON, 2018).

*The Canadian Red Cross.* The Canadian Red Cross is a well-known volunteer-led humanitarian organization. The *Canadian Red Cross Society Act* was passed in 1909 by the Government of Canada. Founded in 1881 by Clara Barton, the International Red Cross aids victims of war and natural disasters throughout the world. There are more than 300 local Canadian Red Cross branches, with more than 20,000 volunteers. The Canadian Red Cross responds both to small local emergencies to help victims (such as in the case of a house fire) and to large natural disasters (such as hurricanes, tornados and earthquakes). In contrast to the American Red Cross, which is the largest supplier of blood and blood products in the United States, in Canada, these services are offered by Canadian Blood Services rather than the Canadian Red Cross. Similar to the American Red Cross, however, the Canadian Red Cross helps thousands of Canadians, who are separated from their families, maintain communication, and offers communities a range of health and safety courses (CPR, First Aid, bullying and abuse prevention, emergency preparedness). The global network of national societies relies on public donations of money, time, and blood. (Canadian Red Cross, n.d.; American Red Cross, n.d.).

# FINANCING HEALTH CARE

## Costs

Health care expenditures in Canada were $253.5 billion in 2018 (or $6,839 per person, see Fig. 3.4), where health spending consumed 11.3% of the GDP. In 2018, the breakdown of national health spending was as follows: hospitals 28.3%, medications 15.7%, and physicians 15.1%, to account for about 60% of total health spending. Employee remuneration is the largest hospital expense (64.1% or about 35 billion dollars) with nursing inpatient services accounting for 19.3% of hospital expenditures (CIHI, 2019c; Figs. 3.3 and 3.4). Hospital expenditures in Canada are about half those of the United States, at $12,865 per person per year. Many other countries spend far less per capita, yet their life expectancy is greater and infant mortality rates are lower (Fig. 3.5; see Table 3.1).

Health care analysts predict that accelerations in health care costs will continue, putting pressure on public and private payers to finance them. Factors driving costs include general inflation; health care cost inflation; application of new and more advanced technologies; growth in the proportion of older persons; government financing of health care services, including long-term care; growth of prescription medication use and costs; misdistribution of health care providers and services; expansion of medical technology and specialty medicine; and other costs associated with providing health care. For example, diagnostic and therapeutic techniques—including computer-aided technology (Box 3.6) and noninvasive imaging (such as magnetic resonance imaging), cardiac surgery, organ transplantation, joint replacements (particularly hips and knees)—enhance the capabilities of medicine while increasing costs.

A combination of the following factors results in hospitals having less time to offer prevention or health-promotion education to individuals: changes in hospital care and use of hospitalists, increased use of outpatient services, shorter inpatient stays, and increased time caring for chronic illness as opposed to acute illness. Moreover, workforce shortages, especially in nursing, increase the use of nonprofessional caregivers, and inadequate resources,

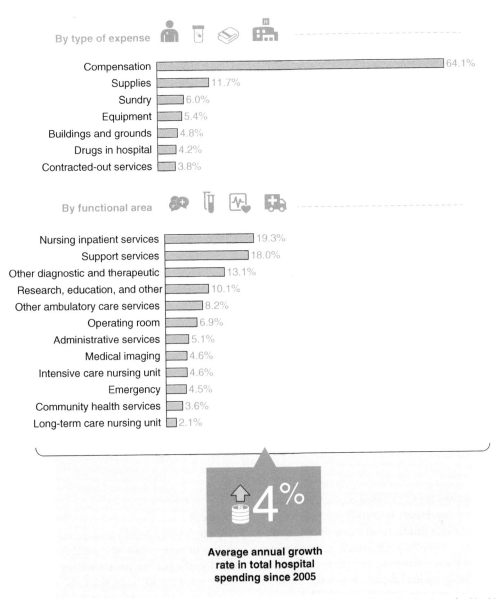

By type of expense

| | |
|---|---|
| Compensation | 64.1% |
| Supplies | 11.7% |
| Sundry | 6.0% |
| Equipment | 5.4% |
| Buildings and grounds | 4.8% |
| Drugs in hospital | 4.2% |
| Contracted-out services | 3.8% |

By functional area

| | |
|---|---|
| Nursing inpatient services | 19.3% |
| Support services | 18.0% |
| Other diagnostic and therapeutic | 13.1% |
| Research, education, and other | 10.1% |
| Other ambulatory care services | 8.2% |
| Operating room | 6.9% |
| Administrative services | 5.1% |
| Medical imaging | 4.6% |
| Intensive care nursing unit | 4.6% |
| Emergency | 4.5% |
| Community health services | 3.6% |
| Long-term care nursing unit | 2.1% |

⬆ 4%

**Average annual growth
rate in total hospital
spending since 2005**

**Fig. 3.3** Hospital Expenditures *National totals exclude Quebec and Nunavut. (Canadian Institute for Health Information. (2019). *What are hospitals spending on? Hospital expenditures, 2017-2018.* Ottawa: CIHI. Retrieved from https://www.cihi.ca/ewhat-are-hospitals-spending-on.)

reimbursement, and numbers of nurses may prevent health care providers from offering the range of health promotion educational efforts.

## Funding Sources

The Canadian people pay for all health care costs. Money is transferred from consumer to provider by various mechanisms. The major sources are the government (federal, provincial/territorial, and local governments collected by taxes), third-party payment (private supplementary insurance), and out-of-pocket support (Figs. 3.6 and 3.7). Health care spending differs considerably across provinces/territories (Fig. 3.8).

## Third-Party Payor Health Benefits

In Canada, *third-party payor* for health benefits includes a range of government and corporation insurance plans. For example,

all provinces/territories have Worker's Compensation Programs that are legislated federally (by the *Government Employees Compensation Act*) and are provincially/territorially administered to protect employees from financial hardship. Employers provide health insurance plans that offer a range of coverage, depending upon the plan the employee chooses. Canadians can purchase private health insurance and are encouraged to do so when travelling between the 13 provinces/territories that have differing health plan coverage, or when travelling outside of the country. Non-Insured Health Benefits (NIHB) is funded by Health Canada First Nations and Inuit Health Branch for eligible members and covers services that are not paid for by private or provincial/territorial insurance or social programs. For example, third-party payors may cover prescription medications, over-the-counter medication, medical supplies heand equipment, mental health counselling, dental care, vision care, and medical transportation, depending on the plan.

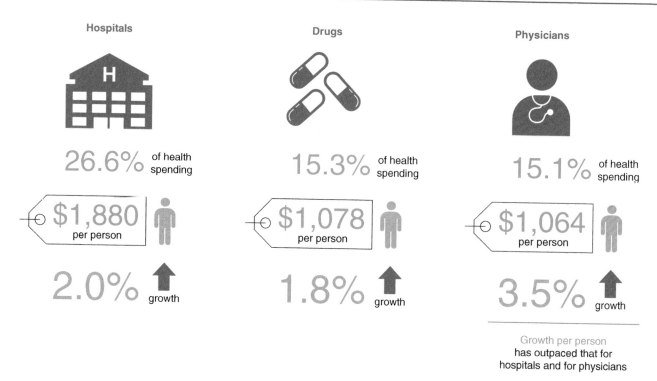

**Fig. 3.4 Health Care Expenditures** (Canadian Institute for Health Information. [2019]. *National Health Expenditure Trends, 1975 to 2019*. Ottawa: CIHI. Retrieved from https://www.cihi.ca/sites/default/files/document/nhex-tren-narrative-report-2019-en-web.pdf.)

Each jurisdiction receives the CHT based on the *CHA*, which sets out the criteria and conditions to qualify for the publicly funded health care insurance funds. Health care spending differs considerably across provinces/territories. Fig. 3.8 provides visual representation of these differences and the overall cost to Canadians. Fig. 3.4 (shown earlier) depicts where the majority of health care dollars are spent. In order receive CHT, jurisdictions must fulfill requirements to qualify for the full CHT cash, which include the following:

- Not-for-profit jurisdictional public administration of health care
- Comprehensiveness—health services provided by hospitals, physicians or dentists in a hospital setting
- Universality for all insured residents
- Portability—coverage if relocating until another Canadian jurisdiction insures the person
- Accessibility in that reasonable access to hospital, medical or dental services in hospital occur
  In addition to:
- Information to the federal Minister of Health, as prescribed
- Recognition of the federal financial contributions
- Extra-billing (billing a person for medical or dental care or user fees) dollar-for-dollar deduction from the federal cash transfer to that jurisdiction will occur, province or territory is required under the *Act*

From 1984 to 1987, $244,732,000 dollars were deducted or refunded to the Government of Canada for extra billing and use fee charges (CIHI, 2016).

## Mechanisms

### Payment

Although some health care providers and other professionals in the private sector are paid on a fee-for-service basis, by third-party private insurance, or by public-supported insurance, most health care workers, including nurses in institutional or community agencies and in the military, receive salaries or are paid by the hour regardless of the amount of care provided. Because nurses are salaried or paid by the hour, the separation of nursing costs from all other health-related costs is difficult. The cost of acute hospital nursing care is typically incorporated in the daily room and board charge in the acute care setting. Without documentation of specific nursing costs, validating the need for skilled nursing services is difficult.

In recent years, RNs and NPs have entered independent practice to provide direct services. Independent nursing practice may be viewed as a logical outgrowth of seeking higher levels of professionalism and autonomy. The regulated health professions acts of some provinces/territories legislatively addresses health professions. Corporations and most nurse regulators have developed self-employed guidelines for nurses. Although a third-party payor may reimburse NPs, and the recently elected government in Alberta made a campaign promise to allow NPs to use fee-for-service billing, not all plans and provider groups support direct payment for nurses' work. Clearly, the nursing practice roles and prescriptive authority of NPs differ between provinces/territories. Incremental steps have been taken to

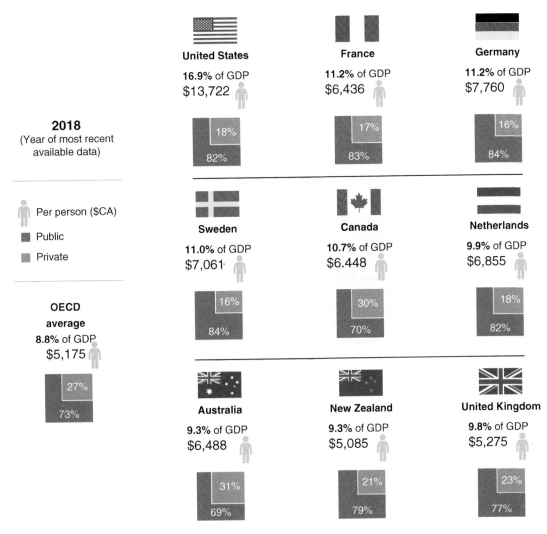

**2018**
(Year of most recent available data)

Per person ($CA)

Public

Private

**OECD average**
**8.8%** of GDP
$5,175

27%

73%

**United States**
**16.9%** of GDP
$13,722

18%

82%

**France**
**11.2%** of GDP
$6,436

17%

83%

**Germany**
**11.2%** of GDP
$7,760

16%

84%

**Sweden**
**11.0%** of GDP
$7,061·

16%

84%

**Canada**
**10.7%** of GDP
$6.448

30%

70%

**Netherlands**
**9.9%** of GDP
$6,855

18%

82%

**Australia**
**9.3%** of GDP
$6,488

31%

69%

**New Zealand**
**9.3%** of GDP
$5,085

21%

79%

**United Kingdom**
**9.8%** of GDP
$5,275

23%

77%

NOTES:

Total current expenditure (capital excluded).

Expenditure data is based on the System of Health Accounts.

**Fig. 3.5** Health Care Spending Comparisons Internationally (OECD Health Statistics 2019, https://www.oecd.org/health/health-data.htm.)

advance the NP role at both the federal level and the provincial/territorial level. Most jurisdictions in Canada have legislation for NPs to practice and prescribe medications without physician oversight. Some provinces/territories have legislated RNs to have prescribing authority for specific disease groups (e.g., diabetes mellitus) and health service needs (e.g., reproductive health or travel medicine) with regulation and legislation that requires a collaborative NP or MD agreement.

## Private Health Insurance

Traditionally, private (third-party) insurers charged employers or individuals annual premiums and provided services on a fee-for-service basis to health care providers. Much of the individual insurance sold today is supplementary to cover non-insured health services. Private health insurance has also been designed to supplement travel associated health expenses in Canada or abroad that are not typically covered by provincial/territorial plans. Provinces/territories vary in supplementing travel funding,

for example, paying for services up to a maximum of $100 per day (Manitoba), and recently the province of Ontario has proposed to end travel associated emergency medical costs of $400 per day as an inpatient and $50 per day for physician services.

***Medicare.*** Medicare is a term used to refer to the federally funded health program previously discussed, which funds dental care in a hospital, inpatient hospital care, and physician services. Out-of-pocket expenses, not funded by medicare, add significantly to Canadians' cost of living. A significant population at risk includes older persons, who may have limited financial resources to seek preventive health services and pharmaceuticals not covered under medicare. Some low-income enrollees may qualify for social assistance health funding services whereas middle-class Canadians may not have supplementary insurance plans through work and also not quality for subsidized services. One specific area missing from medicare benefits that is causing great concern in terms of rising costs is outpatient prescription medications. Federally, the Government of Canada

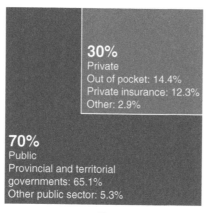 

## BOX 3.6    Health Technology: Digital Health Platforms and Artificial Intelligence

As societal needs for health care resources increase and health human resources become more scarce, technological inventions can provide new options for more efficient and effective health care solutions that engage the patient and take workload pressure off providers. Two such health technologies that are emerging to support health care are digital health platforms and artificial intelligence.

### Digital Health Platforms

Digital health platforms are tools that help improve universal access to essential health services while removing the medical professional as sole broker of health-related knowledge, thereby equalizing the provider–patient relationship toward interactive teamwork with patient engagement in health promotion activities. Some developments are helping traditional medicine to shift focus from treatment to prevention and putting power in the hands of patients. For instance, smartphone applications help support healthy living (e.g., smoking cessation, weight management, mindfulness), while wearable technology (e.g., heart monitors, glucose sensors, watches with biometric sensors) helps to monitor and provide real-time feedback to the patient and/or care provider. Portable diagnostic devices along with wearables transform point of care from clinics, hospitals, and labs to patients themselves. Internet technology supports the connection of patients with care providers, remote consultations with specialists, and online resources to support health education and decision making. Telemedicine and videoconferencing options can help connect patients with care providers by eliminating geographical access barriers. The WHO (2019) published the first guideline on digital health interventions with a goal to identify tools that help maximize people's health while improving system efficiency and data privacy.

### Artificial Intelligence

Artificial intelligence (AI) is an umbrella term for a rapidly advancing division of computer science that is focused on the development of programs to simulate tasks usually requiring human intelligence (e.g., pattern recognition, problem-solving and reasoning), with an aim of improving disease detection, personalized medicine, perfecting standardization and consistency, while improving access and efficiency. For example, AI is being used for pathological differentiation of suspicious lesions, where computer-assisted algorithms for pattern-recognition can be used to detect minor deviations that are not detectable to the human eye, but essential for early detection of disease, thereby supporting speedier treatment initiation.

AI is also central to the algorithms used within computer-assisted delivery of cognitive behavioural therapy for those who experience anxiety and depression. For example, social media–monitoring algorithms can be used to identify posts correlating with those who are most at risk of suicide and then mental health resources can be more quickly notified to investigate the true risk. In 2017, the Canadian federal government dedicated $125 million toward a pan-Canadian AI strategy, with additional funding coming from provincial initiatives. Because of AI's unique application within health care, Health Canada established the Digital Health Review Division within the Therapeutic Products Directorate's Medical Devices Bureau to develop oversight for patient safety.

Sources: World Health Organization (WHO). (2019). *WHO guideline: Recommendations on digital interventions for health system strengthening.* Geneva: World Health Organization. Retrieved from https://www.who.int/reproductivehealth/publications/digital-interventions-health-system-strengthening/en/; Mason, J., Morrison, A., & Visintini, S. (2018). An overview of clinical applications of artificial intelligence. *CADTH: Issues in Emerging Health Technologies, 174.* Ottawa: CADTH; The Medical Futurist. (2018). *How could digital technology make an impact on primary care?* Retrieved from https://medicalfuturist.com.

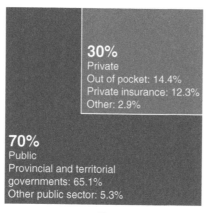
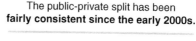
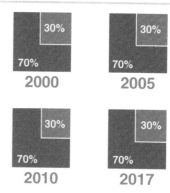

**Fig. 3.6  Public and Private Health Dollar Spending Comparison** (Canadian Institute for Health Information. [2019]. *National Health Expenditure Trends, 1975 to 2019.* Ottawa: CIHI. Retrieved from https://www.cihi.ca/sites/default/files/cument/nhex-trends-narrative-report-2019-en-web.pdf.)

provides prescription medication coverage for about one million Canadians who are members of First Nations and Inuit communities, the Canadian Armed Forces, Veterans Affairs Canada, the Royal Canadian Mounted Police, and offenders in federal correctional institutions. Many middle-class Canadians cannot afford the prescription medications they need. In 2018, the Government created the Canadian Drug Agency to move ahead with a national Pharmacare program. The Canadian Drug Agency will negotiate prescription medication prices on behalf of Canadians to help lower the cost of medications, develop a national formulary, and develop a national strategy for high-cost medications to support more consistent treatment of rare diseases (Health Canada, 2018).

## Pharmaceutical Costs

The spiralling cost of prescription medications continues to add to the complexity of providing adequate health care. Newer medications cost more than the medications they replace and

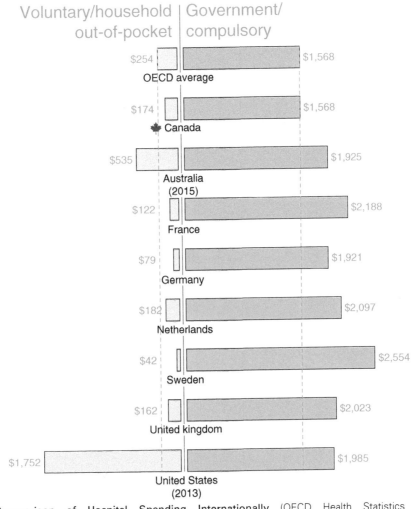

Fig. 3.7 Comparison of Hospital Spending Internationally (OECD Health Statistics 2019, https://www.oecd.org/health/health-data.htm.)

contribute 50% of the increased cost. Increased use of prescription medications adds to an increased cost per day of medications. Consumer demand sparked by American medication advertisements, new indications for use, and increased consumer knowledge of available medications has increased the demand for prescription medications. Increased medication cost is attributed to inflation, more days of therapy per user, greater number of medications per user, cost of research and medication development. Numerous advocacy groups, including the Canadian Nurses Association and the Canadian Nurse Federation of Unions, are urging the federal government to establish a national Pharmacare program to curb costs while opening access to affordable medications for all Canadians.

## The Uninsured: Who Are They?

Canada is well known as being a welcoming country to immigrants with diverse ethnicity, cultures, and languages. Since Canadian Confederation in 1867, the proportion of immigrants in Canada has never fallen below 13% (Statistics Canada, 2017). This proportion has been continually rising over the past 30 years, to 20.7% in 2011. Except for health services, which are funded by the Government of Canada (IFHP), provision of all health care services is the responsibility of provinces/territories, municipalities, or nonprofit organizations.

Migration is reflective of an interconnected world and may be voluntary (e.g., immigration for job opportunity), necessary (e.g., refugee relocation), or involuntary (e.g., displacement resulting from war, climate change, starvation). Migrants may arrive through official processes that require travel documents and health screening (permanent or temporary residency) or by unofficial means (as illegal immigrants, asylum seekers, and refugee claimants) where health screening may not occur (Gushulak, Pottie, Roberts, et al., 2011; MacPherson, Gushulak, & Macdonald, 2007).

Migrants' health is a reflection of many factors, including infectious diseases endemic to their home country or countries travelled through on their way back to Canada, chronic

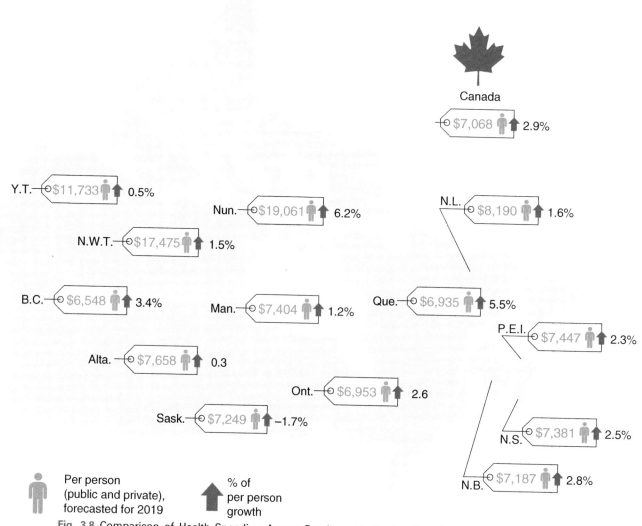

**Fig. 3.8** Comparison of Health Spending Across Provinces/Territories (Canadian Institute for Health Information. [2019]. *National Health Expenditure Trends, 1975 to 2019*. Ottawa: CIHI. Retrieved from https://www.cihi.ca/sites/default/files/document/nhex-tren-narrative-report-2019-en-web.pdf.)

disease consistent with population risk factors, and mental health conditions (e.g., PTSD, depression, anxiety) that result from conflict, displacement, racism, and the stress of assimilating/adapting to their new surroundings, etc. With globalization comes international travel and relocation, which can also lead to fear of imported infectious diseases that were previously eradicated in Canada (e.g., polio) or new diseases (e.g., swine flu) that put vaccinated and unvaccinated Canadians at risk. There are strict expectations for health screening of officially sanctioned immigrants, but those who arrive unofficially may not seek non-emergency-type health care, because those who are new to Canada do not immediately qualify for Canada's public health care coverage. To help mitigate this gap, one community clinic in Toronto, Ontario, offers free health care to refugees and asylum seekers via a network of volunteer health practitioners.

Birth tourism is also increasing as nonresidents of Canada come to deliver a child here, which offers unconditional Canadian citizenship to children born here even if the parents are not Canadian citizens (Ontario Council of Agencies Serving Immigrants, 2017; Bourgon, 2017). Frequently, news headlines address this growing phenomenon, as local residents must seek to deliver at the next closest health care facility because maternity units are full. Compounding this issue is unpaid hospital bills by nonresidents of Canada.

## Unauthorized Immigrants

In Canada, the Immigration and Refugee Board of Canada is responsible for decisions related to asylum claims. The Canada Border Services Agency and office of Immigration, Refugees and Citizenship Canada determine if individuals are eligible to make an asylum claim. The number of asylum seekers is increasing, and in 2018, 19,419 asylum seekers were intercepted by the Royal Canadian Mounted Police and 55,020 at other ports of entry to Canada (Immigration & Citizenship Canada, 2019). Compounding the increase in numbers is the fact that health care funding from the IFHP is limited and is a last resort payer method when there is no other coverage from private insurance or jurisdictional health funding coverage.

Provinces/territories are responsible to provide the health services that are not funded by other sources such as municipalities or nonprofit organizations. In some provinces (British Columbia, Manitoba, Ontario, and Quebec) a 3-month waiting period is imposed for refugees who become permanent residents. Thus eligibility and coverage for health care for newcomers may vary between provinces/territories.

The IFHP provides immigrants with three types of coverage: (1) health care coverage similar to provincial/territorial health insurance plans with some supplemental health care products and services such as prescription medication, limited dental and vision care, home care, and long-term care; (2) health care coverage similar to provincial/territorial health insurance plans, including coverage for hospital services, physician services, laboratory services, diagnostic, and ambulance services; or (3) medications and immunizations are covered only if they are needed to prevent or treat illness that poses a public health risk (Immigration & Citizenship Canada, 2018). Public health or public safety health care coverage includes vaccines, medications, laboratory and diagnostic services, and doctor and hospital services only if they are needed to diagnose, prevent, or treat a disease that poses a risk to public health or a condition of public safety concern.

## THE UNITED STATES HEALTH CARE SYSTEM

The health care delivery system in the United States is a predominantly market-driven, multipayer, heavily private system that is distinct from any other in the world, serving more than 322 million people (US Department of Labor, 2014). It is a massive system that costs approximately $3.0 billion, or $9255 per person (CMS, 2015a). The health care federal reform law called the *Patient Protection and Affordable Care Act (ACA)* was signed into law on March 23, 2010, requiring the largest change in the financing of the American health care system since public Medicare and Medicaid programs were enacted in the 1960s. The law was designed to expand coverage, control cost, and improve the delivery of health care (Kaiser Family Foundation [KFF], 2013). A core component of the ACA is to address the issues of affordability, accessibility, and financing of health care, with focused efforts on meeting the needs of vulnerable populations.

The number of uninsured Americans younger than 65 years of age was estimated to be 46 million in 2008 and rose as a result of the economic downturn and the growing cost of health plan premiums (KFF, 2012). The 2010 ACA is expected to reduce the number of uninsured individuals significantly with the expansion of Medicaid, subsidies to pay premiums in health insurance exchanges, a federal mandate requiring most legal citizens to enroll in an insurance plan or face tax penalties for nonadherence, and a provision allowing children to remain on their parents' employer family insurance until the age of 26 years. Even with all the new options afforded by the ACA, a number of individuals (e.g., undocumented immigrants) will remain uninsured.

## CASE STUDY

### Health Teaching: Using the Internet to Increase Health Literacy

Ella, age 34 years, has been married for 10 years to her husband Joe and recently moved to a new province with their two children, Billy, age 11 years, and Olivia, age 6 years. Joe just started a new position in a government agency and Ella plans to work 3 to 4 days a week as a home health aide. Joe completed a 2-year community college degree, and Ella took a few college courses but never finished her degree. The family is new to a primary care clinic, and Ella asks the nurse for assistance in enrolling with the provincial health care plan. Ella and her husband would like to have a third child in the next year or so. Joe considers himself healthy and active, although he has had recommendations in the past to lose 14 kg (30 lbs.), is borderline hypertensive, and has slightly elevated blood lipid levels. He has a strong family history of coronary artery disease, and his father died of a myocardial infarction at the age of 65. Ella also struggles with her weight and often relies on fast food for quick dinners on the days she works. Their son Billy has attention-deficit–hyperactivity disorder and Olivia has asthma. Both children are above the recommended body mass index for their ages. The family has a home computer with Internet access, and Ella states she is "getting better at using it as her Grade 6 son is learning computer literacy in school and is teaching Mom."

The nurse discusses the family's general health-promotion and health-protection needs and the special needs presented by the diseases that have been identified. She provides some resources for Ella to learn more about the provincial health plan eligibility criteria and consumer-friendly health information websites.

**Reflective Questions**

- What additional information does the nurse need to assess this family's needs?
- What are the priority area teaching needs for this family?
- What community resources might be available to Ella and her family?
- What are some appropriate websites that Ella might find useful?
Guidelines to assist in choosing the appropriate health care:
- Government of Canada—Health care system: https://www.canada.ca/en/health-canada/topics/health-care-systems.html#wb-cont
- Provincial health care coverage: https://www.sunlife.ca/ca/Insurance/Health+insurance/Personal+health+insurance/Provincial+healthcare+coverage?vgnLocale=en_CA
For health care information on multiple topics:
- Health Canada: https://www.canada.ca/en/health-canada.html
- Public Health Agency of Canada: https://www.canada.ca/en/public-health.html
- Mayo Clinic: http://www.mayoclinic.com/

# SUMMARY

The nursing workforce in Canada, composed of more than 400,000 nurses, 48% of health care providers, is the largest segment of the nation's health care workforce (CIHI, 2019a). In order to move health care forward, nurses need to understand the complexity of the health care system—the structures (federal, provincial/territorial, and local) and the financing mechanisms (public and private)—so interventions can be targeted to reduce health inequities, promote health equity, and elevate the level of health and wellness across the population. The Canadian Nurses Association (CNA, 2012) recognizes that a number of barriers exist that prevent nurses from being able to respond effectively to rapidly changing health care settings and an evolving health care system. Nurses need to be proactive in shaping policy that affects the health care system and need a working understanding of the complexity of the health care system to be able to educate individuals and families about health care resources, to coordinate services, and to influence health care policy at the local, provincial/territorial, and national levels. To accomplish this task, nurses need to become and remain well-informed citizens and health care consumer advocates.

A historical perspective and a description of the current health care delivery system in the Canada provides a framework for the analysis of trends, values, and needs related to health. Awareness of global health indicators sets the stage for the nurse to then compare the health of the nation as a whole. The structure and financing of the health care system, both the public sector and the private sector, are complicated. The influence of health reform for provincial/territorial governments, sparks an opportunity for nurses to be key players in engaging effectively to deliver high-quality evidence-informed nursing care.

## Evolve Chapter Features

http://evolve.elsevier.com/Canada/Edelman/healthpromotion/
- Review Questions

# REFERENCES

Alberta Health Services. (2019). *Injury prevention & safety*. Retrieved from https://www.albertahealthservices.ca/injprev/page11930.aspx.

American Red Cross. (n.d.). *About us*. Retrieved from http://www.redcross.org.

Arias, E., & Smith, B. (2003). Deaths: Preliminary data for 2001. *National Vital Statistics Reports, 51*(5), 1–44.

Barua, B. (2017). *Waiting your turn: Wait times for health care in Canada, 2017 report* (pp. 1–98). Retrieved from https://www.fraserinstitute.org/sites/default/files/waiting-your-turn-2017.pdf.

Barua, B., & Jacques, D. (2018). *Comparing performance of universal health care countries, 2018* (pp. 1–66). Retrieved from https://www.fraserinstitute.org/sites/default/files/comparing-performance-of-universal-health-care-countries-2018.pdf.

Barua, B., Palacios, M., & Emes, J. (2017). *The sustainability of health care spending in Canada 2017* (pp. 1–36). Retrieved from https://www.fraserinstitute.org/sites/default/files/sustainability-of-health-care-spending-in-canada-2017.pdf.

Berry, L., & Curry, P. (2012). *Nursing workload and patient care: understanding the value of nurses, the effects of excessive workload, and how nurse-patient ratios and dynamic staffing models can help*. Ottawa: The Canadian Federation of Nurses Unions. Retrieved from https://nursesunions.ca/wp-content/uploads/2017/07/cfnu_workload_printed_version_pdf.pdf.

Bourgon, L. (2017). *Why women are coming to Canada just to give birth*. Maclean's (August 8). Retrieved from https://www.macleans.ca/society/health/why-women-are-coming-to-canada-just-to-give-birth/.

Canadian Centre for Refugee and Immigrant Health Care. (n.d.). Retrieved from https://www.healthequity.ca.

Canadian Federation of Nurses Unions (CFNU). (2018). *Overview of key nursing contract provisions* (pp. 1–2). Ottawa: Author.

Canadian Institute for Health Information (CIHI). (2018). *In pursuit of health equity: defining stratifiers for measuring health inequality—a focus on age, sex, gender, income, education and geographic location*. Ottawa: Author. Retrieved from https://www.cihi.ca/en/health-inequalities.

Canadian Institute for Health Information (CIHI). (2015). *Trends in income-related health inequalities in Canada*. Ottawa: Author. Retrieved from https://www.cihi.ca/en/health-inequalities.

Canadian Institute for Health Information (CIHI). (2016). *National health expenditure trends, 1975 to 2016* (pp. 1–41). Ottawa: Author. Retrieved from http://www.deslibris.ca/ID/10090272.

Canadian Institute for Health Information (CIHI). (2019a). *Regulated Nurses, 2017*. Ottawa: Author. Retrieved from https://www.cihi.ca/en/regulated-nurses-2017.

Canadian Institute for Health Information (CIHI). (2019b). *How much does Canada spend on health care?* Ottawa: Author. Retrieved from https://www.cihi.ca/en/health-spending.

Canadian Institute for Health Information (CIHI). (2019c). *What are hospitals spending on?* Ottawa: Author. Retrieved from https://www.cihi.ca/en/what-are-hospitals-spending-on.

Canadian Museum of History Online Collection. (n.d.). *A brief history of nursing in Canada from the establishment of New France to the present*. Retrieved from https://www.historymuseum.ca/cmc/exhibitions/tresors/nursing/nchis01e.html.

Canadian Nurses Association (CNA). (2015). *Framework for the practice of registered nurses in Canada* (2nd ed.). Ottawa: Author. Retrieved from https://www.cna-aiic.ca/~/media/cna/page-content/pdf-en/framework-for-the-pracice-of-registered-nurses-in-canada.pdf.

Canadian Nurses Association (CNA). (2012). *A nursing call to action: The health of our nation, the future of our health system. National Expert Commission*. Ottawa: Author. Retrieved from https://www.cna-aiic.ca/en/policy-advocacy/national-expert-commission.

Canadian Nurses Association (CNA). (2009). *Position statement: nursing leadership*. Ottawa: Author. Retrieved from https://www.cna-aiic.ca/-/media/cna/page-content/pdf-en/nursing-leadership_position-statement.pdf.

Canadian Paediatric Society. (2019). *Injury prevention, health promotion, caring for kids new to Canada*. Ottawa: Author. Retrieved from https://www.kidsnewtocanada.ca/health-promotion/ijry#the-burden-of-injury-in-the-immigrant-and-refugee-populationGrenier.

Canadian Patient Safety Institute (CPSI). (2016). *Medication incidents: Hospital harm improvement resource.* Ottawa: Author. Retrieved from https://www.patientsafetyinstitute.ca/en/toolsResources/Hospital-Harm-Measure/Documents/Resource-Library/HHIR%20Medication%20Incidents.pdf.

Canadian Public Health Association (CPHA). (n.d.-a.). *History of public health: Acting on the social determinants of health.* Ottawa: Author. Retrieved from https://www.cpha.ca/acting-social-determinants-health.

Canadian Public Health Association (CPHA). (n.d.-b.). 12 *great achievements.* Ottawa: Author. Retrieved from https://www.cpha.ca/acting-social-determinants-health.

Canadian Red Cross. (n.d.). *What is the Red Cross and how do they help?* Retrieved from http://www.redcross.ca/about-us/about-the-canadian-red-cross/what-we-do-infographic.

Carstairs, S. (2010). *Raising the bar: a roadmap for the future of palliative care in Canada.* Ottawa: Senate of Canada. Retrieved from http://www.chpca.net/media/7859/Raising_the_Bar_June_2010.pdf.

Centers for Disease Control and Prevention (CDC). (2015). *Reported tuberculosis in the United States, 2014.* Washington: U.S. Department of Health and Human Services, CDC. Retrieved from http://www.cdc.gov/tb/statistics/reports/2014.

Centers for Medicare & Medicaid Services (CMS). (2015a). *National health expenditure data: NHE projections 2014–2024: Forecast summary fact sheets 7/28/15.* Retrieved from https://www.cms.gov/Research-Statistics-Data-and-Systems/Statistics-Trends-and-Reports/NationalHealthExpendData/NHE-Fact-Sheet.

Chen, A., Oster, E., & Williams, H. (2014). *Why is infant mortality higher in the U.S. than in Europe? NBER working paper no. 20525.* Retrieved from http://www.nber.org.

Colley, R. (2017). Ten years of measuring physical activity—what have we learned? *StatCan Blog.* Retrieved from https://www.statcan.gc.ca/eng/blog/cs/physical_activity.

Community Health and Empowerment Through Education and Research. (2015). *About CHEER.* Retrieved from http://communitycheer.org/about-us/.

Conference Board of Canada. (2019). *Infant mortality.* Retrieved from https://www.conferenceboard.ca/hcp/provincial/health/infant.aspx#top.

Conference Board of Canada. (2017). *Demand for nursing services challenging to meet as Canada's population ages.* Retrieved from https://www.conferenceboard.ca/press/newsrelease/17-03-14/Demand_for_Nursing_Services_Challenging_to_Meet_as_Canada_s_Population_Ages.aspx?AspxAutoDetectCookieSupport=1.

Correctional Service Canada. (2015). *Public health strategy for offenders.* Retrieved from https://www.csc-scc.gc.ca/002/006/phs-eng.shtml.

Department of Finance Canada. (2011). *Canada Health Transfer.* Retrieved from https://www.fin.gc.ca/fedprov/cht-eng.asp.

Department of Justice Canada. (1985). *Privacy Act, R.S.C., 1985, c. P-21.* Retrieved from https://laws-lois.justice.gc.ca/eng/acts/P-21/.

Di Matteo, L. (2019). *Federal transfer payments and how they affect healthcare funding in Canada. EvidenceNetwork.ca.* Retrieved from https://evidencenetwork.ca/federal-transfer-payments-and-how-they-affect-healthcare-funding-in-canada/.

Doherty, R. (2015). Assessing the patient care implications of "concierge" and other direct patient contracting practices: A policy position paper from the American College of Physicians. *Annals of Internal Medicine, 163*(12), 949–952. https://doi.org/10.7326/M15-0366. Retrieved from https://annals.org/aim/fullarticle/2468810/assessing-patient-care-implications-concierge-other-direct-patient-contracting-practices.

Dunlop, M. E. (2015). *Health policy. The Canadian Encyclopedia.* Retrieved from https://www.thecanadianencyclopedia.ca/en/article/health-policy.

Dying with Dignity Canada. (2019). *Get the facts: Bill C-14 and assisted dying law in Canada.* Retrieved from https://www.dyingwithdignity.ca/get_the_facts_assisted_dying_law_in_canada.

Foot, R. (2019). Senate of Canada. *The Canadian encyclopedia.* Retrieved from https://www.thecanadianencyclopedia.ca/en/article/senate.

Freyman, J. G. (1980). *The American health care system: Its genesis and trajectory.* Huntington, NY: Krieger.

Government of Canada. (2000). *Personal Information Protection and Electronic Documents Act, S.C., 2000, c. 5.* Retrieved from https://laws-lois.justice.gc.ca/eng/acts/p-8.6/s.

Government of Canada. (2008). *E-Health (Personal Health Information Access and Protection of Privacy) Act, SBC, 2008, c. 38.* Retrieved from http://www.bclaws.ca/civix/document/id/complete/statreg/08038_01.

Government of Canada. (2016). *Canada's health care system.* Retrieved from https://www.canada.ca/en/health-canada/services/canada-health-care-system.html.

Government of Canada. (2017a). *Health care in Canada: Canada's universal health care system.* Retrieved from https://www.canada.ca/en/immigration-refugees-citizenship/services/new-immigrants/new-life-canada/health-care-card.html.

Government of Canada. (2017b). *Public health practice.* Ottawa: Public Health Agency of Canada. Retrieved from https://www.canada.ca/en/public-health/services/public-health-practice.html.

Government of Canada. (2017c). *For new immigrants—start your life in Canada.* Retrieved from https://www.canada.ca/en/immigration-refugees-citizenship/services/new-immigrants/new-life-canada/health-care-card.html.

Government of Canada. (2017d). *Canada health act R.S.C., 1985.* Retrieved from https://laws-lois.justice.gc.ca/eng/acts/c-6/page-1.html.

Government of Canada. (2018a). *Overview of national data on opioid-related harms and deaths.* Retrieved from https://www.canada.ca/en/health-canada/services/substance-use/problematic-prescription-drug-use/opioids/data-surveillance-research/harms-deaths.html#s1.1.

Government of Canada. (2018b). *Vaccine uptake in Canadian children: Highlights from childhood National Immunization Coverage Survey.* Retrieved from https://www.canada.ca/en/public-health/services/publications/healthy-living/2015-vaccine-uptake-canadian-children-survey.html.

Government of Canada. (2019a). *Canada Health Act Annual Report 2017–2018 [Acts].* Retrieved from https://www.canada.ca/en/health-canada/services/publications/health-system-services/canada-health-act-annual-report-2017-2018.html#s1.

Government of Canada. (2019b). *Measles and rubella weekly monitoring reports.* Retrieved from https://www.canada.ca/en/public-health/services/diseases/measles/surveillance-measles/measles-rubella-weekly-monitoring-reports.html.

Government of Canada. (2019c). *Vaccination coverage goals and vaccine preventable disease reduction targets by 2025.* Retrieved from https://www.canada.ca/en/public-health/services/immunization-vaccine-priorities/national-immunization-strategy/vaccination-coverage-goals-vaccine-preventable-diseases-reduction-targets-2025.html.

Graff Mcrae, R. (2017). *Blurring the line between public and private health care.* Edmonton: Parkland Institute. Retrieved from https://www.parklandinstitute.ca/blurring_the_line_between_public_and_private_health_care.

Gushulak, B. D., Pottie, K., Roberts, J. H., et al. (2011). Migration and health in Canada: Health in the global village. *Canadian Medical Association Journal, 183*(12), E952–E958. https://doi.org/10.1503/cmaj.090287.

Hassen, P., Hoffman, C., Gebran, J., et al. (2006). *The Canadian Patient Safety Institute: Building a safer system and stronger culture of safety.* (5).

Health Canada. (2006). *Nursing issues: Primary health care nurse practitioners.* (Cat. No.: H21-281/4-2006E.) Ottawa: Author. Retrieved from https://www.canada.ca/en/health-canada/services/health-care-system/reports-publications/nursing/nursing-issues-primary-health-care-nurse-practitioners.html.

Health Canada. (2011a). *Health Canada's role in the management and prevention of harmful medication incidents. MedEffect Canada.* Retrieved from https://www.canada.ca/en/health-canada/services/drugs-health-products/medeffect-canada/medeffect-canada-role-management-prevention-harmful-medication-incidents.html.

Health Canada. (2011b). *Activities and responsibilities: about mission, values, activities.* Retrieved from https://www.canada.ca/en/health-canada/corporate/about-health-canada/activities-responsibilities/mission-values-activities.html.

Health Canada. (2016). *Health Canada-a partner in health for all Canadians.* Retrieved from http://www.hc-sc.gc.ca.

Health Canada. (2018). *Canada's Health Care System.* Retrieved from https://www.canada.ca/en/health-canada/services/health-care-system/reports-publications/health-care-system/canada.html.

Health Canada. (2019). *Canada's dietary guidelines.* Ottawa: Author. Retrieved from https://food-guide.canada.ca/en/.

Henkel, G. (2013). Nurse practitioners, physician assistants play key roles in hospitalist practice. *The Hospitalist, 7.* Retrieved from https://www.the-hospitalist.org/hospitalist/article/125734/nurse-practitioners-physician-assistants-play-key-roles-hospitalist.

House of Commons, Standing Committee on Indigenous and Northern Affairs. (2016). *Breaking point: the suicide crisis in indigenous communities.* Retrieved from http://www.ourcommons.ca/Content/Committee/421/INAN/Reports/RP8977643/inanrp09/inarp09-e.pdf.

Immigration and Citizenship Canada. (2018). *Interim Federal Health Program: Summary of coverage.* Retrieved from https://www.the-hospitalist.org/hospitalist/article/125734/nurse-practitioners-physician-assistants-play-key-roles-hospitalist.

Immigration and Citizenship Canada. (2019). *Asylum claims by year.* Retrieved from https://www.canada.ca/en/immigration-refugees-citizenship/services/refugees/asylum-claims/asylum-claims-2018.html.

Institute of Medicine (IOM). (2014). *Dying in America, improving quality and honoring individual preferences near the end of life.* https://doi.org/10.17226/18748.

Jackson, T., Clemens, J., & Palacios, M. (2017). *Canada's Aging Population and Implications for Government Finances* (pp. 1–36). Vancouver: Fraser Institute.

Kaiser Family Foundation (KFF). (2012). *Kaiser Commission on Medicaid and the uninsured.* Retrieved from https://www.kff.org/about-program-on-medicaid-and-the-uninsured/.

Kaiser Family Foundation (KFF). (2013). *Summary of the Affordable Care Act.* Retrieved from http://www.kff.org/health-reform/fact-sheet/summary-of-the-affordable-care-act/.

Keehn, J. (2015). Is 'concierge medicine' worth the extra cost? *Consumer Reports.* Retrieved from https://www.consumerreports.org/cro/health/concierge-medicine.

Khare, S. R. (2017). Family physician hospitalists: the good and the bad. *McGill Journal of Medicine.* Retrieved from https://www.mjmmed.com/article?articleID=20.

MacDonald, D. K. (2016). *Canadian suicide statistics 2016.* Retrieved from http://dustinkmacdonald.com/canadian-suicide-statistics-2016/.

MacPhee, M., Dahinten, V. S., & Havaei, F. (2017). The impact of heavy perceived nurse workloads on patient and nurse outcomes. *Administrative Sciences, 7*(7). https://doi.org/10.3390/admsci7010007.

MacPherson, D. W., Gushulak, B. D., & Macdonald, L. (2007). Health and foreign POLICY: influences of migration and population mobility. *Bulletin of the World Health Organization, 85*(3). Retrieved from https://www.who.int/bulletin/volumes/85/3/06-036962/en/.

Manitoba Health, Healthy Living and Seniors. (2015). *Injury prevention plan: taking steps to prevent injuries in Manitoba.* Winnipeg: Author. Retrieved from https://www.gov.mb.ca/health/mhsip/index.html.

Manitoba Health. (2017). *The Manitoba Health Services Insurance Plan.* Retrieved from https://www.gov.mb.ca/health/mhsip/index.html.

McKeon, F. (2014). Five of Toronto's most exclusive private medical clinics. *Toronto Life* (February 6). Retrieved from https://torontolife.com/style/health-and-beauty/best-private-medical-clinics-toronto/.

Mental Health Commission of Canada (MHCC). (2012). *Changing directions, changing lives: The mental Health strategy for Canada.* Calgary: Author. Retrieved from https://www.mentalhealthcommission.ca/English/resources/mhcc-reports/mental-health-strategy-canada.

Mental Health Commission of Canada (MHCC). (2016). *Advancing the mental health strategy for Canada: A framework for action (2017–2022).* Ottawa: Author.

Mowat, D. L., & Butler-Jones, D. (2007). Public health in Canada: A difficult history. *Healthcare Papers, 3,* 31–36. Retrieved from https://www.longwoods.com.

National Defence & Canadian Armed Forces. (2012). *Injury reduction strategies booklet.* Retrieved from https://www.canada.ca/en/deartment-national-defence/services/benefits-military/health-support/staying-healthy-active/injury-prevention/reduce-injuries-during-sports-and-physical-activity.html.

Nies, M., & McEwen, M. (2014). *Community/public health nursing: Promoting the health of populations* (6th ed.). St. Louis: Saunders.

Nova Scotia Health. (2009). *Promotion and protection, and injury free Nova Scotia. Nova Scotia's renewed injury prevention strategy: Taking it to the next level.* Halifax: Author. Retrieved from https://novascotia.ca/dhw/healthy-communities/injury-prevention-strategy.asp.

Office of the Privacy Commissioner of Canada. (2019). *Personal information transferred across borders.* Retrieved from https://www.priv.gc.ca/en/privacy-topics/personal-information-transferred-across-borders/.

Office of the Privacy Commissioner of Canada. (2018). *Summary of privacy laws in Canada.* Retrieved from https://www.priv.gc.ca/en/privacy-topics/privacy-laws-in-canada/02_05_d_15/.

Ontario Council of Agencies Serving Immigrants. (2017). *My child was born in Canada, can I just stay in Canada?.* Retrieved from https://settlement.org/ontario/immigration-citizenship/immigrating-to-ontario/immigration-categories/my-child-was-born-in-canada-can-i-stay-in-canada/.

Ontario Ministry of Health and Long-Term Care. (2018). *Injury prevention guideline, 2018.* Toronto: Author. Retrieved from http://health.gov.on.ca/en/pro/programs/publichealth/oph_standards/docs/protocols_guidelines/Injury_Prevention_Guideline_2018_en.pdf.

Organisation for Economic Co-operation and Development (OECD). (2018a). *Infant mortality rates.* Retrieved from http://data.oecd.org/healthstat/infant-mortality-rates.htm.

Organisation for Economic Co-operation and Development (OECD). (2018b). *Life expectancy at birth.* Retrieved from http://data.oecd.org/healthstat/life-expectancy-at-birth.htm.

Pan-Canadian Public Health Network. (2013). *Toward a healthier Canada—2013, 2015, 2017 progress report on advancing the federal/provincial/territorial framework on healthy weights.* Retrieved from http://www.phn-rsp.ca/pubs/index-eng.php.

Pan-Canadian Public Health Network. (2016). *About the Pan-Can adian Public Health Network*. Retrieved from http://www.phn-rsp. ca/index-eng.php.

Parachute Canada. (n.d.). *About Parachute's programs*. Retrieved from https://www.parachutecanada.org/programs.

Public Health Agency of Canada (PHAC). (2010). *The pan-Cana dian healthy living strategy: strengthened pan-Canadian health living strategy framework—2010*. Retrieved from http:// www.phac-aspc.gc.ca/hp-ps/hl-mvs/ipchls-spimmvs/ld2-eng.php.

Public Health Agency of Canada (PHAC). (2018a). *Social determinants of health and health inequalities*. Retrieved from https://www.canada. ca/en/public-health/services/health-promotion/popu lation-health/what-determines-health.html.

Public Health Agency of Canada (PHAC). (2018b). *Key health inequalities in Canada: A national portrait (Executive Summary)*. Ottawa: Author. Retrieved from https://www.canada.ca/en/public-health/services/publications/science-research-data/key-health-inequalities-canada-national-portrait-executive-summary.html.

Public Health Agency of Canada (PHAC). (2018c). *A common vision for increasing physical activity and reducing sedentary living in Canada: Let's get moving*. Ottawa: Author. Retrieved from https://www.canada.ca/en/public-health/services/publications/healthy-living/lets-get-moving.html#ex.

Public Health Agency of Canada (PHAC). (2018d). *Pan-Canadian Health Inequalities Data Tool*. Retrieved from https://health-infobase.canada.ca/health-inequalities/data-tool/index.

Public Health Agency of Canada (PHAC). (2016a). *Health status of Canadians 2016, A report of the chief public health officer* (pp. 1–62). Ottawa: Author. Retrieved from http://healthycanadians.gc.ca/publications/department-ministere/state-public-health-status-2016-etat-sante-publique-statut/alt/pdf-eng.pdf.

Public Health Agency of Canada (PHAC). (2016b). *The direct economic burden of socio-economic health inequalities in Canada: An analysis of health care costs by income level* (Cat. No.: HP35-38/2013E-PDF). Ottawa: Author. Retrieved from https://www.canada.ca/en/public-health. html.

Public Health Agency of Canada (PHAC). (2017a, August 30). *Perinatal Health Indicators for Canada 2017* [Research]. Retrieved from https://www.canada.ca/en/public-health/services/injury-prevention/health-surveillance-epidemiology-division/maternal-infant-health/perinatal-health-indicators-2017.html.

Public Health Agency of Canada (PHAC). (2017b). *Obesity in Canadian adults: It's about more than just weight*. Retrieved from https://infobase.phac-aspc.gc.ca/datalab/adult-obesity-blog-en.html.

Public Health Agency of Canada (PHAC). (2008). *Canadian perinatal health report*. Retrieved from http://www.phac-aspc.gc.ca/publicat/2008/cphr-rspc/pdf/cphr-rspc08-eng.pdf.

Public Health Agency of Canada (PHAC) & Pan-Canadian Public Health Network. (2018). *Key health inequalities in Canada: A national portrait (Executive Summary)*. Retrieved from https://www.canada.ca/content/dam/phac-aspc/documents/services/publications/science-research/key-health-inequalities-canada-national-portrait-executive-summary/hir-executive-summary-eng.pdf.

Purdy, N. M. (2011). *Effects of work environments on nursing and patient outcomes*. Thesis. London, ON: Western University. Electronic Thesis and Dissertation Repository. Retrieved from https://ir.lib.uwo.ca/cgi/viewcontent.cgi?article=1140&context=etd.

Registered Nurses' Association of Ontario (RNAO). (2013). *Best practice guideline: Developing and sustaining nursing leadership* (2nd ed.). Toronto: Author. Retrieved from https://rnao.ca/sites/rnao-ca/files/LeadershipBPG_Booklet_Web_1.pdf.

Rao, D. P., Kropac, E., Do, M. T., et al. (2016). Childhood overweight and obesity trends in Canada. *Health Promotion and Chronic Disease Prevention in Canada: Research, Policy and Practice, 36*(9), 194–198. Retrieved from https://www.ncbi.nlm.nih.gov/pmc/articles/PMC5129778/.

Reid, L. (2017). Concierge, wellness, and block fee models of primary care: ethical and regulatory concerns at the public–private boundary. *Health Care Analysis, 25*(2), 151–167. https://doi.org/10.1007/s10728-016-0324-4.

Reid, J., Hammond, D., Rynard, V., et al. (2017). *Tobacco use in Canada: Patterns and trends, 2017 Edition* (pp. 1–112). Retrieved from https://uwaterloo.ca/tobacco-use-canada/sites/ca.tobacco-use-canada/files/uploads/files/2017_tobaccouseincanada_final_0.pdf.

Rowe, J. (2016). Hospitals explore "queuing theory" to improve patient workflows. *Healthcare IT News*. HIMSS Media. Retrieved from https://www.continuumofcarenews.com.

Rutty, C., Sullivan, S. C., Last, J. M., et al. (2010). *This is public health: A Canadian history*. Retrieved from https://cpha.ca/sites/default/files/assets/history/book/history-book-print_all_e.pdf.

Secretariat for the Intersectoral Healthy Living Network (2005). *The integrated pan-Canadian healthy living strategy* (Cat. No. HP10-1/2005). Ottawa: Author. Retrieved from https://www.canada.ca/en/public-health/services/health-promotion/healthy-living/2005-integrated-canadian-healthy-living-strategy.html.

Sheppard, A. J., Shapiro, G. D., Bushnik, T., et al. (2017). *Birth outcomes among First Nations, Inuit and Métis population. Health Reports, 28*(11), 11–16 (Cat. no. 82-003-X). Retrieved from https://www150.statcan.gc.ca/n1/en/pub/82-003-x/2017011/article/54886-eng.pdf.

Special Advisory Committee on the Epidemic of Opioid Overdoses. (2018). *Highlights from phase one of the national study on opioid- and other drug-related overdose deaths: insights from coroners and medical examiners*. Ottawa: Public Health Agency of Canada. Retrieved from https://www.canada.ca/en/public-health/services/publications/healthy-living/highlights-phase-one-national-study-opioid-illegal-substance-related-overdose-deaths.html.

Stanhope, M., & Lancaster, J. (2012). *Public health nursing: population-centered health care* (8th ed.). St. Louis: Mosby.

Statistics Canada. (2017). *Immigration and diversity: Population projections for Canada and its regions, 2011 to 2036*. Retrieved from https://www150.statcan.gc.ca/n1/pub/91-551-x/91-551-x2017001-eng.htm.

Statistics Canada. (2019a). *Table 13-10-0395-01 Leading causes of death, infants*. Retrieved from https://www150.statcan.gc.ca/t1/tbl1/en/tv.action?pid=1310039501.

Statistics Canada. (2019b). *Leading causes of death, total population, by age group*. Retrieved from https://www150.statcan.gc.ca/t1/tbl1/en/tv.action?pid=1310039401.

Statistics Canada. (2019c). *Physical activity, self-reported, adult, by age group*. Retrieved, from https://www150.statcan.gc.ca/t1/tbl1/en/tv.action?pid=1310009613.

Sutherland, J. M., Repin, N., Crump, R. T., et al. (2012). *Reviewing the potential roles of financial incentives for funding healthcare in Canada* (pp. 1–50). Ottawa: Canadian Health Services Research Foundation. Retrieved from http://www.deslibris.ca/ID/236897.

University of Alabama at Birmingham. (2016). *The life of Florence Nightingale. Reynolds historic library*. Retrieved from http://www.uab.edu.

US Department of Labor. (2014). *Bureau of Labor Statistics: Occupational outlook handbook, fastest growing occupations*. Retrieved from http://www.bls.gov/ooh/fastest-growing.htm.

Victorian Order of Nurses (VON). (2018). *History*. Retrieved from http://www.von.ca/en/history.

World Bank. (2019). *Mortality rate, infant (per 1,000 live births)*. Retrieved from https://data.worldbank.org/indicator/sp.dyn.imrt.in.

World Health Rankings. (2018). *World Life Expectancy website.* Retrieved from https://www.worldlifeexpectancy.com/.

World Health Organization (WHO). (2019). *WHO guideline: recommendations on digital interventions for health system strengthening.* Geneva: Author. Retrieved from https://www.who.int/reproductivehealth/publications/digital-interventions-health-system-strengthening/en/.

World Health Organization (WHO). (2015). *Global tuberculosis report 2015* (20th ed.). Geneva: Author.

World Health Organization (WHO). (n.d.-a) *Global health observatory data repository.* Geneva: Author. Retrieved from http://apps.who.int/gho/data/view.main.680.

World Health Organization (WHO). (n.d.-b). *MDGs: Progress made in health.* Geneva: Author. Retrieved from http://www.who.int.

Yanchar, N. L., Warda, L. J., Fuselli, P., et al. (2012). Child and youth injury prevention: a public health approach. *Paediatric Child Health, 17*(9), 511. Retrieved from https://www.cps.ca/en/documents/position/child-and-youth-injury-prevention.

Yousefi, V., & Chong, C. A. K. Y. (2013). Does implementation of a hospitalist program in a Canadian community hospital improve measures of quality of care and utilization? An observational comparative analysis of hospitalists vs. traditional care providers. *BMC Health Services Research, 13*, 204. https://doi.org/10.1186/1472-6963-13-204.

Yousefi, V., & Wilton, D. (2011). Re-designing hospital care: Learning from the experience of hospital medicine in Canada. *Journal of Global Health Care Systems, 1*(3).

# 4

# The Therapeutic Relationship

*Michelle Funk Borgland, RN, MScN, MHR (Palliative Care)*

Originating US chapter by *June Andrews Horowitz, FAAN, CNS-BC, PMH, RN, PhD*

## INTENDED LEARNING OUTCOMES

*After completing this chapter, the reader will be able to:*
- Evaluate values clarification as a prerequisite for effective health promotion.
- Examine the elements and process of communication.
- Analyze differences between functional and dysfunctional communication.
- Develop strategies to promote therapeutic relationships with diverse populations across clinical settings, contexts, and nursing roles.
- Synthesize knowledge of the therapeutic relationship as an essential component of health promotion.

## KEY TERMS

| | | |
|---|---|---|
| 15-minute interview | Interprofessional communication and teamwork | Reciprocity |
| Bullying | Metacommunication | Reflection |
| Communication process | mhealth | Relational practice |
| Countertransference | Milieu | Relationship stages |
| Distorting | Motivational interviewing (MI) | Self-concept |
| Empathy | Nonverbal communication | Self-disclosure |
| Feedback | Output | Self-esteem |
| Feedback loop | Practical reflection | Telehealth |
| Health literacy | Process | Therapeutic use of self |
| Helping or therapeutic relationship | Proxemics | Transference |
| ihealth | Rapport | Values clarification |
| Input | | Verbal communication |

The therapeutic relationship is the milieu (or context, setting) in which nursing care occurs. Nursing practice is shaped by the caregiver's ability to focus on the interests, concerns, and needs of the individual (Stockmann, 2018). Establishing a therapeutic relationship is critical to problem resolution. The nurse–person relationship comprises the key components of knowing each other, reciprocity, respect, and confidence (Errasti-Ibarrondo, Perez, Carasco, et al., 2015). Even in brief interactions, it is critical to communicate a focus on and concern for the person. A 56-year-old woman who experienced an unexpected myocardial infarction recalls that the clinician who made the most impact on her sat quietly at her bedside for a few moments and made eye contact to discuss what was most important about the woman's rehabilitation plan. What made this brief interaction memorable? It was the clinician's attention to the person who was experiencing the health crisis; it was the quiet pause from the acute care arena activity created by sitting, listening, and making eye contact; it was the clinician's focus on what was most important for the woman's recovery. Across delivery settings, the importance of the nurse–person relationship cannot be forgotten or minimized because of time constraints. As the example shared here illustrates, even episodic brief encounters can have profound effects, as shown in this example. Moreover, in today's complex multicultural and global health care arena, nursing's concentration also extends beyond individuals to populations (Fawcett & Ellenbecker, 2015), yet the same critical elements of the relationship remain.

Particularly in health promotion, the nurse–person relationship is the context for care. Health promotion requires sensitivity to each person's goals and values; the individual's and the nurse's. Health Promotion Canada (2018) has detailed competencies that assist health care providers with a toolkit for students, practitioners, managers, and academic institutions (see https://www.healthpromotioncanada.ca/resources/hp-competencies/). These *Pan-Canadian Health Promoter Competencies* build upon the Public Health Agency of Canada's (PHAC) *Core Competencies for Public Health in Canada* (PHAC, 2017), providing greater detail about the knowledge, skills, and abilities that are necessary for the practice of health promotion. They are specific enough to distinguish the work of health promoters among other public health disciplines and reflect the wide variety of settings and structures of health-promotion practice in Canada. The health-promoter competencies respond to several existing challenges, which include the following:

- The relative importance of health promotion increasing (e.g., increased burden of chronic disease, concern for health inequalities)
- Misunderstanding of the role and best use of health-promoter positions
- Diversity of potential training paths
- A lack of consistency in health-promotion position descriptions
- A need to better align training programs and continuing education with workforce needs (Health Promotion Canada, 2018)

## VALUES CLARIFICATION

### Definition

Values are qualities, principles, attitudes, or beliefs about the inherent worth of an object, behaviour, or idea that guide action by sanctioning certain actions and disavowing others. Values and beliefs are essential factors in design and implementation of nursing interventions. To serve the unique and diverse needs of individuals, it is imperative that nurses understand the importance of cultural differences by valuing, incorporating, and examining their own health-related values and beliefs and those of their health care organizations, for only then can they support the principle of respect for persons and the ideal of transcultural care (Beard, Gwanmesia, & Miranda-Diaz, 2015). Cognitive values are those a person ascribes to verbally and intellectually. Active values, in contrast, are those a person physically acts out. Judging the power of a given value by its ability to influence action is important. For example, a nurse may claim to value the worth of all people equally, but may treat individuals of various races differently and provide the most time and concern for those who are racially similar to the nurse. This cognitive value has little power to shape the nurse's behaviour. If the nurse treated people of all races with equal respect, the value would also be active and have great power to motivate behaviour.

Many forces shape values. Passed down from one generation to another, values colour an individual's identity, goals, and sense of personal meaning. Values are embedded in the culture and taught within a family and social context, giving meaning to the life events and happenings outside the family's boundaries (Balzer-Riley, 2017; Shajani & Snell, 2019). To engage in health promotion, the nurse must appreciate that values are culture

---

**BOX 4.1 The Valuing Process**

**Choosing**
- Choosing freely
- Choosing from alternatives
- Choosing after careful consideration of potential outcomes of each alternative

**Prizing**
- Cherishing and being happy with personal beliefs and actions
- Affirming the choice in public, when appropriate

**Acting**
- Acting out the choice
- Repeatedly acting in some type of pattern

---

**BOX 4.2 Techniques for Assisting Individuals to Clarify Values**

**Identify the Individual's Values**
"What is important to you?"
"Which of the following statements sounds most like the way you think?"
"What do you value most in life?"

**Use Reflection to Restate the Value and Make It Explicit**
"In what you've just told me, I hear that it is very important to you that …"
"I understand that you value …"

**Identify Value Conflicts or Conflicts Between Values and Actions**
"What connection does this value have to your current health or illness and to the healthy behaviours, interventions, or treatments needed to maintain or restore your health?"
"How does this particular value affect your behaviour and health?"
"What are some ways that you might put your values into action?"
"Are your actions consistent with your values? If not, then what might you change?"

---

bound and explore how culture, traditions, and practices in a multiethnic and multicultural society influence health-related values. Without this understanding, the nurse is likely to relate to individuals with a limited awareness of their assumptions and inadequate sensitivity to the uniqueness and perspective of the person, family, or community.

Values evolve; they are not static. Life events and social processes can spark a reappraisal of personal values. Values clarification is a method for discovering one's values and the importance of these values (Drolet & Sauvageau, 2016; Raths, Harmin, & Simon, 1978). Values clarification does not tell a person how to act, but it helps people recognize what values they hold and evaluate how those values influence their actions.

Box 4.1 outlines seven steps in the valuing process. The first three steps involve a cognitive process, the next two steps involve the affective or emotional domain, and the final steps involve behaviour (Raths et al., 1978; Stephany & Majkowski, 2012). The nurse uses values clarification to examine personal values and their potential influence on nursing care, and to help people identify their values and reflect on their connection to health-related behaviours. Box 4.2 lists suggestions for putting

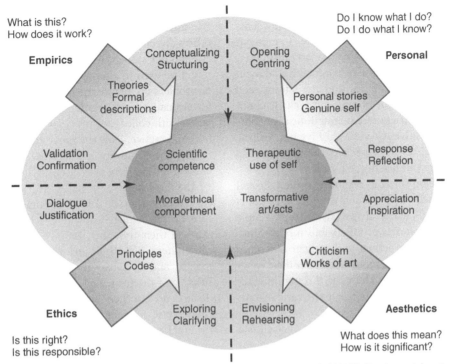

**Fig. 4.1 Fundamental Patterns of Knowing** (Chinn, P. L., & Kramer, M. [2019]. Fundamental patterns of knowing as depicted in *Knowledge development in nursing: Theory and process* [10th ed., Fig 1-2]. St Louis: Elsevier.)

values clarification into action. For a values clarification exercise, try following the steps outlined in Box 4.2 in regard to a personal value. Moreover, values clarification requires exploration of both overt and covert factors that affect our perceptions and actions. The process entails taking a virtual flashlight to shine light on our past and current life experiences to examine the values that shape our attitudes and behaviour.

Values clarification becomes a clinical aim when individuals' values lead to behaviours that conflict with the nurse's value of promoting health. For example, a nurse tells a childbirth education class consisting of pregnant women and their coaches that alcohol use poses serious risks to the fetus. After the class, one woman comments, "Do you really think that having a drink once in a while is bad for the baby? I'm sick of being told that I can't do things because of the baby." In this example, an apparent conflict in values between the nurse and the individual exists. Intervention is needed to examine how this woman's wish for freedom from restrictions clashes with her desire to have a healthy child. Nurses must consider their own values related to health promotion for the individual and the fetus and must weigh the importance of respecting individuals' rights to make decisions about their own health behaviours with potential risks to the fetus. Such value conflicts result in ethical dilemmas. Resolution rests on the nurse's ability to examine conflicting values and available evidence about possible outcomes when fashioning health-promotion interventions. Sharing the evidence to support the clinical recommendation also helps to reduce a judgemental message in the communication and opens communication for discussion about the strength of the evidence

and its practical implications for health behaviours (Waters, Kiviniemi, Orom, et al., 2016).

## Relational Practice

Engaging with patients, families, and communities as nurses is a continual process. How we communicate and "be" with people is a nursing art form. This art form can be called relational practice, as it is essentially how we relate to others in our practice. Nurses develop their relational practice through their ability to navigate the complexity of the human condition, the world, and their nursing practice (Doane & Varcoe, 2015). It is through therapeutic interactions and nursing knowledge that relational interactions occur. Simply, it is the application and embedding of the ways of knowing (Carper, 1978; Fig. 4.1) in the practice area, including ethical knowing, aesthetic knowing, empirical knowing, and personal knowing.

## Values and Therapeutic Use of Self

Therapeutic use of self is the application of one's cognitions, perceptions, and behaviours to create interpersonal encounters that promote health in another person, family, group, or community. Without self-awareness and clarification of values, therapeutic use of self is impaired. Self-concept and self-esteem are interrelated components of individuals' judgements and attitudes about themselves. Self-concept is a mental picture of the self: a composite view of personal characteristics, abilities, limitations, and aspirations. Self-esteem, the affective component of self-perception, refers to how individuals feel about the way that they see themselves. Internalized appraisals from others also influence self-concept and self-esteem.

Self-concept evolves throughout life. From birth, family experiences and parental identification mould the child's sense of identity. Self-esteem is learned from experience. To cultivate children's self-esteem and enable them to have a realistic perception of their strengths and weaknesses, parents should focus on positives, give feedback on abilities and limitations, and provide the child with a sense of belonging and realistic confidence. Positive, rewarding, anxiety-free interactions contribute to security, esteem, and positive self-view. Positive but realistic appraisals from significant others, especially the parents, help the young child to develop this healthy self-view.

The self does not develop solely in response to the reflected appraisals of others. Genetic endowment, experiential opportunities, and the individual's action shape self-concept. People can accept or reject the appraisals of others and modify their behaviour. The ability to control actions and evaluate outcomes of interactions allows individuals to modify and alter their views of self. As such, the self is dynamic, changing through interaction with the outside world and in response to the various maturational and situational crises of life.

The ability to examine, reflect on, and evaluate the self is a uniquely human talent. Self-awareness involves interactions between the self and the external world and the symbolic connections created by the individual. The self includes an unconscious component that is only partially accessible and influences behaviour. Self-awareness is influenced by the degree to which an individual has an accurate concept of all dimensions of the self.

The goal of high self-awareness is reached through three steps. The first step is listening to oneself and paying attention to emotions, thoughts, memories, reactions, and impulses. Frequently, people ignore their feelings and thoughts because they are anxious or because they are in a hurry to accomplish some other task. Without self-reflection, people act automatically and lose some of the meaning of living. To improve the ability of self-reflection, ask questions such as the following:

- What am I feeling now?
- What emotions have I experienced today and in the past day or so? What were my thoughts?
- What events led to these thoughts and feelings?
- What actions did I take? Did my behaviour fit with my thoughts and feelings, or was there a lack of harmony?
- Was I aware of my reactions at the time that they occurred?
- How have I responded in clinical situations lately?
- How did I react in response to a particularly happy, sad, or difficult situation?
- In what way might I alter my actions now?
- What feelings and reactions did I experience while interacting with this individual?

The second step is listening to and learning from others. Feedback from others that conflicts with self-image can produce anxiety. In response, the feedback is ignored or translated incorrectly to preserve self-image and reduce anxiety. However, this pattern of responding limits knowledge of the self and inhibits the ability to examine the appraisals of others, resulting in limited personal growth. Asking reflective questions enables the nurse to use feedback effectively. Helpful questions include "What feedback have I received today?" and "What is the other person trying to tell me now?" A person also can ask others directly for feedback. For example, a student nurse might ask another student how he or she comes across. The feedback might be used to alter aspects of behaviour that are ineffective or problematic before the student nurse asks a faculty member for evaluative feedback. Using clinical supervision and consultation with colleagues provides needed opportunity for reflection on practice. How the nurse comes across to the individual, family, or community is crucial to successful health promotion, making self-awareness and sensitivity to feedback essential.

The third step is self-disclosure; sharing aspects of one's self enriches interpersonal life. Through self-reflection/self-disclosure, people come to know themselves better because they have exposed their thoughts, actions, and feelings for examination with others. Self-disclosure is an indicator of a healthy personality and a strategy for developing one (Steuber & Pollard, 2018). Self-disclosure by one person tends to trigger self-disclosure by another in a reciprocal pattern of interaction. Therapeutic interactions characterized by reciprocity involve a mutual exchange—a pattern of communication between the nurse and an individual, not a one-way intervention from the nurse to the other person. Traditionally, clinicians have been wary of self-disclosure because it may cross a boundary from a professional to a personal relationship. Additionally, the nurse's self-disclosure might burden the individual and shift the focus of attention from the individual to the nurse. Although these guidelines are considered so as to prevent excessive or inappropriate self-disclosure, appreciation that self-disclosure occurs within all human interactions is needed.

Steuber and Pollard (2018) explain that two factors must be taken into consideration: the notion of power, and recognition of the vulnerabilities of patients and families in a health care context. Additionally, the authors cite that nurses decide to self-disclose based on context and the nurse's individual characteristics.

Thus, evidence supports that nurses are not blank screens, robots, or technicians delivering care; individuals value nurses who engage in interactions as real people and who are willing to share information about themselves appropriately and thoughtfully. Seeking consultation from a colleague is helpful whenever a concern arises regarding the limits of appropriate self-disclosure.

Practical reflection (i.e., self-reflection) involves deliberating on one's own thoughts and recollections of events to understand them and to take needed corrective action. In reflection, thoughts are interpreted or analyzed. The process tends to be triggered by a seminal or meaningful event or situation, and the process results in increased understanding or awareness. These insights can then be used in the future when one is faced with a similar event or situation to implement a planned approach. Research outcomes show that self-reflection is associated with lowered practice stress and increased competence among nursing students (Pai, 2015). The process of practical reflection dovetails with steps toward self-awareness previously described and offers complementary helpful tips. First, the nurse recalls an incident when something went wrong. Then, the nurse

- The *public self,* which is shown to others.
- The *semipublic self,* which is seen by others but may be outside the individual's awareness.
- The *private self,* which is known to the individual but is not revealed to others.
- The *inner self,* which is the unconscious portion not known even to the individual because it has anxiety-provoking content.

BOX 4.4  Use Strategies for Communicating Clearly/Enhance Health Literacy Capacity

- *Greet patients warmly.* Receive everyone with a welcoming smile, and maintain a friendly attitude throughout the visit.
- *Make eye contact.* Make appropriate eye contact throughout the interaction.
- *Listen carefully.* Try not to interrupt patients when they are talking. Pay attention, and be responsive to the issues they raise and the questions they ask.
- *Use plain, nonmedical language.* Don't use medical words. Use common words that you would use to explain medical information to your friends or family, such as stomach or belly instead of abdomen.
- *Use the patient's words.* Take note of what words the patient uses to describe his or her illness and use them in your conversation.
- *Slow down.* Speak clearly and at a moderate pace.
- *Limit and repeat content.* Prioritize what needs to be discussed, and limit information to three to five key points and repeat them.
- *Be specific and concrete.* Don't use vague and subjective terms that can be interpreted in different ways.
- *Show graphics.* Draw pictures, use illustrations, or demonstrate what you mean with three-dimensional models. All pictures and models should be simple, designed to demonstrate only the important concepts, without detailed anatomy.
- *Demonstrate how it's done.* Whether doing exercises or taking medicine, a demonstration of how to do something may be clearer than a verbal explanation.
- *Invite patient participation.* Encourage patients to ask questions and be involved in the conversation during visits and to be proactive in their health care.
- *Encourage questions.* Encourage patients to ask questions.
- *Apply teach-back.* Confirm patients understand what they need to know and do by asking them to teach-back important information, such as directions.

experiences the incident again by remembering images and by privately retelling events, statements, outcomes, and associated emotions. Next, the nurse interprets the story of communication that failed by examining expectations, ideals, goals, influences, personal actions, and others' actions that occurred during the event. The last step involves honest inspection of the nurse's own role in the story. Insights gained may be applied to prevent repetition of the problem and to plan future action (Box 4.3).

Why is it important for a nurse to clarify personal values and increase self-awareness? The nurse's values and self-understanding influence behaviour. The self is the nurse's greatest tool: to use the self effectively, the nurse must be fully aware of how it functions. Thus, reflection and self-awareness guide the nurse's practice framework. In addition, sensitivity to individuals' perspectives is required to build a collaborative partnership, the cornerstone of the nurse–person relationship. Helping individuals to explicate their values and direct their actions accordingly toward health-related goals embodies patient-centred care. According to Antonacci, Fong, Sumbly, and colleagues (2018), nurses must be mindful of the various forms of communication and, in doing so, will promote empathic and holistic communication between themselves and their patients, thus promoting a patient-centred approach. Moreover, nurses must "recognize the patient or designee as the source of control and full partner in providing compassionate and coordinated care based on respect for patient's preferences, values, and needs." In today's multicultural society, sensitivity to one's values as a health care provider and those of persons for whom we care becomes crucial to delivery of person-centred effective care (McCaffrey & McConnell, 2015).

## THE COMMUNICATION PROCESS

The communication process is the forum for all thought and relationships shared among people. In conjunction with the use of scientific and technological advances, communication is an essential tool for the nurse to engage in health-promotion interventions. Communication is the foundation for any professional relationship. Nurse–patient communication plays a vital role in the formation and development of the nurse–patient relationship. It is the glue that connects individuals' learning and satisfaction with care (D'Antonio, Beeber, Sills, et al., 2014). Communication is an information exchange between individuals through shared symbols and signs and commonly understood behaviour (Ruesch & Bateson, 1987). This exchange involves all the modes of behaviour that an individual uses, consciously or unconsciously, to affect another person. Communication includes the spoken and written word and nonverbal communication (gestures, facial expressions, movement, body messages or signals, and artistic symbols). Furthermore, communication errors between clinical providers and individuals or their proxies, as well as ineffective communication among, have been identified as a major source of personal and health care delivery safety problems (Box 4.4).

Increasingly, communication is electronic. Telehealth, mobile health (mhealth), or Internet health (ihealth)—the use of telecommunications and data technologies to deliver health care services, including assessment/diagnostic services, treatment, consultation, and health information across platforms—is rapidly growing as a communication/intervention system. Such electronic communication can encompass the spoken and written word, and nonverbal forms of communication. Using technology to engage individuals in clinical communications is already in place, with potential for future development, and brings its own challenges (Haskey, Richmond, Kowalchuk, et al., 2015). Issues of health literacy, as discussed later in this chapter, including access, technology competence, and sensory capacity (such as eyesight and hearing), influence the effectiveness of telehealth as a communication medium.

Thus, clear communication is a major component of promoting an individual's, a family's, and a community's safety and quality care. Yet the format and interface differ from the modes

## INNOVATIVE PRACTICE

### Telehealth/mhealth/ihealth: Therapeutic Relationships in the Age of the Internet

Technological advances have produced rapid changes in communication. Automatic teller machines have replaced human tellers at banks for routine transactions. Voicemail rather than a receptionist routinely answers calls, and messages are recorded electronically. An electronic response to many calls directs the caller to a series of options that may not even include speaking to a person. E-mail, instant messaging, and texting are ubiquitous. Information in many areas is now available via access to a computer and an Internet connection. Wireless Internet (WiFi) access is increasingly used as a perk to lure customers to the local coffee spot and to ease passengers' irritation during long flight delays. Nurses use electronic records and communicate updated information via hand-held devices.

Yet many issues deserve examination as we move into the age of telehealth.

Telehealth or mhealth or ihealth—the use of telecommunications and data technologies to deliver health care services, including diagnostic services, treatment, consultation, and health information—is now omnipresent. Rather than replacing traditional care, telehealth is best understood as a complementary approach to long-distance care delivery, and faster and easily delivered contact. Telehealth has the potential to expand access to care, particularly for individuals receiving home care and those in remote areas, and to contain costs

Technological advances have produced benefits; however, technology can also reduce the need for direct interpersonal contact. Barriers to use include the need for financial investment to establish networks, inadequate reimbursement mechanisms, potential risks to confidentiality with electronic transmission, and licensure issues when care is transmitted across provinces and territories. Challenges include conducting systematic evaluation of outcomes and cost-effectiveness, and ensuring that individuals' economic status and health literacy do not constrain access.

Perhaps the most important threat is that care can become impersonal when face-to-face contact is replaced by an electronic interface. Thus, preserving core nursing values as electronic care systems are created, tested, and implemented is a crucial goal. Innovative practices to safeguard core professional values in the emerging age of telehealth include:

- The avoidance of a "one size fits all" approach through individualized or tailored algorithms and design features specific to the system's use. Moreover, clinician behaviours that facilitate a patient-centred style of communication include using open-ended questions, building partnerships, sharing decision making and information, providing counselling, and using statements of concern, agreement, and approval. This style more successfully addresses individual needs and is associated with greater patient satisfaction, better psychosocial adjustment, and improved health outcomes. Adding opportunities for online questions and answers or an open electronic or telephone chat with a clinician can facilitate tailoring in this delivery approach.
- The development and maintenance of therapeutic relationships by inviting exchanges between the nurse and the person; for example, by creating a series of layered screens that first introduce the nurse (visually and with a biography) and later invite exchanges, feedback, and sharing of experiences and stories from individuals.
- The fostering of individual autonomy by building components that encourage decision making, problem solving, and knowledge development that are timely and specific to the health problem and stage of treatment or management.
- The creation of flexible technology applications that work across a variety of platforms (e.g., computer, smartphone, tablet).

Consider the following questions about telehealth:
- What effects do technological changes have on the therapeutic relationship?
- Will face-to-face interaction become a rare occurrence? In the future, might therapeutic interactions occur primarily via technology, such as voicemail, the Internet, and video-recorded transmission? What advantages and disadvantages will appear with the increasing use of technology in nursing practice?
- What creative approaches may evolve using technology in therapeutic relationships?
- How can electronic communication systems be used in disaster preparedness to alert people at risk and direct actions to increase safety when a human-caused or natural disaster is suspected, imminent, or in progress?

of human communication available until the latter part of the twentieth century and the twenty-first century, and changes will be exponential in the years to come. (For additional discussion, see Innovative Practice.) Social determinants of health can play a crucial role in access to and the effectiveness of Internet-based health information and intervention delivery. Evaluation of Internet-based health education and intervention systems, including access, is a critical goal for translation of research to practice.

In nursing, communication is the cornerstone of a positive nurse–person relationship. Communication refers to a set of strategies and actions to enhance reciprocity, mutual understanding, and decision making. Focusing the clinical discussion on the person's story rather than a version reformulated by the provider is essential to person-centred communication. Box 4.5 highlights strategies associated with person-centred communication based on evidence from the research literature.

Patient-centred communication is one of the key components of patient-centredness when providing care, and represents the most important enabler of patient-centred care (Brouwers, Rasenberg, van Weel, et al., 2017). Studies of patient-centred communication show improved patient satisfaction and

adherence, as well as improved health outcomes, such as reduced levels of discomfort and worry, and better mental health. Furthermore, research findings have indicated that nurses seek communication with individuals that supports openness and engagement of both the nurse and the person to form a bonding factor between them (Tejero, 2011) (Fig. 4.2).

## Function and Process

The following are core functions of communication:
- To obtain and send messages and to retain information.
- To use the information to arrive at new conclusions, to reconstruct the past, and to look forward to future events.
- To begin and to modify physiological processes.
- To influence others and outside events (Ruesch & Bateson, 1987).

Communication transmits information, both interpersonally and intrapersonally, and it provides the basis for action.

The process of communication consists of four components (Watzlawick, Beavin, & Jackson, 1967). Nurses must be able to diagnose communication difficulties in any of these components. Input involves taking in information from outside the individual or group. Once taken in, input must be transformed

## The Mediating Role of Nurse–Patient Dyad Bonding in Patient Satisfaction

### Study Overview

Using a correlational path analytical research design, Tejero (2016) examined the direct and indirect relations of nurse characteristics and patient characteristics to patient satisfaction, as mediated by nurse–patient dyad bonding. A sample of 210 nurses and 210 patients from medical surgery, obstetrics, gynecology, otolaryngology, and ophthalmology units, the trauma ward, and medical critical care units participated in the study. Characteristics of the nurses and patients were gathered through observation, interview, and medical record review. Instruments were used to measure nurse–patient bonding during observation and to measure patient satisfaction with nursing care in the interview. In addition, a checklist was used to collect information on patient complexity, vulnerability, and predictability as well as information on nurse clinical judgement and facilitation of learning.

### Results

The results confirmed the importance of the nurse's role in the formation of a therapeutic dyadic relationship that results in patient satisfaction—a critical part of quality outcomes in health care. Openness and engagement of nurses during interactions were significantly and positively correlated with patient satisfaction. Path analysis showed that nurse facilitation of learning was particularly important in mediating nurse–patient dyad bonding. Nurses' efforts to educate and provide information to patients displayed openness and engagement, which leads to openness and engagement from the patient. The manner, tone, and emotion of the nurse were also shown to affect patient satisfaction.

### Implications

Formation of nurse–patient therapeutic dyadic relationships plays a major role in the quality of patients' experiences. Tejero (2016) stated that a key implication is that the nurse is the healthy individual in the dyad and clinical expert in the interaction, who is obligated to initiate and steer the dyadic relationship toward a therapeutic bond. The findings of this study showed that nurse facilitation of patient learning should be emphasized in practice and in teaching students so as to provide evidence-informed practice and improve patient satisfaction.

Source: Tejero, L. M. S. (2016). Behavioral patterns in nurse-patient dyads: A critical incident study. *International Journal for Human Caring, 20*(3), 129–133. https://doi.org/10.20467/1091-5710.20.3.129.

in some manner to be used. For example, symbols must be translated into words to transmit ideas. The flow and transformation of processed input refers to the way information is analyzed and stored within the individual, or the way it is transmitted from person to person within a human system (group or family) before communication with the external environment occurs. The outcome of information processing, output, involves further exchange with the environment or the other person. A new information exchange is triggered at this point in the cycle by the response called feedback, a monitoring system through which the person or group controls the internal and external responses to behaviour (output) and accommodates these responses appropriately. A feedback loop shows the dynamic nature of communication. Each piece of communication is both a stimulus designed to elicit a response and a response to a different stimulus.

## BOX 4.5 Strategies Associated With Person-Centred Communication

- Permitting people to tell their stories in their own words and chronology.
- Using a conversational interviewing style.
- Being friendly through humour and social conversation, and nonverbal cues such as smiling.
- Eliciting people's views, perspectives, thoughts, wishes, goals, values, and expectations.
- Inquiring about the nature of the person's life.
- Attending to the person's needs.
- Avoiding overemphasis on technical aspects of care and tasks.
- Not being too busy to talk.
- Responding to cues concerning emotional issues and problems.
- Giving information about self-care and participation in decision making.
- Developing mutual understanding.
- Creating collaborative health care plans.
- Showing empathy and concern for the individual's well-being.
- Connecting with individuals through humour, touch, and selective self-disclosure.
- Tuning in to individuals' preferences and style.
- Attending to and advocating individuals' needs.
- Maintaining confidentiality.

Sources: Dziopa, F., & Ahern, K. (2009). What makes a quality therapeutic relationship in psychiatric/mental health nursing: A review of the research literature. *Internet Journal of Advanced Nursing Practice, 10*(1), 1–19; Bolster, D., & Manias, E. (2010). Person-centered interactions between nurses and patients during medication activities in an acute hospital setting: Qualitative observation and interview study. *International Journal of Nursing Studies, 47*(2), 154–165.

When interpersonal communication is analyzed, two types of feedback can be identified: positive (encouraging change) and negative (encouraging homeostasis or no change). Parents' commands to a young child illustrate these types of feedback: positive, "Try that again; you almost had it," and negative, "Don't touch that; it's hot." The first statement shows the parent's attempt to encourage the child to continue new behaviour; the second illustrates an effort to curtail undesired behaviour. Rather than meaning "good" or "bad," positive feedback and negative feedback refer to promotion of system change and stability, which is the process of balancing the direction and magnitude of change. Both types of feedback are needed, depending on the situation.

The situational context of communication is important. The context of communication is the setting's physical, psychosocial, and cultural dimensions. It includes the relationship between the sender and the receiver; their previous experiences, feelings, values, cultural norms, age, and developmental stage; and the physical location.

## Types of Communication

All human communication occurs in three forms: verbal, nonverbal, and metacommunication. Each affects the meaning and influences the interpretation of the message.

### Verbal Communication

Verbal communication is the transmission of messages using words, spoken or written. As symbols for ideas, words impart meaning defined by a specific language. Communicating with language is a critical ability.

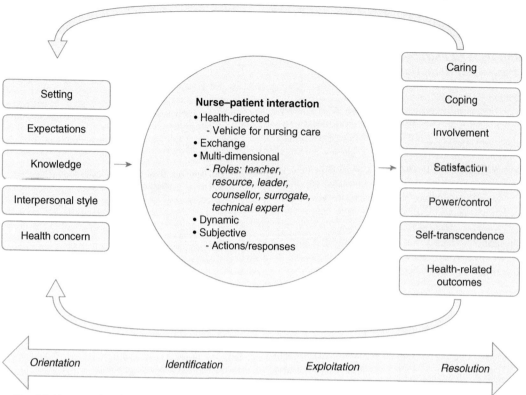

**Fig. 4.2** Nurse–patient interaction has a direct effect on patient satisfaction, and is essential to the provision of nursing care. (From Evans, E.C. [2016]. Exploring the nuances of nurse-patient interaction through concept analysis: Impact on patient satisfaction. *Nursing Science Quarterly, 29*[1], 62-70 [Fig. 1]. https://doi.org/10.1177/0894318415614904.)

People who are deaf or hard of hearing often use sign language to communicate. Signs, similarly to spoken or written words, are used consistently to represent a particular meaning. Words may also be spelled out through finger spelling in a manner parallel to written communication. Braille assists blind and visually challenged people to read. Touch is used to interpret markings that represent letters and words. Sign language and braille blend aspects of verbal and nonverbal communication, but both forms of communication transmit meaning through a consistent language system.

Verbal communication with people who speak a different language poses a challenge. As societies become increasingly multicultural, assistance from specially trained interpreters is essential for the provision of culturally competent care. Most health care facilities, such as major hospitals across Canada, employ interpreters and health care brokers who will guide health care providers in various forms of communication with multicultural patients and families.

Confidentiality issues, the complexity of health information, and the need to validate understandings and reach mutual decisions make it inappropriate to use untrained personnel or relatives to interpret what is meant simply because they are available.

The importance of language development is apparent in its three functions: informing the person of others' thoughts and feelings; stimulating the receiver of a message by triggering a response; and serving a descriptive function by imparting information and sharing observations, ideas, inferences,

and memories (Watzlawick et al., 1967). The ability of verbal communication to fulfill these functions is influenced by many factors, including the communicator's social class, culture, age, milieu, and ability to receive and interpret messages.

## Nonverbal Communication

Nonverbal communication or language encompasses all messages that are not spoken or written. The channels of nonverbal communication are the five senses. Movement, facial and eye expressions, gestures, touch, appearance, and vocalization or paralanguage all constitute nonverbal modes of communication (Blondis & Jackson, 1982). Although all communication has the potential of being misunderstood, nonverbal communication is particularly subject to misunderstanding because it does not always reflect the sender's conscious intent and is highly influenced by culture. Nonverbal messages also tend to be nebulous, without specific beginnings and endings.

Body motion or kinetic behaviour includes facial expression (or facies), eye movements, body movements, gestures, and posture (Blondis & Jackson, 1982). When observing facial expression, the nurse notices the affect or emotion that is communicated. Does the person appear happy or sad; alert, distracted, or sleepy; contented, agitated, angry, or anxious? The degree of emotion expressed should also be noted. Does the person's face express what generally is considered an excessive degree of feeling for the situation, too little, or none at all? Eyes, in conjunction with the movement of other facial muscles, move in ways that convey affect. Eye contact conveys messages of interest or trust; lack of eye contact can imply lack of interest or anxiety; constant eye contact can send a message of hostility.

All of these nonverbal messages are culturally and situationally bound. Nonverbal behaviour, particularly facial and eye expressions, is contextual. For example, in certain circumstances and cultures, avoidance of direct eye contact between some people can be a sign of respect. Yet in other situations and cultures, it can be interpreted as indicative of disinterest, avoidance, or disrespect. Therefore, interpretation requires a cultural lens.

Sign language combines features of both nonverbal and verbal communication. Sign language involves nonverbal communication because, although it uses symbols that are communicated through specific signs, these are enhanced by facial expressions and body postures. However, sign language shares many aspects of verbal communication. It has syntax and grammar, words may be spelled out, and a standard meaning is assigned to specific signs to create symbolic language, just as words share common definitions.

*Importance of nonverbal communication.* Nonverbal communication has great power to transmit information about another's thoughts and feelings; therefore, careful observation is essential. Even silence can be very revealing. The significance of nonverbal communication is best captured by the axiom "actions speak louder than words." Nurses' nonverbal messages that communicate distance from the person, or signal an unfriendly or uncaring attitude, thwart development of a therapeutic relationship (Henry, Fuhrel-Forbis, Rogers, et al., 2012) and thereby render health-promotion efforts unproductive.

## Metacommunication

Besides verbal and nonverbal communication, a phenomenon called metacommunication refers to a message about the message. Watzlawick and colleagues (1967) described metacommunication as the impossibility of not communicating: that is, "one cannot not communicate." Persons transmit a message about what is being communicated even when words are not spoken. Metacommunication is the relationship aspect of communication. In a sense, metacommunication involves reading between the lines or going past the surface content of the message to glean nuances of meaning. When the content and the relationship aspects, or metacommunication aspects, of a message are incongruent, interpreting the communication accurately may be difficult, leaving the receiver uncomfortable and confused.

## Group Process

In group settings, a special type of metacommunication is called process. A basic principle of group theory states that all communication has content and process. Content is what is said; process is the relationship aspect of what is communicated. Group process occurs during every group encounter. Staff meetings and clinically oriented psychoeducation, therapy, and counselling groups always involve group process. For example, consider two individuals in a smoking cessation group who always support each other by agreeing with each other and offering comments or criticism to any group member who disagrees. Although this pairing between the individuals offers them some

protection from anxiety that may result from self-examination and feedback, it isolates them and curtails feedback from others. Examination of this group process is an essential task. The nurse leader and participants can transform this problematic situation into a learning opportunity by identifying the pattern and pointing out the behaviour after it has occurred frequently; helping the pair and other group members consider what needs are being met through this pattern; looking at each person's role in fostering this process (e.g., why other group members have failed to confront the pair); and discussing potential outcomes of changing the behaviour. These steps can be applied in clinical situations when greater self-understanding is a goal.

## Effectiveness of Communication

Understanding what makes communication effective improves the nurse's ability to assess needs and to intervene successfully to promote individuals' health. Steps to functional communication include firmly stating the case, clarifying the message, seeking feedback, and being receptive to feedback when it is received. Implementing these steps to functional communication between nurses and individuals, and between nurses and other care providers, is essential to ensure patient safety and quality care.

To state the case, the sender needs to make the content and the metacommunication congruent; when they conflict, the message is confusing. For example, a nurse is angry with a colleague for making statements to an administrator that undermined the nurse's plans for reconfiguring a health-promotion program in their agency. When the nurse had a chance to speak with this colleague, they exchanged pleasantries without mention of what the nurse thought about the colleague's statements to the administrator. When the colleague asked if something was bothering the nurse, the nurse responded that nothing was wrong. The colleague senses that the nurse's verbal and nonverbal communication did not match; in other words, the content of the message and the metacommunication were incongruent. The colleague was left feeling uneasy, and the nurse failed to express his or her thoughts or to take effective action to rectify the perceived problem with the colleague. To make the communication functional, the nurse needed to bring thoughts and feelings into awareness and reflect on the intended message. Once these steps have been accomplished, the message's content and metacommunication can be adjusted to match, and the nurse's communication is likely to be effective. This example typifies ineffective communications.

To clarify the message, the sender must give a complete message. Important features should be emphasized and specifics of any request must be stated, not assumed. The importance of the message must also be indicated. To illustrate this, a woman mentions to her nurse that it is nearly June. The nurse responds that he has noticed how warm the weather is becoming. On the surface, this communication may seem functional until the intent of the woman's message is considered. She meant to imply that June is the 5-year anniversary of her remission from cancer, and she hoped that her nurse would somehow know that she wanted him to comment on the significance of this anniversary. To make this communication functional, the woman needed to expand the message (e.g., "My anniversary after cancer treatment is coming up"), and then clarify her wish to hear a sensitive response from the nurse (e.g., "This anniversary marks the goal for you to be cancer-free." "What will you do to celebrate?"). Additionally, she needed to show how important the message was (e.g., "I'd really like to do something special to mark this date"). If the nurse had been attuned to the metacommunication in this exchange, he could have clarified this woman's intent and met her need for recognition and dialogue.

One technique for clarifying and qualifying messages is called the "I" statement. Use of "I" statements helps the sender state what he or she wants, feels, thinks, or plans (including likes and dislikes). For example, "I felt unimportant when you forgot to recognize this anniversary" is an "I" statement that the person could have used to communicate effectively. Soliciting such "I" messages is a therapeutic technique to be encouraged.

Questions can clarify and qualify messages, depending on the type of question asked. Open-ended questions tend to elicit descriptive responses rather than one-word answers. For example, the question "Tell me what you did for exercise this week" is likely to yield a more elaborate description of a health behaviour from a person than the question "Did everything go okay with your exercise plan?" However, direct questions that seek a one-word answer are useful when a specific piece of information is sought. "Did you spend 15 minutes or more walking today?" may be a better approach than "What was your activity like today?" when it is important to discuss and promote minimal exercise requirements. Also, for individuals having trouble expressing more than the simplest thoughts, asking direct questions that call for brief replies can be helpful, such as "Did you eat breakfast?" This approach is particularly useful with people who are depressed, regressed, cognitively impaired, or unable to handle complex information or communication at a particular time, or when a specific yes/no response is needed.

Seeking feedback is another element of functional communication. Consensual validation, confirming that both the sender and the receiver understand the same information, calls for the use of the clarification skills just described. In family communication, the parent, as the sender, should model this behaviour for children by asking the child, as the receiver, to explain the sense of the message and how to ask the sender for further explanation. For example, "I want you to clean your room" (message from parent) can be followed by "Tell me how you think you will do that" (validating that the child and the parent agree about what the task entails). This style of seeking validation can be adapted to nurse–nurse or nurse–interprofessional exchanges between colleagues and to therapeutic interactions, and is critical to effective clinical care. Such confirmation in communication is also essential when health-promotion interventions are being provided. Without validating that the person understands the information and its importance, and that the person has a behaviour plan to follow, health-promotion efforts are likely to fail.

Being open to feedback is also crucial. A "no questions" attitude blocks functional communication, whether in the home, classroom, or clinical setting. Children, students, individuals, and even other nurses may be afraid to question anyone in authority or may assume that the person should magically know what is intended or expected. For example, a person may avoid confronting a nurse who fails to explain the clinical plan and then communicates that the person should know how to follow through. Statements by the sender such as "Tell me what you think" and "What is your understanding of what I said?" are helpful in eliciting confirmation of understanding and feedback.

Receiving and sending messages involve many of the same processes. Evaluation of the intent of the message, both the content and the metacommunication, is the first step. The receiver frequently needs to seek clarification and validate understanding of the message for communication to be effective. Clarification of expectations, active exchange of information, power sharing, and negotiation will enhance the quality of nurse–person communication. The outcome is a nurse–person relationship based on trust and partnership, which are critical ingredients of patient-centred care (Adler, Rolls, & Proctor, 2015).

## Interprofessional Communication and Teamwork

Interprofessional communication and teamwork for care design and delivery involve cross-disciplinary education and practice approaches that are now widely promoted as essential to an effective health care system (Lyons, Giordano, Speakman, et al., 2016).

## Factors in Effective Communication
### Listening

Effective listening, an important part of communication, is more than passively taking information. Effective listening is actively focusing attention on the message. Asking questions to explore what is meant helps the listener reach an accurate assessment of the message's meaning.

Many forms of nonverbal communication have been identified that, from a Western or European perspective, commonly convey that the person is listening. These nonverbal communications include direct gazing and eye contact, head nodding, orienting one's body to maintain interpersonal closeness, leaning forward, making facial expressions such as eyebrow animation and smiling, and using brief verbal statements that indicate interest, such as "Please go on" or "Tell me more about that."

For behaviour to communicate that the person is listening also depends on the context and intensity of the activities, and the cultural norms of each person. For example, leaning close to a person might be interpreted as intrusive. Yet the same behaviour could be seen as a sign of support, depending on the context and perspective of those involved. Sensitivity to nuances in communication and validation of meaning can be particularly helpful strategies when the nurse and the person come from different cultural backgrounds.

Reciprocity, the patterning of similar activities within the same interval by two people, can help the nurse communicate a listening stance in an effective way. When the nurse matches nuances of the individual's type and style of behaviour, the chances that the person will interpret the nurse's behaviour as an indication of active listening are increased, and the likelihood of misinterpretation is reduced. Nurses can enhance the quality of their communication, even when encounters are brief, by attending to reciprocity in their interactions and by validating whether or not reciprocity is associated with shared interpretations of meaning.

Poor listening blocks the nurse's understanding of the person. The nurse's failure to listen may be caused by anxiety; focus on other demands; lack of experience, which leads to excessive talking by the nurse; preoccupation with personal thoughts; or lack of practice. Examples of poor listening skills include pseudo-listening, stage-hogging, insulated listening, defensive listening, ambushing, and insensitive listening (Adler et al., 2015). Pseudo-listeners appear to be making eye contact with the speaker but their thoughts and mind are elsewhere (e.g., composing a grocery list in their heads). Stage-hoggers are known to interrupt the conversation with their own examples of the spoken topic, or will attempt to turn the conversation onto themselves as opposed to showing interest in the speaker. Selective listeners do not take in the entire conversation, but instead "select" what they want to hear and only respond to what they wish to address.

When discussing bad news or a poor prognosis with a patient, sometimes the patient may only hear the first few words or phrases when spoken by the nurse. An example of this may be the initial assessment a nurse performs prior to a miscarriage or cancer diagnosis. Difficult news is hard to hear, and people may hear only portions of the information. This is called insulated hearing or listening.

Defensive listening is common with adolescents, as they may believe that their parent or caregiver is trying to get in their business or is being "nosey." Defensive listeners think that someone is attacking them personally and project their insecurities on the speaker. Ambushers hang onto every word from the speaker, gathering information to use against the speaker. One can point out an insensitive listener by reading their body language and other nonverbal cues, such as eye rolling or a genuine disinterest in what the speaker is communicating (Adler et al., 2015).

## Flexibility

Flexibility is a balance between control and permissiveness. In "overcontrol," every message is monitored. In exaggerated permissiveness, anything can be communicated in any way. For communication to be functional, rules are needed about what is appropriate, without rigid prescriptions that inhibit meaningful interchange. For example, the guideline that nurses will not answer questions concerning intimate details of their lives sets an appropriate limit; however, this does not mean that nurses should refuse to answer any question about themselves.

## Silence

Silence between people is often uncomfortable for the nurse who is somewhat insecure about what should occur during a therapeutic encounter. However, silence can be beneficial when used carefully. When one is seeking a verbal response, silence can be perceived as a lack of interest. At other times, silence allows individuals to reflect on what is being discussed or experienced, lets them know that the nurse is willing to wait until they are ready to say more, or simply provides them with comfort and support. Each situation needs evaluation and sensitivity. Rather than asking a flurry of questions to break the silence, the nurse allows the person time to decide when to comment or should make brief comments that do not demand answers, such as "It can be helpful to take time to think about what we've been discussing." Also, comments such as "Try putting your thoughts or feelings into words" and "I am here when you are ready to talk" can help the person to share these thoughts or feelings when silence is blocking rather than improving the communication.

## Humour

Humour is part of being human; it relieves tension, reduces aggression, and creates a climate of sharing. Humour can block communication when it is used to avoid subjects that might be uncomfortable or when it excludes other people. Humour can also inflict emotional pain and communicate negative views or stereotypes about particular individuals or groups through teasing and jokes concerning race, ethnicity, culture, country of origin, occupation, age, sex, sexual activity, or other traits that stand out or are devalued. A direct response to the latent content or message in this type of humour is an effective way to curtail its use and minimize its effect. For example, a response that shows disapproval of the latent message such as "That kind of joke makes me very uncomfortable. I don't find it funny to describe [the specific group in question] that way, and I would like you to stop" will send a clear message and be likely successful in stopping the offensive communication. In contrast, for humour to be helpful the meaning of the humour must be understood and its purpose supportive to the individual. Clarification of the meaning should be used when there is doubt or concern.

## Touch

Touch is an interesting means of nonverbal communication for nurses, who often touch individuals while administering care. The nurse's concern can be expressed by a gentle or soothing application of touch. Nevertheless, in some instances touch is inappropriate. For example, in interactions with individuals who have trauma histories or acute psychiatric disturbances, touch might be misinterpreted. A woman who has been raped might interpret touch during an examination as an attack. Evaluation of the context and meaning of touch to the individual is based on knowledge of that person and interpretation of feedback. Informing the individual about the purpose of touching and asking for permission and feedback are useful techniques to avoid unintended distress or misinterpretation of touching in a clinical encounter.

## Space

Space between communicators varies according to the type of communication, the setting, and the culture. Hall (1973) researched proxemics, the use of space between communicators, and identified four zones of space commonly used in interaction in North America; these are presented in Box 4.6 and Fig. 4.3. It is critically important for nurses to be sensitive to how spatial zones vary across cultures when caring for persons from diverse backgrounds.

Understanding the appropriate distance for a given type of interaction helps the nurse to make nonverbal and verbal communication congruent and to avoid violating spatial norms. Awareness of cultural customs concerning distance is important in shaping communication and interpreting the behaviour of others. When people from different cultures or groups communicate, there may be discomfort about the acceptable distance between them when speaking. Recognition of differences helps the nurse adjust the distance and interpret the meaning of this nonverbal communication.

---

**BOX 4.6   Zones of Space Common to Interaction in North America**

1. *Intimate space:* up to 45.5 cm (18 in.); used for high interpersonal sensory stimulation (see Fig. 4.3A).
2. *Personal space:* 45.5 cm to 1.2 m (18 in to 4 ft); appropriate for close relationships in which touching may be involved and good visualization is desired (see Fig. 4.3B).
3. *Social-consultative space:* 2.7 to 3.6 m (9 to 12 ft); less intimate and personal, requiring louder verbal communication (see Fig. 4.3C).
4. *Public space:* 3.6 m (12 ft) or more; appropriately used for formal gatherings, such as giving speeches (see Fig. 4.3D).

Source: Hall, E. (1973). *The silent language*. Garden City, NY: Doubleday/Anchor Press.

---

Many traits and components discussed in this chapter characterize functional communication. However, communication is a subtle and intricate process. Communication cannot be reduced to a set of parts and principles; its roles and nuances are far more complex and variable. Communicating by language and symbols is a special human ability. Healthy communication enables people to move from being alone to being together—clearly one of the crucial tasks of living. Effective communication is also the foundation for the helping relationship.

### Health Literacy

Clear communication improves the quality of health care encounters. Health literacy—the capacity to read, comprehend, and follow through on health information—is a critical component of health promotion. Increasingly complex health care systems require individuals to assume a high degree of autonomy and employ self-management strategies to achieve their best health. Health literacy is one primary skill that is useful in navigating such complex systems (Jimenez, 2018.).

Nurses also promote health literacy by creating a safe and comfortable environment, sitting to establish eye contact rather than standing when communicating, using visual aids and models to illustrate conditions and procedures, and verifying

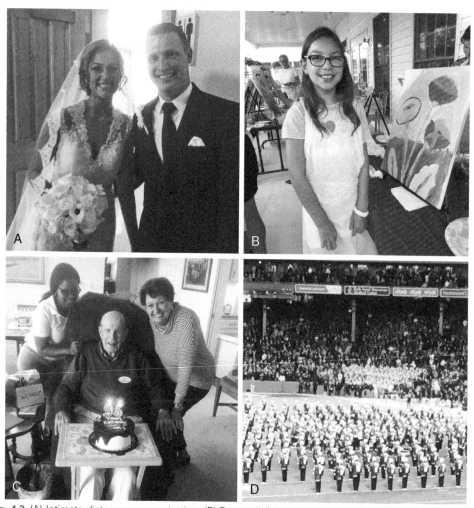

**Fig. 4.3** (A) Intimate distance communication. (B) Personal distance communication. (C) Social-consultative distance communication. (D) Public distance communication.

understanding of care instructions by having individuals then teach the content: that is, using "teach-back" as a strategy (Speros, 2011). Resources are available to help nurses and other clinicians to increase individuals' understanding of health information across health literacy levels. In Canada, the Literacy Volunteers of Quebec published *A Health Literacy Tool Kit for Health Care Providers: Improving Communication with Clients* (see http://www.literacyquebec.org/uploads/1/0/1/0/10106734/introduction_lvq_health_literacy_tool_kit.pdf). This funded kit was authored by Kate Strickland in 2011, who titled her project, *A Teaspoon of Literacy Makes the Medicine Go Down: Facilitating Access to Health and Social Services for People Living with Low Literacy.*

Three key factors regarding health literacy to consider are the educational level of the target audience or users; the reading/comprehension level for materials in online, verbal, or written format; and the native language of the target audience or users. A highly educated target audience generally has high health literacy because of strong command of the native language being used. Research evidence has shown that health information in use may be at a reading level above the comprehension level (i.e., at a Grade 9 level) of the users. Furthermore, nurses need to assess comprehension of all health information and instruction, particularly of complex medical/health information. Developing materials at the Grade 5 or 6 reading level helps ensure that comprehension is very likely across wide ranges of the target audience. Word processing programs and online tools can evaluate the reading level of text. Published materials also are available to help in assessing and developing appropriate content (McKenna & Stahl, 2015). These available resources enable nurses easily to determine the reading level of all health and research materials, and to adjust the level by changing complex terms to more commonly used words with only one or two syllables and simplifying sentences to avoid complex construction with multiple phrases. Finally, adjusting word usage to avoid native colloquialisms will increase understanding among persons whose native language is not being used. Moreover, advocating the development and/or revision of existing materials to reach a Grade 5/6 reading level is an appropriate nursing mandate.

In the emerging age of telehealth, developing strategies for confirming understanding and individualizing methods of communicating health information is increasingly important (see Innovative Practice box, earlier). Health information and even access to appointments are steadily shifting from face-to-face interaction to access by telephone via voice prompts and Internet-based formats. Many factors involved in health literacy can impair individuals' ability to understand and respond to audio and/or visual commands. Consider the array of commands involved in the typical automated telephone system involved in ordering a prescription refill from a typical pharmacy. The individual must select from a list of options; next, multiple numbers must be keyed in that represent prescription numbers listed in small print from a prescription label and birthdays in appropriate format; finally, a variety of confirmations must be entered. Persons with auditory, visual, language comprehension, and/or cognitive limitations may not have adequate capacity to manage

such common health care technologies. Therefore technology competence becomes another component of health literacy to be considered. However, telehealth has seen success in Canada, and in particular in British Columbia with "The Stroke Coach," which is a long-term program to assist stroke survivors with health and behaviour change. This particular telehealth protocol involves a telephone-based and self-management program (Sakakibara, Lear, Barr, et al., 2017).

## THE HELPING OR THERAPEUTIC RELATIONSHIP

A helping or therapeutic relationship is a process through which one person promotes the development of another person by fostering the latter's maturation, adaptation, integration, openness, and ability to find meaning in the present situation (Peplau, 1969; D'Antonio et al., 2014). The therapeutic relationship emerges from purposeful encounters characterized by effective communication. In this relationship the nurse respects the individual's values, attends to concerns, and promotes positive change by encouraging self-expression, exploring behaviour patterns and outcomes, and promoting self-help (Doss, DePascal, & Hadley, 2011). The therapeutic relationship is the foundation of clinical nursing practice (D'Antonio et al., 2014)—the essential element of quality care with every individual in every situation (QSEN, 2012). Techniques, technology, interventions, and contexts differ, but the relational aspect of nursing practice produces a cohesive unity, allowing each nurse to see people holistically and as unique individuals. Although many components of the helping relationship are most germane to relationships that extend over time, the essentials of the helping relationship apply to even brief therapeutic encounters.

No perfect profile or personality of a helping person exists. However, certain traits can be nurtured without thwarting the nurse's unique personality. These characteristics enable the nurse to be an agent of therapeutic care (Peplau, 1963; Stuart, 2012). Box 4.7 lists characteristics associated with therapeutic effectiveness.

### Characteristics of the Therapeutic Relationship

No recipe is available for a successful therapeutic relationship. Techniques and concepts serve only as tools. As a nurse develops

---

**BOX 4.7  Characteristics Associated With Therapeutic Effectiveness**

- Self-awareness and self-reflection
- Openness
- Self-confidence and strength
- Genuineness
- Concern for the individual
- Respect for the individual
- Knowledge
- Ability to empathize
- Sensitivity
- Acceptance
- Creativity
- Ability to focus and confront

and evaluates a helping relationship, be it long term or brief in nature, the following guidelines may be useful.

## Purposeful Communication

Purposeful communication means that the nurse focuses communication toward a particular goal. Social chitchat, communication without a goal, should not make up the bulk of therapeutic interaction. This does not mean that the nurse should never discuss a social topic; nonetheless, there should be some purpose. For example, discussing the weather with a somewhat disoriented older individual serves the purpose of orienting that person to the environment. Discussing the Stanley Cup with a hockey fan may provide valuable assessment data and engage the person in a current topic of social interest. Goals guide the nurse in focusing communication.

## Rapport

Rapport is a harmony and an affinity between people in a relationship. By using many of the traits listed for helping a person, the nurse can establish an atmosphere in which rapport can develop. To let the person know that his or her concerns interest the nurse and that working together may alleviate some of his or her difficulties and encourage growth, it is important to be genuine, open, and concerned.

## Trust

Trust is a necessary component of any helping relationship. Trust is the reliance on a person to carry out responsibilities and promises, based on a sense of safety, honesty, and reliability. Trust is an important component of partnership. The nurse promotes trust by modelling and structuring the relationship appropriately. The following strategies promote trust:

- Anticipating that the individual will do as promised.
- Clearly defining the relationship parameters and expectations, particularly the purpose and specifics of time, place, and anticipated behaviour.
- Being consistent.
- Examining behaviours that interfere with trust.

## Empathy

Empathy is the ability to understand another's feelings without losing personal identity and perspective. Empathic nurses draw on emotions and experiences that enable them to place themselves in the other person's situation. While the person senses increasing understanding and acceptance from the nurse, the individual's distress decreases. Outcomes from research studies are building knowledge about the role that empathic nursing care plays in outcomes. Nurses learn behavioural approaches that enhance empathic relations with people through supervised experiential learning (Haskey et al., 2015). For example, nurses do not empathize by switching the focus of the interaction to themselves or by sympathizing (e.g., "I know exactly how you feel; that happened to me once"). Rather, they use clinical and personal experience to appreciate the individual's feelings and experiences: they try to imagine themselves in the person's situation. Using personal founderstanding based on some shared aspect of experience such as a loss while maintaining boundaries

is the essence of empathy in the helping relationship. With empathic understanding, the nurse acknowledges the affective domain of personal experiences and uses this knowledge to appreciate the person's reactions. Empathy enables the listener to share human experiences as the basis for providing care.

## Goal Direction

A helping relationship is special in its goal-directed nature. Although most human relationships focus on mutual benefit, a helping relationship exists solely to meet some need or to promote the growth of the recipient. Although the nurse may benefit from the interaction, the relationship is centred on the recipient.

Goals are formulated as desired individual behaviours/outcomes. Short-term goals are likely to be achieved within 10 days to 2 weeks; all other goals are long term. All goals should be stated in measurable terms and should focus on a positive change or on the decrease of problematic behaviour/health indicators. Ideally, a person works with the nurse to establish goals. However, some individuals, such as those who are seriously ill, depressed, psychotic, or cognitively impaired, may be unable to establish mutual goals. When an individual is unable to negotiate appropriate goals, the nurse establishes realistic goals and shares them to the degree possible with the person, who is free to participate or to reject efforts to reach these goals. In some circumstances when the care recipient is unable to collaborate regarding care decisions, then a family member or another designee/health care proxy may be the appropriate person for such communication.

## Ethics in Communicating and Relating

Ethical decision making is closely linked with the goal-directed nature of helping relationships. Ethical issues are present in human interactions whenever behaviour may affect others, whenever actions involve conscious choices of methods and ends, and whenever actions can be evaluated in reference to standards of right and wrong (Holmes, 2014). Guidelines that may be adapted as ethical standards for interpersonal communication are highlighted in Box 4.8.

Frequently, the nurse may wish to set goals that the individual does not want to reach; the nurse must remember that the problem belongs to the person, as does the choice of care alternatives. The nurse assists the individual in decision making, with the decision based on the individual's value system. However, the nurse should not take a laissez-faire approach and avoid assisting the person. The nurse's responsibility is to help the individual to examine values, identify conflicts, and prioritize goals and desired health care outcomes. Action follows from understanding values and the best available information. Both the individual and the nurse must bring interpreted facts and personally clarified values to the interaction to establish goals. Recognizing this interplay, the nurse must clarify personal values, subsequently respect the individual's rights, and act to support and protect the integrity of the person, family, group, or community.

Ethical communication also involves safeguarding protected health information. The individual's right to privacy motivated

## BOX 4.8 Guidelines for Ethical Interpersonal Communication

Ethical interpersonal communication involves:
- Being aware and open to changing concepts of self and others.
- Attending to role responsibilities; individual sacrifice, when it is required to make a "good" decision; and emotions, while guarding against letting emotions be the sole guide of our behaviour.
- Sharing personal views candidly and clearly.
- Communicating information accurately, with minimal loss or distortion of intended meaning.
- Communicating verbal and nonverbal messages with congruent meanings.
- Sharing responsibility for the consequences among communicators.
- Recognizing the multicultural context of all communication.
- Respecting the dignity of every person.
- Avoiding coercion and use of power in communicating.
- Being sensitive to gender and cultural contexts of communication and interpretation.
- Building context for intercultural dialogue that is open with conditions of security and mutual respect.
- Eliminating any elements of your communication that denigrates, stereotypes, or devalues patients.
- Facilitating open and accurate communication among professional groups, professionals, staff and families, clinical care unit and department staffs or administrators, and clinical care facilities.

Unethical communication involves:
- Purposefully deceiving.
- Intentionally blocking communication—for example, changing subjects when the other person has not finished communicating, cutting a person off, or distracting others from the subject under discussion.
- Scapegoating or unnecessarily condemning others.
- Lying or deceiving that causes intentional or unintentional harm.
- Verbally "hitting below the belt" by taking advantage of another's vulnerability.
- Violating the standards of practice as set out by the provincial governing bodies and the Canadian Nurses Association (CNA) *Code of Ethics*.

the passage of the *Personal Information Protection and Electronic Documents Act,* which was established in 2004 and which is supported and endorsed by all provincial governing bodies, as well as by the CNA *Code of Ethics*.

Information that is protected by law includes demographic data that relates to the individual's past, present, or future physical or mental health or condition; the provision of health care to the individual, or the past, present, or future payment for the provision of health care to the individual; and information that identifies the individual or for which there is a reasonable basis to believe can be used to identify the individual. Individually identifiable health information includes many common identifiers (e.g., name, address, birth date, Social Insurance Number).

Sharing personal health information (PHI) can be understood on the basis of "need to know" so as to care for the person. Stuart's (2012) concept of the circle of confidentiality provides a helpful guideline to nurses:

*Within the circle, patient information may be shared. Those outside the circle require the patient's permission to receive*

*information. Within the circle are treatment team members, staff supervisors, health care students and their faculty (only if they are working with the patient), and consultants who actually see the patient.*

Adhering to the rules concerning protection of identifiable health information is both an ethical and a legal requirement for the nurse.

## Therapeutic Techniques

Occasionally, clinicians who are novices in establishing helping relationships assume that they are bound to "say the wrong thing" and cause terrible damage to the person, or that they will learn some magical phrases and questions to create instant rapport. No nurse or other professional is so powerful that a "wrong word" will destroy the individual's self-concept or self-esteem. Even people with physical and emotional problems are resilient and have coped, at least to some degree, with a lifetime of stresses. Alternatively, no magical saying exists that the nurse can always plug into an interaction to communicate successfully. Although some techniques are often useful, they must be applied with purpose, skill, and attention to the individuality of each person and to the context of the interaction. The following techniques, therefore, should be viewed as guidelines rather than prescriptions for effective shaping of the therapeutic relationship.

### Focus on the Individual

The first step to therapeutic communication is focusing on the individual and the reason that the interaction is occurring. The nurse is not the focus; the person is. Although an overly business-like style fails to communicate concern and support, delving into one's own personal life to the extent that it diverts attention from the other person's concern is also problematic. Avoiding nurse-directed conversation can be difficult; a useful rule of thumb is to answer or respond to obvious questions and to switch the focus back to clinical concerns when other questions are asked. For example:

Individual (*looks at female nurse's wedding ring*): *"Are you married?"*
Nurse: *"Yes, I am."*
Individual: *"What does your husband do for a living?"*
Nurse: *"Rather than get distracted by a discussion about me, let's get back to planning how you will manage at work."*

Keeping focus on the person's concerns includes identifying the portion of the message that is clear and relevant to the purpose of the interaction, seeking validation, and helping the individual to clarify the rest of the message.

### Help the Individual to Describe and Clarify Content and Meaning

Too often the nurse rushes to offer an interpretation of the nature of the problem and quickly follows up by suggesting a solution. Solving problems efficiently makes the nurse feel effective, important, and powerful; however, the person's needs may not be met. A crucial step in using the therapeutic relationship effectively is to assist the individual to describe a particular experience or concern. Description is enhanced when the nurse prompts the person to clarify the description and interpret its meaning.

Use of who, what, where, and when questions helps the person to clarify and expand the content and meaning of what is communicated. Phrases such as "tell me," "go on," "describe to me," "explain it to me," and "give me an example" are also likely to elicit description of important content and to diminish distracting generalizations and abstractions. By seeking feedback, the nurse helps the individual to explain the meaning further. In clarifying the meaning, the nurse should avoid threatening, detective-like questions. Questions that begin with "why" often increase the person's anxiety because they demand reasons, conclusions, analysis, or causes (Peplau, 1964). Reformulating questions to obtain descriptive data first and then helping the individual to analyze links among events, thoughts, feelings, actions, and outcomes is generally a more helpful approach.

A problem-solving approach by the nurse assists the person to describe and clarify the content and meaning of experience. Sequential steps help the individual to explain events, to change circumstances and responses that interfere with health, and to solve problems (D'Antonio et al., 2014; O'Toole & Welt, 1989; Peplau, 1963). This problem-solving approach can be adapted for use in health promotion to assist the person in problem solving by working through the steps outlined in the Quality and Safety Scenario box. These steps are a useful guideline for keeping the focus of concern on the individual and his or her definition of the problem. Rather than telling the person what is wrong and how to fix it, the nurse's primary goal is helping the person to describe the problem and formulate solutions in partnership. The cyclic nature of the process is illustrated in Fig. 4.4.

## Use Reflection

Reflection is the restatement of what the individual has said in the same or different words. This technique can involve paraphrasing or summarizing the person's main point to indicate interest and to focus the discussion. Effective use of this approach does not include frequent, parrot-like repetition of the individual's statements. Instead, reflection is the selective paraphrasing or literal repetition of the person's words to underscore the importance of what has been said, to summarize a main concern or theme, or to elicit elaborated information. In addition, to verify understanding of health information, the nurse can ask the person to restate what has been communicated. Failure to confirm understanding interferes with desired clinical care outcomes.

## Use Constructive Confrontation

Confronting an individual means that the nurse points out a specific behaviour and then helps the person to examine the meaning or consequences of the behaviour. For example:

Nurse: *"You missed your appointment for the consultation we had scheduled."*

---

### ⚡ QUALITY AND SAFETY SCENARIO

#### *Steps in Promoting Problem-Solving*

**Describe the Experience or Event of Concern**
*Helpful Verbal Nursing Strategies*
"Tell me what happened."
"Describe the experience to me."

**Analyze the Parts of the Experience and See the Relationships to Other Events**
*Helpful Verbal Nursing Strategies*
"What meaning does this have for you?"
"What pattern is there?"

**Formulate the Problem**
*Helpful Verbal Nursing Strategies*
"In what way is this problematic?"
"What do you want to see changed?"

**Validate the Formulation**
*Helpful Verbal Nursing Strategies*
"Do you mean …?"
"Let me tell you what I understand you to be saying."

**Use the Formulation to Identify Ways to Solve or Manage the Difficulty**
*Helpful Verbal Nursing Strategies*
"What would you do the next time?"
"In what way has your view changed?"
"What actions are needed to solve the problem that you've identified?"

**Try Out the Solutions, Judge the Outcomes, and Adjust the Plan Accordingly**
*Helpful Nursing Strategies*
Encourage application in new situations through role playing or through practice in appropriate settings; help the individual cycle through the preceding sequence as needed to evaluate the outcome and make adjustments to the plan.

Source: Peplau, H. E. (1963). Process and concept of learning. In S. Burd, & M. Marshall (Eds.), *Some clinical approaches to psychiatric nursing* (pp. 333–336). New York: Macmillan.

---

Individual: *"Oh, I didn't notice the date."*
Nurse: *"You are usually very aware of time and appointments. What do you think was going on with you that you didn't notice the date this time?"*

This type of confrontation is not an angry exchange but a purposeful way of helping the person examine personal actions and their meaning.

## Use Nouns and Pronouns Correctly

Some individuals have difficulty separating themselves from others or specifying the object or subject in their language. These individuals misuse pronouns by referring to we, us, they, she, he, him, and her, without clearly identifying the referent, and by making vague statements such as "They don't like me. They told me I was useless." Others may use general nouns, such as everyone, people, doctors, and nurses, to avoid clear

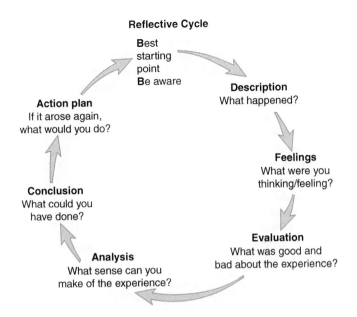

**Reflective Cycle**

**Be**st starting point
**Be** aware

**Description**
What happened?

**Feelings**
What were you thinking/feeling?

**Evaluation**
What was good and bad about the experience?

**Analysis**
What sense can you make of the experience?

**Conclusion**
What could you have done?

**Action plan**
If it arose again, what would you do?

**Fig. 4.4 The Process of Reflection** The reflective process is illustrated here with entry at any point to examine events, associated thoughts, and feelings, and analysis with a goal of understanding the events and one's reactions/actions as well as formulating a plan for responding effectively to similar events in the future.

communication about specific persons. The nurse can clarify the meaning by asking, "Who are they?" or "Who is the person?" Additionally, the nurse must be careful to use separate pronouns when speaking of herself or himself and the individual, particularly when the person has disordered thinking. For example, when communicating with an individual who is confused or exhibits disordered or psychotic thinking, the nurse should say "you" and "I," rather than "us" or "we," to promote clear thinking and communication and to assist the individual to maintain personal boundaries (Peplau, 1963).

Additionally, it is important to understand how people self-identify in terms of their sexual orientation and gender identity. A patient-centred approach encourages nurses to explore and understand an individual's social conditions and how they wish to be addressed (Margolies & Carlton, 2019). Manzer, O'Sullivan, and Doucet (2018) explored the myths and misunderstandings as nurse practitioners in New Brunswick working with LGBTQ2 individuals. Their findings included the importance of the careful use of language in fostering a therapeutic nurse–patient relationship by utilizing neutral language that is more inclusive, such as "partner" or "significant other," rather than traditional language surrounding marriage or boyfriend/girlfriend. They recommended having a non-judgemental attitude and asking the person how they wished to be addressed (such as he, she, or otherwise) to allow the interaction to be as respectful as possible.

### Use Silence

Allowing a thoughtful silence at intervals helps the individual to talk at his or her own pace without pressure to perform for the nurse. Silence also permits time for reflection. Particularly helpful to the depressed or physically ill person, silence can reduce pressure and conserve energy. After several moments, the nurse can ask the person to share some thoughts. For example, "Try putting your thoughts into words," "Tell me what are you thinking or feeling now," or "I'll be here when you feel ready to talk."

### Motivational Interviewing

Motivational interviewing (MI) is a person-centred communication approach used widely in health care and life coaching to assist individuals to make behavioural changes regarding a wide variety of lifestyle and health issues (Barrett & Chang, 2016; Östlund, Wadensten, Krisofferzon, et al., 2015). Key components of MI are:

- Engaging—involving the individual in talking about issues, worries, and desires, and to establish the basis for a trusting relationship.
- Focusing—narrowing the focus to habits or patterns that individuals wish to change.
- Evoking—eliciting motivation for change by increasing the sense of the importance of change, confidence, and readiness to change.
- Planning—developing practical steps that the individual wants to use to create the desired changes.

Nurses can seek training and use many available self-help and life coaching resources for health promotion (e.g., Hall, 2012). For example, *The Life Coach Workbook* (Raymond, 2014) is an example of a self-help book with useful tools that align nicely with MI that could be tailored to specific health care concerns. Such resources have high acceptability and can serve as helpful adjuncts to formal education and treatment/health-promotion guidance from nurses.

Current evidence supports the use of MI as an effective technique that can be taught to health professionals without advanced mental health training to promote desired behavioural change across health problems and settings. For training, use, and evaluation of MI implementation, nurses and other clinicians can use the Motivational Interviewing Skills in Health Care Encounters instrument, a reliable validated assessment tool to evaluate acquisition and use of specific MI skills and principles (Petrova, Kavookjian, Madson, et al., 2015).

### Barriers to Effective Communication

Barriers to effective communication can originate with the nurse, the individual, or both. The most obvious barrier is the nurse's failure to use the types of therapeutic techniques just described. Lack of knowledge or experience can limit the nurse's ability to assess the individual's needs and repertoire of skills. Supervision and study can help the nurse apply the steps of the nursing process by using effective intervention approaches.

Communication is also ineffective when some part of the communication–feedback loop breaks down. Failure to send a clear message, receive and interpret the message correctly, or provide useful feedback can interfere with communication. Diagnosing the source of the communication breakdown, taking steps to correct it, and using knowledge of the communication process and appropriate therapeutic techniques are the nurse's responsibility.

## Anxiety

When the nurse or individual is highly anxious during an interaction, perception is altered and the ability to communicate effectively is curtailed sharply. Defence mechanisms, such as denial, projection, and displacement, reduce anxiety but block understanding of the true meaning of an interaction. Severe anxiety and defence mechanisms distort reality and lead to disordered communication. To enhance interpersonal communication, the nurse identifies the feeling of anxiety and its source and uses anxiety-reducing interventions.

## Attitudes

Biases and stereotypes can limit the nurse's and the individual's ability to relate. When the difficulty is the individual's problem, the nurse can assist by examining those views that interfere with the person's relationships. When it is the nurse's problem, openness in the supervisory relationship to examine personal behaviour is crucial. When the nurse fails to examine his or her attitudes toward the person, negativity may be communicated and perceptions of the interaction may be distorted.

## Bullying in the Workplace

Lux, Hutcheson, & Peden (2014) define bullying as disruptive behaviour, inappropriate behaviour, confrontational, or conflict which can manifest as verbal abuse, physical assault, or sexual harassment or abuse. They also list other words that describe bullying, such as incivility, lateral violence, or horizontal violence. When these disruptive behaviours occur in the workplace, the effectiveness of the work environment greatly decreases, medical errors occur, and the health care team cannot function as a team (Pfeifer & Vessey, 2017). The Canadian Nurses Association (CNA) and the Canadian Federation of Nurses Unions (CFNU) developed a Joint Position Statement titled *Workplace Violence and Bullying,* in which they state: "Health-care organizations report that workplace violence and bullying result in 'a high rate of [nurse] absenteeism, lowered morale, loss of productivity, increased staff turnover, increased sick leave, additional recruitment costs, payouts and legal fees'" (CNA & CFNU, 2018, p. 5).

Incivility and bullying manifest in many forms in the workplace, and may come from patients, patient families, and other dyads. Nurses are responsible for addressing such behaviours in a timely and confidential manner if they witness or are the victim of a bully to both the individual who is bullying and to a manager. Depending on the culture of the workplace, a majority of health care facilities have addressed this phenomenon by implementing codes of professional conduct and by establishing organizational expectations, and through ongoing staff education (Pfeifer & Vessey, 2017). It is of note that posters and visitor boards throughout many health care facilities address the intolerance of bullying or violent behaviour towards health care professions.

## Gaps Between the Nurse and the Individual

Related to attitudinal barriers, differences in gender, age, socioeconomic background, ethnicity, race, religion, or language can block functional communication between the nurse and the individual. These factors can cause differences in perception and block mutual understanding. Newly licensed nurses have attributed communication problems to differences in language proficiency among nurses, including English as a second language, as well as to problems in understanding non–English-speaking individuals (Smith-Miller, Leak, Harlan, et al., 2010). To reduce such gaps, nurses can question unclear verbal or written communications, seek clarification or assistance from translators, and explore the ways in which perceptions may differ and meanings can be clarified (Diversity Awareness and Chapter 2).

Moreover, generation gaps between faculty and student nurses can interfere with effective development of the interpersonal skills required for therapeutic nurse–person relationships (Bhana, 2014). Generation Y students, born from the early 1980s to the late 1990s, constitute a large cohort of current undergraduate/pre-licensure and graduate nursing students. Evidence from the literature demonstrates that this generation benefits from deconstruction pedagogies or interactive teaching strategies such as debates, case studies, role playing, storytelling, journalling, simulations, and webpage links to audio and video page links, rather than more traditional didactic approaches (Bhana, 2014). As younger generations (e.g., millennials), who have been raised with technology at their fingertips, enter nursing, teaching approaches will require ongoing change with use of more technology and interactive approaches. Nonetheless, our students also need to learn how to adapt their technology-mediated modes of communication to the styles and skills of older-generation persons and those who may not have had the same access to technology when communicating with persons in the health care system and in professional situations. So, although faculty members need to be adept at engaging students with a variety of effective strategies, students also need to be coached to use appropriate communication approaches across situations and populations. For example, evidence supports the effectiveness of video feedback, another technological teaching/learning strategy, to enhance the quality of communication, clinical competence, and MI skills of practicing nurses (Noordman, van der Weijden, & Van Dulmen, 2014). Thus, ongoing faculty development and testing of various teaching approaches to help students develop competence in therapeutic communication and relationships is crucial to nursing's future.

## Resistance

Resistance comprises all phenomena that inhibit the flow of thoughts, feelings, and memories in an interpersonal encounter and behaviours that interfere with therapeutic goals. Resistance arises from anxiety when a person feels threatened. To reduce this anxiety, the person implements resistant behaviour to divert the focus, most often in the form of avoidance, such as being late, changing the subject, forgetting, blocking, or becoming angry.

Initially, the nurse should identify the behaviour, whether it is the nurse's or the individual's behaviour, and then attempt to interpret it in the context of the interaction. Exploration of possible threats in the relationship, goals, context, or a particular topic can lead to understanding the source of the resistance and finding the ability to handle these difficulties. Anxiety reduction is often a necessary step in dealing with resistant behaviour.

## 🌐 DIVERSITY AWARENESS

### *Multicultural Context of Communication*

As health care providers, nurses might believe that they have expert knowledge about health promotion and the treatment of illness that will be beneficial to others. Therefore, it seems logical that nurses would select appropriate information to share with individuals to help them maintain health and manage illness or alterations in health status. However, consider the possible influences of cultural differences between the nurse and the individual.

Much of the knowledge generated from nursing-related disciplines and the sciences is rooted in a Western perspective. Particularly in Canada, knowledge is developed and interpreted from the perspective of the dominant cultural group, a white, Anglo-Saxon, Christian point of view. When this perspective remains unexamined, alternative perspectives are ignored and invisible. Nurses who are members of the dominant cultural group may be well-intentioned, but ineffective, when they attempt to engage a person of a different cultural group in a relationship without questioning how culture influences interactions, interpretations of events and information, and beliefs and values concerning health and health care practices. Preconceived ideas about people based on some characteristic or group affiliation, such as racial or ethnic identity, religion, country of origin, gender, or sexual orientation, can interfere with nurses' abilities to relate to people as individuals. At the same time, a lack of knowledge of other cultural groups hampers nurses' understanding of the individual's point of view.

Guidelines for recognizing the multicultural context of communication in therapeutic relationships include the following:
- Make ethnocultural assessment a critical component of every clinical evaluation.
- Allow other people to define themselves.
- Ask the person, and the family as appropriate, about cultural health care practices and traditions.
- Respect cultural practices and traditions while providing opportunity for the person to voice preferences and make choices.
- Respect the language of others and do not assume superiority in language.
- Collaborate with trained translators and health promoters (people with the same ethnic or racial background as the individuals).
- Create intercultural open dialogue based on security and mutual respect.
- Avoid use of racist, sexist, ageist, and other forms of denigrating language.
- Do not perpetuate stereotypes in communication.
- Adapt communication to the uniqueness of the individual.
- Reject humour that degrades members on the basis of gender, race, ethnicity, religion, sexual orientation, country of origin, and so forth.
- Respect the rights of others to have different practices and customs.
- Do not allow injustice to continue through silence.
- Present information clearly, which helps people make informed choices.
- Do not judge values, traditions, and practices on the basis of their similarity to or difference from personal values, traditions, and practices, but judge them on the basis of whether they facilitate human potential.

The following are some issues for the nurse to consider:
- When the nurse works with a person from a different cultural background, what are common barriers to establishing a therapeutic relationship?
- In learning about different cultural groups, is there a risk of creating new stereotypes that interfere with the ability to treat people as unique individuals?
- If the nurse has little or no knowledge about a person's culture, how can the nurse provide meaningful nursing care?
- Are the two previous questions contradictory? How can the nurse meet the different challenges that they imply?
- Research measurements typically are developed from the perspective of the dominant culture. If the nurse wishes to use a standardized instrument to measure clinical or research variables among members of different cultural groups, then what questions about the instrument should the nurse ask, and what problems might the nurse encounter? What would need to be done to determine whether or not an instrument truly measures the same phenomenon across different populations?
- Consider the possible influences of cultural differences between the nurse and the individual. Think of an example of two people from diverse cultural groups who developed a relationship. Examine how they got to know each other and what differences and similarities they uncovered. Did barriers to understanding each other exist? If so, how did they bridge these barriers? What did they learn about themselves? What did they learn about the ways that culture shapes perspective and interactions? Think about how nurses can apply these insights to their relationships with people from cultural groups that differ from their own.
- How would a multicultural perspective change the practice?

#### Reflective Questions
- Write down an incident in which you experienced prejudice or discrimination against yourself. What did you do?
- Next, write about an incident in which you observed prejudice or discrimination directed at someone else by a third party. What did you do?
- Are you satisfied with what you did in both instances above? What do you wish you would have done? What might you do now?
- What efforts have you made, or been involved with, to foster multicultural understanding and cultural humility?
- How do you/would you work with patients and families from diverse cultural backgrounds?

### Transference and Countertransference or Distorting

Transference is reacting to another person in an exchange as though that person were someone from the past. Another term for this process is distorting. Transference, although a concept from the psychoanalytic/psychodynamic tradition in psychiatry and psychiatric nursing, retains relevance today. It is best understood as a process that distorts a current relationship or interaction on the basis of past learning, expectations, and/or relationships. Transference or distorting may involve a host of feelings that generally are classified as positive (love, affection, or regard) or negative (anger, dislike, or frustration). Typical transference reactions involve an important figure from the past such as a mother or father; however, at times, transference may be more general to include all authority figures. Something about another person's characteristics, behaviour, or position, in combination with individual dynamics and context, triggers this response. People in a therapeutic relationship often develop strong transference feelings toward the helping professional, arising from the interaction's intensity and the care provider's authoritative or nurturing role. When transference or distorting reactions interfere with the current relationship (i.e., when reactions are out of proportion to the actual situation such as excessive anger in response to a nurse's suggestion), they require gentle probing by pointing out the reaction and asking about the associated thoughts and feelings, and possible past reactions in similar circumstances (e.g., responses to authority figures). To work with a person's transference reactions effectively, the nurse first helps the person to examine feelings and thoughts about the nurse with a nondefensive or reactive stance. Then, the nurse assists the person to compare and contrast the nurse with people from the person's past to reduce distortions and comprehend the present reality to move forward effectively.

Countertransference is basically the same phenomenon and involves distorting, but it is experienced by the health care provider rather than the person. The nurse experiences many feelings toward the person; these feelings are not problematic, unless they remain unanalyzed and block the nurse's ability to work effectively with the individual. For example, if a nurse has strong feelings about the person and thinks that the person cannot possibly function after discharge without the nurse's assistance, the nurse is likely to distort the person's abilities, encourage a childlike dependency, and interfere with the person's progress. This nurse needs to examine such personal feelings to understand their source. Once understood, countertransference reactions generally cease to interfere with the relationship. Consultation for supervision with an advanced practice psychiatric nurse or other mental health expert is recommended whenever transference or countertransference (i.e., distorting) reactions are persistent and problematic.

### Sensory Barriers

When the individual has sensory limitations, the nurse may need to use extra skill in communicating. Use of the other senses to send or receive messages should be attempted. Special help is often available from trained therapists and teachers; for example, many agencies have access to interpreters for deaf people, and visual aids may be useful. Nurses must be as creative as possible, learn from others who are skilled in alternative forms of communication, and make referrals as necessary. As technology evolves, new communication methods will continue to decrease these barriers. For example, voice recognition software programs assist persons with visual and motor challenges to communicate via text.

### Failure to Address Concerns or Needs

Failure to meet the individual's needs or to recognize the individual's concerns is the most serious barrier to effective interaction. This failure can arise from inadequate assessment, lack of knowledge, inability to separate the nurse's needs from the individual's needs, and confusion between friendship and a helping relationship, including unrecognized or unresolved sexual issues. To correct this problem, the nurse should recognize that a barrier to relating to the person exists. Using the supervisory process to determine the problem's source, the nurse should then take corrective action, such as obtaining more information or knowledge, performing a self-assessment with values clarification, and examining reactions, biases, and expectations. Nurses, particularly novice nurses and those transitioning to a new role (e.g., from staff nurse to nurse practitioner after graduate school), need to *demand* mentorship/clinical supervision that is not tied to performance evaluation. In other words, a supportive mentoring/supervisory relationship with a more senior nurse is a necessary ingredient in helping nurses to be effective. Cost-cutting efforts in today's health care system often neglect such needs. Yet consider the cost of a failed hire or ineffective relationships with care recipients. An argument for

having professional support can be strong. Additionally, nurses can create their own cost-effective professional support systems by creating peer groups and/or engaging their own consultants with a peer group outside the work setting.

### Setting

The setting of a therapeutic interaction can affect the goals and the nature of the communication. The most important aspect of any setting is that the nurse and the individual are able to attend to each other. The nurse's attention to the person helps create this atmosphere. The nurse assesses the influence of factors such as lighting, noise, temperature, comfort, physical distance, and privacy; potentially disturbing factors can be altered or controlled within the limits of the setting. Occasionally the nurse has only minimal control over the setting, as in a busy clinic, health centre, inpatient unit, emergency department, or the individual's home. Although far from the ideal of a quiet, pleasant, well-lit private office, these typical clinical settings can be used effectively by creating a sense of private space. Curtains can be drawn, doors shut, and two chairs pulled to a corner to shape an environment for interaction. When possible, however, nurses seek offices or rooms to establish privacy during significant communication or when imparting important or complex health information. Home settings can also be more comfortable for individuals than for nurses, yet also can provide invaluable context when used. The nurse can also acknowledge verbally that some aspect of the environment, such as an interruption or noise, is bothersome. This strategy shows people that the nurse recognizes possible concentration difficulties and is sharing the environment with them.

### Stages

Therapeutic relationships follow sequential phases, which may overlap, differ in length, or involve issues that appear over time rather than in a set sequence. Orientation (introductory), working, and termination phases have been identified by researchers and clinicians (Shajani & Snell, 2019).

Originally these relationship stages were identified from clinical interactions that developed over a prolonged period. However, they can be observed in brief encounters that are effective: that is, interactions that meet individuals' needs rather than therapeutic interactions that have been reduced to little more than quick question-and-answer sessions. Whether the nurse is engaged in a long-term or short-term relationship with an individual, attention to the relationship stages is important. Brief therapeutic relationships will telescope the stages; therefore it is particularly important that the nurse focuses on meeting the key demands of each relationship phase. It is important to note that individuals may move in and out of direct care episodes, while a therapeutic relationship can be maintained over a longer period. A relationship exists even when the nurse and the individual do not see each other for an extended period, and each encounter occurs within the trajectory of the relationship stages.

### Orientation or Introductory Phase

The orientation or introductory phase begins when the nurse and the individual meet. This meeting typically involves some feeling

---

**BOX 4.9 Key Topics of Discussion During the Orientation or Introductory Phase of the Therapeutic Relationship**

- What to call each other
- Purpose of meeting
- Location, time, and length of meetings
- Termination date or time for review of progress through follow-up
- Confidentiality (with whom clinical data will be shared)
- Any other limits related to the particular setting

---

**BOX 4.10 Interventions for Use During the Termination Phase of the Therapeutic Relationship**

- Let the person know why the relationship is to be terminated.
- Remind the person of the date and how many meetings or appointments are left.
- Collaborate with other staff so that they are aware of how the person is reacting and any special needs that the person may have.
- Help the person to identify sources of support and other people with whom a relationship is possible.
- Review the gains and the remaining goals.
- Discuss the pros and cons experienced during the relationship to help the person develop a realistic appraisal.
- Make referrals for follow-up care as needed.

---

of anxiety; neither party knows what to expect. When the therapeutic relationship is primarily a counselling type of relationship, part of the nurse's role is to help structure the interaction by discussing several topics during the initial meeting and sometimes during the first few meetings. Box 4.9 lists topics appropriate to this phase. Discussion of these issues establishes a contract or pact and involves a mutual understanding of the parameters of the relationship and an agreement to work together.

The orientation stage is a critical juncture in any therapeutic relationship. Without successful transition through the orientation phase, no working alliance will exist and the treatment goals will remain unmet. Consistency, sensitive pacing of communication, active listening, conveying concern and warmth, and paying attention to comfort and control help to establish a connection during the orientation phase. In contrast, inconsistency, unavailability, individual factors associated with trust, nurses' feelings about the other person, confrontation of delusions or strongly held views, and unrealistic expectations hamper relationships.

When the therapeutic relationship is not structured primarily as counselling with a specific number of sessions, the orientation phase may appear less distinct and the topics noted may seem irrelevant. In this case, the nurse can adapt the suggested topics to meet the specific situation. However, except in true emergencies, initial encounters should always include introductions by name, discussion of the purpose, and presentation of a plan for ongoing care or specific follow-up.

### Working Phase

The working phase of the therapeutic relationship emerges when the nurse and the individual collaborate as partners in promoting the person's health. The working phase may last for only a brief time to establish a treatment plan, may last for an established number of sessions, as in brief psychotherapy, or may extend over a longer period if the nurse is the primary care provider, care manager, or long-term caregiver in any setting or context for an individual or family. During the working phase, the relationship is the context through which change occur. Goals are set, and the nurse and the individual work mutually toward their accomplishment. Interventions are tailored to the specific situation and health needs of the person and the family. Solving problems, coping with stressors, and gaining insight are all part of the working phase. The nurse and the individual recognize each other's uniqueness and establish trust as the first step in establishing a working relationship.

Resistant behaviours may be observed during this phase while the nurse and the individual become closer and work on potentially anxiety-producing problems. The person may pull away through the use of defence mechanisms because change can be difficult. Overcoming the resistance becomes an important nursing task.

### Termination Phase

Termination marks the end of the relationship established in the therapeutic contract or negotiated in accordance with the limits of the contract. Ending a relationship can cause anxiety for both the individual and the nurse. Termination represents a loss; therefore, it can trigger feelings of sadness, frustration, and anger. Termination in this case is the loss of a relationship and the loss of future involvement, with its attendant realistic expectations or fantasies. Termination also reawakens feelings of previously unresolved losses, such as a death or divorce.

Working through any feelings related to termination is an important part of clinical care. Some individuals require the nurse's assistance to experience the feelings of loss and to connect present reactions to past real or symbolic losses. Box 4.10 lists additional interventions for use during the termination phase.

Both the nurse and the individual can learn much during termination; the process directs both participants to examine problems and progress in the relationship, feelings, and reactions. The experience also helps the nurse and the individual gain practice in ending relationships and in exploring reactions, which can be most helpful when future losses occur. Nonetheless, major gains can be accomplished with the deadline of termination. Options for follow-up or future treatment as the need determines also require exploration and planning.

### Brief Interactions

Time constraints in practice are unavoidable. Although challenging, brief therapeutic encounters can be meaningful and useful. Limited time is not a valid reason to avoid interviewing or interacting with individuals. Rather, nurses purposefully can structure brief interactions to achieve specific clinical outcomes delineates key ingredients for a 15-minute (or shorter) interview with a family (Box 4.11).

These guidelines for brief interactions with families can be adapted for interviews with individuals. An effective 15-minute (or shorter) interview is feasible if nurses plan to introduce themselves, state the purpose of meeting, validate understanding with the person or the family, clarify parameters such as time, focus and listen, and elicit significant individual and family data. Most important, the goal of the interaction must be realistic and clearly defined. For example, the purpose may be to elicit a family's view of the problem for which the person has sought care or to prioritize problems to be treated. Even when time is limited, the interview is structured to provide an opportunity for the person or the family to engage in dialogue as an active participant in care, and the nurse's attention is completely focused on the individual.

---

### BOX 4.11    Key Ingredients for a 15-Minute (or Shorter) Family Interview

- Use manners to engage or re-engage family members. Make an introduction by offering your name and role. Orient family members to the purpose of a brief family interview.
- Assess significant areas of internal and external structure and function (obtain information from a genogram concerning basic family composition and external support data).
- Ask family members three key questions.
- Commend the family on one or two strengths.
- Evaluate usefulness and conclude.

Source: Shajani, Z, & Snell, D. (2019). Chapter 9: How to do a 15-minute (or shorter) family interview. In *Wright & Leahey's nurses and families: A guide to family assessment and intervention* (7th ed., pp. 255–272). Philadelphia: F. A. Davis.

---

Circumstances also can dictate the need for immediate and instructive communications that command specific actions. For example, during a crisis, directive, clear communication is paramount (such as during disaster-related events). In Canada, between 1980 and 2010, the reported percentages of people affected by disasters were highest for floods (42%) and wildfires (32%), compared with other forms of disasters (Kulig, Edge, & Smolenski, 2014). In their article, the authors emphasize the importance of clear communication during a natural disaster, and that it must be ongoing and continued throughout the phase of a disaster.

Planning in anticipation of human-caused and natural disasters is critical so as to have functional communications systems in place. Such systems increasingly will use various methods of telecommunication. After tragic events have occurred, including shootings on college campuses, efforts to communicate more effectively are paramount. Universities, for example, have responded by instituting systems to communicate rapidly with a large campus community. Widely deployed strategies feature instant text messaging and e-mailing (see Innovative Practice box, earlier).

The following case study presents a detailed scenario of a home visit and questions related to how the nurse can develop a therapeutic relationship with the person. The care plan presents a plan of care for the person, including communication interventions.

---

## CASE STUDY

### A Health-Promotion Visit: Sarah Eustache-Daniel

As part of a health-promotion visit for Sarah Eustache-Daniel and Thomas, her 2-week-old infant, Jessica Wong, a registered nurse, planned to conduct an infant assessment, provide breastfeeding support, teach about normal infant development and care activities, and assess Mrs. Eustache-Daniel's adaptation to motherhood and her postpartum recovery status. Before the visit, Ms. Wong reviewed the clinical information she obtained during Mrs. Eustache-Daniel's hospitalization. Mrs. Eustache-Daniel is a 34-year-old Indigenous primiparous woman who delivered a 3.22 kg (7-pound, 10-ounce) healthy boy (Thomas) after a 12-hour labour. The labour had progressed well without complications. Mrs. Eustache-Daniel received epidural anaesthesia at 6-cm dilatation, and the baby was delivered vaginally. Her husband, Louis Daniel, provided labour support and was present for the delivery. After a 2-day hospital stay, Mrs. Eustache-Daniel was discharged. At discharge, the infant was breastfeeding, had normal newborn examination findings, and weighed 3.40 kg (7 pounds, 5 ounces). Ms. Wong had been impressed by both parents' preparation for the birth. They had attended childbirth classes and read several books about infant development and parenting. Ms. Eustache-Daniel planned to take a 12-month maternity leave from her position as a lawyer in a large practice and had arranged for a child care provider to come to the family's home to take care of the infant beginning 2 weeks before the end of her maternity leave. Mr. Daniel had not planned to take time off from his job because he had recently been promoted to a high-level managerial position in his company that required increased travel and time at work. He was able to postpone a business trip to be present at the delivery and had sent a plane ticket to his mother-in-law so she could come and stay at their home during the first week after Mrs. Eustache-Daniel and Thomas were discharged from the hospital.

During the visit, Ms. Wong first assessed the infant. She incorporated teaching concerning normal infant development and concluded that Thomas was a healthy 2-week-old infant who was feeding well. Thomas's circumcision was healing without complications and he had regained his birth weight.

When Ms. Wong asked how Mrs. Eustache-Daniel was doing, Mrs. Eustache-Daniel hesitated and then responded, "I'm not sure. I'm very glad that Thomas is doing well… but I worry sometimes that I'm not going to be able to do everything right for him. It's funny, but I've spent so many years getting an education and establishing my law career. It was hard work, but I managed to do well. Now a little infant overwhelms me. I don't know how I'll manage this." When Ms. Wong asked Mrs. Eustache-Daniel to talk more about her concerns, Mrs. Eustache-Daniel described how incompetent she felt while her mother was staying with her. "My mother could do everything so easily. I fumbled with every diaper. It felt like she criticized how I did things. When she told me about what she did when she had children, I felt pushed to do things 'her way' and not the way that I had planned. She even wanted to give him a bottle when I was trying so hard to get breastfeeding going. At least the doctor said Thomas had gained enough weight. Thomas's weight gain made me feel like I wasn't a total failure. I couldn't wait for her to go, but I fell apart after she left. I was alone. Louis is out of town until the weekend, and I couldn't get Thomas to stop crying yesterday. I thought I would scream, so I put him down in his crib and I just sat there crying. What's wrong with me? I've never felt so out of control before. I want to be a good mother, but I feel like I can't give any more right now."

In response to Ms. Wong's follow-up questions about mental status, Mrs. Eustache-Daniel described frequently feeling irritated and sad, crying a few times over the previous several days, having difficulty sleeping even when the baby was

## CASE STUDY—cont'd

### A Health-Promotion Visit: Sarah Eustache-Daniel

asleep, feeling fatigued, and being worried about how she would be able to go back to work in only a few weeks. Ms. Wong also inquired about the family's cultural, ethnic, and religious backgrounds. Mrs. Eustache-Daniel responded, "Interesting that you should ask. That's actually another issue right now. I am from Manitoba and my family is Métis and Catholic, but I am not a practising Catholic now.

I added my maiden name to Daniel when I got married, to honour my family. Louis is Protestant, but not really religious. His family comes from Saskatoon. They are very nice and were supportive when we got married. We were lucky that our families accepted us together. I have to admit, though, that we didn't really figure out what we would do about raising the baby. Louis thinks that we'd be hypocrites to have a Catholic christening. Plus, my mother told me that I'd be selfish to go back to work so soon. Can you help me? I feel like I'm going out of my mind and I don't know what to do."

This case study raises a variety of clinical concerns. As the nurse in this encounter, Ms. Wong could begin by considering the following questions.

#### Reflective Questions
- What are my feelings as I listen to her story and her distress? Am I aware of how my values and expectations affect my interaction with this person? How

can I establish a therapeutic relationship to support Mrs. Eustache-Daniel during this stressful period?
- What is the significance of the distress symptoms that Mrs. Eustache-Daniel reported? Given that the period during which many women experience postpartum blues has passed, what is the most appropriate action for referral to obtain a thorough mental status examination for postpartum depression?
- Who is the most appropriate health care provider to evaluate her for postpartum depression, and treat her if it is confirmed? How can I facilitate getting her the care she needs, and can I remain available to her? How can I assist Mrs. Eustache-Daniel meet the infant's developmental needs during this stressful period?
- In what ways do family dynamics, values, and expectations related to differing cultural and religious heritages contribute to the problems described? What can I do to explore these issues further? What strengths can be harnessed? Are there clergy who could be engaged for pastoral counselling? How can I engage support systems to ameliorate rather than exacerbate the difficulties? What can be done to engage both Mr. Daniel and Mrs. Eustache-Daniel in a therapeutic relationship to focus on the couple and parenting concerns, and to involve both partners in treatment strategies?

## CARE PLAN

### Transition to Parenthood: Sarah Eustache-Daniel

#### Nursing Issue
Risk of inadequate parenting related to stress involved in transition to parenthood

#### Defining Characteristics
- Feeling overwhelmed with responsibilities of new parenthood
- Insecurity about tasks of infant care
- Crying
- Sadness
- Feeling out of control
- Difficulty sleeping even when the baby is asleep
- Worry about going back to work soon

#### Related Factors
- Transition from high career achievement to new role as mother
- Differing religious, ethnic, and cultural backgrounds of the two parents and extended families
- Confusion and lack of decisions about religious and cultural traditions to follow for their infant
- Conflicting expectations of extended families, particularly from Mrs. Eustache-Daniel's mother
- Job pressures on Mr. Daniel to travel and be away from home
- Unanticipated social isolation for Mrs. Eustache-Daniel during this postpartum period
- Limited social support (particularly from the husband because of work-associated travel)

#### Expected Outcomes
- Competent mothering and infant care are displayed.
- Mrs. Eustache-Daniel describes her feelings, concerns, and needs.
- Indicators of postpartum depression are evaluated, and referral for follow-up is made for positive findings.
- Social supports are engaged.
- Mrs. Eustache-Daniel and Mr. Daniel successfully negotiate immediate decisions about religious and cultural practice concerning their baby and agree

to use counselling services to work out decisions concerning their child's upbringing and involvement of the extended family.

#### Interventions
- Health information is provided about normal newborn and postpartum adjustment.
- Infant care information is provided on the basis of Mrs. Eustache-Daniel's needs.
- Expectations about postpartum adjustment and parenthood are elicited.
- Health information about postpartum depression is provided, regarding prevalence and common symptoms.
- Personal and family histories are obtained, with a focus on mental health.
- Postpartum depression is evaluated with use of interview questions and an assessment measure, such as the Edinburgh Postnatal Depression Scale (Cox, Holden, & Sagovsky, 1987) or the Postpartum Depression Screening Scale (Beck & Gable, 2001).
- If symptom levels suggest postpartum depression, a referral for mental health evaluation is made. If there are any signs of safety risk to self or others, immediate protective action (e.g., emergency mental health evaluation) is taken.
- Sources of social support are solicited, and specific plans are made to use available support, such as the husband, friends, and hired infant care providers.
- Conflicts and areas of shared values, plans, goals for raising the baby are explored.
- Pros and cons of options for raising the baby are examined in relation to religious, ethnic, and cultural considerations.
- A follow-up plan is made to reassess symptoms of postpartum depression and to discuss ongoing concerns about how to raise the baby with Mrs. Eustache-Daniel and Mr. Daniel.
- Referral is made to local support and psycho-educational programs for interfaith couples.

## SUMMARY

Relating to individuals has many challenges and rewards for nurses. Although some aspects of this work are predictable, each individual and family is unique and provides a chance for the nurse to learn, grow, and help in new ways. This chapter has provided guidelines for developing therapeutic relationships, but these guidelines do not guarantee success or an easy job. The desire and skill of the individual nurse bring this information to life. The blend of the nurse's artistry, humanity, knowledge, skill, and ethics sparks concern and the ability to help another human being communicate effectively: essential components of the nurse–person relationship.

The therapeutic relationship is the primary arena for health promotion. Values clarification, communication, and the helping relationship are its core components. For nurses, applying this knowledge to their varied roles is essential to promoting health and providing quality care.

Increasing use of technology and mounting pressures for cost-effective care are here to stay. In this climate, the importance of the therapeutic relationship is underscored (see Innovative Practice box, earlier). Without a relational context, the care dimension in health care is lost, and health promotion is reduced to standardized, recipe-like prescriptions. Effective health promotion directed to the needs of individuals, families, and communities requires reflection on the value of caring, effective communication, and a helping relationship.

**Evolve Chapter Features**

http://evolve.elsevier.com/Canada/Edelman/healthpromotion/
- Review Questions

## REFERENCES

Adler, R., Rolls, J., & Proctor, R. (2015). Looking out looking in (2nd Canadian ed.). Toronto: Nelson Education Ltd.

Antonacci, R., Fong, A., Sumbly, P., et al. (2018). They can hear the silence: Nursing practices on communication with patients. *Canadian Journal of Critical Care Nursing, 29*(4), 36–39.

Balzer-Riley, J. W. (2017). *Communication in nursing.* St. Louis: Elsevier.

Barrett, K., & Chang, Y. P. (2016). Behavioral interventions targeting chronic pain, depression, and substance use disorder in primary care. *Journal of Nursing Scholarship, 48*(4), 345–353.

Beard, K. V., Gwanmesia, E., & Miranda-Diaz, G. (2015). Culturally competent care: Using the ESFT model in nursing. (2016). *American Journal of Nursing, 115*(6), 58–62.

Beck, C. T., & Gable, R. K. (2001). *Postpartum depression screening scale.* Los Angeles: Western Psychological Services. [Seminal Reference].

Bhana, V. M. (2014). Interpersonal skills development in generation Y student nurses: A literature review. *Nurse Education Today, 34,* 1430–1434.

Blondis, M. N., & Jackson, B. E. (1982). *Nonverbal communication with patients: Back to the human touch* (2nd ed.). New York: John Wiley & Sons.

Brouwers, M., Rasenberg, E., van Weel, C., et al. (2017). Assessing patient-centred communication in teaching: A systematic review of instruments. *Medical Education, 51*(11), 1103–1117. https://doi.org/10.1111/medu.13375.

Canadian Nurses Association (CNA) & Canadian Federation of Nurses Unions (CFNU). (2018). *Joint position statement: Workplace violence and bullying.* Retrieved from https://cna-aiic.ca/~/media/cna/page-content/pdf-en/Workplace-Violence-and-Bullying_joint-position-statement.pdf.

Carper, B. A. (1978). Fundamental patterns of knowing in nursing. *Advances in Nursing Science, 1*(1), 13–24.

Cox, J. L., Holden, J. M., & Sagovsky, R. (1987). Detection of postnatal depression: Development of the 10-item edinburgh postnatal depression Scale. *The British Journal of Psychiatry: Journal of Mental Science, 150,* 782–786. [Seminal Reference].

D'Antonio, P. D., Beeber, L., Sills, G., et al. (2014). The future in the past: Hildegard Peplau and interpersonal relations in nursing. *Nursing Inquiry, 21*(4), 311–317.

Doane, G. H., & Varcoe, C. (2015). *How to nurse: Relational inquiry with individuals and families in changing health and health care contexts.* Philadelphia: Wolters Kluwer Health/Lippincott Williams & Wilkins.

Doss, S., DePascal, P., & Hadley, K. (2011). Patient-nurse partnerships. *Nephrology Nursing Journal: Journal of the American Nephrology Nurses' Association, 38*(2), 115–124.

Drolet, M.-J., & Sauvageau, A. (2016). Developing professional values: Perceptions of francophone occupational therapists in Quebec, Canada. *Scandinavian Journal of Occupational Therapy, 23*(4), 286–296. https://doi.org/10.3109/11038128.2015.1130168.

Errasti-Ibarrondo, B., Perez, M., Carasco, J. M., et al. (2015). Essential elements of the relationship between the nurse and the person with advanced and terminal cancer: A meta-ethnography. *Nursing Outlook, 63*(3), 255–268. https://doi.org/10.1016/j.outlook.2014.12.001.

Fawcett, J., & Ellenbecker, C. H. (2015). A proposed conceptual model of nursing and population health. *Nursing Outlook, 63,* 288–298. https://doi.org/10.1016/j.outlook.2015.01.009.

Hall, E. (1973). *The silent language.* Garden City, NY: Doubleday/Anchor Press. [Seminal Reference].

Hall, P. (2012). *How to be the pilot of your own life: Flying lessons.* Tucson, AZ: Through a Different Lens, LLC.

Haskey, N., Richmond, M., Kowalchuk, J., et al. (2015). Improving the hospital experience: Technology at the bedside. *Canadian Journal of Dietetic Practice and Research, 76*(3), e15–e15.

Health Promotion Canada. (2018). Pan-Canadian health promoter competencies. Retrieved from https://www.healthpromotioncanada.ca/resources/hp-competencies/.

Henry, S., Fuhrel-Forbis, A., Rogers, M. A., et al. (2012). Association between nonverbal communication during clinical interactions and outcomes: A systematic review and meta-analysis. *Patient Education and Counseling, 86*(3), 297–315.

Holmes, P. (2014). Intercultural dialogue: Challenges to theory, practice and research. *Language and Intercultural Communication, 14,* 1–6.

Jimenez, C. (2018). *Health literacy and public health.* Ottawa: Canadian Public Health Association. Retrieved from https://www.cpha.ca/health-literacy-and-public-health.

Kulig, J. C., Edge, D., & Smolenski, S. (2014). Wildfire disasters: Implications for rural nurses. *Australasian Emergency Nursing Journal, 17*(3), 126–134.

Lux, K. M., Hutcheson, J. B., & Peden, A. R. (2014). Ending disruptive behavior: Staff nurse recommendations to nurse educators. *Nurse Education in Practice, 14*(1), 37–42.

Lyons, K. J., Giordano, C., Speakman, E., et al. (2016). Jefferson Teamwork Observation Guide (JTOG): An instrument to observe teamwork behaviors. *Journal Of Allied Health, 45*(1), 49c–53c.

Manzer, D., O'Sullivan, L., & Doucet, S. (2018). Myths, misunderstandings, and missing information: Experiences of nurse practitioners providing primary care to lesbian, gay, bisexual, and transgender patients. *The Canadian Journal of Human Sexuality, 27*(2), 157–170.

Margolies, L., & Carlton, G. (2019). Increasing cultural competence with LGBTQ patients. *Nursing, 49*(6), 34–40.

McCaffrey, G., & McConnell, S. (2015). Compassion: A critical review of peer-reviewed nursing literature. *Journal of Clinical Nursing, 24*(19–20), 3006–3015.

McKenna, M. C., & Stahl, K. D. (2015). *Assessment for reading instruction* (3rd ed.). New York: Guilford Press.

Noordman, J., van der Weijden, T., & Van Dulmen, S. (2014). Effects of video-feedback on the communication, clinical competence and motivational interviewing skills of practice nurses: A pre-test posttest control group study. *Journal of Advanced Nursing, 70,* 2275–2283.

O'Toole, A., & Welt, S. R. (1989). *Interpersonal theory in nursing practice.* New York: Springer.

Östlund, A. S., Wadensten, B., Krisofferzon, M. L., et al. (2015). Motivational interviewing: Experiences in primary care nurses trained in the method. *Nurse Education in Practice, 15*(2), 111–113. https://doi.org/10.1016/j.nepr.2014.11.005.

Pai, H. C. (2015). The effect of a self-reflection and insight program on the nursing competence of nursing students: A longitudinal study. *Journal of Professional Nursing, 31*(5), 424–431. https://doi.org/10.1016/j.profnurs.2015.03.003.

Peplau, H. E. (1963). Process and concept of learning. In S. Burd, & M. Marshall (Eds.), *Some clinical approaches to psychiatric nursing* (pp. 348–352). New York: Macmillan. [Seminal Reference].

Peplau, H. E. (1964). *Basic principles of patient counseling* (2nd ed.). Philadelphia: Smith Kline and French Laboratories. [Seminal Reference].

Peplau, H. E. (1969). Professional closeness: As a special kind of involvement with a patient, client, or family group. *Nursing Forum, 8*(4), 342–360. [Seminal Reference].

Petrova, T., Kavookjian, J., Madson, M. B., et al. (2015). Motivational interviewing skills in health care encounters (MISCHE): Development and psychometric testing of an assessment tool. *Research in Social and Administrative Pharmacy, 11*(5), 696–707. https://doi.org/10.1016/j.sapharm.2014.12.001.

Pfeifer, L. E., & Vessey, J. A. (2017). An integrative review of bullying and lateral violence among nurses in Magnet® organizations. *Policy, Politics, & Nursing Practice, 18*(3), 113–124.

Public Health Agency of Canada (PHAC). (2017). *Core competencies for public health in Canada.* Ottawa: Author. Retrieved from https://www.canada.ca/en/public-health/services/public-health-practice/skills-online/core-competencies-public-health-canada.html.

Quality Safety and Education for Nurses (QSEN). (2012). *Patient centered care.* Retrieved from http://qsen.org/competencies/pre-licensure-ksas/#patient-centered_care.

Raths, L., Harmin, M., & Simon, S. (1978). *Values and teaching.* Columbus, OH: Charles E. Merrill.

Raymond, J. (2014). *The life coach workbook.* London: John Murray Learning.

Ruesch, J., & Bateson, G. (1987). *Communication: The social matrix of psychiatry.* New York: W.W. Norton. [Seminal Reference].

Sakakibara, B., Lear, S., Barr, S., et al. (2017). A telehealth intervention to promote health lifestyles after stroke: The stroke coach protocol. *International Journal of Stroke, 13*(2), 217–222. https://doi.org/10.1177/1747493017729266.

Shajani, Z., & Snell, D. (2019). *Wright & Leahey's nurses and families: A guide to family assessment and intervention* (7th ed.). Philadelphia: F.A. Davis.

Smith-Miller, C. A., Leak, A., Harlan, C. A., et al. (2010). "Leaving the comfort of the familiar": Fostering workplace cultural awareness through short-term global experiences. *Nursing Forum, 45*(1), 18–28.

Speros, C. (2011). Promoting health literacy: A nursing imperative. *Nursing Clinics of North America, 46*(3), 321–333.

Stephany, K., & Majkowski, P. (2012). *The ethic of care : A moral compass for Canadian nursing practice.* Oak Park, IL: Bentham Science Publishers. https://doi.org/10.2174/97816080530491120101.

Steuber, P., & Pollard, C. (2018). Building a therapeutic relationship: How much is too much self-disclosure? *International Journal of Caring Sciences, 11*(2), 651–657.

Stockmann, C. (2018). Presence in the nurse–client relationship: An integrative review. *International Journal for Human Caring, 22*(2), 49–64. https://doi.org/10.20467/1091-5710.22.2.49.

Stuart, G. W. (2012). *Principles and practice of psychiatric nursing* (10th ed.). St. Louis: Mosby.

Tejero, L. M. S. (2011). The mediating role of the nurse-patient dyad bonding in bringing about patient satisfaction. *Journal of Advanced Nursing, 68*(5), 994–1002.

Tejero, L. M. S. (2016). Behavioral patterns in nurse-patient dyads: A critical incident study. *International Journal for Human Caring, 20*(3), 129–133. https://doi.org/10.20467/1091-5710.20.3.129.

Waters, E., Kiviniemi, M., Orom, H., et al. (2016). "I don't know" my cancer risk: Implications for health behavior engagement. *Annals of Behavioral Medicine, 50*(5), 784–788. https://doi.org/10.1007/s12160-016-9789-5.

Watzlawick, P., Beavin, J. H., & Jackson, D. D. (1967). *Pragmatics of human communication: A study of interactional patterns, pathologies and paradoxes.* New York: W.W. Norton. [Seminal Reference].

# 5

# Ethical Issues Related to Health Promotion

*Jane Tyerman, RN, PhD, CCSNE*

Originating US chapter by *Christine Sorrell Dinkins, PhD*

## INTENDED LEARNING OUTCOMES

*After completing this chapter, the reader will be able to:*

- Discuss health promotion as a moral endeavour.
- Describe the relationship of health care ethics to health promotion.
- Analyze the relationship of various ethical theories to the nursing role in health promotion.
- Discuss the historical development and importance to nursing of the codes of ethics.
- Describe contemporary ethical issues in health promotion (e.g., issues related to genetics, genomics, culture, end-of-life decision making).
- Analyze problems related to health promotion using an ethical decision-making framework.

## KEY TERMS

Advocacy
Applied ethics
Autonomy
Beliefs
Beneficence
Civil liberties
Codes of ethics
Confidentiality
Consequentialist
Consent
Descriptive theories
Duty-based theories
Ethical dilemmas

Ethical issues
Ethical (moral) distress
Feminist ethics
Genomics
Genetics
Genetic counselling
Genotype
Informed consent
Justice
Maleficence
Metaethics
Moral
Moral agency

Moral philosophy
Nonmaleficence
Normative theories
Paternalism
Phenotype
Practical wisdom
Preventive ethics
Social justice
Trust
Utilitarian theories
Value theories
Veracity
Virtue ethics

## ? THINK ABOUT IT

### Assisted Suicide or Emotional Support?

A nurse in a clinic is accountable for ongoing assessments of pain management. One of the long-term patients, Ana, has required increasing amounts of narcotics for her pain management over the last year. The nurse has known for more than a year that Ana's husband, Victor, has amyotrophic lateral sclerosis (ALS), or Lou Gehrig's disease. Victor's disease adds a great deal of stress to both their lives, which has had a negative effect on Ana's physical health. The nurse assesses the emotional toll of Victor's illness as part of Ana's pain assessment. During one of these discussions, Ana asks the nurse how much of her narcotic medication her husband would need to take to end his life.

- What are the implications of providing someone, indirectly, with the means to commit medical assistance in dying (MAID)?

- What questions would you have for Ana at this point of the conversation?
- Imagine how she might respond. What would you say or do in response to her answers?
- Do you have any obligations to Victor?
- Do you think you should collaborate with Victor's health care provider?
- What is in Ana's best interests?
- Who or what are your resources?
- Do national nursing organizations have written guidelines about MAID?
- What is the law in your province/territory?
- What should you do?

# HEALTH PROMOTION AS A MORAL ENDEAVOUR

The Canadian Nurses Association (CNA) outlines professional practice expectations and standards of practice founded on the values of the profession; they are articulated in the *Code of Ethics for Registered Nurses* (CNA, 2017). Additionally, provincial and territorial nursing regulatory bodies are legally required to set standards for nursing practice in order to protect the public. Together, these standards or Codes of Ethics provide a succinct statement of ethical values, obligations, and duties of nurses and describes nursing's understanding of its commitment to society and form the foundation of nursing practice in Canada. The code frames how nurses advocate for evidence-informed decision making and best approaches to health promotion; this care can be seen as a moral endeavour. Nurses confront moral issues in the process of attempting to enhance the well-being of a society overall, as well as promoting and protecting health for individual members of a society. Health is considered a human good because it helps people to have a desirable quality of life and achieve life goals. At the level of the individual, health promotion involves providing services that help people achieve their potential.

To set a higher standard of health for all people, it is important to understand the contexts of people's lives. This understanding entails consideration of a variety of factors that can affect a person's health status, such as mental, physical, spiritual, environmental, cultural, social, and genetic factors.

The concept of healthy public policy was originally introduced in the Ottawa Charter for Health Promotion in 1986, and was a tool used to created supportive environments to enable people to live healthy lives by prioritizing health policy at all levels of government (WHO, 1986). Viewing health promotion as a moral endeavour is consistent with the Public Health Agency of Canada's (PHAC) *Declaration on the Prevention and Promotion of Health,* which states (PHAC, 2010):

- Disease, disability, and injury remain a serious concern in Canada, which must be addressed.
- Positive mental health is fundamental to optimal overall health and well-being.
- A large proportion of chronic disease, disabilities, and injuries are preventable or their onset can be delayed.
- A collaboration between government and health partners is needed to reduce and remove disparities in health.
- Ongoing health promotion and disease prevention are needed, even for those who already have disabilities and chronic diseases.

The purpose of health-promotion efforts, as discussed throughout this book, is to ensure that people have access to the tools and strategies to live at the highest level of well-being possible. Health-promotion efforts should address environmental obstacles to human health, such as pollution, marketing of harmful products, and economic disparities. Thus health promotion is not the province of a single discipline but requires intersectoral collaboration of patients, health care providers, institutions, and government working together to create a nurturing environment for achieving health goals.

---

## BOX 5.1  Ethical Practice to Address Broad Societal Issues

Nurses advocate for fair policies and practices by:
- Advocating for publicly administered health systems that ensure accessible, universal, portable, and comprehensive health care services
- Utilizing principles of primary health care for the benefit of the public and the person receiving care
- Recognizing and addressing organizational, societal, economic, and political factors that influence health and well-being within the context of the nurses' role in the delivery of care
- Advocating for a full continuum of accessible health care services, which includes health promotion, disease prevention, and diagnostic, restorative, rehabilitative, and palliative care services in hospitals, nursing homes, home care, and the community
- Recognizing the impact of the social determinants of health and advocating for policies and programs which address them
- Maintaining awareness of major health concerns (e.g., poverty, inadequate housing, food insecurity) while working for social justice and advocating for laws, policies, and procedures to promote equity
- Working with people and advocating for expanding the range of available health care choices
- Collaborating with other health providers and the public to protect human rights, promote health diplomacy, and reduce health inequalities
- Recognizing that vulnerable populations are systemically disadvantaged, which leads to diminished health and well-being, and advocating to improve their quality of life and removing barriers to health care
- Working with governmental agencies to acknowledge the current state of Indigenous health in Canada, and to take actions with Indigenous people to improve their health services
- Supporting environmental preservation and restoration to promote health and well-being
- Maintaining an awareness of broader global health concerns
- Advocating for excellence in palliative and end-of-life care
- Encouraging ethical reflection and working to develop their own and others' awareness of ethics in practice

Source: Canadian Nurses Association. (2017). *Code of ethics for registered nurses* (pp. 18–19). Ottawa: Author.

---

This chapter focuses on understanding the health care provider's moral responsibilities toward individuals and society with regard to facilitating health and well-being, or the relief of suffering. Professional responsibilities are obligations incurred by disciplines that provide a service to society. For example, the *Code of Ethics for Registered Nurses* (CNA, 2017) outlines that issues addressed in nursing involve providing safe, compassionate, competent, and ethical care; promoting health and well-being; promoting and respecting informed decision making; honouring dignity; maintaining privacy and confidentiality; promoting justice; and being accountable. In addition, Box 5.1 describes the ethical endeavours related to broad societal issues. The weblinks for this chapter include a link to the CNA's *Code of Ethics for Registered Nurses.*

Ethical issues focused on health promotion are best viewed as a subset of health care ethics that, in turn, has its roots in moral philosophy and value theory. This chapter discusses factors that can affect health promotion across the life span in diverse health care settings. The development, scope, and limits of ethical theories and perspectives are explored in relation to problems in health promotion. A basic assumption in this chapter is that the anticipation and prevention of ethical problems is a critical component of ethical professional action. A variety of real and hypothetical cases are presented to illustrate how ethical issues relate to health promotion. Strategies to aid nurses in identifying, anticipating, and addressing ethical issues are provided throughout.

The terms *ethical* and *moral* are used interchangeably throughout the chapter. Even though the two concepts are sometimes characterized differently, they have the same root meanings. The term *ethics* is derived from the Greek word *ethos*, meaning customs, conduct, or character. The term moral is derived from the Latin word *mores* and originally referred to doing something from a custom or habit (Sproul, 2015).

## PUBLIC HEALTH ETHICS

### Origins of Applied Ethics in Moral Philosophy

The discipline underlying ethical practice, or applied ethics, is moral philosophy. Moral philosophy is concerned with discovering or proposing what is right or wrong, or good or bad, in human action toward other humans and other entities such as animals and the environment. Singer (1993) described the crucial questions of moral philosophy as "What ought I to do? How ought I to live?" Among the tasks of moral philosophy is that of formulating theories or frameworks to guide action. Using a moral theory to propose and implement appropriate actions in troubling situations guides the decision maker toward good actions and the avoidance of harmful actions.

The theories that emerge as a result of philosophical inquiry about good action are called value theories; they are concerned with either discovering what humans seem to value (descriptive theories) or proposing what they ought to value (normative theories) to achieve predetermined goals. Value theories are based on observations of human behaviour over time and in a variety of settings. Descriptive theories do not tell us what actions we ought to take. They are not directives; they merely tell us how people act toward each other and their environments and what they seem to believe are good or moral actions. Normative theories, in contrast, are concerned with ensuring good actions.

### Types of Normative Ethical Theories

Normative ethical theories are reasoned explanations of the moral purpose of human interactions, or they are believed to be objective truths about good action (divinely given in the case of religious ethics). Actions that are in accord with the foundational principles of the theory are the type of right or good actions we should take given that we believe the principles (e.g., fairness and trust) are valid. What is often called the golden rule is a classic example of a normative principle. The golden rule commits us to treating other people in the manner that we would wish to be treated, given similar circumstances. Normative theories permit judgements about the value of actions on the basis of the extent to which these actions are consistent with the assumptions of the theory. They are key to decision making and relevant for health promotion but may be overlooked by policymakers.

### Consequentialist Theories

The foundational principle of John Stuart Mill's (2002/1861) theory of utilitarianism proposes that actions are good insofar as they aim at yielding the greatest amount of happiness or pleasure or causing the least amount of harm or pain to individuals and overall society. This theory is often formulated as the greatest good for the greatest number. Mill viewed pleasure as a complex concept, with qualitative as well as quantitative aspects. This perspective is consequentialist: it holds that the consequences or intended consequences of actions matter for determining moral worth. Therefore from the consequentialist perspective, any decision about intended actions or interventions must take into account all knowable potential consequences. Among the implications of this type of theory for nurses is the imperative that data gathering must be thorough and complete. Additionally, the provider is accountable for possessing the appropriate skills and knowledge to undertake actions that will promote good. The provider's decision can be evaluated as bad or good to the extent that actions are in accord with the theory: in the case of utilitarianism, "right actions" would be those that are directed toward promoting the greatest good or causing the least harm. The propositions of the theory direct what is needed for moral action or, stated another way, for doing the right thing.

### Duty-Based Theories

Other normative value theories are not as heavily weighted toward producing good consequences. For example, duty-based theories, such as the theory of Immanuel Kant (1724–1804) and those of various religions (Judaism, Christianity, Islam), depend more on adherence to duties than on good consequences. Individuals are viewed as having certain duties that cannot be circumvented, even if deliberately avoiding the duty would result in good outcomes. For religions, these rules are imparted in some way by a divine being.

For Kant, our capacity to reason is what guides moral action. Moral reasoning has been proposed as a model for health promotion (Buchanan, 2006). Kant based his theory on the idea that what separates us from other life forms is our ability to make rules for ourselves using reason. His main rule, whereby each of us can determine for ourselves a moral course of action, is the categorical imperative. It is called the categorical imperative because it applies in all situations (categorical) and is a binding command (imperative). The categorical imperative was framed in several different ways by Kant. One major formulation is as follows: "Act only according to that maxim whereby you can at the same time will that it should become a universal law" (Kant, 1993/1785).

Kant's theory is easier to understand through examples. Kant argued that making a false promise is always wrong even if on some occasions it might produce a good outcome. It is wrong because it is irrational and the promise breaker is making a moral exception for himself or herself. If everyone made a false promise when the immediate outcomes were likely to be positive, humans would lose their ability to trust promises, and this would make promises pointless and ineffective. Thus, making a false promise is irrational (and therefore unethical) because one is making a promise while counting on everyone else to act differently so that promises do not cease to exist. This formulation could thus be stated alternatively as a question to ask oneself before acting: "If I do this act, am I making a moral exception for myself? Am I counting on others to act differently than I am right now?" If a person asked this question before sneaking onto a bus without paying the fare, the answer would be "yes, I am making a moral exception for myself (and therefore should not do this)," because if everyone rode without paying the fare, the bus service could not run anymore!

Another formulation of Kant's categorical imperative is "Act in such a way that you treat humanity, whether in your own person or in the person of another, always at the same time as an end and never simply as a means" (Kant, 1993/1785). Kant calls us all to recognize every human being as a full human being with his or her own ends (i.e., life and goals). To treat someone merely as a means would be to use or ignore that person for one's own purposes. For example, it would be wrong to pretend to be friends with someone just so that person could help us study for a test. The various formulations of the categorical imperative will always lead to the same decision, so when we are deciding on an action, we can choose whichever formulation is easier (or more relevant) to apply in the situation.

## Character-Based Theories

Also referred to as virtue ethics, character-based approaches to ethics centre on the individual agent making the decision. Aristotle (384–322 BCE) argued that being moral was a matter of habits and desires. If a person can learn to desire the right things, then he or she will do the right things. For Aristotle (1985/350 BCE), doing the right thing is all about who you are. If you are a moral person with good ethical thinking skills, you will do the right thing. So, in any given situation, I might ask myself, "What would a good person do in this situation?" or "If I do this, will I be the kind of person I would consider to be a good person?"

Aristotle says that habits help us be moral in two ways. First, they help us put our desires in order: by always acting honestly, for instance, one will begin to form a desire for honest acts, so the habit of acting honestly makes one develop a desire to be honest. Second, habits help us learn how to be moral: the more one acts courageously, for instance, the better one becomes at it. By forming a habit of acting courageously, one is more likely to be able to know what the courageous thing to do is in any given situation, and will be more able to make oneself do it.

The advantage of Aristotle's character ethics is that instead of hard and fast rules to follow, he offers general advice, and thus his ethics is easily applicable to all situations. The drawback comes from the same source though: without any hard and fast rules to follow, it can be hard to look to virtue ethics to determine the right thing to do. Habits can help us learn, in general, how to be courageous, honest, temperate, kind, etc. Also necessary, though, is practical wisdom (phronesis in the original Greek). Aristotle's writings on ethics do not try to tell us what the right thing to do is in any situation. Instead, he describes the skills needed to figure out what to do in any situation. He takes this approach because he believes there is no one right way to act at all times. Any moral decision depends on the situation and the person making the decision.

## Limitations of Moral Theory

Keep in mind that moral theories arise out of a particular perspective or philosophy about the world. They are conceptualized as a result of this perspective and within a historical and political context. The philosophical approach that evaluates value theories or ethical perspectives for their congruence and usefulness in human decision making across environments is metaethics. Philosophers interested in metaethical questions investigate where our ethical principles come from and what they mean. Are they merely social inventions? Do they involve more than expressions of our individual emotions? Metaethics allows us to critique the adequacy of ethical approaches for application across a variety of practice settings and cultural environments. Other sorts of metaethical questions posed by moral philosophers include the following: Are there such things as absolute ethical truths? If so, how do we go about discovering these? If not, what foundations should we use to guide our actions? What is a valid moral theory? Should human values be congruent across settings and cultures?

Religiously based moral theories depend on the idea that good actions are those that obey the laws of a supreme being. However, because the foundational tenets of religions do not consistently mirror each other, what constitutes a moral or morally neutral action from a Jewish perspective may well be morally prohibited from a Roman Catholic perspective. Moreover, even within a religion, the tenets of its different sects or branches may not always lead to the same conclusions about good actions. Nurses and other health care providers need to recognize the influence of religion in people's lives because their duty to provide safe, competent, compassionate, and ethical care extends to an accommodation of religious and cultural values and practices.

As a result of diverse religious and cultural values, there are divergent but strongly held views on what is the good for humans. Many contemporary philosophers have argued that there can be no single approach that permits the identification or resolution of all moral problems (Rachels & Rachels, 2011; Weston, 2010). Even the golden rule can be problematic from a cross-cultural perspective. For example, I might want to be treated as an autonomous being capable of making my own decisions, but a person from Thailand might be more used to family-centred decision making. Treating a patient from Thailand as I would wish to be treated would be a mistake. An understanding of cultural beliefs is necessary for good action in such cases (Diversity Awareness). Health care providers wishing to engage in ethics respectful of diversity may be well served by "listening to the stories of those who are different, who may be unseen, marginalized, and excluded in our healthcare systems" (Sorrell & Dinkins, 2006). If we fail to listen to these stories, we are likely to be oblivious to the harm being done in health care through unwitting oppression of minorities or people from other cultures.

## 🌐 DIVERSITY AWARENESS

### Self-Reflection

The increasingly multicultural society, multiple languages spoken, and diverse set of values presents health care providers with complex assessment and planning problems. Nurses and other health care providers are charged with providing safe, compassionate, competent, and ethical care while honouring dignity of all individuals (CNA, 2017). Cultural humility focuses on the lifelong process of health care providers attaining skills, knowledge, and attitudes to work more effectively and respectfully with people of different cultures, whereas cultural safety moves beyond cultural awareness to focus on understanding the societal and historical context of health inequalities, as well as how interpersonal power imbalances shape health and health experiences (Hart-Wasekeesikaw & Gregory, 2009). Both concepts are critical to effective nursing practice. While it is not possible to know details about every culture as well as the unique differences of each individual, family community, and group within each culture, there are strategies that a health provider can use to ensure that an individual's unique values and particular needs are the focus of health-promotion interventions.

When a particular culture is part of your population base, opportunities should be pursued for learning individual differences in beliefs, values, and needs related to that culture. To facilitate your assessment, think about cultural awareness and cultural safety in practical terms. The following are self-reflection and other considerations for providing culturally safe care:

- What social or historical factors might impact the patient's access to care?
- Could issues with trust influence the therapeutic relationship?
  - How might these trust issues differ between cultures?
- Who has the power in the relationship with the patient?
- Do you believe your patients have the same priorities as you?
- How do your values impact your relationships with patients?
- How does cultural variations in beliefs and values occur?
- As a nurse, would the choices you make be different for yourself or someone you care about?
- What does your body language say about you?
  - How might a patient from another culture interpret your body language?
  - Could your body language be communicating something different from your words?

### Reflective Questions

- What is your definition of culture?
- How could your values negatively impact the care you provide to patients?
- Are care practices taking into consideration the patient's culture, or is care provided in a consistent manner regardless of culture?

Sources: College of Nurses of Ontario. (2019). *Therapeutic nurse-client relationship (Revised 2006)*. Retrieved from https://www.cno.org/globalassets/docs/prac/41033_therapeutic.pdf; Hart-Wasekeesikaw, F., & Gregory, D. M. (2009). *Cultural competence and cultural safety in nursing education: A framework for First Nations, Inuit and Métis nursing*. Ottawa: Aboriginal Nurses Association of Canada. Retrieved from https://www.cna-aiic.ca/~/media/cna/page-content/pdf-en/first_nations_framework_e.pdf.

Additionally, utilitarian theories emerged out of a particular era and as a result of perceived injustices in societal arrangements in England during the turmoil of the Industrial Revolution. Utilitarians such as Jeremy Bentham (1748–1832) and John Stuart Mill (1806–1873) sought frameworks that would permit the rectification of unjust policy decisions and the vast economic inequities within their society. For this reason, such theories have a tendency to privilege the good of the group over the needs of individuals. In health promotion, seeking a balance between good for the group or community and good for the individual can be a particular challenge. Utilitarian theories, in particular, are in danger of favouring the group (the majority) over those who are in fewer numbers (the minority).

The most famous illustration of how our ethical decision making might be determined by our culture and context comes from Plato (~427 to ~347 BCE). In Plato's *Republic* (1992/360 BCE), the character of Socrates describes a cave where prisoners have been shackled since birth, and thus the cave is the only reality they know. The prisoners face a cave wall on which they see shadows cast by the fire behind them, but they cannot turn their heads to see the fire and do not even know it is there. When one prisoner is freed, he journeys upward, first seeing the fire and eventually making it out into the wider world, lit by the light of the sun. Socrates says this prisoner's journey is the moral journey each of us must take. We must recognize that the morals we are taught may just be shadows of the true moral good (represented by the sun in the story).

Health practitioners today should be aware that they are likely most familiar and comfortable with the ideals and morals they have been raised with, and it is not always good to be limited by this perspective. As our society becomes increasingly complex, there are new and emergent ethical issues, such as protection of the environment, use of technology, allocation of scarce resources, and health care reform. Normative ethical theories give each of us means to think for ourselves and reflect on what we believe is right. It is not prudent to adopt one theory to guide actions in every situation related to health promotion. If a moral theory is applied unreflectively, it can lead to actions that are problematic for an individual or group. Health-promotion activities mandate not only a general understanding of the nature of the problem or potential problem but also knowledge of the values, beliefs, needs, and desires of the person or population being served. In addition, it is advisable that individuals look for an action or decision supported by more than one ethical theory—such confluence means that the action or decision will be morally right from multiple perspectives or contexts.

Specific principles derived from ethical theories have proved useful because they highlight salient aspects of complex problems and help to examine implications of different proposed courses of action. Selection of pertinent principles, however, depends both on the context of the problem and on the beliefs and values of the individual or group for which action is needed. For example, imagine a woman who seeks assistance in deciding whether to undergo genetic testing for the breast cancer gene *BRCA2* because several members of her immediate and antecedent families have received diagnoses of breast or associated cancers. She tells her nurse practitioner that she is not sure whether it would be beneficial to be tested. The nurse practitioner, in facilitating the woman's health-promotion efforts, understands that she must use clinical judgement to facilitate the woman's autonomous choice. Understanding the requirements of the principle of autonomy is important in helping the woman make her decision. It is not sufficient, however, to understand the meaning of autonomy and its limits; the nurse practitioner must also know something about the woman's life, values, beliefs, and relationships to provide her with the information and resources necessary for her decision. If the woman is screened and the results are positive for the gene, the woman not only must decide her next actions but also must consider the implications of the results (e.g., how the results affect her children or her decision to have children). The Genomics box presents information on genetic counselling. Individual principles of importance to decision making in health care settings are explored in this chapter. They, along with associated ethical considerations such as professional, feminist, and virtue ethics, underpin a framework of moral decision making for health promotion that is presented at the end of this chapter.

## GENOMICS

### Nurses as Genetic Educators, Researchers, and Counsellors

Nurses have always been important advocates for health care literacy and education. Since the International Human Genome Sequencing Consortium completed the Human Genome Project in 2003, nurses have stepped forward to gain new competencies and assume new roles related to genetics and genomics. In assuming these roles, nurses face ethical, legal, and social implications with patients and community members. These ethical, legal, and social implications require a basic genomic health literacy, as well as an understanding of the expectations of the public. Research strongly suggests that people want to have their genetic sequencing results to better understand their health profile.

The rapidly increasing discoveries in genetics research challenge nurses to gain new competencies so as to be knowledgeable about the often difficult ethical situations related to these discoveries. Genetics involves the study of a single gene's function. Genomics represents a wider view to include all genes in a person, including interactions of the genes with themselves and also the environment (Huddleston, 2013; Kiernan & Vallerand, 2016). Two other terms sound similar but have different meanings. Genotype refers to a set of genes in our DNA that is responsible for a particular trait. Phenotype is the physical expression of that trait, and is determined by interaction between the genotype and the environment. Genotype is an inherited trait; the entire genetic information about an organism is contained in a genotype. Examples of genotypes are the genes responsible for eye and hair colour and the sound of one's voice. Phenotype is what you see; it is the visible expression of the results of the genes combined with the environmental influence on one's appearance or behaviour. Examples of phenotypes are the *visible* or *observable* characteristic of eye and hair colour and the sound of one's voice.

These terms help nurses to understand how the integration of genomic and genetic factors into areas such as biobehavioural research provides new opportunities to understand problems that are difficult to define. For example, Lyon, McCain, Pickler, and colleagues (2011) noted that attempts to study fatigue have "been stymied by the lack of phenotypic clarity." These nurse researchers have studied genetic–genomic approaches that may increase the precision and clarity of the study of fatigue, thus enhancing understanding of mechanisms by which fatigue occurs in various health conditions as a patient symptom. Nurses are making important contributions through integration of genetic–genomic measures into biobehavioural research. This research may lead to better prediction of risk for medical problems, as well as identification of biological markers of symptom onset, progression, and resolution. More research is also needed in examining the relationship between individual genetic–genomic variations and outcomes of nursing interventions so that nurses can use genetic–genomic information to plan nursing interventions. There are potentially many nursing interventions that would be more effective if they were individually tailored to a person's genetic–genomic profile, rather than a "one size fits all" approach (Munro, 2015).

The ever-expanding discoveries in genomics challenge the nurse to be competent in genomic applications to nursing care and knowledgeable in the often difficult ethical issues that arise with these discoveries. There is a need for nurses to position themselves so as to attain advanced knowledge and skills related to their serving as specialized genetic counsellors. For example, medical-surgical nurses need to be aware of all advancements in cancer genetic–genomic practice guidelines in order to educate patients and their families about genetic–genomic testing, specific treatments, and follow-up care to reduce cancer risk and improve patient outcomes (Lacovara & Bohnenkamp, 2018; Santos, Edwards, Floria-Santos, et al., 2013). Although many health care providers have the skills to counsel individuals about genetic testing issues, especially in their fields of expertise, genetic counsellors are an increasingly important resource and are aware of ethical issues to consider in genetic screening.

Genetic counsellors are specially trained master's-prepared individuals. These providers can obtain certification through the Canadian Association of Genetic Counsellors. Genetic counsellors enter the field from a range of backgrounds, including social work, genetics, nursing, and psychology.

Genetic counsellors provide counselling services that are nondirective to avoid coercion or persuasion. Although there is controversy about how directive or nondirective advice should be based on the ethical ideals of autonomy, counsellors strive to be nondirective while at the same time tailoring information to fit the specific needs of people. Because advances in embryo preimplantation genetic testing, as well as in utero fetal testing, permit screening of individuals for certain superior characteristics or the screening out of certain genetic diseases, the perceived need to distance the profession from this issue is understandable.

Ethical issues related to genetic counselling for screening purposes that apply both for genetic counsellors and for other health care providers include the following:

- Understanding the wider context of genetic testing implications (privacy, discrimination, economics, health insurance denials, implications for family members, anxiety and apprehension, and eugenics [striving for perfection], and its associated implications for individuals and society).
- Assisting people to determine the risks and benefits of screening.
- Discussion of expected outcomes, what will be reported from the testing, and potential choices available as results obtained through testing.
- Providing opportunities to enroll in current or future research studies.
- Understanding how cultural differences impact counselling needs.
- Addressing societal issues related to genetic advances, including determining research priorities, justice issues, and discrimination of the genetically disadvantaged.

Sources: Boycott, K., Hartley, T., Adam, S., et al. (2015). The clinical application of genome-wide sequencing for monogenic diseases in Canada: Position statement of the Canadian College of Medical Geneticists. *Journal of Medical Genetics, 52*(7), 431–437; Huddleston, K., (2013). Ethics: The challenge of ethical, legal, and social implications (ELSI) in genomic nursing. *OJIN: The Online Journal of Issues in Nursing, 19*(1), 6; Kiernan, J., & Vallerand, A. H. (2016). Cancer as a platform for genetics education in the undergraduate nursing curriculum. *Journal of Nursing Education, 55*(4), 236–239; Lyon, D. E., McCain, N. L., Pickler, R. H., et al. (2011). Advancing the biobehavioral research of fatigue with genetics and genomics. *Journal of Nursing Scholarship, 43*(3), 274–281; Munro, C. L. (2015). Individual genetic and genomic variation: A new opportunity for personalized nursing interventions. *Journal of Advanced Nursing, 71*(1), 35–41.

## Feminist Ethics and Caring

### Feminist Ethics

Feminist perspectives on ethics derive from the feminist movement's efforts to expose and rectify injustices to women and raise awareness of the dominance of patriarchy in many ethical approaches. The feminist movement perspectives also often include problems common to all oppressed groups. Feminist ethics, emerging as it has out of feminist thought and feminist philosophy, is not another ethical theory as such; rather, it presents a viewpoint on moral problems in health care and other areas of life that have been historically neglected.

Feminist scholars have noted that traditional moral theories, and the principles derived from them, have been unable to adequately capture the nature and origins of health care problems. Feminist critics assert that moral decision making must include an investigation of both hidden and overt power relationships implicit in ethical problems. Additionally, it is important to understand the contexts of situations and the interrelationships of those involved, because human beings are not isolated individuals who may be viewed as totally independent of others. Thus hidden power imbalances in various relationships and situations are an important element in moral decision making. Feminist ethics, then, contributes a perspective that is often missing from traditional ethical approaches and aims to change the way ethical problems are perceived and explored.

The characteristics of feminist ethics include (Green, 2012):

- An understanding that human beings are inseparable from their relationships with others; relationships are the core variable of care.
- A focus on care and responsibility within relationships, rather than rights, rules, and an abstract system of thought.
- A concern with the development of character and attitudes within the context of relationships.
- A concern for the rights and equality of all persons.

Thus, feminist ethics allows a critique of the treatment of individuals in the contexts in which they live. This approach to ethics often focuses on imbalances of power along with oppression attributable to sex, sexual orientation, ethnicity, socioeconomics, politics, and other characteristics. For example, a feminist ethicist might point out that a punitive approach to perinatal substance abuse is not associated with improved outcomes for the fetus; in fact, the fetus may be at greater risk because the possibility of such punishment makes women fearful of accessing health services.

### The Ethic of Care

The feminist ethic of care is an important concept for health promotion because it focuses on the nature of nurse–person relationships and on the context of people's lives. This approach to care has found increasing acceptance in nursing as both a virtue of the nurse and a responsibility of practice in which treatment is offered on a common ground basis that will support people within their relationships. Carol Gilligan's (1982, 2014) research, among that of others, has been instrumental in the acceptance of the concept of care as informing ethics in nursing practice. Gilligan was a graduate student and then colleague of Lawrence Kohlberg, a developmental psychologist. The main focus of Kohlberg's (1981, 1984) body of work was the nature of moral character development, which was informed by Piaget's work on the stages of cognitive development in children. Kohlberg's stages of moral development were derived from longitudinal studies of young men. These moral reasoning studies were designed around the idea that an ability to apply conceptions of justice, rules, and principles to difficult situations denoted the highest achievable level of moral development. Gilligan challenged the reliance on only males in the study of moral reasoning and implemented studies of women's experiences, discovering that women had a moral orientation based on the caring and nurturing of others. In this framework used by women, interrelationships and contexts are critically important in understanding the complexities of a given situation.

The ethic of care calls for a knowledgeable and skillful health care provider to assume responsibility for the unique needs of an individual in all of his or her complexities. Benner, Tanner, and Chesla (2009) define care as "the alleviation of vulnerability; the promotion of growth and health; the facilitation of comfort, dignity or a good and peaceful death," noting that care is "the dominant ethic found in [nurses'] stories of everyday practice."

### Limits of the Ethic of Care

One problem with using care as an ethic of health-promotion practice has to do with individual rights versus the common good. The principles of health ethics at an individual level (autonomy, beneficence, nonmaleficence, and social justice) are not always congruent with ethical issues that occur in the larger community setting, because they are individualistic and patient rights-oriented, to the exclusion of the common good. When the solution to one person's problems affects others, however, the rightness of the action depends on more than the one-on-one caring relationship. The problem remains one of choosing between this person's needs and the needs of others who might be affected by the actions chosen. This problem is resistant to resolution via an ethic of care alone. The problem analysis framework described later combines the ethic of care with other considerations. Both an ethic of care and the principles derived from traditional moral theory may be needed for health promotion.

The purpose of ethical inquiry in health promotion is to gain clarity on actual or potential moral issues arising in the context of health-promotion endeavours and to understand what is expected of the health-promotion agent viewed as a moral agent. Ethical inquiry will not permit the resolution of all problems, because the environments in which health-promotion efforts are conceptualized are incredibly complex. It is impossible to foresee all possible consequences of action, but ethical reasoning can facilitate appropriate and in-depth data gathering, permit the uncovering of hidden agendas and interests, and focus on the most salient aspects of a particular problem, thus enhancing professional judgement.

## PROFESSIONAL RESPONSIBILITY

Professional judgement and ensuing actions are integral to the goal of providing a good for the population of concern. Thus, health promotion is a moral endeavour requiring morally sensitive and knowledgeable agents. But what are the scopes and limits of a nurse's obligations to anticipate, identify, and address morally problematic issues related to the promotion and protection of health for individuals, groups, and society? How do nurses balance their duties to individuals with a duty to society? How are individuals' freedoms (autonomy) balanced with the collective responsibilities owed to society and future generations?

## Accountability to Individuals and Society

### Professions

Although this section focuses on the nursing discipline's mandate to promote health, the discussion can also be applied to the responsibilities of other health providers who assume health-promotion responsibilities. Nursing is a profession insofar as it provides a service to society and is self-governing, and its members are accountable for their actions (CNA, 2017). A significant consequence of professional status is that members can be held accountable for their practice formally by professional licensure organizations. More importantly, they are morally accountable for practicing according to their discipline's implicit or explicit code of ethics. One important characteristic of professions, especially those that provide crucial services to society, is that they have codes of ethics that provide essential elements of their promises of service to society. Codes of ethics provide a normative framework for professional actions. A health care provider implicitly accepts these codes on acquiring membership in the discipline. Thus, each health care provider should establish a personal perspective on ethical practice within the broad framework of professional codes (CNA, 2017).

### Trust

Service professions such as nursing, medicine, and teaching are in part defined by their relationships to those in need of services. This relationship is one of trust. The health care provider has the knowledge and skills to meet an individual's needs or the needs of a group. The potential recipients of services lack the knowledge or ability to anticipate or meet their own needs but trust that the health care provider will keep their best interests as the primary goal and will strive to meet their needs. For example, in the current health care environment in Canada, while people may have timely access to care for emergent or urgent problems (e.g., heart attack, stroke, cancer care), typical wait times for many less urgent problems (e.g., hip or knee arthroplasty, cataract surgery, consultation with a specialist) often exceed established recommendations (Vogel, 2017). Of concern, older people who are not acutely ill often wait months and, on occasion, years in hospitals for assignment into a long-term care facility.

Nurses are responsible not only for promoting health and healing but also for recognizing and addressing barriers to health-promotion activities. The *Code of Ethics* (CNA, 2017) provides a detailed account of the nursing discipline's responsibilities, which describes the social contract between society and the nursing profession and emphasizes the nurse's responsibility to uphold principles of justice, protect human rights, equity and fairness, and promote the public good.

## Codes of Ethics

Codes of ethics are examples of normative ethics in that they prescribe how members of a profession ought to act, given the goals and purposes of the profession related to individuals and society. The provisions of codes of ethics for nurses provide direction and expectations of ethical behaviour. They represent the profession's promises to society. Although the public is not directly involved in the formulation of such codes and, indeed, is for the most part not even aware of their existence, the profession is responsive to the evolving needs of a given society. It can be said that codes of ethics are the tentative end results of a discipline's political process in that they are not static but result from debate and discussion over time among the profession's scholars, leaders, and members.

The current *Code of Ethics for Registered Nurses* presents a central foundation and provides guidance for ethical relationships, behaviours, and decision making to be used with professional standards, best practice, research, laws, and regulations that guide practice (CNA, 2017). A code of ethics tends to offer guidelines not only about responsibilities for ensuring good care but also about responsibilities for recognizing and addressing barriers to service. It also serves as an ethical basis for nurses to advocate for quality practice environments that support the delivery of safe, compassionate, competent, and ethical care. As the societal context in which nurses work is constantly changing, which can significantly influence nursing practice, nurses need to anticipate future health needs and political activity when necessary to ensure health promotion.

## Advocacy

Advocacy, as an expectation of nurses, is strongly reinforced both in the *Code of Ethics for Registered Nurses* and in innumerable scholarly articles. It refers to the "act of identifying a cause and/or recommending a course of action, undertaken on behalf of persons or issues, in order to create equity and better health for all" (CNA, 2017, p. 5). Nurses and other health care providers have a responsibility to speak up on behalf of people whose rights have been compromised or endangered. This is part of the nurse's role because people may not recognize either what is needed to meet their needs or when the care they are receiving is substandard. However, that is not the end of the nurse's responsibilities. Nurses must also consider that specific actions they undertake in the name of advocacy may pose problems for other people who are relying on them for health care services.

For example, Roger LeBlanc, a nurse case manager, is assisting Jim Lightfoot to apply for a special diet allowance in an effort to support his self-management of type 2 diabetes. He is currently living on-reserve in northern Ontario and the nurse manager has identified that he is experiencing food insecurity. The cost of healthy food is inflated in northern communities, with food insecurity being identified as a significant health concern. Roger believes it is a priority for Jim to have access to the healthy food to effectively manage his diabetes, and advocates for his receipt of a government-funded Special Diet Allowance.

This financial diet allowance helps eligible recipients with the extra costs of a special diet for an approved medical condition that (a) is generally considered by the medical community to be an adjunct to the medical treatment, and (b) results in additional costs above that of a normal healthy diet (Ministry of Children, Community, & Social Services, 2018). Because Roger represents other people who would also benefit from this food allowance, his decision to be an advocate for Jim must be weighed against the needs of these other people. A moral responsibility associated with advocacy in health care settings is that the effect of actions on others is considered. When one is advocating extra attention or specialized care for a given person, an injustice may be rendered simultaneously to other people in the nurse's care. Thus, professional advocacy requires a balancing of the health needs of the individual with the health needs of the population (Farrer, Marinetti, Cavaco, et al., 2015).

Advocacy is an ideal of health care professions that requires attention to vulnerable individuals and groups and to broader societal concerns. Moral agency on the part of the nurse requires action and motivation directed to some moral end that is enacted through relationships. Being aware of one's self in relation to others helps to establish the moral choice required to be an advocate for them. Understanding the interdependent nature of individual and social needs facilitates preventive and health-promotion actions on the part of nurses both locally and globally.

In the last decade there has been a shift in global consciousness in both ethics and nursing, in which nursing views ethics in a much broader sense than just direct care provided to individuals (Butts & Rich, 2020). It may encompass such issues as unequal care in communities composed of a large minority population or for undocumented patients. Advocacy may include political activity to address populations of concern. Pre-emptive and sociopolitical advocacy identifies and challenges the source of the ongoing problems. Nurses have moral obligations related to sociopolitical advocacy on behalf of their populations of concern. Roger LeBlanc's obligations include recognizing the problems caused by a chronic shortage of rehabilitation services. His concerns include discovering the source of this problem and joining with others in an attempt to address it at this level. Strategies for solving seemingly intractable problems of health care include collaboration with specialty nursing, medical, or patient advocacy groups, and communication of the issues in both professional and popular media.

Advocacy for health promotion is a concept with broad implications. It includes activities that are directed toward remedying socially based inequities or inadequacies in the health care delivery system. Advocacy can be viewed as an ethic of practice that includes all activities directed toward the person's good. Advocacy carries risks, in that addressing or facilitating the good for individuals or groups may pit nurses against their peers or against potential adversaries who do not share the same professional goals.

The nurse's role of advocacy requires that professional knowledge and judgement be applied to a variety of situations, from the relatively simple to the complex. The CNA's Policy and Advocacy Position Statement emphasized the need for advocacy in nurses through engaging others, acting as a voice on behalf of vulnerable persons/populations, and using evidence to influence policy and practice to create greater equity and health for all (CNA, 2017). This process requires several steps. First, potential or real problems need to be identified and analyzed, often in collaboration with others. Second, appropriate actions need to be formulated and their likely consequences considered. Third, obstacles to action should be recognized and addressed. Finally, actions are performed and evaluated. These basic steps are evident whether the object of health care or health promotion is an individual, a group, or society.

## Problem Solving: Issues, Dilemmas, Risks, and Moral Distress

The nature of health care environments makes it inevitable that difficult decisions will have to be made. However, many of the ethical problems encountered in health-promotion settings are issues rather than dilemmas. Daniel Chambliss (1996), a sociologist who studied nurses in acute care institutional settings, asserts that organizations such as hospitals often give rise to "practical problems, not individual dilemmas." These practical problems are nonetheless moral problems because they interfere with the goals of promoting health, well-being, or the relief of suffering. In both institutional and non-institutional health care settings, obstacles to good care may be caused by health care system arrangements, interprofessional conflicts, and/or lack of resources. Dilemmas are ethical issues of a special sort. Ethical dilemmas are those situations in which a choice must be made between two equally undesirable options, two equally favourable choices, or two choices that are ethically ambiguous (Butts & Rich, 2020).

The goals of health promotion require that both issues and dilemmas be recognized and addressed. The central ethical dilemma in public health often occurs between the needs of the individual and those of the community, and often results in the needs of one being neglected in favour of the other's needs (Holland, 2015). Neglected issues can then become dilemmas. Because nurses are at the front line of providing health care, they are often the first to observe an issue with quality of care or safety. Sometimes this concern may lead the nurse to assume the whistle-blower role—bringing the concern into the open in the hope of effecting change. Various studies have identified whistle-blowing as key in highlighting a need for health reform (Pohjanoksa, Stolt, Suhonen, et al., 2019). There is considerable evidence, however, that the whistle-blower may experience significant negative and harmful consequences, such as being victimized or ostracized by colleagues and administrators or losing employment (Pohjanoksa et al., 2019).

When a nurse is in danger of losing his or her position as a result of advocating better conditions, a balancing of foreseeable risks and benefits to the individual or group is required. The process of decision making in this situation can lead to moral distress. Ethical (moral) distress occurs when a nurse knows the ethically correct action to take, but is unable to act according to their moral judgement (CNA, 2017). Sources of moral distress within the current health care environment include an unsafe work environment due to lack of resources, including human and material, inappropriate staffing complements, negative perceptions of ethical climate, and increased levels of compassion fatigue among nurses (Mason, Leslie, Clark, et al., 2014). There is also an association between the nurse's own distress and the suffering witnessed while providing care (McMillan, 2018). Witnessing suffering conflicts with a moral obligation to reduce suffering. Moral distress can occur when the nurse's values and perceived obligations conflict with the needs and prevailing views of the work environment. With advances in technology, a significant source of moral distress involves the initiation of extensive life-saving actions that are perceived only as prolonging death (Lusignani, Gianni, Re, et al., 2017). Moral distress is correlated with impaired quality of care, and with certain vulnerable populations (Henrich, Dodek, Keenan, et al., 2017). It is also associated with professional burnout and an intention to leave the profession. The framework for making ethical decisions that are discussed later in this chapter includes considerations related to personal security along with preserving integrity.

## Preventive Ethics

Just as preventive health care activities aim to forestall health problems, the practice of preventive ethics aims to forestall ethical problems before they develop. Preventive ethics is an important requirement of health-promotion endeavours that includes individual action by the nurse, as well as social and political activism with other nurses or professional nursing organizations. Preventive ethics requires the health promoter to envision potential problems and institute actions that halt their development. For example, it is possible to extend a dying person's life for a very long time with use of available technology and medications. Although a competent person has the right to refuse treatment and this right is legally recognized as a result of the *Advance Directives for Resuscitation and Other Life-Saving or Sustaining Measures* of 1991, many people become incapacitated before they are able to make their wishes known. In this policy statement, the Canadian Medical Association suggests that persons should articulate their advance directives in two forms: with a written directive and by designating a proxy. All provinces/territories recognize and honour advance directives, but the legally recognized form differs from province to province (Box 5.2). It is important to think about the nurse's role in supporting individuals and their families in end-of-life decision making (CNA, 1998). Much more work needs to be done engaging people in discussion and helping them plan for such eventualities while they are still well. Preventive ethics in this situation entails initiating communication with persons and families before a problem arises. This communication is often missing both in institutional and in primary care settings.

Preventive ethics using a feminist ethics perspective would encourage the addressing of institutional practices to provide more humanistic care and underlying social issues that lead people to overeat, smoke, or be inclined toward violence. For example, preventive ethics would require the investigation of why as a society we have trouble discussing death and dying, and why we find it so hard to have a peaceful or good death. This is best articulated in the long-standing debate surrounding Canadian policy that addresses MAID. Although legal in many countries, it wasn't legal in Canada until 2015, when the Supreme Court of Canada unanimously overturned federal legislature preventing physician-assisted dying, arguing that the old law violated the *Canadian Charter of Rights and Freedoms*. This decision resulted in the 2016 enactment of Bill C-14, Canada's federal law permitting MAID. Despite current federal legislation now being in place, there continues to be uncertainty among some physicians and nurses regarding their rights and obligations, and there is limited access to MAID resulting from challenges with finding health care providers who are willing to provide it (CMPA, 2018).

We need to ask questions about lack of support, lack of resources, resistance from spouses and health care providers, and so on. One strategy for identifying potential ethical problems before they occur or worsen is to examine problematic cases for their antecedents. We should ask fundamental questions about societal arrangements and influences on health trends.

On a local level, nurses and other health promoters need to use clinical judgement in anticipating and forecasting problems before they arise. For example, unrecognized health illiteracy may affect an individual's understanding of his or her rights and entitlements. When a nurse observes that a person and that person's family do not understand either the information that has been given to them or the implications of following a given course of action, the nurse engages in preventive ethics by supplying that information and ensuring that the information is understood. The nurse acts to prevent negative consequences that can arise as a result of poorly understood information. Other examples of opportunities to use preventive ethics include focusing on smoking or childhood obesity. Many problems in health care occur as a result of poor communication or because information has been provided too late for reasoned decision making (Quality and Safety Scenario).

## ETHICAL PRINCIPLES IN HEALTH PROMOTION

Although the tenets of nursing's codes of ethics and standards of practice provide some guidance about the nature of practice and the manner in which services will be provided, they often leave some ambiguity about the best course of action in morally troubling situations. The use of principles derived from a variety of ethical theories, along with feminist insights or an ethic of care, helps to provide further guidance in decision making in morally problematic health situations. Ethical principles provide an important starting point for moral judgement and policy evaluation, but that principles alone are not enough. In other words, principles such as autonomy, beneficence, and justice often serve as helpful starting points in teasing out the tangled elements of complex issues, but taken alone they are usually insufficient for moral problem solving in health care environments. One must decide which principles are important to consider in a given case or situation, and this requires an exploration of the case as discussed in the decision making framework provided later in the chapter.

Additionally, tenets of the CNA's *Code of Ethics for Nurses* and other CNA position statements provide guidance regarding

## BOX 5.2    Preventive Ethics: Patient Self-Determination and Advance Directives

Advance care planning is a process in which patients, their families, and their health care providers discuss the patient's goals, values, and beliefs to document how these should be reflected in future health care choices. It often cannot be predicted whether and when individuals will lose the ability to make their wishes for treatment and care known. Advance care planning is a health-promotion endeavour that can enhance an individual's quality of life, especially while having chronic illness.

In the last two to three decades, great technological and therapeutic advances have been made, with the resulting ability to save the lives of people experiencing catastrophic illnesses and trauma. One effect of these advances, unfortunately, is that sometimes we are successful only in prolonging the dying process. Although it is now recognized that people have a right to refuse treatment to prolong life, critically ill people may lose their ability to articulate their wishes for treatment. Advance directives are a way for people to help ensure that when they become incapacitated, the care and treatment they receive matches their predetermined wishes. At their best, advance directives have the potential to ease the strain felt by loved ones as they strive to make the "right" treatment choices for a friend or relative. Advance directives also guide health providers in their decision making regarding the person in question.

### Types of Advance Directives

There are various forms of advance directives, but the types typically recognized by provincial law in Canada are living wills and power of attorney. Living wills document patient preferences for life-sustaining treatments and resuscitation, whereas a power of attorney documents one's choice of a surrogate decision maker. A major limitation of the living will is that it may not be applicable to every decisional dilemma the patient will actually face. Therefore it is important to also designate a surrogate decision maker who can provide guidance to health care providers in cases where patients are incapacitated and the living will does not apply.

Advance directives are intended to improve communication related to end-of-life care issues and preferences among individuals, health care providers, and proxy decision makers. Although advance directives have great potential, they serve their purpose only to the extent that they are taken seriously as a responsibility of a given institution. Institutions may fail to ensure that a qualified person is available to impart the information or to request personal preferences. It is important for those involved in health promotion to understand and address why people may be reluctant to make an advance directive and why institutions are not diligent in providing information and education. In a 2013 Canadian study of older patients, only 47.9% had completed an advance care plan and only 30.2%

had discussed these wishes with their family doctors (Heyland, Barwich, Pichora, et al., 2013). Although it is considered to be extremely important, Canadians often struggle with legally articulating their wishes and rely on their health care providers to start the conversation. The physician–patient relationship is a key element in satisfaction with end-of-life care (O'Sullivan, Mailo, Angeles, et al., 2015).

### Impediments to the Use of Advance Directives

- Discussions with health care providers about the implications of desired choices have been inadequate.
- People do not want to talk about future incapacity or death. They may have cultural prohibitions about discussing the possibility of serious illness or death.
- Past encounters with the health care system have led to distrust.
- People cannot predict accurately their future preferences and they know too little about what constitutes life support.
- People may change their minds about what they will accept.
- The health care proxy may turn out to be a poor choice or may cause conflicts among other family members or loved ones. The person or family may ask for something that is morally unacceptable.
- Treatments may be specified to which the provider has conscientious objections.
- Documentation may be lost, misplaced, or not accessible in an emergency.
- Written instructions are too vague and open to divergent interpretation to be useful guides.
- Even the most diligent proxy cannot always know what the person would have wanted in the absence of a detailed treatment directive.
- The proxy may make a treatment choice contrary to the person's directive.
- The proxy may make a decision with which the institution or health care provider disagrees.

### Positive Outcomes of Use of Advance Directives

In spite of impediments, research has shown that advanced care planning has resulted in the following positive outcomes:

- Higher rates of completion of advance directives.
- Increased likelihood that clinicians and families understand and comply with a patient's wishes.
- A reduction in hospitalization and intrusive treatments at the end of life.
- Increased utilization of hospice services.
- Increased likelihood that patients will die in their preferred place.

Sources: Detering, K., & Silveira, M. J. (2015). Advance care planning and advance directives. *UpToDate*. Retrieved from http://www.uptodate.com/contents/advance-care-planning-and-advance-directives; Heyland, D. K., Barwich, D., Pichora, D., et al. & ACCEPT (Advance Care Planning Evaluation in Elderly Patients) Study Team. (2013). Failure to engage hospitalized older patients and their families in advance care planning. *JAMA Internal Medicine, 173*(9), 778–787; O'Sullivan, R., Mailo, K., Angeles, R., et al. (2015). Advance directives: Survey of primary care patients. *Canadian Family Physician, 61*(4), 353–356; The Holdings Group. (2012). *The failure of the living will*. Retrieved from http://www.theholdinggroup.org/the-failure-of-the-living-will-2/.

what a nurse's moral responsibilities are in a particular type of situation (CNA, 2003, 2009, 2017). Certain tenets address the responsibilities of the nurse with regard to improving the larger health care environment. These obligations include collaborating with others to "uphold principles of justice by safeguarding human rights, equity and fairness and promoting the public good" (CNA, 2017, p. 15).

## Autonomy as Civil Liberty

In health-promotion settings and endeavours, the concept of autonomy can be understood from two different perspectives. From the vantage point of public health, the extent of individual

autonomy, or freedom of action, may be limited by the duty of protecting the health and safety of the society. From this perspective there is an age-old struggle between civil rights and public safety. Moral questions ask to what degree society is justified in regulating the health and safety of society at large. There is an inevitable tension associated with curtailing civil liberties, or human rights, in the name of safety or health. This tension arises from perceptions that, in most Western contexts, freedom of action is a prerequisite of human flourishing.

Currently there are many indirect threats to the health and safety of our society including, but by no means limited to, bioterrorism and the spread of human immunodeficiency virus/

## ⚡ QUALITY AND SAFETY SCENARIO

**Patient-Centred Care**

Recognize the patient or designee as the source of control and full partner in providing compassionate and coordinated care based on respect for the patient's preferences, values, and needs.

### How Is Health Literacy Related to Ensuring Autonomy in Decision Making for Individuals?

Autonomy is an important ethical principle for health-promotion activities. To ensure autonomy in individual decision making, it is important to assess the individual's health literacy skills. These skills relate to a person's ability to obtain, process, and act on basic health information. Think how difficult it would be for a person with low literacy skills to navigate today's complex health care system. Adequate health literacy is essential for accessing necessary health care services and for fostering effective decision making.

In the process of implementing health-promotion activities, the nurse should first determine whether the person has adequate health literacy skills. This can be assessed with tools such as the Rapid Estimate of Adult Literacy in Medicine-Short Form (REALM-SF) or the Test of Functional Health Literacy in Adults (TOFHLA). It is important however, not to base an approach to health promotion solely on the results of one of these tools, which may not reveal the extent to which health recommendations may be misunderstood. The nurse should take the time to establish a rapport with the individual that includes fostering a sense of trust and openness for the person to ask important questions.

Unrecognized health literacy may interfere with individuals' rights to autonomy in decision making because they may make a decision based on inaccurate information or may automatically accept the decision of the health care provider without deciding for themselves whether or not the decision is appropriate for their individual situation. Thus, it is an ethical obligation of the nurse to make sure that effective communication is implemented. A public health approach founded on health-promotion principles can provide a useful scaffold for assessing the health literacy of persons in the community. This can help to ensure that the person is in control and a full partner in health-promotion decisions that respect his or her preferences, values, and needs.

Source: Guzys, D., Kenny, A., Dickson-Swift, V., et al. (2015). A critical review of population health literacy assessment. *BMC Public Health, 15*, 215.

acquired immunodeficiency syndrome (HIV/AIDS) and medication-resistant tuberculosis. Actions to resolve any of these threats have the potential to impinge on civil liberties; such actions might include, for instance, surveilling citizens or requiring disclosure of disease status. Advances in genetic knowledge present the possibility of discrimination from a variety of sources. It will be difficult to maintain individual privacy, and discrimination based on class or gene profile will be made easier.

The limitations of a publicly funded health care system can also impinge on civil liberties. The behaviour-change approach has been criticized as being too paternalistic, without sufficient regard for the individual's or the group's own perceptions of what is important; this may increase the risk of failed interventions. Prioritizing behaviour change in health-promotion endeavours over the need to address underlying social concerns, such as poverty and other forms of disadvantage, may obscure a focus on the social determinants of health. Rather than focusing on behaviour change, a focus on empowerment may help a person gain control over social and economic factors that contribute to health problems (Tengland, 2016).

## Autonomy as Self-Determination

A second, related, sense of autonomy has to do with individual choice. Autonomy is the moral principle that underlies the concept of informed consent to treatment, interventions, and health-promotion efforts. In Western societies it is probably the most powerful moral principle underlying the treatment of individuals. This principle asserts that people have the ability to reason, and a consequence of the ability to reason is the capacity to make choices. These choices concern both one's own behaviour and how one should act toward others. Although the idea that our ability to reason constitutes the essence of being human originated with Aristotle, Kant (1993/1785) developed this idea in meticulous detail in his work *Grounding for the Metaphysics of Morals*. According to Kant, people are capable of conscious desires and goals and are free agents capable of making decisions and setting goals as guided by their own reason. This principle is a salient consideration in health care settings: it underpins the health provider and promoter–person relationship and the issue of informed consent. However, there is limited agreement about the scope, limits, and strength of this principle. When describing autonomy in the context of health or treatment choices, we should delineate what we mean by autonomy in the context of the problem under discussion. Feminist criticisms of an emphasis on autonomy highlight the problem that our choices necessarily affect others because we are contextual beings inseparable from our relationships with one another.

Respect for human autonomy guides us to permit individuals to make and learn from their own mistakes. Generally, respecting autonomy requires that we permit individuals to make their own decisions, even when these decisions seem to others to be ill-informed. There are exceptions to this rule. Exceptions include those situations in which there is a high risk of serious injury or death and when it cannot be determined whether the person's judgement is impaired. Thus, we make exceptions to the rule of autonomy when we suspect that an individual is not able to reason adequately. A person's reasoning ability may be impaired by psychological or physical conditions, or it may be impaired as a result of incorrect or incomplete information.

In health-promotion activities, respect for autonomy requires that individuals be given the information they need to make choices. Choices can be considered autonomous only if certain criteria are met. The criteria that determine whether or not a person is actually capable of autonomous (voluntary) choice include cognitive maturity, possession of appropriate information to permit decision making, intact mental capacities (the ability to reason logically), the absence of internal or external coercive influences, and the ability to appreciate the risks and benefits of alternative choices. Assessing all such criteria is quite a tall order. And in one sense it may be that nobody acts totally autonomously at any given time because of the influences of entrenched beliefs and values that are derived, for the most part, from our cultural and environmental backgrounds. We have never entirely escaped from Plato's cave. Some of these influences are under conscious control in the sense that we can recognize what values we hold and even revise them if they are dissonant with other values. However, some of these influences are not readily recognizable: they lie beneath the surface of consciousness and are hard to access even if we are willing to try. We all have blind spots; autonomy viewed as informed, uncoerced, and reasoned action is therefore an ideal. Many of us fall short of the ideal.

## Informed Consent

Informed consent to research, treatments, or health-promotion endeavours is a process of ensuring that a person has all of the appropriate information necessary to reach a decision about participation that facilitates autonomous action. Informed consent occurs when a person with substantial understanding, and without substantial control by others, intentionally gives permission or makes choices about care (CNA, 2017). The key phrase is "with substantial understanding." It is important to understand that even after a consent form has been signed, a person has the right to rescind consent in light of additional information and/or changed consequences.

The components of the consent process include determining the person's competency to consent. There must be no physical or mental impairments that hinder the person in question from understanding and processing information. For example, a person with pneumonia who is febrile and confused is probably not capable of making an informed decision until the fever has been reduced and the confusion has cleared. To be substantially informed, a person must be made aware of important details of the proposed intervention, including its nature, purpose, probability of success, and important risks, and must also understand what alternatives (if any) are available. Because this information must be tailored to meet the specific needs of an individual and such a task requires knowledge of the person, an ethic of care is important to understanding a person's unique needs. We can check understanding to a certain extent by asking the individual to articulate how the proposed intervention will facilitate his or her own values and goals. There must be no subtle or overt coercion by professionals or others. Finally, appropriate supports must be available to complete the proposed intervention.

Obtaining consent for any interventions, or for involvement in research, is best viewed as a process that entails ongoing assessment of the person's status and evaluation of needs for further information or support. People may not understand information well when they are in stressful situations or when the information is complex. Thus, we should assess people for and validate understanding on an ongoing basis.

Ensure that all individuals, regardless of age, make informed choices. Although the life span increases in society, nurses must be aware of strategies for ensuring that older persons, who may be less able to advocate their own health needs, participate in the making of informed decisions. More research is needed on ethical problems that confront nurses in caring for older persons in the community.

Adolescence is a period of transition between the dependence and vulnerability of childhood and the autonomy of adulthood. Adolescents are generally considered capable of making decisions related to health-promotion activities, and health care providers have a duty to respect those decisions, provided that doing so does not produce harm to adolescents or others (Coughlin

## RESEARCH FOR EVIDENCE-INFORMED PRACTICE

### Influences on Sexual Decision Making of Late Adolescents

Violence has been identified by the World Health Organization as a major risk to health and well-being. Sexual activity without clear consent is one aspect of violence against adolescents, who are still developing their values and beliefs about sexual activity and sexual norms. In a qualitative research study, DuBois, Macapagal, Rivera, et al. (2015) used an online focus group of adolescent gay and bisexual men (AGBM) to explore the life experiences, motivations, and decision making related to sexual activity. The research question was: What factors inform adolescent gay and bisexual men's decision to have sex or not have sex? In addition, we wanted to examine whether these factors differed by sexual experience. Seventy-five AGBM aged 14–18 years or older were interviewed. They were asked to respond to questions related to reasons to engage in sexual activities, reasons and benefits of abstinence, experiences with peer pressure to have sex, decision making about first sexual experiences, and reasons to stop having sex.

The findings showed that in the decision-making most of the sexual encounters of AGBM were similar to their heterosexual peers, including implied sexual consent, peer pressure, decreased inhibition due to substance use, physical pleasure, and a desire to express love. Unique concerns to this population also included "coming out," safety in identifying same-sex partners, avoidance of sexually transmitted infections (STIs) and HIV. The participants discussed how sexual activity eventually occurred, even when they did not want it, because of pressure from external sources such as peers, culture, media, and one's partner. Interpersonal reasons to stop engaging in sexual activity were identified as feeling "used" for sex and/or "forced to have sex."

The findings from the study provide evidence that both heterosexual and gay/bisexual adolescent decisions involving consent for sexual activity are complex and are influenced by a myriad of personal, interpersonal, and social factors. All individuals have a right to clearly refuse or consent to sexual activity; this is imperative for the promotion of physical, emotional, and sexual health and safety. Nurses and other health care providers who work with adolescents, including the LGBTQ2 community, need to carefully assess sexual behaviours and recognize that all adolescents, regardless of the sexual orientation, are at risk of nonconsensual sexual activity. Sexual violence education should include information on negotiation and communication skills that will help adolescents mediate complicated interpersonal situations. Appropriate educational programs can help to empower young youth through opportunities for increased knowledge and self-confidence.

Source: DuBois, L. Z., Macapagal, K. R., Rivera, Z., et al. (2015). To have sex or not to have sex? An online focus group study of sexual decision making among sexually experienced and inexperienced gay and bisexual adolescent men. *Archives of Sexual Behavior, 44*(7), 2027–2040.

& Canadian Paediatric Society, 2018). Most health-promotion activities do not require formal informed consent. However, it is important to integrate the underlying principles and supporting research related to informed consent to be sure that the selected health-promotion strategies fit individuals' beliefs and values. It is also important to recognize that complex social factors may contribute to adolescents' inability to make well-thought-out decisions (Evidence-Informed Practice).

## Exceptions to Autonomous Decision Making

In some cases, proxy or substitute decision making on behalf of the individual is required (Box 5.3). This term may be referred

## BOX 5.3   Substitute Decision Making

Advance care planning: an ongoing process of reflection, communication, and documentation of personal wishes for future health care decisions in the event the individual becomes incapable of consent to or refusing treatment.

- Written:
  - Living will, advance directive
  - Document details to various degrees what the person will or will not accept
- Substituted judgement:
  - Individual appoints a substitute decision maker who has the legal authority to make health-related treatment decisions in the event that the individual is incapable of making informed decisions
  - Informal (nonappointed significant other)

**Best Interests**

Surrogate chooses the actions that will give the highest overall benefit—may or may not be based on a person's previously expressed desires; a quality of life determination based when possible on knowledge about the person

Sources: Canadian Nurses Association & Canadian Hospice Palliative Care Association. (2015). *The palliative approach to care and the role of the nurse [Joint Position Statement]*. Ottawa: Authors. Retrieved from https://www.cna-aiic.ca/~/media/cna/page-content/pdf-en/the-palliative-approach-to-care-and-the-role-of-the-nurse_e.pdf; Government of Canada. (2017). *Options and decision-making at end of life*. Retrieved from https://www.canada.ca/en/health-canada/services/options-decision-making-end-life.html; Canadian Nurse Protective Society. (2009). Consent of the incapable adult. *InfoLaw, 13*(3), 1–2.

to as *medical proxy, health representative* or *health agent,* or *power of attorney for personal care,* depending on the governing province or territory. Proxy decision making must take into account what is known about the person and must follow a path of action that is most likely to respect that individual's goals and values. Researchers have found that surrogate family members who need to serve as proxies in making decisions for loved ones, often at the end of life, find the decision making overwhelming and extremely stressful (Miller, Morris, Files, et al., 2016). Most surrogate decision makers have had little preparation for making these choices and worry that they are not making the right decision. Nurses and additional support staff (pastor care, social workers) should support these surrogate decision makers as they struggle with making a decision. Iverson, Celious, Kennedy, et al. (2014) described what helps and hampers surrogate decision making (Innovative Practice).

Certain populations are considered less than fully autonomous for a variety of reasons. People with Alzheimer's disease or other physical or psychological disruptions or deficits that prevent adequate comprehension may require proxy decision makers. It is important not to assume, however, that all persons with Alzheimer's disease are incapable of providing informed consent, because many persons in the early stages of the disease are capable of making decisions related to their care (Palmer, Harmell, Pinto, et al., 2017). Incarcerated people are restricted in their choices and may be subject to subtle or not-so-subtle coercion. Children are considered less than fully autonomous because they are not developmentally mature. Additionally, in people with certain mental health disorders, such as psychoses or bipolar disorders, the capacity for decision making may fluctuate. The Canadian Medical Protective

## INNOVATIVE PRACTICE

### Surrogate Decision Making

Most end-of-life health care decisions are made by surrogate decision makers who are under a great deal of stress over their seriously ill family member. Both surrogates and clinicians have various degrees of preparation, knowledge, abilities, or comfort in working effectively with another in making very difficult decisions for someone else.

Iverson et al. (2014) explored surrogate decision makers' challenges in making decisions related to the care of patients in critical care. They interviewed 34 designated surrogates of critically ill patients receiving care in two tertiary care institutions. Surrogates were asked to describe and reflect on their experiences of making health care decisions for others. They identified factors that added to the difficulty in decision making:

- Stress associated with assuming a decision-making role for which they felt unprepared
- Uncertainty of patient outcomes
- Difficulty in communicating with multiple health care providers who would provide different information
- Insufficient knowledge of patients' wishes
- Conflict within the family
- Fatigue resulting from near-constant vigilance in the critical care unit

Social networks that provided access to family and/or friends were helpful in the decision-making process, as they provided surrogate decision makers with emotional and informational support. Nurses were the preferred resource for day-to-day communication and information gathering except when major decisions needed to be made. Most participants perceived that nurses offered compassionate communication and were able to disentangle information that was difficult to understand.

The findings of the study suggest areas where clinicians can intervene to facilitate the processes of surrogate decision making. Stress can be minimized by improving communication between surrogate decision makers and health care providers. Nurses are uniquely poised to intervene to improve communication and reduce surrogates' decision-making anxiety.

Source: Iverson, E., Celious, A., Kennedy, C. R., et al. (2014). Factors affecting stress experienced by surrogate decision makers for critically ill patients: Implications for nursing practice. *Intensive and Critical Care Nursing, 30*(2), 77–85.

Association (CMPA) outlines criteria regarding the minimal capacities needed for competent decision making are "(1) understand the nature and anticipated outcomes of medical treatment and available options; (2) the ability to understand the consequences of refusing treatment; and (3) the capacity to give valid consent" (CMPA, 2016; Evans, 2016). These criteria are generally accepted as a basic minimum. It can be seen from these criteria that some children would be able to understand the implications of a given course of treatment, and adults with cognitive impairments may be deemed competent to make certain decisions. Competency to make autonomous choices is not an all-or-nothing capacity. Competency determinations are, as a rule, made for a given decision or task. Thus, a person may vacillate between competency and noncompetency, depending on either the task at hand (degree of difficulty) or the physical or psychological status during the period when a decision must be made.

When advocating decision making for a cognitively impaired person, consider the risks and benefits of allowing the individual to make his or her own decision. The benefits in terms of self-esteem may well outweigh the risks of many choices. However, if the risk of injury is high and it is obvious that the person is not able to reason effectively, autonomous decision making may not be feasible. In this case, nurses can collaborate with the individual, family members, and other health care providers to arrive at a decision that is best for the individual.

When children are involved, the legal age of majority has become progressively irrelevant in determining capacity to consent, and the concept of maturity has replaced chronological age. Maturity, in a minor, is the extent to which the young person's physical, mental, and emotional development allows for a full understanding of the nature and consequences of the proposed treatment, including the right to refuse treatment (Evans, 2016). When the minor lacks the necessary capacity, it is often the parent or guardian to whom we turn for permission to treat the child. The only exception involves consent to medical assistance in dying, where the patient must be at least 18 years of age and the minor's parent or guardian cannot consent to assistance in dying on the minor's behalf (Evans, 2016). The example of 5-year-old Julianna Snow illustrates how difficult these decisions can be. Julianna had an incurable neuro-degenerative illness and decided that she would rather die at home instead of returning to the hospital for treatment that would likely lead to death or being sedated on a respirator with little quality of life. Julianna's parents honoured this decision and Julianna died. Ethical questions were raised about whether a child of this age could/should be allowed to make an irreversible decision without the maturity to understand the consequences (Cohen, 2015).

For a child's assent to be meaningful, an assessment of the level of maturity and comprehension is required, and information must be provided in language and terms that are appropriate for the developmental level. Conversely, when there is conflict between the decision of the parent and that of the child, the health care provider has a duty to ensure that the parental choice is in the child's best interest. Where there is serious doubt, it may be necessary to involve the courts.

## Confidentiality

Autonomy is also the principle underlying confidentiality. One expression of autonomy is the ability to maintain privacy in one's life (Burkhardt & Nathaniel, 2013). People have the right to decide who can have access to information about them, thus limiting the negative use of personal information by others. Confidentiality is essential in the health care environment because patients trust health care providers with private information in order to receive safe and appropriate care.

Nurses must strive to keep the person's personal information confidential so as to enhance trust within the nurse–person relationship. Therefore, in health care settings, there are strong penalties against breaching confidentiality. In theory, the principle of confidentiality may be overridden only in situations in which extreme harm to self or others is imminent or unless disclosure is required by law. In practice, this can be challenging to enforce, because in medical settings many people have access to the person's information. Private insurance companies may demand access to information before payment for services is made. In outpatient settings, challenges for privacy may occur when personnel

are personally acquainted with the individual. When health care providers are members of the community in which they practice, there may be confidentiality issues associated with the intimate nature of small communities. Nurses and other health-promotion professionals may find themselves being asked by friends and relatives of the person for details about that person's health status. It can be very difficult to respond diplomatically while maintaining the person's privacy. The ethical implications of these threats to confidentiality are many. Thus, it is important for nurses to be aware of potential breaches of confidentiality and to advocate confidential treatment of information for those they serve.

### Personal Information Protection and Electronic Documents Act (PIPEDA)

Established in 2004, the *Personal Information Protection and Electronic Documents Act (PIPEDA)* is the Canadian federal privacy law which applies to all personal data, health-related or otherwise. The purpose is to govern the collection, use, and disclosure of personal information which protects individual privacy of personal information. Once an organization collects data, they become fully accountable and responsible for the protection of all acquired information. Its intent was to ensure that individuals' health information is properly protected, while allowing the flow of information needed to provide and promote high-quality care (including use of information about the person receiving care for research) and to protect the public's health and well-being. PIPEDA was established to protect the privacy of individually identifiable data, including health information, in the face of advances in electronic technology, and to limit the ways in which information is shared. PIPEDA requires adherence to the following legal principles:

- *Accountability.* Organizations are responsible and accountable for the organization's adherence with PIPEDA's principles.
- *Identifying Purpose.* The purpose for the sharing of information will be identified by the organization, at or before the time of collection.
- *Consent.* Knowledge and consent of the individual is required for the collection, use, or disclosure of personal information.
- *Limiting Use, Disclosure, and Retention.* Information is to be used and disclosed only for the purpose for which it was collected.
- *Accuracy and Individual Access.* Minimize possibility of using incorrect information by making it accessible for inspection and correction.
- *Safeguards.* Protection of personal information against loss or unauthorized access, disclosure, copying or modification (Office of the Privacy Commissioner of Canada, 2018).

Additionally, each province and territory has its own legislation to protect a patient's private health information. For example, British Columbia has the *Personal Information Protection Act (PIPA)* and Newfoundland and Labrador has the *Access to Information and Protection of Privacy Act (ATIPPA)* (Lewis, Bucher, Heitkemper, et al., 2019).

### Adolescents: Special Considerations of Confidentiality

Adolescents often present health care providers with very tricky confidentiality issues. As Branje (2018) discusses, adolescence involves a period of rapid biological and psychosocial changes where there is a need to challenge authority in an attempt to assert independence while still needing the help and support of effective parents. Normal developmental needs, along with the results of risk-taking behaviour such as drug and alcohol experimentation and risky sexual activity, mean that teenagers can pose a health-promotion challenge. The task of health promotion is to maintain and facilitate the adolescent's emerging autonomy and confidentiality needs, while mediating between the peer and parental figures who feel that they have a right to information about the adolescent.

Although federal and provincial/territorial laws, as well as ethical considerations, generally serve to protect the privacy and autonomy of adolescents, health promotion involves more than mere protection. It involves facilitating the adolescent's health. Thus, the responsibilities include helping an adolescent to grasp his or her authentic options and rights, facilitating interaction between the adolescent and parents or guardians, maintaining trust, and preserving confidentiality.

On the other hand, clinical judgement (which includes ethical judgement) is important in determining risk. If the risk of preserving the adolescent's privacy is high, on the basis of all pertinent and available evidence such as the presence of sexual or physical abuse, then it may be necessary to report this information to appropriate authorities. Mandatory reporting laws exist. Such laws are important for the general protection of a society's citizens. However, there may be rare occasions when a judgement must be made about whether upholding the legal obligation would cause more harm than good. In such circumstances there are two separate considerations. First, one must decide whether the risk to professional standing and licensure of not following the legally required path is something that the health care provider is willing to assume. The second consideration involves assessing the potential benefits and risks to the person resulting from failure to report. There is no easy resolution for these types of problems. If the situation is not an emergency, it is prudent to solicit appropriate advice from a peer, a counsellor, or an ethics expert or resource. In any case, it remains the professional's ethical responsibility to handle the given situation in a manner that preserves trust and provides ongoing support.

## Veracity

Veracity, or devotion to the truth, is another principle that supports health-promotion activities. People whose health is in question are to various degrees reliant on the person who possesses the knowledge and skills to bring these to bear on their behalf. Veracity, which is fundamental to the nurse–patient relationship, involves providing individuals with factual information about their health care needs to enhance patient decision making (Grace, 2017). Nurses may be tempted to withhold certain details when this is seen as serving the person's best interests or when family members demand it. It is sometimes difficult to determine how much and what types of information will best serve a person's needs. Knowledge of the person's beliefs, values, and lifestyle preferences is essential to the process of supplying adequate information to support autonomous decision making. Withholding information or providing information that is misleading or incomprehensible in an attempt to influence someone to agree to a treatment or intervention conflicts with veracity. It may be tempting to avoid the longer route to resolving such problems (e.g., education, understanding people's motives).

Veracity has some cross-cultural implications, in that some cultures have not traditionally valued truth telling in the case of terminal illness. Decision making about whether or not to honour veracity in such cases must take into consideration what is known about the culture, the particular person, the strength of his or her personal and cultural beliefs, and whether there is evidence about what sorts of things the person would like to know. The absence of veracity may interfere with autonomous action. In the case of terminal illness, it may deprive the person of the ability to plan the remainder of his or her life.

At first glance, veracity appears an easy concept to incorporate into health-promotion interventions. It may sometimes be difficult, in health education endeavours aimed at changing patterns of behaviour in society. Should health care providers just present the facts or should they attempt to persuade people? What are the limits of veracity? Is it permissible to exaggerate the dangers of certain behaviour in the interests of the health of society? These questions cannot be answered within the confines of this chapter but are important to keep in mind when one is assessing the merits of proposed population-based interventions.

## Nonmaleficence

Related to autonomy is the principle of nonmaleficence, which enjoins people not to harm other people. In general society, this principle constrains people from autonomous actions that are likely to harm others. For instance, a 25-year-old individual is allowed to drink alcohol but not to drink and drive because the latter may harm others. In health care settings, this principle prohibits clinicians from harming those to whom they provide services. For health promotion, it means that when activities are being planned on an individual or societal level, possible harms must be minimized. It is often impossible to foresee all the risks of a given course of action, but health care providers who engage in health-promotion endeavours are responsible for foreseeing predictable adverse consequences and taking these potential consequences into consideration. The responsibilities include addressing social or health care policies that are discovered to have unintended effects.

Salas (2015) illustrates how a policy designed to address obesity through use of a mass-media program can have unintended negative health effects. They describe how the public health focus on the obesity epidemic in Canada has been attributed to (1) a heavily individual-focused approach without having the required socioenvironmental policies and programs in place; (2) a minimal focus at interventions aimed at reducing and preventing obesity at a population level; and (3) the inappropriate focus on weight rather than health. Other consequences of this public health approach include excessive preoccupation with weight, leading to eating disorders including excessive dieting; increased weight-based stigma; and negative psychological outcomes, including anxiety and depression. Future public health approaches need to focus on health outcomes rather than weight control, while addressing the individual and system-level determinants of health (Salas, 2015). Teaching about self-esteem and fitness may help people live with obesity in a more holistic, health-focused manner. The Health At Every Size (HAES) approach is gaining increased recognition because it emphasizes self-acceptance and healthy lifestyle practice, regardless of weight changes. Another tool is the Edmonton Obesity Staging System (EOSS), which assesses health based on risk behaviours rather than weight (Bacon & Aphramor, 2011; Sharma & Kushner, 2009).

Unintentional harm is a possibility for actions that are designed to promote health. Risks can be minimized by anticipation of potential negative effects and implementation of measures to control them. Health care providers are responsible for understanding the limits of their knowledge or the data to which they have access. A synthesis of reflection, critical thinking, and knowledge, along with an understanding of the details and context of a situation, is required before one embarks on a course of action aimed at facilitating a person's health or well-being. The overall discomfort encountered by the individual must be the minimum possible to achieve the primary good intended. In other words, the health care provider is accountable for his or her judgement and for providing interventions most likely to bring about the desired result. Thus, more than just the intention not to do harm is required.

Nurses and other health providers can do harm inadvertently through such behaviours as ignorance or incompetence, referral to a provider who is incompetent or inappropriate, or inadequate supervision or training of those under their supervision. However, the duty of nonmaleficence does not mean that nurses are always accountable for foreseeing the consequences of their actions. For example, a course of exercise may be designed for a person who has had a thorough physical examination, but during an exercise session the person faints and fractures his arm. Further testing reveals a previously undetected cardiac anomaly that is subsequently surgically corrected. This is not maleficence; the main objective of the agent was therapeutic, and the event was, if not totally unforeseeable, not identified on routine pre-exercise testing. In this kind of case, we tend to look at the principle behind the action rather than the consequences. The clinician's duty was upheld, even though initially bad consequences were the unintended result. Thus, both deliberate harm and harm caused by indifferent or incompetent decision making should be considered maleficent, but when a competent practitioner evaluates a problem thoroughly in its appropriate context and intervenes with therapeutic intent, and nonetheless there is a partially negative outcome, such action does not violate the concept of nonmaleficence.

## Beneficence

Beneficence is the quality or state of doing or producing good. As a moral principle, beneficence presents us with the duty to maximize the benefits of actions while minimizing harms. There are two related aspects of the moral principle of beneficence in health-promotion settings: actions taken to further the overall health or well-being of the society in general and actions taken to promote the good of a particular individual.

When society formulates rules designed to protect people against the negative effects of their own actions, these rules are considered beneficent. It is important to emphasize, however, that beneficence should be performed in accordance with the person's will or values, and with respect for the person's autonomy. Sometimes rules designed to protect people are described as paternalistic because they override a person's autonomy to disobey them. For example, the legalization of medicinal marijuana remains somewhat paternalistic, as there are many rules governing its access, use, and sale. Paternalism is often justified by the assertion that the persons affected will be better off or protected from harm.

The principle of beneficence, when it overrides an individual's autonomous choice so as to serve that individual's interests, is appropriate when a person lacks the capacity to make personal decisions. Thus, any of the factors discussed earlier that interfere with rational decision making may require the health care provider to beneficently override the individual's decisions. Generally, though, beneficence permits interference only when the risks of the individual's proposed actions are high. This is because autonomy is such a powerful principle in Western societies that a decision to override an autonomous choice is not taken lightly. One may be justified in preventing a person from taking an overdose of sleeping pills or jumping off a cliff because the risks of not doing so are high and, importantly, if the person succeeds there is no possibility of future autonomous actions.

Beneficence, unlike nonmaleficence, is not necessarily a moral requirement of action on the part of societal members toward each other (Grace, 2017). Whether beneficence is viewed as a moral requirement of societal members in everyday life very much depends on philosophical beliefs and the ethical theory or perspective (if any) recognized by the person. Kant (1993/1785), for instance, distinguishes between perfect duties and imperfect duties. Perfect duties must be followed and tend to be defined in negative terms (e.g., "do not lie," "do not steal"); imperfect duties are ones we are called but not bound to follow (e.g., stopping to help someone who is looking for something lost on the sidewalk). An individual is not necessarily morally required to go out of his or her way to help someone unless the person is endangered and assistance would mitigate the danger. In that case, failing to offer assistance could be seen as violating the principle of nonmaleficence. Also, when an individual has responsibility for vulnerable others, such as when parents must use beneficence on behalf of their children, beneficence is required.

In contrast to ordinary members of society, nurses have duties of beneficence because their professional goals involve meeting health care needs and thus are aimed at providing good. For such reasons, beneficence is a moral expectation of nurses. Beneficence is often a difficult principle to use in health-promotion settings, however, because of the dual nature of health-promotion goals—health for individuals and health for communities. As noted earlier, there is often a tension between the two.

A paradox exists when we try to change unhealthy behaviours but do not address the underlying causes of those behaviours.

For example, although smoking cessation programs, including e-cigarettes assist some people to stop smoking, we also should address problems such as companies that aim to gather new smoking recruits from among adolescents. The use of e-cigarettes, or vaping, to quit smoking has become one of the most frequently used smoking cessation methods, but some manufacturers may be attracting adolescents by offering flavoured e-cigarettes, such as cotton candy and cherry flavours (Diemert, Bayoumy, Pelletier, et al., 2019). E-cigarettes heat liquid into an aerosol that is inhaled. The liquid usually contains low levels of nicotine and flavouring that, when used regularly, are addictive and potentially harmful (Canadian Heart and Stroke Foundation, 2018). Education-based health-promotion programs without underlying societal changes are often doomed to fail. Thus, following beneficence, health providers have obligations to address deep-rooted social problems that jeopardize health or are associated with health inequalities.

### Beneficence: Conflict With Autonomy

The principles of beneficence and autonomy sometimes conflict. For example, seat belt rules are ostensibly created to protect people from injury, but they take away autonomous choice. Beneficence may justify overriding the decision of a febrile, confused person who refuses to take her antibiotics for treatment of pneumonia. What is the clinician's responsibility? The duties of beneficence seem to mandate medicating her against her will, ensuring that the good of health is facilitated although violation of the principle of autonomy. The justification for this must include an assessment of her status related to her capacity for autonomous decision making. Preserving the person's life so he or she can make autonomous decisions in the future may be required by beneficence. However, it can be argued that beneficence takes precedence over autonomy only in those cases in which the choice cannot be considered autonomous. First, there has to be evidence that a choice has been made. In this case the choice was between accepting antibiotic treatment versus not accepting antibiotic treatment. Second, the reasonableness (or rationality) of the decision has to be discerned. It must be ascertained whether the person really has grasped the implications of refusing treatment. The reasons given for the treatment refusal, then, should illuminate gaps in information delivery or processing. Finally, it must be determined whether there are any external or internal coercion factors impinging on the decision. Perhaps the person feels she cannot afford the medicine (external), or perhaps she has a mistrust of antibiotics because of a previous experience (internal). When a decision cannot be said to be informed, the principle of beneficence directs us to decide on treatment on the basis of the person's best interests.

### Justice

Justice is an ethical principle of major importance in health-promotion settings. There are various conceptions of justice, and the term is used in a variety of ways. For the purposes of this chapter the discussion is about social justice rather than criminal justice. Social justice includes formal or informal systems within a society that are concerned with disparities in socioeconomic conditions, leading to poor health and fairness in the distribution of goods, such as health, education, food, and shelter (CNA, 2010; De Chesnay & Anderson, 2019). The concept of justice, which is based on human rights and equity, has been central to human understandings of socially significant values for a long time. Justice in health care is a major commitment of nursing, and thus the discipline of nursing is becoming more focused on active engagement in social justice issues.

In democratic societies, the requirements of social justice generally include equitable distribution of the benefits and burdens of societal life. "Justice as fairness" reflects the ideas behind Rawls's (1971 and 1999) *A Theory of Justice*. Rawls identifies two rules that he argues will result in a fair and just society:

> *First: each person is to have an equal right to the most extensive liberty compatible with a similar liberty for others. Second: social and economic inequalities are to be arranged such that they are both (a) reasonably expected to be to everyone's advantage, and (b) attached to positions and offices open to all (Rawls, 1971).*

The goal of public health is to minimize preventable death and disability for all, which is integral to social justice (PHAC, 2008). The emphasis on justice in health care settings is sometimes called the impartialist perspective in that it considers the needs of all who fall under its umbrella. An integral part of social justice involves identifying and improving patterns of systemic disadvantage that undermine the well-being of vulnerable populations. For example, within the Canadian corrections prison system, this view of justice would mandate access to care for prisoners in need. Thus, it would not permit arbitrary obstacles to access (such as requiring good behaviour or favours) that might be presented by prison officers or by other prisoners who wish to exert physical or psychological control. Justice would also require improved access to care for the poor and underprivileged, in terms of both receiving care and having access to transportation or local availability of services.

Social justice stresses the fair disbursement of resources and the sharing of common burdens, which is reflected in health promotion and public health mandates to advance well-being by improving health and focusing on the needs of the most disadvantaged. Although justice might require consideration of the special needs of a disadvantaged group, it does so impartially: that is, it does not distinguish among the particulars of individuals. Each member within the group has an equal right to whatever is proposed. In an economically burdened health care system, injustices occur both at the local level and at the societal level. Because justice viewed as fairness is impartial about individual differences, that moral perspective considered alone is not a perfect tool with which to look at health care disparities and their causes.

Health inequalities are a specific subset of health differences that are important for social justice because they evolve from intentional or unintentional discrimination or marginalization. A core component of social justice infers that there are multiple causes of discrimination, including poverty, substandard housing, inferior education, unhygienic and polluted environments, and social disintegration (Browne, Varcoe, Lavoie, et al., 2016). Nurses and other health care providers need to move beyond thinking about "doing no harm" to identifying and addressing adverse social influences on the health of underprivileged groups and the implications of their consequent poor health (Rogers & Kelly, 2011). This is best exemplified by the Truth and Reconciliation Commission of Canada's *Calls To Action – Health*, which recognize that the current state of health inequities faced by Indigenous people in Canada and communities are a direct result of historical colonial policies and interventions, including Indian residential schools, the Sixties Scoop, and other harmful practices imposed by the federal government (Truth and Reconciliation Commission of Canada [TRC], 2012). In response, in 2016 to 2018, the Government of Canada committed to financial investments to increase the capacity of Indigenous communities for health promotion activities, addressing health-related risk factors and health inequities as a result of intergenerational colonization (TRC, 2012). The goal is to increase access to services, assume self-governance and self-determination of health services, and to address Indigenous social determinants of health.

The combination of justice, feminist concerns about power and oppression, and the acknowledged responsibilities of governments and nurses to promote health permit a comprehensive view of problems associated with health protection and promotion. This view incorporates an ethical approach to problems both for society and for individuals within the society. Social justice is central to the nursing profession because nurses have the moral obligation to include sociopolitical advocacy in their practice (CNA, 2009).

## STRATEGIES FOR ETHICAL DECISION MAKING

### Locating the Source and Levels of Ethical Problems

Most health-promotion problems are moral or ethical issues in the sense that obstacles exist that prevent an individual from living life well or achieving personal goals related to health. Throughout this chapter, discussions of both the larger (societal) and the narrower (individual) perspectives have been emphasized and their relationships highlighted. Sometimes tensions between the two require mediation and may force the health promoter to decide which problem must be addressed first. For example, a nurse at a family practice clinic cares for a teenager who is morbidly obese. At the level of the individual, the nurse is charged with discovering the underlying causes of the obesity (e.g., physical, psychological, contextual) and designing strategies with the individual to help resolve the problem. However, the nurse has responsibilities also to address the issue at the more political level with interested others.

To address health-promotion issues effectively, providers need to possess not only their particular disciplinary expertise and an understanding of ethical language, principles, and perspectives but also a willingness to understand their own values and preconceptions about health and people. Understanding personal philosophy, biases, and values permits one to control for these in the sense of being aware of the influences they have in our interactions with others.

## Values Clarification and Reflection

Gaining confidence in moral decision making is a slow process. The following are suggestions that will guide development related to recognizing and addressing ethical issues.

### Examine Beliefs and Values

Cultivate the habit of examining how your personal values and beliefs relate to the human condition, justice, and responsibility. Be willing to revise your beliefs in line with your professional knowledge base, experiences, or current research findings. For example, how do beliefs that "people get what they deserve" correlate with what we know—for example, that those of lower socioeconomic status have lower levels of health and that poor health interferes with functioning and is associated with depression? How do our attitudes change when we try to place ourselves in the context of the other person's life?

This is not to say that maintaining personal integrity is not important—it is. Maintaining both personal and professional integrity is essential to good practice. Integrity has to do with a sense of wholeness of the self and consistency of actions with truly examined beliefs and values. Nurses have the ethical responsibility to adhere to the values of the profession at all times, in order to uphold the dignity for all (CNA, 2017). The 2017 *Code of Ethics for Registered Nurses* validates the nurse's preservation of integrity in those situations in which he or she feels that personal integrity is compromised. It notes that "if nursing care is requested that is in conflict with the nurse's moral beliefs and values but in keeping with professional practice, the nurse will provide safe, compassionate, competent and ethical care until alternative care arrangements are in place to meet the person's needs or desires" (CNA, 2017, p. 17). In contemplating refusal to provide care on grounds of moral objections, the nurse should ensure that the decision is based on sound ethical principles, not simply on personal beliefs. When opting out of care involves risk to the individual, care must be provided until other arrangements are made to safeguard individual care. Decisions not to participate in a situation cannot be made trivially because of the trust relationship and a nurse's moral accountability for actions. The threat to the nurse's integrity must be serious and the person's well-being must not be jeopardized by the nurse's absence. Other arrangements must be made for care of the person in such circumstances. The nurse who encounters repeated threats to integrity has a responsibility to consider changing the situation in some way. Change efforts may be directed toward institutional policy or may require that an alternative work environment be considered.

A true examination of beliefs and values requires a willingness to admit that they may not always be justifiable; they may be remnants from childhood indoctrination of various sorts. Through self-reflection, nurses should anticipate practices and procedures that would conflict with their beliefs and values, and have a moral obligation to communicate this to employers in advance of the situation. For example, one might hold religious beliefs that conflict with practices or procedures, such as abortion or MAID. An honest and ongoing examination of one's values and biases permits one to control for these beliefs when providing care to diverse persons. Being willing to examine one's beliefs and values—being willing to continue that upward journey out of Plato's cave—is thus a key part of personal and professional integrity.

### The Influence of Personal Beliefs and Values

In addition to examining beliefs and values, we should also think about the influence that these characteristics have on our practice. An understanding of how personal beliefs and values either are congruent or are liable to interfere with the task at hand is crucial to ethical problem solving. In any given situation, the health care provider must ask himself or herself, "What are my beliefs and biases in this situation? How are these likely to influence my actions?" For example, if the home health nurse believes his below-poverty-level, depressed, obese, diabetic patient who smokes is responsible for the poor healing of her leg ulcer, he may be less inclined to work with the person to discover and address the person's goals.

### Reflection on Practice

A third helpful strategy is to reflect on situations afterward to discover what worked, what did not work, and what could be done differently in the future. It is often helpful to interact with peers or other experts after particularly difficult situations to discover alternative perspectives or resources for the purposes of future problem solving. You might ask a peer or mentor to ask you questions to help you think through why you made a particular decision. Or you might practice some reflective writing to help you think through your reasoning and consider whether you would act differently in the future (Dinkins, 2015).

## Decision-Making Considerations

Decision making in health-promotion settings has inescapable moral components. As noted earlier, the nurse has a professional responsibility to further the good for individuals and society. Thus, the careful exercise of experience, skill, and knowledge is warranted when one is trying to formulate the best course of action for a given individual or group, or in resolving societal health-promotion problems. This framework is offered as a way of ensuring clarity about a particular case or situation. Because of the diverse nature of health-promotion activities, no straightforward models of decision making can realistically be applied in all situations. Additionally, decision making is often an ongoing process, and revisions to plans may be required in light of new information. The following are important facets of decision making but do not necessarily occur in the order given.

### Identify the Main Problem or Issue

What level of problem is this: social, group, or individual? If the location of the problem is societal, it will also impact individuals and groups, and a decision has to be made about the order of interventions. Try to determine the main ethical principle involved or whether it is a problem of conflicting principles. For example, after identification of the problem, you may determine that to provide benefit to the person, the person's autonomy must be overridden. Is this a social justice issue? Is it an autonomy issue? What factors led to the problem? Is there coercion or other power imbalance? If so, who has an interest in

maintaining the power imbalance and who gains the most from the imbalance? These are the questions feminist ethics would ask.

### Determine on Whom the Resolution Will Have an Impact

Who has a stake in the issue and in how it will be resolved? Answering this question will permit a determination of whose input is crucial to the decision-making process. Who and what are important considerations (e.g., institutions, individuals, businesses, social policy)? Does this issue result from a failure to predict the consequences of certain social policies?

### Determine the Prevalent Values

What are the values held by all the different players? Are there value conflicts? The value conflicts might be individual versus social, as in the case of a person with tuberculosis who refuses to take his medicines, thus putting at risk members of his family or members of the community. Value conflicts might also be interpersonal among the health-promotion team or they might be personal versus professional. As a general rule, more weight is assigned to the values of the individual who is most likely to be affected by a decision. It is important to consider the influence of culture on values when the issue involves health promotion for culturally diverse groups. It is also important to involve people who can help explain the cultural beliefs, especially when language difficulties are present. A knowledgeable but neutral interpreter may be helpful when liaison between groups is needed.

### Identify Information Gaps

Reflect on whether the decision makers are confident about what they know and do not know, and what they may be overlooking. This determination is not always an easy task. Information may exist that has not yet reached our awareness, or we might fail to ask a question that would reveal important information. How can we be confident about the scope and limits of our knowledge? Clinical judgement is a good tool but it is not foolproof. When doubts exist or the decision is likely to have serious or risky consequences, we need to involve knowledgeable others or try to determine the best places to gain missing information.

### Formulate Possible Courses of Action and Probable Consequences

Courses of action may involve further information gathering, brainstorming, and possibly collaboration with other experts or specialists. Although further data may be needed to resolve problems at the level of individuals or small groups, it is especially necessary to enlist additional help when the issue is one that requires political action to effect policy changes. It may be necessary to recruit community members and leaders or to enlist the political power of specialty groups. Finally, a determination must be made about which proposed courses of action will be the least harmful and the most beneficial. Remember not to look just at likely consequences, however. Consider possible actions from the framework of duty and character as well.

### Initiate the Selected Course of Action and Evaluate the Outcome

Does the actual outcome match the anticipated outcome? If not, what happened that was unexpected? Would this outcome have been foreseeable given more data? Would you do things differently in another similar situation given what you have learned? Does the problem need to be addressed at a different level (institutional or public policy)?

### Engage in Self-Reflection and Peer or Expert Group Reflection

What could you have done differently? Would consulting with others have altered your conception of the problem or your course of action? What insights can you or your peers glean from this that could be appropriate for similar situations in the future? How might continuing education opportunities help you or your peers to address similar problems more appropriately in the future? Would an ethics resource (committee or consultant) be helpful in such situations? Could you use this case as a focused learning experience for your peers and collaborators?

## ETHICS OF HEALTH PROMOTION: CASES

Some cases of special relevance to health promotion are presented next. They are followed by questions that can be answered by individual readers, but they also provide a good starting point for group discussion. Try using the decision-making strategies suggested throughout the chapter as you explore these problems. It is anticipated that you will want more information than is provided. Deciding what extra information would be helpful is an important part of the exercise.

### Case 1: Addressing Health Care System Problems— Elissa Needs Help

Elissa is 38 years old. She recently moved 350 km from her home to a small rural town (population 6000) and separated from her abusive husband in order to escape his continuing threats and to be near her childhood friend. She suffers from persistent, sometimes incapacitating, depression, for which she has received antidepressant medications and counselling, with temporary relief. She has been unable to work and has no extended health insurance. Her friend refers her to the only primary care centre in the area, where she is seen by Jill, one of the two nurse practitioners. As part of her evaluation, Jill discovers that Elissa was abused as a child and has very poor self-esteem. Elissa affirms that her childhood friend is very supportive. Jill believes that longer-term psychological counselling would benefit Elissa and facilitate her well-being, but she also knows that there are no counselling services within a 40-km radius. Elissa has no transportation and no public transportation is available.

- What are Jill's options? What are her responsibilities?
- What actions might Jill pursue both on a local level and on a political level? What are her resources?
- What is the responsibility of the health-promotion disciplines in cases such as this?

### Case 2: She's My Client!—Lilly and "Jake" (a.k.a. Paul)

Shirley, a nurse practitioner, is at a conference when a health care provider colleague discusses a difficult case. One of his patients, "Jake," is HIV positive but refuses any treatment. The health care provider explains that Jake fears that his wife will discover and recognize the names of the medications, because he knows "these drug names are discussed on television all the time." Jake has not told his wife that he is HIV positive and has no intention of ever doing so. There is no requirement under Canada's *Criminal Code* to disclose one's HIV-positive status to partners. Jake firmly believes his condition is his private information and, for now, the couple use condoms for birth control. The health care provider is concerned that Jake will not tell his wife. The health care provider is presenting this case to colleagues to highlight the public awareness campaigns that, to some extent, have affected patient privacy. He argues, "Listen to how they call out your name and the medications at the pharmacy counter."

Shirley recognizes bits and pieces of information and comes to the painful realization that Jake is really Paul, and Paul is the husband of one of her patients, Lilly. Lilly has begun to discuss with Shirley that she wants to get pregnant soon. The town is too small for Shirley to be mistaken. Or is it?

- Is it ethical for the nurse practitioner to ask the health care provider if Jake is Paul?
- Is it ethical for Shirley to tell Lilly she suspects Paul is HIV positive?
- Should this information change how Shirley counsels Lilly about a pregnancy?
- What is in Lilly's best interests? Is Shirley also obligated to consider Paul's interests?
- What resources are available?

### Case 3: Don't Touch My Things! Ms. Smyth and Autonomy

Ms. Smyth, 78 years old, has lived in the same home for 30 years. Never married, she cared for her disabled mother for 15 years. After her mother died, she lived alone on a small pension. She appeared to be well groomed and appropriately dressed when she left her house.

Ms. Smyth was hospitalized for a bowel obstruction, and Joe, a community health nurse, made a follow-up visit after discharge to her home. When Joe arrived at the house, he was overcome with the smell of rotting garbage, urine, and feces. Five small dogs ran back and forth among piles of garbage and magazines, overturned furniture, and discarded appliances. There was no running water, and the bathroom was not functional. Joe told Ms. Smyth that her living conditions were unhealthy and that he would contact a community employer to help her clean her house. Ms. Smyth became very angry and said no one had the right to take her things away.

- Is it ethical for Joe to overrule Ms. Smyth's autonomy in decision making?
- What action is in Ms. Smyth's best interests?
- What action is in the community's best interests?
- What ethical issues are involved in caring for a patient with a hoarding disorder, such as that seen in Ms. Smyth's situation?

## CASE STUDY

### Genetic Screening Programs

A Canadian company has been sequencing the DNA of 20 individuals. With the individuals' consent, the results will be made available to researchers. Each donor will be offered information about genetic variations that might indicate a higher-than-average likelihood of developing a life-threatening condition.

There are hopes that genetic screenings of large populations will change the practice of health care from a focus on treating diseases to preventing them. Some researchers predict the complete sequencing of each human genome will provide routine data to health care providers, much like the common measurements of blood pressure, pulse, temperature, and blood counts today. Other research data show, however, that better predictors of determining the risk of diabetes are asking people about their family history of diabetes, their weight, and their age rather than sequencing their DNA.

#### Reflective Questions

Apply different concepts and theories of ethics in thinking about the following questions.

- What are some of the ethical issues of these DNA analyses?
- What are the responsibilities of health care providers in the genetic screenings of a population?
- What additional components could a community health nurse add to the following plan of care for participants having their DNA sequenced?

Sources: Aiello, L. B. (2017). Genomics education: Knowledge of nurses across the profession and integration into practice. *Clinical Journal of Oncology Nursing, 21*(6), 747–753; Anderson, G., Alt-White, A. C., Schaa, K. L., et al. (2015). Genomics for nursing education and practice: Measuring competency. *Worldviews on Evidence-Based Nursing, 12*(3), 165–175; Hammer, M. J. (2019). Beyond the helix: Ethical, legal, and social implications in genomics. *Seminars in Oncology Nursing, 35*(1), 93–106.

## CARE PLAN

### Genetic Screening Programs

The use of developments in genetics research, including genetic counselling, testing, and screening, as well as advanced therapeutic and reproduction choices, influences the health of both present and future generations throughout the world.

As previously addressed, health care providers have many complex ethical responsibilities in the applications of genetic developments with local, national, and international communities, as well as with individuals and families.

In the following care plan, the community health nurse from the preceding case study addresses aspects of the ineffective management of genetic screenings in a community.

#### Nursing Issue

Lack of community illness-prevention and risk-reduction screening programs.

#### Defining Characteristics

- Community verbalizes desire to manage the genetic screenings and treatment of illness and prevention of sequelae; community verbalizes difficulty with regulation and integration of prescribed regimens for genetic screening and treatment of illness and its effects or prevention of complications.
- Knowledge of risk factors for illness (expected or unexpected) is accelerated.

#### Related Factors

##### Treatment Related

- Complexity of genetic screening and therapeutic regimen
- Complexity of health care
- Financial costs:
  - Actual cost of procedure
  - Side effects
  - Expected (e.g., anxiety)
  - Unexpected (e.g., despair)

##### Situation/Environment Related

- Health and health care needs, multiple and complex, especially for vulnerable population (e.g., unborn children)
- Presence of known and unknown environmental (including occupational) health hazards
- Availability of community resources for screening for risk factors of diseases:
  - Less expensive (e.g., family health histories and physical examinations); more expensive (e.g., genetic screenings)
  - Overall needs and financial resources

#### Expected Outcomes

With the community health nurses' guidance, community members will:

- Evaluate the actual and potential (e.g., significant increases in birth rates) health problems and resources of the community.
- Identify community resources that are needed to promote health and prevent illness, including genetic screenings.
- Participate in program development as needed to improve the effectiveness of the therapeutic regimen management of genetic screening programs.

#### Interventions

- Complete a community assessment, including:
  - Actual and potential health problems and needs
  - Actual and potential resources for health
- Develop an overall program plan for genetic screenings
- Develop a specific program for the genetic screening of an individual, perhaps including the following components:
  - Complete initial interview, individual and family histories, and physical examination with appropriate laboratory studies
  - Generally, discuss the genetic screenings and informed consent, focusing on the concerns of the individual and/or family
- Assess barriers to learning:
  - Physical condition
  - Sensory status (e.g., vision, hearing)
  - Intelligence, learning abilities/disabilities
  - Emotional state(s) (e.g., fears, guilt)
  - Stressors, concerns
- Provide information:
  - Explain needed knowledge and perhaps changes (e.g., lifestyle behaviours)
  - Discuss and add to individual's knowledge of the pros and cons of genetic screening
  - Identify influencing factors to decision making about individual's genetic screening
- Perform screenings (e.g., depression, financial resources)
- Give time to integrate new information, perhaps having a second appointment to:
  - Readdress questions
  - Develop informed consent, including policies on privacy
- Perform actual genetic screening procedure
- Explain results with genetic and reproductive counselling
- Repeat and follow-up as necessary
- Compare the diagnostic criteria for inadequate therapeutic regimen management with other differential diagnoses potentially present in the case study

# SUMMARY

Health promotion is a vast and complex practice area; consequently, the associated ethical challenges are diverse and multilevelled. This chapter has outlined the nature and purpose of health care ethics and related this framework to the responsibilities of Canadian health care providers in health-promotion interventions. Health promotion should be viewed as a moral undertaking of health care providers. After reading this chapter, students will have knowledge of some of the tools and language needed to explore ethical issues, discuss these issues with others, and address problematic issues at both the individual level and the societal level. Perhaps the most important factor to consider is that ethical problems manifesting themselves at the level of the individual almost always have their origins in the broader societal environment.

**Evolve Chapter Features**

http://evolve.elsevier.com/Canada/Edelman/healthpromotion/
• Review Questions

# REFERENCES

Aristotle. (1985). *Nicomachean ethics* (trans. T. Irwin). Indianapolis: Hackett (original work ~350 BCE). [Seminal Reference].

Bacon, L., & Aphramor, L. (2011). Weight science: Evaluating the evidence for a paradigm shift. *Nutrition Journal, 10*(1), 9–21. https://doi.org/10.1186/1475-2891-10-9. [Seminal Reference].

Benner, P., Tanner, C. A., & Chesla, C. A. (2009). *Expertise in nursing practice: Caring, clinical judgment, and ethics* (2nd ed.). New York: Springer. [Seminal Reference].

Branje, S. (2018). Development of parent–adolescent relationships: Conflict interactions as a mechanism of change. *Child Development Perspectives, 12*(3), 171–176. https://doi.org/10.1111/cdep.12278.

Browne, A. J., Varcoe, C., Lavoie, J., et al. (2016). Enhancing health care equity with indigenous populations: Evidence-based strategies from an ethnographic study. *BMC Health Services Research, 16*(1), 544. https://doi.org/10.1186/s12913-016-1707-9.

Buchanan, D. R. (2006). Moral reasoning as a model for health promotion. *Social Science & Medicine, 63*(10), 2715–2726. [Seminal Reference].

Burkhardt, M. A., & Nathaniel, A. K. (2013). *Ethics and issues in contemporary nursing* (4th ed.). Albany, NY: Delmar. [Seminal Reference].

Butts, J. B., & Rich, K. L. (2020). *Nursing ethics across the curriculum and into practice* (5th ed.). Burlington, MA: Jones & Bartlett.

Canadian Heart, & Stroke Foundation. (2018). *E-cigarettes in Canada.* Retrieved from https://www.heartandstroke.ca/-/media/pdf-files/position-statements/ecigarettesincanada.ashx?la=en&hash=8939FF52C37A5E11C551176982F2E4AC5D38D605.

Canadian Medical Protective Association (CMPA). (2016). *Is this patient capable of consenting?* Retrieved from https://www.cmpa-acpm.ca/en/advice-publications/browse-articles/2011/is-this-patient-capable-of-consenting.

Canadian Medical Protective Association (CMPA). (2018). *Medical assistance in dying: Where do we stand two years later?* Retrieved from https://www.cmpa-acpm.ca/en/advice-publications/browse-articles/2018/medical-assistance-in-dying--where-do-we-stand-two-years-later.

Canadian Nurses Association (CAN). (2010). *Social justice ... a means to an end, an end in itself* (2nd ed.). Ottawa: Author. [Seminal Reference].

Canadian Nurses Association (CNA). (1998). *Advance directives: The nurse's role.* Retrieved from https://cna-aiic.ca/~/media/cna/page-content/pdf-en/ethics_pract_advance_directives_may_1998_e.pdf. [Seminal Reference].

Canadian Nurses Association (CNA). (2003). *Ethical distress in health care environments.* Retrieved from https://www.cna-aiic.ca/~/media/cna/page-content/pdf-en/ethics_pract_ethical_distress_oct_2003_e.pdf?la=en.

Canadian Nurses Association (CNA). (2009). *Ethics in practice: Social justice in practice.* Retrieved from https://cna-aiic.ca/~/media/cna/page-content/pdf-fr/ethics_in_practice_april_2009_e.pdf. [Seminal Reference].

Canadian Nurses Association (CNA). (2017). *Code of ethics for registered nurses.* Ottawa: Author. Retrieved from https://www.cna-aiic.ca/-/media/cna/page-content/pdf-en/code-of-ethics-2017-edition-secure-interactive.pdf.

Chambliss, D. F. (1996). *Beyond caring: Hospitals, nurses, and the social organization of ethics.* Chicago: University of Chicago Press. [Seminal Reference].

Cohen, E. (2015). Heaven over hospital. Parents honor dying child's request. *CNN Health.* Retrieved from http://www.cnn.com/2015/10/27/health/girl-chooses-heaven-over-hospital-part-2/.

Coughlin, K., & Canadian Paediatric Society. (2018). *Medical decision-making in paediatrics: Infancy to adolescence.* Retrieved from https://www.cps.ca/en/documents/position/medical-decision-making-in-paediatrics-infancy-to-adolescence.

De Chesnay, M., & Anderson, B. A. (2019). *Caring for the vulnerable: Perspectives in nursing theory, practice, and research.* Burlington, MA: Jones & Bartlett Publishers.

Diemert, L., Bayoumy, D., Pelletier, H., et al. (2019). *E-cigarette use for smoking cessation: Scientific evidence and smokers' experiences.* Toronto: Ontario Tobacco Research Unit.

Dinkins, C. S. (2015). Socratic pedagogy: Teaching students to think like nurses. In J. M. Sorrell, & P. R. Cangelosi (Eds.), *Expert clinician to novice nurse educator: Learning from first-hand narratives* (pp. 97–128). New York: Springer Publishing.

DuBois, L. Z., Macapagal, K. R., Rivera, Z., et al. (2015). To have sex or not to have sex? An online focus group study of sexual decision making among sexually experienced and inexperienced gay and bisexual adolescent men. *Archives of Sexual Behavior, 44*(7), 2027–2040. https://doi.org/10.1007/s10508-015-0521-5.

Evans, K. G. (2016). *Consent: A guide for Canadian physicians.* Retrieved from https://www.cmpa-acpm.ca/en/advice-publications/handbooks/consent-a-guide-for-canadian-physicians#capacity%20to%20consent.

Farrer, L., Marinetti, C., Cavaco, Y. K., et al. (2015). Advocacy for health equity: A synthesis review. *The Milbank Quarterly, 93*(2), 392–437. https://doi.org/10.1111/1468-0009.12112.

Gilligan, C. (1982). *In a different voice: Psychological theory and women's development*. Cambridge, MA: Harvard University Press. [Seminal Reference].

Gilligan, C. (2014). Moral injury and the ethic of care: Reframing the conversation about differences. *Journal of Social Philosophy, 45*(1), 89–106. https://doi.org/10.1111/josp.12050. [Seminal Reference].

Grace, P. J. (Ed.). (2017). *Nursing ethics and professional responsibility in advanced practice*. Burlington, MA: Jones & Bartlett Learning.

Green, B. (2012). Applying feminist ethics of care to nursing practice. *Journal of Nursing Care, 1*, 111. https://doi.org/10.4172/2 167-1168.1000111. [Seminal Reference].

Hart-Wasekeesikaw, F., & Gregory, D. M. (2009). *Cultural competence and cultural safety in nursing education: A framework for first nations, inuit and métis nursing*. Ottawa: Aboriginal Nurses Association of Canada. Retrieved from https://www.cna-aiic.ca/~/ media/cna/page-content/pdf-en/first_nations_framework_e.pdf. [Seminal Reference].

Henrich, N. J., Dodek, P. M., Keenan, S. P., et al. (2017). Causes of moral distress in the intensive care unit: A qualitative study. *American Journal of Critical Care, 26*(4), 48–57.

Heyland, D. K., Barwich, D., Pichora, D., & ACCEPT (Advance Care Planning Evaluation in Elderly Patients) Study Team., et al. (2013). Failure to engage hospitalized older patients and their families in advance care planning. *JAMA Internal Medicine, 173*(9), 778–787. [Seminal Reference].

Holland, S. (2015). *Public health ethics* (2nd ed.). Cambridge, UK: Policy Press.

Huddleston, K. (2013). Ethics: The challenge of ethical, legal, and social implications (ELSI) in genomic nursing. *OJIN: Online Journal of Issues in Nursing, 19*(1). [Seminal Reference].

Iverson, E., Celious, A., Kennedy, C. R., et al. (2014). Factors affecting stress experienced by surrogate decision makers for critically ill patients: Implications for nursing practice. *Intensive and Critical Care Nursing, 30*(2), 77–85. [Seminal Reference].

Kant, I. (1993). Grounding for the metaphysics of morals (3rd ed.) (trans. J. W. Ellington). Indianapolis: Hackett (original work published 1785). [Seminal Reference]

Kiernan, J., & Vallerand, A. H. (2016). Cancer as a platform for genetics education in the undergraduate nursing curriculum. *Journal of Nursing Education, 55*(4), 236–239. https://doi. org/10.3928/01484834-20160316-11.

Kohlberg, L. (1981). In *The philosophy of moral development: Moral stages and the idea of justice. Essays on moral development*. (Vol. 1)San Francisco: Harper & Row. [Seminal Reference].

Kohlberg, L. (1984). In *The psychology of moral development: The nature and validity of moral stages. Essays on moral development*. (Vol. 2)San Francisco: Harper & Row. [Seminal Reference].

Lacovara, J., & Bohnenkamp, S. (2018). Genetic testing in oncology for the medical-surgical nurse. *Medsurg Nursing, 27*(2), 117–121.

Lewis, S. M., Bucher, L., Heitkemper, M. M., et al. (2019). *Medical-surgical nursing in canada: Assessment and management of clinical problems* (4th ed.). Toronto, ON: Elsevier Canada.

Lusignani, M., Gianni, M. L., Re, L. G., et al. (2017). Moral distress among nurses in medical, surgical and intensive-care units. *Journal of Nursing Management, 25*(6), 477–485. https://doi.org/10.1111/ jonm.12431.

Lyon, D. E., McCain, N. L., Pickler, R. H., et al. (2011). Advancing the biobehavioral research of fatigue with genetics and genomics. *Journal of Nursing Scholarship, 43*, 274–281 [Seminal Reference].

Mason, V. M., Leslie, G., Clark, K., et al. (2014). Compassion fatigue, moral distress, and work engagement in surgical intensive care unit trauma nurses: A pilot study. *Dimensions of Critical Care Nursing, 33*(4), 215–225. https://doi.org/10.1097/ DCC.0000000000000056.

McMillan, K. (2018). *A critical organizational analysis of frontline nurses' experience of rapid and continuous change in an acute health care organization (doctoral dissertation)*. Ottawa, Canada: University of Ottawa. Retrieved from https://ruor.uottawa. ca/bitstream/10393/37980/5/McMillan_Kimberly_2018 _Thesis.pdf.

Mill, J. S. (2002). *Utilitarianism* (2nd ed.). Indianapolis: Hackett (originally published 1861). [Seminal Reference].

Miller, J. J., Morris, P., Files, D. C., et al. (2016). Decision conflict and regret among surrogate decision makers in the medical critical care unit. *Journal of Critical Care, 32*, 79–84. https://doi. org/10.1016/j.jcrc.2015.11.023.

Ministry of Children, Community and Social Services. (2018). *Special diet allowance—what heath care professionals need to know*. Retrieved from https://www.mcss.gov.on.ca/en/mcss /programs/social/special_diet_health_care.aspx.

Munro, C. L. (2015). Individual genetic and genomic variation: A new opportunity for personalized nursing interventions. *Journal of Advanced Nursing, 71*(1), 35–41. https://doi.org/10.1111/jan.12552.

Office of the Privacy Commissioner of Canada. (2018). *PIPEDA in brief*. Retrieved from https://www.priv.gc.ca/en/ privacy-topics/privacy-laws-in-canada/the-personal-information- protection-and-electronic-documents-act-pipeda/pipeda_brief/. [Seminal Reference].

O'Sullivan, R., Mailo, K., Angeles, R., et al. (2015). Advance directives: Survey of primary care patients. *Canadian Family Physician, 61*(4), 353–356.

Palmer, B. W., Harmell, A. L., Pinto, L. L., et al. (2017). Determinants of capacity to consent to research on Alzheimer's disease. *Clinical Gerontologist, 40*(1), 24–34. https://doi.org/10.1080/07317115.201 6.1197352.

Plato. (1992). *Republic (trans. C. D. C. Reeve)*. Indianapolis: Hackett (original work ~360 bce). [Seminal Reference].

Pohjanoksa, J., Stolt, M., Suhonen, R., et al. (2019). Whistle-blowing process in healthcare: From suspicion to action. *Nursing Ethics, 26*(2), 526–540. https://doi.org/10.1177/0969733017705005.

Public Health Agency of Canada (PHAC). (2008). *Core competencies for public health in Canada*. Retrieved from http://www.phac -aspc.gc.ca/php-psp/ccph-cesp/pdfs/cc-manual-eng090407.pdf. [Seminal Reference].

Public Health Agency of Canada (PHAC). (2010). *Creating a healthier Canada: Making prevention a priority. A declaration on prevention and promotion from Canada's Ministers of Health and Health Promotion/Healthy Living*. Retrieved from https://www.canada.ca/ content/dam/phac-aspc/migration/phac-aspc/hp-ps/hl-mvs/ declaration/pdf/dpp-eng.pdf. [Seminal Reference].

Rachels, J., & Rachels, S. (2011). *The elements of moral philosophy* (7th ed.). New York: McGraw-Hill. [Seminal Reference].

Rawls, J. (1971 and 1999). A theory of justice. Cambridge, MA: Harvard University. [Seminal Reference].

Rogers, J., & Kelly, U. A. (2011). Feminist intersectionality: Bringing social justice to health disparities research. *Nursing Ethics, 18*(3), 397–407. [Seminal Reference].

Salas, X. R. (2015). The ineffectiveness and unintended consequences of the public health war on obesity. *Canadian Journal of Public Health, 106*(2), e79–e81. https://doi.org/10.17269/cjph.106.4757.

Santos, E. M., Edwards, Q. T., Floria-Santos, M., et al. (2013). Integration of genomics in cancer care. *Journal of Nursing Scholarship, 45*(1), 43–51. [Seminal Reference].

Sharma, A. M., & Kushner, R. F. (2009). A proposed clinical staging system for obesity. *International Journal of Obesity, 33*(3), 289–295. https://doi.org/10.1038/ijo.2009.2. [Seminal Reference].

Singer, P. (1993). *A companion to ethics.* Cambridge, MA: Wiley-Blackwell. [Seminal Reference].

Sorrell, J. M., & Dinkins, C. S. (2006). An ethics of diversity. Listening in thin places. In C. S. Dinkins, & J. M. Sorrell (Eds.), *Listening to the whispers. Re-thinking ethics in healthcare* (pp. 310–314). Madison, WI: University of Wisconsin Press. [Seminal Reference].

Sproul, R. C. (2015). *The difference between ethics and morality.* Ligonier Ministries. Retrieved from http://www.ligonier.org/blog/difference-between-ethics-and-morality/.

Tengland, P. A. (2016). Behavior change or empowerment: On the ethics of health-promotion goals. *Health Care Analysis, 24,* 24–46.

Truth and Reconciliation Commission of Canada (TRC). (2012). *Truth and Reconciliation Commission of Canada: Calls to action.* Retrieved from http://trc.ca/assets/pdf/Calls_to_Action_English2.pdf. [Seminal Reference].

Vogel, L. (2017). Canadians still waiting for timely access to care. *Canadian Medical Association Journal, 189*(9), E375–E376. https://doi.org/10.1503/cmaj.1095400.

Weston, A. (2010). *A practical companion to ethics* (4th ed.). New York: Oxford University Press. [Seminal Reference].

World Health Organization (WHO). (1986). *The Ottawa Charter for Health Promotion. First International Conference on Health Promotion.* Retrieved from https://www.canada.ca/content/dam/phac-aspc/documents/services/health-promotion/population-health/ottawa-charter-health-promotion-international-conference-on-health-promotion/charter.pdf. [Seminal Reference].

# 6

# Health Promotion and the Individual

*Teresa Hannesson, RN, MSN*

Originating US chapter by *Anne Rath Rentfro, RN, PhD*

## INTENDED LEARNING OUTCOMES

*After completing this chapter, the reader will be able to:*

- Define the framework of functional health patterns as described by Gordon (2016).
- Describe the use of the functional health pattern framework to assess individuals throughout the life span.
- Illustrate health patterns of the functional, potentially dysfunctional, and actually dysfunctional categories of behaviour.

- Identify risk factors or etiological aspects of actual or potential dysfunctional health patterns to consider with nursing diagnoses.
- Discuss the planning, implementation, and evaluation of nursing interventions to promote the health of individuals.
- Develop specific health-promotion plans based on an assessment of individuals.

## KEY TERMS

Age-developmental focus
Culturally competent care
Expected outcomes
Functional focus
Functional health patterns
Health status

Individual-environmental focus
Nursing diagnosis
Nursing interventions
Pattern focus
Risk factors

## ? THINK ABOUT IT
### Assessment of Alcohol Consumption

Women have different patterns of alcohol consumption and different thresholds for problem drinking than men. Instruments such as the CAGE questionnaire detect alcohol dependence and would not be a sensitive enough measure for some women, in particular pregnant women, who are less likely than men to be alcohol dependent. The T-ACE instrument provides a measure of alcohol intake patterns more appropriate for women than that derived from the CAGE test (considered Cutting down on drinking, been Annoyed by criticism of drinking, feeling Guilty about drinking, and using alcohol as an Eye-opener). The T-ACE test, developed for use with women, was the first validated screening tool for assessing drinking risk in pregnant women and continues to provide a highly sensitive tool for identifying risk drinking (Bax, Geurtz, & Balachova, 2015; Sokol, Martier, & Ager, 1989). Screening is a useful strategy in health-promotion assessment and intervention (see Chapter 9). A pattern of drinking is established with use of the following questions:

T—How many drinks does it Take to make you feel high?

A—Have you ever been Annoyed by people criticizing your drinking?

C—Have you ever felt you ought to Cut down your drinking?

E—Have you ever had a drink first thing in the morning (Eye-opener) to steady your nerves or get rid of a hangover?

Scores are calculated as follows:

- A reply of more than two drinks to question T is considered a positive response and scores 2 points, and an affirmative answer to question A, C, or E scores 1 point, respectively.
- A total score of 2 or more points on the T-ACE indicates evidence of risk drinking.

Why would a nurse tailor the assessments to individual characteristics of a population? How effectively would this screening tool identify alcohol problems in women other than the pregnant women within the population? Why?

In health-promotion practice, nurses assess patterns and use their assessment to facilitate individual maintenance of well-being or their progression toward wellness. Health and illness within this context reflect changing patterns of the life process. For example, generally, when disorganization or ineffective coping produce fluctuations in patterns that eventually result in illness, a treatment plan is designed to alleviate the symptoms or eliminate the illness altogether. The strategies used in this assessment process focus on identifying abnormalities. Conversely, health promotion aims to maintain effective coping strategies to prevent illness in the first place, therefore requiring different approaches to assessment and planning. One foundational concept in health promotion is strength assessment. Furthermore, a strengths-based nursing approach guides nurses to view patients with a broader, more holistic, perspective that uncovers strengths (Gottlieb, 2014). Holistic nursing provides central unifying themes that connect pattern recognition to person–environment relationships for health promotion throughout the life span. Holism emerges from each of the holistic nursing core values of philosophy, caring process, communication, attunement, healing, cultural diversity, education, research, self-reflection, and self-caring (Dossey, Keegan, & Guzzetta, 2016).

The Public Health Agency of Canada (PHAC) provides strategies and resources that "empower Canadians to improve their health" through identifying health-promotion goals and provides education for prevention (Government of Canada, 2019) (Box 6.1). The Centre for Health Promotion, a division of the PHAC, is responsible for identifying health concerns based on the determinants of health and for developing policy to enhance the health of Canadians. Promoting equitable health outcomes for patients, families, and communities can occur through education and addressing concerns associated with the determinants of health (Andermann, 2016).

Health promotion is not a new concept to nursing. The Canadian Nurses Association (CNA) "believe(s) that nurses have a professional and ethical responsibility to promote health equity through action on the social determinants of health" (CNA, 2017).

Nursing theorists, such as Newman, Rogers, and Levine, recognized that nurses care for well individuals, as well as those who are ill (Endo, 2017; Fawcett, 2015). The International Council of Nurses (2015) defines nursing as encompassing the:

*autonomous and collaborative care of individuals of all ages, families, groups and communities, sick or well and in all settings. Nursing includes the promotion of health, prevention of illness, and the care of ill, disabled and dying people. Advocacy, promotion of a safe environment, research, participation in shaping health policy and in client-centred care, health systems management, and education are also key nursing roles.*

This broad definition provides a foundation for nursing globally using the nursing process: assessment, diagnosis, outcome criteria, process criteria (including planned interventions), implementation, and evaluation. The nursing process, in turn, establishes a useful framework for the health-promotion assessment of the individual.

---

**BOX 6.1    The Public Health Agency of Canada**

**Mission**
To promote and protect the health of Canadians through leadership, partnership, innovation, and action in public health.

**Vision**
Healthy Canadians and communities in a healthier world.

**Values**
- Respect for Democracy
- Respect for People
- Integrity
- Stewardship
- Excellence

**Mandate**
The role of the Public Health Agency of Canada is to:
- Promote health
- Prevent and control chronic diseases and injuries
- Prevent and control infectious diseases
- Prepare for and respond to public health emergencies
- Serve as a central point for sharing Canada's expertise with the rest of the world
- Apply international research and development to Canada's public health programs
- Strengthen intergovernmental collaboration on public health and facilitate national approaches to public health policy and planning

Source: Public Health Agency of Canada. (2019). *Home page.* Retrieved from https://www.canada.ca/en/public-health.html.

---

Nurses typically use assessment strategies, including health promotion, that address interactions among an individual's biophysical, psychosocial, and spiritual states and patterns with the environment. When assessing for primary prevention, the techniques also include generalized health promotion and specific protection from disease, both of which fall within the scope of nursing practice. The active process of promoting health involves targeting the determinants of health such as protection (immunizations, occupational safety, and environmental control) along with lifestyle, value, and belief system behaviours that enhance health.

With health promotion serving as the underlying theme, this chapter addresses nursing assessment of individuals. In most areas of health care, tertiary care and prevention of further disease provide the assessment focus (Hopkins & Rippon, 2015). This tertiary care–focused assessment identifies deficits, thus excluding assessment of overall general health and wellness. The majority of nursing diagnoses approved by NANDA International (formerly the North American Nursing Diagnosis Association) are problem oriented. The NANDA International definition of nursing diagnosis includes human responses to health and reactions to life processes, as well as actual or potential health problems (NANDA International, 2018). One way to address nursing diagnoses in well individuals is to focus on human developmental or maturational tasks. Most approved nursing diagnoses reflect a focus on deficit assessment and problem solving; however, these diagnoses include many life processes that provide the broad base needed for nursing to address strength-based healthy responses or potential for healthy responses (Paans, Müller-Staub, & Nieweg, 2013). Furthermore, concentrating on strengths in the health-promotion setting provides a foundation to help individuals move toward improved health and addresses holism of the individual. Nurses support and enhance the ability of healthy individuals to maintain or strengthen their health.

Current Canadian health care systems continue to use deficit assessment rather than the strength-based approach that is more appropriate for health-promotion settings (Andermann, 2016). Mental health, social work, and nursing, however, embrace a strength-based approach to assessment within the health-promotion context. From using infant competencies to plan care and person-centred approaches for care of people with mental health disorders, nurses incorporate strength-based assessment into their diagnostic process (Hopkins & Rippon, 2015). Although NANDA International has stated that there is a need for work in this area of strength-based assessment and wellness, published material for using wellness diagnoses appears infrequently. The NANDA International taxonomy, however, uses multiple dimensions of human response in the consideration of each diagnosis. These seven dimensions include the status of the diagnosis that considers whether the diagnosis is addressing wellness, risk, or an actual problem (Gordon, 2016). More work is necessary to develop and promote useful language for health-promotion and wellness diagnoses.

Gordon's (2016) framework, which uses a functional health patterns assessment, is one tool that provides a foundation for the construction of the NANDA International nursing diagnosis nomenclature. As NANDA International continues to develop diagnoses for health promotion, Gordon's framework can continue to provide the foundation for these diagnoses. Although there are many frameworks for assessment, Gordon's framework is used throughout this chapter to demonstrate assessment approaches, as well as family and community assessment (see Chapters 7 and 8). In addition, this chapter presents components of the nursing process as they relate to health promotion of the individual.

## ❖ GORDON'S FUNCTIONAL HEALTH PATTERNS: ASSESSMENT OF THE INDIVIDUAL

Nursing assessment determines the health status of individuals. Table 6.1 demonstrates aspects of a complete nursing assessment. Assessment, in this case, refers to collection of data that culminates in problem identification or a diagnostic statement. Effective health assessment considers not only physiological parameters but also how the human being interacts with the whole environment. Behaviour patterns, beliefs, perceptions, and values form the essential components of health assessment when nurses consider the maximal health potential of the individual. Pattern recognition supports our understanding of health of individuals and is reflected in nursing theories such as those initially developed by nursing theorists such as Newman and Rogers (Endo, 2017; Fawcett, 2015).

### TABLE 6.1   Aspects of a Nursing Assessment

| Definition | Deliberate and Systematic Data Collection |
|---|---|
| Components | Subjective data: Health history, including subjective reports and individual perceptions<br>Objective data: Observations of nurse<br>Physical examination findings<br>Information from health record<br>Results of clinical testing |
| Function | Description of person's health status |
| Structure | Organization of interdependent parts describing health, function, or patterns of behaviour that reflect the whole individual and environment |
| Process | Interview, observation, and examination |
| Format | Systematic but flexible; individualized to each person, nurse, and situation |
| Goal | Nursing diagnosis or problem identification<br>Identification of areas of strengths, limitations, alterations, responses to alterations and therapies, and risks |

Historically, conceptual models in nursing have used Gordon's health-related behaviours particularly in regard to formulating a framework to guide assessment. Gordon's 11 functional health patterns interact to depict an individual's lifestyle. Using this framework, nurses combine assessment skills with subjective and objective data to construct patterns reflective of lifestyles. This framework can be applied in any setting where nurses care for individuals and families. Gordon's framework is one mechanism for assessment, but there are limitations associated with this framework, such as its emphasis on subjective data collection.

### Functional Health Pattern Framework

Holism and the totality of the person's interactions with the environment form the philosophical foundations of Gordon's functional health patterns. This foundation provides a context for collecting data that provide information about the entire person and most life processes. By examining functional patterns and interactions among patterns, nurses accurately determine and diagnose actual or potential problems, intervene more effectively, and facilitate movement toward outcomes to promote health and well-being (Gordon, 2016). In addition to providing a framework to assess individuals, families, and communities holistically, functional health patterns provide a strong focus for more effective nursing interventions and outcomes. This stronger focus provides a solid position from which nurses participate as decision makers in health care systems at organizational, community, national, and international levels.

### Definition

Functional health patterns view the individual as a whole being using interrelated behavioural areas. The typology of 11 patterns serves as a useful tool to collect and organize assessment

## TABLE 6.2 Typology of 11 Functional Health Patterns

| Pattern | Description |
| --- | --- |
| Health perception–health management pattern | Individual's perceived health and well-being and how health is managed |
| Nutritional-metabolic pattern | Food and fluid consumption relative to metabolic needs and indicators of local nutrient supply |
| Elimination pattern | Excretory function (bowel, bladder, and skin) |
| Activity-exercise pattern | Exercise, activity, leisure, and recreation |
| Sleep-rest pattern | Sleep, rest, and relaxation |
| Cognitive-perceptual pattern | Sensory, perceptual, and cognitive patterns |
| Self-perception–self-concept pattern | Self-concept pattern and perceptions of self (body comfort, body image, and feeling state); self-conception and self-esteem |
| Roles-relationships pattern | Role engagements and relationships |
| Sexuality-reproductive pattern | Person's satisfaction and dissatisfaction with sexuality and reproduction |
| Coping-stress tolerance pattern | General coping pattern and effectiveness in stress tolerance |
| Values-beliefs pattern | Values, beliefs (including spiritual), or goals that guide choices or decisions |

Modified from Gordon, M. (2016). *Manual of nursing diagnosis* (13th ed.). Sudbury, MA: Jones & Bartlett.

data and to create a structure for validation and communication among health care providers. Each pattern described in Table 6.2 forms part of the biopsychosocial-spiritual expression of the whole person. Individual reports and nursing observations provide data to differentiate patterns. As a framework for assessment, functional health patterns provide an effective means for nurses to perceive and record complex interactions of individuals' biophysical state, psychological makeup, and environmental relationships.

### Characteristics

Functional health patterns are characterized by their focus. Gordon (2016) uses five areas of focus: pattern, individual-environmental, age-developmental, functional, and cultural.

Pattern focus implies that the nurse explores patterns or sequences of behaviour over time. Gordon's term *behaviour* encompasses all forms of human behaviour, including biophysical, psychological, and sociological elements. Pattern recognition, a cognitive process, occurs during information and data collection. Cues are identified and clustered while information is being gathered. Patterns emerge that represent historical and current behaviour. Quantitative patterns such as blood pressure are readily identified, and pattern recognition is facilitated when baseline data are available. As the nurse incorporates a broader range of data, patterns imbedded within other patterns begin to emerge. Blood pressure, for example, is a parameter that falls within both the activity pattern and the exercise pattern. Individual baseline and subsequent readings may present a pattern within expected norms. Erratic blood pressure measurements indicate an absence of pattern. Functional health

pattern categories provide structures to analyze factors within a category (blood pressure: activity pattern) and to search for causal explanations, usually outside the category (excessive sodium intake: nutritional pattern) (Gordon, 2016).

The individual-environmental focus of Gordon's framework refers to environmental influences occurring within many of the patterns. For example, environmental influences in the functional health pattern include role relationships, family values, and societal mores. Personal preference, knowledge of food preparation, and ability to consume and retain food govern the individual's intake. Cultural and family habits, financial ability to secure food, and crop availability also influence food intake. Additionally, the person who secures, prepares, and serves the food controls the nutritional intake for the family. Individuals' internal and external environments influence the health patterns in multiple ways.

Each pattern also reflects a human growth and age-developmental focus (Gordon, 2016). As individuals fulfill developmental tasks, complexity increases. These tasks, however, provide learning opportunities for individuals to maintain and improve their health. Erikson's framework, which organizes specific health tasks for individuals to accomplish at each developmental phase of the life cycle, continues to serve as a framework to assess and plan care (Malone, Liu, Vaillant, et al., 2016). Erikson's eight stages provide the traditional developmental assessment nurses generally use to plan care (Table 6.3). Each stage presents a central task or crisis that must be resolved before healthy growth can continue (Erikson, 1963). Individuals develop their sense of autonomy in early childhood and struggle with the sense of shame and doubt. When this developmental level is achieved or resolved, the child moves on to develop initiative during the next stage.

Both age and developmental stage continue to provide the foundation for contemporary assessment of individuals' health status. Developmental tasks begin at birth and continue until death. By considering current epidemiological data and recommended health behaviours, Gordon's (2016) framework continues to be useful today to explore developmental tasks and their related behaviours for health promotion throughout the life span.

Functional focus refers to an individual's performance level. Other disciplines plan care using functional patterns, but assessment data differ among disciplines (Gomez-Salgado, Jacobsohn, Frade, et al., 2018). Physiotherapists and occupational therapists, for example, focus on physical ability to perform activities of daily living and rely on assessments of independent ability to perform personal activities of daily living to develop their plans. For physicians, genitourinary function refers to frequency or voiding patterns and characteristics of urine, such as colour, odour, and laboratory analysis results. In addition to these factors of genito-urinary function, nurses assess how the particular voiding pattern affects lifestyle, particularly how urinary frequency affects sleep patterns and the ability to perform activities such as shopping or socializing. Additional concerns might include the individual's ability to walk or climb stairs to the bathroom or to manage these activities safely at night. It has been suggested that all health disciplines should use the *International Classification of Functioning, Disability and Health*. Relying on

## TABLE 6.3 Relationship Between Selected Developmental Tasks and Wellness Tasks for Each Stage of the Life Cycle

| Erikson's Eight Life Stages | Havighurst's Developmental Tasks | Examples of Minimal Wellness Tasks for Each Developmental Stage |
|---|---|---|
| 1. Infancy (trust vs. basic mistrust) | Learning to walk<br>Learning to take solid foods<br>Learning to talk<br>Learning to control elimination of body waste | Acquiring ability to perform psychomotor skills<br>Learning functional definition of health<br>Learning social and emotional responsiveness to others and to the physical environment |
| 2. Early childhood (autonomy vs. shame and doubt) | Learning gender difference and sexual modesty<br>Achieving physiological stability<br>Forming simple concepts of social-physical reality<br>Learning to relate emotionally to parents, siblings, and others<br>Learning to distinguish right from wrong and developing a conscience<br>Learning physical skills necessary for ordinary games | Learning about proper foods, exercise, and sleep<br>Learning dental hygiene<br>Learning injury prevention (safety belts and helmets, sunscreen, smoke detectors, poisons, firearms, and swimming)<br>Refining psychomotor and cognitive skills |
| 3. Late childhood (initiative vs. guilt) | Building wholesome attitudes toward self as a growing organism<br>Learning to get along with peers | Developing self-concept<br>Learning attitudes of competition and cooperation with others<br>Learning social, ethical, and moral differences and responsibilities |
| 4. Early adolescence (industry vs. inferiority) | Learning appropriate gender identity: masculine or feminine role<br>Developing fundamental skills in reading, writing, and calculating<br>Developing concepts necessary for everyday living<br>Developing conscience, morality, and scale of values<br>Achieving personal independence<br>Developing attitudes toward social groups and institutions | Learning that health is an important value<br>Learning self-regulation of physiological needs—sleep, rest, food, drink, and exercise<br>Learning risk taking and its consequences (injury prevention) |
| 5. Adolescence (identity vs. role confusion) | Achieving new and more mature relationships with peers and both genders<br>Achieving gender identity<br>Accepting physique and using body effectively<br>Achieving emotional independence of parents and other adults<br>Achieving assurance of economic independence<br>Selecting and preparing for occupation<br>Preparing for marriage and family life<br>Developing intellectual skills and concepts necessary for civic competence<br>Desiring and achieving socially responsible behaviour | Learning economic responsibility<br>Learning social responsibility for self and others (preventing pregnancy and sexually transmitted infections)<br>Experiencing social, emotional, and ethical commitments to others<br>Accepting self and physical development<br>Reconciling discrepancies between personal health concepts and observed health behaviours of others (use of alcohol, drugs, tobacco, firearms, and violence)<br>Learning to cope with life events and problems (suicide prevention)<br>Considering life goals and career plans and acquiring necessary skills to reach goals<br>Learning importance of time to self and world |
| 6. Early adulthood (intimacy vs. isolation) | Selecting and learning to live with a mate<br>Starting a family; managing a home<br>Taking on civic responsibility | Committing to mate and family responsibilities<br>Selecting a career<br>Incorporating health habits into lifestyle |
| 7. Middle adulthood (generativity vs. stagnation) | Accepting and adjusting to physiological changes<br>Achieving adult social responsibility<br>Maintaining economic standard of living<br>Assisting adolescent children | Accepting aging of self and others<br>Coping with societal pressures<br>Recognizing importance of good health habits<br>Reassessing life goals periodically |
| 8. Maturity (ego integrity vs. despair) | Adjusting to decreasing physical strength and health<br>Adjusting to retirement and reduced income<br>Adjusting to death of spouse/life partner<br>Establishing an explicit affiliation with own age group<br>Establishing satisfactory physical living arrangements | Becoming aware of risks to health and adjusting lifestyle and habits to cope with risks<br>Adjusting to loss of job, income, and family and friends through death<br>Redefining self-concept<br>Adjusting to changes in personal time and new physical environment<br>Adjusting previous health habits to current physical and mental capabilities |

Sources: Erikson, E. H. (1998). *The life cycle completed.* New York: W. W. Norton; Hockenberry, M. J., & Wilson, D. (2015). *Wong's nursing care of infants and children* (11th ed.). St Louis: Mosby; Osborn, K. S., Wraa, C. E., Watson, A. S., et al. (2019). *Medical-surgical nursing.* New York: Pearson Higher Education; US Department of Health and Human Services & Centers for Disease Control and Prevention. (2015). *The guide to community preventive services: What works to promote health.* Retrieved from https://www.thecommunityguide.org/.

this classification could promote transdisciplinary communication about functional patterns when used along with the NANDA International taxonomy (Gomez-Salgado et al., 2018).

Culture, age, and developmental and gender norms, considered during assessment, influence development of health patterns. Leininger defines transcultural nursing concepts of cultural care, health, well-being, and illness patterns in different environmental contexts and under different living conditions (Gordon, 2016). Culturally competent care is delivered with knowledge of and sensitivity to cultural factors influencing health behaviour. Complex cultural patterns transmitted from former generations contribute to individuals' health behaviour. Culturally competent care respects the underlying personal and cultural reality of individuals. Given that one may never be fully competent in cultures other than one's own culture, the term *cultural safety* may be more descriptive of the aim. Nurses provide more culturally safe care when they use cultural norms, values, communication, and time patterns in reflective practice (Andrews & Boyle, 2015). The nurse and the individual interact, and the nurse reflects on the interaction and resumes interaction, making changes on the basis of the self-reflection; thus, the nurse is engaging relationally with the individual (Doane & Varcoe, 2015). For example, when one is tuning a piano, the pitch from the piano and that from the tuning fork must match. The tuning continues until the two sounds resonate. When nurses experience emotional and physiological resonance surrounding individuals' sociocultural contexts, such as race, ethnicity, religion, and sexual orientation, they resonate and achieve attunement (Koloroutis & Hanlon, 2017).

The concept of cultural humility is particularly valuable when nurses are caring for people of multiple cultures, such as in an urban setting (Niño, Kissil, & Davey, 2016). Even when the individual and the nurse share ethnic or racial backgrounds, their particular heritage may be quite different. For example, many different ethnic groups speak Spanish from different countries or provinces within a country (Spain, Mexico, Puerto Rico, Cuba, Columbia, etc.), but may have different colloquialisms within their speech and different cultural values and norms. A Spanish-speaking nurse of Mexican heritage may not be culturally competent in caring for a client from Spain. Asian clients will also have diverse languages and cultural values. Cultural humility may be useful in these kinds of settings.

Functional health patterns form a framework that centres on health and can account for cultural factors. Most nursing assessments use functional pattern assessment as a foundation to their practice. Although nursing theoretical and conceptual frameworks differ, the functional health pattern framework is relevant to most conceptual models. In fact, functional health patterns provide the structure used by NANDA International to support nursing diagnosis nomenclature. Nursing classification of interventions and outcome nomenclature also use Gordon's functional patterns as a foundation (Gordon, 2016). The advantages of a functional health pattern framework specific to the practice of nursing include the following:

- It provides consistent nursing language through collecting, organizing, presenting, and analyzing data to determine nursing diagnoses.
- It allows flexibility to tailor content for individuals and situations.

- It suits diverse practice areas (e.g., home, clinic, institution) for assessment of individuals (adult/children), families, or communities.
- It supports theoretical components of nursing service, education, and research by organizing clinical knowledge using nursing diagnoses, interventions, and outcomes.
- It incorporates medical science data while retaining the focus on nursing knowledge and practice.

## The Patterns

Each pattern reflects a biopsychosocial spiritual expression of the individual's lifestyle or life processes from the perspective of both the individual and the nurse. This expression reveals the following elements: a pattern or sequencing of behaviours; the role of the environment (physical surroundings, family, societal, and cultural influences); and developmental influences. The assessment of each pattern includes its status as functional (strengths/ wellness), dysfunctional (actual), or potentially dysfunctional (risk), as well as an indication of the individual's level of satisfaction with the pattern (Gordon, 2016). Nurses continue assessing in more depth to generate an explanation for the problem, to determine remedial actions to take, and to understand the perceived effect of these actions from the individual's perspective. An important goal when assessing each pattern is to determine the impact on determinants of health, the individual's knowledge of health promotion, the ability of the individual to manage health-promoting activities, and the value that the individual ascribes to health promotion with use of an asset-based approach to identify wellness diagnoses. Each pattern is presented in this chapter, with details for nurses to use to assess individuals and determine health-promotion diagnoses using a functional health pattern framework along with a discussion of nursing implications for use of the patterns in health-promotion practice.

## ◆ Health Perception–Health Management Pattern

The health perception–health management pattern involves individuals' health status and health practices used to reach the current level of health or wellness with a focus on perceived health status and meaning of health (Gordon, 2016). When eliciting this information, nurses discover areas for further exploration under other functional health patterns. For example, if the individual reports shortness of breath when mowing the lawn, the nurse stores this information for later retrieval when he or she is assessing activity and exercise patterns or cognitive-perceptual patterns.

Health perception–health management patterns affect lifestyle and ability to function even when individuals do not perceive actual health problems, are unaware of necessary health promotion in the absence of problems, do not feel capable of managing their health, or believe activity on their part is useless to promote health. Health-promoting activities (e.g., adequate nutrition, activity and exercise, sleep and rest), routine professional examinations, self-examinations, immunizations, and safety precautions (e.g., auto safety restraints and locked medicine cabinets) provide this pattern's clues to maintain optimal quality of life.

Assessment objectives for health perception–health management consist in obtaining data about perceptions, management, and preventive health practices (Gordon, 2016).

Exploring values identifies potential health hazards, such as lack of adherence to a prescribed medical or nursing regimen or ability to manage health effectively. In addition to these kinds of assessment cues, nurses identify unrealistic health and illness perceptions and expectations. The transtheoretical model consists of five stages that can be useful in assessing an individual's readiness to change (see Chapter 10). These stages—precontemplation, contemplation, planning/preparation, action, and maintenance—have been used widely in health-promotion programs for diverse populations and multiple age groups with topics ranging from prevention of injury to nutrition-education programs (Doenges, Moorhouse, & Murr, 2015).

Assessment includes the following parameters:
- Health and safety practices of the individual
- Previous patterns of adherence or compliance
- Use of the health care system
- Knowledge of health service availability
- Health-seeking behaviour patterns
- Means to access health care (e.g., financial resources, health insurance, and transportation)

In addition to methods of health management, nurses explore health perceptions as individuals describe their current health status, past problems, and anticipation of future problems associated with health or health care. These findings reveal beliefs about health, perceived susceptibility, self-efficacy, and level of knowledge of health status, taking into account the influence of culture (Andrews & Boyle, 2015) (Diversity Awareness). Health and illness perceptions significantly influence overall direction for care planning. Health beliefs, also discussed later in this chapter in the section Values-Beliefs Pattern, directly impact participation in care. Partnership with providers and attunement is also more likely to yield better attention to self-care, particularly in cultures that value collective responsibility. In addition, individuals from cultures valuing collectivism are more likely to engage in self-care measures when their cultural patterns and social support within families are considered (Ariapooran, Heidari, Asgari, et al., 2018).

It is also important to assess health management practices. In a study about the influence of past health management practices on future health management in posttraumatic brain injury patients, Ulfarsson, Lundgren-Nilsson, Blomstrand, et al. (2014) demonstrated that past health management practices such as use of sick time and employment status influenced their post-traumatic brain injury health management. This study provides some support for the belief that if adherence to a prescribed regimen has not occurred in the past, future adherence is also unlikely. Nurses aim to identify and remedy the causes of the discrepancies between provider recommendations and the individual's implementation of those recommendations. For example, an individual with high blood pressure who has failed to keep follow-up appointments, not taken medication as prescribed, and eaten foods with high sodium content should be assessed to determine whether this evident nonadherence results from a conflict within the value system of the individual (health beliefs); inaccurate information; misunderstanding; inadequate ability to learn, retain, or retrieve information (knowledge deficit); denial of illness (health perception); or inability to access care and/or resources. Variables such as financial resources, transportation difficulties, nutritional preferences, daily activities (individual and family patterns), ability to read written instructions (literacy or visual acuity), and ability to manipulate numbers (numeracy) may affect the individual's behaviours.

◆ **Nutritional-Metabolic Pattern**

Nutritional-metabolic patterns centre on nutrient intake relative to metabolic need (Gordon, 2016). These patterns include individuals' descriptions of food and fluid consumption (history), as well as evidence of adequate nutrition (physical examination). Nurses explore individuals' satisfaction with current eating and drinking patterns, including restrictions, and their perceptions of problems associated with eating and drinking, growth and development, skin condition, and attunement and healing processes.

## DIVERSITY AWARENESS

### Health Perspectives for First Nations in Canada

| TRADITIONAL DEFINITIONS | | TRADITIONAL METHODS | |
| --- | --- | --- | --- |
| Health | Illness | Maintain/Protect Health | Restore Health |
| Total harmony with nature | Human body out of balance | Maintain positive relationship with nature | Drumming |
| Balance between emotional, mental, spiritual, and physical aspects | Result of social or spiritual dysfunction | Treat body with respect | Community support |
| Wellness is an individual responsibility | | Purification acts using water/herbal remedies and rituals | Spiritual healers |
| Values of respect, wisdom, responsibility, and relationships | | Take responsibility for health | Smudging |
| | | | Plant-, animal-, or mineral-based medicines |
| | | | Ceremonies; energetic therapies; or physical/hands-on techniques |

**Reflective Questions**
- How are First Nations perspectives on health and illness similar and different from Western perspectives?
- How does knowing these definitions inform your nursing practice?

Note: There is wide diversity among First Nations groups. Cultural beliefs and language may be quite different from one group to another within the same ethnicity. For more information about these concepts, see First Nations Health Authority (2019): http://www.fnha.ca/.

Intake and supply of nutrients to tissues and organs influence bodily functions and interact with lifestyle. Sufficient food and fluid intake provides energy for performance, which includes both internal physiological functioning and external body movements. Interruption in acquisition or retention of food or fluids offsets balance and significantly alters lifestyle. In addition to individuals' nutrition and metabolism, genetic variation, specific genetic abnormalities, environmental influences, and prenatal nutrition also govern growth rates (Levitsky, 2016).

Assessment within this pattern includes data about typical patterns of food and fluid consumption and adequacy of consumption patterns, along with perceived problems associated with nutritional intake. Assessment should also include access to food; 1 in 6 Canadians are faced with food insecurity on a daily basis (Food Insecurity Policy Research, 2018). Nurses attend to cues to conditions of overweight, underweight, over-hydration, dehydration, or difficulties in skin integrity, such as breakdown or delayed healing. Individuals may also be at risk of developing these problems. Conversely, this pattern may exhibit assets or strengths that can be used to support the health-promotion plan.

The parameters for assessment for this pattern fall into two broad categories of evaluation: nutrient intake and metabolic demand. Intake may be assessed with a 24-hour recall of food and fluid consumption; a listing of dietary restrictions, food allergies, vitamin supplements, and caffeine and alcohol ingestion (when not included in the medication history); and a schedule of eating and drinking patterns. Assessment includes screening individuals for problems associated with swallowing or chewing.

With identified problems, focused assessments include food preferences, feelings about present weight, and eating habits. Intake may be affected when individuals eat alone. Frequent dining out may indicate the need for further exploration within the nutrition area or other functional patterns. Fast food consumption may be the predominant source of nutrients. Consumption patterns may be deficient in essential vitamins or minerals. Food security may also be explored. Who purchases food? Is shopping preplanned with a grocery list? Are financial resources and food budgets adequate? Is food stored properly? Who prepares food? How is food prepared (fried, broiled, steamed, boiled, or baked)?

Metabolic demands differ from individual to individual and vary within the same individual during times of illness, stress, growth, high- or low-activity levels, healing, or recovery. Developmental, physiological, and environmental conditions alter metabolic demands. Appetite and reported changes in weight, skin integrity, attunement, and general healing ability are explored during the interview or health history. Individuals may also report decreased tolerances for hot or cold weather.

Nurses' observations and perceptions play a vital role when they are assessing nutritional and metabolic patterns. Physical examination allows assessment of both the nutrient supply to the tissues and the metabolic needs of the individual. Objective findings serve as indicators to validate subjective reports concerning nutrient intake. Gross metabolic indicators include temperature, height, and weight. Physical examination focuses on skin, bony prominences, dentition, hair, and mucous membranes. Skin and mucous membranes, in particular, use nutrients rapidly and provide excellent indices of nutritional adequacy. Skin assessment includes assessment of colour, temperature, and turgor, and evaluation of any skin lesions, areas of dryness, scaliness, rashes, pruritus, or edema. Mucous membranes are examined for colour, integrity, moisture, and lesions. Dentition is evaluated for structure. Are teeth erupted at normal stages of development? Are teeth firmly implanted? Do dentures fit properly? Additionally, decay and evidence of oral hygiene are evaluated. Healing is assessed when there is evidence of injury. The assessment may also include laboratory information such as levels of fasting glucose, lipids, blood urea nitrogen, creatinine, calcium, and vitamin D.

Although problem identification occurs after assessment of all 11 functional health patterns, a problem in any one area serves as a clue to dysfunction in others. Assessment of one pattern facilitates synthesis and analysis of data collected in other functional health patterns. Nutrition, access to food, and metabolism influence patterns of health management, elimination, activity, sleep, cognition, roles, and stress tolerance and determinants of health (Roncarolo & Potvin, 2016). The values-beliefs pattern may significantly alter all other functional patterns. Sociocultural values and ethnic backgrounds play a major role in the determination of eating patterns. Other areas to consider include eating habits, food preferences, and patterns of nutrient supply and demand across the life span. Raw fruits and vegetables may be fun "finger food" for the toddler, but the older person, especially one with loose dentures or arthritis of the temporomandibular joint, may find these foods intolerable. Older persons may also find gastro-intestinal intolerances that develop over time and were not present in their youth.

A nutritional pattern focus emphasizes educational needs. Assessment aims to demonstrate strengths in functional patterns along with disclosing dysfunctional or potentially dysfunctional patterns. Nutritional health-promotion activities present a strength that provides impetus for similar activities in the other patterns. For example, if balanced nutritional intake improves functional level, individuals may extend their health-promoting behaviours to stress reduction or other behaviours. Understanding food/fluid intake and balance of body requirements helps individuals adjust caloric intake as growth slows to prevent overweight problems during the adult years. Finally, knowledge about recommendations from *Canada's Dietary Guidelines* (Health Canada, 2019) should be explored and information provided to enhance health food choices.

## ◆ Elimination Pattern

Elimination patterns include those related to bowel, bladder, and skin function. Nurses determine regularity, quality, and quantity of stool through subjective reports about methods used to achieve regularity or control and any pattern changes or perceived problems. Perspiration quantity and quality determine excretory skin function (Gordon, 2016).

Elimination pattern significance differs from individual to individual. Many people view elimination patterns as a measure of health and as a sensitive indicator of proper nutrition and stress level. Individuals' perceptions determine whether patterns become problematic or dysfunctional. Misconceptions about regularity exist, particularly of bowel function, and self-treatment commonly occurs to correct perceived problems.

Elimination pattern dysfunction affects interpersonal interactions (Brito-Brito, Oter-Quintana, Martin-Garcia, et al., 2014). Lack of control affects body image (self-perception), activity level, socialization, and sleep patterns. Age, developmental levels, and cultural considerations direct the interview. Pediatric assessment includes toilet training methods, whereas adult assessment may focus on regularity and patterns of dysfunction. In addition to constipation, older persons may begin to develop urinary control problems. Women past childbearing years often develop urinary stress incontinence.

Assessment includes data about regularity and control of excreta (Gordon, 2016). Nurses investigate cues suggesting constipation patterns, diarrhea, or incontinence through focused assessment. Elimination pattern changes, pain, discomfort, and perceived problems receive attention. Data collection includes exploration of the individual's explanation of the problem, methods of self-treatment, and perceived results (Gordon, 2016).

The quantity, quality (colour, odour, and consistency), frequency, and regularity of stool, urine, and perspiration determine the direction of further exploration. Nurses assess excretory mode, time patterns, and control. Encouraging discussion aims to reveal more detailed information about pattern changes, perceived problems, and elimination habits. Examination includes gross screening of specimens, noting the amount, consistency, colour, and odour. Skin assessment includes careful observation and description of wound/fistula drainage.

Transition from nutrition to elimination pattern assessment can occur seamlessly. Fluid intake affects elimination. Dietary fibre affects bowel elimination patterns. Skin integrity heralds concerns about urinary incontinence, leading to additional discussion of elimination patterns. Direct questions about laxatives may be necessary because of the availability of over-the-counter treatments for constipation (Bardsley, 2015). Discrepancies between dietary intake and reported bowel regularity indicate the need for further questioning (Lee, 2015). Laxative dependency in the form of oral supplements, suppositories, or enemas may indicate knowledge deficits in the area of bowel elimination. Health education about normal bowel function, nutritional guidelines to assist the individual in elimination, or implementation of an exercise program may significantly reduce elimination pattern dysfunction. Although overuse of laxatives is generally considered a solution that older persons use to cope with constipation, young adults with bulimia and anorexia should also be assessed for laxative overuse, abuse, and dependency. Furthermore, nurses should explore this issue with parents of children who struggle with constipation. These parents may rely on excess use of stimulant laxatives for the effected child, resulting in chronic laxative use.

Urinary frequency and urinary tract infection (UTI) require health education as well. Several approaches to prevention of UTIs in women have some evidence to support their use (Harvard Women's Health Watch, 2015). Drinking 236 mL (8 ounces) of cranberry juice a day for 6 months to a year, low-dose prophylactic antibiotics, vaginally administered estrogen to promote growth of lactobacilli in postmenopausal women, and probiotic vaginal suppositories containing lactobacilli for premenopausal women have each been shown to be effective in preventing UTI in some women. Presenting symptoms of UTI in both men and women include urinary urgency, urinary frequency, and nocturnal polyuria. Research indicates that prolonged time between urinations is linked to UTIs (Harvard Women's Health Watch, 2015; Nazarko, 2015). Evidence-informed practice guides the nurse in establishing a more suitable elimination routine for the individual.

## ◆ Activity-Exercise Pattern

The activity-exercise pattern centres on activity level, exercise program, and leisure activities. Parameters to explore include movement capability, activity tolerance, self-care abilities, use of assistive devices, changes in pattern, satisfaction with activity and exercise patterns, and any perceived problems (Gordon, 2016). Limitations in movement capabilities or ability to perform activities of daily living significantly alter lifestyle and may affect every other functional health pattern. Mobility and independent functioning in self-care are almost universally valued. Childrearing practices demonstrate this value: parents boast about their infant who walks early, their toilet-trained toddler, and their preschooler who dresses without assistance.

Activity-exercise patterns provide effective indicators for commitment to health promotion and prevention (Fig. 6.1). Exercise's impact on health status has been extensively documented with increased public awareness. Overweightness and obesity, linked to sedentary lifestyle, have reached epidemic proportions worldwide. More than 1.9 billion adults (39%) are overweight, with 13% of the world's population designated as obese (World Health Organization [WHO], 2016). The World Health Organization also regards 41 million children younger than 5 years as either overweight or obese. The obesity epidemic extends from developing countries with undernourished populations to industrialized nations. Worldwide obesity prevalence has tripled since 1975 (WHO, 2016). These statistics are similar within the Canadian population, with 62% of adults self-reporting as being overweight or obese (Statistics Canada, 2018). Modifiable habits such as tobacco use, poor nutrition, and sedentary lifestyle contribute to half of preventable deaths globally (National Research Council & Institute of Medicine, 2015). Assessments, plans, and interventions to prevent obesity have a major impact on global health and health promotion in Canada.

Activity-exercise patterns also indicate energy expenditure and activity tolerance levels. Movement directly affects activities of daily living, along with control of the immediate environment. The environment contributes to mobility as well. For example, individuals living alone in high-crime areas may limit their activity for fear of harm. Factors such as inclement weather, distance from public transportation, lack of outdoor spaces, and negotiating stairways with a cane can also influence decisions about activity (Gebel, Ding, Foster, et al., 2015; Oreskovic, Perrin, Robinson, et al., 2015). Furthermore, global climate change could negatively impact individuals' preference and ability for outdoor exercise

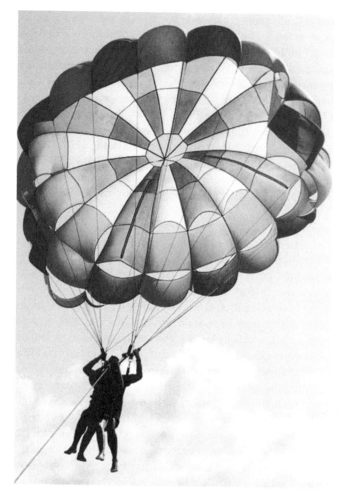

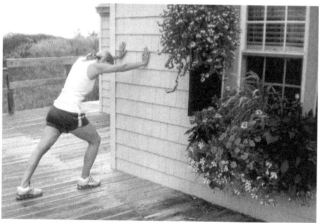

Fig. 6.1 Activity-exercise patterns provide effective indicators for commitment to health promotion and prevention diagrams are from original iteration.

(Wagner, Keusch, Yan, et al., 2016). Environmental barriers significantly impair activity-exercise patterns for individuals with neuromuscular or perceptual disturbances. Moreover, leisure activities provide clues to individuals' value systems (Sahlqvist, Goodman, Jones, et al., 2015). For example, work ethic, socioeconomic status, competitiveness, stage in career, and age influence how individuals perceive leisure and recreational activities.

The objective of assessment within the activity-exercise pattern is to determine the pattern of activities that require energy expenditure. The components reviewed are exercise, activity, leisure, and recreation (Gordon, 2016). The nurse seeks clues to discover strengths and weaknesses within the pattern. Decreased energy levels, perceived problems, coping strategies, changes within the patterns, and associated explanations for these changes are all important clues that require further exploration. Generally, individuals with respiratory or cardiac disease warrant in-depth assessment, and focused assessment is indicated for individuals with neuromuscular, perceptual, or circulatory impairments.

The dimensions to be described and assessed within the activity-exercise pattern include daily activities, leisure activities, and exercise. Daily activities include occupation (position, hours of work or school, and amount of physical exercise versus cognitive or sedentary activities), self-care abilities (feeding, bathing, grooming, dressing, and toileting), and home-management routines (cooking, cleaning, shopping, laundry, and outdoor activities) (Gordon, 2016). Problems within any of these areas require explanation. Is it a problem of energy expenditure, mobility limitations, or decreased motivation caused by depression, grieving, or incongruent values?

Exercise parameters include the type, frequency, duration, and intensity of the individual's regular exercise. Nurses also assess the value the individual places on exercise as a part of determining their (i.e., the individual's) feelings about it. A 24-hour recall of the previous day's activities provides an initial picture of the pattern, whereas each major component addresses specific elements. Weekly logs provide follow-up assessment for suspected problems (Gordon, 2016). In addition to weekly logs, focused assessments include details about modes of transportation. Is a car used for transportation? If public transportation is used, how far away is the route? Are elevators or stairs used more often? Factors interfering with exercise or mobility include dyspnea, fatigue, muscle cramping, neuromuscular or perceptual deficits, chest pain, and angina. As with other patterns, feelings of satisfaction and perception of problems provide valuable indications of dysfunctional or potentially dysfunctional patterns.

Nurses evaluate subjective complaints, such as dyspnea, noting an individual's difficulty with breathing during the interview and physical examination. Examination includes objective circulatory, respiratory, and neuromuscular indicators. Assessment also includes skin colour, skin temperature, apical heart rate, radial heart rate, and blood pressure, as well as respiratory rate, rhythm, depth of inspiration, and effort involved. Gait, posture, and balance are evaluated during ambulation. Muscle tone, strength, coordination, and range of motion provide useful clues to validate reports of activity and exercise. Assistive devices or prostheses are evaluated for proper use, proper fit, and degree of assistance or support provided.

Information obtained during the interview is linked closely to the examination findings. Examination alone may not disclose the invaluable subjective reports of early morning pain and joint stiffness. When appropriate, the nurse may ask the individual to climb stairs or perform self-care activities under observation to assess impairment. Direct observation validates assessment findings and is a valuable technique used by health care educators and home health nurses to evaluate adequate performance of self-care activities, such as dressing, cooking, and insulin administration. Various instruments have been designed to quantify the level of ability or disability. For some individuals, a metabolic activity index, in which each activity is measured according to kilocalories of energy expended per minute, helps to quantify assessment results and plan care.

Developmental norms have been established for infants and toddlers. Milestones such as sitting, crawling, walking, running, and hopping determine a child's development and should be screened in children with use of standardized screening instruments (Canadian Task Force on Preventive Health Care, 2016). Careful assessment of ability, limitations, and interests helps to guide the nurse in a more holistic assessment. Problem identification is reserved for the conclusion of the assessment after all 11 patterns have been constructed. Useful clues within a pattern lead into other pattern areas; however, premature closure of a topic during the examination is avoided. At this point, only tentative diagnoses are possible. Often explanations of problems lie in other functional health patterns. For example, when the individual expresses an inability to perform exercise on a routine basis, barriers may be discovered in another pattern. Barriers may be associated with knowledge deficit, the personal or family value system, overriding priorities, or low value placed on exercise. Is the inability to perform activities a result of general fatigue caused by inadequate or decreased sleep time associated with anxiety, nocturia, pain, or an infant waking every 3 hours for feeding? Are responsibilities associated with caring for several preschoolers and inadequate financial resources to secure a babysitter the cause? The assessment's purpose is to narrow the number of possible explanations.

## ◆ Sleep-Rest Pattern

Perhaps the single most important factor assessed in the sleep-rest pattern is the perception of adequacy of sleep and relaxation. Subjective reports of fatigue or energy levels provide some indication of the individual's satisfaction. People make assumptions about the roles that sleep and rest play in preparing the individual for required or desired daily activities. This pattern becomes extremely important when sleep and rest are perceived as insufficient. Sleep serves a restorative function in most individuals. Sleep deprivation studies provide vivid demonstrations of the need for different types of sleep: light, deep, dream, and rapid eye movement sleep. Again, problems within this pattern may cause problems in other patterns. A person who has difficulty with sleep may be tense and irritable, unable to tolerate stress, more prone to infectious processes, and incapable of making health-promoting relationships. Appetite alterations, elimination difficulties, and activity intolerance may occur (Luyster, Choi, Yeh, et al., 2015). Some degree of cognitive dysfunction generally occurs as well.

The objective when the nurse is assessing the sleep-rest pattern is to describe the effectiveness of the pattern from the individual's perspective (Gordon, 2016). Wide variation in sleep time (from 4 hours to more than 10 hours) does not necessarily affect functional performance; different individuals require different amounts of sleep. Difficulty experienced with sleep

onset, sleep interruptions, and awakening are areas of assessment to consider. The nurse also evaluates disturbances such as dreaming and nightmares, sleepwalking, nocturnal enuresis, and penile tumescence. Counselling, institution of safety measures, or medical referral may be necessary. In addition to sleep, the nurse assesses rest and relaxation according to the individual's perceptions. Activities of the sedentary isolate type, such as reading or crocheting, may be relaxing for some individuals. Passive involvement, as with television viewing, may provide the only source of relaxation for the individual. Daily naps or relaxation exercises (meditation, yoga, or breathing exercises) may also be a part of this pattern.

Assessment parameters of the sleep dimension are divided into two parts: sleep quality and sleep quantity. Sleep quality includes the individual's perception of sleep adequacy, performance level, and physical and psychological state on awakening. Sleep quantity, in addition to focusing on the hours slept each day, is used to build a schedule of sleep times. The nurse assesses the individual for regularity of the time of retiring, time of awakening, and additional periods of sleep throughout the day. Sleep onset, the number of awakenings, and the reasons for awakening provide clues to problems. The dimensions of rest and relaxation include the parameters of the type, frequency or regularity, and duration. The perceived effectiveness of methods used to promote rest is also assessed.

When problems exist, focused assessment that evaluates efficiency of sleep compared with actual sleeping time is warranted. Individuals are conditioned to sleep under certain circumstances, and maintaining bedtime rituals is a distinct advantage in sleep promotion. A person who expects to sleep will usually sleep if such routines are maintained. Nurses assess schedule and routine changes associated with bedtime. When assessing bedtime routines, rituals along with other aids to sleep, such as natural aids (warm milk) or medications (prescription and nonprescription), should be explored. Physical examination includes general appearance, behaviour, and performance changes. As with pain, sleep is a subjective experience. Comprehensive examination, which is beyond the scope of this chapter, may be performed, including polysomnography when indicated. Research indicates that subjective reporting of sleep quality and measures of sleep time closely approximate electroencephalographic findings.

Nursing care focuses on the need to identify evidence of sleep disturbances to design appropriate interventions before sleep deprivation occurs. Frequent awakenings do not necessarily imply sleep interruption. Many individuals awaken numerous times during the night but return to sleep within seconds. These awakenings occur in older persons, who generally spend most of the night in stages of light sleep. The normal developmental pattern of aging does not include deep sleep; therefore, awakenings may not affect the sleep cycles. Older individuals, however, more often have trouble returning to sleep because they experience discomfort or anxiety. Biological rhythm and peak performance time may be helpful to the nurse when he or she is planning health education and return visits. Individuals commonly refer to themselves as morning people or night owls; therefore, patterns of retiring and arising provide clues.

Patterns of sleep and rest in conjunction with subjective reports of physical and mental well-being help determine appropriate interventions.

## ◆ Cognitive-Perceptual Pattern

Cognitive patterns include the ability of the individual to understand and follow directions, retain information, make decisions, solve problems, and use language appropriately. Auditory, visual, olfactory, gustatory, tactile, and kinesthetic sensations and perceptions determine perceptual and sensory patterns. Pain perception and tolerance are analyzed within this pattern area (Gordon, 2016). Capacity for independent functioning is considered a major role of thinking and perceiving. Compensation for cognitive-perceptual difficulties ensures safety. Health requires a balance between the individual and the environment. Decreased levels of cognition or perception require increased levels of environmental control. For example, mentally impaired or sensory-impaired individuals may require sheltered work environments and supervised group living arrangements.

Interrelationships among the individual, the developmental stage, and the environment contribute to several patterns. For example, the behaviour patterns of a 20-year-old high school "dropout" who works in a factory may differ from those of a 20-year-old second-year premedical student. Developmental stage plays a role in cognitive and perceptual abilities as well. Vision and hearing achieve full potential when children reach school age, with 20/30 vision considered normal in preschoolers. Developmental stage determines the ability to solve problems and conceptualize, as described by the theorist Piaget (2003). As adults mature, visual acuity and the senses of hearing, touch, and even taste decline. Cognitive function must be evaluated within the context of the environment (Gordon, 2016). Environmental complexity results in different levels of functioning.

Assessing cognitive-perceptual patterns includes evaluating language capabilities, cognitive skills, and perception related to desired or required activities (Gordon, 2016). Nurses address clues indicating potential problems, particularly sensory deficits, sensory deprivation or overload, and ineffective pain management. Cognitive dysfunction may cause impaired reasoning, impaired judgement, or knowledge deficits related to health practices, as well as memory deficits.

Assessment parameters include hearing and vision test results. Changes in sensation or perception should be noted. In addition to decreased ability or acuity with regard to hearing, vision, smell, and taste, evaluation includes other perceptual disturbances, such as vertigo; increased or decreased sensitivity to heat, cold, or light touch; and visual or auditory hallucinations or illusions. Use and perceived effectiveness of assistive devices, such as hearing aids, eyeglasses, and contact lenses, is also noted.

Discomfort and pain are evaluated further. Useful tools that use pain scales have been designed to record and quantify changes in pain perception (Cunha Batalha, Fernandes, de Campos, et al., 2015). The location, type, degree, and duration of pain provide indicators of possible causes or sources. Relief measures to control pain and their effectiveness both provide data as well as a focus for health education. Attitudes toward pain should be considered. For example, someone may fear that medication is a sign of weakness, concern over potential addiction, or that it will result in a loss of independence. A pharmacological approach may be complemented with non-pharmacological strategies, such as heat or cold applications, distraction (music, reading, television), guided imagery, music therapy, and structured relaxation techniques (Cunha Batalha et al., 2015; Malcolm, 2015). For all individuals, exploring tolerance to pain is appropriate, using questions such as "Do you feel you are particularly sensitive to pain?" and "What level of pain is associated with your (cut, sprain, broken bone, or labour contractions)?"

Other areas of cognitive patterning to be explored include educational level, recent memory changes, ease or difficulty in learning, and preferred method of learning. Even when no problems are apparent or suspected, the nurse may assess these areas in more detail to determine areas of strength for use with health teaching plans.

Objective data are accumulated throughout the interview or assessment process. This data collection begins with the nurse's perception of the individual's general appearance: hygiene and grooming, proper use of clothing, neatness and appropriateness of dress, and indication that these are appropriate to the individual's developmental stage. Language and vocabulary use, the ability to convey an idea with words or with actions when speech is impaired or not yet developed, and grammatical correctness provide clues to cognitive functioning. Amplitude and quality of speech, affect and mood, as well as attention and concentration are all indicative of the individual's mental status. For many individuals, this information is sufficient to relay a sense of the level of understanding, memory, and mentation. Problem-solving abilities can usually be determined when the individual is asked to relate any perceived problems, provide an explanation of the problems and/or actions taken to solve the problems, and describe the results of the actions taken. Because this is a basic assessment in each functional health pattern, the nurse already has an idea of whether thought processes are logical, coherent, and relevant for this individual.

When problems within the cognitive realm do not surface, the information is recorded as part of the objective data or findings of the physical examination. The data to be noted include language; vocabulary; attention span; grasp of ideas; level of consciousness; orientation to person, place, and time; language spoken (whether primary or secondary); and behaviour during the data collection process, including posture, facial expression, and general body movements.

When a problem is apparent or suspected based on age, hereditary factors, or inconsistencies in the assessment data, a focused assessment is essential. Coma scales or functional dementia scales may be appropriate. More commonly, a Folstein Mini–Mental Status Examination (MMSE) is performed to assess orientation, attention, calculation, language (ability to name objects, repeat abstract ideas, and follow commands), and recall (immediate, short-term, and long-term memory). Abilities to read, write, and copy designs can also be assessed.

The examination of a sensory-perceptual pattern evaluates hearing, vision, and areas of pain at a screening level; comprehensive examinations are available and may be indicated. A full neurological assessment is warranted when specific sensory deficits are identified during the examination.

Although completing these assessment areas may seem overwhelming, the time required is generally less than that in most other pattern areas, perhaps because more information relevant to the cognitive-perceptual patterns becomes available as each pattern is assessed. Transition into the cognitive-perceptual pattern from other patterns may be facilitated by referring to a problem already described, with a question such as "Do you generally find it easy to solve problems effectively?" The self-perception pattern follows the cognitive pattern particularly well because mental status measures include feelings and perceptions of the individual regarding self. Mood, affect, and responses to the interviewer, such as eye contact, are indications of self-esteem. Cognitive-perceptual ability greatly influences the ability to function (self-care) or manipulate (activity and exercise) within the environment.

The placement of each of the patterns in a sequence suitable to each nurse, individual, or situation has been discussed. When the cognitive-perceptual pattern is dysfunctional, however, the individual is most likely unreliable as the historian; therefore it is wise to consider this pattern early in the assessment process. Approaching this pattern early saves valuable time and permits the identification of patterns that can be assessed more reliably.

Every person has experienced temporary memory lapses at one time or another. These events alone are not a sufficient basis for judgements. Sequencing of behaviours and clustering of appropriate signals (defining characteristics) are necessary to determine any nursing diagnosis. Equally important is the need to assess all pattern areas before data analysis and problem identification.

Cognitive and sensory ability data guide the nurse in planning care, which is especially apparent in health teaching. Formulation of health teaching plans ideally reflects each individual's preferred method of learning. The effective plan considers the individual's demonstrated developmental level; the ability to store information, retrieve information, and compensate for deficits; and also the neuromuscular and sensory levels necessary for skills development. An individually tailored plan contains mutually developed goals and short-term objectives. Although self-care might be an outcome for any person in whom diabetes mellitus has been newly diagnosed, the behaviours expected of an adult with diabetes will differ from those expected of a child.

### ◆ Self-Perception–Self-Concept Pattern

The self-perception–self-concept pattern encompasses the sense of each individual's personal identity, goals, emotional patterns, and feelings about the self. Self-image and sense of worth both stem from the individual's perception of personal appearance, competencies, and limitations, including the individual's self-perception and others' perceptions. The nurse assesses physical, verbal, and nonverbal cues (Gordon, 2016).

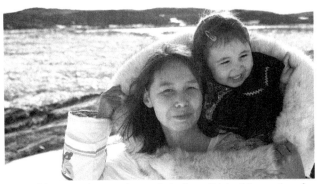

**Fig. 6.2** Most people care about what others think of them; therefore, the support of significant others, such as a mother supporting a grandchild, affects their self-perception–self-concept pattern. (iStockphoto/RyersonClark.)

The significance of the sense of self to the whole person is best exemplified by personal experiences. Individuals who feel good about their self-worth look and act differently from those who feel unable to accomplish anything worthwhile. Self-concept changes may affect patterns of eating, sleeping, communication, and activity.

The individual's developmental level affects and is affected by this pattern. One of the tasks identified during the later phases of Erikson's developmental framework, described previously, is building wholesome self-esteem. Delays in self-esteem and self-concept development affect progress toward subsequent tasks (Blakely-McClure & Ostrov, 2016) (see Table 6.3).

Family climate and relationship patterns provide the environmental impact that influences the self-concept pattern (see Chapter 7). People who are closely associated with the individual affect that person's self-esteem. Most people care about what others think of them; therefore, the support of significant others affects the self-perception–self-concept pattern (Philips, 2015; Tranväg, Petersen, & Näden, 2015) (Fig. 6.2).

The assessment objective in this pattern area is to describe each individual's patterns and beliefs about general self-worth and feeling states (Gordon, 2016). The nurse looks for clues that indicate identity confusion, altered body image, disturbances in self-esteem, and feelings of powerlessness. Nurses often identify anxiety, fear, and depression states that are responsive to nursing interventions (Webb, Wood-Barcalow, & Tylka, 2015).

The nurse notes the general appearance and effect of each individual, which may have been assessed as part of a formal mental status examination. Low self-esteem may be indicated by head and shoulder flexion, lack of eye contact, and mumbled or slurred speech. Anxiety or nervousness might be revealed through extraneous body movements such as foot shuffling or tapping, facial tension or grimace, rapid speech, voice quivering, twitches or tremors, and general restlessness or shifts in body position. Any of these indicators demands further exploration to determine underlying problems for each individual.

Self-concept influences each individual's interaction with others. In their study of 74 graduating college students, Wilt, Bleidorn, and Revelle (2016) linked meaning in life (MIL) to psychosocial functioning and self-concept at a time when the participants were embarking on a major life transition. The concept of MIL incorporates the belief that life is comprehensible and existence is important. Participants in this study who interacted with their family and friends had a higher level of MIL than those participants who experienced graduation and academic life without such interactions (Wilt et al., 2016).

Because the information in this pattern is personal, sharing the information may actually facilitate the process of goal setting and intervention planning when the nurse possesses strong communication skills and a caring attitude.

## ◆ Roles-Relationships Pattern

The roles-relationships pattern describes the position assumed and the associations engaged in by the individual that are connected to that position. The individual's perception is a major component of the assessment, and exploration of the pattern includes each individual's level of satisfaction with roles and relationships.

The need for relationships with other people is universal. Dossey and colleagues (2016) have identified basic needs for communication, fellowship, and love in high-level wellness. The ability to communicate with other people in a meaningful way greatly affects the whole person. The understanding of health as the harmonious balance between the individual and the environment indicates the major role that relationships with others play in health. Developmental hypotheses about readiness propose that attainment of each stage is required to progress to the next stage. For example, a person can become immersed in a relationship of genuine intimacy only after self-identity has stabilized. Developmental tasks that promote family development have also been identified similarly by Duvall and Miller, as noted by Gilbert (2015) (see Chapter 7). The emphasis within these models is on the individual's relationships within the nuclear family.

The objective of the roles-relationships pattern assessment is to describe an individual's pattern of family and shared circumstances, with the associated responsibilities. The individual's perception of satisfaction with the established relationship contributes to this assessment. Loss, change, and threat produce the major problems within this pattern. Clues indicative of impaired verbal communication, social isolation, alterations in parenting, independence-dependence conflicts, dysfunctional grieving, and potential for violence are pertinent.

Assessment focuses on family, work, and community roles and relationships. Within the family, assessment parameters include the family structure, tasks performed, social support systems, and other dynamics, such as decision making, power, authority, division of labour, and communication patterns. Parenting or marital difficulties and family violence issues are explored. The roles of student and employee are explored to determine specific occupation or position, along with work responsibilities and work environment. Parameters such as stress, safety, and health factors should be included (see the Case Study and the Care Plan at the end of this chapter). Financial concerns, job security, and retirement plans are elicited. Activity-rest patterns elicit information about time commitments, leisure activities,

and physical exercise; therefore, the assessment at this point addresses the impact of these factors on the roles-relationships pattern. Community roles and relationships indicate involvement within the neighbourhood and other social groups, such as the level of socialization and the amount of social support available. Within all three components (family, work or school, and community) the individual is asked to describe the level of satisfaction with the roles and relationships.

Threat of change, actual change, and loss are areas to be explored further. In addition, family or work roles alone may not cause stress, but combining them may cause difficulties, as with the working mother or travelling husband and father.

Objective data for assessment within this pattern are usually unavailable unless the nurse makes a home visit or sees the individual in the company of significant others in some other capacity. Family interaction and communication patterns are noted whenever possible. Cognizant of meaningful relationships within the family, the nurse identifies potential problems, such as those that occur with the college student away from home, the individual who travels or moves frequently, and sole family survivors when older people outlive their family members and friends (Gilbert, 2015). The relationships among the functional health patterns are clearly apparent in light of the developmental stages. Difficulties within the self-concept pattern and difficulties with relationships often appear together. Relationships affect the whole person; therefore, problems in the roles-relationships pattern may be exhibited in other areas, such as sleep, appetite, self-perception, and sexuality.

## ◆ Sexuality-Reproductive Pattern

The sexuality-reproductive pattern describes the individual's sexual self-concept, sexual functioning, methods of intimacy, and reproductive areas. Data collection combines subjective information, nursing observations, and physical examination. Normal development and perceived satisfaction combine to provide the elements of this pattern (Gordon, 2016).

Sexuality is the behavioural expression of sexual identity. The importance of this pattern area to the individual's life and health is closely related to the self-perception and the relationships patterns. Body image, self-concept, and role and gender identity are linked to sexual identity. This concept of sexual self and the individual's relationships pattern indicate the level and the perceived satisfaction of sexual functioning. Sexual functioning involves, but is not limited to, sexual relations with a partner. Reproductive patterns are equally significant to this pattern assessment, the whole individual, and the family and community (see Chapters 7 and 8).

As discussed, individual development influences reproductive capacities; these include genotype, secondary sex characteristics, genital development, phenotype, ego integrity, and the family life-cycle stage (Gilbert, 2015). The environment also plays a part in expression of the sexuality-reproductive pattern. Cultural and family norms may contribute to the expression of sexuality and combine with other factors, such as the family's financial stability, to influence reproductive patterns (Sutherland, Rehman, Fallis, et al., 2015). Norms within society may create issues in expressions of sexuality. During the assessment process, nurses consider the continuum of sexual identity expression, including heterosexuality, bisexuality, and transgender, gay, or lesbian sexuality. The information gathered guides the health-promotion plan in those who inquire about their sexual identity. Cochran, Bjorkenstam, and Mays (2016) indicate that sexual orientation influences the risk of death in their analysis of National Health and Nutrition Examination Survey data. Heterosexual participants ($n = 14,521$) were more likely to experience lower death risk than their nonheterosexual counterparts ($n = 1045$). These findings were consistent with the view that sexual orientation–related health disadvantages create this disparity in death risk. Nurses should remain informed about sexual orientation health disadvantages, such as mental distress, tobacco use, binge drinking, and lack of health insurance.

One objective of assessment in this pattern is to describe behavioural problems or difficulties (Gordon, 2016). Equally important is assessing the individual's knowledge of sexual functioning and preventive health practices, such as breast and testicular self-examination, Papanicolaou tests, effective contraceptive use, and avoidance of infection. Clues are evaluated for potential or actual sexual dysfunction. Through cultural safety, recognizing diversity of sexuality within the LGBTQ2 community will help to reduce health inequities in this population (Butler, McCreedy, & Schwer, 2016).

The following parameters are assessed: sexual self-concept, which may be derived from information collected in the self-perception–self-concept and the roles-relationships patterns; sexual functioning, with the nurse noting evidence of some form of intimacy, the level of sexual activity or libido, and the effect of health or illness on sexual expression; and reproductive patterns, in which the nurse collects data pertinent to health-promotion factors, such as feelings related to aging, preventive practices, and knowledge of sexual functioning. For women, reproductive pattern assessment would also include information about menstruation, such as onset, duration, and frequency, date of last menstrual period, discomfort, and menopause, as well as information about reproductive stage, such as pregnancy history and birth control methods. Male concerns with sexuality tend to be overlooked, but questions regarding physical changes, changes in functioning, and intimacy concerns must be assessed in order to ascertain a holistic view of the individual.

The level of satisfaction with sexual self-concept, sexual functioning, and reproduction is also explored. Difficulties such as ineffective or inappropriate sexual performance, discharges, infections, venereal disease, discomfort, and history of abuse are evaluated. Focused assessment to collect additional information is warranted with sexual dysfunction or trauma. Physical examination evaluates genital development and secondary sex characteristics. Signs of intimacy between partners, such as holding hands and hugging, are noted.

People may feel threatened by discussion of topics in this pattern; the depth of exploration is governed in part by the individual's wishes. Dialogue is encouraged but may be postponed until a firm and trusting relationship is established. A clear representation of the individual's knowledge and use of preventive

⚡ **QUALITY AND SAFETY SCENARIO**

### Using Quality Improvement Techniques in Indigenous Primary Health Care

Improving the quality of health promotion was explored in four primary health centres in Australia. These centres served Indigenous people of Australia. The researchers aimed to describe the scope and quality of health-promotion activities and introduce health-promotion interventions. The findings suggest that quality-improvement projects can improve the delivery of evidence-informed health promotion by engaging front-line health practitioners in redesign of systems. In addition to medical care, primary health centres that have health promotion as a core function should also deliver counselling, preventive medicine, health education and promotion, rehabilitative services, antenatal and postnatal care, and maternal and child care programs. Often, organizational support for such core functions is inadequate. This study attempted to engage the centres in a systems approach to quality improvement to address the organizational components that hindered health-promotion delivery. The researchers used an iterative action research strategy to explore current practice, introduce best practices, and engage physicians, nurses, Indigenous health workers, and administrative staff in the action plan to redesign health-promotion delivery systems within the four primary health centres.

Source: Percival, N., O'Donoghue, L., Lin, V., et al. (2016). Improving health promotion using quality improvement techniques in Australian Indigenous primary health care. *Frontiers in Public Health, 4*, 53.

practices facilitates planning for health promotion. Although sex education is usually associated with school programs, information and discussion about sexuality is just as important for adults of all ages. Sex education is a key element of parenthood classes. Improved understanding of sexuality and sexual function leads to discovery and increased satisfaction.

### ◆ Coping–Stress Tolerance Pattern

Gordon (2016) describes the coping–stress tolerance pattern as a depiction of general coping and the individual's ability to effectively manage stress. This pattern includes the individual's ability to process life crises and to resist disruptive factors that will influence self-integrity of ego, mode of conflict resolution, stress management, and accessibility to necessary resources (Quality and Safety Scenario).

The ability to manage stress effectively in life is a learned behaviour. Stress is a necessary part of life; without it there is no motivation to grow. Vulnerability to stress may be linked to individuals' coping strategies, such as avoidance behaviour (Gorka, LaBar, & Hariri, 2016). Stress is exacerbated by accumulation of minor irritations. Stress is inherent not in the event but in the individual's perception of that event. Whereas one individual may experience stress from missing a bus and can think only of being 10 minutes late, another will consider the same event an opportunity to spend 10 minutes reading the newspaper. This difference in perception may represent the different values used to identify sources of stress or it may represent coping strategies.

For purposes of assessing this pattern, coping, which is considered the individual behavioural response to stress, includes both problem-solving ability and use of defence mechanisms. Coping is viewed not as a single act but as a process incorporating many behaviours. The function of coping is to deal with the threat or emotional distress of an event. Coping effectiveness is assessed from the individual's perspective and from the nurse's observation of the individual's ability to function in the presence of actual or potential stressors in the environment.

The perception of stress and the ability to manage it depend on personal development, the amount of stress previously experienced, the current level of stress within the environment, and the sources of social support. For example, an older person may experience many stresses during life and manage them effectively, but now coping may no longer be possible because too many stressors are present, such as physical incapacitation, fixed income, fear of illness or injury, and lack of transportation (Bielderman, Schout, de Greef, et al., 2015; Boehm, Chen, Williams, et al., 2015). In addition, this person may no longer have a social support system, which has been associated with promotion of health. Determining individuals' stress tolerance and past coping patterns becomes the objective of assessment for this functional pattern. Clues to difficulties in managing past and current stressors and changes in the effectiveness of a coping pattern help to determine personal coping capacity.

The following assessment parameters are included: the coping task, including the physical, psychological, and socioeconomic stimuli with which the individual must cope; coping style, or the tendency to use a specific style, such as approach oriented, avoidance oriented, or nonspecific; coping strategies, including specifics; and coping effectiveness. Coping strategy may be divided into information seeking, direct action (fight or flight), inhibition of action, or use of social support. Individual resources include the variety of coping mechanisms used by the individual, the flexibility of these mechanisms, and the health-promotion value associated with each of them. For example, in their study of problem-solving intervention with 166 stroke rehabilitation clients, Visser, Heijenbrok-Kal, Van't Spijker, and colleagues (2016) report that their problem-solving intervention improved task-oriented coping and general health-related quality of life. However psychosocial health-related quality of life associated specifically with stroke in their sample did not seem to improve.

Stress tolerance patterns elicit the amount of stress effectively processed in the past. Use of anticipatory coping is assessed along with whether the individual knows how to cope, but does not cope (production deficit), or simply does not know how to cope (skill deficit). Other indicators of value within this pattern are discussed in the section Self-Perception–Self-Concept Pattern. Objective data of concern include physical signs of restlessness, irritability, and nervousness, such as increased heart rate, blood pressure, and perspiration. Evidence of coping ability and tolerance to stress are found in every other functional health pattern. Stress also affects the other patterns, thereby resulting in health problems such as insomnia, weight loss, and poor concentration (Dossey et al., 2016; Gordon, 2016).

Health can be promoted through early intervention to reduce stress. Coping patterns and stress tolerance in the past may uncover unhealthy coping behaviour, such as smoking and alcohol consumption, which needs to be replaced by alternative coping strategies. Stress-reduction workshops would be helpful

## INNOVATIVE PRACTICE

### The Humor Potential, Inc.

The Humor Potential, Inc., is a company that provides resources, products, and seminars for stress management with the use of humour. Company president Loretta LaRoche is a recognized expert on stress management, emphasizing the importance of balancing daily living experiences with humour. The Humor Potential offers seminars and lectures to health care providers, schools, corporations, other organizations, and the general public. The company also produces television programs. One television program, *The Joy of Stress*, was nominated for an Emmy Award.

Books, prints, audiotapes and videotapes, and other products dealing with humour can be purchased from Loretta LaRoche's website. The collection consists of audiotapes and videotapes that have been developed for corporate meetings and training. An example is *Lighten Up!* This is a videotape and action guide that increases productivity by reducing stress. A catalogue is available for e-mail, fax, phone, and mail orders.

**Contact Information**
The Humor Potential Inc.
Corporate Offices
50 Court Street
Plymouth, MA 02360
Website: http://www.lorettalaroche.com
Telephone: 800-99-TADAH (800-998-2324)

Based on data from the Humor Potential, Inc. Retrieved from http://www.lorettalaroche.com.

for most of the population because the future undoubtedly holds stressful events, some of which may be overwhelming without coping strategies. The Innovative Practice box includes information about a unique company that offers stress-management interventions. Dossey and colleagues (2016) offer categories for stress management: social engineering strategies, such as time management or planned change; personality engineering strategies, such as assertiveness training or cognitive rehearsal; and altered states of consciousness, such as meditation or relaxation. Planning based on the assessment of all functional health patterns to help determine a coping pattern should include these kinds of strategies.

## ◆ Values-Beliefs Pattern

The values-beliefs pattern describes values, including the individual's spiritual values, beliefs, and goals. This pattern also includes perceptions of what is right, what is good, and conflicts that beliefs or values impart. Each of the 11 patterns addresses the value systems of individuals, their family, and society. Individual beliefs or values develop over time and govern life through personal experiences and family and societal influences (Bielderman et al., 2015; Boehm et al., 2015). The objective in assessing this pattern is to determine the basis for health-related decisions and actions (Gordon, 2016). Individuals engage in preventive health behaviour when a threat to wellness or health status exists. Several other health belief models expand on this concept by including other motivations, such as personal values and environmental influences. Clues to conflict within the individual's value system or between the person's value system and that of the family or society are explored.

The dimensions of assessment include the individual's values, beliefs, or goals that guide choices or decisions that are related to health. The nurse collects information while exploring each pattern, while summarizing, clarifying, and securing additional information. Specifically, values and beliefs about self, relationships, culture, and society are appraised. Individuals' beliefs, goals, and purposes of life are reviewed, along with any conflicts, perceived philosophies, and philosophies of the family, culture, and society. Sources of strength, such as a higher being or significant individual practices, are explored, including spiritual and religious beliefs and preferences. Past goals and expectations are assessed through the individual's satisfaction. The nurse must identify the individual's goals and expectations concerning health, clarifying them to help the individual achieve them. To be effective, health-promotion interventions are based on the individual's value system and health beliefs (Dossey et al., 2016). The brevity of this discussion is not an indication of the importance that the values-beliefs pattern plays in the assessment of the individual. Individual values play a role in all the patterns.

## INDIVIDUAL HEALTH PROMOTION THROUGH THE NURSING PROCESS

The nursing process—the systematic approach to reduce or eliminate the individual's health problem—is accomplished in several steps, the first being the collection of necessary data. With the individual, the nurse analyzes the data, identifies a nursing diagnosis, projects outcomes, prescribes interventions, and evaluates effectiveness. Reassessment, reordering of priorities, new goal setting, and revising the plan continue as part of the process toward outcome attainment (Carpenito-Moyet, 2016).

### Collection and Analysis of Data

Assessment is a systematic technique for learning as much as possible about the individual. The main purposes in collecting data from a new individual is to see whether health problems exist and to identify the individual's health goals. Data collection includes biographical data, such as age, sex, and the purpose of the visit. This process is followed by assessment of the previously outlined 11 functional health patterns. Subjective reporting, nursing observations and perceptions, and the physical examination findings are assessed and recorded. The remaining discussion focuses on nursing diagnosis.

### Problem Identification

As the concept of problem identification evolved, most nurses have distinguished *nursing diagnosis* as the most useful label. Diagnosis is a careful examination and analysis of the facts to provide a basis for nursing intervention. Nursing diagnosis is the naming of individual, family, and community responses to actual or potential health problems or life processes (Gordon, 2016; NANDA International, 2018). Nursing diagnoses provide the basis for selection of nursing

interventions to achieve outcomes for which the nurse is accountable (Gordon, 2016). Leadership from NANDA International has provided standardization of the descriptions of human responses that nurses manage. Although Wang, Yu, and Hailey (2015) describe issues associated with the use of the NANDA International taxonomy, such as inadequacy of terms to describe complex nursing care and nurses' reluctance to incorporate these diagnoses into their documentation language, the NANDA International taxonomy remains the most widely used standardized language for nursing diagnoses.

Gordon (2016) proposes the accepted format of nursing diagnosis that lists the problem, cause, and signs and symptoms, or defining characteristics, for each diagnosis accepted for clinical testing. The NANDA International taxonomy uses a multiaxial framework for nursing diagnoses, including diagnostic concept (e.g., parenting), acuity (e.g., altered), unit of care (e.g., individual), developmental stage (e.g., adolescent), potentiality (e.g., at risk of), and descriptor, for creation of the diagnostic statement (NANDA International, 2018). The Research for Evidence-Informed Practice box discusses how this nursing classification system compares with a non-nursing system.

### RESEARCH FOR EVIDENCE-INFORMED PRACTICE

#### Sexual Health Promotion for Ethnic-Minority Adolescent Women

Evidence-informed strategies should be used to promote individuals' health. Adolescent sexual health-promotion efforts may be inaccessible and lack confidentiality. Multiple interrelated risks develop among adolescents, requiring multifaceted health-promotion strategies. Champion, Young, and & Rew (2016) aimed to explore these issues in their study exploring psychological distress, violence, and substance use among Black (n = 94) and Mexican American (n = 465) adolescent women with a history of risky sexual behaviour. These adolescent women self-reported psychological distress, sexual risk behaviour, sexually transmitted infection (STI), personal and friend/peer substance use, alcohol use, and violence. Substance-using friends, physical violence, and STI were highly associated with personal substance use in these adolescent women. Alcohol users were five times more likely than nonalcohol users to use other substances.

Adolescents in this study self-reported adverse sexual health outcomes, including initial and repeated unplanned pregnancies, human immunodeficiency virus (HIV) infection, and other STIs. Predictors of substance use in these women were ethnicity, friend substance use, physical violence history, STI history, and history of alcohol use. Nurses should consider social determinants, including demographic, educational, environmental, and behavioural components, in their assessment of specific adolescent populations such as ethnic minority females. The authors recommend that nurses integrate these complex health inequities into their health-promotion practice. They aim for their findings to guide health-promotion strategies in primary care settings for women experiencing multiple health inequalities.

Source: Champion, J. D., Young, C., & Rew, L. (2016). Substantiating the need for primary care–based sexual health promotion interventions for ethnic minority adolescent women experiencing health disparities. *Journal of the American Association of Nurse Practitioners, 28*(9), 487–492.

In discussions of problems, the meaning of the problem must be clearly defined and identified. The concept as used in this text refers to Gordon's (2016) proposition that a health problem is defined as a dysfunctional pattern and that nursing's major contribution to health care is in preventing and treating such a pattern. A pattern is dysfunctional when it represents a deviation from established norms or from the individual's previous condition or goals. A dysfunctional pattern is a problem when it generates therapeutic concern on the part of the individual, others, or the nurse and when it is amenable to nursing therapies.

As patterns are assessed, the nurse proposes several hypotheses regarding functional or dysfunctional labelling. At the completion of the assessment, conclusions must be drawn. The possibility exists that all patterns are functional, that some are functional, and that others are dysfunctional or potentially dysfunctional. Functional refers to wellness and optimal health. Dysfunctional patterns, indicating some health problems, may be present in the absence of disease; that is, nursing care may be needed for health promotion and health maintenance, not health restoration. The case history of Antonio in Chapter 1 effectively illustrates the multiple nursing care needs of an individual who is not ill. In potentially dysfunctional patterns, sufficient evidence exists or enough risk factors are present to indicate that a pattern dysfunction will likely occur if interventions are not made. Early identification of potential problems is possible through systematic data collection and analysis.

## Contributing Etiological Factors

To plan care the nurse must first determine what has caused the actual or potential health problem: its contributing etiological factors. The etiological factors of most dysfunctional patterns lie within another pattern or patterns. Although cause is never an absolute within human sciences, the projection of outcomes or goals must be based on probable causes. Interventions then focus on mediating or resolving the probable causes. Most often, many factors are involved, and problems are said to relate to rather than be a result of these factors. Potential problems are not actual problems but risk states; therefore, they have no specific cause and are identified when risk factors are present. Nursing intervention is directed toward risk reduction through education to improve nutrition, prevent accidents, and so forth.

## Diagnostic Variables

The ability to arrive at an accurate diagnosis, even when comprehensive data are unavailable, is governed primarily by the nurse's clinical knowledge. Experience improves the effectiveness when nursing is performed as a scientific process. Nursing requires the gathering of information, interpreting it based on normative values, organizing and grouping information on the basis of healthy findings, identifying the problem, and then planning appropriate goals and interventions. Difficulties are encountered when there are no available norms that occur frequently in the psychosocial assessment components. Use of the 11 interdependent functional health patterns helps to solve these difficulties. By focusing on each

of these areas, nurses find it easier to recognize whether a problem does or does not exist. Any change within the pattern may be a sign of dysfunction or an unhealthy but stabilized behaviour. For example, a sign of dysfunction might be a 2-year-old child who is still not walking; developmental growth is a major factor in activity patterns of infants, toddlers, and children.

The use of physiological parameters clearly demonstrates the idea of a stabilized dysfunctional pattern, but equal attention must be given to psychological development. For instance, a 26-year-old man who lives with his mother and gives no indication of independent decision making should be evaluated. It should be apparent that assessment information primarily comes from the initial contact with the individual and the database, which is generally the case in health-promotion activities. However, in any acute situation or emergency, quick assessment of the major problems is given high priority on a hierarchy-of-needs basis, and the full nursing assessment is postponed temporarily. For further understanding of the nursing diagnosis, the nurse is referred to those authors who discuss the development of diagnoses, the diagnostic process, and specific details of each accepted diagnosis (Carpenito-Moyet, 2016; Gordon, 2016; NANDA International, 2018).

## Planning the Care

In the nursing process, planning is the proposal of diagnosis-specific treatment to assist the individual toward the goal, or expected outcome, of optimal health. The individual's goals and the determined nursing diagnosis provide the basis for planning. Clear goals and diagnoses are critical to development of an effective plan of care. The nursing process identifies the following purposes of the planning phase: to assign priority to the problems diagnosed; to specify the behavioural outcomes or goals with the individual, including the expected time of achievement; to differentiate individual problems that can be resolved by nursing intervention, those that can be handled by the individual or family member, and those that should be handled with or referred to other members of the health team; to designate specific actions, the frequency of these actions, and the short-, intermediate-, and long-term results; and to list the individual's problems (nursing diagnosis) and nursing actions (frequency and expected outcomes, or goals) on the nursing care plan or blueprint for action (Carpenito-Moyet, 2016). This plan provides the direction for individual and nursing activities and is the guide for the evaluation. There are many research studies involving outcomes from which nurses can draw to increase the effectiveness of the care they provide.

## Implementing the Plan

Implementation consists of the actions necessary to fulfill the goals for optimal health; it is the enactment of the nursing care plan to elicit the behaviours described in the proposed individual outcome. The selection of a nursing intervention depends on several factors: the desired individual outcome, the characteristics of the nursing diagnosis, the research base associated with the intervention, the feasibility of implementing the intervention, the acceptability of the intervention to the individual, and the capability of the nurse (Carpenito-Moyet, 2016). A nursing interventions classification is being developed. As discussed in Unit 1, a critical component of effective communication is the accurate interpretation of the individual's information. This feedback process continues throughout all phases of the nursing process; the nurse continues to collect data to modify the plan as needed and does not blindly implement the care plan. The most frequently used nursing interventions in health promotion are screening, education, counselling, and crisis intervention. All these interventions require strong communication abilities from the nurse. Checklists and screening instruments may be used to document nursing assessment and help to ensure transmission of reliable and quality information for patient-centred care. Implementation requires transdisciplinary collaboration in the analysis and plan. Computerized data entry, information systems, and electronic medical records may facilitate communication; however, ongoing interaction with other health care providers is essential for collaboration.

## Evaluating the Plan

The process of analyzing changes experienced by the individual occurs in the evaluation phase of the nursing process, with the nurse examining the relationships between nursing actions and the individual's goal achievement. The nursing process emphasizes that evaluation is always considered in terms of how the individual responds to the plan of action (Toney-Butler & Thayer, 2019). As discussed, the nursing diagnosis (or health problems) and the goal (or expected outcome) guide the evaluation of the nursing care plan. Many variables influence outcomes: the interventions prescribed by the health care providers, the health care providers themselves, the environment in which the care is received, motivation, the individual's genetic structure, and the individual's significant others (Genomics). The task for nursing is to define which outcomes are sensitive to nursing care so as to identify the expected and attainable results of nursing care for each individual (NANDA International, 2018). Families and patients are partners in the process of client-centred care (Spruce, 2015). Documentation of all components of the nursing process in the individual's health care record is then performed (Toney-Butler & Thayer, 2019).

## GENOMICS

### Genome British Columbia

Genome British Columbia "lead academia, government and industry to develop world-class genome sciences that deliver social and economic benefits to British Columbia, Canada and beyond" (Genome British Columbia, 2019). One such initiative is research into hereditary connections with those who have been diagnosed with cancer. They provide hereditary genetic testing that helps individuals learn what cancers they may develop. Screening provides information of potential risks and what types of preventive measures are available to counteract risks. Research has provided more sensitive testing to genetic disorders. For example, one panel test can now screen for 17 genes, which is both cost saving in time and money.

Source: Genome British Columbia. (2019). *Home page*. Retrieved from https://www.genomebc.ca/.

## CASE STUDY

### Spiritual Distress: Cindy

Cindy is a single 28-year-old woman. Cindy studies nursing and shares an apartment with two friends. She was having increasing difficulties with her course work and was placed on academic probation. Cindy became concerned about the effect of stress on her ability to finish her studies and on her future career. She grew increasingly nervous and began to ask, "Will I ever be okay?" and "Will I ever be able to finish school and function as a nurse?" Cindy expressed her fear of weakness and feelings of isolation, loneliness, helplessness, and loss of control. These feelings began to find expression in anger related to this major life disruption. She verbalized her anger at God for allowing this to happen to her. Her incapacity deprived her of her normal outlets for expressing and finding support for such concerns. Cindy was unable to participate in the practices of her faith, in which she had previously found strength in facing life's challenges. Her inability to concentrate and her growing feeling of lethargy added to her frustration. Expressing these fears and concerns was difficult for Cindy. The nurse, however, developed a trusting relationship with Cindy, permitting her to express her fears, anxieties, and concerns. Based on the nurse's assessment, the nursing diagnosis of spiritual distress was formulated.

Reflective Questions

- What differential diagnoses should the nurse consider?
- Describe other individuals you know who have experienced spiritual distress.
- How does distress with spirituality affect social determinants of health?
- What health- promotion strategies could be used with Cindy?

## CARE PLAN

### *Spiritual Distress: Cindy*

**Nursing Issue**

Spiritual distress resulting from a threat to well-being, loss of meaningful role, and separation from religious and family ties.

**Defining Characteristics**
- Experiences a disturbance in the belief system.
- Demonstrates discouragement or despair.
- Chooses not to practice religious rituals.
- Shows emotional detachment from self and others.
- Expresses concern, anger, resentment, and fear, related to a major life disruption.

**Related Factors**
- Threat to well-being from change in role as a student and fear of failure.
- Loss of meaningful role as a student.
- Separation from religious and family ties.

**Expected Outcomes**
- Person will verbalize a greater sense of purpose, meaning, and hope.
- Person will express feelings of anger verbally and will discuss anger with another person.

**Interventions**
- Take time to be present and available to listen to the individual.
- Convey a nonjudgemental attitude.
- Encourage the individual to verbalize feelings.
- Pray with the individual as indicated.
- Engage the individual in values clarification.
- Encourage the individual to acknowledge feelings of anger and to acknowledge and name any other feelings experienced.
- Reassure the individual that it is acceptable to feel anger toward a supreme being.
- Encourage honest dialogue with a peer whom the individual trusts.
- Offer consultation with an appropriate spiritual advisor.
- Inform the individual of religious resources.

## SUMMARY

Data relevant to the health-promotion activities of the individual focus primarily on the assessment of the current health status so that the nurse can identify problem areas, or areas of dysfunction, within the individual's health and lifestyle pattern. This process is a fundamental first step and precedes all other components of the nursing process. Without a clear picture of the problem, nursing activities are fruitless. Gordon's (2016) functional health pattern framework provides guidance for the individual assessment. The focus of each pattern includes the age-developmental influences exerted, cultural and environmental roles played, functional ability displayed, and behavioural patterns specific to each individual. The interaction between internal mechanisms and the environment is assessed through these 11 functional health patterns. When assessing each pattern, the nurse must understand the pattern definition, the significance of the pattern to the whole individual, the developmental influences, the environmental role, the assessment objectives, the assessment parameters and indicators, and the nursing implications. Assessment is essential to all components of the nursing process in health promotion for the individual.

**Evolve Chapter Features**

http://evolve.elsevier.com/Canada/Edelman/healthpromotion/
- Review Questions

## REFERENCES

Andermann, A. (2016). Taking action on the social determinants of health in clinical practice: A framework for health professionals. *Canadian Medical Association Journal, 188*(17–18), E474–E483. https://doi.org/10.1503/cmaj.160177.

Andrews, M. M., & Boyle, J. S. (2015). *Transcultural concepts in nursing care* (7th ed.). New York: Wolters Kluwer.

Ariapooran, S., Heidari, S., Asgari, M., et al. (2018). Individualism, collectivism, social support, resilience and suicidal ideation among women with the experience of the death of a young person. *International Journal of Community Based Nursing and Midwifery (IJCBNM), 6*(3), 250–259.

Bardsley, A. (2015). Approaches to managing chronic constipation in older people within the community setting. *British Journal of Community Nursing, 20*(9), 444–450.

Bax, A. C., Geurtz, C. D., & Balachova, T. N. (2015). Improving recognition of children affected by prenatal alcohol exposure: Detection of exposure in pediatric care. *Current Developmental Disorders Reports, 2*(3), 165–174.

Bielderman, A., Schout, G., de Greef, M., et al. (2015). Understanding how older adults living in deprived neighbourhoods address aging issues. *British Journal of Community Nursing, 20*(8), 394–399. https://doi.org/10.12968/bjcn.2015.20.8.394.

Blakely-McClure, S. J., & Ostrov, J. M. (2016). Relational aggression, victimization and self-concept: Testing pathways from middle childhood to adolescence. *Journal of Youth and Adolescence, 45*(2), 376–390.

Boehm, J. K., Chen, Y., Williams, D. R., et al. (2015). Unequally distributed psychological assets: Are there social disparities in optimism, life satisfaction and positive affect? *PLoS ONE, 10*(2), e0118066. https://doi.org/10.1371/journal.pone.0118066.

Brito-Brito, P. R., Oter-Quintana, C., Martín-García, A., et al. (2014). Case study: Community nursing care plan for an elderly patient with urinary incontinence and social interaction problems after prostatectomy. *Journal of Nursing Knowledge, 25*(1), 62–65. https://doi.org/10.1111/2047-3095.12021.

Butler, M. M., McCreedy, E., & Schwer, N. (2016). Lesbian, gay, bisexual and transgender populations. In *Improving cultural competence to reduce health disparities*. Rockville, MD: Agency for Healthcare Research and Quality (US).

Canadian Nurses Association (CNA). (2017). *Code of ethics*. Retrieved from https://www.cna-aiic.ca/~/media/cna/page-content/pdf-en/code-of-ethics-2017-edition-secure-interactive.

Canadian Task Force on Preventive Health Care. (2016). Recommendations on screening for developmental delay. *Canadian Medical Association Journal, 188*(8), 579–587. https://doi.org/10.1503/cmaj.151437.

Carpenito-Moyet, L. J. (2016). *Nursing diagnosis: Application to clinical practice* (15th ed.). Philadelphia: Lippincott Williams & Wilkins.

Champion, J. D., Young, C., & Rew, L. (2016). Substantiating the need for primary care–based sexual health promotion interventions for ethnic minority adolescent women experiencing health disparities. *Journal of the American Association of Nurse Practitioners, 28*(9), 487–492.

Cochran, S. D., Bjorkenstam, C., & Mays, V. M. (2016). Sexual orientation and all-cause mortality among adults aged 18 to 59 years, 2001–2011. *American Journal of Public Health, 106*(5), 918–920. https://doi.org/10.2105/AJPH.2016.303052.

Cunha Batalha, L. M., Fernandes, A., de Campos, C., et al. (2015). Pain assessment in children with cancer: A systematic review. *Revista De Enfermagem Referéncia, 5*, 119–127. https://doi.org/10.12707/RIV14013.

Doane, G. H., & Varcoe, C. (2015). *How to nurse: Relational inquiry with individuals and families in changing health and health care contexts*. Philadelphia: Wolters Kluwer/Lippincott Williams & Williams.

Doenges, M. E., Moorhouse, M. F., & Murr, A. C. (2015). *Nursing diagnosis manual: Planning, individualizing and documenting client care* (5th ed.). Philadelphia: F.A. Davis.

Dossey, B. M., Keegan, L., & Guzzetta, C. E. (2016). *Holistic nursing: A handbook for practice* (7th ed.). Boston: Jones & Bartlett.

Endo, E. (2017). Margaret Newman's theory of health as expanding consciousness and a nursing intervention from a unitary perspective. *Asia-Pacific Journal of Oncology Nursing, 4*, 50–52. https://doi.org/10.4103/2347-5625.199076.

Erikson, E. H. (1963). *Childhood and society*. New York: Norton.

Fawcett, J. (2015). Evolution of science of unitary human beings: The conceptual system, theory development and research and practice methodologies. *Visions, 21*(1), 10–16.

First Nations Health Authority. (2019). Home page. Retrieved from http://www.fnha.ca/.

Food Insecurity Policy Research. (2018). Home page. Retrieved from https://proof.utoronto.ca/food-insecurity/.

Gebel, K., Ding, D., Foster, C., et al. (2015). Improving current practice in reviews of the built environment and physical activity. *Sports Medicine, 45*(3), 297. https://doi.org/10.1007/s40279-014-0273-8.

Genome British Columbia. (2019). *Home page*. Retrieved from https://www.genomebc.ca/.

Gilbert, P. (2015). When it hurts: Too young or too old. *Journal of Nursing Care, 4*(228). https://doi.org/10.4172/2167-1168.1000228.

Gomez-Salgado, J., Jacobsohn, L., Frade, F., et al. (2018). Applying the WHO international classification of functioning, disability and health in nursing assessment of population health. *International Journal of Environmental Research & Public Health (IJERPH), 15*(10), 2245. https://doi.org/10.3390/ijerph15102245.

Gordon, M. (2016). *Manual of nursing diagnosis* (13th ed.). Sudbury, MA: Jones & Bartlett.

Gorka, A. X., LaBar, K. S., & Hariri, A. R. (2016). Variability in emotional responsiveness and coping style during active avoidance as a window onto psychological vulnerability to stress. *Physiology & Behavior, 158*, 90–99. https://doi.org/10.1016/j.physbeh.2016.02.036.

Gottlieb, L. N. (2014). Strengths-based nursing: A holistic approach to care, grounded in eight core values. *American Journal of Nursing, 114*(8), 24–32.

Government of Canada. (2019). *Centre for Health Promotion (CHP)*. Retrieved from https://www.canada.ca/en/public-health/services/health-promotion/centre-health-promotion.html.

Harvard Women's Health Watch. (2015). When urinary tract infections keep coming back. *Harvard Women's Heaslth Watch, 23*(1), 5.

Health Canada. (2019). *Canada's dietary guidelines for health professionals and policy makers*. Retrieved from https://food-guide.canada.ca/static/assets/pdf/CDG-EN-2018.pdf.

Hopkins, T., & Rippon, S. (2015). *Head, hands and heart: Asset-based approaches in health care*. London: The Health Foundation.

International Council of Nurses. (2015). *Definition of nursing*. Retrieved from https://www.icn.ch/nursing-policy/nursing-definitions.

Koloroutis, M., & Hanlon, T. (2017). *Cultivating connection: The magic of attuning, wondering, following and holding*. Minneapolis: Creative Health Care Management. Retrieved from https://chcm.com/thought-leadership/cultivating-connection-magic-attuning-wondering-following-holding/.

Lee, A. (2015). Combating the causes of constipation. *Nursing & Residential Care, 17*(6), 327–331.

Levitsky, L. L. (2016). Nutrition and growth–a multitude of manifestations and room for further investigation. *Current Opinion in Endocrinology, Diabetes and Obesity, 23*(1), 48–50. https://doi.org/10.1097/MED.0000000000000223.

Luyster, F. S., Choi, J., Yeh, C.-H., et al. (2015). Screening and evaluation tools for sleep disorders in older adults. *Applied Nursing Research, 28*(4), 334–340. https://doi.org/10.1016/j.apnr.2014.12.007.

Malcolm, C. (2015). Acute pain management in the older person. *Journal of Perioperative Practice, 25*(7/8), 134–139.

Malone, J. C., Liu, S. R., Vaillant, G. E., et al. (2016). Midlife eriksonian psychosocial development: Setting the stage for late-life cognitive and emotional health. *Developmental Psychology, 52*(3), 496–508. https://doi.org/10.1037/a0039875.

NANDA International. (2018). *Nursing diagnoses: Definitions and classifications* (11th ed.). Oxford: Wiley-Blackwell.

National Research Council, & Institute of Medicine. (2015). *Measuring the risks and causes of premature death: Summary of workshops*. Washington: The National Academies Press.

Nazarko, L. (2015). Solve the case: Urinary frequency and recurrent urinary tract symptoms. *Nurse Prescribing, 13*(9), 458–463.

Niño, A., Kissil, K., & Davey, M. P. (2016). Strategies used by foreign-born family therapists to connect across cultural differences: A thematic analysis. *Journal of Marital and Family Therapy, 42*(1), 123–138. https://doi.org/10.1111/jmft.12115.

Oreskovic, N. M., Perrin, J. M., Robinson, A., et al. (2015). Adolescents' use of the build environment for physical activity. *BMC Public Health, 15*(1), 1596–1603. https://doi.org/10.1186/s12889-015-1596-6.

Paans, W., Müller-Staub, M., & Nieweg, R. (2013). The influence of the use of diagnostic resources on nurses' communication with simulated patients during admission interviews. *Journal of Nursing Knowledge, 24*(2), 101–107.

Philips, A. (2015). Diabetes and relationships: How couples manage diabetes. *Practice Nursing, 26*(6), 298–301. https://doi.org/10.12968/pnur.2015.26.6.298.

Piaget, J. (2003). *The psychology of intelligence*. London: Taylor and Francis.

Roncarolo, F., & Potvin, L. (2016). Food insecurity as a symptom of a social disease, analyzing a social problem from a medical perspective. *Canadian Family Physician, 62*(4), 291–292.

Sahlqvist, S., Goodman, A., Jones, T., et al. (2015). Mechanisms underpinning use of new walking and cycling infrastructure in different contexts: Mixed-method analysis. *International Journal of Behavioral Nutrition and Physical Activity, 12*(24). https://doi.org/10.1186/s12966-015-0185-5.

Sokol, R. J., Martier, S. S., & Ager, J. W. (1989). The T-ACE questions: practical prenatal detection of risk-drinking. *American Journal of Obstetrical Gynecology, 160*(4), 863–870. [Seminal Reference].

Spruce, L. (2015). Back to basics: Patient and family engagement. *AORN Journal, 102*(1), 33–39.

Statistics Canada. (2018). *Health fact sheet: Overweight and obese adults, 2018*. Ottawa: Author. Retrieved from https://www150.statcan.gc.ca/n1/pub/82-625-x/2019001/article/00005-eng.htm.

Sutherland, S. E., Rehman, U. S., Fallis, E. E., et al. (2015). Understanding the phenomenon of sexual desire discrepancy in couples. *Canadian Journal of Human Sexuality, 24*(2), 141–150. https://doi.org/10.3138/cjhs.242.A3.

Toney-Butler, T. J., & Thayer, J. M. (2019). Nursing process. *StatPearls*. National Library of Medicine/NIH. Retrieved from https://www.ncbi.nlm.nih.gov/books/NBK499937/.

Tranväg, O., Petersen, K. A., & Näden, D. (2015). Relational interactions preserving dignity experience. *Nursing Ethics, 22*(5), 577–593. https://doi.org/10.1177/0969733014549882.

Ulfarsson, T., Lundgren-Nilsson, A., Blomstrand, C., et al. (2014). A history of unemployment or sick leave influences long-term functioning and health-related quality-of-life after severe traumatic brain injury. *Brain Injury, 28*(3), 328–335. https://doi.org/10.3109/02699052.2013.865274.

Visser, M. M., Heijenbrok-Kal, M. H., Van't Spijker, A., et al. (2016). Problem-solving therapy during outpatient stroke rehabilitation improves coping and health-related quality of life randomized controlled trial. *Stroke; a Journal of Cerebral Circulation, 47*(1), 135–142. https://doi.org/10.1161/STROKEAHA.115.010961.

Wagner, A. L., Keusch, F., Yan, T., et al. (2016). The impact of weather on summer and winter exercise behaviors. *Journal of Sport and Health Science, 8*(1), 39–45.

Wang, N., Yu, P., & Hailey, D. (2015). The quality of paper-based versus electronic nursing care plan in Australian aged care homes: A documentation audit study. *International Journal of Medical Informatics, 84*(8), 561–569. https://doi.org/10.1016/j.ijmedinf.2015.04.004.

Webb, J. B., Wood-Barcalow, N. L., & Tylka, T. L. (2015). Assessing positive body image: Contemporary approaches and future directions. *Body Image, 4*(6), 130–145. https://doi.org/10.1016/j.bodyim.2015.03.010.

Wilt, J., Bleidorn, W., & Revelle, W. (2016). Finding a life worth living: Meaning in life and graduation from college. *European Journal of Personality, 30*(2), 158–167. https://doi.org/10.1002/per.2046.

World Health Organization (WHO). (2016). *Global strategy on diet, physical activity, and health*. Retrieved from https://www.who.int/dietphysicalactivity/strategy/eb11344/strategy_english_web.pdf.

# 7

# Health Promotion and the Family

*Leslie Graham, RN, MN, PhD(c), CNCC, CHSE, CCSNE*

Originating US chapter by *Anne Rath Rentfro, RN, PhD*

## INTENDED LEARNING OUTCOMES

*After completing this chapter, the reader will be able to:*

- Describe three theoretical approaches to the study of families.
- Assess a family throughout the life span using the functional health pattern framework.
- Describe an example of the clinical data to collect in each health pattern during each family developmental phase.
- Provide two examples of behavioural changes (functional, potentially dysfunctional, and actually dysfunctional) within the health patterns of families.

- Describe developmental and cultural characteristics of the family to consider when identifying risk factors or etiological factors of potential or actual dysfunctional health patterns.
- Plan, implement, and evaluate two nursing interventions in health promotion with families.
- Evaluate a specific health-promotion plan based on family assessment, nursing diagnosis, and contributing risks or etiological factors.

## KEY TERMS

Developmental theory

Ecomap

Family

Family developmental tasks

Family function

Family health status

Family nursing interventions

Family pattern

Family resilience

Family risk factors

Family strengths

Family structure

Family theory

Genogram

Risk-factor theory

Systems theory

 **THINK ABOUT IT**

### *Caring for Older Persons*

Adult family members, who may have health problems of their own, find themselves caring for their older parents as well as grandchildren. Increased life expectancies combined with increased age at the birth of the first child present adults with the caring for older parents along with young children (Boyczuk & Fletcher, 2016). This population, known as the sandwich generation, is expected to become more prevalent in the coming years. An increasing number of parents of young adults provide financial support or provide care for grandchildren younger than 18 years, at the same time care for an older parent aged more than 65 years (Boyczuk & Fletcher, 2016).

- What are the implications of this growing situation for individuals? For families? For communities? For the nation?
- How will this trend affect individual lives personally and professionally?
- How does multigenerational caring affect family finances?

A family consists of a group of interacting individuals related by blood, marriage, cohabitation, or adoption who interdependently perform relevant functions by fulfilling expected roles. Relevant family functions include practices and values placed on health. Family health practices, whether effective or ineffective, encompass activities performed by individuals or families as a whole to promote health and prevent disease. How well families complete developmental tasks and how well families, including individuals within a family, generate health-promoting behaviours determine a family's potential for enhancement of family health practices.

How family members relate to one another influences their understanding of behaviour, which is demonstrated in the family's structural, functional, communication, and developmental patterns (Perry, Hockenberry, Lowdermilk, et al., 2013). Families provide the structure for many health-promotion practices;

## TABLE 7.1   Variety of Family Structures

| Configuration | Positions in Family |
|---|---|
| Single parent (separated, divorced, or widowed) | Mother or father, sons(s), daughter(s) |
| Unmarried single parent (never married) | Mother or father, sons(s), daughter(s) |
| Unmarried cohabitating couple | Two adults living together in a long-term relationship that resembles marriage |
| Unmarried parents | Two adults, sons(s), daughter(s) |
| Commune family | Mothers, fathers, adults, shared son(s), daughters(s) living together |
| Stepparents | Adults with son(s), daughter(s) from previous marriage |
| Adoptive family | Adults who provide a permanent home to son(s) and/or daughter(s) through a legal process |
| Family of choice | Adults with selected partners and family members |
| Married couple | Two cohabitating adults living in a recognized legal union |
| Same sex couple | Two persons of the same gender sharing an intimate, romantic, or sexual relationship |
| Married parents | Mother and father, son(s), daughter(s) |
| Nuclear family | Mother and father, son(s), daughter(s) |
| Gay, lesbian, transgender family | Adults and children living together with one or more members of the group who identifies as gay, lesbian, or transgender |
| Immigrant family | Adults and children living together with one or more members of the group who is an immigrant |
| Biracial or multiracial family | Mother, father, adults, or children include two or more races |
| Transracial family | Mother, father, adults, or children include at least one member who is born of one race and decides to represent themselves as another race |
| Blended family | Mother, father, adults, or children represent members from previous unions |
| Joint-custody family | Adults living with children who are legally awarded to both biological parents |
| Conditionally separate families | A family member is separated from the family but remains a significant member of the family (military service, incarceration, distant employment, hospitalization) |
| Extended family | Significant family members beyond the nuclear family that may include grandparents, aunts, uncles, and other adults who live nearby or in one household |
| Foster family | Adults, serving as provincial/territorial ministry-approved caregivers, for children placed into a ward, group home, or private home |
| Grandparent(s) | Grandchildren, son(s) and/or daughter(s)<br>Grandmother and/or grandfather |

Modified from Brown, S. L., Manning, W. D., & Payne, K. K. (2016). Family structure and children's economic well-being: Incorporating same-sex cohabiting mother families. *Population Research and Policy Review, 35*(1), 1–21; Government of Ontario. (1990). *Child & Family Services Act*. Retrieved from https://www.ontario.ca/laws/statute/90c11; Edwards, J. O. (2009). *The many kinds of family structures in our communities*. Retrieved from https://www.scoe.org/files/ccpc-family-structures.pdf.

therefore, family assessment informs health promotion and disease-prevention planning. Within families, children and adults are nurtured, provided for, and taught about health values by word and by example. Family members first learn to make choices to promote health within the family structure (Table 7.1). Appreciating how families make decisions and encouraging family participation in all aspects of care from acute care to health promotion helps families and individuals acquire new behaviours (Parkinson, Gallegos, & Russell-Bennett, 2016).

Families influence children's lifestyle choices. If the child is exposed to healthy living, then they are more likely to adopt healthy living practices (Stanhope, Lancaster, Jakubec, et al., 2017). Through family planning, parents assume the responsibility of caring for their children. Prenatal care and breastfeeding give infants a healthy start. Nutritious diets support physical growth and development. Children first observe and learn behaviours within their family. Patterns of nutrition, activity, oral hygiene, and coping develop at early ages, supported by the example of family members. Patterns of alcohol consumption and tobacco

use are similarly established within families. Learning about human development fosters a healthy self-concept, including positive awareness of the family member's sexuality. Promoting self-esteem and reinforcing positive behaviours also strengthen the health of children. Primary care providers support positive behaviours by offering family members evidence-informed health-promotion and disease prevention services, such as anticipatory guidance for developmental tasks, immunizations, screening for early detection, and appropriate counselling.

This chapter uses family theory, systems theory, developmental theory, and risk-factor theory to guide the nursing process with families. The 11 functional health patterns described in Chapter 6 establish the structure for interview questions during data collection. The analysis phase of the nursing process categorizes these data within stages of family development, and from the analysis, nursing diagnoses are formulated. *Family health* is a term that is used to refer to family functioning in terms of coping skills. Healthy families with effective coping strategies foster autonomy within the family unit, supporting each family member's needs and unique interests (Stanhope et al., 2017). The planning phase begins when family goals and objectives are stated. The family, the nurse, or another health professional facilitates implementation. Later in this chapter, four types of interventions for health promotion and disease prevention are discussed: increasing knowledge and skills; increasing strengths; decreasing exposure to risks; and decreasing susceptibility. Nurses assume various roles throughout the stages of family development, and these roles are also presented. Evaluation of a family plan considers outcomes that are specific, objective, and measurable and that rely on the family's subjective interpretation of concerns and probability of success, as well as that at the population level (Maurer & Smith, 2014).

## THE NURSING PROCESS AND THE FAMILY

The nursing process when promoting the health of families includes the family as a group and the interactions among family members. The US National Center on Parent, Family, and Community Engagement (NCPFCE) views the entire family as the participant that guides assessment from a holistic framework (NCPFCE, 2018). Partnerships with families begin with an assessment (NCPFCE, 2018). The home is a natural environment for health-promotion encounters, although the process may occur in other settings as well. Different age groups (infants, children, and older persons) are likely to be present in the home. Nurses observe physical surroundings first hand during home visits. For example, household safety hazards are observed directly. Nurses also monitor family unit rituals, roles, and interpersonal interactions. Generally, the nurse contacts the family and establishes an appointment time for visiting the family. Including each family member in the visit provides a broad perspective. During visits, the nursing process develops mutually with families; it is not a treatment done for the family. Families collaborate with nursing in all phases of the process. Guidelines for home visits are presented in Box 7.1.

Comprehensive family assessment provides the foundation to promote family health (NCPFCE, 2018). Several factors influence family assessment, such as nurses' perceptions about family constitution; theoretical knowledge; norms; standards; and communication abilities during visits. In addition to factors that pertain to the nurse, familial factors also influence assessments, such as family cooperation, mutual agreement to work toward goals, and family ability to recognize the relevance of health-promotion plans. Useful health-promotion family assessments involve listening to families, engaging in participatory dialogue, recognizing patterns, and assessing family potential for active, positive change (NCPFCE, 2018).

The assessment phase of the nursing process seeks and identifies information from the family about health-promotion and disease-prevention activities. To obtain this information, nurses follow family progress through developmental tasks and identify strengths in the family's ability to generate behaviours associated with disease prevention. The approaches considered in this chapter include the developmental framework, strength-based assessment, and the risk-factor estimate. Developmental phases for families as proposed by Duvall and Miller (Duvall, 1988; Duvall & Miller, 1985), strength-based assessment using a standardized tool (e.g., Calgary Family Assessment Model [CFAM]) proposed by

### BOX 7.1  Guidelines for Home Visits to Promote Health and Prevent Disease

**Planning the Visit**
- Make arrangements for a convenient time at which the greatest number of family members can attend the meeting.
- Study information regarding the family from agency records, referral forms, and other sources.
- Contact the family to make initial introductions and to state the purpose of the visit.
- Obtain appropriate supplies and teaching aids for visits.
- Maintain safety of the nurse by visiting in pairs and by having a cell phone close by.

**Making the Visit**
- Offer an introduction and explain the purpose of the visit.
- Establish trust through respectful interactions.
- Identify the family's request for assistance.
- Include all family members in the discussion. Understand the situation from the family's perspective.
- Identify appropriate activities for health promotion and disease prevention.
- Make a contract with the family that states specific goals and objectives that the family wants to reach.
- Think about safety before and during the visit.
- Identify and respond to health and home safety issues.
- Terminate the visit with specific instructions and information about the next visit: when it will occur, what will happen, who will be present, and what the family must accomplish before then.
- Carry through promptly on agreements made.
- Document the home visit according to employer requirements and regulatory standards.

Source: College of Nurses of Ontario (CNO). (2018). *Therapeutic nurse–client relationship,* Revised 2006. Retrieved from http://www.cno.org/globalassets/docs/prac/41033_therapeutic.pdf.

Shajani and Snell (2019), and risk-factor appraisal (Stanhope et al., 2017) can be used to guide nurses through the steps of the nursing process when they are working with families. Fig. 7.1 is a diagram that outlines the categories and subcategories of the CFAM.

### The Nurse's Role

Nurses collaborate with families using a systems perspective to understand family interaction, family norms, family expectations, effectiveness of family communication, family decision making, and family coping mechanisms. The nurse's role in health promotion and disease prevention includes the following tasks:
- Become aware of family attitudes and behaviours toward health promotion and disease prevention.
- Act as a role model for the family.
- Collaborate with the family to assess, improve, enhance, and evaluate family health practices.
- Assist the family in growth and development behaviours.
- Assist the family in identifying risk-taking behaviours.
- Assist the family in decision making about lifestyle choices.
- Provide reinforcement for positive health-behaviour practices.
- Provide health information to the family.
- Assist the family in learning behaviours to promote health and prevent disease.
- Assist the family in problem solving and decision making about health promotion.

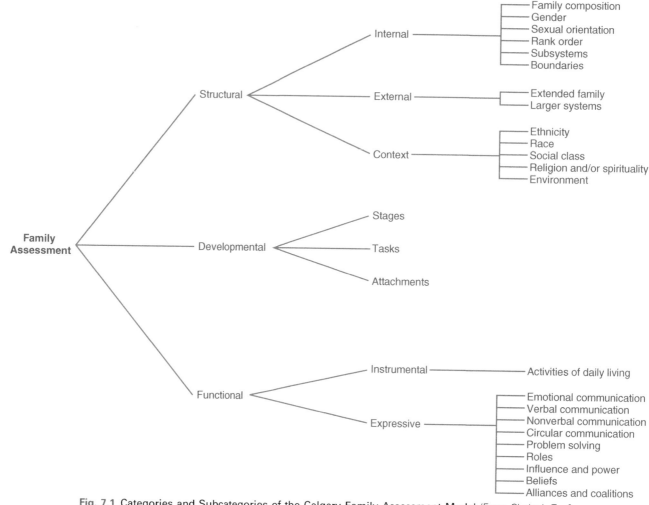

**Fig. 7.1** Categories and Subcategories of the Calgary Family Assessment Model (From Shajani, Z., & Snell, D. [2019]. *Wright and Leahey's nurses and families: A guide to family assessment and intervention,* 7e. F. A. Davis Company, Philadelphia, PA; with permission.)

- Serve as a liaison for referral or collaboration between community resources and the family.

Nurses use family theoretical frameworks to guide, observe, and classify situations. Nursing roles for families in various stages of development are presented in Table 7.2.

## FAMILY THEORIES AND FRAMEWORKS

Family theory stems from a variety of interrelated disciplines (Atkin, Corder, Goodyear, et al., 2015). Family systems theory explains patterns of living among the individuals who comprise family systems. In systems theory, behaviours and family members' responses influence patterns. Meanings and values provide the vital elements of motivation and energy for family systems. Every family has its unique culture, value structure, and history. Values provide a means for interpreting events and information, passing from one generation to the next. Values usually change slowly over time. Families process information and energy exchange with the environment through values. For example, holiday food traditions may be changed slightly by a daughter-in-law, whose own

daughter may then adjust the traditional recipe within her own nuclear family.

System boundaries separate family systems from their environment and control information flow. This characteristic forms a family internal manager that influences and defines interactions and relationships with one another and with those outside the family system. The family forms a unified whole rather than the sum of its parts—an integrated system of interdependent functions, structures, and relationships. For example, one drug-dependent individual's health behaviour influences the entire family unit.

Living systems are open systems. As living systems, families experience constant exchanges of energy and information with the environment. Change in one part or member of the family results in changes in the family as a whole. For example, loss of a family member through death changes roles and relationships among all family members. Change requires adaptation of every family member as roles and functions assume new meanings. Changes families make are incorporated into the system.

When the system is the family, issues can be clarified by family processes, communication interaction among family members, and family group values. In Bowen's family systems

**TABLE 7.2   Possible Nurse's Roles in Health Promotion and Disease Prevention Through Stages of Family Development**

| Stage | Possible Nursing Role |
|---|---|
| Couple | Counsellor on sexual and role adjustment<br>Teacher of and counsellor on family planning<br>Teacher of parenting skills<br>Coordinator for genetic counselling<br>Facilitator in interpersonal relationships |
| Childbearing family | Monitor of prenatal care and referrer for problems of pregnancy<br>Counsellor on prenatal nutrition<br>Counsellor on prenatal maternal habits<br>Emotional support for amniocentesis<br>Counsellor on breastfeeding<br>Coordinator with pediatric services<br>Supervisor of immunizations<br>Referrer to social services<br>Assistant in adjustment to prenatal role |
| Family with preschool or school-age children | Monitor of early childhood development; referrer when indicated<br>Teacher of first-aid and emergency measures<br>Coordinator with pediatric services<br>Counsellor on nutrition and exercise<br>Teacher of dental hygiene<br>Counsellor on environmental safety in home |
| Family with adolescents | Facilitator in interpersonal relationships<br>Teacher of risk factors to health<br>Teacher of problem-solving issues regarding alcohol, smoking, diet, and exercise<br>Facilitator of interpersonal skills with adolescents and parents<br>Direct supporter of, counsellor on, or referrer to mental health resources<br>Counsellor on family planning<br>Referral for sexually transmittable infection |
| Family with young or middle-aged adults | Participant in community organizations involved in disease control<br>Teacher of problem-solving issues regarding lifestyle and habits<br>Participant in community organization involved in environmental control<br>Case finder in home and community<br>Screener for hypertension, Pap test, breast examination, mental health, and dental care<br>Counsellor on menopausal transition |
| Family with older persons | Facilitator of interpersonal relationships among family members<br>Referral for work and social activity, nutritional programs, homemakers' services, and nursing home<br>Monitor of exercise, nutrition, preventive services, and medications<br>Supervisor of immunization<br>Counsellor on safety in home<br>Counsellor on bereavement |

Modified from Australian College of Nursing. (2015). *Community & primary health care nursing position statement*. Retrieved from https://www.acn.edu.au/wp-content/uploads/position-statement-community-primary-health-care-nursing.pdf.

theory, birth order is considered an important determinant of behaviour. In addition, family patterns of behaviour differentiate one family from another (Stanhope et al., 2017; Vedanthan, Bansilal, Soto, et al., 2016). When an individual family member expresses behaviours that differ from the learned family pattern, differentiation of self occurs. Interaction among family members and the transmission of these interaction patterns from one generation to the next provide the framework for the family systems approach (Rothenberg, Hussong, & Chassin, 2016).

The framework for health promotion introduced by Murdaugh, Parsons, and Pender (2019) recognizes the family as the unit of assessment and intervention because families develop self-care and dependent-care competencies; foster resilience among family members; provide resources; and promote healthy individuation within cohesive family structures. Furthermore, because the family often provides the structure for implementation of health promotion, family assessment becomes an integral tool to foster health and healthy behaviours (Murdaugh et al., 2019).

## THE FAMILY FROM A DEVELOPMENTAL PERSPECTIVE

Building on Erikson's (1998) theory of psychosocial development, Duvall and Miller (1985) identified stages of the family life cycle and critical family developmental tasks. Although Duvall's classification has been criticized for its middle class

## BOX 7.2 Characteristics and Indicators of Healthy Families

**Nurturing RELATIONSHIPS**
- Maintains trust traditions and shares quality time.
- Communications are open and members listen to each other.
- Respectful of individuality.

**Establishing ROUTINES**
- Maintains routines that promote health patterns of nutrition, hygiene, rest, physical activity, and sexuality.
- Maintains routines to promote safety and injury prevention; health protection; disease prevention; smoking and alcohol or substance abuse, and/or violence.
- Establishes patterns to promote mental health: interacting, communicating, and expressing affection, aggression, sexuality, and similar interactions.

**Maintaining EXPECTATIONS**
- Maintains morale and motivation, rewarding achievement, meeting personal and family crises, setting attainable goals, and developing family traditions, loyalties, and values.

**ADAPTING to challenges**
- Evolves during crises and respects each member of the group.
- Promotes strategies to make decisions about health and illness.
- Shares power appropriately among family members.
- Is receptive to outside assistance/interventions when necessary.

**Connecting to COMMUNITY**
- Family table time and conversation occur regularly.
- Members act as interactive caregivers across the life span to socialize children and adolescents, to participate in the community, and to support members as they age.

Sources: Modified from Search Institute. (2016). *Family strengths.* Retrieved from Stanhope, M., Lancaster, J., Jakubec, S., & Pike-MacDonald, S., et al. (2017). *Community health nursing in Canada* (3rd ed.). Toronto: Elsevier Canada.

homogeneity and lack of diversity in family forms, this conceptual model helps to anticipate family events and has formed the basis for more contemporary developmental models (Duvall & Miller, 1985). Knowing a family's composition, interrelationships, and particular life cycle helps nurses predict the overall family pattern. Box 7.2 lists characteristics of healthy families. From Duvall's perspective, most families complete these basic family tasks. Each family performs these tasks in a unique expression of its personality. Progression through the stages occurs in a linear fashion; however, regression may occur and families may experience tasks in more than one stage at a time (Duvall & Miller, 1985). Specific tasks arise as growth responsibilities during family development. Failure to accomplish a developmental task leads to negative consequences. For example, intimate partner violence or child abuse or neglect may result in intervention by police, welfare, the Children's Aid Society, health department, or other agencies. Life-cycle tasks build upon one another. Success at one stage is dependent on success at an earlier stage. Early failure may lead to developmental difficulties at later stages.

As families enter each new developmental stage, transition occurs. Families move through new stages as a result of events ranging from marriage (heterosexual, same-sex), gay and lesbian relationships, childbirth, lone-parent families, joint custody, or remarried families; to adolescents maturing into young adults and leaving the home; to the aging years.

Each new developmental stage requires adaptation with new responsibilities. Concurrently, developmental stages provide opportunities for families to realize their potential. Nurses anticipate change through analysis of progress through each stage. Each new stage presents opportunities for health promotion and intervention. Family developmental stages, although reflective of traditional nuclear families and extended family networks, also apply to nontraditional family configurations (Coyne, Grafton, & Reid, 2017; Stanhope et al., 2017). A family systems approach addresses the interaction of these multiple family configurations. For example, couples may marry and bring children from a previous marriage to a blended family that works toward achieving developmental tasks of couples along with family stages for the children. Both the couple and their children possess values and beliefs from the past that must integrate within the present union. Childless couples present developmental tasks that are different from those proposed for couples with children. One family conceptual model proposed by Vedanthan and colleagues (2016) illustrates the multiple connections of interdependence among family systems, shared environment, parenting style, caregiver perceptions, and genomics to promote cardiovascular health.

Nurses collect data to determine progress toward family developmental task attainment during the family assessment. Use of assessment tools include gathering factors that strengthen and protect the family such as the Canadian Family Assessment Tool, Friedman Family Assessment Model, and the McGill Model of Nursing and provide more robust information (Harper Browne, 2014; Stanhope et al., 2017). These newer assessment tools focus on the assessment of family assets and social network resources that families currently use. These kinds of assessments intend to build on strengths at particular developmental stages to promote healthy family environments. Assessment of family developmental stages entails use of guidelines to analyze progress toward developmental tasks, family growth, and health-promotion needs.

## THE FAMILY FROM A STRUCTURAL–FUNCTIONAL PERSPECTIVE

Families consist of both structural and functional components. Family structure refers to family composition, including roles and relationships, whereas family function consists of processes within systems as information and energy exchange occurs between families and their environment.

## THE FAMILY FROM A RISK-FACTOR PERSPECTIVE

Family risk factors can be inferred from lifestyle; biological factors; environmental factors; social, psychological, cultural, and spiritual dimensions; and the health care system. As outlined in the Antonio case study in Chapter 1, lifestyle habits such as overeating, drug dependency, high sugar and cholesterol intake, and smoking influence health outcomes. Biological risk factors may include the elements of genetic inheritance, congenital malformation, and intellectual disability. To fully explore environmental risk factors that influence family function, nurses explore work pressures, peer pressure, stress, anxieties, tensions, and air, noise, or water pollution. Social and psychological dimensions such as crowded living conditions, isolation, or rapid and accelerated rates of change are areas to consider when nurses are assessing family risk factors. Cultural and spiritual aspects may include traditions of preventing illness such as daily prayer and meditation practices. Other family traditions, such as inclusion of complementary therapies, or rituals such as female genital mutilation, need to be explored (Simpson, Robinson, Creighton, et al., 2012). Finally, health care system factors such as overuse, underuse, inappropriate use, or accessibility are considered in the family risk assessment.

To reduce risk factors, nurses help families focus on influencing health behaviours of their members. Society glamorizes many hazardous behaviours through advertising and mass media promotions that minimize negative health consequences. Families influence their members to weigh the consequences of risk-taking behaviour. Awareness of risk factors may prompt families to reduce modifiable risk factors. Healthy behaviour, including use of preventive health care services, is a significant area of family responsibility.

Traditionally, epidemiology has used levels and trends of mortality and morbidity rates as indirect evidence of health. Data such as infant mortality rates, stillbirth rates, and leading causes of death have long been used as indicators of collective community health. Healthy family functioning links the family life-cycle stages with specific risk factors. Epidemiology often describes a disease association in terms of risk. Health risks can be physiological or psychological. Physiological risks arise from genetic background, whereas psychological risks include those related to low self-image. Risks also arise from environmental considerations, including the physical environment and socioeconomic condition (Gray, 2018). Risk-factor theory considers families a pivotal part of the environment and also an important support system used to decrease health risks for individuals. As young family members mature developmentally and seek more independence from the family, peers may influence risk to compete with family values.

Risk estimates calculate differences between two groups: one with the risk factor and one without it. The frequency of deaths, illnesses, or injuries with some specific risk factor compared with those for another group without the risk factor, or the population as a whole, determines the risk estimate. Some diseases (e.g., sickle cell anemia in Black-Canadian families and Tay–Sachs disease in families of Ashkenazi Jewish descent) occur more frequently in certain families and can be identified by carrier screening (Azimi, Schmaus, Greger, et al., 2016). Other recessive genetic disorders (e.g., cystic fibrosis and Gaucher's disease) have decreased in incidence with prenatal carrier screening with genetic counselling in couples with suspect family histories (Azimi et al., 2016). Azimi and colleagues (2016) compared current strategies that target specific high-risk families to next-generation DNA sequencing (NGS) that provides high-level sensitivity and specificity for carrier screening. They developed a mathematical model to screen individuals for 14 recessive disorders commonly recommended for screening in targeted populations. The mathematical model provides support to transition from traditional lower-accuracy genotyping to more accurate NGS techniques focused on the most prevalent disorders (Azimi et al., 2016). Other diseases such as iron-deficiency anemia may not be attributed to a specific genetic background. The natural history of a chronic disease predisposes family members to greater risk, but specific causes may be difficult to identify. Well siblings, particularly adolescents, may be affected. Kramer-Kile, Osuji, Larsen, et al. (2014) describe the phases that individuals and families may experience as they progress through chronic illness adaptation from the time before the disorder is recognized through a stable adjustment phase to the final relinquishment of life interest and activities.

The probabilities of risk to the family's health may also change depending on the family's activities in health promotion and disease prevention. Risk to the family's health focuses on three main areas: (1) biological and age-related risks, (2) environmental risks, and (3) behavioural risks (Stanhope et al., 2017). Stages of family development are also used to classify risk factors. Age-specific developmental stages, along with their associated age-specific health risks, are given in Table 7.3, which displays periods during which families become most sensitive to certain problems, with corresponding key times for health promotion and disease prevention. The risk behaviours highlighted include tobacco and alcohol use, inadequate nutrition, overuse of medications, unsafe driving habits, stress, and relentless pressure to achieve. Habits learned in family settings help to develop individual lifestyle behaviours. Overlying risk assessment of the family is a broad understanding of the context in which the family is situated. Structural inequalities such as poverty, food insecurity, unemployment, and isolation (geographic or social) must be considered (Stanhope et al., 2017).

## ❖ GORDON'S FUNCTIONAL HEALTH PATTERNS: ASSESSMENT OF THE FAMILY

Gordon's (2016) 11 functional health patterns help organize basic family assessment information. Patterns form the standardized format for family assessment using a systems approach with emphasis on developmental stages and risk factors. Assessment includes evaluation of dysfunctional patterns within families, with corresponding details in one or more of the other interdependent patterns (see Chapter 6).

The presence of risk factors predicts potential dysfunction. Developmental risk and risk arising from dysfunctional health patterns increase whole family risk (see Table 7.3). Gordon (2016) interprets risk states as potential problems. To formulate clinical judgement for real or potential health challenges, nurses identify problems along with their associated and etiological factors. Influencing factors may precede or occur concurrently

## TABLE 7.3    Family Stage: Specific Risk Factors and Related Health Problems

| Stage | Risk Factors | Health Problems |
|---|---|---|
| Beginning childbearing | Lack of knowledge of family planning<br>Adolescent marriage<br>Lack of knowledge concerning sexual and marital roles and adjustments<br>Low-birth-weight infant<br>Lack of prenatal care<br>First pregnancy before age 16 years or after age 35 years<br>History of hypertension and infections during pregnancy<br>Rubella, syphilis, gonorrhea, and acquired immunodeficiency syndrome (AIDS)<br>Genetic factors<br>Lack of safety in home | Premature baby in family<br>Birth defects<br>Birth injuries<br>Unintentional injury and accidents<br>Sudden infant death syndrome (SIDS)<br>Sterility<br>Pelvic inflammatory disease<br>Fetal alcohol syndrome<br>Intellectual disability<br>Injuries<br>Birth defects<br>Underweight |
| Family with school-age children | Generational pattern of using social agencies as way of life<br>Multiple, closely spaced children<br>Low family self-esteem<br>Children harmed as result of parental frustration<br>Repeated infections, accidents, or hospitalizations<br>Parents immature, dependent, and unable to handle responsibility<br>Unrecognized or unattended health problems<br>Strong beliefs about physical punishment<br>Toxic substances unguarded in the home | Behaviour disturbances<br>Speech and vision problems<br>Communicable diseases<br>Dental caries<br>School problems<br>Learning disabilities<br>Injuries<br>Chronic diseases<br>Homicide<br>Violence |
| Family with adolescents | Health inequities<br>Lifestyle and behaviour patterns leading to chronic disease<br>Lack of problem-solving skills<br>Family values of aggressiveness, competition, rigidity, and inflexibility<br>Risk-taking behaviours<br>Conflicts between parents and children<br>Pressure to live up to family expectations | Violent deaths<br>Unwanted pregnancies<br>Sexually transmitted infections (STIs)<br>Gang-related activities<br>Bullying behaviours<br>Substance abuse |
| Family with middle-aged adults | Hypertension<br>Smoking<br>High cholesterol levels<br>Genetic predisposition<br>Use of oral contraceptives<br>Menopause<br>Cancer | Cardiovascular disease, principally coronary artery disease and cerebrovascular accident (stroke)<br>Diabetes<br>Unintentional injuries and accidents<br>Homicide<br>Birth defects<br>Mental illness<br>Periodontal disease and loss of teeth<br>Substance abuse<br>Hormone replacement therapy<br>Breast cancer<br>Prostate cancer<br>Lung cancer<br>Colorectal cancer |
| Family with older persons | Age<br>Medication interactions<br>Metabolic disorders<br>Pituitary malfunctions<br>Cushing's syndrome<br>Hypercalcemia<br>Chronic illness<br>Retirement<br>Loss of spouse<br>Past environments and lifestyle | Mental confusion<br>Reduced vision<br>Hearing impairment<br>Hypertension<br>Acute illness<br>Infectious disease<br>Influenza<br>Pneumonia<br>Injuries such as burns and falls<br>Death without dignity<br>Osteoporosis |

Sources: Canadian Nurses Association (CNA). (2005). *The built environment, injury prevention, and nursing.* Retrieved from https://cna-aiic.ca/-/media/cna/page-content/pdf-en/bg1_built_environment_e.pdf?la=en&hash=F6F5222F75BF847B79441C507A8447B5FBA5R79C; Public Health Agency of Canada (PHAC). (2017). *The Chief Public Health Officer's report on the state of public health in Canada 2017.* Retrieved from https://www.canada.ca/content/dam/phac-aspc/documents/services/publications/chief-public-health-officer-reports-state-public-health-canada/2017-designing-healthy-living/PHAC_CPHO-2017_Report_E.pdf; Stanhope, M., Lancaster, J., Jakubec, S., et al. (2017). *Community health nursing in Canada* (3rd ed.). Toronto: Elsevier Canada.

with the problem and are used to plan care. Interventions aim to modify influencing factors to promote positive change.

Family history begins with the health perception–health management pattern. Exploring issues within this pattern first provides an overview to help locate where problems exist in other patterns and to determine which problems require more thorough assessment. Interviewing from the family's perspective helps families define situations. The roles-relationships pattern defines family structure and function. The remaining nine patterns address lifestyle indicators.

## ◆ Health Perception–Health Management Pattern

Characteristics of family health perceptions, health management, and preventive practices emerge with assessment of the health perception–health management pattern. The Canadian Health Survey on Children and Youth is currently being conducted (Statistics Canada, 2019) to contribute additional information to help identify health-promoting behaviours of families. Data collected in the Health Survey on Children and Youth include information about health practices such as food and sleep behaviours, use of electronic devices, physical activity, and social practices. The intent of the survey is to provide information on a broad range of child and family health measures such as emotional and mental health, access to health care, family activities, neighbourhood safety, and support. This supports the development of evidence-informed programs and policies to improve the well-being of children and youth living in Canada (Statistics Canada, 2019). These assessment indicators also provide data to guide the remaining functional health pattern assessment. Patterns overlap, and findings in one pattern may encourage further assessment in another pattern. The following are some research questions that concern family health promotion:

- What are the chief concerns of parents and other adults in the household about their children's development, learning, and behaviour?
- How do children's health status and the health practices (physical activity and smoking behaviour) of the adults compare?
- What health-related behaviours, such as eating three meals a day at regular times, eating breakfast every day, exercising for a minimum of 2 or 3 days a week, sleeping for 7 to 8 hours each night, and abstaining from smoking, are practiced by the family?
- How safe are homes, schools, and neighbourhoods from the perspective of the family?
- What are the emerging trends for health challenges facing the family: for example, vaping?

Health practices differ from family to family. Families identify and perform health-maintenance activities based on their beliefs about health. Exploration during the assessment also includes the following areas:

- What is the family's philosophy of health? Does each family member hold similar beliefs? Do family members practice what they believe?
- In what negative behaviours or lifestyle practices, such as smoking, alcohol, and drug abuse, does the family engage?
- What chronic disease risk behaviours are exhibited within the family?

- Are risk factors present for infections, such as lack of immunization, lack of knowledge of transmittable diseases, and poor personal hygiene?
- Are risk factors for bodily injury, accidents, or substance abuse present in the home?
- Do older persons know what medications they are taking and the reasons for their using them?
- Does the family discard outdated medications or those not used?
- What unattended health problems exist?
- Is there a history of repeated infections and hospitalization?
- Is the home understimulating or overstimulating?
- Where does the family obtain health and illness care?
- Is the family engaged in a dental program?
- How does the family describe previous experiences with nurses and other health care providers?

## ◆ Nutritional-Metabolic Pattern

The nutritional-metabolic pattern depicts characteristics of the family's typical food and fluid consumption and metabolism (Gordon, 2016). Included in it are growth and development patterns, pregnancy-related nutritional patterns, and the family's eating patterns. Risk factors for obesity, diabetes, anorexia, and bulimia are identified.

Dietary habits, learned within the family context, involve behavioural patterns central to daily life. Keeping a diary of intake for a week is a useful strategy for assessing family food and fluid intake patterns. Assessment notes both meals shared with the whole family as well as additional consumption by individuals. Recent research provides evidence that family meal sharing is associated with healthier eating habits. For example, Utter, Denny, Robinson, and colleagues (2013) report that family meal sharing in their sample of New Zealand adolescents ($n = 9101$) was positively associated with higher well-being scores, lower depression scores, and fewer risk-taking behaviours. In a follow-up report of this same population, Utter, Denny, Denny, and colleagues (2016) found the same positive associations with better nutritional indicators (fruit and vegetable intake), better mental health indicators (fewer depressive symptoms), and stronger family connections in adolescents who knew how to prepare food compared with those adolescents without the cooking abilities. However, the adolescents with cooking ability were more likely to have higher body mass index (BMI).

Exploration during nutrition pattern assessment includes the following areas:

- What kinds of foods are typically consumed?
- Who eats together at mealtimes?
- How is food viewed (reward/punishment)?
- Is there adequate storage and refrigeration?
- How is food purchased?
- How is food prepared?
- Who prepares food?

## ◆ Elimination Pattern

The elimination pattern describes characteristics of regularity and control of the family's excretory functions (Gordon, 2016). Bowel and bladder function and environmental factors such as

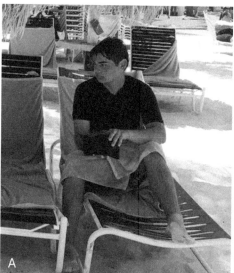
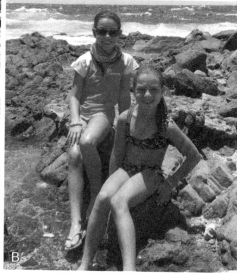

**Fig. 7.2** Family outings can be (A) leisurely and restful, or (B) adventurous and exciting.

waste disposal in the home, neighbourhood, and community that influence family life are considered in this pattern.

Questions are phrased according to the age-specific developmental stage of the family. For example, when the nurse is attempting to determine whether there is a problem in the preschool stage, it would be appropriate to ask whether the child is being toilet trained. In families with adolescents, the nurse may ask how often individuals have bowel movements and whether there have been any changes from usual patterns. The nurse may ask older person members whether they have any problems with constipation. Issues that particularly concern older people include constipation, diarrhea, polyuria, and incontinence, as well as use of antacids and constipation-relieving medications and strategies. The nurse evaluates whether use of these strategies is appropriate or possibly contributing to poor health.

### ◆ Activity-Exer cise Pattern

The activity-exercise pattern represents family characteristics that require energy expenditure (Gordon, 2016). The nurse reviews daily activities, exercise, and leisure activities. Families create settings for individual members to be physically active, sedentary, or apathetic toward physical activity. The quantity of sedentary activities such as television and video game screen time is explored.

Exploration during assessment of this pattern includes the following areas:

- How does the family exhibit its beliefs about regular exercise and physical fitness being necessary for good health?
- What types of daily activities include physical exercise and who does what with whom?
- What are the television viewing habits of children?
- How are other screen-viewing activities (computers, video games) incorporated into the daily routines?
- How often do children exercise?
- How are these activity and exercise factors related to children's health?
- What does the family do to have fun (Fig. 7.2)?

### ◆ Sleep-Rest Pattern

Rest habits characterize the sleep-rest pattern (Gordon, 2016). Without the restorative function of sleep, individuals exhibit decreased performance, irritability, and decreased tolerance for stress, and may rely on alcohol or other chemicals to induce sleep. Regular, sufficient sleep patterns are linked to better mental status, including learning and decision making. Most families have sleeping patterns, although in some families these patterns may not be readily apparent. It is important to elicit the data about sleep and rest from the family's perspective.

Assessment of the sleep-rest pattern includes the following:

- What are the usual sleeping habits of the family?
- How suitable are they to the age and health status of the family members?
- What are the usual hours established for sleeping?
- Who decides when and how children go to sleep?
- Do family members take naps or have other regular means of resting or relaxing?
- How early does the family rise? What are the patterns related to bedtime and rising?
- Do all family members have the same general sleep-rest pattern?
- Is there a family member with sleep disruption?
- What are the sleeping arrangements?

### ◆ Cognitive-Perceptual Pattern

The cognitive-perceptual pattern identifies characteristics of language, cognitive skills, and perception that influence desired or required family activities (Gordon, 2016). Specifically, this pattern concerns how families access information to make decisions, how concrete or abstract the thought processes are, and whether the decisions focus on present or future issues. Decision making in families is associated with power in family functioning. Highly educated families usually have greater repertoires for problem solving. Power and ability to solve problems are linked to leadership; family leaders must be acknowledged if nursing interventions are to be implemented.

Cognitive-perceptual pattern assessment includes the following:

- How does the family access and interpret information, especially about health (e.g., newspaper, books, computer, television, or radio)?
- What are the usual family reading patterns and strategies used for ongoing learning (e.g., continuing education programs)?
- What kinds of materials does the family read to the children?
- How does the family usually make decisions about health promotion and disease prevention?
- How do family members contribute to the decision-making process?
- How knowledgeable is the family about risk factors and developmental milestones?
- How are choices made regarding lifestyle?
- How knowledgeable are family members about correct information?
- How do family members acquire information?
- How accurate are the information sources used to make health-promotion choices?
- How do family members describe whether their health behaviour is constructive or destructive?
- How do family members recognize signs and symptoms of deteriorating health?
- How do family members decide when medical attention is necessary?
- Who makes the decisions about when to seek health care?
- What factors contribute to delays from the time of onset to the time of treatment?
- How long do families wait before seeking care?
- What are some of the cues that signal to families that care is needed?
- How is professional care accessed?
- What type of health care is generally used (health maintenance for immunizations well-child care or emergency/urgent care facilities)?
- How are decisions made about the use of over-the-counter medications or the use of alternative or traditional health practices?

## ◆ Self-Perception–Self-Concept Pattern

The self-perception–self-concept pattern identifies characteristics that describe the family's self-worth and feeling states (Gordon, 2016). Rapport between the family members and the nurse facilitates disclosure. Families have perceptions and concepts about their image, their status in the community, and their competencies as a family unit. Families manifest these perceptions through shared aspirations, values, expectations, fears, successes, and failures. Relationships in families determine the amount of sharing that occurs. Situations affecting one member influence perceptions of the entire family group. How each member describes the family often gives clues to the family self-concept.

Exploration during assessment includes the following:

- How is this family similar to or different from other families?
- How does this family perceive itself to be similar to and different from other families?

- What special assets does each member contribute to the family?
- What changes would each member like to see occur in the family?
- What kinds of feelings do family members have for each other?
- Describe the general tone of feelings in the family. Is the tone indifferent, secretive, angry, or open?
- How does the family think it assimilates into the neighbourhood and community?
- How does the family handle stress and crisis situations?
- How does the family experience changes in the way it feels about itself?
- How does the family describe the events that led to a change?

## ◆ Roles-Relationships Pattern

The roles-relationships pattern identifies characteristics of family roles and relationships (Gordon, 2016). Both structural and functional aspects of the family are assessed. Structural aspects of families include each member's name, age, sex, education, occupation, and role in the family. Traditionally, families have been described as nuclear and extended. The traditional nuclear family consists of husband, wife, and children, with an extended family that would include aunts, uncles, cousins, and grandparents. Today there are many varieties of nuclear and extended families. Stanhope et al. (2017) describes various contemporary family structures: traditional nuclear family, extended families, lone-parent families, stepfamilies, cohabiting families, gay and lesbian families, grandparent-headed families, foster families, and living-apart-together families. Traditional nuclear family structure has been influenced by societal changes, such as the women's movement, employment of mothers, divorce, and remarriage. Exploration of family origin and genetic heritage completes family identification data collection. Cultural practices in the home may or may not reflect the family's genetic heritage; therefore, it is important to explore the diversity of cultural and ethnic practices during the family assessment (Andrews & Boyle, 2015).

The American Academy of Pediatrics regards the family as the most enduring link to health for children. For example, findings from the Early Childhood Longitudinal Study, Birth Cohort ($n = 5000$), maternal health behaviours at each phase of early development (9 months, 2 years, 4 years, 5 years) indicated the importance of the mother–child relationship in health promotion (Prickett & Augustine, 2016). Statistics Canada (2016) released a consensus report stating that just over one-third of young adults still live with their parents. This phenomenon has consistently increased since 2001, citing economic and cultural norms as the reason.

Schoon, Jones, Cheng, and colleagues (2012) suggest that children in the United Kingdom experiencing poverty for the first 5 years of life are at higher risk of impaired cognitive development than those who do not experience poverty. These data indicate the need to identify family structure for poverty-related factors to determine those families at risk and effectively intervene (see Figs. 7.2 through 7.4). Family structure and function influence family stability and pose a challenge to the nurse in health promotion and disease prevention.

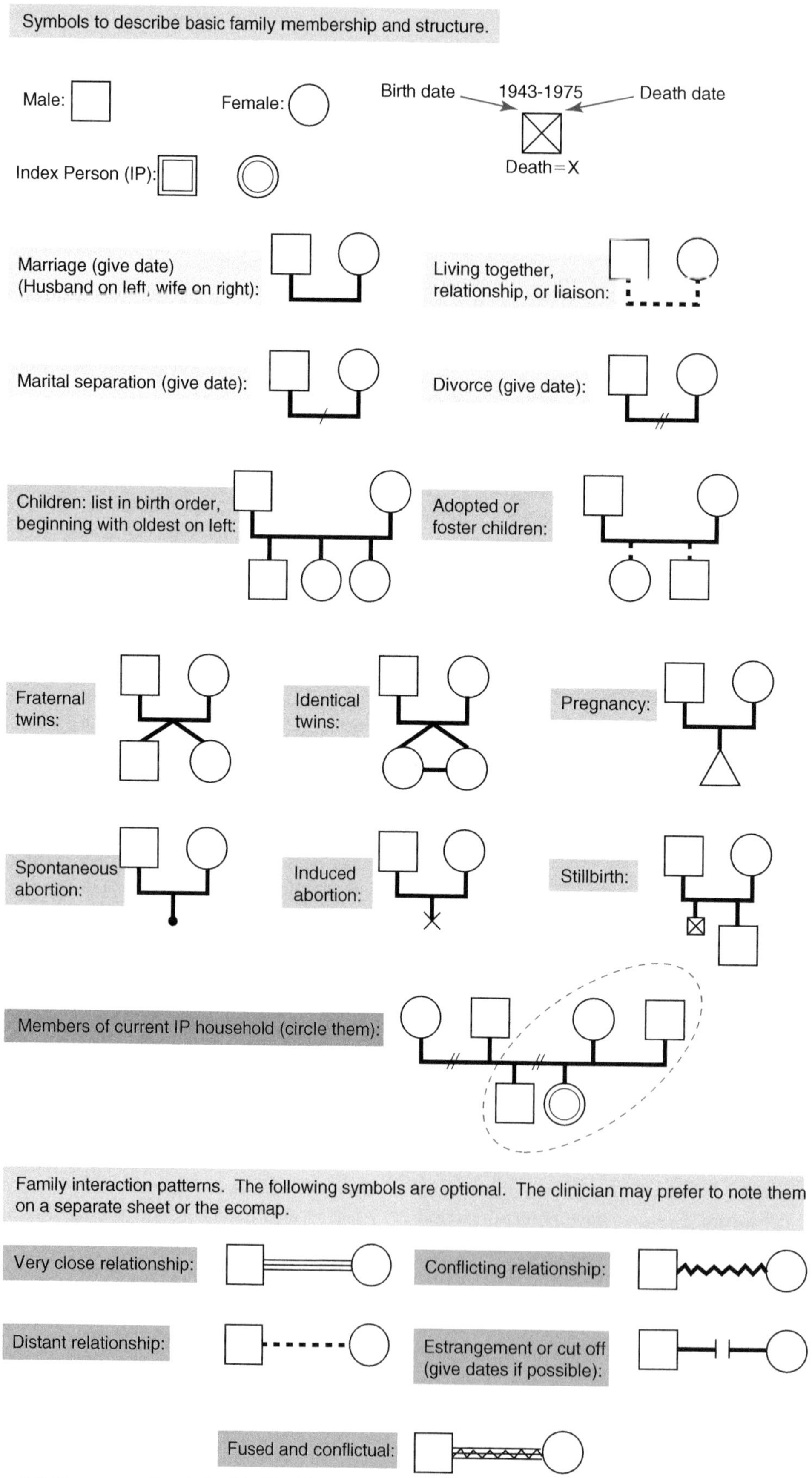

**Fig. 7.3 Genogram Symbols** (Modified from McGoldrick, M., Gerson, R., & Petry, S. [2008]. *Genograms: Assessment and intervention* [3rd ed.]. New York: Norton.)

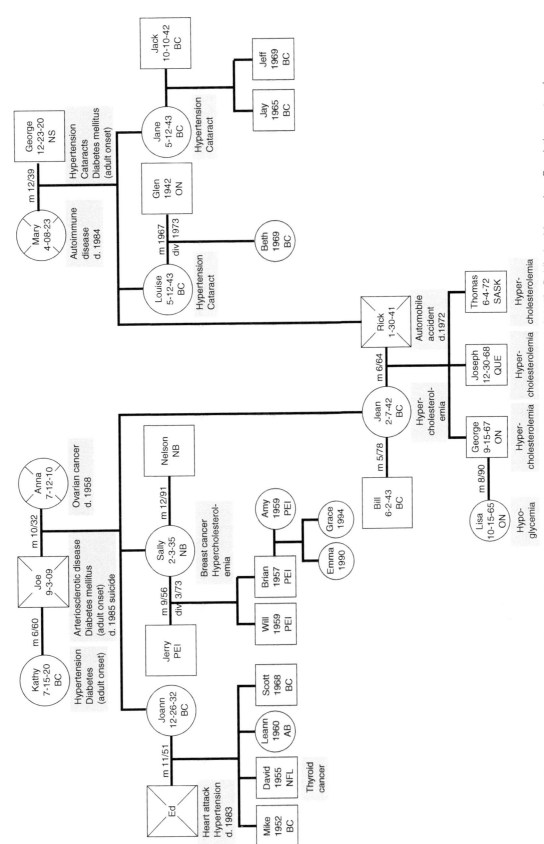

**Fig. 7.4  Genogram of the Graham Family** (Modified From Stanhope, M., & Lancaster, J. [2015]. *Public health nursing: Population-centered health care in the community* [9th ed., p. 632]. St. Louis: Mosby.)

Divorce and remarriage involve a complex transition that requires the disintegration of one family structure and reorganization to another (Hiyoshi, Fall, Netuveli, et al., 2015). How parents cope during situational crises, as well as after the divorce, is a significant variable in long-term individual and family adjustment. See the case study at the end of this chapter for the presentation of a stepfamily situation. Developmental levels of children, individual temperaments of children, and quality of environmental support for children all contribute to family response to crises. For example, Fiese and Bost (2016) explore how families' responses impact obesity risk in children. They link family system factors, such as family meal routines and distress during meals, with the biological risk of obesity.

A family resilience framework may be useful to promote strategies for prevention efforts aimed at strengthening families as they face life challenges. Masten and Monn (2015) describe an integrated method for understanding and promoting resilience in children and families. Family disruption has been associated with substance abuse and psychosocial maladjustment in adolescents and young adults. Family supports are associated with adherence, and substance abuse may decrease healthy social support systems. Moreover, both family dissolution and family disruption may be associated with substance abuse, alcohol consumption, and externalizing behaviours such as theft, property destruction, fighting, and assault (Masten & Monn, 2015). The current literature provides support for the importance of the roles-relationships patterns in the development of health-promoting behaviours (Gordon, 2016; Masten & Monn, 2015).

Family organization influences performance of health-promotion and disease-prevention functions. For example, a single parent without an extended family network may be in need of more community resources to help raise the children. A two-parent family living near its extended family may need less support to raise children, but family members may need to know about growth and developmental stages and immunization schedules. Individuals may experience a variety of family structures in one lifetime. A person may be part of a nuclear family as an infant, a lone-parent family after the parents have divorced, a stepparent family after the mother or father has remarried, and an unmarried couple family when the person is one of two adults who share a household. The person brings the values and beliefs about health promotion and disease prevention that were practiced in previous unions to each new family configuration. Divergent values may result in conflicting expectations unless the new union forms a set of integrated values and beliefs. The current trend away from the nuclear family with the extended family may influence the general direction of the health care system and the strategies used to promote health with other family configurations.

Certain health-promotion issues are of particular concern to the nurse while he or she is assessing family health promotion and disease prevention. Family violence is a health problem that threatens the integrity of families. Family violence has far-reaching consequences both in the short term and longer term. These consequences range from physical and mental health challenges to further victimization, and significant economic challenges. According to Burczycka and Conroy (2018),

family violence is most often perpetrated against girls and women. In fact, women were victims of intimate partner homicide four times more often than males. As a global health concern, intimate partner violence has a deleterious effect on the victim, physically, emotionally, and financially, but also impacts children who may witness acts of violence (Burczyca & Conroy, 2018). It is known that underreporting of family violence for a variety of reasons (stigma, young children) makes it challenging to address this issue (Government of Canada, n.d.). The role of the family dysfunction and support is also linked to bullying behaviour (Kann, McManus, Harris, et al., 2015). Furthermore, bullying within families among siblings also occurs (Berry & Adams, 2016).

Family violence includes child abuse, intimate partner violence, and elder abuse, with women being victimized more often during pregnancy. Death in pregnancy is often associated with domestic violence (Alhusen, Ray, Sharps, et al., 2015). Health promotion and violence prevention require a complex set of skills. Nurses use approaches to reduce violence-related injuries and deaths by acquiring the role of advocate and helping to eliminate victim blaming (Research for Evidence-Informed Practice). It is also recommended that nurses implement routine universal screening for all females over the age of 12 (Registered Nurses Association of Ontario [RNAO], 2012). Explorations to assess families for health promotion and violence prevention may include the following:

- What formal positions and roles does each of the family members fulfill?
- What roles are considered acceptable and consistent within the family's expectations? What kind of flexibility in roles occurs when needed?
- What informal roles exist? Who plays informal roles and with what consistency?
- What purpose do the informal roles serve?
- How are the family social support networks associated with health and development?
- Who were the role models for the couples or single people as parents?
- Who were the role models for marital partners and what were their characteristics?
- How does the family manage daily living? How are the household tasks divided?
- How are problems handled? How are problems with children handled?
- Who is employed outside the home?
- Who takes care of the children when both parents are employed outside the home?
- How does the family care for its ill members? How does it care for its older members?
- Are behaviours appropriate for family stages of development?
- Is decision making allocated to the appropriate members?
- Does the family respond appropriately to its members' developmental needs? Is there fair distribution of tasks among family members?
- Is the family's emotional climate conducive to growth and development?
- Is there a connection between family and community crime?

### Perspectives on Regional Differences in Intimate Partner Violence in Canada

This qualitative study examined intimate partner violence within rural and northern communities in Canada. The intent of the study was to provide perspectives from community service providers and academic researchers in order to gain insight into the unique needs of survivors of intimate partner violence. Interviews were conducted with 10 participants from geographically diverse regions of Canada. The results revealed the challenges experienced by survivors of intimate partner violence from each region, such as access to services within rural and remote locations. Themes emerged around lack of transportation to access services; housing and economic issues for survivors to escape unsafe living conditions; gender inequality, particularly for earning power; intermittent and inconsistent access to services (i.e., policing positions that were unfilled, leaving gaps in service); and research challenges such as definition of terms (i.e., rural, northern, remote) and vastness of the geographic landscape.

Source: Zorn, K., Wuerch, M., Faller, N., et al. (2017). Perspectives on regional differences and intimate partner violence in Canada: A qualitative examination. *Journal of Family Violence, 32*(6), 633–644. https://doi.org/10.1007/s10896-017-9911-x.

In their study of 413 adolescents, Hardaway, Sterrett-Hong, Larkby, and colleagues (2016) provide evidence that family relationships protect adolescents from harm in violent communities. They report that interaction with the extended family and parental engagement act as resources for youth who are exposed to violence in their neighbourhoods. These findings indicate that nurses working with families should encourage parents to maintain open communication within the family and that parents should enlist additional support from their extended family members as a larger network of positive influence for their children.

When this initial assessment reveals possible neglect, abuse, or violence, further assessment is warranted with a branched assessment that may include the following assessment parameters and questions:

- What cues are present to indicate chemical abuse?
- Who are the significant adult members of the household? (Determine the presence of a boyfriend/girlfriend.)

High-quality evidence-informed intervention is based on a systematic approach to assessment. For example, quality intervention for victims of intimate partner violence can be planned in advance to promote the safety and well-being of the victims (Quality and Safety Scenario).

### Genogram

A genogram, or family diagram, represents the family's biological risk for health challenges and associated patterns between the generations. This useful technique gathers data on at least three generations, including the current one; their parents, grandparents, aunts, and uncles; and their children. The genogram describes family characteristics including, gender, age, relationships, health challenges, and mortality. Fig. 7.3 depicts accepted genogram symbols, with a sample genogram of the fictional Graham family portrayed in Fig. 7.4 (Stanhope et al., 2017). The Graham family genogram shows a variety of family structures,

### Domestic Violence: Intimate Partner Violence

If the person is still in the relationship:
- Think of a safe place to go if an argument occurs—avoid rooms with no exits (bathroom) or rooms with weapons (kitchen).
- Think about and make a list of safe people to contact.
- Keep a cell phone with you at all times.
- Memorize all important numbers.
- Establish a "code word" or "sign" so that family, friends, teachers, or coworkers know when to call for help.
- Think about what to say to the partner if he/she becomes violent.
- Remind the individual that he/she has the right to live without fear and violence.

If the person has left the relationship:
- Change the phone number.
- Screen calls.
- Save and document all contacts, messages, injuries, or other incidents involving the batterer.
- Change locks, if the batterer has a key.
- Avoid staying alone.
- Plan how to get away if confronted by an abusive partner.
- If a meeting is necessary, have it in a public place.
- Vary the routine.
- Notify school and work contacts.
- Call a shelter.

If the individual is leaving the relationship or thinking of leaving, that person should take important papers and documents to facilitate application for benefits or take legal action. Important papers include social insurance cards, health cards and birth certificates for self and children, marriage license, leases or deeds, chequebook and bank card, credit cards, bank statements and charge account statements, insurance policies, proof of income (pay stubs), and any documentation of past incidents of abuse (e.g., photos, police reports, medical records).

The National Clearinghouse on Family Violence provides information on all aspects of family violence, including a referral service for organizations (Contact: 613-957-2938; email: ncfv-cnivf@phac-aspc.gc.ca).

including changes resulting from marriage, divorce, death, and childbearing. This information highlights family health patterns to use for anticipatory health guidance: for example, in the case of the Graham family, hypertension, type 2 diabetes, cancer, and hypercholesterolemia. Family histories provide the unique perspective of family risk of inherited diseases as well as the influence of lifestyle (Murdaugh et al., 2019). Although *My Family Health Portrait* (https://www.hhs.gov/sites/default/files/familyhistory/portrait/portraiteng.pdf) takes a more traditional approach to family history, encouraging families to visit the website helps them explore their own family history. Resources for this continuously evolving topic of genomics can be found at the National Human Genome Research Institute (http://www.genome.gov/HealthProfessionals/), and online genetics education resources can be found at the US National Institute of Health's National Genetics Research Institute at http://www.genome.gov/10000464. The Genomics and Family Assessment box explores how family assessment incorporates genomics. New technology is emerging in personal genetic testing for home use, but efficacy has yet to be established for scientific rigour.

## GENOMICS AND FAMILY ASSESSMENT

Family assessment is the first line of assessment for genetic testing. Family assessment encompasses both genetic and environmental risks shared among family members. Family assessment provides the foundation for the complex process of genetic assessment, which includes nondirective genetic counselling to facilitate the balance of risk versus benefit (Wilson & Nicholls, 2015).

In order to foster family time, two-thirds of the Canadian provinces have instituted a Family Day holiday, usually during the month of February. Other provinces have a similar holiday; however, it may have a name of significance to the people of that particular province. Multiple tools have now been designed to facilitate gathering and sharing information in preparation for use in an electronic health record (EHR) environment. The design of these tools is intended to improve quality, while decreasing disease burden and cost.

Evidence supports multiple genomic interventions that are derived from accurate family assessment. A number of conditions have been identified as tier 1 disorders. Tier 1 designation indicates that genomic and family health history synthesized studies support implementation of the evidence into practice. Currently, the following disorders that rely on accurate family assessment are classified as tier 1:

### Breast/Ovarian Cancer

- Hereditary breast and ovarian cancer in women (see the Genomics box in Chapter 6):
  - *BRCA1* and *BRCA2* genes related
  - Deleterious mutation of the *BRCA* gene
- Chemoprevention of breast cancer

### Colorectal Cancer

- Newly diagnosed colorectal syndrome (test for Lynch's syndrome; see the Genomics box in Chapter 6)
- Known Lynch's syndrome in family
- Metastatic colorectal cancer (*KRAS* gene, cetuximab, panitumumab)
- Invasive colorectal cancer (carcinoembryonic antigen–related cell adhesion molecule 5)

### Cardiovascular Disease

- Familial hypercholesterolemia (DNA testing and low-density lipoprotein cholesterol concentration measurement)
- Cholesterol screening

### Other

- Osteoporosis screening in women—parental history of hip fracture
- Hereditary hemochromatosis–family health history, especially siblings
- Newborn screening of 31 core conditions

Other tier 1 genomic applications, in addition to family assessment, could be used to reduce morbidity among affected people and their families (Douglas & Dotson, 2015).

Adding family health history to meaningful use standards for EHRs may also decrease the gaps between the evidence and how it is implemented in practice. Promoting the importance of family assessment through education and policy may facilitate identification of at-risk families (Kolor & Khoury, 2015).

Sources: Douglas, M. P., & Dotson, W. D. (2015). *Evidence matters in genomic medicine—round 2*. Retrieved from http://blogs.cdc.gov/genomics/2012/08/23/evidence-matters-in-genomic-medicine-round-2/; Kolor, K. & Khoury, M. J. (2015). *Evidence matters in genomic medicine–round 3: Integrating family health history into preventive services*. Retrieved from http://blogs.cdc.gov/genomics/2012/09/27/evidence-matters-in-genomic-medicine-round-3/; Wilson, B. J., & Nicholls, S. G. (2015). The Human Genome Project, and recent advances in personalized genomics. *Risk Management and Healthcare Policy*, (8)2, 9–20. https://doi.org/10.2147/RMHP.S58728.

## Ecomap

The ecomap, which is similar to the genogram, uses pictorial techniques to document family organizational patterns with visual clarity. First a genogram is constructed for a family or household, beginning with a circle in the centre of the page. Outside the circle, smaller circles are drawn and labelled with the names of significant people, agencies, and institutions with whom the family interacts. Lines are drawn from the family household to each circle. Solid lines indicate strong relationships. Dashed lines reflect fragile or tenuous connections. Slashed lines signify stressful relationships. Arrows can be drawn parallel to the lines to indicate the direction for the energy flow or for resources (Stanhope et al., 2017). Fig. 7.5 shows an ecomap for the fictional Graham family. Both the genogram and the ecomap provide useful information and can be incorporated into family systems assessment (O'Brien, 2014; Tramonti & Fanali, 2015). The ecomap helps to overcome the issues of the genogram encountered when one is assessing nontraditional families. The ecomap uses a functional rather than a structural approach to the assessment of family roles and function to determine social risk and characteristics of the community.

## Sexuality-Reproductive Pattern

Sexuality is the expression of sexual identity. The sexuality-reproductive pattern describes sexuality fulfillment (Gordon, 2016), including behavioural patterns of reproduction.

This pattern also includes perceptions of satisfaction or disturbances in sexuality, sexual relationships, reproduction (including contraception), and developmental changes throughout the life span, such as menarche and menopause. The sexuality-reproductive pattern addresses transmission of information within the family about sexuality, as well as sexuality for the couple, including their sexual relationship, perception of problems, manner in which problems are handled, and actions taken to solve problems (Gordon, 2016). Information transmission during childhood is an important area to explore to better understand how issues related to sexuality and gender identity are addressed within the family (Gordon, 2016).

Topics to explore during the assessment may include the following areas:

- How do the adults in the family communicate their needs to each other?
- How do family members commit to, love, and care for each other, as well as fulfill their obligations and responsibilities toward one another?
- How do the adults in the family view marriage, parenthood, and their relationship as lovers?
- How does the family address family planning and birth control?
- How do family members participate in the choice of family planning and contraceptives used?

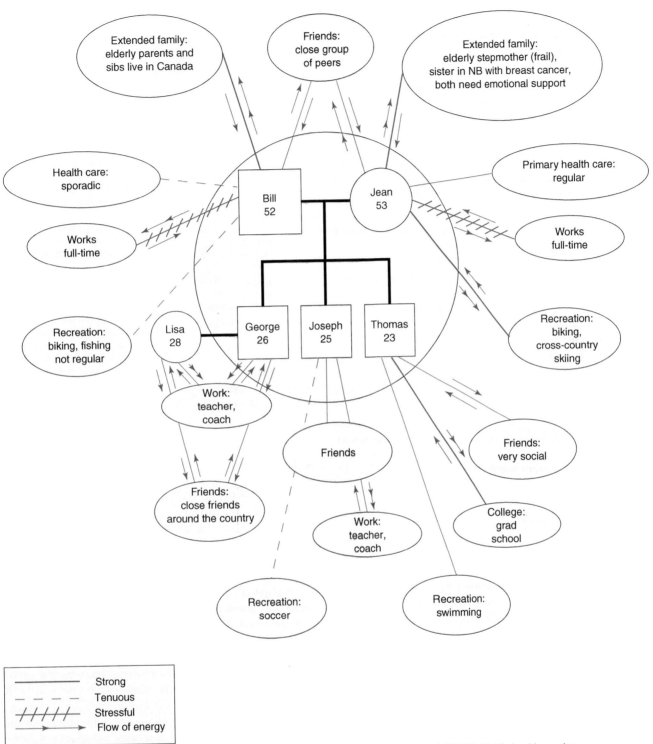

**Fig. 7.5 Ecomap of the Graham Family** (From Stanhope, M., & Lancaster, J. [2012]. *Public health nursing: Population-centered health care in the community* [8th ed., p. 636]. St. Louis: Mosby.)

When needed, complete pregnancy histories include sexual practices and partners, the number and ages of children, the number and outcome of pregnancies (including live births, miscarriages, spontaneous/therapeutic abortions), and the birth control methods used. Nurses also observe the comfort levels the adults demonstrate when discussing their own sexuality, or if an adult seems uninformed when discussing sexual subjects with children. Because of the impact that sexual relationships within the family have on children, exploring the variety of sexual practices within heterosexual, same-sex, and bisexual relationships in the family is an important part of health-promotion assessment (Perry et al., 2013). The onset of the use of EHRs in many settings provides an opportunity to systematically assess and intervene to provide best practices and eliminate disparities in these populations (Donald & Ehrenfeld, 2015).

## ◆ Coping–Stress Tolerance Pattern

The coping–stress tolerance pattern helps to depict the family's adaptation to both internal and external pressures (Gordon, 2016). On a daily basis, family members generate energy to face evolving needs. Society continually compels families to adapt to new situations. Survival and growth depend on coping mechanisms as families face external demands required to move from one developmental stage to the next. The family's ability to cope with everyday living demands determines family success. Family relationships support coping or generate more stress. Life events, such as divorce, moving, or developmental stages of the life cycle, and economic hardships, such as loss of a job, provoke stress and mobilize family coping strategies. Exploration of coping and stress tolerance includes the following assessment areas:

- How does the family cope with stressful life events?
- What experiences have family members had with chemical abuse?
- What strengths does the family have and use to counterbalance the stresses?
- What stressful family situations are experienced?
- How does the family view the association between stress and children's health and development?
- How does the family make appraisals of the situations, and are they realistic?
- Describe the family's resources. How do family members use knowledge or links to family networks or community resources?
- What kinds of dysfunctional adaptive strategies are used, such as chemical abuse or violence?

## ◆ Values–Beliefs Pattern

The values-beliefs pattern characterizes the family's perspective and attitudes about life meanings, values, beliefs, and spirituality and the way these issues affect behaviour (Gordon, 2016). Assessment, planning, and intervention are based on these attitudes. Assessment of this pattern enhances the interpretation of family behaviour. Exploration of values and beliefs includes the following assessment areas:

- What are the values and beliefs held by the family?
- How flexible are rules?
- How do family members interact (calm, aggressive, competitive, or rigid)?
- How do family members view spirituality?
- Describe the cultural or ethnic group with which the family identifies. What family practices are consistent with the norms of that ethnic group? How are the practices inconsistent with these norms?
- What are the family's traditions and practices?
- How do the significant cultural beliefs affect health or illness?
- Describe the role that religion plays in the family on a regular basis and during times of stress. How does the family rely on religious practices?
- How does the family perceive its competency during a crisis?
- What are the family goals, and do members perceive that they are attaining these goals?
- How are value conflicts demonstrated within the family?

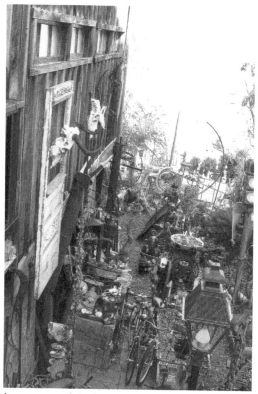

**Fig. 7.6** Assessment of the home includes environmental assessment of the yard.

- How do identified family values affect the health status of the family?

Spirituality, defined as life purpose and connection with others, affects health. The metaphysical and transcendental phenomenon of spirituality, as well as the religious and nonreligious systems of belief within families, should be assessed (Denham, Eggenberger, Young, et al., 2015). How well families communicate their unconditional love and forgiveness for injury or betrayal may contribute to physical symptoms within families. Clearly, spirituality and social skills promote health and prevent disease.

Data collected in the 11 functional patterns reveal ideas about family health-promotion and disease-prevention practices. Risks to healthy family functioning may be identified in each pattern. Risk factors may be found in more than one area. For example, passive smoke from one family member's cigarettes may be identified as an environmental risk factor in the home. However, the family's reaction to passive smoking determines the family members' perceived susceptibility, their perceived severity of the problem, and whether they will make a change in the environment to promote family health. The pattern indicates high risk if chronic asthma is described during the family history. In this situation, several other pattern areas support the finding. The nurse determines each risk behaviour along with its effects on the others.

## ENVIRONMENTAL FACTORS

The environment also influences family health and well-being. The home, neighbourhood, and community constitute the family environment. Assessment includes exploration of the following home environment areas (Fig. 7.6):

- What type of dwelling is it (condominium, single dwelling, low-income apartment, or temporary shelter)?
- How has the family acquired the home (purchase, rental)?
- What is the condition of the home (interior/exterior: glass, garbage, broken stairs, peeling paint, inadequate insulation, inadequate lighting on stairs, or broken fixtures)?
- Are the number and type of rooms adequate for the size of the family?
- How satisfactory are the furnishings to meet the needs of the family (enough chairs and beds, and a kitchen table)?
- How comfortable is the temperature (warm in winter and cool in summer, insulated)?
- How adequate is lighting for reading, sewing, and other activities?
- How adequate is the water supply (sufficient/clean/fluoridated/polluted)?
- Does the family have access to a telephone, and are emergency numbers available?
- How safe are the kitchen sanitation and refrigeration capabilities?
- How adequate are the bathroom sanitation facilities, water supply, toilet, and towels and soap?
- Are the sleeping arrangements adequate for family members, considering age, gender relationships, and spatial needs?
- How adequate is the plan for escape in an emergency (smoke detectors/escape route/plan inside the home)?
- What are the arrangements for and knowledge of first aid (directions posted for poisons, burns, lacerations, and other first-aid needs)?
- What signs of rats, mice, or cockroaches are present inside or outside the home?
- What are the family's impressions about the home? How do the family members describe the adequacy of their living space for privacy, their own interests, and status?
- How are chemicals stored in the home (out of reach of children)?
- How is safety ensured in the home? What safety issues are evident?

The areas to explore for neighbourhood assessment are as follows:

- What is the condition of the dwellings and streets (maintenance/deterioration)?
- How and when is the garbage collected?
- What is the incidence of violent crime, burglaries, and automobile accidents?
- What kinds of industry are nearby and do they produce air pollution or toxic waste?
- What are the social class and ethnic characteristics of the neighbourhood?
- What are the occupations and interests of the families in the neighbourhood?
- What is the population density?
- How available and accessible is public transportation? Why is public transportation not used if it is available?

Exploration during assessment of the community includes the following areas:

- What resources, such as schools, church, transportation, shopping, and recreational facilities, are available for family use?
- How accessible are the health facilities, such as health care provider's office, clinic, hospital, gym, swimming pool, natural food store, and weight-reduction clinic?

By driving or walking around the area, the nurse can obtain neighbourhood and community data. Other sources of information include the family, health professionals, teachers, business people, and others who work in the area. Official resources, such as the Canadian Community Health Survey (http://www23.statcan.gc.ca/imdb/p3Instr.pl?Function=assembleInstr&Item_Id=839130) allow a glimpse into a broad range of self-reported information about the individual's health status and use of health services.

## ANALYSIS AND NURSING DIAGNOSIS

### Analyzing Data

After completing the data collection, the nurse and the family analyze the data. Several approaches are used to analyze health data, including systems theory, developmental theory, and risk-estimate theory. A systems approach categorizes families as open or closed, with permeable or rigid boundaries determining both structural and functional components of family systems.

Developmental theory approaches families from the perspective of tasks and progression through cycles. Nurses analyze data to identify accomplishment of family life-cycle stages and family tasks needed to function successfully. Family developmental needs are determined considering the wide variety of family structures and functions in society. Although most family models are based on nuclear family structures, additional family structures should be explored as indicated by current population trends (Brown, Manning & Payne, 2016; Coyne et al., 2017; Stanhope et al., 2017). The stages of family development guide the baseline data analysis. Gaps, missing data, or conflicting information is identified and clarified.

### Couple Family

The first stage of family development begins when adults define themselves as a family, regardless of the legal status. When individuals move from their family of origin to a new couple relationship, adaptation to role expectations of a partner becomes a developmental task for each individual. Establishing a mutually satisfying adult relationship that converges with the kinship network is one family developmental task. Adjustment for couples includes learning how to weave together two personalities, two life histories, and two aspirations of growth. Decisions in this stage include whether adults are gainfully employed, how money is managed, where they live, how they socialize with friends and other family members, patterns of sexual activities, and whether the couple has decided to have children. Determining how to divide household tasks of cooking, washing, cleaning, and shopping occurs either consciously or subconsciously.

Developmental tasks that integrate health practices and habits into the couple's lifestyle require consideration during analysis. Health behaviour constitutes particular actions to promote health and prevent disease. Examples of health-promotion and disease-prevention activities may include maintaining well-balanced rest, exercise, diet, and contraception; smoking-cessation programs; wearing seat belts; and directing activities toward self-actualization. Each individual brings values and beliefs to the relationship. Practices from the family of origin and values from personal experiences combine to form the adult beliefs of the individual. Achieving mutually satisfying relationships also depends on couples' conflict management. Strategies that stem from congruent value systems facilitate couple's adjustment. When couples use divergent strategies, problem solving tends to be less effective.

## Childbearing Family

Decisions about adding children to the family commit couples to more complex long-term responsibility. Family development and primary health needs change to focus on additional members. To analyze the learning needs of couples with a pregnant member, nurses consider aspects of decisions and motivations involved with the pregnancy. With lone-parent families (usually mothers) becoming increasingly common through divorce, death, adoption, or the choice to have a child, analysis of family function addresses these diverse family structures (Atkin et al., 2015; Coyne et al., 2017; Stanhope et al., 2017).

Attitudes and practices in society regarding sexuality have influenced the incidence of sexually transmitted infections (STIs), such as genital herpes, gonorrhea, and syphilis. Acquired immunodeficiency syndrome (AIDS), first described in 1981, poses a threat to the family and society, in addition to affected individuals. Human immunodeficiency virus (HIV) is transmitted through heterosexual, same-sex, or oral sexual intercourse, as well as through direct contact with infected blood, shared needles during intravenous drug use, and perinatal transfer from infected mothers to their infants. Prevention of HIV transmission requires abstinence from and modification of relevant behaviours.

Risk factors associated with sexuality include lack of knowledge of safer sexual practices, the reproductive system, and personal hygiene; lack of prenatal care; pregnancy before age 16 years; pregnancy after age 35 years; a history of hypertension or infection during pregnancy; and unplanned or unwanted pregnancy.

Risk factors for premature pregnancies and unsatisfying marriage consist of ignorance about, or values regarding, family planning; adolescent age; and sexuality and role adjustment problems. In unplanned pregnancies, adolescent parents put themselves and their developing child at risk. Lack of knowledge of prenatal care, childbirth, and childrearing practices compounds the risks for both the mother and the child. Parents who are unable to perform parenting roles risk an unsatisfying relationship and inappropriate developmental growth for this beginning stage of the family life cycle. If couples decide to remain childless, learning needs include information about contraception.

The birth or adoption of a child begins a new family unit. Family members adjust to new roles as the unit expands in function and responsibility. As described more fully in the next section, parents' history as a dyad and their experiences in other groups, particularly their families of origin, influence the development of the triad (Diversity Awareness). Accommodating

### DIVERSITY AWARENESS
#### Preconception Care

Preconception care is a significant health-promotion opportunity for the whole family. The importance of this care has been recognized by the Public Health Agency of Canada's *Preconception Care* document (PHAC, 2017). The goal of preconception care is to improve the health of the parents in order to improve maternal and child health outcomes.

One important area of preconception care is evaluating a couple's genetic history as documented on the standard family genogram. Further evaluation should be considered for couples who are related outside marriage or who have ethnic backgrounds such as Mediterranean, Black, or Ashkenazi Jew, and for women older than 35 years or younger than 16 years who have preexisting medical conditions. Couples who have family histories of any of the following health problems should be referred for further genetic testing and counselling: cystic fibrosis, hemophilia, phenylketonuria, Tay–Sachs disease, thalassemia, sickle-cell disease or trait, birth defects, or developmental delay.

#### Reflective Questions
- Examine your thoughts, values, and beliefs surrounding genetic testing to identify chromosomal abnormalities, such as trisomy 21.
- Consider the value of prenatal testing and explore your beliefs concerning risk versus benefit of this form of genetic testing.

Sources: Johnson, K. A., Floyd, R. L., Humphrey, J. R., et al. (2014). *Action plan for the National Initiative on Preconception Health and Health Care (PCHHC). A report of the PCHHC Steering Committee.* Retrieved from http://www.cdc.gov/preconception/documents/ActionPlanNationalInitiativePCHHC2012-2014.pdf; Public Health Agency of Canada (PHAC). (2017). *Chapter 2: Preconception care. Family-centred maternity and newborn care: National guidelines.* Retrieved from https://www.canada.ca/content/dam/phac-aspc/documents/services/publications/healthy-living/maternity-new-born-care/maternity-newborn-care-guidelines-chapter-2-eng.pdf.

new members disrupts family equilibrium. As a group, families explore ways to meet each other's needs, to minimize differences, and work together. First-time parents often feel a lack of emotional support during the first several months of parenthood. Some, but not all, new parents have available family leave policies that may facilitate this transition. Without a family network or friends, the first days after the birth or adoption may be difficult. Parents may care for the child proficiently, but may need assistance to grow in the parenting role. If parents are both employed outside the home, they may encounter difficulty with the routines of baby care and being confined to the house more for child care. Anxiety about the adequacy of income may cause parents to increase their work hours to increase their income. Exhaustion for both parents is common from working full-time while providing child care as the infant develops. Single parents, usually mothers, carry these same burdens alone. Emotional support may be limited, particularly if one has not found satisfaction in parenthood. The families of origin or other support systems, such as self-help groups, neighbours, or friends, assist family members as they struggle to adapt to a new member. King, Boyd, and Thorsen (2015) reported their findings from a US longitudinal study (Adolescent and Adult Health). Their structural equation modelling indicated that perceived family belonging for adolescents of stepfather families ($n = 2085$) was strongly associated with the perceived quality of parent relationships, particularly with both the stepfather and the birth mother. Nurses facilitate processes within families of origin, families of choice, or other support systems to promote health in the newly formed family unit.

Some parents thrive during the period when an infant needs almost constant care and nurturing. These parents find support in a network of family and friends. Couples who find satisfaction in parenthood seem to realize that parental influence begins at birth and is the single most important factor in the child's physical, emotional, and cognitive development. The parents' ability to assume responsibility depends on a complex array of factors: their own maturity; how they were nurtured as children; their conceptions about self, culture, social class, and religion; their relationship with each other; their values and philosophy of life; their perceptions of and experiences with children and other adults; and the life stresses they have experienced.

In analyzing the needs of childrearing families, nurses consider many factors, including providing for physical health, economic support, and nurturing actions that are vital to learning and social development of children. In analyzing couples' needs during this stage, nurses recognize the importance of interactions among the triad. Observing decision making helps nurses determine family functioning, member roles, and effectiveness of family members. Risks associated with role relationships include working parents with insufficient resources for child care, abuse or neglect of children, multiple closely spaced children, low family self-esteem, children used as scapegoats for parental frustration, immature parents who are dependent and unable to handle responsibility, and strong beliefs about physical punishment or obedience.

## Family With Toddlers/Preschool Children

Families may have more than one child, each growing and developing at an individual pace. Preschool children place great demands on families. Families adjust to each new member with space and equipment for expansion. The needs and interests of preschool children influence home environments. Nurses assess the quality of the home environment for whether children have healthy amounts of stimulation-promoting opportunities. Safety balanced with exploration by the child results in health-promoting home environments. Rather than removing children from the kitchen or garden, finding ways to include them in a cooking or planting activity provides learning experiences. Other environmental influences affecting the child's rate and style of development include religious practices, ethnic background, education, and discipline techniques.

Evidence increasingly demonstrates the link between environment and health. Home environments that contain contaminated air, water, or food increase health risks. For example, lead poisoning, a preventable disease that continues to affect thousands of children, often results from lead paint and other factors in the home, such as water. In Canada, all paint produced since 1992 is lead-free. In addition, gasoline has been sold unleaded since 1990 (O'Grady & Perron, 2011). Lead levels have declined over the past 30 years due to the removal of lead from gasoline, paints, and solder used in food cans. Government regulations have contributed to this decline (O'Grady & Perron, 2011).

Health promotion needs for young children include proper foods, adequate exercise and sleep, and dental hygiene. Parents teach children through modelling and use of positive reinforcement. Family developmental tasks include adjusting to fatigue resulting from parenting demands. Nurses explore alternatives to relieve parents. Parents need time for themselves, individually and as a couple (e.g., to exercise, socialize), while knowing their children are safe with a responsible person. Economic restraints may limit relaxation time away from the children. Sharing child care with friends and the family provides one source of support for new parents.

## Family With School-Age Children

A family with children in school may have reached its maximal size in numbers and interrelationships. The parents' major problem during this stage is the dichotomy between pursuing self-interests and finding fulfillment in producing the next generation. Family developmental tasks revolve around goals of reorganization to prepare for the expanding world of school-age children. School achievement becomes a critical task for socialization. Viewing social and educational goals from the perspective of family culture and parents' defined goals becomes particularly important during this developmental stage. For example, many opportunities for health education exist in schools, including influencing healthy beliefs and behaviours. However, school health programs focus on problems such as tobacco and substance abuse with messages aimed at problems and crises rather than pursuit of healthy behaviours. The family's influence over health practices at home and in school is both by teaching children ways to assess and manage risky situations and by describing the benefits to expect when healthy behaviours are practised.

As children's activities broaden away from the home, another important developmental task for both the parent and the child becomes "letting go." Parents become involved in community groups such as the parent–teacher association, scout groups, sports teams, and other volunteer organizations. Encouraging children to join family discussions about their heritage can foster understanding of self within the family network (Fig. 7.7). Children exposed to unsafe home environments are at risk of disruptive behaviours, difficulties adapting to the learning environment, and learning disabilities. Parents who cannot manage their children in growth-promoting ways soon experience energy depletion and may turn to dysfunctional relief from parenting (e.g., drug and alcohol abuse).

## Family With Adolescent Children

Parents with adolescent children may experience a late pregnancy, resulting in care for an infant while other children in the family are in school. A new family member at this stage may be a source of joy or frustration for the family. The overall goal with adolescent members is to loosen family ties to allow greater responsibility and autonomy in preparation for adulthood. Although each member of the family strives to achieve individual developmental tasks in the midst of social pressures, the family as a whole has tasks to accomplish. Strengthening the marital relationship to build a foundation for future family stages is a critical task during this time.

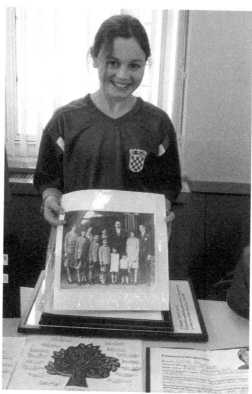

**Fig. 7.7** A school-age girl learns about her family heritage and presents this information through a school project.

Open communication is often difficult during this stage, partly because of the differing developmental tasks of adolescents and adults. Adolescents seek their own identity, and adults attempt to facilitate adolescent decision-making processes. Choices about values and lifestyles may differ. Adolescents may challenge family values and standards. Although parents maintain some authority, adolescents tackle their own desires and needs. Adolescents want to do what their friends do, have their own cars, and make their own money to spend in ways that they see fit. Parents who give adolescent members opportunities to experience social, emotional, and ethical situations with others are providing learning opportunities to enhance their sense of autonomy and responsibility. As adolescents become mature and emancipated, families face balancing freedom with responsibility. Health problems in this age group include violent deaths, including suicide, injuries, and alcohol and drug abuse. Contributing risk factors involve lack of problem-solving skills, family values of aggressiveness and competition, socioeconomic factors, peer relationships, rigid and inflexible family values, risk-taking behaviours, and conflicts between parents and children. Environmental risk–related violent deaths and injuries are influenced by substance abuse/misuse, the highway system, automobile manufacturers, and the legislation of standards of safety. Adolescents may also engage in risky sexual behaviours such as having multiple sex partners and failure to use protection during sexual activities (Government of Canada, 2012). Families rely on public health officials and nurses' efforts as advocates to reduce environmental risks.

Families support adolescents in this stage of development by including them in decision making and ensuring that they understand the positive and negative consequences of their choices. Family values of winning at all costs, aggressiveness, and competition may need to be explored during this period. Adolescents may discard these values if they are no longer applicable. Considerable change in adolescent values produces conflict and poses a threat to family cohesiveness. Families may place pressure on adolescents to conform to family values. In matters of adolescent safety, parents should approach issues in an individual manner, maintain open channels of communication through use of open-ended questions, and listen to concerns expressed by the young adult (Government of Canada, 2012).

Families with adolescents experience identity crises for the adolescent, the adults, and the family as a whole. All experience periods of transition as adolescents move from childhood to adulthood, while adults progress beyond parenthood. Adolescents struggle to find independent identities that remain connected to their family. Adults, in midlife, must resolve their own adolescent fantasies to move toward an identity for their remaining life.

### Family With Young Adults

Families with young adults act as a launching centre when children begin to leave home. As children leave home, parents relinquish their parenting roles of many years, to return to the marital dyad. The couple builds a new life together while maintaining relationships with aging parents, children, grandchildren, and in-laws. Couples focus on redefining relationships during this stage. As children mature, they no longer need a primary caregiver, often their mother, in the same way as they did during childhood. When mothers/caregivers devote years to raising children, their role and purpose within the family changes. This transition from a life with children as the priority to redefining life with new or renewed interests (e.g., career, community service) may require assistance and support from the entire family. Careers at this stage may become more stable. Developmental tasks at this stage for the family's adults require focus on future prospects. In addition to individual changes occurring at this stage, families with young adults may experience other pressures. Aging parents and adult children may require financial or emotional support. Financial and emotional responsibilities to other family members hinder the couple's ability to focus on their relationship during this developmental phase. Health-promoting activities to be focused on during this stage include coping with pressures of social roles and occupational responsibilities, maintaining health tasks to promote healthy aging, and reassessing life goals.

### Family With Middle-Aged Adults

Families consisting of only two members are able to enhance self-concept and support their relationship during middle age. Usually children have left home and adults experience a sense of freedom and well-being. Some relationships, by this stage, have reached a level of security, stability, and meeting each other's needs. Parenting pressures diminish, allowing parents to enjoy the accomplishments of their children and grandchildren. Middle-aged adults usually have an established network of friends/acquaintances and seek participation in neighbourhood rituals and events. Economic security and personal self-esteem may be at a peak.

In contrast, some relationships falter at this time. With young adults successfully launched, the parents may experience a quieting of the home with less activity, known as the "empty nest." When individuals are unprepared for this stage, they might seek opportunities to enhance self-concept from outside of the family. With parenting roles now complete, adults may develop feelings of inadequacy or begin new relationships, start new families, or resort to substance abuse. In addition, this life phase may include becoming grandparents, parenting grandchildren, coping with the needs of middle-aged children, and caring for older persons (children, siblings, or parents).

Health tasks in this developmental stage require new awareness of susceptibility or vulnerability to health problems. Couples adjust their lifestyle and habits to cope with health risks. Losses promote health problems, and at this stage couples begin to cope with deaths among family and friends, along with declining income. If either member has developed physical or mental illness, the other adjusts to the resultant physical and mental impairments, redefining self-concept.

Middle-aged families face a host of risk factors leading to three prevalent causes of death: heart disease, cancer, and cerebrovascular accident (stroke). Family lifestyle may decrease risks by placing a high value on being physically active, refraining from smoking, maintaining adequate nutritional habits, and following the recommended drinking guidelines of no more than two drinks per day for women and three drinks per day for men (Canadian Centre on Substance Use & Addiction, 2018). Lifestyle habits that are transmitted through role modelling have a greater influence on the younger members of the family than any verbal edict. Middle-aged members positively influence their health if they are able to choose environments low in water and air pollution and free from crippling stress factors such as excessive noise, traffic, and overcrowding. Family members can also apply pressure on key members of the community to decrease risks in the environment.

## Family With Older Persons

Retirement affects many aspects of life, particularly on interpersonal relationships for couples and individual family members. Besides decreased work hours, retirement also means reduction in income and fixed incomes for most people. Adjusting living standards to retirement income and being able to supplement this income with wage-earning activity is one task of the family with older persons. Other tasks during this stage include ensuring a safe and comfortable home environment, preparing for end of life, and adjusting to the loss of a spouse and making meaning of the grief process (MacKinnon, Smith, Henry, et al., 2016). In their qualitative pilot study, MacKinnon and colleagues (2016) reported that participants ($n = 12$) used group intervention (meaning-based group counselling) to establish effective coping strategies, adapt to their loss, and reframe life goals.

Health promotion aims to maintain functional ability, limit the effects of disabling conditions, and maintain quality of life. Older people may fear becoming helpless, feeling useless, and

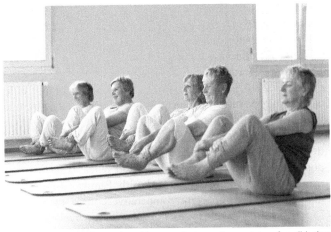

Fig. 7.8 As with all people, older people hope for a state of well-being that allows them to function at their highest capacity physically. (iStockphoto/SilviaJansen)

being incapable of caring for themselves. When analyzing risk factors in the aging family, nurses look for the couple's ability to function well enough to carry out normal roles and responsibilities. As with all people, older people hope for a state of well-being that will allow them to function at their highest capacity physically, psychologically, socially, and spiritually (Fig. 7.8). Many older people remain in their own homes, and most of these individuals are robust, healthy, and completely independent. Assuming that most older people prefer to remain in their own homes, assessment of the family for this age group should consider predictors of independence or those factors that indicate a need for institutionalized care such as assisted living, adult day care, or nursing homes. In their report of a longitudinal 22-year study of 1032 Finnish adults aged from 73.1 to 92.3 years (average age 83.5 years), Salminen, Vire, Viikari, and colleagues (2017) reported that falling several times a year, absence of nearby assistance, diminished cognitive function, and both high or low BMI significantly increased the likelihood of institutionalization. These findings highlight the importance of assessing fall risk, social support networks, cognitive function, and maintaining an ideal body weight in families with older persons.

Ego integrity (the union of all previous phases of the life cycle) is the challenge in this stage and demands successful aging through continued activity. Having gone through the various stages of family development, the couple accepts what they have done as their own. At this time, they may need family or professional support to pursue other interests or maintain former activities to feel needed and useful.

The nurse and the family jointly analyze the information, comparing the family's data with documented norms of health promotion and disease prevention in older persons. Norms or expected values can be derived from the family's baseline information of 11 functional pattern areas, knowledge of growth and development for all age groups and the family as a whole, risk-factor estimates, and population norms. Population norms specify normal ranges for these groups. For example, age is associated with various risk factors; some disorders are so common that they are referred to as diseases of the older person. In certain diseases, such as lung cancer, there is a long period of exposure. Risk increases with cumulative exposure; therefore, the incidence and prevalence of diseases increase with age.

*Sexuality.* Because of the popular perception that older persons are asexual, their sexual concerns may be disregarded (Salladay, 2016). The strength of sexual desire of the older woman may be more influenced by age, education, and attitude than by biomedical factors.

General population norms for values, beliefs, self-perception, or role relationships may be less available than physical population norms. Cultural, ethnic, and religious factors contribute to values and beliefs about health. Family baseline information provides important comparative criteria for analysis. Family records provide useful information when available. The first contact assessment provides baseline information for subsequent comparison and evaluation of progress. Whether the family perceives situations to be problematic should also be considered in the analysis phase. Nurse and family perceptions about problems may differ.

## Cultural Sensitivity

Cultural sensitivity and respect for individual beliefs forms a foundation for the nursing process of assessing, planning, intervening, and evaluating (see Chapter 2 for more detail). With changing trends in families and shifts in diversity within society, cultural sensitivity, cultural humility, and cultural safety become priorities for family assessment and nurses. Pandit, Chen-Feng, Joo Kangm, and colleagues (2014) define "sociocultural attunement (SCA) as the ongoing process of experiencing clients' emotions around the intersection of sociocultural contexts (i.e., gender, race, ethnicity, religion, sexual orientation, age, etc.)." Their definition of sociocultural attunement was derived from a study that developed a working model of SCA in which 13 therapists and five couples participated in a total of 25 therapy sessions. Four cycles of qualitative analysis resulted in a working model for the SCA process. The process of SCA these researchers designed includes three recursive phases: the initial guiding lens, sociocultural interpretation, and patient and therapist resonance (Pandit et al., 2014).

Cultural values, such as those connected to nutrition, influence most health-promotion practices. As globalization occurs, diversity will also expand, and competent care for Indigenous populations and migrating populations will be needed (Giger, 2014). Culturally humble care increases the efficacy of health promotion for all families, particularly families from within vulnerable populations (Giger, 2014).

## PLANNING WITH THE FAMILY

Intervention planning stems from a comprehensive complete assessment and analysis. The plan's purpose aims for behavioural change in families to promote health or prevent dysfunction. As in the assessment phase, family members play an active role in the planning process. Family responsibility for personal health status enhances the success of behavioural change outcomes. The planning process involves several steps, with the nurse and family identifying the following:

- Order of priority for problems or potential problems.
- Items that can be managed by the nurse and the family and items that must be referred to others.
- Actions and expected outcomes.

The nursing plan provides direction for implementation and the framework for evaluation (see the Care Plan at the end of this chapter).

As mentioned, a family's health status can be diagnosed as functional, potentially dysfunctional, or dysfunctional. Functional family health status warrants verification by the nurse with a plan for periodic re-evaluation that is formulated jointly. Plans to continue healthy lifestyle behaviours are reinforced. The nurse provides specific information requested by the family, such as immunization schedules, growth and development milestones, and recommended dietary allowances. In working with healthy families, the nurse controls the assessment and analysis phases of the nursing process. If the health status is judged functional, then planning health-education materials, scheduling periodic examinations, and providing accessibility of the nurse remain professional responsibilities. Implementation and evaluation of health-promotion activities become family responsibilities.

In health-promotion and disease-prevention settings, life-threatening situations rarely occur; however, when such situations do occur, they become the highest priority for intervention. For other identified potential or actual problems, the nurse relies on the family to decide which problem or potential problem to approach. After the ordering of priorities has been established, the family and nurse determine who will work on the problem. Problems or potential problems to be resolved by the nurse are identified separately from those requiring referral or family intervention. Problems for the family to address or those the family is already managing are considered strengths and are acknowledged and supported by the nurse. For example, when there is consistency among values and actions, physical fitness, weight management, and ability to cope with stress, the family is already taking informed and responsible action in these areas. The extent to which family members can provide their own health promotion and disease prevention will depend on their knowledge, skills, motivation, and orientation toward health.

Problems that need medical, legal, or social attention are referred to appropriate agencies. The nurse should provide a directory of community resources in the event that referrals are needed. Nursing intervention requires clearly stated actions that are purposeful, moral, capable of being accomplished, and adapted to the particular life situation, beliefs, and expectations of the family.

### Goals

Goals are statements describing desired outcomes. Family outcome statements include expected family behaviours, circumstances for exhibited behaviours, and criteria for determining performance. Health-promotion goals reflect a desire to function at a higher level of health and to grow beyond maintaining health or preventing disease.

# IMPLEMENTATION WITH THE FAMILY

The implementation phase is dynamic. As the nurse and family work together, new information is used to adapt and change the plan as necessary. Family nursing interventions aim to assist families in performing functions that members cannot perform for themselves. In health promotion and disease prevention, nurses assist families to improve their capacity to act on their own behalf. Ten studies were identified in a systematic review of the literature about family interventions (Deek, Hamilton, Brown, et al., 2016). This review linked reduced readmission rates, emergency department (ED) visits, and anxiety levels and family-centred interventions. Evidence to support the use of family-centred interventions, including active learning strategies, transitional care, and appropriate follow-up in families with chronic conditions, was presented.

Families may know that they engage in risk-taking behaviours through smoking, substance misuse, and engaging in a stressful lifestyle. As the nurse explains the rationale behind the proposed changes, families may choose to deny how they jeopardize their future health and continue their risk-taking behaviours. Factors that the nurse has not considered may cause the family's resistance. For example, families may have more pressing basic needs such as food, clothing, and housing.

Federal legislation known as the *Canada Health Act* was passed in 1984 to promote the health of Canadians. In 1995, federal cash and tax transfers were converted to single block transfers to the provinces to provide health care funding. Universal health care in Canada is based on five basic tenets: universal coverage, accessibility, portability, comprehensive care for all, and public administration (Government of Canada, 2018; see Chapter 3). This ensures that all insured residents of Canada are entitled to receive health services, including hospital care, health care provider services, and care provided by surgical dentists.

Health promotion and disease prevention may not have been part of the family's life experiences, giving the nurse the educational task to try to change attitudes and values by expanding the options for families to consider health promotion. Four types of nursing interventions appear in health promotion and disease-prevention planning: increasing knowledge and skills; increasing strengths; decreasing exposure; and decreasing susceptibility. Increasing knowledge and skills to improve family capacity for health promotion and disease-prevention behaviour may be the primary strategy. Use of this strategy helps families make informed choices about healthful lifestyle behaviours and eliminate harmful environmental influences that affect health. Improved knowledge aims to create awareness as the nurse and family work together to uncover actual or potential problems. Nurses recognize particular families at risk and move toward motivating and supporting behavioural change in these families. Innovative Practice presents an example of one program that provides education and support to people with cancer and their families.

Family strengths or forces that contribute to family unity and solidarity foster the development of inherent family potential (Carrascosa, 2015). These factors include:

- Physical, emotional, and spiritual factors
- Healthy childrearing practices and discipline
- Meaningful and clear communication
- Support, security, and encouragement
- Growth-producing relationships and experiences
- Responsible community relationships
- Growth with and through children
- Self-help and acceptance of help
- Flexibility in family functions and roles
- Mutual respect for individuality
- Crisis as a means for growth
- Family unity and loyalty and intrafamily cooperation
- Adaptability of family strengths

In recent years, a shift of family health care from an illness or problem and deficiency focus to a strength-based focus has occurred (Aston, Price, Etowa, et al., 2015; Gottlieb, 2013). Multiple models in nursing view families as systems and base their assessment and nursing process on strengths rather than deficits. These models of nursing provide the framework to assess and plan care using family strengths and resources (Carrascosa, 2015). Family members develop and maintain health-promoting behaviours by using commitment, appreciation, affection, positive communication, time together, a sense of spiritual well-being, and ability to cope with stress and crisis. Multiple assessment tools are available for nurses to use to generate discussion among family members about their strengths. Aston and colleagues (2015) describe the importance of corresponding nursing interventions to support and further develop the family dynamics of socialization, support, and nurturance.

Families with significant strengths may need to learn new, unfamiliar skills for mastering a specific technique, such as meditation, and to apply new tools for decision making. These families rarely require ongoing supervision or support of sustained interventions aimed at changing their coping patterns, communication, or role behaviour. They may be highly capable of seeking and using information. Assisting functional families may simply involve providing information in terms that can be understood and offering opportunities to ask questions and

## INNOVATIVE PRACTICE

**Wellspring**

Wellspring, a national network of community-based centres, provides programs and services for people who are experiencing cancer—both patients and caregivers. Each Wellspring centre offers similar programs at each site, tailored to meet the needs of the community it serves. Each of the 11 sites, in addition to an online centre, offers programs to help cope with a cancer diagnosis. Programs range from financial matters to rehabilitation from physical effects of cancer to psychological impact.

**Contact Information**

*Wellspring*
4 Charles Street East
4th Floor, Suite 400
Toronto, Ontario M4Y 1T1
Toll-free: 1 888 939-3333 Fax: 416-961-3721
E-mail: dawn@wellspring.ca
Website: https://wellspring.ca/downtown-toronto/register/#!1

clarify information. Unit 4 contains individual chapters devoted to many of the strategies commonly used in health-promotion intervention, such as health teaching and counselling.

Decreasing exposure to risk factors may include enhancing parents' ability to assess and adjust their behaviour to their child's temperament. Parents with limited literacy may need assistance to learn to respond constructively to their child's communication attempts. Health promotion includes teaching parents to avoid exposure to risks—for example, to use adequate restraints in automobiles, to protect their toddler from wandering into dangerous streets, and to supervise children to avoid falls and hazardous materials.

Although no substitute can be found for continuous supervision of a child, homes can be made safer if common hazards are moved out of children's reach. This effort includes storing all cleaning solutions and medications beyond children's reach; erecting barriers in front of exposed heaters, high windows, and stairways; keeping pots and pans turned inward on the stove; fencing-in a yard or a swimming pool; and teaching children to avoid dangerous areas. Becoming aware of peeling paint and toxic chemicals that parents might carry home from the job on their clothing can also protect the child.

Decreasing susceptibility means educating families about prevention principles. Families who realize how diseases are spread are better able to avoid transmission from person to person; through air, water, and food; and by insects and the rodents on which insects live. Health promotion includes emphasizing the role of personal hygiene and cleanliness to avoid infection. Families who know signs and symptoms that require medical attention and how to treat minor illnesses are better able to maintain healthy environments.

Murdaugh and colleagues (2019) cite research that demonstrates how perceived susceptibility predicts preventive behaviour. Perceived susceptibility is the family's estimated subjective probability that a specific health problem will be encountered. Family members' perceptions of health risks and their susceptibility to them will determine how they change their behaviour. If the family members experiencing obesity believe that obesity and a high BMI is a threat to the health of the family, the family members are more likely to react positively to the changes suggested by the nurse than is a family who perceives no health threat. Nurses who introduce threat as a motivator to action are morally obligated to reduce the threat by meaningful and purposeful interventions. Table 7.2 (earlier in the chapter) lists various nursing roles used in the implementation stage.

## EVALUATION WITH THE FAMILY

The purpose of evaluation is to determine how the family has responded to the planned interventions and whether these interventions were successful. Goals and objectives that are stated in specific behavioural terms will make evaluation much easier than when they are given in general terms. The criteria used to evaluate interventions—such as weight change, increased lung capacity from an exercise program, and lower pulse rate as a result of relaxation exercises— are simple to measure. Other results of health promotion and disease prevention are not as easy to measure but must be considered in the evaluation step of the nursing process. When considering such factors as values, beliefs, self-perceptions, or role relationships, the nurse may base the evaluation on whether the family indicates that the interventions were successful. Additionally, the family's baseline data are used as comparative criteria in evaluation. The nurse reassesses the situation and compares the new information with that on the original assessment to determine whether change has occurred.

The following five measures of family functioning can be used to determine the effectiveness of interventions: changes in interaction patterns; effective communication; ability to express emotions; responsiveness to needs of members as individuals; and problem-solving ability. Using these measures, the nurse returns to the original assessment of the family's functioning and compares current observations with previous data. These characteristics of family functioning continue to provide a useful framework even today, when family structures are becoming more diverse and the nuclear family is becoming less prevalent (Brown et al., 2016; Coyne et al., 2017; Stanhope et al., 2017).

When, during the planning phase of the nursing process, the nurse has identified the criteria (norms and standards) for the desired outcomes, these outcomes are the basis of evaluation. Data from the family that describe the behaviour of family members relative to the desired outcomes determine whether the nursing care was successful. With the criteria stated, the goals and objectives outline how the family can demonstrate a successful outcome and the behaviour change expected to result from nursing intervention. The more objective and measurable the desired outcome is, the more reliable the results of evaluation will be.

After the goals and objectives have been reached, the problem no longer exists. If evaluation shows the nursing actions did not achieve the goals or objectives, the nurse must review the nursing process to determine whether there were gaps in the assessment data, errors in analysis or nursing diagnosis, or alternative interventions that might have been considered. The nurse also needs to review the process with the family to determine whether the family members have contributed to outcome failure. Finally, the agency employing the nurse may be another factor; if intervention is costly or a shortage of staff exists, then health promotion and disease prevention may have low priority.

## CASE STUDY

### Family Member With Alzheimer's Disease: Mark and Jacqueline

Mark and Jacqueline have been married for 30 years. They have grown children who live in another province. Jacqueline's mother has moved in with the couple because she has Alzheimer's disease. Jacqueline is an only child and always promised her mother that she would care for her in her old age. Her mother is unaware of her surroundings and often calls out for her daughter Jackie when Jacqueline is in the room. Jacqueline reassures her mother that she is there to help, but to no avail. Jacqueline is unable to visit her children on holidays because she must attend to her mother's daily needs. She is reluctant to visit friends or even go out to a movie because of her mother's care needs or because she is too tired. Even though she has eliminated most leisure activities with Mark, Jacqueline goes to bed at night with many of her caregiving tasks unfinished. She tries to visit with her mother during the day, but her mother rejects any contact with her daughter. Planning for the upcoming holidays seems impossible to Mark, because of his wife's inability to focus on anything except her mother's care. Jacqueline has difficulty sleeping at night and is unable to discuss plans even a few days in advance. She is unable to visit friends and is reluctant to have friends visit because of the unpredictable behaviour of her mother and her need to attend to the daily care.

#### Reflective Questions

- How do you think this situation reflects Jacqueline's sense of role performance?
- How do you think that Jacqueline may be contributing to her own health challenges?

## CARE PLAN

### Family Member With Alzheimer's Disease: Mark and Jacqueline

#### Nursing Issue

Potential for reduced role performance related to caring for a family member with Alzheimer's disease.

#### Defining Characteristics

- Feeling exhausted
- Inability to complete tasks
- Feeling loss of usual or expected relationship with care receiver
- Increased stress or nervousness about the future
- Preoccupation with care routine
- Withdrawal from social contacts or change in leisure activities

#### Related Factors

- Illness severity of care receiver
- Increasing needs of care receiver
- Addiction or codependency of caregiver or care receiver
- Conflicting role demands
- Caregiver health impairment
- Unpredictable illness course or instability in the care receiver's health
- Psychological or cognitive problems in the care receiver
- Caregiver not developmentally ready for caregiving role
- Marginal family adaptation or dysfunction before the caregiving situation began
- Marginal coping patterns of caregiver
- Providing direct, ongoing care in the community
- History of poor relationship between caregiver and care receiver
- Care receiver who exhibits deviant, bizarre behaviour
- Incontinence in the care receiver

#### Expected Outcomes

- Caregiver distinguishes obligations that must be fulfilled from those that can be controlled or limited.
- In conjunction with the nurse, the caregiver develops a plan of care for the individual.
- Caregiver receives and accepts appropriate levels of support from family members, friends, and others.
- Caregiver describes help available from informal and formal support systems in the community and takes steps to obtain help.

#### Interventions (I) and Evaluations (E)

- I: Assess the level of the caregiver's stress. E: Use a screening tool.
- I: Assist the caregiver in developing a realistic plan of care, considering the care receiver's abilities and limitations; the plan will require modification as the person decompensates. E: Develop a realistic plan of care.
- I: Foster autonomy of care receiver, to the greatest extent possible, in social and self-care activities such as bathing, dressing, dining out with friends, and playing cards. E: Care receiver performs basic self-care activities.
- I: Facilitate a family meeting to help the primary caregiver seek assistance from other family members. E: Primary caregiver delegates care for respite.
- I: Support the caregiver and family members as they adjust to the degenerative nature of the disease; be aware that over time the stress associated with caring for the person increases. E: Caregiver and family demonstrate coping measures as care receiver's health deteriorates.
- I: Identify community resources that may offer the caregiver relief from constant supervision of the individual (home health aides, respite care, and adult day care). E: Caregiver connects with community resources.
- I: Help the caregiver contact informal sources of support, such as church groups, extended family, and community volunteers. E: Caregiver contacts support groups.
- I: Encourage the caregiver to attend an Alzheimer's disease support group. E: Caregiver attends support group.
- I: Refer the caregiver to the Alzheimer Society of Canada. E: Caregiver contacts Alzheimer Society of Canada.

*I*, Implementation; *E*, evaluation.

# SUMMARY

Learning about health promotion and disease prevention begins at birth, with the family providing the stimulus for incorporating health in the value system of its members. From a systems perspective, the family has both structure and function; relevant functions include values and practices related to health. The effective execution of health-related functions involves the family's progression through its developmental tasks and its ability to generate low-risk-producing behaviours associated with disease prevention.

Developmental and risk-estimate theories can be applied effectively to the nursing process with the family. The nurse uses functional patterns (an inherent part of both theories) to collect data for assessment. After organizing information on family life-cycle stages for analysis with the family, the nurse writes the nursing diagnosis and plans, implements, and evaluates the interventions used to promote health and prevent disease in the family.

## Evolve Chapter Features

http://evolve.elsevier.com/Canada/Edelman/healthpromotion/
- Review Questions

# REFERENCES

Alhusen, J. L., Ray, E., Sharps, P., & Bullock, L. (2015). Intimate partner violence during pregnancy: Maternal and neonatal outcomes. *Journal of Women's Health*, 24(1), 100–106. https://doi.org/10.1089/jwh.2014.4872.

Andrews, M. M., & Boyle, J. S. (2015). *Transcultural concepts in nursing care* (7th ed.). New York: Wolters Kluwer.

Aston, M., Price, S., Etowa, J., et al. (2015). The power of relationships exploring how public health nurses support mothers and families during postpartum home visits. *Journal of Family Nursing*, 21(1), 11–34. https://doi.org/10.1177/1074840714561524.

Atkin, A. J., Corder, K., Goodyear, I., et al. (2015). Perceived family functioning and friendship quality: Cross-sectional associations with physical activity and sedentary behaviours. *International Journal of Behaviour Nutrition and Physical Activity*, 12(1), 23. https://doi.org/10.1186/s12966-015-0180-x.

Azimi, M., Schmaus, K., Greger, V., et al. (2016). Carrier screening by next generation sequencing: Health benefits and cost effectiveness. *Molecular Genetics & Genomic Medicine*, 4(3), 292–302. https://doi.org/10.1002/mgg3.204.

Berry, K., & Adams, T. E. (2016). Family bullies. *Journal of Family Communication*, 16(1), 51–63. https://doi.org/10.1080/15267431.2015.1111217.

Brown, S. L., Manning, W. D., & Payne, K. K. (2016). Family structure and children's economic well-being: Incorporating same-sex cohabiting mother families. *Population Research and Policy Review*, 35(1), 1–21. https://doi.org/10.1007/s11113-015-9375-8.

Boyczuk, A., & Fletcher, P. (2016). The ebbs and flows: Stresses of sandwich generation caregivers. *Journal of Adult Development*, 23(1), 51–61. https://doi.org/10.1007/s10804-015-9221-6.

Burczycka, M., & Conroy, S. (2018). *Family violence in Canada: A statistical profile*. Retrieved from https://www150.statcan.gc.ca/n1/pub/85-224-x/2010000/aftertoc-aprestdm2-eng.htm.

Canadian Centre on Substance Use and Addiction. (2018). *Canada's low risk alcohol drinking guidelines*. Retrieved from http://www.ccsa.ca/Resource%20Library/2012-Canada-Low-Risk-Alcohol-Drinking-Guidelines-Brochure-en.pdf.

Carrascosa, L. L. (2015). Ageing population and family support in Spain. *Journal of Comparative Family Studies*, 46(4), 499–516. https://doi.org/10.3138/jcfs.46.4.499.

Coyne, E., Grafton, E., & Reid, A. (2017). Understanding family assessment in the Australian context: What are adult oncology nursing practices? *Collegian (Royal College of Nursing, Australia)*, 24, 175–182 doi:10.1016.01.001.

Deek, H., Hamilton, S., Brown, N., et al. (2016). Family-centered approaches to healthcare interventions in chronic diseases in adults: A quantitative systematic review. *Journal of Advanced Nursing*, 72(5), 968–979. https://doi.org/10.1111/jan.12885.

Denham, S., Eggenberger, S., Krumwiede, N., et al. (2015). *Family-focused nursing care*. Philadelphia: F. A. Davis.

Donald, C., & Ehrenfeld, J. M. (2015). The opportunity for medical systems to reduce health disparities among lesbian, gay, bisexual, transgender and intersex patients. *Journal of Medical Systems*, 39(11), 1–7. https://doi.org/10.1007/s10916-015-0355-7.

Douglas, M. P., & Dotson, W. D. (2015). Evidence matters in genomic medicine—round 2. Atlanta: Centers for Disease Control and Prevention. Retrieved from http://blogs.cdc.gov/genomics/2012/08/23/evidence-matters-in-genomic-medicine-round-2/.

Duvall, E. M. (1988). Family development's first forty years. *Family Relations*, 37, 127–134. [Seminal Reference].

Duvall, E., & Miller, B. (1985). *Marriage and family development* (7th ed.). New York: Harper Collins. [Seminal Reference].

Erikson, E. H. (1998). *The life cycle completed*. New York: W. W. Norton. [Seminal Reference].

Fiese, B. H., & Bost, K. K. (2016). Family ecologies and child risk for obesity: Focus on regulatory processes. *Family Relations*, 65(1), 94–107. https://doi.org/10.1111/fare.12170.

Giger, J. (2014). *Transcultural nursing* (6th ed.). St. Louis: Elsevier. [Seminal Reference].

Gordon, M. (2016). *Manual of nursing diagnosis* (13th ed.). Sudbury, MA: Jones & Bartlett.

Gottlieb, L. (2013). *Strengths-based nursing care: Health and healing for the person and family*. New York: Springer. [Seminal Reference].

Government of Canada. (2012). Chapter 10: Substance use and risky behaviour. *The health of Canada's young people: A mental health focus*. Retrieved from www.canada.ca/en/public-health/services/health-promotion/childhood-adolescence/publications/health-canada-young-people-mental-health-focus/risk.html. [Seminal Reference].

Government of Canada. (2018). *Canada Health Act*. Retrieved from https://www.canada.ca/en/health-canada/services/health-care-system/canada-health-care-system-medicare/canada-health-act.html.

Government of Canada. (n.d.). *Family violence initiative*. Retrieved from. https://www.canada.ca/en/public-health/services/health-promotion/stop-family-violence/initiative.html.

Gray, K. (2018). From content knowledge to community change: A review of representations of environmental health literacy. *International Journal of Environmental Research and Public Health*, 15(466), 1–17. https://doi.org/10.3390/ijerph5030466.

Hardaway, C. R., Sterrett-Hong, E., Larkby, C., et al. (2016). Family resources as protective factors for low-income youth exposed to community violence. *Journal of Youth and Adolescence, 45*(7), 1309–1322. https://doi.org/10.1007/s10964-015-0410-1.

Harper Browne, C. (2014). *The strengthening families approach and protective factors framework: Branching out and reaching deeper.* Washington, DC: Center for the Study of Social Policy. Retrieved from https://cssp.org/wp-content/uploads/2018/11/Branching-Out-and-Reaching-Deeper.pdf.

Hiyoshi, A., Fall, K., Netuveli, G., et al. (2015). Remarriage after divorce and depression risk. *Social Science & Medicine, 141*(9), 109–114. https://doi.org/10.1016/j.socscimed.2015.07.029.

Kann, L., McManus, T., Harris, W., et al. (2015). Youth risk behaviour surveillance United States. *Morbidity and Mortality Weekly Report, 63*(4), 1–172. https://doi.org/10.15585/mmwr.ss6506a1.

King, V., Boyd, L. M., & Thorsen, M. L. (2015). Adolescents' perceptions of family belonging in stepfamilies. *Journal of Marriage and Family, 77*(3), 761–774. https://doi.org/10.1111/jomf.12181.

Kolor, K., & Khoury, M. J. (2015). *Evidence matters in genomic medicine–round 3: Integrating family health history into preventive services.* Atlanta: Centers for Disease Control and Prevention. Retrieved from http://blogs.cdc.gov/genomics/2012/09/27/evidence-matters-in-genomic-medicine-round-3/.

Kramer-Kile, M., Osuji, J., Larsen, P., et al. (2014). *Chronic illness in Canada: Impact and intervention.* Burlington, MA: Jones & Bartlett Learning. [Seminal Reference].

MacKinnon, C., Smith, N., Henry, M., et al. (2016). A pilot study of meaning-based group counseling for bereavement. *OMEGA-Journal of Death and Dying, 72*(3), 210–233. https://doi.org/10.1177/0030222815575002.

Masten, A. S., & Monn, A. R. (2015). Child and family resilience: A call for integrated science, practice, and professional training. *Family Relations, 64*(1), 5–21. https://doi.org/10.1111/fare.12103.

Maurer, F. A., & Smith, C. M. (2014). *Community/public health nursing practice: Health for families and populations* (5th ed.). St. Louis: Saunders. [Seminal Reference].

Murdaugh, C., Parsons, M., & Pender, N. (2019). *Health promotion in nursing practice* (8th ed). Boston: Pearson.

National Center on Parent, Family, and Community Engagement (PFCE). (2018). *PFCE Understanding family engagement outcomes: Research to practice series.* Retrieved from https://eclkc.ohs.acf.hhs.gov/family-engagement/article/understanding-family-engagementoutcomes-research-practice-series.

O'Brien, V. (2014). Responding to the call: A conceptual model for kinship care assessment. *Child & Family Social Work, 19*(3), 355–366. https://doi.org/10.2147/RMHP.S58728. [Seminal Reference].

O'Grady, K., & Perron, A. (2011). Reformulating lead-based paint as a problem in Canada. *American Journal of Public Health, 101*(S1), S176–S187. https://doi.org/10.2105/AJPH.2011.300185. [Seminal Reference].

Pandit, M. L., Chen-Feng, J., Joo Kangm, Y., et al. (2014). Practicing socio-cultural attunement: A study of couple therapists. *Contemporary Family Therapy, 36*(4), 518–528. https://doi.org/10.1007/s10591-014-9318-2. [Seminal Reference].

Parkinson, J., Gallegos, D., & Russell-Bennett, R. (2016). Transforming beyond self: Fluidity of parent identity in family decision-making. *Journal of Business Research, 69*(1), 110–119. https://doi.org/10.1016/j.jbusres.2015.07.025.

Perry, S., Hockenberry, M., Lowdermilk, D., et al. (2013). *Maternal child nursing care in Canada* (1st Canadian ed.). Toronto: Elsevier Canada. [Seminal Reference].

Prickett, K. C., & Augustine, J. M. (2016). Maternal education and investments in children's health. *Journal of Marriage and Family, 78*(1), 7–25. https://doi.org/10.1111/jomf.12253.

Public Health Agency of Canada (PHAC). (2017). Chapter 2: Preconception care. From *Family-centred maternity and newborn care: National guidelines.* Retrieved from https://www.canada.ca/content/dam/phac-aspc/documents/services/publications/healthy-living/maternity-newborn-care/maternity-newborn-care-guidelines-chapter-2-eng.pdf.

Registered Nurses of Ontario (RNAO). (2012). *Woman abuse: Screening, identification and initial response.* Retrieved from https://rnao.ca/sites/rnao-ca/files/BPG_Woman_Abuse_Screening_Identification_and_Initial_Response.pdf. [Seminal Reference].

Rothenberg, W. A., Hussong, A. M., & Chassin, L. (2016). Intergenerational continuity in high-conflict family environments. *Development and Psychopathology, 28*(1), 293–308.

Salladay, S. A. (2016). Sex in the nursing home. *Journal of Christian Nursing, 33*(1), 13. https://doi.org/10.1097/CNJ.0000000000000233.

Salminen, M., Vire, J., Viikari, L., et al. (2017). Predictors of institutionalization among home-dwelling older Finnish people: A 22-year follow-up study. *Aging Clinical and Experimental Research, 29*, 499–505. https://doi.org/10.1007/s40520-016-0530-9.

Schoon, I., Jones, E., Cheng, H., et al. (2012). Family hardship, family instability, and cognitive development. *Journal of Epidemiology and Community Health, 66*, 716–722 doi: 10.10.1136/jech.2010.121228. [Seminal Reference].

Shajani, Z., & Snell, D. (2019). *Wright & Leahey's nurses and families: A guide to family assessment and intervention* (7th ed.). Philadelphia: F. A. Davis.

Simpson, J., Robinson, K., Creighton, S., et al. (2012). Female genital mutilation: The role of health professionals in prevention, assessment, and management. *British Medical Journal, 344*(7848), 1–7. https://doi.org/10.1136/bmj.e1361. [Seminal Reference].

Stanhope, M., Lancaster, J., Jakubec, S., et al. (2017). *Community health nursing in Canada* (3rd ed.). Toronto: Elsevier Canada.

Statistics Canada. (2016). *Young adults living with their parents 2016.* Retrieved from https://www12.statcan.gc.ca/census-recensement/2016/as-sa/98-200-x/2016008/98-200-x2016008-eng.cfm.

Statistics Canada. (2019). *Canadian health survey on children and youth—2019.* Ottawa: Author. Retrieved from http://www23.statcan.gc.ca/imdb/p3Instr.pl?Function=getInstrumentList&Item_Id=1209093&UL=1V&2017.

Tramonti, F., & Fanali, A. (2015). Toward an integrative model for systemic therapy with individuals. *Journal of Family Psychotherapy, 26*(3), 178–189. https://doi.org/10.1080/08975353.2015.1067531.

Utter, J., Denny, S., Denny, S., et al. (2016). Adolescent cooking abilities and behaviours: Associations with nutrition and emotional well-being. *Journal of Nutrition Education and Behaviour, 48*(1), 35–41. https://doi.org/10.1016/j.jncb.2015.08.016.

Utter, J., Denny, S., Robinson, E., et al. (2013). Family meals and the well-being of adolescents. *Journal of Paediatrics and Child Health, 49*, 906–911. https://doi.org/10.1016/j.jneb.2015.08.016. [Seminal Reference].

Vedanthan, R., Bansilal, S., Soto, A. V., et al. (2016). Family-based approaches to cardiovascular health promotion. *Journal of the American College of Cardiology, 67*(14), 1725–1737. https://doi.org/10.1016/j.jacc.2016.01.036.

Wilson, B. J., & Nicholls, S. G. ( (2015). The Human Genome Project, and recent advances in personalized genomics. *Risk Management and Healthcare Policy, 8*, 9–20. https://doi.org/10.2147/RMHP.S58728.

# 8

# Health Promotion and the Community

*Maureen M. Ryan, RN, MN, PhD*

Originating US chapter by *Anne Rath Rentfro, RN, PhD*

## INTENDED LEARNING OUTCOMES

*After completing this chapter, the reader will be able to:*

- Define and describe the concepts of community and community health promotion.
- Describe the 11 functional health patterns and explain how they are used for data collection to assess communities.
- Evaluate community characteristics that require supportive measures.
- Identify developmental aggregates of potential or actual dysfunctional health patterns.
- Explain methods of community data collection and sources of information.
- Describe a method of planned change for the community.
- Discuss the planning, implementation, and evaluation of nurses' health-promotion interventions with communities.
- Develop a health-promotion plan based on community assessment (including resources), nursing diagnoses, and other contributing factors.

## KEY TERMS

Advocate
Ambient
Community
Community diagnosis
Community evaluation
Community health promotion
Community nursing intervention
Community outcomes
Community pattern

Demography
Developmental theory
Focus groups
Function of a community
Health promotion
Interview data
Key informants
Lobbying
Lobbyist

Measurement data
Observation data
Policy decision making
Population
Structural foundations of a community
Systems theory
Windshield survey

---

### ❓ THINK ABOUT IT

#### Teenagers: Drinking and Driving

In a small rural community, seven teenagers have died in substance misuse-related car accidents within the past 3 months. Alcohol and drug education is taught during the first year at the local high school, but driver's education classes are not offered because the school cannot afford the program. Parents within this community are extremely concerned.

- What information must be acquired before a community diagnosis is made?
- What community health-promotion ideas could be recommended based on the information provided?

Social trends creating interest for health promotion in Canada include the opioid crisis, disparities in access to promote sustain health, increasing incidences of childhood obesity, mental health and well-being, the prevention of communicable diseases, and the changing population (see Chapter 2). As baby boomers entered older age beginning in 2011, the older population continues to expand and will grow more in the next two decades (Fig. 8.1). The proportion of those older than 80 years is also increasing as the Canadian older population continues to age (Fig. 8.2). These changes in the rates of the oldest old contribute to a growing number of older people with functional decline in our communities. Community assessment for health promotion will need to consider the health needs of aging populations more thoroughly, particularly home health that allows people to remain at home with community supports to augment functional decline. Currently, older people also tend to have more chronic diseases and consume larger portions of health care resources than people in other age groups (Fig. 8.3). This aging population will require more home services than previous generations because of increased life span and the concurrences of health problems (including altered levels of functioning).

Community health nurses support the health and well-being of individuals, families, groups, communities, populations, and systems (CHNC, 2019). A general understanding of community is a group of people who live, learn, work, and play together. Another way to think about community is by boundary, either geographic or political. For example, school, workplace, neighbourhood, and even the global or virtual community. *Aggregate community* is a term used to describe a group of people with similar interests, culture, beliefs, or intent (Stanhope, Lancaster, Jakubec, et al., 2017).

People are integral to any conceptualization of community; human beings give each community shape, character, and form. People are often characterized by their age, sex, socioeconomic status, education level, occupation, religion, ethnicity, and with whom they share a household. Individual health is reflected in each community through each person's contribution to its statistical rates and cultural and psychological makeup. At the same time, the community contributes to the health of individuals through the provision of services, security and protection, and relational opportunities that sustain well-being and capacity to promote health. This chapter focuses on community and health promotion, exploring the ways a community health nurse practices.

Globalization has affected communities. Swift methods of travel and Internet communication impact community health

(Petersen, Wilson, Touch, et al., 2016; Young, Tabish, Pollock, et al., 2016). Communities globally are exposed to emerging communicable diseases such as Zika virus disease, Ebola fever, severe acute respiratory syndrome (SARS), human immunodeficiency virus (HIV)/acquired immunodeficiency syndrome (AIDS), and pandemics of tuberculosis and influenza (Petersen et al., 2016). For example, in 2016 the World Health Organization declared Zika virus disease a global emergency because of its associated serious newborn neurological disorders (microcephaly) and Guillain–Barré syndrome, and more than 50 countries reporting cases (http://www.who.int/emergencies/zika-virus/situation-report/28-april-2016/en/). Infected female mosquitos transmit most Zika virus infections. Although sexual intercourse, blood transfusions, and perinatal transmission have been proposed as alternative means of contracting the virus, among mothers who delivered infants ($n = 35$) with microcephaly, 74% remembered rashes in the first or second trimester (21 in the first trimester). Most infected individuals (80%) experience few symptoms. The symptoms, such as fever, malaise, rash, conjunctivitis, headache, and muscle and joint pain, occur about 1 week after the insect bite, then last for about 1 week after onset (Petersen et al., 2016). Public health nurses play a key role in alerting the public to possible infections through health promotion and by responding to outbreaks detected through surveillance and assessment.

Disparities in health across the world are associated with poverty, industrialization, violence, social disruption, education, food access, and maternal health. Even in developed countries with health resources, disparity occurs. Universal health insurance coverage helps to eliminate barriers to receiving health care; however, geography remains a potential barrier to access. Rural communities are often disadvantaged, with higher mortality rates in both men and women related to poorer socioeconomic conditions and access to health services (Pampalon, Hamel, & Gamache, 2010). Compared with urban Canadians, rural people have increased prevalence of smoking and obesity and lower levels of protective dietary practices and physical activity. In addition, mortality rates as a result of circulatory

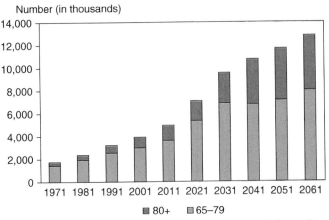

**Fig. 8.1** Proportion of Population Aged 65 Years and Over, Canada, 1971–2061 (From Statistics Canada. [2016]. *Research highlights on health and aging.* Retrieved from https://www150.statcan.gc.ca/n1/pub/11-631-x/11-631-x2016001-eng.htm.)

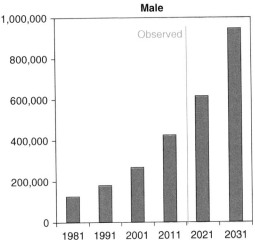
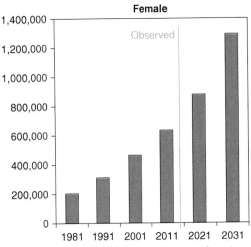

**Fig. 8.2** Community-Dwelling Seniors Aged 80 and Over, Canada, 1981–2031 (From Statistics Canada. [2016]. *Research highlights on health and aging.* Retrieved from https://www150.statcan.gc.ca/n1/pub/11-631-x/11-631-x2016001-eng.htm.)

disease, respiratory disease, accident, and suicide are generally higher in rural communities (Canadian Institute for Health Information [CIHI], 2006). Community health nurses play a key role in advocating at the policy level for equitable access to health resources.

Methods of data collection and sources of information about communities differ from individual sources. Systems theory, developmental theory, and assessing for identifiable risks to health and well-being inform community nursing practice. Developmental theory refers to a variety of explanations of phases of human development—physical, psychosocial, cognitive, and spiritual dimensions—based on descriptive research studies. Systems theory provides an overall framework to connect and integrate community data. Epidemiological data highlights increased risks of disease or infection in populations. Geographical mapping provides data on community resources and access. These, among other sources of information, assist the community health nurse determine possible threats to health and well-being in communities. Diverse communities require comprehensive assessment techniques that gather information about the unique characteristics of the population (e.g., cultural health practices or use of herbal remedies).

Gordon's (2016) functional health patterns provide the assessment framework for this textbook. Although other community assessment strategies are used in Canada, Gordon's (2016) patterns can be used to align community assessment findings with those of individuals, families, and groups, to engage in health promotion. An example of a data collection guide is presented to facilitate the comprehension, synthesis, and application of observation data, interview data, focus groups, and measurement data. An example of data analysis, nursing diagnosis, planning, implementation, and evaluation follows, along with a description (Table 8.1).

## COMMUNITY HEALTH NURSING PRACTICE

General systems theory (described in Chapter 7) fits well with health promotion and the socioecological/socioenvironmental

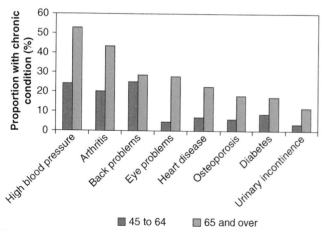

**Fig. 8.3** Chronic Conditions in More Than 10% of the Population Aged 65 or Over (From Statistics Canada. [2016]. *Research highlights on health and aging.* Retrieved from https://www150.statcan.gc.ca/n1/pub/11-631-x/11-631-x2016001-eng.htm.)

view of health. The Canadian community-as-partner (CCAP) model holds community systems and related social and ecological environments as being central to collaborative nursing assessment and intervention processes. While there are other models that Canadian community health nurses may choose to guide their practice, in this chapter the CCAP, combined with the Canadian Community Health Nursing Professional Practice Model and Standards of Practice (CHNC, 2019), are referenced. Community health nurses work with the Canadian CCAP model to "assist the community to attain, regain, maintain and promote health," beginning with assessment through evaluation of interventions (Vollman, Anderson, & McFarlane, 2017, p. 216). Community health assessment begins with becoming acquainted with a community and the diverse people who live, work, and play within it.

The approach to assessment is systematic and the purpose is—in partnership with community stakeholders—to collect, analyze, and present data to determine the health of the community, and utilize these evidences to inform community nursing. No single method of data collection will provide a complete picture of a community; therefore, the nurse will often use multiple methods of primary and secondary data collection. In strength-based approaches and Gordon's functional pattern approach, the nurse begins with locating and describing the strengths of the community, followed by noting areas where nursing can help strengthen the community.

Gordon's (2016) health-related patterns provide a useful guide to collect observation, interview, and measurement data. Health-related patterns depend on community settings, assessment focus, and the preference of each community. Assessing all pattern areas provides a basic data set to analyze and use for comparison during evaluation (see Chapter 6).

Known risks to health (e.g., exposure to contaminated drinking water) and stage of development also influence community health patterns. For example, health concerns may occur in one pattern area, such as the increased age-related factor of teenage pregnancy (sexuality-reproductive pattern). Data from other areas may reveal that parental opposition (values-beliefs pattern) tends to restrict healthy sexuality at home and limit supportive sex education in schools and communities (coping–stress tolerance pattern). Attempting to restrict sex education or "ignoring" sexuality as a healthy part of development at home or in schools, community, and primary care may increase the number of unplanned pregnancies in young people or, alternatively, may provide minimal community supports for its young people of childbearing age to promote their health and well-being. Information from several pattern areas may form clusters that suggest community health is determined by more than individual assessments (see Chapter 6).

## THE COMMUNITY HEALTH NURSE'S ROLE

In Canada, community health nursing practice is described as combining nursing knowledge, social science, and public health science with home health and primary health care (CHNC, 2019). Alongside community health nurses, public health and home health nurses provide care in the community. Public health

## TABLE 8.1   Implementation of Community Health Plans With Objectives and Rationale

**Nursing Issue:** Potential for increasing the incidence of fatal motor vehicle accidents in high school population as a result of substance misuse and driving.

**Goal:** North High School population will have reduced incidence (at least 20%) of fatal motor vehicle accidents related to substance misuse by December.

| Objective | Plans | Rationale |
|---|---|---|
| 1. Community will have access to information about incidence of fatal motor vehicle accidents and substance misuse-related arrests of its high school population for the past 5 years by March. | Interview local police about the incidence of fatal automobile accidents and substance misuse in the community. Interview parents of deceased high school students, students, teachers, physicians, clergy, and emergency department personnel about the incidence of the problem and suggested measures for decreasing the incidence; suggest that interviews be shared at a high school, school, and community social media sites (e.g., Twitter, Facebook). Have several people write to the community newspaper and social media sites commenting on the broadcast and the problem. | *Unfreezing.* For change to occur, the community has to become dissatisfied with the status quo and sense a need for change. *Empiric-rational strategy.* People are rational; discussion of facts can result in support for change. Important elements for preventing the problem include educating the public and having key community leaders discuss their views; concern lends credibility and is necessary for action. People tend to listen to those with informal power. Keeping the issue before the community can raise consciousness. |
| 2. Community will take action to inform the high school students about responsible drinking/drug use and driving by June. | Suggest to the school principal and the school board the creation of a task force of community residents to plan a health program on individual accountability and making responsible choices regarding substance use for high school students. Conduct focus group discussions with the task force and develop collaborative group goals and strategies. The task force should include teachers, students, parents, clergy, police, nurses, and physicians. The task force will locate evidence-informed content about healthy choices regarding substance use alongside resources to build capacity to make healthy choices, integrate it into the curriculum, and recommend that community members, such as a nurse, be involved in delivery and evaluation of the content. | *Changing.* Moving to a new level; community involvement will influence acceptability of changes. Community residents like to be involved in decision making. It is important to establish trust and collaboration among community groups; this opens communication channels between adolescents and the health community. Community involvement facilitates acceptance of change. |
| 3. Community will implement an educational program for its high school population related to use of substances and individual responsibility delivered yearly. | Implement educational content in high schools. | *Refreezing.* Moving to level of change brought about by community forces. Educational strategies built around the concept of community responsibility to locating and provide resources to augment adolescent capacity to make informed choices are essential elements in promoting health and well-being of young adults (Das, Salam, Arshad, et al., 2016; Steinka-Fry, Tanner-Smith, & Hennessy, 2015). |

nurses in Canada carry out the functions of promoting, protecting, and preserving public health, for example, by participating in *population health* assessment and surveillance, and through emergency preparation and response to local, national, and international threats to public health safety. Population health assessments that are informed by epidemiology and other evidences locate risk factors that determine the health of individuals or aggregate communities. Public health nurses intervene at various levels of the population health-promotion model, including helping individuals to develop personal skills, creating supportive environments, reorienting health services, and building healthy public policy. Home health nursing is specialized nursing care that is delivered at home within the community or in a community setting, focusing on the treatment of diseases or conditions that require medical intervention and care coordination.

Key to community health nursing is the recognition of the political, cultural, and environmental contexts of health, and a commitment to equity and social justice. Complex and dynamic communities, with their increasing public involvement in health and health policy, highlight the importance of community-engaged partnerships with nurses to build community capacity in order to respond to health and well-being challenges of community members and influence healthy public policy. For example, active participation in environmental issues, such as lobbying for safe drinking water, provides an avenue for nurses to promote healthy environments by influencing policy.

Harmful substances in the environment contribute to up to 33% of global environmental disease, including pollution-related diseases, and foodborne and waterborne diseases (CNA, 2005). In Canada, the growth of urban populations into farmland has resulted in the increase of air pollutants and a thinning ozone, which in turn has increased the numbers of diagnosed melanomas (CNA, 2005, 2017). Toronto Public Health estimates that upwards of 1300 Toronto residents per year die prematurely and 3500 Torontonians are hospitalized because of air pollution from transportation sources (Toronto Public Health, 2016). Environmental contaminant exposure is higher in children, particularly children living in poverty where living conditions increase their exposure, related to geographic location and less resources. Community health nurses are in a position to identify patterns of symptoms related to the environment and act accordingly. Moreover, the community health nurse as partner is able to translate information about environmental health risks to the community members.

Community nursing practice requires a broad knowledge base derived from health-promotion theories and models in practice, primary health care, population health promotion models, and social and ecological determinants of health (CHNC, 2019) (Figs. 8.4 and 8.5). The community-as-partner model (Vollman, 2017) emphasizes nursing action on the determinants of health, and the importance of public engagement in decisions impacting community health.

## Influencing Health Policy

The primary responsibility of the nurse is to the individual, family, group, or community being served. A major portion of the nurse's role is to be an advocate not only for the individual but also for social justice in health care delivery. Nurses advocate for the right of all Canadians to have access to health care, to participate in decisions about their health and well-being, and to work at a political systems level to ensure equitable distribution of health-promoting resources.

Health and the environment are integrally connected; therefore, nurses who engage in partnership with communities' assessment through planning facilitate the capacity to health potential of those communities they serve. Involvement that includes attention to policy decisions and political action affects broader aspects of environmental, biophysical, and socioeconomic conditions of homes, schools, workplaces, communities, and health care delivery. For example, nurses could take active roles joining any one of the advocacy campaigns located on the Canadian Nurses for Health and the Environment (http://cnhe-iise.ca/issues.html). By

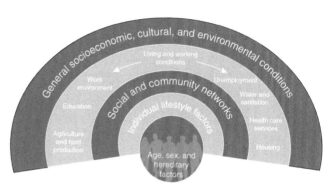

**Fig. 8.4 Wider Determinants of Health Model** (From Dahlgren, G., & Whitehead, M [1991]. *Policies and Strategies to Promote Social Equity in Health.* Stockholm, Sweden: Institute for Future Studies. https://www.iffs.se/policies-and-strategies/.)

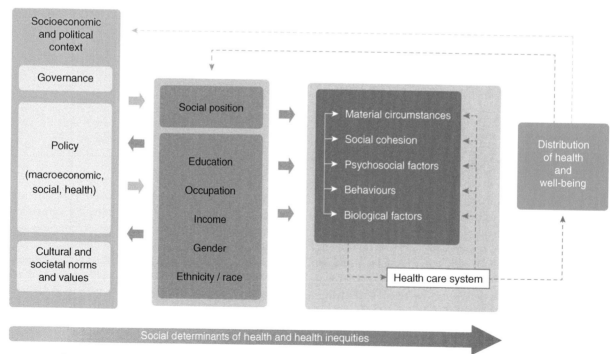

**Fig. 8.5 Social Determinants of Health and Health Inequities** (From Commission on the Social Determinants of Health [CSDH]. [2008]. *Closing the gap in a generation: health equity through action on the social determinants of health.* Retrieved from https://www.who.int/social_determinants/thecommission/finalreport/en/.)

virtue of their numbers, nurses—who constitute the largest group of health care providers in Canada—have tremendous potential to influence decision making.

Participation in policy decision making requires that nurses take a proactive stance to determine needs before a problem arises. Policy development and change occur on many levels, from within the nurse's agency or work group to the community, provincial/territorial, and national levels. At the institutional level, clinical decisions influence policy, as do management issues. The nurse examines the rationales underlying existing or planned policy and determines their current relevance. Nurses, by virtue of their education and experience, develop communication skills and apply change theory to influence policy.

Health-related decision making often results from legislation at the local, provincial/territorial, or national level. Laws—rules enforced by a ruling authority by which society is governed—and regulations—agency or department rules developed to implement laws—define the services offered. Politics influence change and provide an arena for nursing to participate in shaping the future of health care. Political involvement may include voting, communicating with local representatives, supporting candidates, contributing time or financial support, and running for city, municipal, provincial/territorial, or federal office. Voting, after nurses have become well informed on current issues and candidates, and serving on local and provincial/territorial committees are important ways for nurses to be actively involved.

In addition, knowing local representatives, informing them about health care issues, and advising them as to their constituents' needs are other ways nurses become involved. Legislators are influenced by the information that they receive and by the sources of that information. Nurses have a wealth of knowledge about health care. The process of seeking to influence legislators' views and votes is called lobbying. When an individual is employed to lobby, he or she is known as a lobbyist and is required to register as the representative of a special interest group. The Canadian Nurses Association (CNA), located in Ottawa, Ontario, employs nurse lobbyists, as do many politically grounded organizations. Individual nurses, however, can support colleagues who represent nursing's interests and who run for political office. The CNA regularly engages in campaigns during elections to inform nurses about candidates' platforms related to health, and provides "Take Action" guides that assist nurses in calling for action on health-related issues. Membership in professional and community groups provides nurses with the collective voice to influence public policy.

Communicating with a politician is essential and can be done by phone, writing a letter, personal visits, or email correspondence. Politicians have staffs of experts in various areas, and each legislator is assigned to committees. The healthy public policy process is iterative, beginning with setting an agenda, forming a policy, making a decision, implementing, and evaluating the new policy. Community nurses can bring community health problems to the attention of politicians (agenda), provide evidences to support change (forming a policy), and thus influence decision making. In their day-to-day work, community nurses are implementing and evaluating policy that contributes to health. It is important for nurses to advocate and lobby to inform policymakers as issues arise, including providing evidence and giving professional testimony. Nurses who are politically aware extend the collective nursing voice to its full potential.

History has taught us that health and the promotion of health is political. In 1974, the publication of *A New Perspective on the Health of Canadians* (called the Lalonde Report) proposed that health was influenced by biology, lifestyle, and environment as well as by health services. The report gained international attention as being the first to challenge reliance on biomedical health services as the only contributor to the health of people, leading to a convening of the World Health Organization (WHO) member states and the *Declaration of Alma-Ata* (WHO, 1978). The Alma Ata declaration emphasized the principles of social justice, equity, public participation, appropriate technology, and intersectoral collaboration. Canada responded by developing a framework for health promotion and introducing it during the first WHO international health promotion in Ottawa in 1986 with the aim of "achieving health for all" (WHO, 1986). Seven global health conferences followed, and there continued to be national and international efforts to promote health and well-being for all people. Health promotion is recognized as the process in which people collectively work to create conditions that sustain health and address social and economic conditions that affect a population's health (Raphael, 2010). Globally, health promotion is the process of recognizing health as a resource for everyday life and enabling people to reach a state of complete physical, mental, and social well-being (WHO, 2009). Community nurses' roles in health promotion include the recognition that some determinants of health exist beyond individual lifestyle choices.

Community health nurses in Canada began to integrate health promotion into their practice, aligning it with the Ottawa Charter for Health Promotion strategies (WHO, 1986) to:

- Build health public policy
- Create supportive environments
- Strengthen community actions
- Develop personal skills
- Reorient health services

Within these five strategies, the community health nurse moves from individual interventions through to political action, determining at which system level health-promotion interventions will have sustainable impact. In 2011, the 25th anniversary of the Ottawa Charter for Health Promotion, Lamarre (2011) reminded us that that the core values that inform the practice of community health promotion include the following:

- A sociological model of health that recognizes the cultural, economic, and social determinants of health
- A commitment to equity and social justice
- A respect for cultural diversity and sensitivity
- A dedication to sustainable development
- A participatory approach to identifying needs and setting priorities for action
- Planning, implementing, and evaluating practical and feasible solutions

## METHODS OF DATA COLLECTION

Nurses obtain community assessment data through observation, individual interviews, focus groups, town hall meetings, and measurement (e.g., survey). These methods are used in various combinations to ensure the validity of the information. Obtaining data through observation—often referred to as the windshield survey approach to assessment—includes the use of the senses (sight, touch, hearing, smell, and taste) to determine community appearances. These appearances include the types and condition of residential dwellings and their people and also physical and biological characteristics, such as animal and plant life, temperature, transportation, sounds, and odours. Some communities have a characteristic "flavour." A community's physical characteristics influence health. What type of space is available? Children need space to run and play; young and middle-aged adults require space for recreation and exercise. What spatial barriers exist? Where is this space located in relation to traffic and schools? What does the air feel and smell like? What does the water taste like?

Community nurses obtain abundant subjective data by simply walking or riding around a community. Data obtained by observation provide important clues about the community, its actual or potential health problems, and its strengths. Technological advances such as the use of geographical information systems (GIS) enhance nurses' ability to assess communities. The ability to link health-related survey and census data to small or large geographic areas through GIS facilitates the study of health inequities and directs the nurse to the system level of intervention. In Canada, one in three children through adolescence are overweight (OW) or obese (OB) (Rodd & Sharma, 2017). From a survey of adolescents in a Canadian city, 65% of adolescents reported purchasing food from fast food outlets or convenience stores more than once per week (He, Tucker, Gilliland, et al., 2012). Using GIS, He and colleagues then mapped postal codes of the adolescents—a 1-km line (walking distance) was used to construct a radius around the adolescents' homes and school. The Network Analysis functions in GIS located the number of fast food outlets and convenience stores within the 1-km radius of home and school. The study revealed that fast food density (more than 3 fast food outlets close to home or school) increased the likelihood of adolescents to purchase fast food more than once per week. This important information directs the community health nurse to not only strengthen capacity of adolescents to make healthy food choices but also points to the importance of environmental capacity to support healthy choices. Analysis of observation data generates hypotheses about next steps in data collection.

Interview data, the most common source of information from people, include verbal statements from community residents, key community officials, health care personnel, and various community agency staff. Key informants provide useful ways to learn how members perceive their community. Key community leaders often provide important information about community health concerns, necessary health resources, and community strengths, along with particular health beliefs and community health goals. Community residents provide useful information about their perceptions of health, health concerns, and needs, as well as their perceptions of the availability, accessibility, and acceptability of health services. Health agency personnel provide data about health resources, the population served, availability, and perceptions of concerns and needs. Developing a basic set of questions in advance enhances the relevance of interview data.

Community participation is key to assessment and planning. Through dialogue with stakeholders and community members, the community nurse participates in the prioritizing of needs and deciding where to take action (Frerichs, Lich, Dave, et al., 2016; Vollman, 2017). Strategies initiated by engaged community members empower community partners and enhance the ability to apply evidence-informed strategies.

Measurement data use instruments to quantify data during information collection. Measurement data include population statistics, pollution indices, morbidity and mortality rates, census statistics, and epidemiological data. These data can be accessed by the Internet or locally in community libraries; health departments; environmental protection agencies; schools; police and fire departments; local health system agencies; and town, city, or provincial/territorial planning offices. Publicly supported agencies share their information, and community nurses readily use such data.

## SOURCES OF COMMUNITY INFORMATION

Census information available from Statistics Canada (http://www.statcan.gc.ca), and also found in libraries and public agencies, is the most complete source for population information. The Canadian Census is completed once every 5 years and has over 350 active surveys on virtually all aspects of Canadian life. Community agencies and local planning commissions, project statistics, and developmental trends are how nurses understand population patterns and dynamics. Many communities and provinces also have databases available for public use.

The complete Canadian environmental record can be obtained from https://yourenvironment.ca. The government of Canada collects data on environment and natural resources (https://www.canada.ca/). Municipal and provincial public health departments monitor water, food, and sanitation systems. Community nurses' role in safeguarding of natural resources is protecting communities from industrial toxins. In areas that use well water, testing should be performed regularly. Community health nurses can participate in interventions to promote testing to assure the safety of water used in home. For example, Nova Scotia and areas across the northern United States risk exposure to arsenic that occurs naturally in the groundwater (Chappells, Campbell, Drage, et al., 2015). Private well users should be testing their well water regularly to determine if their water is safe and prevent related threats to health. Guided by a knowledge-to-action (KTA) process, community health nurses could intervene with multiple stakeholders to ensure sustainable multisystem-level interventions. According to Graham, Logan, Harrison, and colleagues (2006), turning knowledge into action requires that a range of stakeholders engage in identifying what is already known about effective solutions to the situation at hand, in this case arsenic in groundwater. The next step, to ensure sustainable interventions (action) within multiple community systems, requires adapting what is known to the community context, identifying barriers to applying the knowledge, followed by promoting sustainable effective actions. A community health nurse in Nova Scotia would reach out to community stakeholders to assess which knowledge gaps exist. Strategies to gather necessary information will include home visits, town hall meetings, and environmental home assessment planning to assess knowledge about the water issue and how to ensure healthy water. Action strategies include long-term initiatives such as training in water testing, and treatment; low-cost or no-cost convenient testing stations; and mandatory regulated enforced testing at the point of property transfer or when new wells are constructed (Chappells et al., 2015).

Public health departments, along with school administrators, provide school health information. Town, city, or county administrators provide information about land use, boundaries, housing conditions, utilities, and community services. Community newspapers and social media sites supply information about community dynamics, health-related concerns, cultural activities, and community decision making. The documentation techniques for community observation, interview, and measurement data are similar to those used for individuals and families. A triple-column format that separates the data obtained with each method facilitates recording.

## COMMUNITY FROM A SYSTEMS PERSPECTIVE

Systems consist of interrelated, interacting parts or components within boundaries that filter both the type and the rate of input and output (Frerichs et al., 2016). Similar to how families form systems (see Chapter 7), communities viewed as systems have both structure and function. Assessment of communities begins by identifying key characteristics of the people who populate the community. The study of populations is referred to as demography. A population is a group defined as an aggregate of people who share similar personal or environmental characteristics. Demography provides information about population characteristics—such as size and racial composition, along with the distribution of age, sex, marital status, nationality, language, religious affiliations, education, and occupation. Demographic data provide the basis for analysis and a means to identify groups who may be more at risk than others for health concerns. Such information also provides direction for health-promotion strategies. For example, examination of the age distribution over several years reveals important population shifts with associated needs for additional health-promotion activities. The increasing numbers of individuals older than 65 years require changes in community health priorities that reflect this group's needs. Comparing demographics between communities enables nurses to make inferences about the health of community members. Examples of useful comparisons are rural versus urban, affluent versus poor, and diverse versus homogeneous. The next step is to recognize that people are in reciprocal interaction with their structural environment.

### Structure

The structural foundations of a community consists of multiple systems with which people interact.

Community leadership provides direction for both health-promotion and health-protection activities; therefore, community assessment includes identifying what resources are available to promote and support health and well-being, and identifying where there are gaps in resources or barriers to access.

### Function

Assessing the function of a community refers to the ways that community systems and subsystems interact to make decisions about the allocation of health-promoting and health-protection resources. Community health nurses advocate for a strengths-based and capacity-building approach to resource development and allocation. In partnership with community members, a community health nurse enacts social justice-promoting equity in decision making and distribution of health resources, often empowering community members, and facilitating social, environmental, and political change. These multifaceted functions require expertise in communication and interpersonal relations.

### Interaction

Interactions amongst community systems contribute to community systems' ability to protect and promote the health and well-being of community members. For example, certain human-activity patterns negatively alter natural environmental patterns, which in turn influence human health patterns. Gordon's (2016) assessment framework focuses on 11 health-related functional patterns that assume community and environment interaction from a systems perspective.

## COMMUNITY FROM A DEVELOPMENTAL PERSPECTIVE

A framework based on developmental theory can also be used to identify existing or potential health problems for particular age groups in communities. Community nurses, focusing on the total community population, use a developmental, age-correlated approach to identify health-promotion and health-protection activities.

Community nurses engage with community groups to co-create health resources that recognize differences in development and, thus, promote health and wellness. For example, adolescent single mothers of infants are often characterized as being at risk for emotional and physical health problems. However, community health nurses have demonstrated that with developmentally informed intensive support that is inclusive of emotional support, accessible health care, and programs that recognize their strengths and partner with mothers to meet their identified needs (e.g., allow them to continue their education and peer relationships), the potential for health problems is reduced (Ontario Centre of Excellence for Child and Youth Mental Health, 2014). Accidents are the greatest threat to children's health; therefore, accident-prevention activities become a priority for communities with a young population. Age-related risk factors associated with individuals and families can be extended to include community groups based on the demographics of the community.

# COMMUNITY FROM A RISK-FACTOR PERSPECTIVE

A risk factor may be an individual attribute, a characteristic, or an exposure that *determines* the likelihood of developing a disease or injury (WHO, 2019a). The influence of various risk factors differs from person to person and from group to group because of genetic composition, geographical location, lifestyle patterns, access to health-promoting resources, socioeconomic status, and education level. Some communities may be at high risk from a single risk factor, such as insufficient immunizations or exposure to asbestos in drinking water. Risk factors synergistically influence each other and have a cumulative effect on communities. Health inequity, social inequality, and environmental injustice increase community vulnerability and call for a nurse to partner with the community to remediate risk and advocate for equitable public policy (Research for Health-Informed Practice).

Communities, therefore, experience substantial differences in developing strength and meeting challenges to health and well-being. Community health nurses recognize that risks to health and well-being are multifactorial and correlational, and move beyond individual biology. For example, risk factors such as air pollution, smoking, and forms of radiation in various combinations may be related to high rates of lung cancer, emphysema, and bronchitis in a community. Similarly, a lack of culturally safe resources, or fear and mistrust by community members as a result of prior treatment to engage with health-promoting resources increases risk. The potential to identify risk factors and to provide relevant health-related resources forms one way for community health nurses to determine health-promotion and health-protection activities.

# ❖ GORDON'S FUNCTIONAL HEALTH PATTERNS: ASSESSMENT OF THE COMMUNITY

A variety of functional health pattern assessments may be used with communities. In this textbook, Gordon's (2016) functional health reference assessment is exemplified and may augment other assessments described in the literature.

## ◆ Health Perception–Health Management Pattern

The health perception–health management pattern identifies data about community health status, health-promotion and disease-prevention practices, and community members' perceptions of health (Gordon, 2016). Residents may perceive a threat to the health of members relating to issues reported in the media. Community health nurses provide information and education to address perceived health issues and develop community health management plans. For example, the opioid crisis in Canada is a complex public health issue that is related to the high rates of opioid prescribing and the development of strong synthetic opioids, such as fentanyl, in the illegal drug supply.

## ⚡ RESEARCH FOR EVIDENCE-INFORMED PRACTICE

### Supporting the Health, Resilience, and Well-Being of Indigenous Youth

Hatala, Peral, Bird-Naytowhow, and colleagues (2017) used a community-based participatory research (CBPR) approach to better understand how community might support processes of resilience and well-being among urban Indigenous youth in Canada. CBPR relies on relationships that shape the research process, so that perspectives of community members are heard and generate knowledge that leads to social change. This is particularly important as meaningful engagement with youth can increase the scope, significance, and usefulness of research findings. Moreover, harmful practices as a result of colonization and racist othering of Indigenous peoples have contributed to a lack of trust of researchers, because past studies led to horrific public policy (e.g., residential schools).

In this study, the researchers engaged in ceremonies of relationship that recognized the sacredness of the stories the youth were sharing, helped build a relationship with youth and community members, and acknowledged that Indigenous ways of knowing and being are equally recognized throughout the research process. Examples of ceremonies included the opportunity for smudging, and talking circles that provided a safe place for youth and other community members to discuss experiences and directions in the research process. With a view to capacity building and empowerment, youth chose how and what data was collected, what parts of their stories could be shared outside the talking circle, and the ways that stories would be shared.

When relationships and trust were established, 28 youth agreed to be interviewed in a semi-structured interview. They shared their stories about how they managed moments of distress in their lives. It was recognized by the researchers that Indigenous youth lived alongside systemic social inequities and traumas resulting from racism, colonization, high rates of substance misuse, interpersonal violence, and suicide. While contemporary research with youth suggests that future-oriented youth are more likely to consider the consequences of their immediate behaviours and make choices in the present that will lead to a favourable outcome in the future, the question remained whether Indigenous youth, in the face of many challenges to health and well-being, could imagine a future for themselves.

Themes were identified in the interview data, and then presented to the youth for further reflections. A second round of interviews further refined the thematic interpretation. This study suggests that there are three ways in which Indigenous youth are supported: nurturing a sense of belonging, developing self-mastery, and fostering cultural continuity. Moreover, when these three processes are in place, youth exhibit more resilience toward immediate challenges by locating a place for themselves in the future.

Sources: Bird-Naytowhow, K., Hatala, A., Pearl, T., et al. (2017). Ceremonies of relationship: Engaging urban Indigenous youth in community-based research. *International Journal of Qualitative Methods, 16*, 1–14; Hatala, A., Peral, T., Bird-Naytowhow, K., et al. (2017). "I have strong hopes for the future": Time orientations and resilience among Canadian Indigenous youth. *Qualitative Health Research, 27*(9), 1330–1344.

From January to July 2016, more than 2000 deaths were reported (Government of Canada, 2019), sparking a public concern. Community nurses provided education and opioid-response education to strengthen community capacity in responding to the crisis.

Valuable information can be elicited by nurses conducting focus group discussions and by interviewing key community members about their health concerns and issues. Mortality and morbidity statistics and other public health information sources provide measurement data (see Chapter 2).

## ◆ Nutritional-Metabolic Pattern

The nutritional-metabolic pattern identifies data relevant to community consumption habits as reflected in accessibility and availability of food stores and subsidized food programs for infants, children, and older persons. Community well-being, which depends on adequate dietary habits, food intake, and supply of nutrients, is influenced by culture, the presence or absence of kitchen facilities, and adequate plumbing.

Community assessment includes the collection of data by driving or walking through the community while using all five senses; it provides information about grocery stores, fast-food establishments, ethnic shopping facilities, and street corner vendors. Even affluent and developed countries contain areas without adequate access to food, or "food deserts," places where fresh food is not available. Income and food insecurity are highly correlated. Food insecurity, affecting 12% of Canadian households in 2014, has grown with the growth in the urban poor population (Tarasuk, Mitchell, & Dachner, 2017). Children are significantly impacted by poor nutrition because their physiology is ever-changing and requires supportive nutrients. Poverty is the main contributor to household food insecurity. Social programming to reduce poverty is necessary and is located at the provincial/territorial and federal levels of government. Municipal responses such as "good food boxes," community gardens, food charters, and efforts toward buying local, healthy organic foods are also helpful (Collins, Power, & Little, 2014). Government programs, private soup kitchens, and food donations by houses of worship also provide information about nutritional patterns of communities.

## ◆ Elimination Pattern

The elimination pattern identifies environmental factors, including exposure to pollutants in the community through contaminated soil, water, and air, and the food chain. This pattern further classifies environmental factors into the two broad categories—physical and biological. Alterations in environmental processes threaten the health and integrity of communities, necessitating health-promotion and health-protection activities. For example, humans eliminate most endocrine-disrupting chemicals, pharmaceuticals, and personal care products into the environment (Noguera-Oviedo & Aga, 2016). Antibiotics and hormones from animals and fish also contaminate the environment. Groundwater, drinking water, surface water, and treatment plant effluents can be affected. Furthermore, some contaminants transform into contaminants that are more toxic than the original substance. For example, the antiviral acyclovir is excreted as a transformed product that is more toxic than the original drug (Schlüter-Vorberg, Prasse, Ternes, et al., 2015).

Physical agents include geological, geographical, climatic, and meteorological aspects of the community. Certain population groups are particularly susceptible to acute respiratory disease and aggravated asthmatic episodes when the air quality is poor (Solomon, Morello-Frosch, Ziese, et al., 2016). For example, when schools are located in high-pollution or high-traffic areas, children are exposed to polluted air. In addition, when home cooking devices pollute home air, families are exposed to polluted air (Pillarisetti, Mehta, & Smith, 2016). Use of solid fuel combustion such as wood or coal for cooking inside produces polluted home air. Community health nurses can use the Household Air Pollution Intervention Tool to plan interventions (Pillarisetti et al., 2016). Depending on resources, community collaborations, and partnerships, the community health nurse may use a variety of possible interventions to eliminate home air pollution from solid fuel cooking indoors. These interventions include simple chimney stoves with adequate exhaust, stoves with fan-assisted combustion, and/or clean fuel (Pillarisetti et al., 2016).

The geographical locations of communities, and major waterways, highways, or mountains located within communities, act as barriers to access to health facilities. Inaccessibility of health care services also hinders health in at-risk groups. Knowledge of climatic conditions provides clues to susceptibility to illness resulting from temperature or humidity in certain populations.

Biological agents include living things—such as plants, animals and their waste products, disease agents, microbial pathogens, and toxic substances—that can be hazardous to health. For example, Lyme disease, viral hepatitis, pneumonia, influenza, and the large number of diseases associated with childhood continue to be threats to community health. Observation, focus groups, and interviews with key community members reveal information concerning elimination patterns. Environment and Climate Change Canada (http://www.canada.ca/en/environment-climate-change.html.) and the Centers for Disease Control and Prevention (http://www.cdc.gov/globalhealth/countries/canada) provide excellent resources for community health nurses.

## ◆ Activity-Exercise Pattern

The activity-exercise pattern identifies physical activities and recreational options within communities. Science and technology have increasingly influenced productivity while simultaneously reducing or eliminating physical work. Consequently, physical activity no longer occurs during the work day for most community members, leaving leisure time as the only time for physical activity. Physiological evidence demonstrates that physical activity improves many biological measures associated with health and psychological functioning. Regular physical activity and musculoskeletal fitness are important for healthy, independent living as people grow older. Physical activity reduces the risk of many diseases, including obesity, heart disease, hypertension, cancer, osteoporosis, and diabetes mellitus.

Observation, focus groups, and interviews provide clues to a community's ability to provide cultural and recreational activities. Furthermore, noting whether the community has evidence of recreational facilities or is a "built community" with physical activity options (such as bike/walking trails), assessing transportation options, and observing community development that encourages walking should be included in the community assessment of the activity-exercise pattern.

## ◆ Sleep-Rest Pattern

The sleep-rest pattern identifies a community's rhythm of sleeping, resting, and relaxing. Some towns never close, with stores, traffic flow, and recreational facilities operating during both day and night hours. This ongoing activity produces unpleasant disturbances, such as unwanted noise, that may be harmful to community well-being. Excessive noise from highways or airplanes produces physiological or psychological problems eliciting responses ranging from mild irritation to pain or permanent hearing loss. Although noise cannot be eliminated, efforts to minimize and control it are possible. Observation, focus groups, and interviews provide clues to this pattern.

## ◆ Cognitive-Perceptual Pattern

The cognitive-perceptual pattern identifies information about community capacity to identify and respond to community health issues as they arise. Subsystems that provide environmental supports are informed by and rely upon policy decision making and resource allocation processes. Community assessment includes assessing how people interact with the systems in their environment, including how useful they perceive those resources to be in addressing their health needs. The effectiveness of all promotion strategies relies on the partnership between the community nurse and the community (Vollman et al., 2017).

Approaches to planning a partnership with a community include engaging in community social action to assist those adversely impacted by policy; promoting collective actions to bring community preferences to policymakers; and analyzing data and engaging with other health services to set goals and deliver programs. Information is gathered from community members and service providers.

## ◆ Self-Perception–Self-Concept Pattern

The self-perception–self-concept pattern identifies self-worth and personal identity of communities. Characteristics such as image, status, and perceived competency with problem solving indicate community self-concept. Housing conditions, buildings, and cleanliness reflect community image. School systems, crime rates, accidents, and opinions about whether the community is considered a good place to live suggest community perception of self-worth. Competency with social and political issues as well as community spirit creates positive self-evaluation. Community pride facilitates development of innovative health programs. Emotional tone (fear, depression, or positive emotional outlook) relates to findings in other pattern areas. For example, tensions in the cognitive-perceptual pattern (conflict between groups concerning health issues) may explain a general feeling of fear among the residents. Data are obtained through observation, focus groups, and interviews.

## ◆ Roles-Relationships Pattern

The roles-relationships pattern identifies communication styles along with formal and informal relationships. Of particular concern are roles and relationships affecting community ability to realize health potential. Patterns of crime, racial incidents, and social networks form indices of human relationships in communities. Publicizing health promotion becomes more effective when patterns of official communication are used.

Health program success depends on support from prominent community members. Community members involved in health programs help identify other key community leaders. Use of media and other mass information programs improves communication, the flow of health information, and the number of community members reached. Interviews, television, the Internet, and newspapers are examples of ways to obtain and convey information.

## ◆ Sexuality-Reproductive Pattern

The sexuality-reproductive pattern identifies reproductive data of communities, which is reflected in live birth statistics, mothers' ages, ethnicity, and marital status. This information provides clues to the health-promotion needs of a particular community group. Premature infant rates, low-birth-weight infants, and abortion rates, as well as neonatal, infant, and maternal death rates, reflect reproductive patterns of communities. Such information identifies at-risk groups on the basis of particular characteristics associated with these rates. Mismatches between existing health services, health education, and community health statistics also indicate health concerns. Availability of sex education in schools, the levels of intimate-partner and child abuse, and the number of sex-related crimes also indicate health-promotion issues. Minutes of meetings, health records, statistical data, and public documents provide sources for these data.

## ◆ Coping–Stress Tolerance Pattern

The coping–stress tolerance pattern identifies the community's ability to cope or adapt. Communities respond to stress in different ways, some of which might threaten their integrity. Community responses reveal the group coping patterns. Communities develop abilities to exchange goods, services, goals, values, and ideals to survive and to promote community health. Community efforts to obtain goods from the environment, contain goods within the environment, retain goods within the community, and dispose of goods play significant roles in influencing health. Examples of resources that communities obtain from the environment to promote health include local, state, or federal funding; health services; health-related workforce personnel; new knowledge; and technological advances. Some communities obtain abundant health care services; however, primary services often remain inadequate or nonexistent. Lack of available health services, or lack of ability to obtain them, characterizes community health needs. Examples of problems communities may attempt to control include sex-related crimes, diseases, substance abuse, industry, hazardous waste in the water supply, and noxious chemicals in the air.

Community coping patterns aim to retain certain health-protection services, such as immunization services for children and adequate health facilities. Coping efforts may also include strict zoning laws and housing codes or certain values such as sex education within the home. Expendable goods of communities include industrial and human wastes. Data can be obtained through minutes of meetings, public documents, health surveys, statistical data, and health records.

## TABLE 8.2   Stages of Change

| Stages | Community Stages | Interventions |
|---|---|---|
| Precontemplation | Community does not recognize a problem, know the consequences to health and well-being, or feel a need to change | Community assessment; strategize on how and for whom sharing the assessment will have the biggest impact |
| Contemplation | Community recognizes problem and contemplates change and preventive changes | Raising awareness |
| Planning or preparation | Community members intend to participate in the process of changing the problem | Building networks |
| Action | Health-promoting activities commence; policies are changed to support the change as needed | Actions are taken |
| Maintenance | Problem has changed for more than 6 months; community members seek out ways to ensure sustainability of the change | Consolidating efforts |

Modified from Prochaska, J., Redding, C. & Evers, K. (2015). The transtheoretical model and stages of change. In K. Glanz, B. Rimer & K. Viswanath (Eds.), *Healthy behaviour: Theory, research and practice* (5th ed., pp. 125–148). San Francisco: Jossey Bass.

## ◆ Values-Beliefs Pattern

The values-beliefs pattern identifies the community values and beliefs. Such information provides clues for health-promotion and health-protection efforts valued by the community. Values underlie decisions about community health education and tax support for schools, hypertension screening for the public, disease-prevention programs, or well-child clinics. Traditions, norms, and cultural and ethnic groups share values and beliefs in communities. Data can be obtained through focus groups, town hall meetings, and through interviews with key community members and health-related personnel.

## ANALYSIS AND DIAGNOSIS WITH THE COMMUNITY

A community nurse draws some conclusions based on the evidence collected and health promotion–population health-informed reasoning. Often times, analysis leads to more data collection as trends and patterns in health are compared and contrasted to evidences about population health. A community diagnosis includes statements about what is working well for the community members and ideas about what may be strengthened and changed to promote optimal health and well-being. An example of a clinical scenario about a particular community is presented in the case study and care plan at the end of this chapter. Table 8.2 presents an example of one way to think about partnering with a community using Prochaska's stages of change.

## Organization of Data

Charts, figures, and tables graphically display population distributions, morbidity and mortality data, or vital statistics to pinpoint significant community concerns with actual or potential health problems along with health-related responses to these concerns. Another valuable organizational technique—mapping—facilitates simultaneous analysis of several variables. Overlap of the locations of environmental hazards, densely populated areas, health-promotion services, and major highways becomes apparent. Poor environmental conditions; the distribution of illness, disease, and death rates; and accessibility of health-protection and health-promotion activities for the population appear at a glance with dotted scatter maps. Use of maps requires knowledge about the community's population base. Less-populated rural areas with fewer health facilities or fewer neonatal deaths in a community with fewer women of childbearing age are examples of how population statistics influence interpretation of mapping techniques. Use of the community-as-partner assessment wheel provides a one-page summary of strengths and challenges in a community. Gordon's (2016) 11 pattern areas facilitates analysis of community data. Several guidelines, presented next, help community nurses analyze population data.

## Guidelines for Data Analysis
### Check for Missing Data
The complexity, size, and number of community characteristics prohibit all possible facts about the health-related pattern areas being gathered; however, missing or insufficient data that indicate areas for further assessment should be identified. Additional assessment may determine specific approaches or a particular community diagnosis. Examples of missing data in community assessment include pollution indices, links between health resources and population groups, accessibility to resources, and morbidity statistics. Dates for census data used should be noted.

The nurse examines community data for incongruities and conflicting information. For example, a key community official might deny the existence of pollutants in the water supply, whereas newspaper reports of health department water analysis findings indicate otherwise. The nurse evaluates such inconsistencies before identifying existing or potential health concerns.

### Identify Patterns

Clues about a community pattern emerge from subjective and objective data gathered. During this stage, community nurses make decisions, begin to formulate diagnostic hypotheses (ideas and tentative judgements about possible health concerns), identify community groups that might be at risk, and establish probable causes or relationships. Ideas generated from this activity direct the search for additional clues in the data to confirm, reject, or revise hypotheses. Judgements about hypotheses continue to support patterns in the data.

To narrow the huge list of possible community health-promotion and health-protection concerns, community nurses formulate broad problem statements based on the health-related pattern areas (Gordon, 2016). For example, the community nurse differentiates among elimination problems (e.g., noxious chemicals), coping and stress-tolerance problems, and health perception–health management problems (e.g., high teenage mortality rate from motor vehicle accidents). Developing these general categories facilitates analysis.

## Apply Theories, Models, Norms, and Standards

Analysis of community data requires extensive knowledge of developmental, age-related risks, as well as theories and concepts of nursing, public health, and epidemiology. Such a broad foundation enables nurses to identify additional clues in health-related patterns that contribute to community nursing diagnoses and intervention. Developmental approaches form a basis to identify groups with potential health concerns. Age groups differ in susceptibility; therefore, nurses examine community resources directed toward highly susceptible groups. For example, community data that show increases in the number of live births among older women indicate a need for health-promotion services for this group. If community data show increasing numbers of aging citizens, nurses explore the availability and accessibility of existing health services for this older group.

Analysis of data for common personal or environmental characteristics also occurs. For example, select groups may be at risk on the basis of a shared health concern, such as substance abuse, lack of immunizations, unsafe housing conditions, high exposure to asbestos or noxious chemicals, or inadequate health services. In addition, community literacy contributes to health-promotion activity development methods used by nurses to establish educational programs. A low-literacy level limits community member's ability to use all available resources.

Environmental information is readily available on the Internet. Databases and search engines provide useful information about environmental hazards and other environmental problems in communities. Prevention of disease worldwide depends on the dissemination of global environmental health information (WHO, 2019b). Analysis of data relies on standards developed nationally or globally. For example, community data regarding air quality can be compared with provincial/territorial or national ambient air quality standards to determine health. In this context, the term *ambient* refers to outside air in a town, city, or other defined region. In Canada, air-monitoring stations are generally located in each province. The Canadian Air and Precipitation Monitoring Network (CAPMoN), operated by Environment and Climate Change Canada (ECCC), is designed to study the regional patterns and trends of atmospheric pollutants such as acid rain, smog, particulate matter, and mercury, in both air and precipitation. The goal of this network is to serve as a resource for publicly available data to use for analysis and research. Data are continually monitored and updated (ECCC, 2018). Current information about community resources enables more effective strategies to prevent risk factors and avoid health problems. Internet access facilitates identification of gaps in health-promotion and health-protection services.

## Identify Strengths and Health Concerns

Interpretation of community data occurs with regard to community concerns, community strengths, and feasibility studies. Community nurses make judgements and inferences about community health, community responses to health situations,

**TABLE 8.3 Examples of Community Strengths and Concerns**

| Strengths | Concerns |
|---|---|
| Well-child clinic available | Unavailable |
| Feeding program accessible to older persons | Inaccessible |
| Sex education in schools acceptable | Unacceptable |
| Family planning services accessible | Inaccessible |
| Fluoridated water system | Nonfluoridated water system |
| Open communication | Dysfunctional communication |
| Interagency cooperation | Dysfunctional transactions |
| Adequate kitchen and plumbing facilities | Inadequate |
| High interest of key leaders in health promotion | Lack of interest |

and population needs. Other systems of assessment base decisions on community strengths. It is important to note that assessment data provide the nurse with information about possible or actual problems in the community. The use of strength-based approaches to assessment emphasizes strengths and integrates health-promotion and health-protection activities into a person's plans. For example, a community may have nutritional feeding programs for older persons, women, and children that are underutilized. Community members may not use them because communication is inadequate. Examples of community strengths and concerns are shown in Table 8.3.

## Identify Causes and Risk Factors

Identification of risk factors guides community nursing actions. Some risk factors signify immediate health concerns, such as a polluted water supply, whereas other risk factors indicate potential problems, such as lack of knowledge of childhood disease prevention. Nurses consider whether community risk factors can be altered, eliminated, or regulated through nursing actions. Nurses modify risk factors when possible by using strategies such as health education (Diversity Awareness).

## Community Diagnosis

Community assessment, as previously described, culminates in a community nursing diagnosis. Community data are summarized and analyzed considering how the social determinants of health interact and impact the health of community members. Existing strengths, health concerns, and potential health concerns (risk factors) are identified and compared with other community systems and evidence about community health. Inferences are then written as a diagnostic statement, which typically has four parts describing:
1. The community or population of focus
2. Actual or potential community strengths or challenges to supporting health and well-being
3. Factors of influence on the strength or challenge to health
4. Evidences gathered to support that diagnostic statement

*Example:* children at risk of health challenges related to obesity (*population of focus*); influenced by low family income (*challenge*), influencing diet intake, unsafe park and recreation areas in the neighbourhood (*factors of influence*), evidenced by census data reporting income, a windshield survey of the neighbourhood, and public health research reports (*evidences gathered*).

## ⊕ DIVERSITY AWARENESS

### *Promoting Health and Wellness for Community Youth in Northern Canada*

Mental health and wellness is one of the most pressing issues for Indigenous youth in Canada today. A recent public health survey revealed that suicide rates are 6.5 times higher in places with a concentration of Inuit people, 3.7 times higher for First Nations people, and 2.7 times for Métis people (Minister of Health, 2018). The Truth and Reconciliation Commission of Canada (TRC) (2015) reported about the devastating effects of historical colonization practices toward Indigenous people in Canada, particularly the generational effects of residential schools. Examining high rates of suicide in communities is but one indicator of the effects of trauma on communities. For many survivors, addressing post-trauma begins with a process of healing themselves, their communities, and nations, and relies on the revitalization of Indigenous cultures, languages, spirituality, laws, and governance systems (TRC, 2015).

Community nurses are well-positioned to engage with communities who embark on this healing journey. The nurse is responsible for understanding the effects of colonizing practices on community members, and how that history impacts the ways in which health and well-being of Indigenous community members is described and supported.

The following case example demonstrates how community members identified the need to instill programs to assist youth, informed by evidences from health research and Indigenous knowledges about healing and health.

#### Case Example

The Eight *Ujarit*/Rocks model was developed to promote the health and well-being of youth in Nunavut during a critical stage of adolescent development (Healey, Noah, & Means, 2016). *Ujarit* is the Inuktitut word for rocks. Symbolizing a solid rock foundation, eight modules were developed and grounded in research, best practice and community perspective (see The Eight *Ujarit*/Rocks Model, later in this box). The intervention modules reflect the social context, language and values of the population (Inuit youth) for whom it was designed. The modules were delivered through a camp program that demonstrates a positive impact beyond the camp experience into the community. Early evaluation data reveal that youth, families, and their community improved relationships in family, community, and to the land (Healey et al., 2016). Key to this program is that the model was developed by the community and reflected community values.

#### *Reflective Questions*

Cultural humility refers to the nurse's ability to relate to aspects of cultural identity that are most important to others. When working with communities, diversity in knowledge about health and how to promote health are recognized and respected. The following questions invite you to think about your own cultural values and how they may impact on your work with communities:

*   How do the TRC findings inform your ideas about the health and well-being of Indigenous people?
*   How might a nurse who is working with an Indigenous community demonstrate cultural humility?

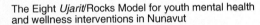
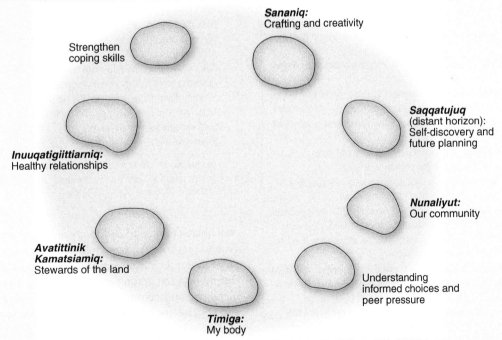

The Eight *Ujarit*/Rocks Model for youth mental health and wellness interventions in Nunavut

Strengthen coping skills

*Sananiq:* Crafting and creativity

*Saqqatujuq* (distant horizon): Self-discovery and future planning

*Inuuqatigiittiarniq:* Healthy relationships

*Nunaliyut:* Our community

*Avatittinik Kamatsiamiq:* Stewards of the land

Understanding informed choices and peer pressure

*Timiga:* My body

The Eight *Ujarit*/Rocks Model. (Figure from Healey, G., Noah, J., & Mearns, C. (2016). The eight *Ujarait* (Rocks) model: supporting Inuit adolescent mental health with an intervention model based on Inuit knowledge and ways of knowing. *International Journal of Indigenous Health, 11*(1), 92–110.)

## ⚡ QUALITY AND SAFETY SCENARIO

### *Workplace Violence*

The following are some recommendations to minimize workplace violence:
* Encourage public awareness campaigns.
* Develop workplace policies and plans.
* Adopt a zero-tolerance workplace violence policy.
* Apply preventive law enforcement policies.
* Perform background checks on employees.
* Study government agencies that make workplace violence a priority.
* Provide proper training for employees, supervisors, and managers about warning signs of violent behaviour.
* Encourage a workplace culture that facilitates healthy relationships, creative problem solving, and voicing concerns while discouraging a hostile environment.
* Expect nonautocratic leadership styles.
* Prevent/minimize negative coworker behaviour.
* Encourage social support (listening, recognition) for employees to succeed at their work.
* Implement strategies to minimize absenteeism, turnover, and low performance.
* Implement strategies to encourage participatory management.
* Ensure protection of the abused person when domestic violence or stalking occurs in the workplace.
* Develop and distribute clear and comprehensive legal and legislative guidelines.
* Evaluate programs and strategies after they have been implemented. Suggestions for approaches included the following strategies:
* Educational efforts should reflect cooperative efforts by employers, unions, and advocacy groups.
* Enact multidisciplinary no-threats/no-violence policies and prevention plans.
* Violence prevention training should occur regularly and include practicing the plan.
* The work space and policies should provide a physically secure work environment.
* Preventive measures should be established, including documenting incidents, planning antiviolence strategies, and conducting threat assessments.
* Systems should be developed for the monitoring of incidents of workplace violence.
* Resource lists should be maintained and include social service, mental health, legal, and other agencies that provide assistance.
* Training programs should extend community policing concepts to workplace violence. Government or private organizations should develop training materials for small employers. Employers should keep the abuser out of the workplace (e.g., screening telephone calls, making the victim's work space physically more secure, instructing security guards or receptionists).
* Employers should provide resources for emotional, financial, and legal counselling. Clear, comprehensive, and uniform legal guidelines should be distributed widely.
* Incentives for employers should be identified and instituted.

Source: Modified from Cowie, A. K. (2016). Some predictors of workplace violence. *From Science to Practice: Organizational Psychology Bulletin, 2*(1), 13–14.

## 🖐 INNOVATIVE PRACTICE

### *Intervention Techniques to Prevent and Diffuse Workplace Violence*

Lanza, Ridenour, Hendricks, and colleagues (2016) reported their findings from a research study exploring the benefits of an innovative community intervention to prevent and diffuse workplace violence. The community meetings used a format (the violence-prevention community meeting [VPCM]) designed to minimize violence and promote nonviolent problem solving and acting with civility. Their study included patients and staff on seven locked psychiatric units in the US Veterans Health Administration. During 21 weeks, each site had a VPCM during the middle 7 weeks, with 7 weeks before the VPCM and 7 weeks after the VPCM. After the VPCM, aggression rates dropped. In addition to innovative strategies such as the VPCM, the following techniques may also be useful:
* Recognize warning signs, which include changes in mood, personal hardships, mental health issues (e.g., depression, anxiety), negative behaviour (e.g., untrustworthy, lying, bad attitude), verbal threats, and history of violence.
* Do not limit at-risk behaviour to a standard profile.
* Environments should be designed to detect signs of impending violence and to prevent violence with security cameras, key card access, administrative controls, and behavioural strategies.
* Reporting systems should be confidential and seamless.
* Stay calm; create a relaxed environment and speak calmly.
* Separate the individual from the group, if possible.
* Use nonthreatening body language; build trust and strengthen the relationship.
* Keep your verbal communication simple, clear, and direct; be open and honest.
* Reflect on the person's message to allow time for clarification, allow the person to verbalize, listen attentively, and stop what you are doing and give full attention.
* Ask for examples to help illustrate the points that are being made. Carefully define the problem, exploring it with open-ended questions.
* Silence allows the individual time to clarify thoughts.
* Monitor the tone, volume, rate, and rhythm of your speech.
* Seek opportunities for agreement.
* Be creative and open to new ideas.

Source: Lanza, M., Ridenour, M., Hendricks, S., et al. (2016). The violence prevention community meeting: A multi-site study. *Archives of Psychiatric Nursing, 30*(3), 382–386.

contributes to quality and safety and how leaders might intervene to prevent or diffuse violence.

Community diagnoses and problem structuring facilitate communication among community health professionals, team members, and community members through the use of clear and concise nomenclature with development of diagnostic categories using both inductive and deductive reasoning specific to community nursing (Frerichs et al., 2016). Diagnoses may be written or stated according to the structural and functional aspects of a community.

Structural aspects include those related to the population, such as the demographic characteristics of groups with similar characteristics (preschool children, adolescents, or a high school population). Functional aspects include those related to the psychosocial, physiological, or spiritual health patterns,

Diagnostic statements form the basis for planning, implementing, and evaluating nursing approaches to health challenges. The Quality and Safety Scenario and Innovative Practice boxes provide an overview of how workplace violence such as decision making (cognitive-perceptual pattern) or communication links among health care resources (roles-relationships pattern). Functional health patterns guide data collection about health concerns. Structural and functional aspects of the community provide a framework for diagnostic statements (see Chapter 6).

## PLANNING WITH THE COMMUNITY

Community health planning begins with nurses participating with community members to design goals to resolve existing or potential health concerns. For example, high rates of childhood diseases in the community require goals aimed at decreasing rates. Identification of specific or potential health concerns with planned actions to achieve desired community outcomes provides the framework and data for community evaluation.

### Purposes

The following are major purposes of the planning phase:

- Prioritization of problems and identification of diagnoses through assessment
- Differentiation of problems resolved through nursing actions from those best resolved by others
- Reduction or elimination of disparities in health experienced by community members, improving quality of life, strengthening community action on the determinants of health
- Formalization of a community nursing care plan (see the Care Plan at the end of this chapter) that includes written problems, actions, and proposed outcomes

The planning phase culminates in a community nursing plan that provides the framework for evaluation. Once developed, the plan is implemented. The costs associated with the delivery of health services and personnel, as well as the financial resources available, often influence the priorities for implementation. Community health nurses often act as advocates for communities who are not receiving the health-promoting resources and services they require. High-priority issues often include programs directed toward protecting the health of community members, for example, the prevention of infectious agents.

Community participation in health planning contributes to a strengths-based approach to determining which resources the community requires to address challenges to health and well-being. Communities are composed of diverse groups of people with varied capacity to access health resources.

During the planning phase, nurses determine those problems most amenable to community nursing intervention. Community nurses differentiate problems nursing can resolve from those health concerns that could best be managed by an intersectoral and/or interprofessional approach to addressing community concerns. Nurses partner with other health-related systems in the community to address threats to health, for example, calling attention to poor sanitation or the absence of community recreational facilities to community.

Community nurses identify goals with the community, develop measurable objectives, and participate in actions to achieve improved health and well-being. Evaluation in community intervention is continual, as more information is gathered with each community contact. Health planning emphasizes promoting and protecting population health; therefore problems, solutions, and actions require participation by community members, groups, and systems. Community nurses plan and implement health-promotion plans at the level of greatest impact. Following the Ottawa Charter mentioned earlier in this chapter, the community health nurse may engage with individuals or groups to develop personal skills and create supportive environments. However, reorienting health services and contributing to the building of health-oriented public policy through community actions may result in the community health nurse contributing to change at the community system or larger political system.

### Planned Change

Community health interventions that depend on active decisions by individuals to change their lifestyles (reducing alcohol consumption or quitting smoking) become the central focus of effective risk reduction programs (Brown, Todd, O'Malley, et al., 2016).

Health-promotion theorists attempt to explain why some groups of people effectively participate in certain health programs or make lifestyle changes, whereas others do not. Pender, Murdaugh, and Parson's (2014) theory of health promotion identifies critical concepts for understanding how individuals change their health behaviour, suggesting that if a health threat is believed to be serious enough, community members will assume more responsibility for their own health, become more active in adopting healthy lifestyles, and utilize resources in the community to achieve healthy behaviours. However, health promotion *only* as risk reduction may present a limited view of health if the social contexts within which individuals are asked to make lifestyle choices and changes are overlooked or ignored. Recognition of the structural determinants of health embedded within economic, class, cultural, and gender-based patterns of social relationships assist the community health nurse to locate at which system level community-oriented change ought to take place. Table 8.1 provides one example of a community-oriented, health-promotion plan that targets change at multisystems levels. Examples of various rationales in Table 8.1 show how nurses incorporate important concepts of planned change into community-based health-promotion plans.

Communication and collaborative relationships amongst community stakeholders remain an essential aspect of planning. Local newspapers, local bulletins, and school correspondence to parents provide avenues to communicate with the community about health-promotion plans. Other community-based actions, such as those for nursing involvement with community coalitions that seek to address growing concerns with substance misuse in the community, can be used effectively to influence change within the larger systems such as healthy public policy. A community health nurse plans change across multiple systems levels, working within the intersections of community systems.

## TABLE 8.4 Potential Barriers to Health-Promotion Programs Uptake, With Nurse Responses

| Barrier | Nurse Response |
| --- | --- |
| Lack of communication: opportunity for input into the health-promotion program or opportunity to participate | Communicate through community newsletters, newspapers, posters in high schools and community centres, and social media sites: offer opportunities throughout the development and implementation of the program |
| Misinformation regarding time and place of healthy activity | Disseminate valid information |
| Fear of unknown | Inform, listen to community member concerns, encourage ideas, support introduction of new information in a culturally respectful manner |
| Need for security | Transparency in intentions and methods used |
| No desired or perceived need to change behaviours | Provide information, demonstrate impacts of change, and answer questions |
| Cultural or religious beliefs or vested interests threatened | Enlist key community leaders in planning change; modify intended change to fit with community concerns |
| Inaccessibility | Focus activities near the largest target population and in an area accessible by public transportation; advocate for assistance to access resources |

## IMPLEMENTATION WITH THE COMMUNITY

In collaboration with community members or other health team members, the community health nurse implements the health-promotion plan. Involving key community members, in the assessment and planning process, is crucial for success. To ensure involvement, activities must be accessible. For example, schedule meetings in accessible areas, offer child care services and provide light refreshments. Identify clearly what the community perceives as health-promotion needs. Maintain open communication—provide clear and correct information at regular intervals, and if necessary, amend the proposed health-promotion plan as necessary to ensure that community members' needs are being respected.

Perceived resistance to health-promotion and health-protection activities provides useful feedback to modify, as necessary, community interventions. Collaborating with communities ensures that the community needs are being met and facilitates change during the implementation phase. Table 8.4 lists possible barriers to community participation and offers ways for nurses to respond.

Community nurses promote health in multiple community settings (schools, industry, public and health agencies, and ambulatory care settings). Nursing centres provide nursing faculty, staff, and students with unique opportunities to assess health and to plan, implement, and evaluate care (including holistic health promotion and primary health care) for individuals, families, and communities with unmet health care needs (Harvey, Fisher, & Green, 2012). The complexity of health-promoting actions differs from one community to another. As plans evolve, nurses learn more about the community and their own responses, strengths, limitations, and abilities to cope or adapt (Subica, Grills, Douglas, et al., 2016). Although implementation takes an action focus, it also includes assessment, planning, and evaluation activities to monitor actions taken to resolve, reduce, eliminate, or control the health concern.

## EVALUATION WITH THE COMMUNITY

During the evaluation phase of the process, community nurses in partnership with the community gather information to determine whether planned actions achieved desired outcomes. Nurses take overall responsibility for the process; however, collaborating with community members and allied health team members in the process produces comprehensive results. For example, if implemented plans intend to reduce the incidence of fatal motor vehicle accidents, nurses guide the process to obtain community indicators and outcomes data, requisite community actions, and expected outcomes achieved from joint collaboration with community stakeholders.

Community nurses approach the dynamic process of evaluation in a purposeful, goal-directed manner (Stanhope, Lancaster, & Jakubec (2017)). The frequency of evaluation depends on the situations, changes expected, and objectives. Evaluation intervals differ depending on immediate, intermediate, and long-range goals. The evaluation process continues until community goals are realized or modified.

Evaluation results indicate the need for reassessment, revision, or modification of plans. In partnership with community stakeholders, community health nurses reassess, plan new approaches, and implement and evaluate revised plans, ensuring that the health-promotion plan is collaborative, inclusive, and equitable.

Workable, cost-effective programs of community health promotion are necessary to achieve health for all community health members. Nurses play an important role in providing evidence to support effective community health plans. Historically, documentation of effective health-promotion activities has been limited (Maurer & Smith, 2014; Pender et al., 2014). Effectiveness is determined through research studies that include analyses and outcomes evaluation of home-based and community-centred nursing interventions designed to meet the health and well-being of all the community, particularly those who experience barriers to health care resources.

## CASE STUDY

### Community Efforts to Improve Resources for LGBTQ2 Adolescents

Lesbian, gay, bisexual, transgender, and questioning/queer (LGBTQ2) youth are at increased risk for smoking, alcohol consumption, illicit drug use, HIV risk behaviours, teen pregnancy, discrimination, violence victimization, depression, and suicidal ideation and attempts (Eisenberg, Mehus, Saewyc, et al., 2018). The community health nurse is aware that strengths and supports in the community promote positive health comes for LGBTQ2 youth. In particular, there is evidence to suggest that inclusive education, gay–straight alliances, and antibullying in policies in schools provide critical support (Coulter, Birkett, Corliss, et al., 2016). The nurse was contacted by several concerned parents of a local high school Parent Advisory Council who wished to make their school a safe and healthy school for everyone. One parent expressed concern that her child had experienced some bullying in school, which they believed was related to a lack of understanding of LGBTQ2 youth. When she had taken her concern to the parent advisory group, although supportive, they were unsure how to address the problem.

The school offered health courses twice between Grade 7 and Grade 12. Within the context of these two health courses, most of the materials were focused on promoting safe sexual health practices for heterosexual youth (e.g., risks associated with sexually transmitted infections, risk of pregnancy, and the influence of alcohol and drugs on consent). The nurse thinks that perhaps meeting with parents and teachers is a good place to begin to assess the school community's commitment to making the school a safe and positive space for all students. In the meeting, the nurse suggests engaging youth leaders in a social marketing approach.

#### Reflective Questions
- How could the school members, including parent advisory members, approach its goal to improve resources for LGBTQ2 youth and create a safe and positive space?
- How might the community group approach this issue with the support of all youth in the school?

## CARE PLAN

### Community Efforts to Improve Resources for LGBTQ2 Adolescents

#### Nursing Issue
Risk of ineffective community coping as a result of lack of knowledge about and support for LGBTQ2 youth, as evidenced by recent research outlining the resources needed to ensure schools are safe, equitable, and health promoting.

#### Defining Characteristics
- Absence of support for LGBTQ2 teenagers
- Absence of programs for promoting and supporting gay–straight alliances
- Absence of antibullying policies related to sexual orientation
- Community conflicts over how to or when to teach adolescent and preadolescent children about diversity in sexual preference
- Failure of all youth to perceive the long-term effects of bullying and socially isolating behaviours
- High incidence of anxiety, depression, or mental health impacts in youth experiencing bullying and social marginalization
- High rate of school drop outs of youth who do not feel safe at school and/or school becomes a source of anxiety and fear
- Lack of access to preferred pronouns or other non-hetero visuals in the school (e.g., rainbow flag)
- Lack of community awareness about health-promotive and supportive programs

#### Related Factors
- Community members' lack of knowledge about the effects of overlooking LGBTQ2 youth needs in schools
- Inadequate school resources to support LGBTQ2 youth
- Lack of adequate communication patterns and community cohesiveness regarding strategies to support LGBTQ2 youth

#### Interventions
- Assess teenagers' knowledge of LGBTQ2 and the harmful effects of non-acceptance to determine their educational needs.
- Work with schoolteachers and parents and LGBTQ2 to develop LGBTQ2 resources.
- Work closely with individual adolescents who are LGBTQ2 to assess their needs and provide care.
- Implement an outreach and health-promotion program to raise the school community members' awareness of the need to make schools a safe place to learn.
- Consider taking the following five steps:
  - Work with teachers, school psychologists, counsellors, school nurses, students, and the parent–teacher association to determine the extent of bullying or other harmful practices.

- Encourage local LGBTQ2 youth groups and social service organizations to feature presentations on how to support LGBTQ2 youth in class and in school spaces.
- Contact representatives of local corporations to ask for funding for educational programs.
- Help community members (school nurses, counsellors, and teachers) recognize the importance of listening attentively and remaining nonjudgemental.
- Establish clubs for LGBTQ2 in the community. The goal of these clubs is to foster self-esteem. During club meetings, members should have the opportunity to openly discuss difficult questions, and how to respond to bullying or other harmful peer encounters.
- Encourage all adolescents to participate in peer-support networks (gay–straight alliances) where they can openly discuss social and dating pressure and other issues related to sexuality, to allow them an opportunity to express their feelings openly and obtain support from peers.
- Encourage community members to establish school-based clinics in which teens can have access to sexual health materials.
- Develop a list of supportive community resources for LGBTQ2 youth.
- Encourage school community members to implement a campaign to provide information to adolescents, parents, and community members about the problems associated with not supporting LGBTQ2 youth.
- Work with school community members to evaluate the effectiveness of the resources developed and assist in modifying it as needed to ensure its effectiveness and promote the program as a model for preventive health.
- Collect statistical data from the schools to analyze the bullying, school dropout rates, to help evaluate the effectiveness of the prevention program.

#### Intended Outcomes
- School and community members express awareness of the needs of LGBTQ2 youth.
- Community members express the need to develop and evaluate supportive resources for LGBTQ2 youth.
- Community members develop and implement plans to address bullying, provide safe spaces, and support LGBTQ2 youth in the classroom (e.g., use of pronouns).
- Community members evaluate the success of the plan in meeting goals and objectives.
- Community members continue to revise the plan to support LGBTQ2 youth as necessary.

## SUMMARY

Challenges to health and well-being are not inevitable events experienced equally among a community's members. Community health nurses understand the dynamic and complex nature of determining health and collaborative health promotion with communities (Fig. 8.6). Community nurses, through partnership with the community, contribute to reducing the risks associated with disease, premature death, and injury as well as engaging in health-promoting activities with a view to achieving health and well-being for all community members. Community health nurses may use various theoretical frameworks to assess health-related patterns, and engage with communities to understand their health concerns. In partnership with the community, the nurse collaborates, advocates, and informs at multiple systems levels to ensure equity.

Nurses use principles of planned change to increase community awareness of health, and to promote health and healthy public policy. Communities are complex, diverse, culturally unique and geographical impacted. Community nurses connect health-promotion actions to specific community phenomena, providing scientific evidence to support nursing actions in the community.

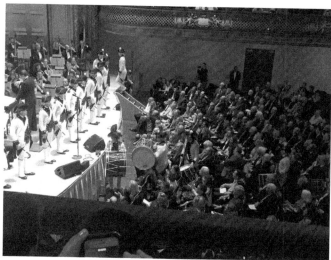

**Fig. 8.6** Communities Come Together for the Enjoyment of One of Their Traditional Holidays (iStockphoto/Thinkstock.)

### Evolve Chapter Features

http://evolve.elsevier.com/Canada/Edelman/healthpromotion/
- Review Questions

## REFERENCES

Bird-Naytowhow, K., Hatala, A., Pearl, T., et al. (2017). Ceremonies of relationship: Engaging urban Indigenous youth in community-based research. *International Journal of Qualitative Methods, 16,* 1–14. https://doi.org/10.1177/1609406917707899.

Brown, T. J., Todd, A., O'Malley, C., et al. (2016). Community pharmacy-delivered interventions for public health priorities: A systematic review of interventions for alcohol reduction, smoking cessation and weight management, including meta-analysis for smoking cessation. *BMJ Open, 6*(2):e009828. https://doi.org/10.1136/bmjopen-2015-009828.

Canadian Institute for Health Information (CIHI). (2006). *How healthy are rural Canadians? An assessment of their health status and health determinants.* Ottawa: Author.

Canadian Nurses Association (CNA). (2005). *The ecosystem, the natural environment and health and nursing: A summary of the issues.* Ottawa: Author.

Canadian Nurses Association (CNA). (2017). *Position statement: Nurses and environmental health.* Ottawa: Author. Retrieved from https://www.cna-aiic.ca/~/media/cna/page-content/pdf-en/nurses-and-environmental-health-position-statement.pdf.

Chappells, H., Campbell, N., Drage, J., et al. (2015). Understanding the translation of scientific knowledge about arsenic risk exposure among private well users. *The Science of the Total Environment, 505,* 1259–1273. https://doi.org/10.1016/j.scitotenv.2013.12.108.

Collins, P., Power, E., & Little, M. (2014). Municipal-level responses to household food insecurity in Canada: A call for critical, evaluative research. *Canadian Journal of Public Health, 105*(2), e138–e141.

Commission on the Social Determinants of Health (CSDH). (2008). *Closing the gap in a generation: Health equity through action on the social determinants of health. Final report of the commission on social determinants of health.* Geneva: World Health Organization.

Community Health Nurses of Canada (CHNC). (2019, revised). *Canadian community health nursing professional practice model & standards of practice.* Retrieved from https://www.chnc.ca/standards-of-practice.

Coulter, R., Birkett, M., Corliss, H. L., et al. (2016). Associations between LGBTQ-affirmative school climate and adolescent drinking behaviors. *Drug and Alcohol Dependence, 161,* 340–347. https://doi.org/10.1016/j.drugalcdep.2016.02.022.

Dahlgren, G., & Whitehead, M. (1991). *Policies and strategies to promote social equity in health.* Stockholm, Sweden: Institute for Future Studies. Retrieved from https://www.iffs.se/policies-and-strategies/.

Das, J., Salam, R., Arshad, A., et al. (2016). Interventions for adolescent substance use: An overview of systematic reviews. *Journal of Adolescent Health, 59,* 561–575.

Eisenberg, M., Mehus, C., Saewyc, E., et al. (2018). Helping young people stay afloat: A qualitative study of community resources and supports for LGBTQ adolescents in the United States and Canada. *Journal of Homosexuality, 65*(8), 969–989. https://doi.org/10.1080/00918369.2017.1364944.

Environment and Climate Change Canada (ECCC). (2018). Canadian air and precipitation monitoring network (CAPMoN). Retrieved from http://data.ec.gc.ca/data/air/monitor/networks-and-studies/canadian-air-and-precipitation-monitoring-network-capmon/.

Frerichs, L., Lich, K. H., Dave, G., et al. (2016). Integrating systems science and community-based participatory research to achieve health equity. *American Journal of Public Health, 106*(2), 215–222. https://doi.org/10.2105/AJPH.2015.302944.

Gordon, M. (2016). *Manual of nursing diagnosis* (13th ed.). Sudbury, MA: Jones & Bartlett.

Government of Canada. (2019b). *Infographic: Opioid-related harms in Canada: December 2018.* Retrieved from https://www.canada.ca/en/health-canada/services/publications/healthy-living/infographic-opioid-related-harms-december-2018.html.

Graham, I., Logan, J., Harrison, M., et al. (2006). Lost in knowledge translation: Time for a map? *Journal of Continuing Education in the Health Professions, 26*(1), 13–24. https://doi.org/10.1002/chp.47.

Harvey, S. T., Fisher, L. J., & Green, V. M. (2012). Evaluating the clinical efficacy of a primary care–focused, nurse-led, consultation liaison model for perinatal mental health. *International Journal of Mental Health Nursing, 21*(1), 75–81.

Hatala, A., Peral, T., Bird-Naytowhow, K., et al. (2017). "I have strong hopes for the future": Time orientations and resilience among Canadian Indigenous youth. *Qualitative Health Research, 27*(9), 1330–1344. https://doi.org/10.1177/1049732317712489.

Healey, G., Noah, J., & Mearns, C. (2016). The eight *Ujarait* (rocks) model: Supporting Inuit adolescent mental health with an intervention model based on Inuit knowledge and ways of knowing. *International Journal of Indigenous Health, 11*(1), 92–110. https://doi.org/10.18357/ijih111201614394.

He, M., Tucker, P., Gilliland, J., et al. (2012). The influence of local food environments on adolescents' food purchasing behaviours. *International Journal of Environmental Research and Public Health, 9*, 1458–1471. https://doi.org/10.3390/ijerph9041458.

Lamarre, M. C. (2011). 2011…a year of celebrations. *Global Health Promotion, 18*(4), 3–4.

Lanza, M., Ridenour, M., Hendricks, S., et al. (2016). The violence prevention community meeting: A multi-site study. *Archives of Psychiatric Nursing, 30*(3), 382–386. https://doi.org/10.1016/j.apnu.2016.01.003.

Maurer, F. A., & Smith, C. M. (2014). *Community/public health nursing practice: Health for families and populations* (5th ed.). St. Louis: Saunders.

Minister of Health. (2018). *Key health inequalities in Canada: A national portrait.* Ottawa: Government of Canada. Retrieved from https://www.canada.ca/content/dam/phac-aspc/documents/services/publications/science-research/key-health-inequalities-canada-national-portrait-executive-summary/hir-full-report-eng.pdf.

Noguera-Oviedo, K., & Aga, D. S. (2016). Lessons learned from more than two decades of research on emerging contaminants in the environment. *Journal of Hazardous Materials, 316*, 242–251. https://doi.org/10.1016/j.jhazmat.2016.04.058.

Ontario Centre of Excellence for Child and Youth Mental Health. (2014). *Evidence in sight: Supporting young as risk mothers and their children.* Toronto: Canada.

Pampalon, R., Hamel, D., & Gamache, P. (2010). Health inequalities in urban and rural Canada: Comparing inequalities in survival according to an individual and area-based deprivation index. *Health & Place, 16*(2), 416–420.

Pender, N. J., Murdaugh, C. L., & Parsons, M. A. (2014). *Health promotion in nursing practice* (7th ed.). Upper Saddle River, NJ: Pearson.

Petersen, E., Wilson, M. E., Touch, S., et al. (2016). Rapid spread of Zika virus in the Americas—implications for public health preparedness for mass gatherings at the 2016 Brazil Olympic Games. *International Journal of Infectious Diseases, 44*, 11–15. https://doi.org/10.1016/j.ijid.2016.02.001.

Pillarisetti, A., Mehta, S., & Smith, K. R. (2016). HAPIT, the Household Air Pollution Intervention Tool, to evaluate the health benefits and cost-effectiveness of clean cooking interventions. In E. A. Thomas (Ed.), *Broken pumps and promises: Incentivizing impact in environmental health* (pp. 147–169). Cham, Switzerland: Springer International Publishing.

Prochaska, J., Redding, C., & Evers, K. (2015). The transtheoretical model and stages of change. In K. Glanz, B. Rimer, & K. Viswanath (Eds.), *Healthy behavior: Theory, research and practice* (5th ed.) (pp. 125–148). San Francisco: Jossey Bass.

Raphael, D. (2010). Setting the stage: Why quality of life? Why health promotion. In D. Raphael (Ed.), *Health promotion and quality of life in Canada: Essential readings* (pp. 1–13). Toronto: Canadian Scholars Press.

Rodd, C., & Sharma, A. (2017). Prevalence of overweight and obesity in Canadian children 2004 to 2013: Impact of socioeconomic determinants. *Paediatric Child Health, 22*(3), 153–158. https://doi.org/10.1093/pch/pxx057.

Schlüter-Vorberg, L., Prasse, C., Ternes, T. A., et al. (2015). Toxification by transformation in conventional and advanced wastewater treatment: The antiviral drug acyclovir. *Environmental Science and Technology Letters, 2*(12), 342–346. https://doi.org/10.1021/acs.estlett.5b00291.

Solomon, G. M., Morello-Frosch, R., Zeise, L., et al. (2016). Cumulative environmental impacts: Science and policy to protect communities. *Annual Review of Public Health, 37*(3), 83–96. https://doi.org/10.1146/annurev-publhealth-032315-021807.

Stanhope, M., Lancaster, J., Jakubec, S., et al. (2017). *Community health nursing in Canada* (3rd ed.). Toronto: Elsevier Canada.

Steinka-Fry, K., Tanner-Smith, E., & Hennessy, E. (2015). Effects of brief alcohol interventions on drinking and driving among youth: A systematic review and meta-analysis. *Journal of Addiction & Prevention, 3*(1), 11–16.

Subica, A. M., Grills, C. T., Douglas, J. A., et al. (2016). Communities of color creating healthy environments to combat childhood obesity. *American Journal of Public Health, 106*(1), 79–86. https://doi.org/10.2105/AJPH.2015.302887.

Tarasuk, V., Mitchell, A., & Dachner, N. (2017). *Household food insecurity in Canada 2014. Toronto: Research to identify policy options to reduce food insecurity (PROOF).* Retrieved from http://proof.utoronto.ca.

Toronto Public Health. (2016). *Path to healthier air: Toronto air pollution burden of illness update.* Retrieved from http://www.toronto.ca/health/reports.

Truth and Reconciliation Commission of Canada (TRC). (2015). *Honouring the truth, reconciling for the future: Summary of the final report of the Truth and Reconciliation Commission of Canada.* Retrieved from http://trc.ca/assets/pdf/Honouring_the_Truth_Reconciling_for_the_Future_July_23_2015.pdf.

Vollman, A. (2017). A model to guide practice. In A. Vollman, E. Anderson, & J. McFarlane (Eds.), *Canadian community as partner: Theory and multidisciplinary practice* (4th ed.) (pp. 203–217). Philadelphia: Wolters Kluwer.

Vollman, A., Anderson, E., & McFarlane, J. (Eds.). (2017). *Canadian community as partner: Theory and multidisciplinary practice* (4th ed.) Philadelphia: Wolters Kluwer.

World Health Organization. (1986). *Health and Welfare Canada & Canadian Public Health Association. Ottawa charter for health promotion.* Ottawa: Author.

World Health Organization (WHO). (1978). *Declaration of Alma-Ata: International conference on primary health care, Alma-Ata, USSR, 6–12 September 1978.* Geneva: Author.

World Health Organization (WHO). (2009). *Milestones in health promotion: Statements from global conferences.* Geneva: Author.

World Health Organization (WHO). (2019a). *Health Impact Assessment (HIA).* Retrieved from https://www.who.int/hia/evidence/doh/en/.

World Health Organization (WHO). (2019b). *Quantifying environmental health impacts.* Retrieved from https://www.who.int/quantifying_ehimpacts/en/.

Young, S. K., Tabish, T. B., Pollock, N. K., et al. (2016). Backcountry travel emergencies in Arctic Canada: A pilot study in public health surveillance. *International Journal of Environmental Research and Public Health, 13*(3), 276. https://doi.org/10.3390/ijerph13030276.

9

# Overview of Growth and Development Framework

Laurie Peachey, RN, PhD

Originating US chapter by *Elizabeth Connelly Kudzma, CNL, MPH, WHNP-BC, DNSc*

## INTENDED LEARNING OUTCOMES

*After completing this chapter, the reader will be able to:*
- Define the terms growth, development, and maturation.
- List factors that influence growth in an individual.
- Explain the importance of growth and development theory as a framework for assessing and promoting health.
- Outline Erikson's theory of psychosocial development.

- Differentiate Piaget's and Vygotsky's theories of cognitive development.
- Compare Kohlberg's and Gilligan's theories of cognitive moral development.
- Analyze individual growth and development, distinguishing normal and abnormal processes.

## KEY TERMS

Cephalocaudal
Denver Developmental Screening Test
Development
Developmental patterns
Differentiation
Erikson's theory of psychosocial development
Gilligan's theory of moral development
Growth
Growth charts
Growth patterns

Kohlberg's theory of moral development
Learning
Looksee Checklist (NDDS)
Maturation
Piaget's theory of cognitive development
Proximodistal
Scaffolding
Vygotsky's theory of cognitive development
Zone of proximal development

---

## ? THINK ABOUT IT

### Vaccine Issues and Controversies

A 4$^1/_2$-year-old child begins to scream as the nurse approaches with her "kindergarten immunization." The mother tries to comfort her child, as she turns anxiously to the nurse and states, "I've heard vaccinations can be dangerous. No wonder she's frightened. Are they really necessary?"
- What influence might the mother's anxiety have on the child's behaviour?
- What approaches and information can the nurse have for the mother?
- What resources might the mother use to review recommendations for childhood vaccinations?
- What approaches can the nurse take to gain the child's cooperation?

Unit 3 introduces growth and development as a framework for health assessment and promotion throughout the life

span. Understanding human growth and development facilitates nursing assessment of health knowledge and behaviour. Furthermore, health education is more effective when the nurse acknowledges and incorporates growth and developmental needs, as well as the individual's prior understanding of and beliefs about health and health-related concepts.

Growth and development theory is incorporated in nursing practice. Throughout Unit 3, specific topics and objectives in the application of health promotion will be examined in chapters appropriate to the age and individual developmental level in the life span under discussion. Although these objectives will serve as guides for the promotion of health care at each level, the topic "access to health services" crosses all levels and the entire life span. In Canada, provinces and territories must administer and deliver health care services with insurance plans that are

## TABLE 9.1   Growth and Development

### Developmental Periods at a Glance

| Period | Age | Characteristics |
|---|---|---|
| Infant | Birth to 12 months | Fully dependent on others for basic needs<br>Ends as infant begins to explore environment, walks alone, and develops basic communication skills |
| Toddler | 12 months to 3 years | Motor development progresses significantly<br>Child achieves a degree of physical and emotional autonomy while maintaining a close identity with the primary family unit |
| Preschool child | 3–5 years | Child has increased interest in and involvement with peers and may have social interactions with many people |
| School-age child | 5–12 years | Marked by entry to elementary school; interests turn away from family toward peers |
| Adolescent | 12–18 years | Period of transition, adjustment, and personal exploration; ends when adolescent demonstrates readiness to assume full adult responsibilities of financial, emotional, and social independence |
| Young adult | 18–35 years | Establishing an occupation or career, finding and learning how to live with a partner, and starting and rearing a family |
| Middle-aged adult | 35–65 years | Being established in a marriage, an occupation or career, and a community; may continue to be a time of transition; adjusts to physiological changes of middle age |
| Older person | >65 years | May be a time of continued involvement in work and active socializing; adjusts to decreased physical strength and health; retirement; reduced income; decreasing independence; and deaths of spouses, friends, and self |

expected to meet national principles set out under the *Canada Health Act*. In turn, the provincial and territorial government plans must provide all insured persons with reasonable access to medically necessary hospital and physician services, without financial or other barriers (Government of Canada, 2019). Although access to health care services is achieved using technology and telemedicine in northern and rural Canada, these areas face challenges and barriers of being underserviced.

Without access to health services, health promotion cannot occur, and a person has difficulty achieving and maintaining health. This chapter focuses on the study of health promotion at individual developmental levels by exploring basic concepts foundational to growth and development, as well as providing an overview of representative theories of development. Each of the following nine chapters provides health-assessment and health-promotion strategies appropriate for selected age groups across the life span. The age groups described are the prenatal period, infant, toddler, preschool child, school-age child, adolescent, young adult, middle-aged adult, and older person (Table 9.1).

## OVERVIEW OF GROWTH AND DEVELOPMENT

A fuller understanding of growth and development has continued to expand with advances in science. Currently, the genomic era is intersecting with the digital age, and nursing educators are racing to integrate genomic content (Read & Ward, 2016). The contribution of genomic knowledge to growth and development is huge, and there is an explosion of findings on genetic and long-term impacts of early development on later health and health-related behaviours.

Individuals continue to evolve throughout the life span, and developmental transitions occur beyond childhood and adolescence, extending into the early, middle, and later adult years. Aging adults are receiving increased attention as the average life expectancy increases, and the adult population older than 85 years has become the fastest growing age group, providing new challenges for health protection and promotion.

## Growth

Growth refers to a quantifiable change in structure size. In the body this change increases the number and/or size of the cells, resulting in an increase in the size and weight of the whole, or any of its parts. During childhood, physical changes in height, weight, and head circumference, or growth parameters, are measured and recorded regularly. Growth refers to both the obvious changes in the whole individual and to the increases (and, as we age, decreases) in the size of specific organs and systems. The health history and physical assessment of an individual should include all body systems and should emphasize systems undergoing the most change. Table 9.2 outlines growth as it occurs throughout the body systems and life span. The growth of some systems, such as the skeletal and muscular systems, is more influenced by sex, whereas the growth of other systems, such as the nervous and respiratory systems, is less dependent on sex. Growth changes that occur in young, middle-aged, and older persons should be noted. Thinking of growth only as it applies to infants, children, and adolescents misses important changes that occur from conception and throughout all the stages of adulthood.

Influences on an individual's potential for growth include genetic factors, prenatal and postnatal exposures, nutrition, and environmental factors (see the Case Study and Care Plan at the end of this chapter). Other influences include emotional health and traditional cultural practices that influence childrearing, lifestyle, and health care practices (Diversity Awareness). Although much of the potential for growth is primarily determined by individual genetics, health and environmental exposures influence the attainment of that potential (Centers for Disease Control and Prevention [CDC], 2011a,b). The timing of contact with environmental hazards and stressors may determine to a great extent the amount and kind of effects of these influences. If a pregnant mother is exposed to a virus in utero (e.g., the Zika virus), the developing fetus is more vulnerable than either the mother or an older child, especially during the first trimester, when all organs systems

(Text continues on page 202)

## TABLE 9.2 Growth and Development

### Growth Changes Throughout the Life Cycle

| Overview of Developmental Changes | Prenatal Period | Infancy | Childhood | Puberty and Adolescence | Adulthood | Middle Age | Old Age |
|---|---|---|---|---|---|---|---|
| **Heart and Circulatory System** | | | | | | | |
| Action of heart and circulatory system is under the control of autonomic nervous system. Throughout life cardiac rate is responsive to organ needs and emotional states (fear, anxiety, tension, depression) | Heart formed and begins to beat about third week | Heart grows somewhat more slowly than rest of body (weight doubled by 1 year, body weight triples). Grows steadily during childhood. With birth, considerable change in paths and relative volumes of blood flow, reflected in loss of certain fetal structures and changes in heart and major vessels | | At puberty, heart takes part in rapid growth, reaching mature size with rest of body | Heart weight remains relatively constant after age 25 years (only organ other than prostate that does not decrease in weight with age). Capacity to increase rate and strength of beat during physical work is diminished with aging. Cardiac strength lessens with age, whereas expenditure of energy is more than in youth | | |
| | Heart rate high, ≈150 beats/min | Heart rate falls steadily throughout childhood | | | At maturity, women have slightly higher pulse rate than men, 65 beats/min (girls' temperature remains stationary, higher than boys'); men maintain same pulse rate in maturity (slightly lower body temperature than women) | | |
| | | 130 beats/min | 70–80 beats/min | 60 beats/min in adolescence, rate differs with sex | | | |
| | | Heart rate more variable during childhood—regular | | | | | |
| | | Not until middle childhood does peripheral blood picture become same as adult | | | | | |
| **Urinary System** | | | | | | | |
| Parallels growth as a whole. Proportion of body water and solids follows pattern related to growth—tendency for human organism to dry out as life progresses. Function of kidneys, with other organ systems, is to help in regulation of internal environment of body | Young fetus is approximately 90% water. Urinary system begins in first month | Newborn is approximately 70% water. Urinary system does not complete full development until end of first year. All renal units immature at birth; thus, fluid and electrolyte imbalance occurs readily. Kidney function adequate at birth if not subjected to undue stress | Composition of urine in healthy child (after age 2 years) changes very little as child matures; thus renal function and urinalysis can be used as monitor of well-being | | Adult is approximately 58% water. Glomerular filtration rate decreases by approximately 47% from age 20 to age 90 years | | |

Continued

## TABLE 9.2   Growth and Development—cont'd

### Growth Changes Throughout the Life Cycle

| Overview of Developmental Changes | Prenatal Period | Infancy | Childhood | Puberty and Adolescence | Adulthood | Middle Age | Old Age |
|---|---|---|---|---|---|---|---|
| **Digestive System** | | | | | | | |
| As a whole, grows as total body grows, although evidence suggests that various parts of gastrointestinal system undergo separate periods of growth, maturity, and senescence | Before birth nutrients are supplied through placental circulation; digestion and absorption do not occur in gastrointestinal tract | Stomach size increases rapidly in first few months, then grows steadily throughout childhood | | | All actions of gastrointestinal tract (food intake, digestion, absorption, elimination) not only respond to physiological needs but from birth to old age are also sensitive to tensions and anxiety | | |
| | | | | Spurt of growth at puberty | | | |
| | | Digestive apparatus immature at birth (food passes through rapidly, reverse peristalsis common). Acidity of gastric juices varies over life span; low during infancy, rises during childhood, plateaus approximately age 10 years, rises during puberty. Free gastric acid (HCl) more marked in boys | | | Data suggest generalized atrophy of entire gastrointestinal tract with advancing age. Nutritional needs differ according to individual variation—decreasing metabolism—tone of large intestine may become impaired until decrease with senescence (also diminished taste) | | |
| | Salivary glands small at birth | Increase rapidly during first 3 months; reach relative adult proportions by age 2 years | | | | | |
| **Special Senses** | | | | | | | |
| Most are well developed at birth, although their association with higher centres comes about gradually during early life and diminishes with advancing age | Begin very early in embryonic development—3–6 weeks | Sense of touch is developed first, then hearing and vision. Vision: infant can perceive simple differences in shape but not complex patterns (greater proportion of total growth before birth); various dimensions of vision develop at various ages, eye muscles function at mature level in first year, fusion begins at 9 months until 6 years; refractive power changes over life cycle—hyperopia increases until eyeball reaches adult size (≈8 years), then reverses trend toward emmetropia; postpubertal years—toward myopia until 30 years, when myopia decreases and hyperopia increases | | | | | |

## Adipose Tissue

| | | | | | | | |
|---|---|---|---|---|---|---|---|
| Although adipose tissue differs greatly among individuals, an overall lifetime pattern exists. Fat accumulation differs greatly with body build and constitution. Relationship between caloric intake, amount of exercise, and utilization or accumulation of fat is not yet fully understood but is the basis of much interrelated research | Accumulates rapidly before birth; peaks at seventh gestational month. Premature infant may look wrinkled and scrawny because of lack of adipose tissue | Increases rapidly during first 6 months | Decreases from first to seventh year in both sexes | Begins to increase slowly to puberty. Fat begins to accumulate slowly and continues to accumulate uninterrupted in girls, producing feminine curves, and accounts for much of weight gain | Some girls become slim after full maturation; many maintain approximately the same amount of adipose tissue as at puberty | Typically, both sexes tend to gain weight in their 50s and 60s but do not maintain the same body contours of earlier years at same weight (increased deposit on abdomen and hips) | Usually fat stores are lost after the seventh decade in both sexes. Sharpness in contours, increasingly prominent bony landmark |
| | | | Sex differences are not noted in body shape of prepubescent children | | Deposition of fat differs in body—amount decreases sharply at time of maximal growth spurt (increased weight caused by increase in muscle mass and bones) | After full maturation, fat accumulation begins | |

## Lymphoid Tissue

| | | | | | |
|---|---|---|---|---|---|
| Lymphoid tissue is scattered widely throughout the body and includes lymph nodes, tonsils, adenoids, thymus, spleen, and lymphocytes of blood; follows unique pattern of growth, rapid in infancy and begins to atrophy at puberty | Begins during last month of uterine life—crosses placenta at levels equal to mother's and remains for several months after delivery | Grows most rapidly during infancy and childhood, reaching maximal size a few years before puberty; parallels development of immunity | | Atrophies and is smaller in volume at full maturity than during childhood | Thymus is small and difficult to locate in older people |
| | | Increased incidence of disease with increasing age of child | | | |

Continued

## TABLE 9.2   Growth and Development—cont'd

### Growth Changes Throughout the Life Cycle

| Overview of Developmental Changes | Prenatal Period | Infancy | Childhood | Puberty and Adolescence | Adulthood | Middle Age | Old Age |
|---|---|---|---|---|---|---|---|
| **Respiratory System** | | | | | | | |
| Growth parallels that of total body. Respiratory apparatus is a highly organized system of organs under nervous system and hormonal regulation, which functions in coordination with rest of body. Sex difference in gas exchange becomes apparent during puberty | Before birth, air sacs do not contain air; oxygen is supplied through maternal circulation | When umbilical cord is cut, infant must use own breathing apparatus—breathing irregular at first, both in rate and in depth—fast in infancy and gradually slowing through childhood until maturity is reached | | | No sex difference in respiratory rate at any time of life | | |
| | | | | | | Basal metabolic rate declines (rate higher in men than in women) | |
| | | Respiratory exchange gradually becomes more efficient as life advances. Actual volume of air inhaled with each breath increases as lung size expands with general body growth. Vital capacity and maximal breathing capacity rise gradually in both sexes, increasing more in boys during puberty; adult men have more efficient respiratory exchange, are capable of greater feats of muscular exertion without exhaustion than women | | | | | |
| **Skeletal System** | | | | | | | |
| Bone growth passes through successive stages of development from connective tissue to cartilage to osseous tissue; completion of calcification indicates end of growing period and is thus a useful measure of growth rate and physiological maturity. Most growth ceases during adolescence | Follows cephalocaudal law of development; 70% of head growth before birth; bones of hands and wrist laid down in cartilage | | Reserved during growth spurt | | Maximal height in early 20s to 30s | Gradual decline until onset of senescence | |
| | | After first year, legs grow fastest, 66% of total increase in height; the longer puberty is delayed, the greater the leg length | | | | Thinning of vertebral disks beginning in middle years; most rapid in last decade | |
| | | Trunk fastest growing, 60% of total increase | | Length of trunk and depth of chest reach peak growth | | | |
| | | At birth, shafts of metacarpals are ossified (and visible by radiography); carpal bones begin to ossify | | Growth of both sexes is nearly even until onset of puberty in girls first (≈10 years). Boys begin ~2 years later, but growth is markedly greater. Peak in height comes before peak in weight | | Spinal column shortens (osteoporosis) with thinning vertebrae—shortening of trunk with long extremities—reversal of growth proportions in infancy | |

## Muscle System

Number of striated muscle fibres is roughly the same in all humans. Tremendous difference in size, not only from fetus to adult but also among adults, is caused by ability of individual muscle fibres to increase in size

| | | | | | |
|---|---|---|---|---|---|
| Muscle formation begins early, assuming final shape by end of second month | Increases rapidly during infancy but slowly during childhood | | With onset of puberty, muscle strength is greater in boys (when muscle growth is stimulated by testosterone) | Muscle mass continues to increase gradually—maximal strength attained in early adulthood—then declines slightly—according to use and genetic constitution. Will increase in bulk and strength as used until onset of senescence | |
| | Growth in both sexes is same in childhood | | Greatest increase begins in puberty, muscle size precedes muscle strength in boys | | Atrophy and loss of muscle tone |
| | Increase in muscle size means increasing strength in children; increase in skill is more intimately related to maturation of nervous system | | | | |

## Nervous System

Growth and maturation of central and peripheral nervous systems (brain, spinal cord, peripheral nerves, many sense organs) reflected by changing size of head

| | | | | | |
|---|---|---|---|---|---|
| Growth very rapid during intrauterine development; head grows at greater rate than rest of body | In first year has all the brain cells, which will continue to increase in size; number and complexity of axons, dendrites, and synapses will continue to increase | | | Function continues with use | Depletion of fully functioning brain cells, whether they are lost, shrink, or lose connections |
| | All neural tissues grow rapidly during infancy and early childhood | | (No neural growth spurt at puberty) | | Decrease in myelin sheath, impulses decrease; slowed down speed of action and reaction |
| | Brain grows rapidly after birth, reaching 90% of total size by age 2 years | By middle childhood almost reaches adult size | Slow increase to full maturity | Brain weight decreases with age | |
| Segmented spinal nerves are mature, fully myelinated, and functioning at term (e.g., knee jerk), but acquisition of myelin in cortex, brainstem, and spinal cord is closely correlated with observed behaviour (myelination of this tract follows cephalocaudal, proximodistal rules) | | | | | Taste less acute, less discriminatory with advancing age |
| Equipment for sense of taste and smell present at birth and perhaps most acute at that time | | | | | Structural changes in central nervous system result in impaired perception |

Continued

## TABLE 9.2  Growth and Development—cont'd

### Growth Changes Throughout the Life Cycle

| Overview of Developmental Changes | Prenatal Period | Infancy | Childhood | Puberty and Adolescence | Adulthood | Middle Age | Old Age |
|---|---|---|---|---|---|---|---|
| **Reproductive System** | | | | | | | |
| Organs of reproductive system show little increase during early life but rapid development just before and coincident with puberty. Maturation and fulfillment of reproductive functions of maturity (in female) are followed by involution in later years | Genital organs form during uterine life; uterus undergoes growth spurt before birth (hormonal stimulation from mother) | Female sex organs well formed but not functioning at birth (but have full quota of sensory nerves) | Quiescent during childhood | Maturation at puberty (menstruation) | | | Involution after menopause |
| | | Uterus undergoes involution to half its birth weight | Regained size by age 10–11 years | | | | |
| | | In males, testes, as with ovaries, remain dormant and small, not even growing in proportion to rest of body (with sensory nerves) | Until puberty, interstitial cells of Leydig reappear and secrete testosterone, so testes and penis continue to increase in size; pubic hair appears | Adult size at puberty | | | Begins to atrophy with advancing age |
| | Mammary glands develop in both sexes during fetal life | Enlargement of breasts at birth (both sexes) | Nonsecretory during childhood until puberty | Development rapid | Enlarge during pregnancy, developing alveoli | Maximum increase with pregnancy | Atrophy with advanced age |
| | Sex hormones: until puberty girls and boys produce male hormones (androgens) and female hormones (chiefly estrogens) in small and roughly equal amounts | | | | | | |
| **Integumentary System** | | | | | | | |
| Includes skin and its appendages and adnexa (nails, hair, sebaceous glands, eccrine and apocrine sweat glands). Although all skin is similar, this organ shows considerable variability in different parts of body (and from individual to individual) and varies greatly during life span | Hair, skin, and sebaceous glands fully formed in utero | Skin contains all its adult structures at birth but immature in function | Matures slowly until puberty (children prone to rashes) | Rapid spurt in maturation of skin and all its structures | | | Changes in skin most obvious sign of aging (exposure and environmental conditions) |

| | | Regenerative and growth power decrease and skin loses elasticity |
|---|---|---|
| | Lanugo begins to decrease before birth and continues regression for a few weeks postnatally | Replaced by body hair, less extensive distribution; marked difference in type and distribution of hair at puberty |
| | Activity of sebaceous glands decreases after birth | Increases rapidly at puberty (more prone to acne) |
| **Endocrine System** Consists of a number of glandular structures scattered throughout body. Although small in size, their hormones influence all growth and development of whole organism | Immaturity of entire endocrine system puts infant at a disadvantage if required to adjust to wide fluctuations in concentration of water, electrolytes, glucose, and amino acids. All are interrelated, but each organ develops at its own rate:<br>• Thyroid—increases in size from midfetal life to maturity; slightly larger in boys than girls; growth spurt at adolescence<br>• Adrenals—after birth decrease in size and this continues throughout first year, increase again during childhood (but smaller than at birth); spurt at puberty, reaching maturity with rest of body; greater increase in male gonads and testes and female ovaries (endocrine glands as well as reproductive organs), follow genital type of growth pattern<br>• Hypophysis, or pituitary gland—produces or stimulates hormones that influence growth<br>• Parathyroid—produces hormones that maintain homeostasis of calcium and phosphorus<br>• Islets of Langerhans—dispersed throughout pancreas; produce insulin and glucagon | With age, decline occurs in all endocrine gland functions |

NOTE: This table indicates only general trends in growth and development; it is not all inclusive. No distinct ages, absolute values, or ranges of normal variations are intended in this table.

Source: Modified from a format originally developed in Sutterly, D. C., & Donneley, G. F. (1973). *Perspectives in human development: Nursing throughout the life cycle*. Philadelphia: J. B. Lippincott. Further modified from Papalia, D. E., & Feldman, R. D. (2011). *Experience human development* (12th ed.). New York: McGraw Hill. Physiological adaptations updated from McCance, K. L., Huether, S. E., Brashers, V. L., et al. (2014). *Pathophysiology: Biological basis for disease in adults and children*. St. Louis: Mosby.

## 🌐 DIVERSITY AWARENESS

### Childhood Lead Poisoning, Refugee Families, and Internationally Adopted Children

Whereas Canada and the United States have made tremendous progress in eliminating some of the more significant sources of lead (lead paint was banned in 1978; leaded gasoline was phased out in the early 1990s), lead poisoning remains a significant threat to today's children. Lead exposure results in behaviour and learning problems, decreased intelligence, attention problems, lower academic achievement, impaired growth, poor eye–hand coordination, and hearing loss. The World Health Organization (WHO) (2010) now uses a reference level of 5 mcg/dL to identify children with lead exposure, and this reference value is lower than in past years. As a consequence, more children will likely be identified as having lead exposure. The WHO emphasizes that lead poisoning is a totally preventable disease. During the past two decades, public health and provider efforts have resulted in a >90% decline in the overall number of children affected in Canada and the United States. It would be important for Canadian health care providers to also learn from the Flint, Michigan, water contamination crisis that started in April 2014 in the United States, as it clearly illustrates the importance of lead testing during childhood and prompt treatment of children who demonstrate high lead levels (Bosman & Smith, 2016).

Refugees and internationally adopted children, especially from resource-poor countries, may be found to have elevated lead levels in their body when they arrive in Canada.

An often-overlooked risk is the use of warm, hot, or boiled tap water from contaminated pipes. Many feel that heating the water removes contaminants, although any heat mobilizes the lead and makes it easier to absorb. This is also true of pottery that is heated by cooking in it, placing heated fluids in it, or heating it in a microwave oven. Although typical instruction pamphlets teach that tap water should be run for a full minute before it is consumed, they fail to state that the water consumed should come from the cold tap if it is to be consumed.

When screening for lead poisoning in children, the nurse should ask about the use of traditional remedies, pottery, imported foods, and candies, as well as the use of boiled or hot tap water. In addition, the nurse should encourage a diet with less fat, because lead is retained in fat, and a greater vitamin C, calcium, and iron intake, which reduces the amount of lead in the body.

For more information about the health effects of lead on children, or how to identify children with elevated lead levels visit the following webpages:

* Health Canada: Lead Information Package (https://www.canada.ca/en/health-canada/services/environmental-workplace-health/environmental-contaminants/lead/lead-information-package-some-commonly-asked-questions-about-lead-human-health.html)
* Caring for Kids New to Canada (https://www.kidsnewtocanada.ca/screening/lead)
* National Safety Council: Lead Poisoning Is Not Yesterday's News (http://www.nsc.org/learn/safety-knowledge/Pages/Lead-Poisoning-Prevention.aspx)
* CDC: What Do Parent's Need to Know to Protect Their Children (http://www.cdc.gov/nceh/lead/faq/acclpp/blood_lead_levels.htm)
* US Environmental Protection Agency: Protect Your Family From Exposure to Lead (http://www.epa.gov/lead/protect-your-family)
* Environmental Protection Agency: Learn About Lead (http://www.epa.gov/lead/learn-about-lead)
* Natural Resources Defense Council: Environmental Threats in the Latino Community (http://www.nrdc.org)

#### Reflective Questions

* Children with lead poisoning often have no symptoms. A child can be poisoned and show no outward signs. What is the nurse's best action to determine if the child has been exposed to lead poisoning?
* What are the possible sources of lead poisoning in a child's home?

From Bosman, J. & Smith, M. (2016). Gov. Rick Synder of Michigan apologizes in Flint water crisis. *New York Times*, January 19. Retrieved from http://www.nytimes.com/2016/01/20/us/obama-set-to-meet-with-mayor-of-flint-about-water-crisis.html?r=00; World Health Organization. (2010). *Childhood lead poisoning*. Retrieved from https://www.who.int/ceh/publications/leadguidance.pdf.

are in a stage of rapid growth and development. Teens who fracture a limb at the bone's growth plate also have more difficulty healing than older teens and young adults who have completed their growth spurt.

### Growth Patterns

Expected growth patterns exist for all people. Growth is not steady or uniform throughout life. The periods of extremely rapid growth—childbearing period, infancy, and adolescence—are contrasted with slower rates of growth during the toddler, preschool, and school-age periods. Infants typically double their birth weight by 6 months of age and triple their birth weight by 1 year of age. The well-known early adult "growth spurt" in height typically occurs early in adolescence for girls and later in adolescence for boys.

Different parts of the body increase in size at different rates. For example, during early life the head is the fastest-growing section, followed by the trunk, and then the arms and legs. Newborns' heads account for one-quarter of their overall length, as opposed to adults' heads, which account for one-ninth of their overall height. The growth changes in proportions of body parts from infancy to adulthood are demonstrated in Fig. 9.1.

### Growth Charts

Growth is one of the most important indications of a child's overall health and well-being. Accurate growth assessment depends on precise measurement of growth parameters with proper equipment, correct and consistent techniques, careful plotting of measurements, and thoughtful interpretation of the data. A collaborative statement advisory group was formed to include the Dietitians of Canada, the Canadian Paediatric Society (CPS), the College of Family Physicians of Canada (CFPC), and the Community Health Nurses of Canada (CHNC). In their collaborative expert panel statement, the authors advocate consistent practices for monitoring growth and assessing patterns of linear growth, and weight gain in children to support health child growth and development (Dietitians of Canada, CPS, CFPC, & CHNC, 2010). On the basis of input from an expert panel in the collaborative statement, the advisory group recommended that health practitioners in Canada use the 2006 World Health Organization (WHO) international growth charts for children from birth to 24 months and continue to use the revised 2000 CDC growth charts (including the body mass index [BMI] and the 3rd and 97th percentiles) for children aged 2 to 20 years. This recommendation was based on

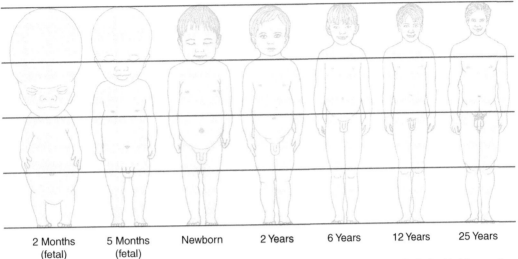

**Fig. 9.1** Changes in Body Proportions from Birth to Adulthood (From McKinney, E. S., Smith Murray, S., James, S. R., et al. [2017]. *Maternal child nursing* [5th ed.]. St Louis: Saunders.)

2 Months (fetal)   5 Months (fetal)   Newborn   2 Years   6 Years   12 Years   25 Years

the fact that WHO growth charts were compiled from healthy breastfed infants living in optimal conditions and achieving the greatest potential of growth possible, which was recognized as the desired standard against which to compare the growth of all other infants (CDC, 2010). In creating the WHO growth charts, researchers gathered data from six countries (Brazil, Ghana, India, Norway, Oman, and the United States) using longitudinal and cross-sectional methods (Mei & Grummer-Strawn, 2011). The exceptional strength of the WHO growth charts is that they are globally representative (Ziegler & Nelson, 2012). The CDC and the WHO growth charts both describe weight for age, length (or stature) for age, weight for length, and BMI for age, and include the 5th and 95th and the 3rd and 97th percentiles (CDC, 2010). The WHO and the CDC growth charts for each sex with percentile curves can be viewed at the CPS website: (https://www.cps.ca/en/tools-outils/who-growth-charts). These charts have been used by pediatricians, nurses, and parents to compare infant, child, and adolescent growth since 1977.

When one is assessing growth data for use in the growth charts, it is important to remember that a single measurement taken at one point in time, although helpful in providing a baseline, does not allow the best assessment of a child's growth. Serial measurements plotted over time on a growth chart best reflect a child's pattern of growth. Slowed growth, plateaus, or decreases in height, weight, and head circumference, as well as rapid increases, raise questions for health care providers about the adequacy of a child's nutritional intake, disease states, neglect, or emotional problems. See Research for Evidence-Informed Practice on the use of the new growth charts and young children.

## Concept of Development

Development refers to change and expansion of ability and advancement in skill from a lower to a more advanced capability. In contrast to growth, which is a quantitative or precisely measurable change, development is a qualitative change. Qualitative changes are more challenging to describe because

they cannot be easily measured in precise units. Development has best been conceptualized as a process that can be assessed because it follows certain sequencing or patterns, although the timing of this advancement is individual.

### Developmental Patterns

All individuals follow similar developmental patterns, with one stage of development building on and leading to the next. Early development proceeds as follows:

- Cephalocaudal, from head to toe
- Proximodistal, from midline to periphery
- Differentiation follows a pattern: simple to complex, and general to specific

The following are examples of patterns of development:

- Cephalocaudal: infants advance in neck and head control before controlling the movements of the extremities.
- Proximodistal: infants' central nervous systems develop before peripheral nervous systems.
- Differentiation: infants use a whole-hand grasp before learning the finer control of the pincer grasp, and they coo or babble before they speak.

Although the sequence of development is predictable, the exact timing of the sequencing depends on the individual. Individuals develop at their own rate, on their own schedule. For example, infants creep and crawl before they walk, and their primary teeth erupt in a predictable sequence, but each will walk and develop primary teeth on an individual schedule. However, there are guidelines or parameters that assist parents and health care providers in assessing whether children are progressing in an acceptable developmental sequence within a reasonable time frame. Areas of assessment usually focus on personal and social, gross and fine motor, and language development. The Denver Developmental Screening Test, which was revised in 1992 (now known as Denver II), is a screening tool that assists health care providers in monitoring children's development in each of these areas from birth to 6 years of age. In Ontario, the Looksee Checklist (NDDS) tool is utilized with the intent for parents to observe their children and check off a list of 12–22 items with a

## ⚑ RESEARCH FOR EVIDENCE-INFORMED PRACTICE

### *Comparing the New Growth Charts: Prediction of Future Obesity From Childhood Weight Status*

The Canadian Paediatric Society (CPS), the Centers for Disease Control and Prevention (CDC), and the World Health Organization (WHO) growth charts use the same indicators for growth, and comparative studies have been done to indicate differences when each chart is used. These studies are critical to provide better support for public health prevention efforts addressing the increasing prevalence of childhood obesity (Mei & Grummer-Strawn, 2011).

From the beginning, it was recommended that, when the WHO growth charts are used to screen individuals for abnormal or unhealthy growth, the narrower ranges of the 3rd and 97th percentiles should be used instead of the 5th and 95th percentiles, respectively. This would identify fewer children as underweight as slower growth among breastfed infants is normal within the first 6 months.

Rapid weight gain during the first year of life is predictive of obesity in 2-year-olds to 3-year-olds, and there is need to promote parental awareness regarding the actual weight of their children (Vallejo, Cortes-Rodrigues, & Colin-Ramirez, 2015). Maalouf-Manasseh, Metallinos-Katsaras, and Dewey (2011) also reported that gaining weight more rapidly in the first year than directed by the WHO growth charts may be an early sign of later obesity.

Ziegler and Nelson (2012) observed in their comparative studies that the weight percentiles of the WHO growth charts were higher in the first 6 months and lower between 6 and 24 months when compared with the same age range

CDC percentiles. Their conclusion was explained not only by their appreciating that breastfed infants grow somewhat slower than formula-fed infants but also by their realizing the attrition rate of low-weight-gaining breastfed infants that occurred when data were being compiled for the WHO growth charts.

Whereas the WHO growth charts may be used for national and international observations of malnutrition, it is imperative that additional data be obtained before the WHO standards can be applied for local public health interventions. The low weight of the WHO growth charts should not be used to misclassify a child as overweight or obese with the use of corrective interventions (Ziegler & Nelson, 2012).

Although the new WHO growth charts furnish health care providers and researchers with an improved tool to assess and track the growth of children from birth to 24 months of age, care must be taken not to misinterpret the results for each individual child. As indicated by the evidence presented, it is too early to use the WHO growth chart as the magic bullet of early identification of and intervention for future obesity in children during the first year of life. Mothers' underestimation of the weight of their own children was common in both overweight and children of normal weight (Vallejo et al., 2015). Continued investigation in this area is promising for planning of health care education to counter factors contributing to the child and later adult obesity epidemic.

Sources: Maalouf-Manasseh, Z., Metallinos-Katsaras, E., & Dewey, K. G. (2011). Obesity in preschool children is more prevalent and identified at a younger age when WHO growth charts are used compared with CDC charts. *Journal of Nutrition, 141*, 1154–1158; Mei, Z., & Grummer-Strawn, L. M. (2011). Comparison of changes in growth percentiles of US children on CDC 2000 growth charts with corresponding changes on WHO 2006 growth charts. *Clinical Pediatrics, 50*(5), 402–407; Vallejo, M., Cortes-Rodrigues, B. A., & Colin-Ramirez, E. (2015). Maternal underestimation of child's weight status and health behaviors as risk factors for overweight in children. *Journal of Pediatric Nursing, 30*(6), e29–e33; Ziegler, E. E., & Nelson, S. E. (2012). The WHO growth standards: Strengths and limitations. *Current Opinion Clinical Nutrition Metabolic Care, 15*(3), 298–302.

"yes" or "no." The NDDS was first formed in 1993 as a result of concern from Northern Ontario agencies around the number of children being identified with developmental needs after the age of 3. The NDDS screening tool is designed to be implemented by parents and to be time efficient in promoting early identification of issues and providing a path towards early intervention. The NDDS also coincides with the immunization schedule, as well as key developmental stages (First Words, 2019).

Social expectations can influence developmental tasks with expectations that an individual achieve certain landmarks during each period of development. However, the age at which a child is expected to master certain developmental tasks is determined partly by cultural expectations. Some cultures are comfortable with breastfeeding their children well into childhood, whereas others expect the transition to self-feeding with a cup much earlier. When assessing a child's abilities, nurses are aware that a child who has never been given the opportunity to learn or master a skill may be developmentally capable but fails when tested. For example, a child who is capable of learning colours or numbers can do so only if taught, just as the child who was breastfed well into childhood, never having been offered a cup, may well be developmentally capable of drinking from a cup but probably will fail in early attempts.

Development is closely interrelated with the concepts of both learning and maturation. Learning is the process of gaining specific knowledge or skills that result from exposure, experience, education, and evaluation. Maturation is an increase in competence and adaptability that reflects understandings in

the complexity of a structure that makes it possible for that structure to begin to function or to function at a higher level. Maturation of a structure, system, or individual refers to the emergence of the genetic potential of that structure, system, or individual. Learning cannot occur unless the individual is mature enough to understand and control behaviour. Children can be toilet trained only when their bodies have matured to the point of developing internal and external sphincter control. Earlier attempts will be frustrating for both the child and the parent.

Growth and development are complex, interrelated processes that are influenced by and, in turn, influence the health of an individual. The nurse who understands this relationship is aware of the need for age-specific health-assessment, health-protection, and health-promotion strategies (Quality and Safety Scenario).

## THEORIES OF LIFE-SPAN DEVELOPMENT

Specific aspects of development of the person have been studied for centuries. Many theories of development are used in the study of individuals throughout the life span; the nurse may wish to refer to a text on developmental psychology to become familiar with some of these theories. In this unit, theories are discussed to gain a holistic view of the progression of individual development throughout the life span. These theories were originally advanced by Erikson, Piaget, Vygotsky, Kohlberg, and Gilligan. Whereas these theories can assist in understanding

## QUALITY AND SAFETY SCENARIO

### Anticipatory Guidance

The nurse is often in a position to provide anticipatory guidance to parents, which involves teaching parents ways to handle a situation before it becomes an issue or problem. Knowledge of normal growth and development provides a foundation for this teaching. For example, the toddler period is one of intense exploration of the environment, when locomotion is the major gross motor skill acquired. The nurse, knowing the number one cause of death in toddlers is accidents, provides the following teaching to the parents of a child who is entering the toddler period:

- Use a federally approved car restraint/car seat and check for proper installation and placement.
- Supervise a child closely near any source of water, including buckets, bathtubs, toilets, and especially swimming pools.
- Move pot handles toward the back of the stove and use the back burners whenever possible.
- Place toxic substances in a locked cabinet and have the poison control contact number easily accessible. Avoid the use of syrup of ipecac unless advised by a poison control representative to use it.
- Move a toddler from the crib to a bed.
- Provide barriers on open windows.
- Decrease water temperature to avoid scald burns from tap water.
- Avoid foods that pose a choking hazard such as nuts, hard candies, raisins, fresh carrots, whole grapes, chewing gum, hot dogs, and fish with bones.
- Guard against the toddler running into the street when walking and playing outside.

### TABLE 9.3  Growth and Development
**Erikson's Eight Stages of Human Development**

| Age Group | Psychosocial Stage | Lasting Outcomes |
|---|---|---|
| 1. Infancy | Basic trust versus basic mistrust | Faith and hope |
| 2. Toddler stage | Autonomy versus shame and doubt | Self-control and will-power |
| 3. Preschool stage | Initiative versus guilt | Direction and purpose |
| 4. School age | Industry versus inferiority | Method and competence |
| 5. Adolescence | Identity versus role confusion | Devotion and fidelity |
| 6. Young adulthood | Intimacy versus isolation | Affiliation and love |
| 7. Middle adulthood | Generativity versus stagnation | Production and care |
| 8. Older personhood | Ego integrity versus despair | Renunciation and wisdom |

Modified from Erikson, E. H. (1995). *Childhood and society* (35th anniversary ed.). New York: Norton; Erikson, E. H., & Erikson, J. M. (1998). *The life cycle completed.* New York: Norton.

Although each of the conflicts is predominant at a certain stage in life, it is important to recognize that all the conflicts exist in each person, to some extent, at all times and that a conflict, once resolved, may emerge again in appropriate situations. For example, the renunciation and wisdom of old age is accomplished by a person reflecting on the crises of early development and coping with the physical and mental changes of aging (Perry, Ruggiano, Shtompel, et al., 2015). These stages are summarized in Table 9.3 and are discussed more fully in the chapters on each developmental age group. See the case study at the end of this chapter about a potentially disabled infant girl and how hospitalization could affect her stage of psychosocial development.

### Cognitive Development

Another aspect of development is cognitive development. Jean Piaget, a Swiss psychologist, also trained in biology and philosophy, is well known for his theory of cognitive development. He viewed children as biological organisms interacting with their environment, and his theory contends that cognitive development reflects children's attempts to make sense of their worlds. Piaget developed his cognitive theory by observing his own children (Piaget, 1950). Hence, the major criticism of his work is that he underestimated children's capabilities and gave little or no consideration to cultural differences. Lev Vygotsky, a Russian contemporary, was also trained in both the physical sciences and psychology. His theory of cognitive development maintains that a child's development cannot be separated from the social and cultural context in which it occurs. He also credited children with more innate ability to learn and emphasized the importance of language (Vygotsky, 1986). The theories of Piaget and Vygotsky are presented in more detail in the following sections.

### Cognitive Development: Piaget's Theory

Jean Piaget's theory of cognitive development is concerned primarily with structure rather than content, with how the individual mind works rather than with what it does. Piaget uses the word scheme to describe a pattern of action or thought. A scheme is used to take in or assimilate new experiences or may be modified or accommodated by new experiences. Each person

developmental tasks, they are not definitive, and individuals may exhibit variations and stage activities may overlap. It is important to remember that these theories are oriented specifically to postcolonial Western society and, in many cultures, such as Indigenous people in Canada, these theories may not apply as expectations of milestones across the life span. Indigenous ways of knowing reflect the unique cultures, aspirations, and needs of First Nations, Inuit, and Métis children across Canada. Indigenous child care is ideally rooted in distinct Indigenous cultures, languages, and knowledge to honour the foundation from which children shape their identity and the essential components of their well-being (Government of Canada, 2018).

### Psychosocial Development: Erikson's Theory

Erik Erikson described the development of identity of the self through successive stages that unfold throughout the life span (Erikson, 1968, 1995; Erikson & Erikson, 1998). Although he studied with Freud and supported the psychosexual theory of development, Erikson's theory of psychosocial development is based on the need of each person to develop a sense of trust in self and others and a sense of personal worth. Erikson described a healthy personality in positive terms, not merely through the absence of disease.

According to Erikson, psychosocial development is composed of critical stages, each requiring resolution of a conflict between two opposing forces (e.g., intimacy versus isolation). Each stage depends on the preceding stage, which must be accomplished successfully for the person to proceed. Erikson's use of a psychosocial framework acknowledges the influence of socialization and the environment but maintains that it is ultimately the individual who must master each of the conflicts.

## TABLE 9.4  Growth and Development

### Piaget's Stages of Cognitive Development

| Stage | Age | Characteristics |
|---|---|---|
| Sensorimotor | Birth to 2 years | Begins with a predominance and reliance on reflexes that permit the body to learn |
| | | Reflexes decrease, and voluntary acts develop |
| | | Imitation predominates |
| | | Thought is dominated by physical manipulation of objects and events |
| | | Develops the concept of object permanence and the ability to form mental representations |
| Preoperational | 2–7 years | Advancing use of language and movement |
| | | Development of egocentric, animistic, and magical thinking |
| | | Uses representational thought to interpret and learn, not in terms of general properties but in terms of the relationship or use to themselves |
| | | No cause-and-effect reasoning |
| | | Thought is dominated by the senses—what is seen, heard, or experienced |
| Concrete operations | 7–11 years | Mental reasoning processes assume logical approaches to solving concrete problems, including cause and effect |
| | | Collecting; mastering facts |
| | | Can consider other points of view |
| | | Thought influenced by social contacts |
| | | Language is perfected |
| Formal operations | 11–15 years | True logical thought and manipulation of abstract concepts emerge |
| | | Morality established |

Modified from Piaget, J. (1959). *Language and thought of the child.* New York: Routledge; Piaget, J., & Inhelder, B. (2000). *The psychology of the child.* New York: Basic Books; Schuster, C. S., & Ashburn, S. S. (1992). *The process of human development: A holistic life span approach* (2nd ed.). Boston: Lippincott.

is striving to maintain a balance, or equilibrium, between assimilation and accommodation (Phillips, 1975; Piaget, 1950).

Piaget described the stages of cognitive development throughout the developmental years. Through a natural unfolding of ability, the child acquires sequentially predictable cognitive abilities. Given adequate environmental stimuli and an intact neurological system, the child gradually matures toward full conceptualized reasoning. Piaget's theory of cognitive development encompasses the time from birth to approximately 15 years of age. Each of the four distinct stages is summarized in Table 9.4 and is discussed more fully in the specific chapters on each developmental age. Piaget suggests that quantitative, but no further qualitative, changes in cognitive function occur after approximately age 15 years. Although more recent developmental theorists may dispute some of Piaget's findings, this scheme of cognitive development assists the nurse in assessing growth and development in children and adolescents (Carey, Zaitchik, & Bascandziez, 2015).

## Cognitive Development: Vygotsky's Theory

One of the significant differences between the cognitive theories of Piaget and Vygotsky is that Piaget believed that development precedes learning. Piaget proposed that a level of cognitive development must be reached *before* learning can occur. Vygotsky thought that by viewing development and learning in this way, adults would teach to the lowest ability, aiming instruction at those mental functions or intellectual operations that had already matured in the child (Wink & Putney, 2002). In contrast, Vygotsky proposed that learning precedes development. He states that learning pulls development, which is in stark contrast to Piaget, who felt children are not capable of learning something until they are developmentally ready.

Vygotsky argued that, while learning may be similar among children at certain times or phases of development, it is not identical in all children because of their differing social and cultural experiences (Vygotsky, 1978). He felt Piaget overemphasized the intellectual and biological universality of developmental stages. Vygotsky was more interested in the cultural and social influences on learning and development, as well as how individual children actively internalize what they learn from others. For Vygotsky, development begins as an interpersonal process of "meaning making," which then becomes an individualized process of "making sense." There are no predetermined levels of development; rather, experience is in the front—leading and expanding development in unlimited ways.

Although Vygotsky's theory of cognitive development is less known to health care providers, educators have embraced his theory, especially what he refers to as the zone of proximal development. The zone of proximal development is the distance between the actual developmental level and the potential developmental level (Wink & Putney, 2002). In this zone, children are pulled toward new learning through their interaction with others and the environment. The guidance given by others in this zone is referred to as scaffolding. According to Vygotsky, all people need to understand not only the way in which an individual learns and develops but also the social, cultural, and political context within which that learning and development occur. This difference can profoundly impact how the nurse approaches teaching and learning (Innovative Practice).

## Moral Development: Kohlberg's Theory

Another aspect of cognitive development is the development of moral thinking and judgement. Lawrence Kohlberg's theory of moral development is based on interviews that focused on hypothetical moral dilemmas such as: Should a man steal an expensive medication that would save his dying wife? This question forms the basis of Kolhberg's classic Heinz dilemma. From interviews

## INNOVATIVE PRACTICE

### The Digital Landscape

The Canadian Paediatric Society (CPS, 2017) recommends *no screen time (television/video/computer/tablet/phone) for children younger than 2 years* and recommends limits on screen time for children older than 2 years. The CPS reports that active, not passive, adult–child communication is important to expand learning experiences for children (Boyce, Riley, & Patterson, 2015). Recent studies have associated television watching with decreased language development. A study of 329 children ranging in age from 2 to 48 months found that even audible television that decreased the child's exposure to discernible adult speech led to decreased child vocalizations and delayed speech development (Christakis, Gilkerson, Richards, et al., 2009). In a similar study, television viewing by itself was significantly negative for the child younger than 2 years, but this negative result disappeared with the inclusion of two-sided adult–child conversations (Zimmerman, Gilkerson, Richards, et al., 2009). Previous studies reported that infants and toddlers learn faster and better when they are able to interact with adults, rather than just watch and listen (Boyce et al., 2015).

A later study of 3- to 5-year-olds refined these findings and indicated that the amount of television viewing negatively affected vocabulary and executive functioning, but this affect disappeared when the home learning environment was removed as a background variable (Blankson, O'Brien, Leerkes, et al., 2015). A systematic review (Carson, Kuzik, Hunter, et al., 2015) of 37 studies of cognitive development in healthy children from birth to 5 years reported that the type of sedentary behaviour, particularly television screen time as opposed to reading, may have differential effects on cognitive development. This study reported that further studies need to investigate the whole range of cognitive domains (language, spatial skill, executive function, and memory) to fully investigate the relationship between cognitive development and television viewing. Since the American Academy of Pediatrics (AAP) guidelines were introduced in 2013, there has been an explosion in the use of digital devices, including iPads, tablets, and smartphones, and applications created for young children. Professional policy advice in this area may lag behind digital innovation (Brown, Shifrin, & Hill, 2015). The nurse needs to convey to parents that the evidence supporting the recommendation for less television viewing for children from birth to age 5 years is evolving as this is studied further and access to digital devices increases.

- How can nurses talk to parents about the recommendation for television viewing for children younger than 2 years?
- How can nurses use the results of this study when teaching parents that face-to-face interaction and two-way conversations with their children promote cognitive development more than watching television, videos, or other virtual media?
- How can the nurse support parents to role model appropriate behaviours regarding online politeness and use of media?
- How can nurses reinforce a focus that content matters and content quality is more influential than the media platform?

Sources: Blankson, A. N., O'Brien, M., Leerkes, E. M., et al. (2015). Do hours spent viewing television at ages 3 and 4 predict vocabulary and executive functioning at age 5? *Merrill-Palmer Quarterly, 61*(2), 264–289; Boyce, J. S., Riley, J. G., & Patterson, L. G. (2015). Adult-child communication: A goldmine of learning experience. *Childhood Education, 91*(3), 169–173; Brown, A., Shifrin, D. L., & Hill, D. L. (2015). Beyond 'turn it off': How to advise families on media use. *AAPNews, 36*(10). Retrieved from http://www.aappublications.org/content/36/10/54; Canadian Paediatric Society (CPS). (2017). *Screen time and young children: Promoting health and development in a digital world.* Retrieved from https://www.cps.ca/en/documents/position/screen-time-and-young-children; Carson, V., Kuzik, N., Hunter, S., et al. (2015). Systematic review of sedentary behavior and cognitive development in early childhood. *Preventive Medicine, 78*, 115–122; Christakis, D. A., Gilkerson, J., Richards, J. A., et al. (2009). Audible television and decreased adult words, infant vocalizations, and conversational turns. *Archives of Pediatric and Adolescent Medicine, 163*(6), 554–558; Zimmerman, F. J., Gilkerson, J., Richards, J. A., et al. (2009). Teaching by listening: The importance of adult-child conversations to language development. *Pediatrics, 124*(1), 342–349.

with boys, Kohlberg developed his theory, which is outlined in Table 9.5 (Kohlberg, 1969, 1981). The three stages of moral development—preconventional, conventional, and postconventional—were based on Piaget's theory of cognitive development and emphasize the ethics of rights and justice. Progression through the successive stages of moral development generally occurs during the school-age, adolescent, and young-adult years. Beyond the young-adult years, stabilization or increased consistency of thought and perhaps an increased correlation between moral judgement and moral action occur (Kohlberg, 1981).

### Moral Development: Gilligan's Theory

Carol Gilligan's theory of moral development (Gilligan, 1982, 2013; Gilligan, Ward, & Taylor, 1988) suggests that the process of moral development differs in women. While a doctoral student, Gilligan conducted research with Lawrence Kohlberg at Harvard University. She discovered that Kohlberg's original research was conducted with only men and that women often scored lower in Kohlberg's scaling of moral levels. She asserted that women were not inferior in their moral development, just different. In developing her own research with women, she proposed an alternative theory of moral development, which, like Kohlberg's, has three stages (Table 9.6). Gilligan concluded that the transitions between stages are based on changes in one's

**TABLE 9.5   Growth and Development**

### Kohlberg's Stages of Moral Development

| Stage | Goal |
|---|---|
| Preconventional | Avoiding punishment |
|  | Gaining reward |
| Conventional | Gaining approval |
|  | Avoiding disapproval |
| Postconventional | Agreeing upon rights |
|  | Establishing personal moral standards |
|  | Achieving justice |

Source: Kohlberg, L. (1981). *The philosophy of moral development* (Vol. 1). San Francisco: Harper & Row.

sense of self rather than on changes in cognitive development, as Kohlberg proposed. Gilligan more clearly differentiated the "voice of care" from the "voice of justice." She also reported that women think and act more from a base of caring and relationships than do men, who are more inclined to think in terms of justice, rights, and rules. The voice of justice promotes legislative policies (e.g., immigration) and development of codes of ethics (McThomas, 2015); the voice of caring speaks to the importance of social relationships, which directs health practitioners to pay more attention to individual moral situations (Campbell, 2015).

## TABLE 9.6  Growth and Development

### Gilligan's Stages of Moral Development (for Women)

| Stage | Characteristics | Goal |
|---|---|---|
| Preconventional | What is practical to others and best for self, realizing connection to others | Individual survival |
| Conventional | Sacrifices wants and needs to fulfill others' wants and needs | Self-sacrifice is goodness |
| Postconventional | Moral equal of self and others | Principle of nonviolence: do not hurt self or others |

Sources: Gilligan, C. (1982). *In a different voice: Psychological theory and women's development.* Cambridge, MA: Harvard University Press; Gilligan, C. (2013). *Joining the resistance.* Malden, MA: Polity Press; Gilligan, C., Ward, J. V., & Taylor, J. M. (Eds.). (1988). *Mapping the moral domain: A contribution of women's thinking to psychology and education.* Cambridge, MA: Harvard University Press.

## BEHAVIOURAL BIOLOGICAL DEVELOPMENT

All the preceding theories discuss the importance of experience and environmental exposure on behaviour and learning. One of the fundamental questions in the nature versus nurture debate is understanding how environmental stress (physical and behavioural) alters biological development (epigenetics). Evidence in animals and from human epidemiological studies indicates that experiences and the environment change the functioning of genes, and thus provide a basis for a model of gene–environment interaction. Early life experiences and social exposures may alter the way in which genes direct cell activities (Genomics); early life adversity, including living in poverty, appears to result in DNA changes in the brain and other body tissues (Szyf, Tang, Hill, et al., 2016). Recent studies suggest that even parental experiences can affect the behaviour of children; brain plasticity theory describes brain cell development that can potentially modify ways individuals learn and experience their outside environment. This has implications for physical disease as well as attention and behavioural and mental health disorders, and even the transmission of behavioural traits to the next generation (Szyf, 2015) (see Genomics box).

## GENOMICS

### Epigenetics

- What is epigenetics?
- What are the associations between environmental stressors and physical and behavioural disorders?
- How can stressors, including poverty, affect more than one generation?

Epigenetics is the scientific investigation of the capacity of cells to react differently to variations in environmental stimuli that are not related to the DNA code itself. The term epigenetics means "above genetics." Variations in cell response were historically attributed to changes in DNA gene sequences and the manufacture of cellular proteins with RNA transcription. However, this description does not fully explain why cells sharing identical DNA sequences can have differing appearances and effects. Some of this was attributed to cell mutations or alternative forms of genes (alleles). Again, this did not fully explain the full variety of appearances seen. Further scientific investigations showed that in two cells having identical DNA, the genes may be expressed differently. Cells are capable of regulating gene expression via the presence of regulatory proteins that wrap around DNA and RNA and can change cell function negatively or positively. Some of these regulatory proteins may turn off (repress) or silence cell function (methylation). Methylation and cell regulatory proteins are stable and heritable and separate from DNA genomic patterns. Epigenetic investigations have shown that these regulatory changes can be long-lasting and passed from one generation to the next. Stressors and/or maltreatment affecting one generation may have lasting behaviour effects on subsequent generations. It is estimated that many of these epigenetic regulatory changes occur early in childhood and brain development (before the age of 3 years), and that poor early development influences risks of adult diseases (diabetes, obesity, heart disease, mental health, and addiction problems) (Szyf et al., 2016; van Dijk, Molloy, Varinli, et al., 2015). There are also associations with attention deficit disorders, learning problems, and acquisition of language and numeral skills. Studies have linked poverty to brain impairment in early child development (Boivin, Kakooza, Warf, et al., 2015). Whereas this science is in its infancy, and it is difficult to study human generational effects, there is no question that various stressors and physical and learning disorders affecting parents and children may be a problem for the next generation (Szyf, 2015), even when the original precipitating stressors are removed.

Sources: Boivin, M. J., Kakooza, A. M, Warf, B. C., et al. (2015). Reducing neurodevelopmental disorders and disability through research and interventions. *Nature, 527*(7578), S155–S160; Szyf, M. (2015). Nongenetic inheritance and transgenerational epigenetics. *Trends in Molecular Medicine, 21*(2), 134–144; Szyf, M., Tang, Y., Hill, K. G., et al. (2016). The dynamic epigenome and its implications for behavioral interventions: A role for epigenetics to inform disorder prevention and health promotion. *Translational Behavioral Medicine, 6*(1), 55–62; van Dijk, S. J., Molloy, P. L., Varinli, H., et al. (2015). Epigenetics and human obesity. *International Journal of Obesity, 39*, 85–97.

## CASE STUDY

### Birth of a Disabled/Chronically Ill Child: Avery

Avery is a 33-year-old woman pregnant with her third child; her other two children are aged 5 and 10 years. At 26 weeks' gestation, Avery is hospitalized for contractions. Despite pharmacological attempts to stop labour, Avery's labour continues to the active phase. Avery and her partner just learned that a baby born this prematurely may have many problems, including cerebral palsy. As the perinatologist leaves the room, Avery turns to the nurse and starts to cry.

*Reflective Questions*

- What is the nurse's role when the parents learn a child has a chronic disease and/or disability?
- What can the nurse anticipate for these new parents during the labour? At the birth of the baby?

- What can the nurse anticipate in the first 2 weeks after birth? Over the baby's first year of life? Over the first 5 years?
- How will this child's growth, development, and goals for health promotion be affected? What about those of the parents? What about those of the siblings?
- What factors might contribute to Avery's development of chronic sorrow?
- If Avery becomes depressed, how might this affect the growth and development of the new baby? What effect might this have on her relationship with her partner? What effect might her depression have on her other children?
- What will be the impact of this child's disabilities on the siblings?
- How might the nurse intervene to lessen the effects of chronic sorrow?

## CARE PLAN

### Birth of a Disabled/Chronically Ill Child: Avery

**Nursing Issue**

Persistent sorrow (parental) related to missed opportunities and unending care-giving for a new child

**Definition**

A cyclical, recurring, and potentially progressive pattern of pervasive sadness experienced (by a parent, caregiver, individual with chronic illness or disability) in response to continual loss, throughout the trajectory of an illness or disability

**Defining Characteristics**

- Parental expression of disparity between preconceived notions of parenting and reality
- Parental expression of an ongoing or recurrent sense of sadness or loss
- Parental expressions of negative feelings (e.g., anger, depression, disappoint-ment, emptiness, frustration, self-blame, helplessness, hopelessness, loneli-ness, overwhelmed) that are often triggered by health care crises or conflict with expected social norms for child or family

**Related Factors**

- Change in family structure
- Change in parental role expectation
- Parental coping styles

**Goal**

- Assist family unit to attain, maintain, or regain optimal health

**Expected Outcomes**

- Grief resolution: *adjustment to actual or impending loss.* For example, parents verbalize reality of loss, progress through stages of grief, decreasing preoccupation with loss, verbalize acceptance of loss, resolve feelings about loss.

- Hope: *optimism that is personally satisfying and life-supporting.* For example, parents express inner peace, expectation of a positive future.
- Psychosocial adjustment: *adaptive psychosocial response of an individual to a significant life change.* For example, parents set realistic goals, maintain pro-ductivity, verbalize optimism about present, use effective coping strategies, report feeling socially engaged.

**Nursing Interventions**

- Grief work facilitation: *helping another cope with painful feelings of actual or perceived responsibility.* For example, listen to expression of grief, encourage identification of fears, and assist in identifying modifications that are needed in their lifestyle.
- Hope inspiration: *Enhancing the belief in one's capacity to initiate and sustain actions.* For example, help identify areas of hope in their lives, demonstrate hope by recognizing the disability or illness as only one facet of the child, and provide parents with opportunities to be involved with support groups, especially with other parents of children who are disabled/chronically ill who have transcended.
- Coping enhancement: *assisting a person to adapt to perceived stressors, changes, or threats that interfere with meeting life demands and roles.* For example, provide an atmosphere of acceptance, seek to understand each par-ent's perspective of the situation, appraise and discuss alternative responses to the situation, foster constructive outlets for negative feelings, assist the parents to identify positive strategies to deal with limitations, and manage necessary lifestyle changes.
- Resiliency promotion: *assisting individuals, families, and communities in development, use, and strengthening of protective factors to be used in coping with environmental and societal stressors.* For example, encourage positive health-seeking behaviour, facilitate development, and use neigh-bourhood resources.

Sources: Bulechek, G. M., Butcher, H. K., Dochterman, J. M., et al. (Eds.) (2013). *Nursing interventions classification (NIC)* (6th ed.). St Louis: Mosby; Johnson, M., Moorhead, S., Bulechek, G., et al. (2011). *NANDA, NOC, and NIC linkages* (3rd ed.). St Louis: Mosby; Kao, B., Plante, W., & Lobato, D. (2009). The use of the impact on sibling scale with families of children with chronic illness and developmental disability. *Child: Care, Health and Development, 35*(4), 505–509; Masterson, M. K. (2010). *Chronic sorrow in mothers of adult children with cerebral palsy: An exploratory study.* Doctoral dissertation (UMI AA13408137). Kansas State University; Marcella-Brienza, S., & Mennillo, T. (2015). Back to work: Manager support of nurses with chronic sorrow. *Creative Nursing, 21*(4), 206–210; Moorhead, S., Johnson, M., Maas, M., et al. (Eds.). (2013). *Nursing outcomes classification (NOC)* (5th ed.). St. Louis: Mosby; Patrick-Ott, A., & Ladd, L. D. (2010). The blending of Boss's concept of ambiguous loss and Olshansky's concept of chronic sorrow: A case study of a family with a child who has significant disabilities. *Journal of Creativity in Mental Health, 5,* 74–86.

## ▌ SUMMARY

Individuals make many choices that affect their health each day, and a number of factors influence how these choices are made. The stage of growth and development, as well as the context in which learning occurs, influences how individuals experience different situations and realize the choices available. Understanding the most widely used theories of human growth and development assists nurses to have a clear understanding of the challenges an individual is likely to encounter, as well as the skills the individual is likely to need, for successful growth, development, and maturation throughout the life span. Theories provide nurses with frameworks, resources, and comparisons for health assessment, promotion, and intervention.

**Evolve Chapter Features**

http://evolve.elsevier.com/Canada/Edelman/healthpromotion/

- Review Questions

## REFERENCES

Blankson, A. N., O'Brien, M., Leerkes, E. M., et al. (2015). Do hours spent viewing television at ages 3 and 4 predict vocabulary and exec-utive functioning at age 5? *Merrill-Palmer Quarterly, 61*(2), 264–289.

Boivin, M. J., Kakooza, A. M., Warf, B. C., et al. (2015). Reducing neurodevelopmental disorders and disability through research and interventions. *Nature, 527*(7578), S155–S160.

Bosman, J., & Smith, M. (2016). *Gov. Rick Synder of Michigan apolo-gizes in Flint water crisis.* New York Times. January 19. Retrieved from http://www.nytimes.com/2016/01/20/us/obama-set-to-meet-with-mayor-of-flint-about-water-crisis.html?r=00.

Boyce, J. S., Riley, J. G., & Patterson, L. G. (2015). Adult-child communication: A goldmine of learning experience. *Childhood Education, 91*(3), 169–173.

Brown, A., Shifrin, D. L., & Hill, D. L. (2015). Beyond 'turn it off': How to advise families on media use. *AAPNews, 36*(10). Retrieved from http://www.aappublications.org/content/36/10/54.

Paediatric Society (CPS), Canadian (2017). *Screen time and young children: Promoting health and development in a digital world.* Retrieved from https://www.cps.ca/en/documents/position/screen-time-and-young-children.

Campbell, T. (2015). Voicing unease: Care ethics in the professionalization of social care. *The New Bioethics, 21*(1), 33–45. https://doi.org/10.1179/2050287715Z.00000000065.

Carey, S., Zaitchik, D., & Bascandziez, I. (2015). Theories of development: In dialog with Jean Piaget. *Developmental Review, 38*, 36–54. https://doi.org/10.1016/j.dr.2015.07.003.

Carson, V., Kuzik, N., Hunter, S., et al. (2015). Systematic review of sedentary behavior and cognitive development in early childhood. *Preventive Medicine, 78*, 115–122.

Centers for Disease Control and Prevention (CDC). (2010). Use of World Health Organization and CDC growth charts for children aged 0–59 months in the United States. *MMWR. Recommendations and Reports, 59*(rr09), 1–15. [Seminal Reference].

Centers for Disease Control and Prevention (CDC). (2011a). CDC health disparities and inequalities report—United States, 2011. *MMWR. Recommendations and Reports, 60*(Suppl), 1–116. [Seminal Reference].

Centers for Disease Control and Prevention (CDC). (2011b). Ten great public health achievements—United States, 2001–2010. *MMWR. Recommendations and Reports, 60*(19), 619–623. [Seminal Reference].

Christakis, D. A., Gilkerson, J., Richards, J. A., et al. (2009). Audible television and decreased adult words, infant vocalizations, and conversational turns. *Archives of Pediatric and Adolescent Medicine, 163*(6), 554–558. [Seminal Reference].

Dietitians of Canada, Canadian Paediatric Society, College of Family Physicians of Canada, & Community Health Nurses of Canada. (2010). *Promoting optimal monitoring of child growth in Canada: Using the new WHO growth charts.* Retrieved from https://www.cps.ca/uploads/tools/growth-charts-statement-FULL.pdf. [Seminal Reference].

Erikson, E. H. (1968). *Identity, youth, and crisis.* New York: Norton.

Erikson, E. H. (1995). *Childhood and society* (35th anniversary ed.). New York: Norton. [Seminal Reference].

Erikson, E. H., & Erikson, J. M. (1998). *The life cycle completed.* New York: Norton. [Seminal Reference].

Gilligan, C. (1982). *A different voice: Psychological theory and women's development.* Cambridge, MA: Harvard University Press. [Seminal Reference].

Gilligan, C. (2013). *Joining the resistance.* Malden, MA: Polity Press. [Seminal Reference].

Gilligan, C., Ward, J. V., & Taylor, J. M. (Eds.). (1988). *Mapping the moral domain: A contribution of women's thinking to psychology theory and education.* Cambridge, MA: Harvard University Press. [Seminal Reference].

Government of Canada. (2018). *Indigenous early learning and child care framework.* Retrieved from https://www.canada.ca/en/employment-social-development/programs/indigenous-early-learning/2018-framework.html.

Government of Canada. (2019). *Canada's health care system.* Retrieved from https://www.canada.ca/en/health-canada/services/health-care-system/reports-publications/health-care-system/canada.html.

Kohlberg, L. (1969). Continuities and discontinuities in childhood and adult moral development. *Human Development, 12*, 93–120. [Seminal Reference].

Kohlberg, L. (1981). *The philosophy of moral development* (Vol. 1). San Francisco: Harper & Row. [Seminal Reference].

Maalouf-Manasseh, Z., Metallinos-Katsaras, E., & Dewey, K. G. (2011). Obesity in preschool children is more prevalent and identified at a younger age when WHO growth charts are used compared with CDC charts. *Journal of Nutrition, 141*, 1154–1158. [Seminal Reference].

McThomas, M. (2015). Engendering attitudes toward immigration policy: The impact of justice and care. *Public Integrity, 17*(2), 177–188. https://doi.org/10.1080/10999922.2015.1000772.

Mei, Z., & Grummer-Strawn, L. M. (2011). Comparison of changes in growth percentiles of US children on CDC 2000 growth charts with corresponding changes on WHO 2006 growth charts. *Clinical Pediatrics, 50*(5), 402–407. [Seminal Reference].

Perry, T. E., Ruggiano, N., Shtompel, N., et al. (2015). Applying Erikson's wisdom to self-management practices of older adults. *Research on Aging, 37*(3), 253–274. https://doi.org/10.1177/0164027514527974.

Phillips, J. L. (1975). *The origins of intellect: Piaget's theory* (2nd ed.). San Francisco: W. H. Freeman. [Seminal Reference].

Piaget, J. (1950). *The psychology of intelligence.* London: Routledge and Kegan Paul. [Seminal Reference].

Read, C. Y., & Ward, L. D. (2016). Faculty performance on the genomic nursing concept inventory. *Journal of Nursing Scholarship, 48*(1), 5–13. https://doi.org/10.1111/jnu.12175.

Szyf, M. (2015). Nongenetic inheritance and transgenerational epigenetics. *Trends in Molecular Medicine, 21*(2), 134–144. https://doi.org/10.1016/j.molmed.2014.12.004.

Szyf, M., Tang, Y. Y., Hill, K. G., et al. (2016). The dynamic epigenome and its implications for behavioral interventions: A role for epigenetics to inform disorder prevention and health promotion. *Translational Behavioral Medicine, 6*(1), 55–62. https://doi.org/10.1007/s13142-016-0387-7.

Vallejo, M., Cortes-Rodrigues, B. A., & Colin-Ramirez, E. (2015). Maternal underestimation of child's weight status and health behaviors as risk factors for overweight in children. *Journal of Pediatric Nursing, 30*(6), e29–e33.

van Dijk, S. J., Molloy, P. L., Varinli, H., & Members of EpiSCOPE, et al. (2015). Epigenetics and human obesity. *International Journal of Obesity, 39*, 85–97.

Vygotsky, L. S. (1978). *Mind in society: The development of higher psychological processes.* Cambridge, MA: Harvard University Press.

Vygotsky, L. S. (1986). *Thought and language.* Cambridge, MA: MIT Press.

Wink, J., & Putney, L. (2002). *A vision of Vygotsky.* Boston: Allyn & Bacon. [Seminal Reference].

Words, First (2009). Nipissing District developmental screening tool. Retrieved from https://firstwords.ca/nipissing-district-developmental-screening-tool/.

World Health Organization (WHO). (2010). *Childhood lead poisoning.* Retrieved from https://www.who.int/ceh/publications/leadguidance.pdf. [Seminal Reference].

Ziegler, E. E., & Nelson, S. E. (2012). The WHO growth standards: Strengths and limitations. *Current Opinion in Clinical Nutrition and Metabolic Care, 15*(3), 298–302. [Seminal Reference].

Zimmerman, F. J., Gilkerson, J., Richards, J. A., et al. (2009). Teaching by listening: The importance of adult-child conversations to language development. *Pediatrics, 124*(1), 342–349. [Seminal Reference].

# 10

# The Prenatal Period

*Kaitlyn Hall, RN*

Originating US chapter by *Susan Scott Ricci, CNE, MEd, MSN, ARNP*

## INTENDED LEARNING OUTCOMES

*After completing this chapter, the reader will be able to:*

- Differentiate fetal development and the newborn transition to extrauterine life.
- Analyze changes in the maternal system during pregnancy on the basis of their influences on pregnancy adaptation.
- Interpret the role of the nurse in promoting the physical, mental, and spiritual health of the childbearing family.
- Compare and contrast fetal complications caused by maternal drinking, smoking, drug use, and viral exposure during pregnancy.
- Outline the nursing role during labour and birth with a focus on the physical, emotional, spiritual, and educational needs of the woman giving birth and her family.
- Evaluate the influence of factors such as ethnicity, legislative priorities, and the sociopolitical context of the health care delivery system on prenatal and childbirth care and the needs of families.

## KEY TERMS

Acquired immunodeficiency syndrome (AIDS)
Amniocentesis
Amniotic membranes
Anemia of pregnancy
Apgar scoring system
Bacterial vaginosis
Bradycardia
*Candida albicans*
Cervical effacement
*Chlamydia*
Chloasma
Chorionic membranes
Chorionic villi
Colostrum
Conception
Congenital defect
Cytomegalovirus (CMV)
Dilation
Diversity
Down syndrome
Embryo
Endometrium
Estrogen
Fertilization
Fetal alcohol spectrum disorder
Fetal alcohol syndrome
Fetal heart monitor
Fetus

First stage of labour
Fourth stage of labour
Fundus
Gestation
Gestational hypertension
Gonococcus (GC)
Group B streptococcus
Hepatitis B virus (HBV)
Herpes simplex
Human chorionic gonadotropin (hCG)
Human immunodeficiency virus (HIV)
Infant mortality rate (IMR)
Infertility
Labour
Lamaze
Linea nigra
Meconium
Miscarriage
Neonatal abstinence syndrome
Obesity
Pica
Placenta
Polyhydramnios
Positive signs of pregnancy
Prejudices
Premature delivery
Presumptive signs of pregnancy
Preterm birth

**THINK ABOUT IT**

### *First Pregnancy Labour*

Laura, currently 41 weeks into her first pregnancy, is admitted at 2:00 a.m. to the hospital with uterine contractions occurring every 8 minutes since midnight. Her cervix is dilated to 2 cm and is 80% effaced, and her station is –3. Her husband is out of town on a business trip, and Laura's neighbour has accompanied her to the hospital. Although Laura attended prenatal classes with her husband, she is anxious about the labour. She says to the nurse, "My back is about to break, I have so much bottom pressure, and I wanted to go natural, without medication and all this high-technology stuff, including the monitor."

- On the basis of your knowledge of ethical and legal principles of care, how would you as a caregiver appropriately respond to Laura's needs with labour and birth?
- What factors in Laura's database would support the use of the fetal heart monitor? What factors would not support use of the monitor?
- What political, legal, ethical, and other factors might be relevant to the widespread use of monitors in Canadian maternity units today?
- How does the use of fetal heart rate monitoring fit into a health-promotion approach to labour and birth?

The process of conception, pregnancy, and birth involves a complex interaction of many factors, including the physiological and psychological changes in the woman and family and the development of a fetus into a viable newborn. The nurse's role during the pregnancy cycle should encompass evidence-informed practice recommendations for effective health-promotion interventions prenatally, intranatally, and postnatally to improve maternal and newborn health outcomes. The focus of this chapter is on the pregnant woman, her family, and the developing fetus. The nurse must consider all three entities when seeking to promote a healthy pregnancy and healthy family system after birth.

## BIOLOGY AND GENETICS

Cells are the basic units of life. Pregnancy begins with fertilization, the fusion of a sperm from a male and an egg from a female. Each one contains half of the genetic material to form a new individual. Fertilization is the first embryonic event in a series that culminates in the birth of an infant. The physical changes during pregnancy include natural processes involving fertilization of the egg by the sperm, implantation of the fertilized egg into the uterus, embryonic or fetal growth and development, placental development and function, and maternal changes related to the pregnancy process.

### Duration of Pregnancy

Pregnancy begins with the union of a sperm and an egg, a process called fertilization. Under normal healthy circumstances, a full-term pregnancy lasts approximately 9 solar months, 10 lunar months, or 40 weeks. An accurate estimated date of delivery is determined by use of Nägele's rule. One does this by adding 7 days to the date of the first day of the last normal menstrual period and subtracting 3 months. A usual pregnancy consists of 9 months, divided into three equal periods called trimesters. Often these trimesters form the basis for discussion of expected fetal and maternal changes during pregnancy.

### Fertilization

The union of a sperm and an egg requires several crucial factors, many of which are not fully understood. When a sperm cell penetrates an egg in the ampulla of the fallopian tube, the beginning of a human being (called a *zygote*) results. Early cell divisions occur while the zygote is slowly being transported through the fallopian tube toward the uterus. Additional division of zygotic cells results in more differentiated structures that eventually produce an embryo and, subsequently, a fetus.

An absence of one or more critical factors may cause infertility (failure of the couple to become pregnant despite usual sexual activity in a period of 1 year). For example, both a sperm cell and an egg cell must be mature and in the fallopian tube for approximately 5 hours for union of the sperm and egg to occur (the process of conception). The sperm must be of uniform size, be normally formed, possess high motility, and have an ability to secrete enzymes that dissolve the membrane surrounding the egg. Cellular changes within the egg prevent other sperm from entering the ovum after the sperm penetrates it (Mattson & Smith, 2015). The woman attempting pregnancy must have a certain basal body temperature and fallopian tubes free of adhesions or obstructions. A woman will likely conceive within 24 hours after ovulation.

### Implantation

The process of attachment and placental formation is called implantation. A pregnancy has not occurred until successful implantation has happened. The placenta is an organ that serves to prevent the direct exchange between the blood of the fetus and the blood of the mother. It also functions as an endocrine gland, manufacturing and secreting hormones that play a vital role in maintaining the pregnancy. Transplantation of the fertilized egg in the uterine cavity after its trip through the fallopian tube requires approximately 6 days (Mader & Windelspecht, 2015). Once the zygote reaches the uterus, it stays there for up to 5 days, receiving nutrition from the endometrium, the inner lining of the uterus (El-Mazny, 2014). The process of fertilization and implantation triggers the production of large amounts of the hormone progesterone, which stimulates the formation of endometrial cells known as the decidua, meaning "to shed." The decidua provides nutrition for the embryo, a term that defines the growing conceptus up to 8 weeks of age.

## Fetal Growth and Development

Much is known about the stages of physical development in each structural system of the embryo. However, metabolic functions, particularly those relevant to the endocrine and neurological systems, are less well defined. Appropriate fetal development depends on these events occurring in a specified period and order during each trimester of pregnancy. If this does not occur, an abnormality in structure or function (a congenital defect) may result. This defect may be noted at birth, did not occur at conception (called a genetic defect), but most likely resulted from some disruption that occurred after conception and during fetal development.

## Placental Development and Function

After implantation of the zygote, the placenta develops through an integration of embryonic and decidual cells. The chorionic membranes and amniotic membranes, which surround the fetus throughout gestation, also begin to form. The amniotic fluid, manufactured by the amniotic membrane, supports the developing fetus and protects it from injury.

The basic structure of the placenta allows maternal–fetal blood exchange to nourish the fetus and allow excretion of fetal waste products. Throughout most of gestation, increasing placental development allows maternal blood to flow through the intervillous spaces and fetal blood to flow through the chorionic villi (Cunningham, Leveno, Bloom, et al., 2014). The unique structure of the placenta permits the exchange of certain molecules but prevents fetal and maternal blood supplies from mixing for most of the pregnancy. Substances with larger and heavier molecules (such as heparin or insulin) normally do not pass through the placenta to the fetus, but lighter molecules (such as anaesthetic gases, oxygen, carbon dioxide, and electrolytes) readily cross the placenta. Due to the difficulty involved in predicting exactly which substances will cross the placenta, the nurse needs to encourage pregnant women and those contemplating pregnancy to avoid any substance that might cause harm to the fetus.

The placenta manufactures and secretes four hormones throughout pregnancy. The primary hormones produced by the placenta are estrogen, progesterone, human chorionic gonadotropin (hCG), and human placental lactogen (hPL). Estrogen's role is to increase uterine blood flow and increase uterine and breast growth. Progesterone maintains the uterus in a quiet state throughout the pregnancy to prevent labour contractions occurring too early. The main role of hCG is to sustain estrogen and progesterone production in early pregnancy, and it is also the hormone detected in pregnancy tests. hPL ensures adequate fetal nutrition, increases insulin resistance, and stimulates production of growth hormones (King, Brucker, Fahey, et al., 2015).

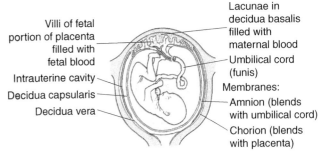

**Fig. 10.1** Relationship of Fetus, Placenta, Membranes, and Uterus During Gestation (From Lowdermilk, D., Perry, S., Cashion, K., et al. [2016]. *Maternity and women's health care* [11th ed.]. St. Louis: Mosby.)

The fetus, which continues to gain strength and maturity during the later weeks of gestation, generally rests its head in the lower maternal pelvis by the end of pregnancy (Fig. 10.1). The membranes protect the fetus from infection and act as a container for the amniotic fluid. As birth begins, the membranes may rupture, causing the loss of amniotic fluid and stronger uterine contractions, reflective of the labour process. If the membranes rupture more than 24 hours before birth, uterine infection and potential fetal harm may result.

As gestation nears completion, placental function gradually decreases, which may serve as a stimulus for the onset of labour. When pregnancy continues beyond 42 weeks, or 2 weeks beyond the calculated due date, placental function decreases even more, posing concerns about the well-being of the fetus (Blackburn, 2014).

The discussion of fetal development provides only a brief glimpse of the prenatal period. It is also important to address maternal changes and culmination of the prenatal period, labour, and birth.

## Maternal Changes

A woman experiences various physiological effects based on a combination of hormonal and mechanical changes during pregnancy. Hormonal influences tend to increase as the pregnancy progresses. The mechanical (hemodynamic) changes reach a peak in the seventh or eighth month and then gradually decline as the pregnancy nears completion (Cunningham et al., 2014). Clinical symptoms will manifest themselves during this peak stress time.

### Signs of Pregnancy

A woman may assume that she is pregnant because she has skipped her menstrual period or experiences nausea and vomiting, changes in breast sensations and size, or increased urinary frequency (presumptive signs of pregnancy). Presumptive signs of pregnancy are the least reliable indicators of pregnancy because any one of them can be caused by conditions other than pregnancy. If she suspects she is pregnant, the woman should undergo a pregnancy test. If it is performed too early, a home pregnancy test may produce a false negative result attributable to a low level of human chorionic gonadotropin (hCG). This hormone, produced by the placenta and found in a pregnant woman's urine and blood,

## BOX 10.1   Signs of Pregnancy and Time of Occurrence

**Presumptive**

- Breast changes (e.g., tenderness) (3–4 weeks)
- Fatigue (12 weeks)
- Urinary frequency (6–12 weeks)
- Nausea and vomiting (4–14 weeks)
- Amenorrhea (4 weeks)
- Quickening (16–20 weeks)

**Probable**

- Enlargement of the uterus (12–14 weeks)
- Softening of the uterine isthmus (Hegar sign) (6–12 weeks)
- Bluish or cyanotic colour of cervix and upper vagina (Chadwick sign) (6–8 weeks)
- Softening of the cervix (Goodell sign) (5 weeks)
- Ballottement of the fetus (16 –28 weeks)
- Positive test result for hCG in the maternal urine or blood serum (4–12 weeks)
- Changes in skin pigmentation (chloasma and linea nigra) (2nd half of pregnancy)

**Positive**

- Detection of fetal heart tones by auscultation, ultrasonography, or a Doppler scan (8–17 weeks)
- Palpation of fetal body parts with Leopold manoeuvres (19–22 weeks)
- Fetal movements visible and detected by examiner (late pregnancy)
- Radiological or ultrasonographic demonstration of fetal parts (6–16 weeks)

hCG, Human chorionic gonadotropin.

triggers a positive pregnancy result. These home pregnancy tests have a high degree of accuracy (97%), if the instructions are followed exactly. If the pregnancy test is positive, a prenatal visit should be scheduled to estimate gestational age and for the woman to receive appropriate pregnancy counselling, which should include taking folic acid supplementation to prevent neural tube defects (NTDs), if she has not already started taking it preconceptually. All women of reproductive age should supplement their diet before conception with 0.4 to 1.0 mg of folic acid daily as part of their multivitamins. The incidence of NTDs (~10 in 1000 live births in Canada) has fallen since the inclusion of folic acid supplementation and food fortification, but recent research suggests folic acid supplementation is underused because of low adherence (Ami, Bernstein, Boucher, et al., 2016; Chitayat, Matsui, Amitai, et al., 2016). As the pregnancy progresses, the woman may experience presumptive signs of pregnancy, which are subjectively experienced; probable signs of pregnancy, which are objectively observed by the health care provider; and positive signs of pregnancy, which are positive signs that verify that a pregnancy exists (Box 10.1). During the first trimester of pregnancy, using sophisticated testing with ultrasound, health care providers can determine fetal presence and placental adequacy early in pregnancy. This technology, which uses high-frequency sound waves that bounce off the fetus and are interpreted by a computer, allows visualization of the fetus and gestational structures throughout pregnancy (Norwitz & Schorge, 2015).

Nausea and vomiting in pregnancy occurs in 50% to 90% of women, and there is a tendency for many health care providers to minimize it. Health Canada has approved doxylamine-pyridoxine (Diclectin) to treat nausea and vomiting in women whose symptoms have not abated with a change in diet or other nonmedical treatments. It is a delayed-release medication containing a combination of doxylamine (antihistamine) and pyridoxine (vitamin $B_6$). The major side effect is drowsiness (Health Canada, 2016b).

### Adaptive Changes of Other Systems

In addition to pregnancy-related changes in the reproductive system, adaptive changes in other body systems occur. The urinary system undergoes the following dramatic changes during gestation:

- A 50% increase in glomerular filtration rate occurs related to the influences of estrogen and progesterone.
- Ureters increase in diameter by 25% secondary to progesterone influence.
- Urinary output increases by approximately 80% related to the total body water increase.
- Bladder capacity increases to approximately 1500 mL to accommodate extra fluids.

The cardiovascular system changes also begin in early in pregnancy and are as follows:

- Cardiac output increases by up to 50% to meet the demands of pregnancy.
- Total blood volume increases by up to 45% during pregnancy. Physiological anemia of pregnancy may result because of a greater increase in the volume of plasma compared with the volume of red blood cells.
- Heart rate increases by 10 beats per minute to compensate for the increase in blood volume.

Respiratory system changes include the following:

- Tidal volume (volume of air inspired) increases by 30% to 40%, to increase the effectiveness of air exchange. Total oxygen consumption increases by approximately 20%.
- The diaphragm is displaced upward secondary to the enlarging uterus and causes shortness of breath during the last trimester.

Increased elasticity and softening of connective tissue of the musculoskeletal system cause the following changes during pregnancy:

- The joints relax, especially the pelvic joints that support the pregnancy and create pliability at the time of birth.
- Lumbar and dorsal curves of the spine increase late in pregnancy and contribute to low back pain and the waddle of pregnancy.
- Separation of the symphysis pubis occurs secondary to the influence of the hormone relaxin.

Changes also occur in the integumentary system and include the following:

- Hormonal changes and stretching of the connective tissue of the abdomen, attributable to an enlarging uterus, lead to stretch marks (striae gravidarum).
- A narrow, brownish line (linea nigra) divides the abdomen, running from the umbilicus to the symphysis pubis. The linea nigra fades after the pregnancy ends.

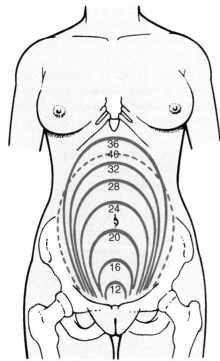

**Fig. 10.2** Upper Level of Enlarging Uterus by Weeks of Normal Gestation With a Single Fetus (From Seidel, H. M., Ball, J. W., Dains, J. E., et al. [2015]. *Mosby's guide to physical assessment* [8th ed.]. St. Louis: Mosby.)

- An increase in pigmentation caused by melanocyte-stimulating hormone causes darkened areas on the face, termed the mask of pregnancy (chloasma).

The gastrointestinal system undergoes dramatic changes, such as the following:

- The enlarging and space-occupying uterus cramps the intestinal region, causing a slowing of peristalsis and an increase in the emptying time of the stomach.
- Relaxin causes a decrease in gastric motility, leading to constipation.
- Frequent "heartburn" results from reflux of stomach contents into the esophagus secondary to upward displacement of the stomach and a relaxed gastroesophageal sphincter (King et al., 2015; Tharpe, Farley, & Jordan, 2016).

### Reproductive System

The effects on the reproductive system include changes in the uterus, breasts, vagina, vulva, and ovaries. The prepregnant uterus is approximately the size of a closed fist. The uterus at term has the capacity to contain a 3.2 to 4.5 kg (7 to 10 lb) infant and the placenta. As the uterus enlarges, the fundus (the upper uterine segment) moves higher in the abdomen (Fig. 10.2). The breasts begin enlarging early in the pregnancy, and in late pregnancy they may secrete small amounts of colostrum, a precursor of mature breast milk. *It is important to note that a pregnant woman should not express colostrum in early pregnancy, as it increases the risk for preterm labour* (Forster, Jacobs, Amir, et al., 2014). In late pregnancy, a woman may be advised by her obstetrician or midwife to express colostrum, as it can be useful for regulating the blood sugar levels of hypoglycemic newborns,

newborns with cleft lips or palates, and postpartum women experiencing early breastfeeding issues. The vagina and vulva receive a greater blood supply and appear darker (cyanotic) as a result. Some women will notice an increase in vaginal secretions and experience a whitish discharge (Mattson & Smith, 2015).

Hormones such as hCG and estrogen, secreted by the placenta and the fetus, create an optimal intrauterine environment for the fetus and stimulate many changes in the pregnant woman's body. The developing fetus contributes to the provision of an adequate environment for its own growth and nourishment, despite the possibility of creating discomforts for the pregnant woman.

### Preconception Care of Women

Preconception health promotion is a primary intervention that benefits reproductive-age women and their potential children. Prenatal care has been used as secondary prevention to improve the health of the woman during her pregnancy, but by the time prenatal care has generally started at weeks 8 to 12, a considerable amount of fetal development has already occurred. The fetus is most sensitive to maternal health and environmental exposures from weeks 4 to 10 of pregnancy, and many women may not know they are even pregnant then. The current Canadian recommendations on preconception health and health care (Public Health Agency of Canada [PHAC], 2017a) include the following:

- Women trying to conceive should take 400 mcg (0.4 mg) of folic acid per day.
- They should engage in 150 minutes of moderate to vigorous physical activity per day.
- They should limit alcoholic beverages to two glasses per day, 10 per week, to maintain optimal health.
- All women trying to conceive should have their immunizations up to date.

The key points introduced included that preconception health is a gateway for broader conversations about women's wellness and that health practices and policies with an individual focus have finite success (PHAC, 2017a).

Not all couples who seek preconception care are able to conceive on their own. Conception requires ovulation of a mature ovum, normal fallopian tubes, the presence of progressively motile sperm in the female reproductive tract, and an endometrium favourable for implantation. For many couples, the experience of fertility problems and aspects of the care with uncertain outcomes can be stressful and distressing. Infertility is defined as a failure to conceive after 1 year of regular and unprotected sexual intercourse. Infertility affects 1 in 6 (16%) Canadian couples (Health Canada, 2013b). Frequently, couples will seek treatment for their infertility issues and undergo testing that may include a semen analysis, assessment of ovulation, evaluation of tubal patency, and tests for ovarian reserve (Galliano & Pellicer, 2015). The nurse's role is that of support and education of the couple. The nurse can assist in educating the couple about the various methods to treat infertility and allow them to make their own decision as to which method is best for them. Infants conceived through in vitro fertilization (IVF) technologies have a higher risk of genetic abnormalities, being part of a multiple pregnancy, and being born prematurely (Green, Darbyshire, Adams, et al., 2015). The nurse must be knowledgeable to be able to respond to questions that will come up throughout the treatment experience. One of the greatest risks of assisted reproduction is the risk of obtaining a multiple pregnancy after intrauterine insemination with more than one embryo. Compared with a single pregnancy, the risks of a multiple pregnancy include iron- and folate-deficiency anemia, gestational hypertension, pre-eclampsia, polyhydramnios, gestational diabetes, and a high surgical birth rate (De Sutter, 2015). Most couples need a great deal of emotional support, and it is important for the nurse to be able to act as an advocate for them, particularly those using gestational surrogacy as a means of achieving parenthood.

Surrogacy is an arrangement in which a woman carries and gives birth to a child for another couple. The fundamental nature of families has changed over the years, whereby gestational surrogacy as an option for infertile couples is widely accepted. Gestational surrogacy, where the surrogate is not genetically related to the embryo, has become the norm. Surrogate motherhood is treated as a form of adoption in many countries: the birth mother and her partner are presumed to be the parents of the child, whereas the intended parents have to adopt the infant once it is born. In Canada, compensated surrogacy is not legal under the *Assisted Human Reproduction Act* (2004), which specifies that reimbursement may only be owed to the surrogate mother for pregnancy and birth-related fees (Government of Canada, 2018). For example, the intended parents are not required to pay for the surrogate woman's time off work related to pregnancy complications.

Preconception care before a pregnancy implies health-promotion activities that are conducted before a pregnancy occurs to address risk factors across the life span—including during adolescence. Although most pregnancies during adolescence are unintended, health behaviours initiated during this period can have a great impact, not only on future reproductive outcomes but also on present and future health.

Preconception care offers an effective and efficient means to reduce complications of pregnancy for both the mother and her newborn. Women should be made aware that certain preconception interventions may improve not only the outcomes of pregnancy but also the overall health of the woman. The following interventions may be included:

- Folic acid supplementation to reduce the risk of NTDs
- Rubella vaccination to reduce the risk of severe congenital defects
- Diabetes management to reduce the risk of birth defects threefold
- Hypothyroidism management to promote healthy fetal neurological development
- Hepatitis B vaccination for at-risk women to prevent chronic liver disease
- Human immunodeficiency virus (HIV)/acquired immunodeficiency syndrome (AIDS) screening and treatment to prevent transmission to the fetus
- Healthy diet instruction throughout pregnancy
- Physical activity needs throughout pregnancy

- Substance use and medication safety
- Intimate partner violence screening
- Counselling women about immunizations for themselves and their infants
- Assessment of chronic health conditions such as diabetes, hypertension, and thyroid disease
- Screening and treatment for sexually transmitted infections (STIs) to reduce the risk of ectopic pregnancy and/or fetal anomalies
- Oral antiepileptic medication management to minimize birth defect potential
- Cessation of acne treatment with isotretinoin (Accutane) to prevent defects
- Smoking cessation counselling to reduce negative perinatal outcomes
- Screening and treating of depression to reduce the risk of postpartum depression
- Elimination of alcohol use to prevent fetal alcohol spectrum disorders (PHAC, 2017a)

As a group, nurses are challenged to effectively translate the concept of preconception care to all women in their practice setting. By informing women that existing health conditions and medications can affect pregnancy outcomes, nurses can provide a positive environment for the woman's future pregnancy and improve overall health practices.

### Normal Discomforts of Pregnancy

Changes in the woman's body during pregnancy support a nursing diagnosis of *alteration in comfort with relevant interventions* for most women. Women may feel a sense of relief that other pregnant women have these concerns and that interventions exist to increase their comfort at various points during gestation. Particularly for those experiencing a first pregnancy, the nurse serves as a valuable support person to help expectant couples adjust to the challenges and discomforts of pregnancy, a goal for the earlier-stated diagnosis.

### Teaching the Woman About Changes to Expect in the Body During Pregnancy

In addition to serving as a caregiver, advocate, and support person, the nurse serves as a teacher throughout the pregnancy care process. Health teaching that is responsive to an individual's concerns about pregnancy may occur in the clinic, physician's office, or other care environments. Nursing interventions should address recommended professional practice guidelines for education during the prenatal period to prevent complications for the family. For example, the nurse may offer textbooks, pamphlets, DVDs, and referrals to websites and other media to increase a couple's knowledge of fetal, maternal, and family changes during gestation and then encourage and answer any questions based on the material. Going beyond one-to-one teaching, the nurse may also refer couples to early pregnancy and Lamaze childbirth preparation classes to enlarge their social support network and increase knowledge of labour and birth. Throughout the care process, the nurse is sensitive to the cultural and ethnic beliefs and behaviours of the individual or family. For instance, Indigenous women may seek prenatal

| TABLE 10.1 | Cultural Values Related to Pregnancy and Birth |
|---|---|
| Indigenous Canadians | In many nations, women are expected to seek prenatal care with pregnancy; some nations accept late care. Indigenous women are encouraged to eat according to *Canada's Food Guide—First Nations, Inuit, and Métis*. Dialogue with women in the tribal community is important to maximize pregnancy and birth process. Meditation, self-control practice, and Indigenous plants (herbal teas) are used for discomforts of pregnancy and birth. Kin are present to support women in labour; breastfeeding is encouraged after birth |
| Arab Canadians | Pregnancy is a normal event; women may not access prenatal care because of that belief. Much family support is given to pregnant woman to allow maximal rest and minimal work. They rely on family members for support. They are very modest about care, especially with an opposite-sex health care provider. |
| Chinese Canadians | Pregnant women are discouraged from engaging in moderate to vigorous physical activity to prevent risk of harm to the fetus, stillbirth or miscarriage. Avoid use of language that could be considered taboo. A warm diet is encouraged to strengthen the womb and certain meats may be avoided (Cantonese). |

NOTE: General ideas about beliefs and behaviours of each of these cultural groups have been given with no intent to stereotype all individuals who represent these groups' beliefs or behaviours. It is important that the nurse integrate cultural perspectives in care, because culture influences health practices. Becoming aware of how culture influences individual behaviour and thinking allows the nurse to plan the best care for the patient. Sources: Callister, L. (2011). Global and cultural perinatal nursing research: Improving clinical practice. *Journal of Perinatal & Neonatal Nursing, 25*(2), 139–143. doi:10.1097/JPN.0b013e318215d7c1; Haas, A. (2011). Cultural diversity in childbirth education. *Midwifery Today with International Midwife, 97*, 39; Health Canada. (2010). *Eating well with Canada's food guide—First Nations, Inuit and Métis*. Retrieved from https://www.canada.ca/en/health-canada/services/food-nutrition/reports-publications/eating-well-canada-food-guide-first-nations-inuit-metis.html; Lewallen, L. (2011). The importance of culture in childbearing. *Journal of Obstetric, Gynecologic, and Neonatal Nursing, 40*(1), 4–8. doi:10.1111/j.1552-6909.2010.01209; Purnell, L. D. (2014). *Guide to culturally competent health care* (3rd ed.). Philadelphia: F. A. Davis; Spector, R. E. (2012). *Cultural diversity in health & illness* (8th ed., pp. 101–137). Upper Saddle River, NJ: Prentice Hall; Yeo, T. R. (2013). *Chinese birth rituals*. Retrieved from http://eresources.nlb.gov.sg/infopedia/articles/SIP_2013-05-14_113920.html.

and postpartum support from a midwife through the National Aboriginal Council of Midwives [NACM] (NACM, 2019). Indigenous midwives are trained in women's health and reproduction, provide prenatal education, promote breastfeeding and parenting, and advocate for equitable access to health care. Indigenous midwives incorporate native language, tradition, and oral cultures into their practice and strive to keep the birth within the woman's community (NACM, 2019). Indigenous birthing centres are also available to Indigenous pregnant women in Canada. It is important for nurses to be knowledgeable of the beliefs and behaviours of other cultures to protect the pregnant woman and her baby by providing individualized care (Table 10.1). A summary of perinatal care guidelines is provided in Table 10.2.

Prenatally, pregnant women experience a wide variety of physiological adaptations. Nurses must possess a broad and deep understanding of these changes, combined with accurate and early risk assessment to identify deviations. This knowledge base is vital for nurses caring for women during the childbearing cycle.

## Total Weight Gain

Total weight gain during pregnancy reflects not only the growth of the baby and placenta but also the growth of the uterus and breasts, the storage of maternal fat, and the increased amounts of blood and other body fluids. Achieving the recommended weight gain will require individualized attention and support from a woman's care providers, as well as her family and community. In addition, the Internet, social media, and eHealth technologies provide unprecedented opportunities to efficiently reach and educate influential family members, friends, and the media. Utilization of these modalities can quickly transform unhealthy cultural norms and prevent significant morbidity among generations of at-risk women and children (Chang & Moniz, 2015).

The PHAC (2011b) guidelines advise that healthy women at a normal weight for their height (body mass index [BMI] of 18.5–24.9 kg/m$^2$) should gain 11.3 to 15.8 kg (25 to 35 pounds) during pregnancy. Underweight women (BMI less than 18.5 kg/m$^2$) should gain more (12.7 to 18.1 kg [28 to 40 pounds]), and overweight women (BMI of 25–29.9 kg/m$^2$) should gain less (6.8 to 11.3 kg [15 to 25 pounds]. Obese women (BMI greater than 30 kg/m$^2$) should limit their gain to 4.9 to 9.07 kg (11 to 20 pounds). Overweight and obese women are at increased risk of pregnancy complications that include abortion, gestational diabetes, hypertension, pre-eclampsia, thromboembolism, surgical birth, and postpartum weight retention. Despite the serious health implications of obesity in pregnancy, the current level of awareness of such risks among childbearing women is limited (Liat, Cabero, Hod, et al., 2015).

Ideally, all women with a BMI greater than 30 kg/m$^2$ should be provided with accurate and accessible information about the risks associated with obesity in pregnancy at a preconception visit. Most women are highly motivated to have healthy infants, which could be a key factor for nurses when having health-promotion discussions informing women of the risks of obesity in pregnancy and how to promote healthy lifestyle choices preconceptually and between pregnancies.

## Labour and Birth

Pregnancy culminates with labour and giving birth. Giving birth is a life-changing event, and the care that a woman receives during labour has the potential to affect her both physically and emotionally for a long period. The process of giving birth elicits a significant emotional response from the delivering family. A description of the events of a usual labour and birthing process must occur to establish a background for considering the physiological changes in the mother and the infant.

Several theories offer explanations for the cause of labour. Many factors likely interact, including uterine distension,

## TABLE 10.2 Perinatal Care Guidelines

| First Trimester | Second Trimester | Third Trimester | Labour Stages | Postpartum |
|---|---|---|---|---|
| Complete assessment to identify risk factors | Assess adaptation to pregnancy and fetal well-being | Review physiological changes | Admission to birthing facility | Complete a head-to-toe physical assessment: breasts, uterus, bladder, bowels, lochia<br>Emotional status<br>Circulatory status<br>Episiotomy |
| Awareness of subtle or overt physical, sexual, or emotional abuse | Update health history | Monitor changes related to pregnancy | *First stage:*<br>Complete maternal/fetal assessments<br>Determine labour progress<br>Assist with comfort measures<br>Monitor fetal heart rate<br>Support family in their efforts<br>Praise efforts | Assess mother for postpartum blues/depression |
| Assess physical and psychosocial progress in adaptation to pregnancy | Continue to recognize cultural influences | Assess expectant family's readiness for labour, birth, and parenting role | *Second stage:*<br>Offer encouragement<br>Assist with pushing efforts<br>Document activities | Encourage bonding and attachment |
| Inquire about physical changes and discomforts; explain causes and identify appropriate relief measures | Encourage informed decision making and positive health care practices | Review finalized birth plan | *Third stage:*<br>Provide care as needed<br>Document time of placental delivery<br>Administer medications as ordered | Demonstrate breastfeeding techniques |
| Provide anticipatory guidance appropriate for the woman's individual needs<br>• Educational needs: hazards during pregnancy<br>• Use of drugs, alcohol, and smoking | Review potential risk factors and when to report them<br>Ensure community referrals/resources as needed.<br>Educational needs:<br>Oral hygiene<br>Nutritional needs | Identify community resources available to the family<br>Explain any diagnostic tests ordered. Meet educational needs: needs for newborn care | *Fourth stage:*<br>Monitor vital signs, palpate fundus, assess bladder status<br>Encourage parental–infant interaction<br>Monitor newborn's well-being<br>Provide perineal care, food, fluids<br>Provide family support | Provide anticipatory guidance needed for the family<br>Educational needs:<br>Nutrition<br>Fatigue<br>Child care |
| Seat belts, high-risk behaviours<br>Warning/danger signs to report<br>Nutrition and weight management<br>Sexuality | Safety issues in workplace<br>Discomforts of pregnancy<br>Relief of common discomforts of pregnancy<br>Prepared childbirth classes | Monitoring fetal movements<br>Strategies to cope with discomforts<br>Promote family safety<br>Including partner in process<br>Childbirth preparation | | Immunizations<br>Sexuality<br>Family planning<br>Breast engorgement<br>Family adaptation<br>Follow-up care needed<br>Danger signs to report<br>Sibling readiness for new member<br>Self-care activities |

Sources: King, T. L., Brucker, M. C., Kriebs, J. M., et al. (2015). *Varney's midwifery* (5th ed.). Burlington, MA: Jones & Bartlett Learning; Macones, G. (2015). *Management of labor and delivery* (2nd ed.). Somerset, NJ: Wiley-Blackwell; Norwitz, E. R., & Schorge, J. O. (2015). *Obstetrics and gynecology at a glance* (4th ed.). Malden, MA: Blackwell Publishing.

mechanical irritation, progesterone deprivation, placental aging and hormones, and posterior pituitary activity. Labour usually begins at approximately 40 weeks of gestation, suggesting that hormonal control similar to that regulating the menstrual cycle also contributes to its onset (Cunningham et al., 2014).

Labour may be divided conveniently into the following four distinct stages:

- Dilation stage—lasts from the onset of true labour contractions to complete dilation of the cervix. It is divided into three phases: latent (0–3 cm dilation); active (4–7 cm dilation); and transition (8–10 cm dilation).
- Pushing stage—lasts from complete dilation (10 cm) of the cervix to birth.

- Placental stage—lasts from the time of birth of the newborn to delivery of the placenta and membranes, which can range from 2 to 15 minutes.
- Recovery stage—defined as the first 4 hours after childbirth, where physiological and psychological adjustments begin to occur.

The first stage of labour starts with regular timing of uterine contractions and ends with complete dilation (opening) and cervical effacement (thinning of the cervix). The signs of beginning labour include those listed in Box 10.2. The cervix, the lower portion of the uterus, must dilate from a closed position (0 cm) to a totally open position (10 cm in diameter). During the first stage, the cervix must also completely efface

## BOX 10.2 Signs of Beginning Labour

- Bloody show or loss of the mucous plug that seals cervical canal during pregnancy
- Regular uterine contractions
- Contractions increasing in intensity, duration, and frequency
- Palpable hardening of the uterus during contractions
- Pain in the lower back radiating to the front of the abdomen

or shorten from a length of 1 to 2 inches to a barely palpable (paper-thin) thickness. For most women, painless Braxton Hicks contractions throughout pregnancy cause some cervical dilation and thinning, or at least cervical softening, before the onset of active labour.

During the first stage of labour, the presenting part of the fetus begins to press on the cervix, lower uterine segment, and nerve endings around the cervix and vagina. Women's responses to this process differ; pain thresholds, cultural perceptions, and responses to pain differ among labouring women (see Table 10.1). The fundus, the active contractile part of the uterus, becomes thicker as labour progresses, retracts the lower uterine segment and cervix, and helps push the fetus toward the cervix and eventually through the vagina for birth (Macones, 2015). The first stage lasts an average of 8 to 12 hours for women experiencing a first birth and somewhat less for women having a second or additional child. On the basis of a labouring woman's needs, various pain medications, nonpharmacological measures, Lamaze breathing, and other distractive techniques may alleviate the discomfort associated with first-stage labour. Periodic vaginal examinations by the nurse or other health care provider can indicate a labouring woman's cervical dilation, effacement, and descent of the fetus into the birth canal (a concept called station). In a full-term pregnancy, loss of the amniotic membrane usually increases pressure of the fetal head against the cervix, making dilation and effacement more efficient, and tends to augment the labour process.

During the second stage of labour, the fetus descends through the lower birth canal toward the woman's perineum. It is the time elapsing from the full cervical dilation to the birth of the newborn. The upper uterine segment greatly thickens, and the abdominal muscles assist in the descent and expulsion of the fetus. Cultural practices may support pushing from a squatting or upright position and not in supine. Nurses must acknowledge that the maternity health care system has a unique culture that may clash with the cultures of many of our care recipients. For many women there is an overwhelming urge to bear down during uterine contractions at this time. The fetal head accommodates to the mother's pelvis and vaginal structure and finally, the head becomes flush with the vaginal opening on the woman's perineum. The woman at this point actively pushes to expel the newborn.

The third stage of labour begins after the birth of the newborn and lasts until placental expulsion. Placental separation usually occurs within 2 to 30 minutes after completion of the second stage. After delivery of the placenta, the health care provider examines the placenta to determine that all placental tissue is intact and to detect any abnormalities that could affect the infant's condition and adaptation to extrauterine life.

The fourth stage of labour generally consists of the first 2 hours after childbirth, during which the mother faces the greatest risk of postpartum hemorrhage. An expected blood loss of 250 mL to 500 mL may cause the mother to experience a moderate decline in blood pressure, but nurses should not wait or rely on this change to intervene (Pavord & Maybury, 2015). The mother may also experience an increase in pulse rate (tachycardia) to compensate for blood loss during the early postpartum period. The care plan at the end of this chapter addresses the nurse's role in managing the stages of labour.

### Overview of Care

Professional members of the health care team (nurses, midwives, physicians) play an important role in labour and birth, but a woman's family, partner, or significant other (i.e., husband, friend, family) also inherently contributes to her care during labour and birth, particularly in certain cultures (see Table 10.1). Many practitioners suggest that the expectations and beliefs of a birthing couple have a great effect on how the woman fulfills the mothering role. Therefore, the nurse needs to collaborate with the people who care for the pregnant woman to meet that family's needs during pregnancy, labour, and childbearing.

With increasing numbers of LGBTQ2 couples deciding to start families of their own, and the availability of alternative methods of conception, these couples are coming in contact more with nurses and health care providers throughout the birthing process (preconception, pregnancy, and postpartum periods). Nurses need to have a better understanding of their needs and ways to improve the overall experience for this population. Many challenges that lesbian, gay, bisexual, and transgender couples face include making complex childbearing decisions, navigating a health care system designed for heterosexual couples, and confronting barriers such as uncertain legal rights. Changes in health care settings to address the needs of this population might include the need to display equality signs, use of gender-neutral language on medical records, in-service education for all health care personnel to confront any heterosexist bias, and discussion of privacy issues throughout the perinatal period (Ellis, Wojnar, & Pettinato, 2015; Holley & Pasch, 2015).

The importance of the nurse's knowledge, caregiving, and support cannot be underestimated during the first stage of labour. Active emotional and physical nursing support decreases the length of many women's labours, use of analgesics and anaesthetics, and number of operative deliveries, and may help women reach their birthing goals (World Health Organization [WHO], 2016a). Provided that they are accepted by a woman's culture, independent nursing interventions to increase comfort (e.g., giving backrubs or massages, offering ice or warm fluids by mouth, assisting with ambulation and position changes, and providing a clean and dry environment) may help the labouring woman cope with the challenges of labour. Many women will request medication to diminish the pain of labour and birth, and the nurse may need to review the options for medication with each woman or couple. During the first stage, the mother must not bear down as this may cause cervical swelling; often, active nursing support and distractive techniques, such as breathing and visual refocus, can prevent pushing before the second stage of labour. A woman may depend on the nurse to model breathing techniques to relieve labour discomfort. The nurse may need to explain usual interventions during this stage of labour, including the use of a fetal heart monitor (a machine that detects and records fetal heart rate and activity during labour), intravenous fluids, a digital blood pressure machine, and a urinary catheter. Open and clear communication among the health care providers, the labouring woman and her significant others, particularly during frequent and difficult uterine contractions, will improve coping before the pushing stage begins.

Contemporary childbearing has benefited from many medical and technical advances, but the current high rate of maternity care interventions may bring about many disadvantages for the healthy majority. Current understanding suggests that safely avoiding unneeded interventions would be wise. Promoting and supporting physiological births, which are low-technology health and wellness approaches to childbearing, would yield better outcomes. Today, physiological childbearing refers to childbearing conforming to healthy biological processes. Evidence-informed research reveals that physiological childbearing facilitates better outcomes by promoting fetal readiness for birth and safety during labour, enhances labour effectiveness, provides physiological help with labour stress and pain, promotes maternal and newborn transitions, and optimizes breastfeeding and maternal–infant attachment (Buckley, 2015). Selected physiological principles include limiting use of maternity care interventions, providing prenatal care that reduces stress and anxiety in women, fostering the physiological onset of labour, not artificial intervention, encouraging hospital admission in active labour, providing privacy and reducing anxiety in labour by continuous support, making nonpharmacological pain measures available, using pharmacological measures sparingly, fostering spontaneous vaginal births, and supporting continuous skin-to-skin contact between the mother and the newborn and early breastfeeding after birth (Lewitt, 2015).

During the second stage of labour, the woman needs reassurance and support for her pushing efforts. Constant reinforcement and education by the nurse about labour progress, fetal heart monitor tracings, and other interventions will give the mother and her support system the guidance needed to give birth to the infant. Throughout labour, the nurse considers the specific cultural and ethnic needs to support nursing assessment and positive responses to labour by the childbearing family.

Active nursing support during the third and fourth stages of labour includes observing the woman for excessive vaginal bleeding after the placenta has been expelled, assisting the woman in breastfeeding her new baby, monitoring vital signs, and implementing uterine massage if the uterus becomes boggy or fails to contract over the placental site. Emotional support during assessments and delivery of information to explain the rationale for assessments are also important nursing roles supported by professional practice standards.

Current hospital guidelines call for mother–baby dyad care on postpartum units. Nurses must therefore be competent in caring for both populations and be able to share a large amount of information in a short time (typically 1–3 days) to prepare mothers for discharge. Although teaching and support related to breastfeeding take priority, other topics nurses must address before discharge include bathing, car seat safety, jaundice, safe sleep, postpartum mood disorders, and nutrition for both the mother and the baby. Having a standard discharge checklist and pamphlets to give the mother to read will help nurses ensure a successful transition from the hospital to the home.

Throughout the entire labour and birth process, the nurse carefully observes the labouring woman and fetus so that she can detect any difficulties with the progress of labour or with maternal or fetal health. Problems may include unusual fetal or uterine activity, the presence of meconium (fetal stool) in the amniotic fluid, fetal tachycardia (heart rate greater than 160 beats per minute) or fetal bradycardia (heart rate less than 110 beats per minute) in a full-term infant, and fetal heart rate decreases with uterine activity during labour (Mattson & Smith, 2015). These events must be reported immediately to the health care provider, with a complete oral and electronic description of the event. The nurse must be aware that abnormal fetal and maternal signs and patterns may be related to factors such as maternal diabetes or hypertension; the type, timing, or dosage of labour medications; uterine contraction pattern; maternal or fetal infections; maternal anemia; pre-eclampsia; the presence and character of amniotic fluid; bleeding in the pregnant woman or fetus; or early gestational age of the infant (Spong, 2015).

Our major role as nurses is to provide safe and evidence-informed care to promote optimal birth outcomes for all women. Nurses need to remember there is more than one way to provide this care. Nurses are educated to assess every woman as an individual and to plan care with mutual goal setting for the best outcomes. By assisting all people seeking care from diverse cultures and by adopting our practices as much as possible to embrace the cultural traditions of others, we will enhance the childbearing experience and promote the health of women, newborns, and families.

## CHANGES DURING TRANSITION FROM FETUS TO NEWBORN

Most newborns experience a smooth transition from intrauterine to extrauterine life. The fetus-to-newborn transition is complex and depends on several factors, including maternal health and chronic medical conditions, the status of the placenta, gestational duration, the presence of fetal anomalies, and birthing room care. When difficulty occurs, however, the newborn's viability depends on the nurse's understanding of the fine balance of chemical, physiological, and anatomical changes that occurs as it makes the transition to postnatal life (Swanson & Sinkin, 2015).

### Nursing Interventions

Nursing activities during this adaptation process include assessments and interventions aimed at specific protection of the infant and prevention of complications. Cold stress should be

## TABLE 10.3 Apgar Scoring

| Sign | SCORE 0 | 1 | 2 |
|------|---------|---|---|
| Heart rate | Absent | Slow (<100) | >100 |
| Respiratory effort | Absent | Weak cry, hypoventilation | Good strong cry |
| Muscle tone | Flaccid, limp | Some flexion of extremities | Active motion, extremities well flexed |
| Reflex irritability | No response | Grimace | Cry |
| Colour | Blue, pale | Body pink, extremities blue | Completely pink |

Sources: Bier, D., Mann, J., Alpers, D. H., et al. (Eds.). (2015). *Nutrition for the primary care provider*. Basel: Karger Medical and Scientific Publishers; Whitney, E. N., & Rolfes, S. R. (2015). *Understanding nutrition* (14th ed.). Boston: Cengage Learning.

avoided by the newborn being kept dry and warmly dressed and by avoidance of environments that cause heat loss. Overall, the nurse should minimally disturb, but maximally observe and document, the newborn's behaviour during reactive periods.

### Apgar Score

Assessment of the newborn after the first few hours of life is essentially the same as assessment of the young infant (see Chapter 11). One technique, specific to timing after birth, is the Apgar scoring system. This scoring system has historically been used to provide a simple clinical measure to evaluate the newborn's general condition at birth. The Apgar score, obtained at 1 and 5 minutes of age, may be obtained again at 10 minutes of age until the infant's condition has stabilized. A total score is calculated by the addition of the values allotted to the categories noted in Table 10.3. The highest possible score is 10 and a score of 8 to 10 indicates that the baby is adapting well. The Apgar score does not predict the neurological development of an infant but may relate to the infant's risk of illness or death during the first year of life, which is important information for parents of an infant with a low Apgar score (Apgar, 2015).

### Sex

Sex differences occur in fetal growth. Generally, boys grow faster than girls in the third trimester, and at birth boys are slightly heavier, are longer, and have a larger head circumference than girls (Lissauer, Fanaroff, Miall, et al., 2015). Although more boys are conceived, they tend to be aborted spontaneously more often than girl embryos; the two X chromosomes possessed by female embryos may protect them from the early hazards of pregnancy. After birth, boys continue to have a lower survival rate than do girls (Stevenson, Cohen, & Sunshine, 2015).

### Race and Culture

Race may affect the health of the fetus in several ways. For example, Black women are more likely to have fraternal twin pregnancies than White women (Cunningham et al., 2014). Because their organs are less mature, twin fetuses face an increased risk of premature delivery as a result of gestational factors in the mother. Currently, Canada is 180th in the world ranking for infant mortality rate (IMR), with a rate of 4.5 per 1000 live births (Central Intelligence Agency, 2017). This rate reflects the number of infants who die before the end of their first year of life and is the leading indicator of a nation's health. It reveals the higher IMRs and low-birth-weight outcomes of other ethnic minority populations in Canada. This rate illustrates the complex sociopolitical issues that produce birth outcomes in Canada and those needing attention to reduce the IMR.

Race is also a factor in the frequency of certain genetic and congenital malformations (Genomics). For example, more babies of Indigenous descent have cleft palates (an opening in the oral palate) than do Black babies (Tewfik, Karsan, & Kanaan, 2015). Cleft palates have also been shown to be more prevalent in populations of low socioeconomic status, which must be considered by the nurse when advocating for equitable access to health care for Indigenous people in Canada (Pawluk, Campaña, Gili, et al., 2014). Black babies have higher rates of sickle cell anemia (abnormally shaped red blood cells) than White babies, because individuals of African descent are higher carriers of the sickle cell gene (Sickle Cell Disease Association of Canada, 2016).

A woman's socioeconomic background may also influence the health of her fetus on the basis of a link to socioeconomic status. For increasing numbers of homeless pregnant women, income may support family survival needs but not prenatal care. Minority-group pregnant women may have fewer economic resources to obtain a nutritious diet or early and consistent high-quality prenatal care.

### Genetics

The science of genetics has expanded recently to genomics (the science that studies genes that make up the human genome). The completion of the mapping and sequencing of the human genome led to the expansion of research technologies that are now used to identify genetic and genomic factors that have an influence on people's health. Genetic influences affect the survival and later well-being of the child through several known mechanisms. Down syndrome (trisomy 21) remains the most recognized and most commonly occurring example of an extra chromosome. Extra chromosomes, deleted chromosomes, or translocations usually cause multiple malformations incompatible with life, causing early loss of the fetus via spontaneous abortion. Single malformations in an otherwise normal fetus (e.g., clubfoot, cleft palate, or NTD) probably result from a combined effect of many genes (March of Dimes, 2015). These defects, found at birth, may be surgically corrected or managed during the child's life. Invasive techniques of amniocentesis, chorionic villus sampling, and chromosome analysis have expanded genetic counselling options and interventions for women facing possible fetal genetic defects. Nurses now will have to deal with the challenges of the explosion of genomic information to provide personalized health care based on genomics. The nurse, as a vital member of the health care team, needs to assist in informing these women and couples of genetic and high-risk screening resources when family history or other factors indicate that a fetal genetic defect may be likely.

## GENOMICS

### *Genetic Testing May Lead to Ethical Dilemmas*

Prenatal genetic testing provides important opportunities for assessment of genetic risk and diagnosis. However, some genetic tests do not identify all the possible gene mutations that can cause a particular condition, or they have limited predictive value. Because some genetic tests may not provide all the information that families may want, the test may subsequently require difficult decisions without providing full information. As an example, a cystic fibrosis carrier test can identify couples who are both carriers. When the cystic fibrosis mutations are identified in the parents, prenatal diagnosis can be performed to determine whether a fetus has inherited a cystic fibrosis gene mutation from each parent. Knowing that a fetus has inherited two cystic fibrosis mutations, however, does not, at this time, predict the severity of the disease in the infant. For couples in this situation, the ethical dilemma involves the decision to continue or to end a pregnancy without having knowledge of the severity of the disorder.

#### Should the Information Be Obtained if No Treatment or Intervention Exists?

Genetic testing can lead to specific treatments or interventions for some conditions but not for others. This is the case with some disorders that can be detected in expanded newborn screening. When phenylketonuria is identified, dietary intervention allows individuals with this condition to lead healthy and productive lives. Currently, however, not all conditions can be adequately treated. Genetic testing for some conditions, for which there are no treatments, might have the potential to cause psychological harm, stigmatization, and discrimination. Genetic testing for Huntington's disease, a progressive motor and cognitive disorder with onset in midlife, is one example. There are no effective treatments or preventive measures currently available. Thus choosing to have genetic testing for Huntington's disease is highly personal, and it is recommended that individuals consider extensive pretest counselling. These tests may lead to decisions that cannot be reversed and are based on a woman's best guess as to what would be the best course of action for her and her family. The dilemma that occurs then is whether a newborn should be tested for disorders that we cannot treat.

Ethical decision-making models/frameworks are valuable tools that can assist nurses in addressing ethical dilemmas. Principles of autonomy, informed consent, privacy/confidentiality, beneficence, nonmaleficence, and justice are applicable to use in the ethics involved in genetic testing. These principles should be sensitive to human needs, should be responsive to contextual considerations, and should emphasize the uniqueness of each situation.

- What might be the nurse's role in assisting the family in the decision-making process?
- What assurances can be made regarding privacy and confidentiality of the genetic information to prevent future employment or health insurance discrimination?
- What resources are available to nurses to keep current on prenatal genetic testing?

## ❖ GORDON'S FUNCTIONAL HEALTH PATTERNS

Box 10.3 provides an example of a pregnancy assessment using Gordon's (2016) functional health patterns.

### ◆ Health Perception–Health Management Pattern

On the basis of her culture and life experience, a woman may view pregnancy as an illness, as a completely natural and healthy state, or as a combination of the two. This perception will influence her view of her changing body, her attitude toward the usual discomforts of pregnancy, such as fatigue or backache, her choice of health-oriented or illness-oriented care, and her decision to seek prenatal care. The woman who sees herself as healthy and pregnancy as a normal part of her life will most likely seek a health care provider with a similar outlook. Another woman with the same perception may seek help from a socially approved group, as defined by her culture, and avoid standard Western medicine during pregnancy. Generally, women with a positive view of pregnancy will continue with active participation in their respective social circles and careers. However, the woman who sees her pregnancy as a time of illness may use this as a reason to withdraw from her work and social obligations.

A woman's acceptance of her pregnancy influences her health-management practices and choices. The woman who denies, or has strong negative feelings about her pregnancy, may fail to eat properly, get enough rest and exercise, breastfeed, or seek prenatal care. A woman may deny a pregnancy because she never intended to become pregnant despite having sexual intercourse without birth control. Approximately 50% of Canadian pregnancies are unintended, particularly among vulnerable aggregates such as adolescents, women older than 40 years, women with low income, and women who lack health care access, cultural acceptance, and education, experience sexual violence, and lack financial resources to purchase or use contraceptives (Oulman, Kim, Yunis, et al., 2015). These women, faced with an unplanned or a closely spaced pregnancy, may expose a fetus to alcohol, tobacco, and sexually transmitted infections (STIs), abuse a child who was never wanted, or fail to obtain follow-up care for a high-risk child (i.e., experience complications from childbirth) (PHAC, 2017a).

Nurses encounter women with reproductive health needs and concerns in all practice settings and play an important role in caring for them as an integral member of the health care team. The nurse who works with a pregnant population must be sensitive to a wide range of views expressed by these women and work with each to effectively manage their pregnancies. For example, Indigenous women may sometimes not access early prenatal care because of the limited number of health care centres in their community, secondary to geographical isolation (National Collaborating Centre for Aboriginal Health [NCCAH], 2011). The nurse must target interventions that focus on this group's needs and beliefs while adhering to professional practice standards that will improve their outcomes.

### ◆ Nutritional-Metabolic Pattern

A woman's nutritional status should be assessed preconceptually with the goal of optimizing maternal and fetal health. Pregnancy-related dietary changes should begin before conception, with

## BOX 10.3 Assessment for Pregnancy According to Gordon's Functional Health Patterns

*Health perception–health management pattern.* Aware of, or participates in management of pregnancy, or both; expects an uncomplicated pregnancy on the basis of the woman's or significant other's active involvement in her own care; able to state complications of pregnancy that mandate physician notification; engages in health-promotion behaviours specific to pregnancy.

*Nutritional-metabolic pattern.* Follows diet changes of pregnancy as recommended by nurse; has appropriate weight for height and has gained adequate weight for gestational age of pregnancy; eats three meals a day and two snacks (afternoon and evening), focusing on increased amounts of vegetables and fruits; drinks healthy fluids, including at least eight glasses of water per day; has elastic skin turgor.

*Elimination pattern.* Experiences occasional constipation from progesterone influence of gastro-intestinal peristalsis relaxation, usually corrected by increased fluids, nightly walking, and more diet roughage; voids 7 to 10 times a day, depending on amount of fluids consumed; no known hemorrhoids or difficulty in elimination; voiding without excess frequency, urgency, or burning; understands signs of UTI.

*Activity-exercise pattern.* Walks three times a week for 20 minutes without reports of unusual fatigue or soreness; active at home with housework and at work teaching in a primary school; swam two times a week before pregnancy and moved to current residence.

*Sleep-rest pattern.* Generally, sleeps 7 to 8 hours a night; has increased total daily sleep somewhat with fatigue of pregnancy—naps for 1 hour on weekends and 30 minutes after work; sleeps on side and with two pillows for comfort; uses no sleep aids; generally able to relax and initiate sleep without difficulty; occasionally has headache at end of workday and takes acetaminophen (Tylenol) for relief or listens to soft music after work.

*Cognitive-perceptual pattern.* Realizes the need to decrease work activity and increase rest periods as she nears end of pregnancy; answers questions in appropriate tone and words during pregnancy visits; has intact memory (alert and remote); reads about pregnancy and early parenthood to prepare for the birth.

*Self-perception–self-concept pattern.* States she is excited about pregnancy after 1 year of trying to conceive; well groomed, wears maternity clothes because "I want to"; believes she looks "nice" because of pregnancy.

*Roles-relationships pattern.* Lives with husband of 3 years; visits extended family, 100 km away, every month; shares family roles with husband, accepts this balance; has many friends who support her pregnancy; perceives extensive employee and employer support with pregnancy and time off after delivery.

*Sexuality-reproductive pattern.* States, "I have a satisfying love life and enjoy my husband"; before pregnancy, engaged in sexual intercourse four to five times a week with desire to become pregnant; with pregnancy and fatigue, has intercourse generally two to three times a week, with pattern acceptable to both partners; no known STIs in past or present.

*Coping–stress tolerance pattern.* Concerned about fatigue affecting performance as primary school teacher; walks three times a week for 20 minutes to "centre myself and feel good"; smiles often, good sense of humour; supportive family excited about her pregnancy.

*Values-beliefs pattern.* Protestant religion; prays daily and gains strength from religion.

**Other Data**

- Medication history:
  Prenatal vitamin, one tablet each morning
  Ferrous sulfate, one tablet each morning
  Acetaminophen (Tylenol) 650 mg for occasional headaches
- Physical examination:
  162 cm (5 feet, 4 inches) tall
  Weight 63.5 kg (140 lb) (at 14 weeks of pregnancy; weight gain of 2.26 kg [5 lb] with pregnancy)
  29 years of age
  Pupils equally round and reactive to light and accommodation
  Temperature 36.7°C (98.2°F); pulse 76 beats per minute; respiration 16 breaths per minute
  Blood pressure 114/78 mmHg right arm (sitting, left arm)
  Peripheral pulses equal, strong bilaterally
  Skin warm, dry, elastic turgor; mucous membranes intact, moist; alert, oriented

Sources: Modified from Gordon, M. (2010). *Manual of nursing diagnosis* (12th ed.). Sudbury, MA: Jones & Bartlett Learning; Peterson, R. (2012). *Clinical companion for fundamentals of nursing* (8th ed.). St. Louis: Mosby.
*STIs,* Sexually transmitted infections; *UTI,* urinary tract infection.

needed modifications during pregnancy and lactation. Most nutritional requirements of pregnant and lactating women can be met by their consumption of a variety of foods according to government-endorsed guidelines. Massive amounts of literature support the importance of optimal nutrition during pregnancy for maternal and fetal well-being. The key components of nutritional management during pregnancy include consumption of a variety of foods, appropriate weight gain, appropriate micronutrient supplementation, physical activity, and avoidance of alcohol, tobacco, and other harmful substances. Maternal malnutrition before and during pregnancy may exert a teratogenic effect on the fetus. A teratogen is an agent that causes either a functional or a structural disability in the organism as a result of exposure to that agent (Merriam-Webster, 2015). Teratogens principally affect the central nervous system (CNS) of the fetus, leading to impaired intelligence and performance later in life. They are discussed more in the Environmental Processes section later in the chapter.

Various factors influence the quality of nutritional requirements for positive fetal development and birth outcome. Fetal development suffers in cases of adolescent pregnancy or in pregnancies of older women who experience poor nutrition between and during several pregnancies. Maternal nutritional deficiencies during a woman's own fetal, infant, and childhood periods also contribute to the development of structural and physiological disadvantages to supporting a growing fetus. For example, women who are severely underweight before pregnancy often experience higher rates of low-birth-weight infants and preterm labour than do women of appropriate prepregnant weight (Cunningham et al., 2014). Inherited maternal stature and pelvic development may influence pregnancy and efficiency of labour and delivery. A lack of income to buy healthy food may also exist, and sometimes cultural values related to food intake influence the quality of nutrition during pregnancy.

To meet increased metabolic, energy, and structural needs for pregnancy, it is recommended that a pregnant woman increase her intake by approximately 350–450 calories each day, resulting in a total weight gain of approximately 11.33 to 15.87 kg (25 to 35 pounds) (Health Canada, 2009a) (Fig. 10.3). These calories should be added through the selection of nutritious foods from diverse food groups as recommended by Canada's *Prenatal Nutrition Guidelines*. If at the end of 20 weeks of gestation the woman has not gained at least 4.5 kg (10 pounds), she risks delivering an ill infant with fetal growth restriction. This risk also exists when a woman continues to gain insufficient weight throughout the pregnancy or in a woman who was underweight or overweight before pregnancy. Although the rate of gain and the total gain during pregnancy differ among women, a correlation exists between an erratic pattern of weight gain or a too-rapid weight

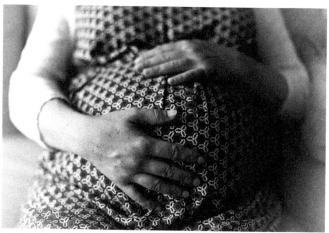

**Fig. 10.3** Many practitioners recommend a weight gain of 11.33 to 15.87 kg (25 to 35 pounds) for pregnant women at normal weight for their height. (iStockphoto/gevende.)

gain and a lack of fetal well-being (Bier, Mann, Alpers, et al., 2015). The nurse advises the pregnant woman and her family to eat a well-balanced diet.

The nurse encourages the pregnant woman to drink 8 to 10 glasses of water per day to develop amniotic fluid and prevent urinary tract infections (UTIs) often seen with pregnancy. The nurse may also need to encourage the woman to modify her diet to include more fibre and roughage to avoid constipation during pregnancy (Table 10.4).

Protein requirements during pregnancy increase to approximately 70 g per day, or a daily increase of 25 g above normal (Whitney & Rolfes, 2015). This ensures an adequate supply of amino acids for fetal growth and development, blood volume expansion, and maternal tissue growth. Other protein sources, such as cheese, cream soups, puddings, tofu, and yogurt, may be better tolerated by women from other cultural backgrounds. Animal protein and less-expensive legume sources provide protein and, if combined with other healthy food sources, provide high-quality meals (e.g., tuna and rice, peanut butter, and whole-wheat bread). Protein foods cost more than other foods; therefore, the nurse may need to teach pregnant couples about economical ways to meet protein needs for fetal development.

Mineral intake must also increase during pregnancy. Increased protein intake usually provides the extra needed essential minerals, particularly phosphorus and calcium. The rapid deposit of calcium in fetal bones and teeth during the third trimester of pregnancy requires adequate maternal calcium stores from early pregnancy and continued calcium intake to prevent maternal bone demineralization. Other calcium sources include green, leafy vegetables and calcium-fortified foods, sources more acceptable to cultures with a history of lactose intolerance (African, Mexican, and some European groups).

| TABLE 10.4 | Nutritional Needs for Pregnant and Lactating Women | | | |
|---|---|---|---|---|
| **Nutrient** | **Pregnancy** | **Lactation** | **Sources** | **Comments** |
| Calories | +300 | +500 | Eat a variety from all food groups | Begin to increase calories in second and third trimesters |
| Protein | 70 g | 70 g | Lean meat, fish, eggs, poultry, milk, and dairy products | Supports fetal growth and development; formation of placenta and amniotic fluid; and expanded blood volume |
| Calcium | 1000 mg/day | 1000 mg/day | Milk, cheese, dark green leafy vegetables, nuts, and dried fruit | Women with low calcium intake require calcium supplements with vitamin D |
| Iron | 27 mg/day | 9 mg/day | Lean meats, dark green leafy vegetables, eggs, whole grain, dried fruit, and shellfish | Provides iron for fetal liver storage, which sustains infant for first 4–6 months of life |
| Folic acid | 600 mcg | 500 mcg | Fresh green leafy vegetables, liver, peanuts, whole-grain breads, and cereals | All women of childbearing age should take 400 mcg of folic acid daily to prevent neural tube defects in first trimester |
| Fats | 30% of daily calories | 30% of daily calories | Low-fat dairy products and lean cuts of meat | Provide a valuable source of energy for the body during pregnancy |
| Carbohydrates | 7–11 servings daily | 7–11 servings daily | Dairy products, fruits, vegetables, whole-grain cereals, and breads | Provide fibre necessary for proper bowel functioning. Carbohydrate intake needs to be sufficient to prevent ketoacidosis from protein use for energy |

NOTE: Canada's *Prenatal Nutrition Guidelines* are based on the 2007 Canada's Food Guide recommendations. Although the food guide was updated in 2019, the *Prenatal Nutrition Guidelines* continue to reflect the 2007 Eating Well with Canada's Food Guide. The guidelines reflect Health Canada's recommendations for prenatal nutrition and continue to be used as a reference for health professionals.
Sources: Health Canada. (2009). *Prenatal nutrition guidelines for health professionals*. Retrieved from https://www.canada.ca/en/health-canada/services/publications/food-nutrition/prenatal-nutrition-guidelines-health-professionals-background-canada-food-guide-2009.html; Thompson, J., & Manore, M. (2012). *Nutrition: An applied approach* (3rd ed.). San Francisco: Benjamin Cummings.

Sufficient iodine intake by pregnant and lactating women is crucial for thyroid hormone production, which contributes to the offspring's neurocognitive development. Approximately one-third of pregnant women are marginally deficient in iodine. The WHO calls for pregnant and lactating women to use iodized salt and take a supplement of 250 mcg of iodine daily, which typically is not contained in prenatal vitamins. As processed and convenient foods make up a large portion of Canadian diets today, women need to be informed that the salt used in them is not iodized (WHO, 2009).

A woman who eats a well-balanced diet should gain sufficient vitamins and minerals for maternal and fetal needs during pregnancy. However, most health care providers recommend that the pregnant woman include 16–20 mg of elemental iron daily to benefit both herself and the fetus, particularly during the last trimester. Anemia of pregnancy is a global health problem affecting nearly half of all pregnant women worldwide. High fetal demands for iron, increased erythrocyte mass, and, in the third trimester, expanded maternal blood volume, render iron deficiency the most common cause of anemia of pregnancy. In certain geographical populations, human pathogens such as hookworm, malarial parasite, and HIV are important factors contributing to anemia of pregnancy. The hemoglobinopathies—sickle cell disease and thalassemia—represent diverse causes of anemia of pregnancy, requiring specialized care. Iron-deficiency anemia is common among pregnant women, and anemia contributes to hemorrhage, postpartum infection, and preterm birth. Anemia occurs more often among pregnant adolescent, Black, and older White women (Cantor, Bougatsos, Dana, et al., 2015; Health Canada, 2009b).

There are almost universal recommendations for periconceptual folic acid supplementation to prevent NTDs. NTDs are congenital malformations that include anencephaly, encephalocele, and spina bifida caused by the failure of fusion of the neural tube, which normally closes between the 22nd and 28th days after conception (at an average of 40–42 days after the first day of the last menstrual period). The occurrence of NTDs differs among the population, ranging between 8 and 10 per 1000 births, and there is an approximately 3% chance that a woman will deliver a second baby with an NTD (Ami et al., 2016). According to the WHO, increased consumption of folic acid can decrease the risk of NTD to 0.6 per 1000 births (Cordero, Crider, Rogers, et al., 2015). To decrease the risk of NTD, it is recommended that all women capable of becoming pregnant should begin taking a folic acid supplement (Health Canada, 2018b). The goal is that every woman could start her pregnancy with an optimal folate status. Evidence-informed research thus supports that women planning pregnancy and those in their first trimester take 0.4 mg of folic acid in a daily multivitamin supplement to prevent NTDs and anemia. This is particularly important for women with multiple gestations, who experience a greater risk of anemia.

Fats and carbohydrates must supply the caloric requirements during pregnancy. Although increased protein intake provides more calories, the body-building requirements of pregnancy and fetal growth demand most of the added protein. Fats and carbohydrates remain the most important sources of energy and essential vitamins and minerals. Supplemental vitamins and minerals, although not known to cause maternal or fetal harm if taken in reasonable doses, probably cost the pregnant woman more to meet the nutritional needs of pregnancy than does a well-balanced diet.

The practice of pica, a psychobehavioural disorder characterized by the ingestion of nonfood substances such as dirt, clay, laundry starch, ashes, plaster, raw rice, paint chips, coffee grounds, and ice, may negatively influence the quality of a pregnant woman's nutrition during pregnancy. No one knows what causes these cravings, but a combination of biochemical, psychological, and cultural factors may be at work. Pica in humans can be classified by the type of ingested substance. The three main substances consumed by pregnant women are soil or clay (geophagia), ice (pagophagia), and laundry or corn starch (amylophagia). Other pica cravings include burned matches, stones, charcoal, mothballs, soap, sand, plaster, coffee grounds, baking soda, paint chips, and glue (Jyothi, 2015). Common in rural pregnant Black women, this practice may contribute to iron-deficiency anemia and interfere with nutrient absorption, particularly among women of lower economic status. Other potential complications may include lead poisoning, fecal impaction, nutritional deficiency, preterm labour, low-birth-weight infants, and anemia in the infant (Ezzeddin, Zvoshy, Noroozi, et al., 2015). Pica is thought to occur as a result of an iron deficiency that leads to the craving and/or a carryover from behaviours practiced in Africa (Mattson & Smith, 2015). The nurse completes a nutritional assessment on all pregnant woman. The nurse identifies instances of pica and suggests a culturally sensitive diet that will better meet the needs of the woman and her developing fetus. It is essential that the nurse remains nonjudgemental but stresses the importance of an adequate diet, folic acid, iodine, and iron supplements, and the dangers of pica.

The best time to teach a woman about prenatal nutrition is before she becomes pregnant. Most women do not seek prenatal care until they suspect pregnancy. Therefore, the nurse often delivers information about optimal nutrition to the pregnant woman after critical fetal development has already begun. If all school-aged children received nutrition information as part of their kindergarten through Grade 12 curriculum (a primary prevention approach), women might have better overall personal nutrition established through lifestyle practices of individuals and families that would support high-quality prenatal nutrition later in their lives. Without such a primary prevention approach, secondary prevention intervention during pregnancy occurs through laboratory monitoring of iron levels, assessment of the woman's feelings of well-being, determination of the woman's actual intake of essential nutrients, and assessment of her pattern and total weight gain during the pregnancy. The nurse alerts the pregnant woman and her family to the documented high amounts of cholesterol, calories, sodium, and fat, and low amounts of iron and calcium that these foods contain so as to improve nutritional intake during pregnancy.

In 2019, Health Canada unveiled *Canada's Dietary Guidelines*, the revised version of Canada's Food Guide, a tool used to support healthy nutrition and healthy living (Health Canada, 2019). *Canada's Dietary Guidelines* recommend consuming plenty of vegetables and fruits, drinking water rather than sugary beverages, consuming high-protein foods, and choosing whole gain options when possible. The Eat Well Plate is a simple guide to help consumers visualize how the portions of each food group should appear on their plate (Government of Canada, 2019a). To build a healthy meal, the Eat Well Plate suggests that consumers choose fruits, vegetables, whole grains, low-fat dairy products, and lean protein foods to get essential nutrients without excess calories. The strategies for creating such a plate include filling half your plate with fruits and vegetables, using whole grains when possible (e.g., 100% whole-grain cereals, breads, and pasta), switching from whole milk to skim or 1% milk, and choosing a variety of protein sources (e.g., seafood, small portions of lean meat and poultry, and beans). It also recommends that women should avoid shark, swordfish, king mackerel, or tilefish when they are pregnant or breastfeeding (Health Canada, 2017b). These fish contain high levels of mercury and should be avoided. In summary, the *Prenatal Nutrition Guidelines* (which are based on the 2007 Canada Food Guide) are as follows:

- *Fruits and Vegetables*—seven to eight servings daily. Eat one dark green and one orange vegetable per day that have little or no added sugars, and limit juice intake.
- *Grain Products*—six to seven servings daily (include barley, brown rice, and quinoa).
- *Milk and Alternatives*—two servings of low-fat or nonfat milk, yogurt, or cheese daily. Have 500 mL of milk each day to ensure adequate vitamin D intake.
- *Meat and Alternatives*—two servings daily. Select meat alternatives when possible. Select lean meats and remove the skin from the meat prior to consumption) (Government of Canada, 2019a; Health Canada, 2019).

See Chapter 21 for more information on nutrition, including *Canada's Dietary Guidelines*.

## ◆ Elimination Pattern

### Fetus

The fetus accomplishes all essential elimination functions through the placenta. Carbon dioxide, water, urea, and other waste products pass through the placenta to be eliminated by the mother's body. By the end of the first trimester, the fetus swallows, makes respiratory movements, and urinates. However, these abilities become truly functional only after birth.

### Pregnant Woman

The pregnant woman experiences changes in her elimination pattern because of the enlarging uterus and hormonal influences. These changes (urinary frequency during the first and third trimesters, constipation, and hemorrhoids) cause normal, minor discomforts. Anticipatory guidance by the nurse helps the pregnant woman cope with these changes and prevents complications of pregnancy. For example, teaching the pregnant woman commonsense measures (Innovative Practice) may prevent UTIs, typically a problem that is more common during pregnancy. With a known correlation between UTIs and

premature labour, a focus on preventing and managing these infections must occur during pregnancy.

## ◆ Activity-Exercise Pattern

### Fetus

Early spontaneous movements of the fetus may be reflexive, stimulated by passive uterine movement. Ultrasonographic observation of fetal movement shows repetitive movements early in pregnancy; at approximately 16 weeks, the pregnant woman feels these movements, termed quickening. By the end of the second trimester, fetal movement occurs less frequently because of lack of space in the uterus. The woman and her partner look forward to the regular daily cycle of movements, indicators of fetal well-being. An absence of or a dramatic increase in fetal movements for more than 8 hours may indicate fetal distress. The nurse routinely teaches a pregnant woman to count the number of fetal movements each day, typically starting at

---

### INNOVATIVE PRACTICE

#### Evidence-Informed Practice for Preventing Urinary Tract Infections (UTIs) and Promoting Genitourinary Health

- Increase fluid intake to approximately 8 to 10 glasses per day; plain water is best to flush the body's systems of potential toxins; drink a glass of water before sexual intercourse to allow urinary output afterward to prevent UTIs.
- Avoid bladder irritants such as caffeine products, alcohol, artificial sweeteners, spicy foods, and carbonated beverages.
- Make urination a regular habit; avoid waiting to urinate until bladder is full.
- Urinate before and after sexual intercourse to cleanse the urethra and empty the bladder.
- Be aware that vigorous or frequent intercourse may contribute to increased risk of UTIs.
- Maintain consistently good perineal hygiene, including wiping from front to back after urination and defecation.
- Take all prescription medications given for UTIs, even when the symptoms of the infection have been alleviated.
- Drink cranberry juice to acidify the urine or take cranberry pills; these products may relieve some of the symptoms of a UTI. Cranberry *(Vaccinium macrocarpon)* has demonstrated anti-inflammatory, antiadhesive, and antioxidant properties.
- Seek health care advice for a vaginal infection, which may contribute to development of a UTI.
- Nurses need to be aware that most UTIs are caused by *Escherichia coli*, and most women may be asymptomatic. Obtaining a urine specimen and culture is needed with any degree of suspicion of a UTI.
- Approximately half of UTIs in pregnancy occur in women with pre-existing asymptomatic bacteriuria, and these UTIs have poor outcomes, including preterm rupture of membranes, preterm birth, neonatal infection, pre-eclampsia, maternal anemia, amnionitis, and maternal septic shock.
- The nurse should assess the woman for increased risk of developing a UTI: congenital or structural abnormalities of the genitourinary system, previous surgery to the genitourinary system; pregnancy; previous UTIs; high intake of carbonated beverages; and poor intake of water.

Sources: Matuszkiewicz-Rowińska, J., Małyszko, J., & Wieliczko, M. (2015). Urinary tract infections in pregnancy: Old and new unresolved diagnostic and therapeutic problems. *Archives of Medical Science, 11*(1), 67–77, doi:10.5114/aoms.2013.39202; Sheerin, N. S. (2015). Urinary tract infection. *Medicine, 43*(8), 435–439, doi:10.1016/j.mpmed.2015.05.007.

28 weeks' gestation, and to report any decrease in fetal activity to the health care provider.

## Pregnant Woman

The physical changes during pregnancy and the rigours of labour and delivery require that a pregnant woman be in the best physical condition of her life. Fortunately, many pregnant women view pregnancy as a normal, natural state, and they often participate actively in physical activities or sports enjoyed before pregnancy. Generally, a woman should avoid high-risk sports, such as sky diving and high-altitude climbing, because these could cause trauma to the fetus from low oxygen pressure or a maternal fall. Nurses encourage each woman to choose activities on the basis of her interests, comfort, and good judgement. When a sport or activity causes exhaustion or pain, it should be modified or discontinued. Later in pregnancy, the woman should be encouraged to choose safe physical activities because of changes in her centre of gravity attributable to the enlarging uterus and in the musculoskeletal system.

The woman with a sedentary lifestyle before pregnancy should slowly increase her activity level during pregnancy. A daily swim or 30-minute walk provides a good introduction to a regular exercise program. Regular exercise contributes to joint flexibility, increased cardiovascular and gastro-intestinal fitness, decreased uterine tone for an efficient labour, fewer pregnancy discomforts, weight control and a lower risk of diabetes by maintaining glycemic control, and overall feelings of well-being in the pregnant woman (PHAC, 2011b). For the self-directed woman, prenatal classes or a consumer-oriented book of prenatal exercises will facilitate an adequate exercise program. For most women, group exercise with other pregnant women is more enjoyable than exercising alone. The benefits of physical activity in the general population are established, and research suggests regular physical activity following childbirth is linked to improved health outcomes. However, many women do not resume prepregnancy exercise levels. The nurse encourages women to enter a structured diet that follows *Canada's Dietary Guidelines* and an exercise program to help women lose weight after childbirth (Spencer, Rollo, Hauck, et al., 2015).

In an uncomplicated pregnancy, a couple may continue their usual sexual activity. However, threatened abortion or a history of abortion in the first trimester, early rupture of membranes, and other complications may call for restrictions on sexual intercourse or orgasm.

## ◆ Sleep-Rest Pattern

### Fetus

Electroencephalographic studies have shown four cyclical states of activity in the fetus: complete wakefulness, drowsy wakefulness, rapid eye movement sleep, and quiet sleep. Evidence suggests that a diurnal (day-night) pattern exists during the fetal period. Sleep is required for somatic and brain growth and development. Sleep-wake patterns change with CNS maturation. In one research study, the median relative percentage of time spent in a quiet state was 26%. The median duration of time spent in a quiet state was 15.7 minutes within a 1-hour recording. Both quiet states and active states were established in

84% of the fetuses studied (Piontelli, 2015). Infant development entails increasing amounts of quiet sleep as well as increasing periods of quiet alertness. Both states require remarkable neural organization; thus, sleep-wake patterns are an excellent window to the infant's neurological status.

## Pregnant Woman

Fatigue reflects the significant physical and emotional changes occurring in the pregnant woman. The nurse counsels a woman that fatigue usually subsides by the fourth month but may return later in pregnancy. Rest breaks during the day and 8 hours of sleep each night help prevent fatigue and increase the pregnant woman's comfort. The nurse encourages each pregnant woman to rest when her body signals it is tired because of the rapidly growing fetus and the woman's needs for physical renewal. This encouragement must be directed particularly toward working women, who may need a physician's note for their employer that validates the need for rest during the workday.

Women experience significant sleep disruption and inadequate sleep throughout pregnancy. Many pregnant women do not sleep well because they need to urinate several times a night during the first and third trimesters. In addition, some women experience positional discomfort in late pregnancy that prevents effective sleep and, therefore, increases their fatigue. Fatigue may influence a woman's evaluation of her role as a pregnant woman, her body changes, and her cultural beliefs related to her ability to succeed in pregnancy. The nurse helps the woman express her thoughts and feelings and find ways to support better sleep and rest patterns (e.g., sleeping upright in a chair at night for easier breathing).

## Fetus

During the prenatal period, although motor functions lag behind, all fetal sensory systems function or nearly function. These systems include vision, hearing, taste, smell, touch, and proprioceptive and vestibular senses (Blackburn, 2014). The fetus with all senses intact experiences the discomfort of pregnancy and the pain of labour contractions. The visual system matures relatively late in gestation, especially compared with the tactile, olfactory, and auditory systems. Although capable of seeing by 30 weeks of age, the fetus has little opportunity to use this ability in utero because of the absence of light (Blackburn, 2014). After approximately 25 weeks, pregnant women note that their babies respond to a loud, sudden noise. Some pregnant women and their partners offer sensory stimulation to the fetus by singing or rubbing the woman's abdomen. This parental behaviour may assist in the bonding process between the parent and the baby. Thus the nurse may wish to include this kind of information in prenatal teaching sessions.

## Pregnant Woman

Physical and psychological processes remain closely intertwined as pregnancy progresses. Psychological stresses and normal emotional growth affect the physical status of the pregnancy, interactions of the family members, and the eventual relationship between the mother and the infant. When considering the emotional aspects of pregnancy, the nurse

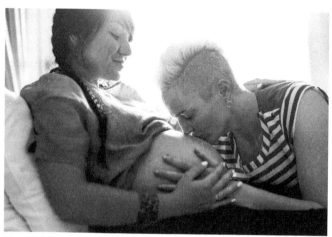

Fig. 10.4 The pregnant woman enjoys time with her family while pregnant. (iStockPhoto/Rawpixel.)

recognizes that the woman's personality, environment, physical state, family, and sociocultural and spiritual background affect the ways in which she handles the psychological changes (Fig. 10.4).

Two major categories of psychological influences are normal psychological growth required of parents to emotionally and physically prepare them for parenthood, and internal or external stressors on the pregnant woman that decrease her ability to provide the best environment for the developing fetus. The pregnant woman undergoes many cognitive changes that ultimately result in her psychological readiness for motherhood.

*Emotional changes.* Hormonal and other physical changes assist the woman in the psychological work of pregnancy. Progesterone level increases can affect the woman's general mood, causing her to be more introverted and passive. These mood changes help her to focus her energy on the growing child and her own growth and development. In addition to hormonal changes, the presence, growth, and movements of the fetus become more a part of the woman's experiential self. According to Rubin (1984), the classic researcher on maternal–infant bonding, the pregnant woman receives immediate sensations of touch, motion, and weight from the fetus that she can share only partially with others. These support a maternal feeling of separateness and uniqueness that causes the woman to turn inward. She frequently worries that the shift in energy away from the world toward herself and her child may cause her to lose contact, drift away from valued relationships, and lose feelings of competence in her areas of achievement. She spends time analyzing her experiences and their possible influence on her effectiveness as a future parent. She constantly studies the qualities of human relationships and shows increased sensitivity and perceptiveness to many people. To others, the woman may seem overly sensitive and analytical during pregnancy (Stockwell, 2015).

Although a woman's mood varies on the basis of a variety of factors and at different times during the pregnancy, many women experience wide mood swings, emotional lability, irritability, and changes in sexual desire. Physical discomforts, hormonal changes, feelings about altered body image, cultural considerations, work and relationship adjustments, and demanding cognitive maturational processes may also cause these emotional changes.

Rubin's classic work stimulated nurses to look beyond the physiological and pathological aspects of childbearing to the intricate process of becoming a mother, and to identify areas for providing help. Current research identifies two simultaneous processes in the transition to motherhood: engagement and growth, and transformation. Engagement is making a commitment and being engrossed in mothering through active involvement in the child's care. At the same time, the woman's engagement leads to the woman's growth and transition as she becomes a mother. The bond between a mother and her newborn is one of strength, power, and potential (von Mohr, Mayes, & Rutherford, 2017).

Current descriptions for the stages in the process of establishing a maternal identity in becoming a mother include the following:

- Commitment, attachment, and preparation for the pregnancy
- Acquaintance, learning, and physical restoration during the first 6 weeks after birth
- Moving toward a new normal from 2 weeks to 4 months

Nurses can promote the maternal–newborn bond through encouraging skin-to-skin contact, breastfeeding, eye contact, and newborn massage during the first hour after childbirth.

*Stressors influencing development.* The mother's age, fears related to a previous fetal loss, feelings about the pregnancy, life situation and culture, degree of stress, loss of control at times, and unintended pregnancy, the presence of other children, and the influence of loved ones may serve as stressors that influence the ways in which the mother completes the developmental tasks of motherhood. Women with unwanted pregnancies have multiple risk factors and would benefit from targeted interventions (Hall, Kusunoki, Gatny, et al., 2015; Mori, 2015). A young pregnant woman facing the additional developmental task of adolescence may have difficulty incorporating the pregnant body or the role of mother into her still undefined self-image. Cognitively, she may still be unable to make plans for the baby or even accept the pregnancy until she feels the baby move. Anticipatory guidance is critical when an adolescent faces overlapping developmental challenges of age and pregnancy.

On the other hand, a pregnant woman older than 35 years may feel more isolated by her situation than does the pregnant woman in her 20s. Frequently established in career and family, the older pregnant woman needs to learn to balance her growth and development in these valued areas with her new sense of self. Fears related to being considered at high risk because of age may increase her anxiety and ambivalence about the pregnancy, even if she was previously infertile. As a first-time mother, she may worry about managing the physical demands of labour and delivery, sleeplessness of motherhood, the chances of having an abnormal child, and the need to juggle conflicting life responsibilities and relationships.

A woman with other children moves through the developmental tasks differently from a woman who is pregnant for the first time. Even with a desired pregnancy, the woman may worry about incorporating the new infant into her relationships and managing the time needed for a new baby. She may have fears and anxieties about labour and delivery because of a previous negative experience. She may be much more aware of the problems involved with caring for a new infant and may not be excited about another pregnancy experience that demands a redefinition of motherhood or additional childrearing expenses.

### ◆ Cognitive-Perceptual Pattern

#### Developmental Tasks

Rubin (1984) describes four major developmental tasks that a woman seeks to accomplish as she learns to become a mother: ensuring safe passage through pregnancy and childbirth; ensuring acceptance of the child by significant people in her family; binding to her unknown child; and learning to give of herself. According to Rubin, all four tasks must be confronted simultaneously, but each task assumes greater priority at certain times than do other tasks. Each woman works through these tasks on the basis of her unique style, cultural values, and life priorities. At the end of pregnancy, however, all tasks must be integrated to create a presentation, similar to a tapestry (Rubin, 1984).

#### Ensuring Safe Passage

- The woman engages in a variety of prenatal care options appropriate to her culture and life experience. For example, pregnant Inuit women rely on older same-culture women to give prenatal care and advice and may rely little on prenatal classes or visits.
- The woman becomes more protective of herself and the fetus by avoiding crowds, revolving doors, small spaces, and people believed to place the mother at risk. She tires of being pregnant but fears the effect of delivery on her safety and that of her child (Rubin, 1984; Solchany, 2013). Although sharing fears and desires with her partner, family, or health care provider helps, only the safe delivery of a normal child can fully free a pregnant woman from her fears to meet this developmental task (Solchany, 2013).

#### Ensuring Acceptance of the Child

- The woman must believe that her child will be accepted into her family based on her definition of family. According to Rubin (1984), the partner's receptivity to the child is particularly important, and many women fantasize about the sex of their child on the basis of a partner's preference.
- The woman frequently judges her partner's degree of receptivity to the infant by the amount of love and attention that she, herself, receives from him during her pregnancy.
- She may desire support from other women, rather than her partner, on the basis of her life experience, values, and cultural background.

#### Binding to Her Unknown Child

- This task is the most complex cognitive process for the pregnant woman (Rubin, 1984). To accomplish this task, the woman must integrate the fetus as an integral part of herself but also as a separate being. Completion of this task occurs with birth of the baby.

- Initially, the woman fantasizes about the baby through associative images: when she eats an egg, she thinks of the baby. Fantasies in the second and third trimesters relate more specifically to what the child will be like; the woman may imagine the baby in little girl or little boy clothes.
- During the eighth month the woman begins nesting activity by preparing the nursery and thinking increasingly of the baby as an external reality in her home.

#### Learning to Give of Herself

- Although the actual mothering activity occurs after birth, the learning process to become a mother begins during pregnancy.
- The woman begins the task by examining what she will gain and lose by becoming a mother.
- She then explores the meaning of giving by examining how others give to her and to others and how she has given to others in the past (Rubin, 1984).
- Gifts for herself and the baby represent meaningful manifestations of her own and others' acceptance of her motherhood and her ability to give to her child and develop her identity as a mother (Rubin, 1967; Solchany, 2013).

### ◆ Self-Perception–Self-Concept Pattern

To develop a maternal identity, the woman must first accept the pregnant body image. Initially, she may show ambivalence based on her need to "fit" the pregnancy with her perception of self. She may dislike the physical changes of pregnancy or gladly "show off" her pregnant body to others. During the second trimester, however, the woman frequently begins to feel more positive about her changing womanly image as she feels the baby move, and increased amounts of estrogen and progesterone enhance her sense of vitality, inner peace, and acceptance. Her body begins to look pregnant, and generally, others respond positively to this change (Solchany, 2013).

By the third trimester, however, the woman frequently tires of the pregnancy. Her sense of awkward moments supersedes feelings of well-being. She may experience uncomfortable, sleepless nights, the constant need to urinate, Braxton Hicks contractions, and other discomforts. Some women experience infant movement or mild contractions as pleasurable, sensual sensations, whereas others find them extremely uncomfortable. By pregnancy's end, these women yearn to have their former body boundaries back, to hold the baby in their arms, or to have someone else carry the baby.

After birth, the woman gradually sees the infant more and more as a separate individual, dependent on her care. The mother starts to bond with her baby on the basis of her self-perception. If she feels good about herself, she will show love toward the infant; when she feels ugly or unlovable, she may make uncomplimentary remarks about the infant's appearance (Rubin, 1984; von Mohr et al., 2017).

#### Maternal Role

The pregnant woman's personality, maturity level, and psychological development influence her readiness to assume the role of a mother. The way in which society in general and her culture in particular perceive motherhood and the role of women, as well as the way in which her own views mesh with these perceptions, will affect the ease of the transition. The family situation, the availability of peer role models, and the relationship with her mother are also significant. Internalization of the mother role occurs only after the birth, when the woman interacts with the infant in a reciprocal relationship (Solchany, 2013).

### Nursing Interventions

The woman may feel overwhelmed by her feelings and thoughts during pregnancy. Although others acknowledge her physical changes, only she experiences the psychological changes of excitement, ambivalence, or confusion associated with being pregnant.

During prenatal assessment, the nurse should address expected cognitive changes and self-image issues with each pregnant woman and respond nonjudgementally to concerns expressed in this area. In one-to-one sessions or group prenatal classes, women and their partners should be encouraged to discuss their ideas and feelings related to the emotional and relationship changes expected during pregnancy, because these changes influence the future intimate relationship.

Education on, and practice of, the maternal role and being a mother, is an effective intervention in increasing self-confidence in caring and maternal identity. During their transition to motherhood, pregnant women want attentive, proactive, professional psychosocial support from nurses. They expect nurses to oversee the transition period and to be capable of supporting them in dealing with changes in pregnancy and in preparing them for birth and motherhood.

### ◆ Roles-Relationships Pattern

The pregnant family changes throughout the pregnancy and postpartum period as each family member explores and responds to new roles and relationships. A pregnant woman without a partner may feel isolated during pregnancy and depend on family or friends as she adjusts to her situation.

The partner of the pregnant woman faces many new situations that influence that person's parental development. The pregnant woman may seem to be a different person to others because of her emotional response to the pregnancy, introspection, fantasies, need for more rest, and changes in sexual drive. The partner may feel a rivalry with the fetus and baby because the mother is devoting increasing amounts of time to the baby. He may resent the attention that she receives during the pregnancy and the additional demands that she may make on his time. He may experience more financial pressure because of baby expenses and his partner's need to stop working on a short-term or long-term basis. These perceptions may lead him to abuse his partner, possibly causing poor pregnancy and newborn outcomes (Quality and Safety Scenario). The nurse assesses each pregnant woman for abuse and intervenes appropriately to protect the safety and health of the family during gestation.

### Infant Loss and Grief

After the loss of an infant, parents are likely to experience an emotional response called grief. Grief is the normal response to interpersonal loss and it is experienced by everyone differently (Goldstein, Lederman, Lichtenthal, et al., 2018). Families

experience increased difficulty coping with the loss of an infant when it is unexpected, there is a history of loss, or when they feel unprepared. Loss can result in role confusion and a lack of trust in others. It is important for families to seek bereavement support from their health care provider and specialized support programs (Goldstein et al., 2018). For example, MyGrief.ca is a program created by the Canadian Virtual Hospice (CVH) to help individuals understand their grief, move through the grieving process, and learn about self-care and coping (CVH, 2016). Nurses can support families during the grieving process by actively listening to their feelings and concerns, being mindful of their language, and allowing for therapeutic silence (Canadian Paediatric Society [CPS], 2018). For instance, if the family had named the infant, use the given name when conducting postmortem care.

The male partner may be concerned about his ability to fulfill the father role and support his wife or significant other. His fathering role models may be limited because of a lack of contact with his own father or because he spends time with men who are not actively parenting. He may never have held a baby before and may worry that he might drop or harm his own child. If his partner experiences pregnancy complications, he may feel guilty about causing the pregnancy. Table 10.5 gives a more complete list of both the father's and the mother's emotional responses to a first pregnancy. The nurse must work with the pregnant family to help the family adapt to a first pregnancy, because this one affects how the family will cope with subsequent pregnancies.

Children in the family also experience role changes during and after the pregnancy. The very young child, unaware of the concept of a new baby before the infant arrives, may experience a changed relationship with his pregnant mother. She may have less time to play, be more irritable from fatigue, or limit or stop active play late in pregnancy because of increased awkwardness and concern about her safety. After the baby has arrived, the child may be kept away from both the baby and the mother by well-meaning friends and relatives, have to share parents with others, or may want to breastfeed from the mother as the baby does. When permitted to see the newborn, the child may be admonished to "be careful" or "don't touch the baby." Thus, a young child may not accept the baby with open arms.

The older child understands the newborn's significance more clearly but still experiences apprehensions about the effects of the baby on the family. Older children may have been told that they will become a big brother or sister, but does this mean they will lose toys and time with their parents and have to give up a private bedroom? Older children may worry about their mother, who seems more tired, less available, and perhaps even sick at times. Her enlarging abdomen may appear frightening. With help from the nurse, parents can make pregnancy an exciting time of learning and growing for the family (Box 10.4). Chapter 12 discusses the sibling relationship in greater detail.

In extended families, expectant grandparents also experience changes during the pregnancy of their daughter or daughter-in-law. The maternal grandmother, seeing her daughter assume the

## QUALITY AND SAFETY SCENARIO

### Birth Outcomes in Pregnant Women Who Are Abused

Nurses and other providers who deliver health care to women must address the issue of abuse of the pregnant woman by an intimate partner. Intimate partner violence is a significant public health problem, with negative physical and psychological outcomes. It has been associated with increased levels of STIs, preterm labour, low-birth-weight infants, anxiety, substance abuse behaviours, and postpartum depression (Alhusen, Ray, Sharps, et al., 2015). Consider the following research study and the questions that follow to understand the issue further.

Several studies have attempted to identify risk factors associated with experiencing violence during pregnancy. However, all these studies compared women who were abused during pregnancy with non-abused pregnant women. To further the understanding of risk factors for experiencing violence during pregnancy, it may be useful to investigate factors that differentiate female victims of intimate partner violence who were and were not victimized during pregnancy. This will allow us to shed light on unique aspects of pregnancy violence. In addition, the current study examines risk factors using a nationally representative sample. The risk factors identified included young age, less than a high school education, unemployment of mother and/or father, dissatisfaction with relationships, alcohol abuse, and violence in the family of origin; unmarried status increased the risk of violence during pregnancy, but the relative risk was even greater if the women separated or divorced while pregnant; paternal uncertainty and accusations of infidelity have been associated with an increased risk of violence among pregnant women (Slep, Foran, Heyman, et al., 2015). Male partners may develop paternal assurance tactics, such as the use of violence to establish control, to combat paternal uncertainty, and to increase the probability that the children they raise are their own and there is no infidelity on the part of the woman. Patriarchal domination has also been linked to an increased risk of violence against women. Pregnancy may symbolize a time when the woman assumes more control over her own body and may represent a degree of independence from her male partner; violence against the pregnant partner may represent a male partner's attempt to reassert control. Many women who are abused during pregnancy have reported that their partners attempt to socially isolate them from family, friends, and other social support systems. Most women reporting physical violence during pregnancy are also victims of verbal abuse and psychological aggression. Psychological abuse may be the predominant form of abuse during pregnancy in some cultures. Women who had a partner with a drinking problem were more than three times as likely to be abused during pregnancy compared with women whose partner did not have a drinking problem.

The health outcomes of violence against pregnant women include substance use, poor mental health, inadequate weight gain, and inconsistent prenatal care (Alhusen et al., 2015). A number of violence-related injuries also include cuts, bruises, fractures, concussions, dental injuries, stab wounds, vaginal bleeding, and persistent headaches. Mental health issues include depression, stress, distress, fearfulness, anxiousness, and feelings of isolation. Possible health outcomes of violence against pregnant women for the neonate include low birth weight, preterm birth, and death (Alhusen et al., 2015).

#### Nursing Implications

Overall, this study indicates a need for nurses to screen women for high-risk factors prenatally, to be aware of the health risks secondary to violence, and to tailor nursing interventions supportive of pregnant women facing abuse. Nurses need to be aware of the issues surrounding pregnancy violence and have the ability to provide pregnant women with the resources and information necessary to ensure their safety.

#### Reflective Questions

- How do the current health care system and the sociopolitical context of care in Canada contribute to the high numbers of pregnant women facing abuse from their intimate partners?
- What kind of interventions do you believe would be effective for these abused women?
- How should the federal government create laws that ethically and legislatively address the problem of intimate partner abuse during pregnancy?

Sources: Alhusen, J. L., Ray, E., Sharps, P., et al. (2015). Intimate partner violence during pregnancy: Maternal and neonatal outcomes. *Journal of Women's Health, 24*(1), 100–106. doi:10.1089/jwh.2014.4872; Brownridge, D. A., Taillieu, T. L., Tyler, K. A., et al. (2011). Pregnancy and intimate partner violence: Risk factors, severity, and health effects. *Violence Against Women, 17*(7), 858–881. doi:10.1177/1077801211412547; Slep, A. M. S., Foran, H. M., Heyman, R. E., et al. (2015). Identifying unique and shared risk factors for physical intimate partner violence and clinically-significant physical intimate partner violence. *Aggressive Behavior, 41*, 227–241. doi:10.1002/ab.21565
STIs, Sexually transmitted infections.

mother role, may now view her daughter as a rival because they are both mothers. The grandparents may be reminded of their own aging, resenting when their advice about pregnancy and parenting goes unheeded. A positive outcome of a pregnancy may be a new closeness between the woman and her mother if the woman turns to her mother to seek advice and share feelings. The nurse may encourage expectant parents to use pregnancy as a transition time for their own parents, which can enhance extended family cohesion in the future.

During and after birth, each family member begins to establish an emotional attachment to the imagined or real new baby. Research shows that when the mother has a strong support system to develop deep feelings of attachment to the fetus, she will most likely attach to the baby after birth. Therefore the nurse assesses the support system of each pregnant woman and implements primary and secondary interventions to increase family bonding with a new baby.

### ◆ Sexuality-Reproductive Pattern

The pregnant woman's body image and merging of this body image with her definition of femininity greatly influence her feelings about her sexuality. For a previously infertile couple, achieving pregnancy may be a blessed event, despite the need for technology that affects a woman's concept of self and femininity and a man's concept of self and masculinity. The reflections of others, particularly those of a pregnant woman's husband, partner, or friend, help a woman to accept changes in her body, leading to better adjustment in their sexual relations.

On the other hand, women may experience different sexual feelings during pregnancy. Some women experience an increase in desire, but many worry about intercourse during pregnancy, fearing that it will cause miscarriage, infection, or an early birth. Other women may experience nausea during pregnancy or simply lack sexual interest. Physical discomfort, fatigue, and awkwardness as well as fear of membrane rupture, infection, or

## TABLE 10.5    Possible Responses to First Pregnancy

| Phase of Pregnancy | Father's Response | Mother's Response |
| --- | --- | --- |
| First trimester | Fear of losing wife or child<br>Self-doubt as a future father<br>May develop new hobby outside of partner as way of distancing self | Loss of interest in coitus<br>Possible less sexual effectiveness<br>Sleepiness and chronic fatigue<br>Nausea<br>Increased dependence<br>Feels ambivalent toward reality of pregnancy<br>Anxious about process of labour and prospect of caring for a child<br>Worries about miscarriage<br>Becomes aware of physical changes in her body<br>May develop a closer relationship with her mother with a common experience of motherhood |
| Second trimester | Increased respect<br>Awe as quickening comes<br>Names for fetus coined<br>May give partner extra attention she desires<br>Feeling of change, accepting the reality of the pregnancy | Solemnity, hilarity, and playfulness about fetal movements<br>Talks about and with fetus<br>Increased eroticism<br>Expects partner to demonstrate interest in caring for her and baby<br>Feels movement and thinks of child as an individual |
| Third trimester | Fear of coitus hurting fetus<br>Abstinence difficult<br>Envy or pride, or both, at wife's creativity<br>Concern about identity as a "father"<br>Worry about birth<br>Keen awareness of male–female differences<br>May show a greater level of tenderness and protectiveness | Abstinence (often recommended by physician)<br>Sleepiness<br>Backache<br>Abdominal discomfort<br>Sexual isolation<br>Heightened sense of femininity<br>Assembles items needed for care of infant and selects possible names |
| Postpartum period | Eagerness to resume marital relations<br>Concern over endangering wife's recovery<br>Sense of triumph in becoming a father<br>Tenderness toward wife and baby | Pain and fear of harm from too early coitus<br>Low eroticism<br>Concern about effect on husband of continued abstinence<br>Sense of completion as a mother |
| Pregnancy as a whole | Increased romanticism<br>Increased nurturance<br>Increased family life participation<br>Financial stress<br>Concern about lack of skills in baby care | Increased romanticism<br>Increased optimism<br>Family roles replacing marital emphases<br>Fear of miscarriage or problems with baby<br>Pride of accomplishment<br>Emotional stress, feeling overloaded |

Sources: Golian Tehrani, S., Bazzazian, S., & Dehghan Nayeri, N. (2015). Pregnancy experiences of first-time fathers: A qualitative study. *Iranian Red Crescent Medical Journal, 17*(2), 12271–12273. doi:10.5812/ircmj.12271; Nierenberg, C. (2015). Mood swings & mommy brain: The emotional challenges of pregnancy. *Live Science*. Retrieved from http://www.livescience.com/51043-pregnancy-emotions.html; Poh, H. L., Koh, S. S. L., Seow, H. C. L., et al. (2014). First-time father' experiences and needs during pregnancy and childbirth: A descriptive study. *Midwifery, 30*(6), 779–787. doi:10.1016/j.midw.2013.10.002.

### BOX 10.4    Nursing Strategies to Help Parents Prepare Siblings for the Neonate

- Explain the pregnancy and birth appropriate to the child's age.
- Answer all the child's questions.
- Use relevant literature to educate the child about the coming baby.
- Encourage discussion and questions by talking about the new baby during relaxed family times rather than during busy, rushed times.
- Have the child participate in decisions, such as choosing a name, clothes, and toys for baby.
- When sibling classes are available as part of the childbirth education process, encourage parents and the child to attend.
- Suggest that the child go with the mother during clinic or office visits.
- Allow and discuss negative comments about the pregnancy or baby.
- Encourage the child to make drawings or give small gifts to the baby when it is born.

harm to the fetus may also diminish the woman's interest in sexual relations. Sexual dissatisfaction of the couple may result from restrictions in sexual positions, pain on penetration, increased vaginal discharge, breast tenderness, or the other physical discomforts of pregnancy such as fatigue and heartburn. In some cases, the enlarging uterus will require the couple to modify the positions for intercourse, particularly during the latter part of pregnancy. The couple's feelings about the woman's changing body may alter their sexual relationship. The nurse's first step in primary prevention intervention in this area is to support the couple's needs and to relate, in a sensitive fashion, accurate information that facilitates couple intimacy during pregnancy.

Some women experience a decreased desire for sexual intercourse but an increased desire for holding, touching, and other signs of physical affection from their husbands or partners.

The nurse encourages the couple to explore other activities for mutual sexual satisfaction.

In summary, the nurse can use the following guidelines concerning sexual activity:

- Sex is generally considered safe in pregnancy.
- Abstinence should be recommended only for women who are at risk of preterm labour, multiple gestation, premature rupture of membranes, unexplained vaginal bleeding, or antepartum hemorrhage because of placenta previa.
- There is little evidence to show that sex at term may help induce labour, but this practice is considered safe in women with low-risk pregnancies (Zakšek, 2015).
- The resumption of intercourse postpartum should be dictated by a woman's level of comfort.

### ◆ Coping–Stress Tolerance Pattern

Physical and psychological adaptations of the woman to pregnancy affect her perception of stressors and her ability to cope with all aspects of her life. Even normal discomforts of pregnancy may be stressful for a woman, mandating her to modify her usual routine to cope more effectively. Anxiety tends to be high during the first trimester as the woman adapts to pregnancy and anticipated life changes. During the second trimester the woman feels less anxious, but anxiety returns during the third trimester with impending labour and delivery. Throughout pregnancy women may demonstrate their anxieties through psychosomatic complaints and behaviours, such as nausea and vomiting after the first trimester, excessive eating, food cravings, sleeplessness, and fainting. Realistically, every pregnant woman probably experiences some degree of stress. However, many women have considerable stress or ongoing stress—such as poverty, marital difficulties, or unsatisfactory living or working conditions, that influences their coping abilities.

A pregnant woman's anxieties may be reflected in her dreams and fantasies. Many pregnant women report dreams about their babies being deformed or dead, themselves dying, or a family member being injured. Many women at the end of their pregnancies express fears about body mutilation with delivery. Other women may manifest their anxiety by smoking, drinking, or using drugs (legal or illegal), all of which can harm the fetus. Prenatal depression and/or anxiety has been associated with excessive activity and growth delays in the fetus, as well as prematurity, low birth weight, disorganized sleep, and less responsiveness to stimulation in the neonate. Infants of depressed/anxious mothers have difficult temperaments; later in development, attentional, emotional, and behavioural problems have been noted during childhood and adolescence, as well as chronic illnesses in adulthood. Caring for a newborn requires energy, patience, and emotional presence, which are all lacking in a depressed mother (Rode & Kiel, 2016). The nurse must direct a pregnant woman who is not coping well to relevant resources for assistance. The nurse must also assess each woman's progress in taking on the mothering role as the pregnancy nears term. This information can be shared with the postpartum nursing staff to encourage discussion in this important area.

The nurse encourages the pregnant woman to use tension-relieving strategies such as listening to soft music, using humour, crying, sleeping, talking to a friend, meditating, exercising, and fantasizing during times of stress. These strategies are safe for the fetus and provide relief from many normal tensions and anxieties during pregnancy and afterward. Overall, the nurse plays a key role by responding nonjudgementally and promoting the coping of women during pregnancy.

### ◆ Values-Beliefs Pattern

Although pregnancy has been described as the fulfillment of the deepest and most powerful wish of a woman, this fulfillment often coincides with a woman's fear of losing part of herself. She gives up some relationships and pleasures to assume other anticipated satisfactions. She may find that she values friendships with other mothers now, whereas before pregnancy her friendships focused on work or school colleagues. She may discover, much to her husband's confusion, that she values different qualities in him than she did before anticipating birth. Her husband may also experience a shift in his values.

Pregnant women and their partners may experience changes in their spiritual values. For women with strong spiritual needs related to their cultural backgrounds, spiritual interventions will help them integrate various dimensions of their lives, develop the ability to parent successfully, and find meaning in the changes and goals of pregnancy. Seen as a mystical event or miracle, conception may lead to an increased faith in God or a favourite saint. Non-religious couples may start to attend church after the baby's birth because they want religion to be part of their child's life. Religious beliefs may influence a woman's decision to undergo certain tests or procedures, such as amniocentesis or abortion. Some women may feel forced to reproduce because their religious or cultural mores forbid contraception or encourage large families. In these groups, each pregnancy may be seen as another unwanted, but unavoidable, burden or may be valued because having more children signifies a stronger family.

## ❖ ENVIRONMENTAL PROCESSES

### ◆ Physical Agents

A healthy infant is the outcome of most pregnancies. However, genetic abnormalities and environmental hazards may cause fetal harm, spontaneous abortion (natural loss of conceptive products), or minor or serious congenital defects. Diagnostic methods that identify an early pregnancy or a fetal loss may assist couples in practicing healthy decisions to prevent loss or congenital abnormalities. The best time for a fetal scan is at 18 to 20 weeks of gestation (Rayburn, Jolley, & Simpson, 2015). This knowledge, gained before giving birth, permits expectant couples and the health care delivery team to access resources for improving the baby's life or to support a grieving family if the baby is not expected to live. With progress made in diagnostic tools and the Human Genome Project, some couples may be able to prevent fetal defects or manage them during pregnancy to improve the quality of their baby's life after birth (see the Case Study at the end of this chapter). Unfortunately, even when no genetic or congenital defects exist, the fetus may still be injured during the process of labour and delivery and face a lesser quality of life.

Teratogens are environmental agents that cause spontaneous abortions or congenital defects. Unlike genetic abnormalities, which occur only at conception, environmental agents may affect the developing infant at any point during gestation. Fetal organs have critical periods of development, and if affected at that time by a teratogen, the infant may have a defect in that organ system. Teratogens normally do not cause a congenital defect during the first 14 days after conception. However, the embryo may be lost later during early gestation (a spontaneous abortion). Therefore, as a primary prevention strategy, any woman contemplating or attempting pregnancy should be counselled to avoid teratogens that might cause fetal loss or damage.

## Physical Factors and Diagnostic Tools

Modern diagnostic tools, such as ultrasonography, amniocentesis, blood sampling, chorionic villus sampling, and alpha-fetoprotein screening, have been used to identify a number of fetal problems. Certain risk factors, some of which may be found in the family history, or maternal and paternal age, maternal illness, or previous fetal abnormalities, may indicate the need for these diagnostic tools during a woman's pregnancy. These tools commonly identify problems related to abnormal size or rate of fetal growth, chromosomal abnormalities, NTDs, and fetal lung immaturity. The nurse, in consultation with the health care team, must participate in providing informed consent to women before these diagnostic tools are used.

In Canada, prenatal screening is available to all pregnant women and is voluntary (Genetics Education Canada Knowledge Organization [GECKO], 2019c). If a woman decides to have prenatal screening and a second trimester ultrasound, there is a higher chance of detecting congenital abnormalities and genetic conditions. In Canada, reproductive genetic carrier screening is available, and the family health history–based risk assessment is considered to be the gold standard for the initial assessment of heredity conditions (GECKO, 2019a). This tool has been replicated and adapted to consider the biological parent's ethnic backgrounds. Expanded carrier screening is also available, and looks beyond an individual's family health history and ethnic background; it uses next-generation sequencing to assess more than 100 genes at a time. This testing is not covered by provincial health care plans (GECKO, 2019b). Other screening tools used in Canada can assess for familial hypercholesterolemia, hereditary cancers, and hereditary hemochromatosis.

## ◆ Biological Agents

Biological processes in the fetal environment, which include infections and other health problems of the mother, may affect fetal growth and development. A pregnant woman who acquires an asymptomatic viral infection may not seek health care because she believes that the fetus will not be harmed. However, viral agents may cause fetal damage early in pregnancy. The woman with a health problem, such as diabetes,

may also cause fetal damage if she fails to adhere to her health care provider's directives.

When the nurse discusses with pregnant couples the effects of biological processes on the fetus, she must emphasize that the timing of the maternal infection or illness is critical to predicting fetal defects. Maternal infections during the first trimester of pregnancy may cause severe fetal defects or death, depending on the organism. Infections later in pregnancy may also seriously affect the fetus, but less often. Unfortunately, pregnancy renders many women more susceptible to viral illness, supporting an argument for all women of childbearing age to be fully immunized. Many vaccines (measles, mumps, rubella, and polio) cannot be given during pregnancy because of potential risk to the fetus, but others present no risk (tetanus and diphtheria). A TORCH (*t*oxoplasmosis, *o*ther agents, *r*ubella, *c*ytomegalovirus, *h*erpes simplex; other infections include *Treponema pallidum*, hepatitis viruses, HIV, varicella, parvovirus B19, and enteroviruses) screen may be done to detect the presence of teratogenic perinatal infections: toxoplasmosis, hepatitis B, rubella, cytomegalovirus infection, and herpes simplex (Table 10.6). TORCH infections are major contributors to prenatal, perinatal, and postnatal morbidity and death. Evidence of infection may be seen at birth, in infancy, or years later. For many of these pathogens, treatment or prevention strategies are available, but early recognition, including prenatal screening, is essential.

### Toxoplasmosis

Toxoplasmosis is caused by a protozoan that infects people through consumption of undercooked meat, handling of feces of cats that become infected by eating infected rodents and birds, and exposure to contaminated soil, in countries outside Canada (College of Family Physicians of Canada [CFPC], 2014b). An infected pregnant woman is usually asymptomatic but may have flulike symptoms or mild to severe upper respiratory tract symptoms believed to be unrelated to an infection. Vertical transmission from an infected pregnant woman to the fetus predominantly occurs when infection is acquired for the first time during pregnancy. Overall, approximately one-third of infected pregnant women give birth to an infant with toxoplasmosis, and the risk of vertical transmission rises sharply with gestational age at maternal infection. However, fetuses infected during an early pregnancy period are much more likely to show clinical signs of infection, such as chorioretinitis, hydrocephalus, or intracranial calcification (King et al., 2015). Approximately 60% of maternal infections acquired during the third trimester will result in fetal infection, which might manifest itself as rashes, enlarged lymph nodes and liver, inflammation of the heart, pneumonia, jaundice, or severe CNS damage after birth or years later (CFPC, 2014b). Nurses can offer some simple hygiene suggestions that reduce the risk of infection. For example, humans can acquire toxoplasmosis from eating undercooked or raw meat (especially lamb and pork), from being exposed to contaminated soil or water, or from consuming uncooked vegetables. Clearly, nurses should advise pregnant women to cook meat thoroughly and wash and scrub vegetables well, especially those eaten raw. Pregnant women should use good handwashing hygiene, avoid eating raw meat,

| TABLE 10.6 | TORCH Perinatal Infections | | | |
|---|---|---|---|---|
| Infection | Agent | Source | Fetal–Neonatal Risks | Comments |
| **T**oxoplasmosis | Protozoan *Toxoplasma gondii* | Raw or undercooked meat; unpasteurized goat's milk; feces of infected cats | Fetal growth restriction, hydrocephaly, seizures, neurological and cognitive effects, chorioretinitis, intracranial calcifications | Instruct mother to not eat undercooked or raw meat; avoid exposure to cat litter |
| **O**ther/hepatitis B | Hepadnavirus | Blood or blood products; sexually transmitted via body fluids | Generally asymptomatic, but majority become chronically infected | Newborn should receive HBIG within 12h after birth and hepatitis B vaccine postpartum |
| **R**ubella | Rubella virus | Direct or indirect contact with droplets of infected person | CNS defects, developmental delay, deafness, cataracts, IUGR, microcephaly, cardiac defects, glaucoma | Screen all pregnant women with rubella antibody titres |
| **C**ytomegalovirus | Herpes virus | Transmitted by droplet infection from person to person | Microcephaly, fetal growth restriction, CNS abnormalities, deafness, blindness, jaundice, gastro-intestinal defects, seizures | Prevention of maternal primary infection in early pregnancy; stress good personal hygiene |
| **H**erpes simplex | HSV-1 and HSV-2 | Sexually transmitted infection to mother; fetus contacts it during birth from genital lesions | Intense herpetic lesions on eyes, mouth, and skin; keratitis; conjunctivitis | Practice safer sex; careful handwashing; surgical birth if active lesions |

*CNS,* Central nervous system; *HBIG,* hepatitis B immune globulin; *HSV-1,* herpes simplex virus type 1; *HSV-2,* herpes simplex virus type 2; *IUGR,* intrauterine growth restriction.

Sources: Neu, N., Duchon, J., & Zachariah, P. (2015). TORCH infections. *Clinics in Perinatology, 42*(1), 77–103. doi:10.1016/j.clp.2014.11.001; Smith, B. (2015). Neonatal-perinatal infections: An update. *Clinics in Perinatology, 42*(1), 77–104. doi:10.1016/j.clp.2014.12.001; Suliman, S., & Seopela, L. (2015). Congenital and neonatal infections: Review. *Obstetrics and Gynecology Forum, 25*(2), 27–32. Retrieved from https://journals.co.za/content/medog/25/2/EJC169136#related_content.

wear gloves when gardening, and avoid handling cats or cleaning cat litter boxes to avoid exposure to *Toxoplasma.*

## Syphilis

Syphilis is an STI that can be transmitted through oral, anal, or vaginal contact. An infected mother transfers syphilis, caused by a bacterium, to her fetus. The causative organism, *Treponema pallidum,* can be transferred across the placenta and can infect the developing fetus as early as at 9 weeks of gestation. The risk of vertical transmission and infection in the newborn is directly related to the stage of maternal syphilis during pregnancy; transmission occurs more frequently during primary or secondary syphilis in the mother than during latent stages of the disease. Although syphilis is preventable and treatable, the number of congenital and neonatal syphilis cases has increased in the last several years (Health Canada, 2018a). Maternal risk factors for acquiring syphilis include homelessness, HIV-positive status, single marital status, and a history of STIs. Maternal syphilis has been associated with complications such as polyhydramnios, spontaneous abortion, and preterm births. Fetal complications such as fetal syphilis, fetal hydrops, prematurity, fetal distress, and stillbirth also occur. Neonatal complications can include congenital syphilis, seizures, neonatal death, and late sequelae (Singh, Levett, Fonseca, et al., 2015). The infant may be born with localized mucocutaneous lesions, nasal congestion, anemia, and generalized septicemia, but may appear healthy at birth only to have symptoms appear later. Routine testing of high-risk women for syphilis at the first prenatal visit and during the third trimester and antibiotic treatment (benzathine penicillin G) for affected women and their partners have reduced the number of infants with congenital syphilis (King & Brucker, 2016).

## Rubella

In Canada, the incidence of rubella occurring in pregnancy is rare, because most women are immunized against it with the measles, mumps, and rubella (MMR) vaccine (Canadian Paediatric Society, 2015). The risk of vertical transmission from a nonimmune mother with primary rubella infection in the first trimester of pregnancy is considerably high, at 80% to 90%. Beyond the first 12 weeks of gestation, fetal organogenesis is nearly complete, and deafness may be the only consequence in the infected infant. Deafness, cataracts, and cardiac defects are the classic congenital anomalies associated with a rubella infection (Silasi, Cardenas, Kwon, et al., 2015). The symptoms of rubella may cause the mother to think she has a minor viral infection, but rubella during the first trimester may cause improper fetal development of the ears, eyes, and heart, and deafness. No treatment exists for an infected fetus; however, a pregnant woman may receive the vaccine to protect future pregnancies if she has no history of rubella infection. After giving birth, new mothers often receive the vaccine before being discharged, with a recommendation to avoid pregnancy for at least 3 months to prevent fetal harm from the vaccine.

## Cytomegalovirus

Cytomegalovirus (CMV) is a virus in the herpes virus family and is a leading cause of congenital infections and long-term neurodevelopmental disabilities among children. Contacts with young children have been identified as the main source of virus transmission to mothers. It is the most common infection that can cause serious fetal complications. CMV infects an estimated 0.2% to 2.4% of all infants born in Canada (Health Canada, 2011b). Most mothers infected with CMV have mild, often nonspecific symptoms, but their infants may experience hearing loss, blindness, enlarged liver and spleen, seizures, intracranial calcifications, and neurodevelopmental disabilities (Kovacs & Briggs, 2015). Unfortunately, no means exist to prevent or manage this viral infection. Perhaps an immunization similar to that for rubella will be developed in the future. Until vaccines and nontoxic antiviral agents are available, hygienic measures are important as prophylaxis and should be emphasized by all nurses to their prenatal patients.

### Herpes Simplex Virus

Herpes simplex virus infections remain extremely common today, with many people unaware that they have the disease. Herpes is lifelong infection that has the potential for transmission throughout the life span (King et al., 2015). Herpes simplex may cause spontaneous abortion or fetal neurological damage. Infants infected at birth may show localized or generalized disease, with symptoms of vesicular skin lesions, microcephaly, hydrocephalus, chorioretinitis, conjunctivitis, seizures, respiratory distress, or gastro-intestinal bleeding. These symptoms may cause newborn death. An infant delivered vaginally by a woman with active genital herpes has a 50% to 70% chance of being infected (Health Canada, 2013a), supporting a decision for a Caesarean delivery for any women with active vaginal or perineal herpes lesions. Risk factors for the transmission of herpes from the mother to the newborn have been detailed. The pregnant woman who acquires genital herpes as a primary infection in the latter half of pregnancy, rather than before pregnancy, is at greatest risk of transmitting this virus to her newborn. This is true for both herpes simplex virus type 1 (HSV-1) and herpes simplex virus type 2 (HSV-2) (Kovacs & Briggs, 2015). Generally, an antiviral agent is recommended during pregnancy for treatment of viral lesions. The nurse educates the infected woman about comfort measures at this time, including ways to keep the lesions dry and application of comfort measures to reduce the pain of the lesions (Queenan, Spong, & Lockwood, 2015).

### Zika Virus Disease

Zika virus is transmitted to humans primarily through the bite of an infected *Aedes* species mosquito during the daytime. The most common symptoms of Zika virus disease are fever, rash, headaches, bone pains, joint tenderness, and conjunctivitis. The illness is typically mild, with symptoms lasting for several days to a week after the person has being bitten. Up to 80% of people infected with the virus have no symptoms (Health Canada, 2016a). The virus is in the Caribbean, as well as parts of Central America and South America. The virus has been reported to be spread through blood transfusions and sexual contact and can also be passed from a pregnant woman to her fetus, and has been linked to a serious birth defect of the brain termed microcephaly. Health Canada, the WHO, and other scientific organizations are working to understand this possible link.

In 2016, the WHO (2016b) declared Zika virus a public health emergency of international concern. The Centers for Disease Control and Prevention (CDC) recommends abstaining from oral, anal, or vaginal sexual contact with anyone who

has travelled to areas with active infections. Pregnant women are also discouraged from travelling to regions with active infections (Health Canada, 2016a). At this time there is no vaccine given to prevent Zika virus disease or antiviral medication to treat the infection. Prevention measures would include better housing construction, use of insect repellents, wearing long-sleeved shirts and pants, regular use of air conditioning, use of window screens, avoidance of travelling to mosquito-infested areas, and state and local mosquito control efforts.

### Chlamydia, Gonococcus, Group B Streptococcus, Bacterial Vaginosis, and *Candida albicans*

Infections caused by chlamydia, gonococcus, group B streptococcus, and yeast (*Candida albicans*) may occur in the woman's vagina or cervix, infecting the infant during a vaginal birth. Chlamydia, the most common bacterial STI, appears most often among poor women with little access to care. Although few symptoms are seen, infection may cause preterm labour, premature rupture of membranes, low-birth-weight infants, or newborn conjunctivitis or pneumonia. Routine treatment of the newborn's eyes after birth with erythromycin or other effective antibiotic ointment destroys the organisms. Maternal gonococcus (GC) infection can be transmitted to the newborn from the mother's genital tract at the time of birth and can cause ophthalmia neonatorum, a systemic neonatal infection, maternal endometritis, or pelvic infection. The risk of transmission from an infected mother to her infant is nearly 50% (PHAC, 2017b). Newborn infants often receive an antibiotic ointment in the eyes to prevent GC infection. Screening at 35 to 37 weeks of pregnancy for group B streptococcus infection has been recommended because this infection causes preterm rupture of the amniotic membranes, preterm labour, fetal respiratory distress syndrome, fetal septicemia, and meningitis (Michihata, Yamamoto, & Mukaigawa, 2015; Society of Obstetricians and Gynaecologists of Canada [SOGC], 2019a). Bacterial vaginosis may also cause preterm labour (Sangkomkamhang, Lumbiganon, Prasertcharoensook, et al., 2015). *Candida albicans,* the cause of a common vaginal fungal infection, may also cause an oral infection called thrush in the newborn. Routine assessment of pregnant women, and occasionally their sexual partners (GC), for these bacterial and yeast infections must occur during pregnancy so that treatment can occur and prevent fetal infection at the time of birth.

### Human Immunodeficiency Virus

*Acquired immunodeficiency syndrome.* The CPS and the SOGC recommend that all pregnant women be tested for HIV infection, ideally at the first prenatal visit (CPS, 2019; SOGC, 2019b). Any woman in a high-risk group (e.g., intravenous drug users, women who have bisexual partners or multiple sexual contacts, women with a history of STIs, women who engage in sex for money or drugs, or Black or Latin American women living in poverty) should be tested for antibodies to HIV. For the HIV-positive woman or one who engages in high-risk sexual practices, counselling must occur before conception. Counselling should include both the direct effect of the virus on pregnancy and the effect of pregnancy on HIV disease progression. Although unclear, it appears that HIV infection becomes worse during pregnancy because of a woman's altered immune status. Some early pregnancy discomforts, such as fatigue, anorexia, and weight loss, may mask the early symptoms of HIV infection and thus postpone a definitive diagnosis.

Infants born to HIV-positive women who have taken antiretroviral medications during their pregnancy, in whom the virus is undetectable, and who have avoided breastfeeding have a less than 1% perinatal transmission rate (CPS, 2019). Affected infants may not be seropositive for HIV for many months after birth and then later develop the disease. The use of antiretroviral medications throughout pregnancy has improved the prognosis of an HIV-positive woman and has decreased viral transmission to the fetus, although the medication remains expensive and may be inaccessible for women who do not receive prenatal care.

The pregnant woman who has acquired immunodeficiency syndrome (AIDS) or who is HIV positive should be carefully monitored by a health care team for opportunistic infections that occur frequently. The nurse can be instrumental in helping this woman coordinate her contacts with care providers, answering her questions, and working as a member of the team to provide optimal care for the woman and her child. Frequently, the pregnant woman with AIDS does not seek care because of fears of being reported for her disease. Involving the woman in continuous prenatal care decreases her risk of preterm rupture of membranes, problems with fetal growth, postpartum infection, drug and alcohol abuse, and difficulty in addressing sociocultural barriers to a better life (Money, Tulloch, Boucoiran, et al., 2014).

Although important in decreasing the transmission of any disease, astute preventive measures are mandatory for nurses who are exposed to HIV-infected body fluids, such as blood, amniotic fluid, and vaginal secretions (standard precautions should be followed). All health care providers must follow hospital and birth centre policies regarding the use of gloves and gowns and the disposal of needles and other potentially contaminated equipment to prevent the transmission of this disease in particular.

## Hepatitis B

Hepatitis B virus (HBV) is a serious global public health problem, with more than 2 billion people infected and more than 1 million deaths occurring annually because of cirrhosis and liver carcinoma (Reddy, Venkateswarlu, Umadevi, et al., 2015). HBV infection remains a significant concern during pregnancy because it affects the maternal liver and has a high fetal transmission rate (Castillo, Murphy, & van Schalkwyk, 2017). High-risk groups for HBV infection include women from Asia, Indigenous peoples, as well as health care workers, intravenous drug users, and women with multiple sexual partners (Health Canada, 2011a). On the basis of the large number of infected women who fail to show symptoms until liver damage has occurred, all pregnant women early in pregnancy and those at risk should be screened routinely for HBV (Queenan et al., 2015). HBV immunization (three injections over a period of 6 months) may be given before or during pregnancy to a mother who is

seronegative (Health Canada, 2017a). Since the HB vaccine is a routine immunization in Canada and received during childhood, many women may already have immunity. According to Jhaveri (2015), most women harboring HBV transmit it vertically through the placenta to the fetus or through contaminated urine, feces, saliva, or vaginal fluids during birth. Many women carrying HBV deliver prematurely, and some infants may have acute hepatitis or later develop liver cancer.

## Other Health Concerns

Pregnant women may also develop any of the infections of nonpregnant women. For example, pregnant women frequently experience upper respiratory tract and gastrointestinal tract infections, adding to the discomforts of pregnancy. However, there is no evidence the viruses causing these infections have a teratogenic effect on the fetus.

Fever frequently occurs with illness. A high temperature for a prolonged time (hyperthermia) in a pregnant woman may harm the fetus, especially during the first trimester. Some literature indicates that fever is associated with miscarriages, low birth weight, stillbirths, and preterm births (Silasi et al., 2015). Whether the fever or an underlying illness causing the fever has created the problem must be determined. Some reports have also correlated prolonged use of a sauna or hot tub, causing hyperthermia, with birth defects such as microcephaly, anencephaly, and hypotonia (Biswas, Banerjee, Sanyal, et al., 2015). Until health care providers understand this issue better, the nurse should advise pregnant women to avoid prolonged sauna or hot tub use and spending time with people who are ill or carrying disease. When a pregnant woman develops a fever, she should be advised to contact her health care provider immediately.

Pregnant woman may have other health problems that influence their physiological processes and thus harm the developing fetus. In Canada, the maternal mortality rate was 8.3 per 100,000 deaths in 2018 (Statistics Canada, 2019). The top three causes of maternal deaths in Canada during these years were diseases of the circulatory system, postpartum hemorrhage, and hypertension. Between 2008 and 2010, there were 7.8 deaths per 10,000 deliveries in Canada (PHAC, 2011a).

*Diabetes.* Diabetes mellitus is approaching epidemic proportions worldwide, and the effects and treatment of it are still not well understood by the medical community. Diabetes may exist before pregnancy (pre-existing diabetes) or start during pregnancy (gestational diabetes), affecting both the mother and the fetus. Pregnancy increases the need for maternal insulin to balance the woman's blood glucose level. Currently, the Canadian Diabetes Association (CDA) recommends that all pregnant women complete a glucose tolerance test between 24 and 28 weeks of gestation to identify abnormal blood glucose utilization and the need for additional monitoring (CDA, 2018). Complications from diabetes during pregnancy include polyhydramnios (excessive amniotic fluid volume), acidosis, increased rate of infection, vascular complications, and increased risk of pregnancy-induced hypertension. Because of an increased incidence of intrauterine death after 36 weeks of gestation attributable to an aging placenta, close monitoring in the last month is essential. Neonatal complications from diabetes include hypoglycemia, respiratory distress syndrome, hyperbilirubinemia, and hypocalcaemia. Infants of mothers with diabetes also have a higher incidence of congenital anomalies, such as a heart lesion or meningocele (Langer, 2015). The diabetic pregnant woman needs close health care team supervision and ongoing health teaching, including diet and exercise management, to control her disease effectively for an optimal pregnancy outcome.

*Heart disease and hypertension.* The physiological changes that occur in pregnancy can place extra demands on cardiac function. Cardiac disease complicates approximately 1–4% of all pregnancies in the Canada (Malin & Wallace, 2019). Heart disease and hypertension are two serious maternal cardiovascular problems during pregnancy. Rheumatic heart disease, a common problem that affects more than 34 million people annually, contributes to heart failure, threatening the lives of both the mother and the fetus. The greatest tragedy of all is that it is eminently preventable (Carapetis, 2015). The fetus may require preterm birth to prevent complications. Chronic hypertension, seen more frequently in first-time mothers older than 35 years, increases the chances of stillbirths, preterm births, pre-eclampsia, chronic hypertension, and development of gestational hypertension, which increase both maternal and infant mortality rates. Mothers with these problems must be monitored closely throughout pregnancy to prevent complications (Raio, Bolla, & Baumann, 2015).

*Rh blood group incompatibility.* Rh blood group incompatibility, which is a rare occurrence today because of implementation of anti-D immune globulin prophylaxis given to the mother prenatally and postnatally, sometimes affects fetal development. This problem usually occurs when the mother has Rh-negative red blood cells and the fetus has Rh-positive red blood cells, inherited from a father who has Rh-positive blood. In this disorder, maternal antibodies develop, cross the placental membranes, and destroy the Rh-positive red blood cells of the fetus. Depending on the severity of the response, the infant may develop various levels of hyperbilirubinemia after birth or may die in utero from the anemia of erythroblastosis fetalis (hemolytic disease of the newborn).

All women should be assessed for blood type, Rh factor, and development of antibody to Rh-positive cells at their first pre-natal care visit and again at 24 to 28 weeks of pregnancy unless the father of the baby is Rh negative (Moise, 2015). Rh incompatibility between a mother and a future fetus may be prevented by administration of Rho(D) immune globulin (WinRho) to a Rh-negative mother at 28 weeks of gestation and within 72 hours after birth. The immunization prevents the mother's sensitization to fetal Rh-negative cells by inactivating fetal red blood cells in the mother before she can develop an antibody response. The ideal injection time is after the mother's first birth of an Rh-positive infant, miscarriage, or therapeutic abortion. The incompatibility generally does not occur during the first pregnancy, and the immunization prevents problems with later pregnancies.

## Chemical Agents

Substance abuse in pregnancy remains a major public health problem. The use and abuse of alcohol and other mind-altering drugs has political, legal, socioeconomic, health, mental health, and familial impact felt widely around the world. Certain prescription medications and illicit drugs ingested by the mother may be teratogenic to the fetus. The tragic experience with the tranquilizer medication thalidomide, which caused limb deformities during the early 1960s, led to a recommendation that medications should be avoided during pregnancy unless absolutely necessary (Research for Evidence-Informed Practice). The fact remains, however, that during the most critical early weeks of fetal development and growth, when many women do not know they are pregnant, ingested medication may seriously affect the fetus. Depending on fetal gestational age and drug metabolism, medications may alter the placenta itself or directly affect development and growth of the fetus. The substances that most commonly cause congenital defects are prescription medications, over-the-counter (OTC) medications, street drugs, nicotine (cigarettes), caffeine, and alcohol. Pregnant and postpartum breastfeeding mothers can learn about medication safety in prenatal classes, consulting with their primary care provider and through online resources (Best Start, 2018).

### Prescription Medications

Women frequently become pregnant while taking medications for illnesses diagnosed before pregnancy, such as hypertension, or they may receive medication to treat an illness acquired during pregnancy, such as a UTI. Some of the more common medications that have been studied for fetal effects include antibiotics and anticonvulsants.

Most short-term and usual-dose antibiotics do not cause fetal harm. The tetracyclines are harmful to baby teeth formation because they combine with calcium ions and are deposited in deciduous teeth (causing discoloration) and bones (inhibiting bone growth and causing deformities) (King & Brucker, 2016). Primary teeth seem most affected, but when the antibiotic is given near the time of delivery, the permanent teeth may also be damaged.

On the basis of our current state of knowledge, the vast majority of antibiotics do not cause serious harm to the unborn child if used properly and at the appropriate doses during pregnancy. The treatment with an antibiotic that is contraindicated does not justify termination of pregnancy. However, ultimately, no medicine, including antibiotics, can be described as absolutely safe (Doulatram, Raj, & Govindaraj, 2015).

The prevalence of antiepileptic medication use in pregnant women is very low. Although their main indication is for management of epilepsy, antiepileptic medications are increasingly being used in the treatment of bipolar mood disorders, migraine, and neuropathic pain syndrome, which means their prevalence will increase (Tomson & Klein, 2015). The effects of anticonvulsants on the fetus have been documented thoroughly. Women with seizure disorders have carried infants to term while being treated with hydantoin, barbiturates, and other antiseizure medications. Infants born to mothers taking hydantoin (Dilantin) may have fetal hydantoin syndrome, reflected

## RESEARCH FOR EVIDENCE-INFORMED PRACTICE

### Substance Use in Pregnancy

***Objective.*** To improve awareness and knowledge of problematic substances (alcohol, tobacco, illicit substances of opioids, amphetamine-type stimulants, cocaine, marijuana, and unprescribed prescription medications) used in pregnancy and to provide evidence-informed recommendations for the management of this challenging clinical issue for all health care providers.

***Options.*** This guideline reviews the use of screening tools, general approach to care, and recommendations for clinical management of problematic substance use in pregnancy.

***Outcomes.*** Evidence-informed recommendations for screening and management of problematic substance use during pregnancy and lactation.

***Evidence.*** Medline, PubMed, CINAHL, and the Cochrane Library were searched for articles published from 1950 with use of the following keywords: substance-related disorders, mass screening, pregnancy complications, pregnancy, prenatal care, cocaine, cannabis, methadone, opioid, tobacco, nicotine, solvents, hallucinogens, and amphetamines. The results were initially restricted to systematic reviews and randomized controlled trials/controlled clinical trials. A subsequent search for observational studies was also conducted because there are few randomized controlled trials in this field of study. Articles were restricted to human studies published in English.

#### Recommendations

- All pregnant women and women of childbearing age should be screened periodically for alcohol, tobacco, and prescription and illicit drug use.
- When testing for substance use is clinically indicated, urine drug screening is the preferred method. Informed consent should be obtained from the woman before maternal drug toxicology testing is ordered.
- The 5As of intervention (ask, advise, assess, assist, and arrange) can be a useful framework for encouraging women to quit substance use.
- Pregnant women may require a medically supported inpatient setting to assist them in their recovery from substance abuse.

- Policies and legal requirements with respect to drug testing of newborns may differ by jurisdiction, and caregivers should be familiar with the regulations in their region.
- Health care providers should use a flexible approach to the care of women who have substance use problems, and they should encourage the use of all available community resources.
- Women should be counselled about the risks of periconception, antepartum, and postpartum drug use.
- Women seeking help should be provided with counselling and substance abuse treatment option referrals.
- Smoking cessation counselling should be considered as a first-line intervention for pregnant smokers. Nicotine replacement therapy and/or pharmacotherapy can be considered if counselling is not successful.
- Methadone maintenance treatment should be a standard of care for opioid-dependent women during pregnancy. Other slow-release opioid preparations may be considered if methadone is not available.
- Opioid detoxification should be reserved for selected women because of the high risk of relapse to opioids.
- Opiate-dependent women should be informed that neonates exposed to heroin, prescription opioids, methadone, or buprenorphine during pregnancy are monitored closely for symptoms and signs of neonatal withdrawal (neonatal abstinence syndrome).
- The risks and benefits of breastfeeding should be weighed on an individual basis because methadone maintenance therapy is not a contraindication to breastfeeding.

***Nursing implications:*** Using these guidelines, nurses can assist in helping pregnant women improve access to health care, and assistance with appropriate addiction care leads to reduced health care costs and decreased maternal and neonatal morbidity and mortality.

Source: Wong, S., Ordean, A., & Kahan, M. (2011). Substance use in pregnancy. *Journal of Obstetrics & Gynaecology Canada, 33*(4), 367–384. Retrieved from https://www.jogc.com/article/S1701-2163(16)34855-1/pdf.

in microcephaly, developmental delay, cleft lip and palate, and congenital heart disease. Barbiturates, such as phenobarbital, may cause newborn addiction. Women with seizure disorders should discuss their medication requirements with their physicians before becoming pregnant and have close health care team monitoring throughout pregnancy.

### Over-the-Counter Medications

Pregnant women frequently choose to treat minor illnesses with OTC medications. Research on acetylsalicylic acid (aspirin) and acetaminophen (Tylenol) indicates that both medications are safe in the recommended dosages. However, aspirin alters platelet function and may cause maternal and newborn bleeding if taken close to delivery. Acetaminophen can be toxic to the liver. Certain ingredients in common cold remedies have been associated with fetal irritability (King & Brucker, 2016). Ibuprofen has been known to prolong labour on the basis of its antiprostaglandin effect. Any medication may harm a fetus, so all should be avoided during pregnancy unless prescribed by the health care provider.

The nurse includes information on the known and probable effects of medications on the fetus in prenatal teaching of couples. Discussion of herbal treatments is included, because

little research exists on their effects and interactions with OTC and prescribed medications. The nurse recognizes that many cultural groups use these nontraditional medications because they believe that they will effectively manage pregnancy-related concerns. The nurse may need to encourage an individual to reconsider the use of herbs when evidence exists that these may harm the fetus or mother.

### Drug Abuse

Given the prevalence of drug use and abuse in our society, it is imperative that nurses be able to recognize, manage, and refer as appropriate substance abuse problems for their care recipients. Substance abuse during pregnancy poses a significant risk because all substances consumed by the mother pass freely through the placenta, and thus the fetus as well as the mother experiences substance use, abuse, and addiction. All pregnant women and women of childbearing age should be screened periodically for alcohol, tobacco, and prescription and illicit drug use.

Maternal use of narcotics, tranquillizers, cocaine, amphetamines, marijuana, and other drugs may cause serious health problems to both the mother and the unborn child. These drugs represent an enormous cost to society by causing increased risks of low-birth-weight infants and preterm infants, as well as deficits in child development, if the mother ingests them during pregnancy (Foray & Foster, 2015).

*Narcotics.* Long-term narcotic use during pregnancy is increasing in prevalence. Signs of narcotic withdrawal in the newborn include tremors, irritability, hyperactivity, vomiting, diarrhea, sweating, poor feeding, and possibly convulsions. No evidence suggests withdrawal in infants whose mothers used cocaine or amphetamines, although there is an increased risk of preterm births, neonatal irritability, placental abruption, premature rupture of membranes, and fetal distress (Kremer & Arora, 2015). Frequent maternal marijuana use during pregnancy may cause fetal immunological problems, but evidence conflicts with an unclear impact. Current research has shown that some infants born to women who used marijuana during their pregnancies display altered responses to visual stimuli, increased tremulousness, and a high-pitched cry, which could indicate problems with neurological development (Foray & Foster, 2015). With Canada's legalization of marijuana in October 2017, there may be additional implications for mothers and their infants (Public Health Ontario, 2018). To avoid these problems, nurses must recognize women who abuse drugs and assist them in seeking appropriate help. This task may be difficult because drug abusers often try to hide their habit, fear being reported to the police, and may be unable to change their lifestyle without extensive intervention.

Drug and substance misuse is a serious public health issue in Canada, especially among women of childbearing age. The problem of drug abuse during pregnancy has affected women in all communities, races, and cultures and of all ages and socioeconomic levels. As a result, many infants are born exposed to illicit substances in utero, are addicted, and develop the complex disorder known as neonatal abstinence syndrome. This is a drug withdrawal syndrome that most commonly occurs after an in utero exposure to addictive prescriptive or illicit drugs, such as opioids, which has been increasing in prevalence during the last decade (McQueen & Murphy-Oikonen, 2016). Infants with neonatal abstinence syndrome have prolonged hospital stays; they experience serious medical complications and their treatment is very costly. Any prenatal substance abuse can have lifelong consequences for the newborn.

For early identification of newborns needing interventions, the nurse should observe newborns with a history of maternal drug abuse for the following: hyperactivity, shrill cry, muscle tension, tremors, seizures, sneezing, yawning, restless sleep, disorganized suck, vomiting, diarrhea, poor feeding, tachypnea, scratches on face, flushing, and sweating. Supporting care for these infants with neonatal abstinence syndrome includes placing them in a quiet area with dim lights, using a tight swaddling position on the side or back, using calming techniques and rocking, clustering infant-care activities with gentle handling, encouraging non-nutritive sucking, providing small, frequent feedings, and administering pharmacological medications as ordered to control withdrawal symptoms.

Nurses need to possess knowledge in the area of chemical dependency, as many women continue to consume nonprescribed medications during pregnancy. Additionally, knowledge of how to recognize symptoms of withdrawal in infants during the immediate newborn period can lead to improved outcomes if they are treated appropriately during their withdrawal period. Nurses can also help children learn about the negative effects of consuming alcohol and other illicit drugs, especially during pregnancy. By understanding child development and appropriate strategies for teaching children, nurses can play an important role in the prevention of alcohol and illicit drug use among women during pregnancy.

*Alcohol.* Alcohol is the most widely used recreational substance worldwide. Many women in today's society drink alcohol regularly. Research has demonstrated that alcohol is a teratogen—a substance that can cause abnormal development in a growing fetus—as it crosses the placenta readily. Recognition of the effects that even low levels of prenatal alcohol exposure can have on the physical and cognitive development of a child led to the coining of the umbrella term fetal alcohol spectrum disorder (FASD). Fetal exposure to alcohol throughout pregnancy may cause fetal alcohol syndrome (FAS) or FASD, a collection of symptoms including intrauterine growth restriction (IUGR), increased risk of facial anomalies, structural brain abnormalities, mental health problems, attention-deficit/hyperactivity disorder, and developmental delays. It is clinically proven that alcohol consumption during all stages of pregnancy puts the fetus at risk of being born with lifelong alcohol-related brain damage (Jarmasz, Basalah, Chudley, et al., 2017). Recent studies have reported symptoms of fetal alcohol disorder in children whose mothers may have consumed just a couple of drinks a day at certain stages of pregnancy. Numerous studies have shown that no safe level of alcohol use exists during pregnancy; therefore, alcohol consumption should be avoided during this time and when conception is being attempted. The consequences of prenatal alcohol exposure are often grave, inhibiting both physical and intellectual development, societal acceptance, and adult success. The evidence is clear—alcohol can be more damaging to the developing fetus than heroin, cocaine, or any other drug, producing by far the most serious neuro-behavioural effects in the fetus. Prenatal alcohol exposure is the leading preventable cause of intellectual disability in Canada. In Canada, 9 in 1000 babies are diagnosed with FASD (Government of Canada, 2017). During prenatal appointments, the nurse may utilize the T-ACE screening tool to help identify a woman's risk of alcohol abuse during pregnancy (Chang, Fisher, Hornstein, et al., 2010). Overdrinking during pregnancy is defined as having more than seven alcoholic beverages per week, and more than three on one occasion. By utilizing this screening tool, nurses can better plan health teaching and make referrals to supportive community services. Nurses can support population health by raising awareness of the risks of drinking during pregnancy and support abstinence from teratogenic substances. By raising awareness, the nurse supports future generations by fostering a healthy start in life.

*Nicotine.* In Canada, it is estimated that approximately 16% of pregnant women smoke during their pregnancies. Carbon monoxide and nicotine from tobacco smoke may interfere with the oxygen supply to the fetus. Nicotine also readily crosses the placenta, and concentrations in the fetus can be as much as 15%

higher than maternal levels. Nicotine concentrates in fetal blood, amniotic fluid, and breast milk. Combined, these factors can have severe consequences for the fetuses and infants of mothers who smoke (Foray & Foster, 2015). The Centre for Addiction and Mental Health (CAMH) recommends that clinicians ask all pregnant women about tobacco use and provide an augmented, pregnancy-tailored counselling framework for engaging women in smoking cessation discussions (CAMH, 2010):

- Ask the woman about tobacco use.
- Advise the woman to quit through clear, personalized messages.
- Assess the woman's willingness to quit.
- Assist the woman to quit.
- Arrange follow-up and support.

Evidence indicates that maternal smoking causes increased rates of spontaneous abortion and ectopic pregnancy, decreased fertility, fetal growth restriction, increased numbers of low-birth-weight or preterm infants, placental abnormalities, vaginal bleeding, congenital anomalies, perinatal death, and premature rupture of the membranes (Banderali, Martelli, Landi, et al., 2015). The best advice for pregnant mothers or women considering pregnancy is to cease all use of tobacco products, decreasing smoking if the woman is a heavy smoker, and avoiding places where smoking occurs. The Prevention of Gestational and Neonatal Exposure to Tobacco Smoke (PREGNETS) is a network that offers resources to both health care providers and pregnant and postpartum women using tobacco (Nicotine Dependence Clinic, 2019). The website's resources include self-help tips for smoking cessation, frequently asked questions, and informational pamphlets. The nurse should also understand the context of smoking in a woman's life and the complexity of her choice to quit smoking, so as to propose solutions to decrease fetal exposure to nicotine (Research for Evidence-Informed Practice).

*Caffeine.* Caffeine is a widely consumed psychoactive substance. It is a stimulant found in tea, coffee, cola, chocolate, and some OTC medications. Caffeine is an addictive substance. Gene mutations have been found in laboratory animals exposed to moderate amounts of caffeine; however, these defects have not been found in human beings. One study found an association between excess caffeine intake (>300 mg daily) and a higher risk of low-birth-weight infants (James, 2015). Until additional research clarifies the relationship between caffeine intake and fetal effects, nurses should teach pregnant women to avoid excess caffeine intake.

## ◆ Chemical Agents

The influence of chemicals on human development remains unclear. Some natural substances found to be teratogenic in animals, but not necessarily in human beings, include insect and bacterial toxins, insecticides, herbicides, and fungicides, including dichlorodiphenyltrichloroethane (DDT). Fish is a source of several nutrients that are important during pregnancy for healthy fetal development, including iodine, omega-3 polyunsaturated fatty acids, and vitamins A, D, and $B_{12}$. Recent studies involving pregnant women who eat large amounts of fish with high mercury levels (shark, swordfish, king mackerel, canned tuna, or tilefish) support evidence that mercury negatively affects fetal development, particularly brain development, and may be associated with preterm labour (Starling, Charlton, McMahon, et al., 2015). Women can safely eat up to 12 ounces of cooked fish weekly. Some studies report stillbirths, abortions, preterm births, and developmental delays in fetuses exposed to lead. This area needs more study, particularly with more women working in traditional male workplaces where there are environmental contaminants. Nurses assess and provide women in their first trimester with information on environmental agents

## ⚡ RESEARCH FOR EVIDENCE-INFORMED PRACTICE

### Nicotine Replacement Therapy in Pregnancy

Maternal tobacco smoking during pregnancy is the most significant preventable cause of poor health outcomes for women and their babies, with morbidity resulting from placental abruption, miscarriage, stillbirth, prematurity, low birth weight, neonatal or sudden infant death, and asthma. Frequently, clinicians use nicotine replacement therapy (NRT) in attempts to help pregnant smokers stop smoking. However, although NRT is an effective smoking cessation treatment for nonpregnant smokers, its efficacy and safety in pregnancy have not been demonstrated adequately.

The purpose of this study was to determine the efficacy and safety of NRT with or without behavioural support when used to support smoking cessation in pregnancy.

*Design, setting, and participants.* In a systematic review of randomized controlled trials in which NRT was used with or without behavioural support to promote smoking cessation, trials providing unequal behavioural support to different trial groups were excluded. Included were randomized controlled trials with designs that permitted independent effects of any type of NRT (e.g., patch, gum) for smoking cessation to be isolated. Five trials were identified that met the criteria, giving a total of 525 enrolled pregnant smokers.

*Findings.* There is currently some evidence to demonstrate that NRT used by pregnant women for smoking cessation is either effective or safe for long-term use. Although birth outcomes were generally better among those infants born to women who had used NRT, none of the observed differences reached statistical significance. By ensuring that the only difference between the arms of the included trials was the provision of NRT to all participants, the independent effects of NRT that are of most importance to clinicians were isolated. Clinical guidelines assume that when pregnant women are heavily dependent on nicotine, use of NRT will be less harmful to them and their babies than continued smoking; however, these findings have not produced evidence for this assumption. Additional studies are needed to determine the safety and efficiency of NRT.

*Nursing implications.* In the absence of sufficient evidence for either the effectiveness or the safety or long-term use of NRT in pregnancy, nurses should perhaps emphasize the importance of the use of proven, behavioural strategies to promote smoking cessation in pregnancy to ensure optimal outcomes.

Sources: Dhalwani, N. N., Szatkowski, L., Coleman, T., et al. (2015). Nicotine replacement therapy in pregnancy and major congenital anomalies in offspring. *Pediatrics, 135*(5), 859–867. doi:10.1542/peds.2014-2560; Prochaska, J. J. (2015). Nicotine replacement therapy as a maintenance treatment. *JAMA, 314*(7), 718–719. doi:10.1001/jama.2015.7460.

that are potentially damaging throughout gestation and counsel them on ways to avoid exposure.

### Medications Given During Childbirth

The final time that the fetus encounters medications through the mother is during the birthing process. Many women desire medications for labour discomforts, and usually only medications deemed safe and monitored closely during labour and birth have been used (e.g., epidural anaesthetics, opiate agonists in small doses). Some analgesic medications administered during labour can cause neonatal sedation and respiratory depression and can influence the rate and quality of the infant's adaptation to extrauterine life. Studies of visual attentiveness and sucking behaviour, as well as neurological tests and electroencephalography, suggest that fetal depressant effects may last as long as days after birth (Halpern & Garg, 2015).

### Mechanical Forces

The amniotic fluid reservoir protects the fetus during pregnancy and during mild to moderate trauma to the mother's abdomen. However, major trauma to the mother's abdomen, such as that sustained in a severe car accident, may cause maternal bleeding, preterm labour, and other concerns. The nurse instructs the pregnant woman in the proper way to wear both a lap belt and a shoulder harness to protect her and her fetus while driving. All women in the second and third trimesters should be encouraged to seek medical care following an accident believed to influence the health of mother or fetus.

The uterus, another mechanical force, also influences the fetus. Near the end of pregnancy, the fetus outgrows the uterus and becomes moulded by it, particularly in cases of multiple pregnancy. Some children have congenitally dislocated hips from uterine pressure and fetal position in utero. Most deformities resolve either naturally or with repositioning after birth. Fetal malposition cannot be prevented; therefore, the neonate is assessed for problems and support is provided to the parents about the newborn's appearance.

The actual labour and birth process represents the final mechanical force. Few newborns experience injury during this process, and those who do usually recover with limited effect. It is difficult to predict and prevent birth traumas, such as when delivery of an infant who is larger than expected requires vacuum extraction, which may injure the child. In these cases, on the basis of health care team assessment, the mother may undergo Caesarean section to protect herself and the baby.

### Radiation

Radiation exposure during pregnancy has been debated for years, but various experiences are continuing to show that there are increasingly negative effects on the growing fetus, as well as effects later in life. Scientific evidence indicates that exposure to X-rays, especially early in pregnancy during organogenesis, may cause chromosomal changes, spontaneous abortion, growth restriction, microcephaly, fetal loss, or malignancy later in life (Abdalla & Elshikh, 2015). The fetus is most sensitive to radiation effects between 8 and 15 weeks of pregnancy, and thus should be spared any radiation exposure during that period (Gök, Bozkurt,

Guneyli, et al., 2015). The literature supports a greater incidence of leukemia in children of women exposed to X-rays during pregnancy compared with children whose mothers were not exposed. Unless the benefits of radiographic information clearly outweigh the risks of exposing the fetus to X-rays, these examinations should not be performed during gestation. If radiography is deemed necessary, the wearing of a lead apron, use of as low a radiation dose as possible, and application of other recommendations made by the US National Council on Radiation Protection and Measurements should be used to protect the developing fetus.

## ❖ DETERMINANTS OF HEALTH

### ◆ Social Factors and Environment
#### Community and Work

More women now work outside the home, either in careers or in jobs needed for family economic survival. As each woman considers or experiences pregnancy, she will need to ask herself questions that will optimize her pregnancy outcome. These questions include the following: Is my work strenuous or possibly dangerous to my baby because of exposure to toxic substances? Do I need to work for long periods, influencing my need for rest? Will workplace stressors influence my coping with pregnancy and my family needs?

A safe workplace environment (one that does not involve exposure to hazardous substances or organisms and provides adequate breaks for worker rest and body movement) will allow a pregnant woman to work until her baby is due, unless her health becomes impaired. The nurse helps each woman assess the safety of her workplace and suggests ways to decrease hazards in that setting. These hazards include exposure to viruses, fungi, industrial products (hydrocarbons or pesticides), second-hand smoke, radiation emitted by medical diagnostic equipment, air pollutants, and asbestos, and the possibility of workplace violence, mental and physical stress, and even noise pollution. The nurse encourages the pregnant worker to consider workplace ergonomics, addressing how the current work space will meet her changing physical needs.

Some employers in Canada have been designated creators of "family friendly" work environments, because they have willingly made accommodations to support breastfeeding and pregnant workers and their families. These accommodations allow women to prioritize their pregnancy and family needs. Evidence indicates that such approaches reduce pregnancy complications and increase work productivity. Although few in number, family friendly employers offer health-promotion programs focusing on healthy nutrition, stress management, and exercise for employees, who experience better health outcomes.

As a rule, however, too few employers support flexible work schedules for prenatal care visits, rest periods for pregnant workers, or removal of vending machines to support optimal nutrition for pregnant working class women. Some working women, regardless of status, believe that once they announce their pregnancy, they will face workplace pressure to stop working or change positions in the company to suit their gestational needs. On the basis of experience, some employers fear that their pregnant employees will overuse sick time or seek a reduced workload.

In a recent study of pregnancy within the workplace, two factors were identified that may be challenging. In many workplaces, pressures on women to "ignore" pregnancy and to "push on" through sickness and exhaustion may relate to certain workplace cultures referred to as "male norms." The partiality for male norms could be seen as creating problems for these pregnant women, who feel obliged to downplay their "inherent femaleness" by minimizing their pregnancy so as to fit in with workplace notions of reliability and presence.

Secondly, health advice on pregnancy might also be difficult to implement within women's workplaces because of underlying assumptions, reflected in health advice, that women's care is most appropriately performed in the home. It is significant that health guidance on pregnancy care work makes little reference to place and offers slender guidance on how pregnancy care work might be implemented at work. Common sense suggests that instructions about napping during the day and using ice packs to relieve hemorrhoids would be entirely inappropriate within most workplaces, whatever the occupation of the pregnant woman (Fox & Quinn, 2015).

Research suggests that pregnant women are discriminated against in the workplace and that a significant number of new mothers leave the workforce. The pregnant woman must deal with these situations by being factual and assertive about her ability to continue working. National law dictates that it is illegal to discriminate against a woman because she is pregnant. If a woman believes that she has been treated unfairly because of her pregnancy, she may pursue the issue legally or become active in local women's rights organizations to gain support. However, when a woman leaves a job that did not support her pregnancy, she often gives up accrued leave time or takes a lower salary in another job. These outcomes influence her choices during pregnancy and early parenting.

Workplaces differ greatly in allowing leave time during and after pregnancy. Federal legislation, the *Employment Standards Act*, entitles new parents 61 to 63 weeks of paid leave and up to 17 weeks of paid leave for women who have medical problems during pregnancy (Ontario Ministry of Labour, 2019). Ideally, a woman who desires children should explore the issue of leave during a job interview, but many women fail to do this until they are already pregnant. A woman often requires written verification from her physician if she needs a leave of absence from her job attributable to pregnancy complications. Although she may wish to return to work shortly after giving birth, due to financial reasons, the woman is counselled to allow sufficient time to regain her strength and adapt to parenting. The nurse may help the couple make reasonable decisions related to locating resources for child care, exploring "shared time" with other new mothers or part-time employees (e.g., middle-age adults caring for their older parents), or finding ways of balancing work and family needs. Although some women may return to work early, the majority of Canadian women take maternity leave for 12 to 18 months following birth.

## Culture and Ethnicity

With the increasing diversity in Canadian populations, nurses are challenged to develop culturally competent skills that meet the social, cultural, and linguistic needs of those for whom they care. Cultural competence is not static and requires frequent relearning and unlearning about diversity. Nurses must acknowledge the implications of their own "cultural lens" and continuously reflect on their own assumptions, biases, and stereotypes. Nurses must adopt an attitude of open-mindedness and respect for all cultures. Cultural groups have unique ideas and beliefs related to pregnancy, childbirth, and childbearing that must be understood by the nurse so as to render individualized care to each pregnant woman.

Nonconscious stereotyping and prejudice contribute to racial and ethnic disparities in health care. Contemporary training in cultural competence and cultural safety is insufficient to reduce these problems because even educated, culturally sensitive nurses can activate and use their biases without being aware they are doing so. Research in social psychology shows that, over time, stereotypes and prejudices become invisible to those who rely on them. Automatic categorization of an individual as a member of a social group can unconsciously trigger the thoughts (stereotypes) and feelings (prejudices) associated with that group. This implies that, when activated, implicit negative attitudes and stereotypes shape how nurses evaluate and interact with minority groups. This makes minority group care recipients uncomfortable and discourages them from seeking or adhering to treatment (Tucker, Arthur, Roncoroni, et al., 2015).

Nurses need to be very cognizant of their stereotyping and prejudices and "park them at the door-stop" before interacting with minority women. Have nurses ever thought about why pregnant women do not seek prenatal care or do not return for follow-up care once they have encountered a negative reception? If nurses would reverse roles with minority women and just imagine how it feels to encounter negative attitudes when needing health care, perhaps biased attitudes would change dramatically (Canadian Nurses Association [CNA], 2019).

Nurses need an awareness of how culture, tradition, and acculturation may affect the women for whom they provide care, as this is the first step toward understanding diverse cultural behaviour. The next step is for nurses to be aware of the three "levels" of culture when offering health advice and planning health care for various diverse groups:

- The *primary* level of culture refers to rules that are known by all and obeyed by all and may be almost unconsciously performed by women (e.g., health, healing, and health-belief systems, or how illness, diseases, and their causes are perceived by that specific culture).
- The *secondary* level is the underlying rules and guidelines known by the group but not generally relayed to outsiders. This may include taboos and rituals relating to behaviour, which may be followed depending on the individual.
- A *tertiary* level is visible to the outsider, such as traditional dress, foods, and religious ceremonies (Darnell & Hickson, 2015).

Intercultural caring by nurses is complex. However, nurses need to have a positive attitude and demonstrate acceptance of different cultures. This can be achieved by nurses taking the stance of respecting and understanding diversity, as well as acknowledging any barriers such as culture. Nursing support may assist the individual in adjusting both her needs and those of the culture she represents to experience a satisfactory pregnancy.

The nurse has an obligation to read about and seek information on cultures encountered in practice and to become active in community organizations that represent cultures whose members get prenatal care from the nurse. Above all, the nurse must be open to a variety of viewpoints, judging them not against personal beliefs but rather in relation to the general concept of health promotion and today's goal to provide culturally competent care to a variety of cultural groups. All nurses want to deliver care that is inclusive—that is, sensitive to the care seeker's and the family's needs—and that respects the values of their health beliefs and practices. To do this, nurses need to learn about the most common minority cultures with which they interact (Diversity Awareness).

## ◆ Levels of Policy Making and Health

Both legislative actions and social movements influence childbearing. In some countries, such as China, the government decrees the number of children a couple may have and imposes economic or social sanctions to enforce these restrictions. Although Canadians may have as many children as they desire, various coalitions lobby strongly for families. The *Canadian Labour Code* validates the federal government's commitment to prioritizing family issues by giving new parents time off from work during the early months of parenthood, while supporting these individuals' professional work goals and needs (Government of Canada, 2019b).

The Canadian government remains concerned about the health of pregnant women and ways to decrease fetal and infant morbidity and mortality. Many countries provide universal access to prenatal care and some provinces have health departments and community health centres offering free or low-cost prenatal services. These prenatal services are especially beneficial for women who are pregnant and newcomers to Canada, or for women who do not have a provincial health insurance plan number (Ontario Council of Agencies Serving Immigrants, 2017; Ontario Ministry of Children, Community and Social Services, 2019). Fortunately, in some provinces such as Ontario, newcomers are not required to have provincial insurance coverage to access midwifery support. Many ethnically diverse populations, in particular Indigenous people in Canada, may lack a level of education that supports understanding of health-related information (low health literacy) for family health promotion (Crengle, Luke, Lambert, et al., 2018). Educating women during the childbearing cycle is particularly important to increase the chances of families obtaining and understanding health-promotion information for healthier behaviours (First Nations Health Authority, 2019).

With the nurse's help in data collection, consumers should be encouraged to express their views and opinions on pregnancy and parenting topics to their elected governmental representatives. Over the past two decades in Canada, the average

## 🌐 DIVERSITY AWARENESS

### *Nursing Roles in Providing Culturally Competent Care*

In recent years, greater emphasis has been placed on nurses recognizing and appreciating diversity so as to acquire cultural competency. Cultural competency is the ability of nurses to reflect their awareness of a group's values, beliefs, customs and norms when developing care plans for their patients (Cope, 2015). Cultural knowledge is the most important construct of cultural competence for nurses, being crucial for the accurate appreciation of a care recipient's worldview. Delivery of culturally competent care implies that a nurse acknowledges and acts on the unique history that a pregnant woman and her family bring to a health care interaction. The essence of both the patient-centredness and competence for the nurse is the importance of seeing the woman as a unique individual. The nurse supports culturally competent care by:

- Recognizing that cultural diversity exists and affects the process and outcome of health care
- Respecting people as unique individuals who, by their differences from the majority, bring a broadened definition of appropriate health care
- Using data gained from a cultural assessment for completion of a care plan
- Encouraging cultural behaviour that protects the biopsychosocial, spiritual, and safety needs of the individual
- Gaining insight into the nurse's own beliefs and values about people who may be different from or have needs different from those of the majority or those of the nurse's own culture; understanding how these beliefs and values influence the outcomes of health care delivery with childbearing families
- Recognizing the values of the health care system reflected in the customs and practices of birthing facilities
- Providing interpreters to improve communication between the individual and health care providers
- Becoming literate in languages, customs, and cultural practices of people commonly seen in the health care environment
- Developing cultural humility by maintaining an interpersonal stance as it relates to the other person from a different culture
- Recognizing and valuing the diversity of those seeking care and entering all therapeutic relationships acknowledging that nurses are always in the process of learning and growing

#### Reflective Questions

- How do you support culturally competent care in terms of a male physician performing a pelvic exam on a Middle Eastern woman?
- What must a nurse consider when providing culturally competent prenatal care to an Indigenous woman?

Sources: Foronda, C. L., Baptiste, D., Reinholdt, M. M., et al. (2016). Cultural humility: A concept analysis. *Journal of Transcultural Nursing*, *27*(3), 210–217. doi:10.1177/104365915592677; Garneau, A. B. (2016). Critical reflection in cultural competence development: A framework for undergraduate nursing education. *Journal of Nursing Education*, *55*(3), 125–132. doi:10.3928/01484834-20160216-02.

hospital stay postpartum has decreased from 5 days to an average of 2–3 days, due to the increasing cost of obstetrical care (Canadian Institute for Health Information, 2006; Lemyre, Jefferies, & O'Flaherty, et al., 2018). The length of a woman's stay may be lengthened by 12–24 hours, depending on complications present that are related to the delivery method (vaginal or Caesarean), abnormal laboratory test results for mother or baby, or an unanticipated NICU (neonatal intensive care unit) admission. Despite the cost of care, longer hospital stays have been proven to help health care providers identify potential problems in the mother or the baby before discharge, such as difficulty breastfeeding (Benitz, 2015).

## Economics

When the pregnant woman begins prenatal care, personal financial resources influence the kind of care she receives, the need to remain employed during or after a pregnancy, the acceptance of her pregnancy, her nutritional status, and other choices. The expenses of planning and experiencing a pregnancy may determine whether the woman or her family faces a financial crisis. The nurse needs to understand the financial history and priorities of the couple because this information will affect access to and use of prenatal care.

The nurse inquires in a sensitive fashion about a woman's or a couple's finances to make appropriate referral to resources for care (e.g., social assistance or disability programs). The Canadian Prenatal Nutrition Program (CPNP) provides nutrition counselling, food vouchers, prenatal vitamins, and breastfeeding support to vulnerable pregnant women across Canada (PHAC, 2015). Patients who are struggling with poverty, are adolescent mothers, are using substances, or are experiencing social isolation, are all eligible to access the CPNP. During prenatal visits, the nurse may help a woman or family plan a budget for food and other essential requirements based on individual family needs, cultural values, the need for a healthy diet during pregnancy, and income level. Local food banks and second-hand clothing and baby supply stores may provide needed items for these families. Occasionally, women may access free transportation and child care at the prenatal clinic if the nurse provides information about this program.

## ◆ Health Services/Delivery System

Options for care during pregnancy range from medical-based care by a health care provider to more health-promotion–focused care by a nurse practitioner or midwife. In Canada, 10.8% of all Canadian births were supported by midwives (Canadian Association of Midwives, 2018a). Midwives have a long tradition that includes watchful waiting, sharing empirical knowledge, protecting the normal, nonmedicalized birth process, and engaging in research to incorporate the findings into evidence-informed practice. Midwifery is distinguished by characteristics that define a partnership with women by listening, being sensitive to cultural, sexual, and generational needs, encouraging shared decision making, and practicing patience to be "with women" during their most vulnerable periods (King et al., 2015).

In Canada, registered midwives provide support to women in their early stages of pregnancy up until 6 weeks postpartum (Canadian Midwifery Regulators Council [CMRC], 2019). They provide the pregnant woman the opportunity to decide if she would like to labour and deliver her child at home or at the hospital. Postpartum, midwives attend in-home and in-office visits with their patients and will provide 24/7 support to the new family. Several national organizations provide oversight for practicing midwives. The CMRC is the professional group of authorities that regulate registered midwives in Canada, and the College of Midwives (COM) is the membership organization responsible for setting the standards in midwifery education and practice (CAM, 2018b). The CAM believes that midwifery care should be available to all Canadians, regardless of ethnic background or socioeconomic status. They also recognize the National Aboriginal Council of Midwives as the representative for Indigenous midwifery care in Canada.

A pregnant woman may prefer the support of a doula during her pregnancy and postpartum. A doula is a certified professional who provides non-medical support to women during their pregnancy and postpartum (Association of Ontario Doulas, 2019). A doula can support with comforting the woman during labour and delivery, support the initiation of breastfeeding and make referrals to other health care providers or services in the community as needed. Geographical availability of options, finances, previous experience, partner's preference, cultural or social acceptability of certain options, and pre-existing or newly recognized risk factors will influence a woman's choice of care. Because of her culture and the belief that pregnancy is not an illness, a woman may not seek Western medical prenatal care, but rather may rely on individuals from her culture to provide care until the actual labour, when she will go to a hospital.

Unless complications arise, a woman generally chooses where she will labour and give birth and the extent of labour and birthing process intervention. The movement toward home birth that began during the early 1970s continues to meet some women's needs for a more family-oriented, natural, health-focused experience. However, most couples choose a hospital birth setting because of the availability of emergency equipment and personnel in the case of complications. The nurse helps expectant couples become aware of the care and birthing alternatives to make an informed choice for a positive labour and birth experience. Women who lack resources to access the health care delivery system and teaching by the nurse during regular prenatal visits are generally less able to make informed decisions that affect their childbearing experiences.

Many expectant couples also make an informed choice about the actual process of labour and birth by developing a birth plan—those components of care and intervention that the couple desires for the birth experience. A birth plan can include selecting the delivery location, pain relief options, delivery positions, and preferred postpartum feeding method (Solchany, 2013). A pregnant woman and her partner may choose natural childbirth or a method of analgesia or anaesthesia. The nurse helps the pregnant woman and her partner choose the most appropriate method by providing information about options and encouraging questions about each option. Collaboration between the nurse and the woman or couple in meeting their birth plan goals is important because research shows that women remember their labour and birthing experiences for a long time. A positively viewed birth experience may support a couple's involvement as active health care consumers, thus facilitating the future health of their family.

The nurse may encourage the pregnant couple or woman to attend prenatal classes. These provide valuable information and preparation for birth for many couples. The International Childbirth Education Association and many local groups offer a variety of classes for the expectant couple. These classes may include information on how to have a healthy pregnancy, birthing positions, Caesarean birth, breastfeeding, postpartum care, and newborn care (SOGC, 2019c). Involvement of older children in the birth experience may also increase sibling bonding.

## ❖ NURSING APPLICATION

Teaching the pregnant woman and her partner during the prenatal period is the most important role of the nurse. Even the woman who has previously given birth or who has a high degree of education may need or want information from the health care team that will assist her family to adapt effectively to changes of pregnancy to support a healthy birth outcome.

To provide appropriate teaching, the nurse performs a comprehensive assessment that involves the entire family. Assessment, the first step in the nursing process, allows the nurse to determine maternal and fetal physical and psychological risks, the woman's informational base for pregnancy and birth, and cultural and family needs. Assessment should also include physical, spiritual, emotional, and sociocultural inspection and recognition of abuse. Battering increases during pregnancy and may be detected by physical, emotional, behavioural, and history assessment of the woman. Pregnant women at high risk of abuse include adolescents, those with low incomes, and those with a history of alcohol or drug abuse, as well as those with a partner with a similar history (Bohra, Sharma, Srivastava, et al., 2015; Copelon, 2004). In cases of suspected abuse, the nurse, in consultation with other members of the health care team, provides support and resources for the woman to make an informed decision about protecting herself and her fetus during pregnancy. The nurse may also want to refer the woman to a professional counsellor for a brief counselling outreach intervention or abuse shelter for personal safety (Jewkes & Penn-Kekana, 2015).

As discussed in this chapter, assessment may also be made by use of Gordon's (2016) functional health patterns, a common conceptual framework for clinical assessment (see Box 10.3). Data used in the assessment process will likely be collected during the prenatal visit and may change, depending on life occurrences of the pregnant woman. A woman may be defined as high risk during her pregnancy if she experiences heavy bleeding, premature labour, elevated blood pressure, or extreme anxiety; if there is fetal distress; or if the woman shows unexpected behaviour or symptoms. After noting these high-risk conditions, the nurse should refer the pregnant woman to an obstetrical specialist or other resources for pregnant women and their families (see the Case Study at the end of this chapter).

After a complete assessment during each prenatal visit, the nurse develops a teaching plan for the individual. Throughout the prenatal course, the nurse collaborates with the woman and her partner to assess their learning and support needs. For example, literature on bottle feeding or breastfeeding may be provided to help a woman decide on a method, and books, videos, and websites may help couples understand more about birth, and therefore feel that they have more control during labour and in meeting their birthing goals. If the woman plans to attend group prenatal classes, the nurse should coordinate her teaching content and process with those expected in the classes, thereby preventing undue repetition. The nurse teaching prenatal classes should also provide a list of topics to participants in the class to share with their health care providers. A woman may be knowledgeable in some areas, and the nurse can use this knowledge as a foundation for further individualized teaching. Box 10.5 covers relevant topics to be covered by the nurse during prenatal care interactions with pregnant women (CFPC, 2014a). These topical areas relate to nursing interventions discussed earlier in this chapter. Basic handouts detailing danger signs of pregnancy can be posted in the home to consult if the woman experiences unexpected complications of pregnancy.

---

### BOX 10.5    Topics for Prenatal Care Teaching

- Rationale for and interpretation of physical findings and laboratory results
- Value of keeping appointments
- Danger signs that should be reported
- Breast care to prepare for lactation
- Breastfeeding versus bottle feeding
- Exercise and rest
- Fetal growth and development
- Physical and psychological changes during pregnancy and relief measures
- Effects of smoking, drinking, and drugs on the fetus
- Nutrition
- Work and play
- Body mechanics
- Personal hygiene
- Sex during pregnancy
- Preparation for labour and birth
- Superstitions and old wives' tales
- Signs of impending labour
- Supplies and preparations for the baby
- Partner's and siblings' responses

## CASE STUDY

### Active Labour: Susan Wong

Mrs. Wong, a first-time mother, is admitted to the birthing suite in early labour after spontaneous rupture of membranes at home. She is at 38 weeks of gestation with a history of abnormal alpha-fetoprotein levels at 16 weeks of pregnancy. She was scheduled for ultrasonography to visualize the fetus to rule out an open spinal defect or Down syndrome, but never followed through. Mrs. Wong and her husband disagreed about what to do (keep or terminate the pregnancy) if the ultrasonography indicated a spinal problem, so they felt they did not want this information.

#### Reflective Questions

- As the nurse, what priority data would you collect from this couple to help define relevant interventions to meet their needs?
- How can you help this couple if they experience a negative outcome in the birthing suite? What are your personal views on terminating or continuing a pregnancy with a risk of a potential anomaly? What factors may influence your views?
- With the influence of the recent Human Genome Project and the possibility of predicting open spinal defects earlier in pregnancy, how will maternity care change in the future?

#### Prediction of Human Disease

An organism's complete set of DNA is called its genome. Virtually every single cell in the body contains a complete copy of the approximately 3 billion DNA base pairs, or letters, that make up the human genome. The Human Genome Project (completed in 2003), conducted by the National Human Genome Research Institute, produced a very high-quality version of the human genome sequence that is freely available in public databases. Researchers have been able to use DNA sequencing to search for genetic variations and/or mutations that may play a role in the development or progression of a range of diseases. Clearly, there are implications and ethical considerations for the health sciences here. Along with the important information uncovered by the Human Genome Project, a great controversy arose. Even though blood tests are now available for the detection of various fatal diseases such as Huntington's disease, cystic fibrosis, and colon cancer, many people would rather live with uncertainty than know they have an incurable life-threatening disease. Sadly, the tests, which have been developed, are to detect the disease and not cure it.

Another consideration is the use of genetic information by existing and prospective employers. Imagine a situation where employment preference is given to those who can demonstrate they are "genetically free" of future diseases that might limit their capacity to work. Still, three major unsolved problems in perinatal and neonatal health are preterm birth; the neonatal consequences of vaginal versus Caesarean birth; and neonatal gastrointestinal disease, specifically necrotizing enterocolitis. Hopefully, soon, the Human Genome Project's research will be able to address all three problems and improve pregnancy outcomes.

In just one decade, the Human Genome Project has sparked an explosion of information that has proved useful to basic and clinical scientists. We must remain cautious as to how and when this new information and technology are used in the future to ensure they are used for the betterment of humankind.

## CARE PLAN

### Nursing Management for Stages of Labour: Susan Wong

**Nursing Issue**
Inadequate coping as a result of active labour status

**Defining Characteristics**
- Initiation of labour at 2:00 a.m. with spontaneous rupture of membranes
- First-time mother who did not attend childbirth classes
- Supportive spouse
- Current gestational age of 38 weeks
- Contraction pattern defined as moderate intensity, frequency every 2 minutes, 60 seconds in duration
- After 6 hours of labour, 4 cm dilated, 100% effaced, and stage active phase
- Moaning, moving around in bed, and stating, "I can't take this much longer; it hurts too much!"

**Related Factors**
- Prenatal history of abnormal alpha-fetoprotein levels at 16 weeks
- Prenatal care since 12 weeks pregnant
- History of depression while in university
- Works as an engineer with large manufacturing firm
- Gravida 1, parity 0
- Recent resident of city; moved from East Coast approximately 4 months ago
- 25 years of age, Asian family history, married for 1 year

**Expected Outcomes**
- Mother will state level of pain to be less than 4 on a scale of 1 to 10 during labour.
- Mother will successfully use visual imagery techniques, massage, and slow deep breathing for relaxation during labour.
- Mother will state early in labour at least three ways to cope effectively with pain and will implement these strategies as relevant.
- Fetus will demonstrate an expected heart rate pattern and will experience no compromise during labour.
- Mother and family will verbalize their needs during labour and delivery to the health care team.

**Interventions**
- Assess level of labour discomfort every 20 to 30 minutes, and, as needed, according to pain scale rating of 1 to 10.
- Implement and document nursing interventions (backrubs, heat and cold applications, position changes, back pressure and massage, and birth pool therapy, among others) to relieve labour discomforts.
- Assess cultural beliefs with labour and delivery management and implement interventions as needed to meet practice standards.
- Provide teaching about labour and delivery progress and breathing, visual imagery, and massage techniques that may decrease labour discomfort.
- Provide verbal and nonverbal reassurance during labour.
- Teach about fetal response during labour and rationale for nursing interventions to support fetal health, such as use of left side position to increase placental blood flow.
- Throughout labour, answer any questions from the mother and family members about needs and responses to labour process.
- Involve family members as much as possible during labour and as requested by the mother to improve her ability to cope.

# SUMMARY

Dramatic changes occur during pregnancy: a new life forms and develops and the expectant family members (mother, father, siblings, and other close members) experience major changes in their roles and relationships with each other. Although all fetal development processes, changes in pregnant women's bodies, and role transitions among family members share common elements, each family uniquely experiences pregnancy because of life experience and personal values. The focus is the entire family, although the nurse most often deals directly with the pregnant woman. The nurse provides valuable resources and information that the family may use to meet its specific needs. The overall nursing goal involves assisting each family to have a healthy pregnancy and birth outcome, to lay the foundation for satisfactory parenting and family life.

## Evolve Chapter Features

http://evolve.elsevier.com/Canada/Edelman/healthpromotion/
- Review Questions

# REFERENCES

Abdalla, I., & Elshikh, M. (2015). Effect of radiation on pregnancy. *International Journal of Medicine and Medical Sciences, 7*(5), 98–101. https://doi.org/10.5897/IJMMS2013.0894.

Alhusen, J. L., Ray, E., Sharps, P., et al. (2015). Intimate partner violence during pregnancy: Maternal and neonatal outcomes. *Journal of Women's Health, 24*(1), 100–106. https://doi.org/10.1089/jwh.2014.4872.

Ami, N., Bernstein, M., Boucher, F., et al. (2016). Folate and neural tube defects: The role of supplements and food fortification. *Paediatric & Child Health, 21*(3), 145–149. https://doi.org/10.1093/pch/21.3.145.

Apgar, V. (2015). A proposal for a new method of evaluation of the newborn infant. *Anesthesia & Analgesia, 120*(5), 1056–1059. https://doi.org/10.1213/ane.0b013e31829bdc5c.

Association of Ontario Doulas. (2019). *AOD—Scope of practice.* Retrieved from http://www.ontariodoulas.org/scope-of-practice.

Banderali, G., Martelli, A., Landi, M., et al. (2015). Short and long term health effects of parental tobacco smoking during pregnancy and lactation: A descriptive review. *Journal of Translational Medicine, 13*(327), 1–7. https://doi.org/10.1186/s12967-015-0690-y.

Benitz, W. E. (2015). Hospital stay for the healthy term newborn infants. *Pediatrics, 135*(5), 948–953. https://doi.org/10.1542/peds.2015-0699.

Best Start (2018). *Prenatal education program.* Retrieved from http://en.beststart.org/resources-and-research/prenatal-education-program.

Bier, D. M., Mann, J., Alpers, H. H. E., et al. (2015). *Nutrition for the primary care provider.* Basel: Karger Medical and Scientific Publishers.

Biswas, J., Banerjee, K., Sanyal, P., et al. (2015). Fetomaternal outcome of pyrexia in pregnancy: A prospective study. *International Journal of Women's Health and Reproductive Sciences, 3*(3), 132–135. https://doi.org/10.15296/ijwhr.2015.28.

Blackburn, S. T. (2014). *Maternal, fetal, and neonatal physiology: A clinical perspective* (4th ed.). Philadelphia: Elsevier Health Sciences. [Seminal Reference].

Bohra, N., Sharma, I., Srivastava, S., et al. (2015). Violence against women. *Indian Journal of Psychiatry, 57*(6), 333–338. https://doi.org/10.4103/0019-5545.161500.

Buckley, S. (2015). Executive summary of hormonal physiology of childbearing: Evidence and implications for women, babies, and maternity care. *The Journal of Perinatal Education, 24*(3), 145–153. https://doi.org/10.1891/1058-1243.24.3.145.

Canadian Association of Midwives (CAM). (2018a). *Midwifery-led births per province and territory.* Retrieved from https://canadianmidwives.org/2018/08/08/midwifery-assisted-births/.

Canadian Association of Midwives (CAM). (2018b). *Midwifery regulation.* Retrieved from https://canadianmidwives.org/midwifery-regulation/.

Canadian Diabetes Association. (2018). *Diabetes and pregnancy.* Retrieved from http://guidelines.diabetes.ca/cpg/chapter36.

Canadian Institute for Health Information. (2006). *Giving birth in Canada: The costs.* [Seminal Reference] http://publications.gc.ca/collections/Collection/H118-38-2006E.pdf.

Canadian Midwifery Regulators Council. (2019). *Midwifery in Canada.* Retrieved from http://cmrc-ccosf.ca/midwifery-canada.

Canadian Nurses Association (CNA). (2019). *Position statement: Promoting cultural competence.* Retrieved from https://cna-aiic.ca/~/media/cna/page-content/pdf-en/ps114_cultural_competence_2010_e.pdf.

Canadian Paediatric Society (CPS). (2015). *Rubella (German measles) in pregnancy.* Retrieved from https://www.caringforkids.cps.ca/handouts/rubella_in_pregnancy.

Canadian Paediatric Society (CPS). (2018). *Supporting and communicating with families experiencing a perinatal loss.* Retrieved from https://www.cps.ca/en/documents/position/perinatal-loss.

Canadian Paediatric Society (CPS). (2019). *HIV infection in pregnancy: Identification of intrapartum and perinatal HIV exposures.* Retrieved from https://www.cps.ca/en/documents/position/hiv-in-pregnancy.

Canadian Virtual Hospice (CVH). (2016). *How to use mygrief.ca.* Retrieved from http://www.mygrief.ca/mod/page/view.php?id=193.

Cantor, A. G., Bougatsos, C., Dana, T., et al. (2015). Routine iron supplementation and screening for iron deficiency anemia in pregnancy: A systematic review for the US preventive services task force. *Annals of Internal Medicine, 162*(8), 566–576. https://doi.org/10.7326/m14-2932.

Carapetis, J. R. (2015). The stark reality of rheumatic heart disease. *European Heart Journal, 36*(18), 1070–1073. https://doi.org/10.1093/eurheartj/ehu507.

Castillo, E., Murphy, K., & van Schalkwyk, J. (2017). No. 342-hepatitis B and pregnancy. *Journal of Obstetrics and Gynaecology Canada, 39*(3), 181–190. https://doi.org/10.1016/j.jogc.2016.11.001.

Central Intelligence Agency. (2017). Country comparison: Infant mortality rate. *The world factbook.* Retrieved from https://www.cia.gov/library/publications/the-world-factbook/rankorder/2091rank.html.

Centre for Addiction and Mental Health (CAMH). (2010). *Canadian smoking cessation: Clinical practice guideline.* Retrieved from https://www.nicotinedependenceclinic.com/en/canadaptt/PublishingImages/Pages/CAN-ADAPTT-Guidelines/CAN-ADAPTT%20Canadian%20Smoking%20Cessation%20Guideline_website.pdf. [Seminal Reference].

Chang, G., Fisher, N. D. L., Hornstein, M. D., et al. (2010). Identification of risk drinking women: T-ACE screening tool or the medical record. *Journal of Women's Health, 19*(10), 1933–1939. https://doi.org/10.1089/jwh.2009.1911. [Seminal Reference].

Chang, T., & Moniz, M. H. (2015). Pregnancy and weight gain: We have observed enough. *Obstetrics & Gynecology, 126*(1), 215. https://doi.org/10.1097/aog.0000000000000939.

Chitayat, D., Matsui, D., Amitai, Y., et al. (2016). Folic acid supplementation for pregnant women and those planning pregnancy: 2015 update. *The Journal of Clinical Pharmacology, 56*(2), 170–175. https://doi.org/10.1002/jcph.616.

College of Family Physicians of Canada (CFPC). (2014a). *Pregnancy—during pregnancy. Taking care of you and your baby.* Retrieved from https://www.cfpc.ca/Pregnancy/.

College of Family Physicians of Canada (CFPC). (2014b). Toxoplasmosis and pregnancy *Canadian Family Physician, 60*(4), 334–336. Retrieved from http://www.motherisk.org/prof/updatesDetail.jsp?content_id=1076. [Seminal Reference].

Cope, D. G. (2015). Cultural competency in nursing research. *Oncology Nursing Society, 42*(3), 305–307. doi:0001986791.

Copelon, R. (2004). Violence against women: The potential and challenge of a human rights perspective. *Women's Health Journal, 2*(3), 62–67 [Seminal Reference].

Cordero, A. M., Crider, K. S., Rogers, L. M., et al. (2015). Optimal serum and red blood cell folate concentrations in women of reproductive age for prevention of neural tube defects: World Health Organization guidelines. *Morbidity and Mortality Weekly Report, 64*(15), 421–423.

Crengle, S., Luke, J. N., Lambert, M., et al. (2018). Effect of a health literacy intervention trial on knowledge about cardiovascular disease medications among Indigenous peoples in Australia, Canada and New Zealand. *BMJ Open, 8*(1), 1–11. https://doi.org/10.1136/bmjopen-2017-018569.

Cunningham, F. G., Leveno, K. J., Bloom, S. L., et al. (Eds.). (2014). *William's obstetrics* (24th ed.) New York: McGraw-Hill Medical Education. [Seminal Reference].

Darnell, L. K., & Hickson, S. V. (2015). Cultural competent patient-centered nursing care. *Nursing Clinics of North America, 50*(1), 99–108. https://doi.org/10.1016/j.cnur.2014.10.008.

De Sutter, P. (2015). The challenge of multiple pregnancies. In R. Mathur (Ed.), *Reducing risk in fertility treatment* (pp. 1–17). London: Springer.

Doulatram, G., Raj, T. D., & Govindaraj, R. (2015). Pregnancy and substance abuse. In A. D. Kaye, N. Vadivelu, & R. D. Urmaneds (Eds.), *Substance abuse* (pp. 453–494). New York: Springer.

Ellis, S. A., Wojnar, D. M., & Pettinato, M. (2015). Conception, pregnancy, and birth experiences of male and gender variant gestational parents: It's how we could have a family. *Journal of Midwifery & Women's Health, 60*(1), 62–69. https://doi.org/10.1111/jmwh.12213.

El-Mazny, A. (2014). *Human reproduction: Basic anatomy and physiology.* Charleston, SC: Amazon CreateSpace. [Seminal Reference].

Ezzeddin, N., Zvoshy, R., Noroozi, M., et al. (2015). The association between postpartum depression and pica during pregnancy. *Global Journal of Health Science, 8*(4), 120–126. https://doi.org/10.5539/gjhsv8n4p120.

First Nations Health Authority. (2019). *Healthy pregnancy and early infancy.* Retrieved from http://www.fnha.ca/what-we-do/maternal-child-and-family-health/healthy-pregnancy-and-early-infancy.

Foray, A., & Foster, D. (2015). Substance use in the perinatal period. *Current Psychiatry Reports, 17*(91), 1–11. https://doi.org/10.1007/s11920-015-0626-5.

Forster, D. A., Jacobs, S., Amir, L. H., et al. (2014). Safety and efficacy of antenatal milk expressing for women with diabetes in pregnancy: Protocol for a randomized control trial. *Obstetrics and Gynaecology, 4,* 1–9. https://doi.org/10.1136/bmjopen-2014-006571.

Fox, A. B., & Quinn, D. M. (2015). Pregnant women at work: The role of stigma in predicting women's intended exit from the workforce. *Psychology of Women Quarterly, 39*(2), 226–242. https://doi.org/10.1177/0361684314552653.

Fetal behavioral states. In A. Piontelli (Ed.), (2015). *Development of normal fetal movements: The last 15 weeks of gestation* (pp. 87–98). Milan: Springer.

Galliano, D., & Pellicer, A. (2015). Potential etiologies of unexplained infertility in females. In *Unexplained infertility* (pp. 141–147). New York: Springer.

Genetics Education Canada Knowledge Organization (GECKO). (2019a). *Carrier screening in Canada.* Retrieved from https://geneticseducation.ca/point-of-care-tools-2/reproductive-genetic-carrier-screening-in-canada/.

Genetics Education Canada Knowledge Organization (GECKO). (2019b). *Expanded carrier screening.* Retrieved from https://geneticseducation.ca/point-of-care-tools-2/expanded-carrier-screening/.

Genetics Education Canada Knowledge Organization (GECKO). (2019c). *Guide to understanding prenatal screening tests.* Retrieved from https://geneticseducation.ca/public-resources/prenatal-and-preconception-genetics/guide-to-understanding-prenatal-screening-tests/#diagnostic.

Gök, M., Bozkurt, M., Guneyli, S., et al. (2015). Prenatal radiation exposure. *Proceedings in Obstetrics and Gynecology, 5*(1), 1–10. Retrieved from http://ir.uiowa.edu/pog/.

Goldstein, R. D., Lederman, R. L., Lichtenthal, W. G., et al. (2018). The grief of mothers after sudden unexpected death of their infants. *Pediatrics, 141*(5), 1–9. https://doi.org/10.1542/peds.2017-3651.

Gordon, M. (2016). *Manual of nursing diagnosis* (13th ed.). Burlington, MA: Jones & Bartlett Learning.

Government of Canada. (2017b). *Fetal alcohol spectrum disorder.* Retrieved from https://www.canada.ca/en/health-canada/services/healthy-living/your-health/diseases/fetal-alcohol-spectrum-disorder.html.

Government of Canada. (2018). *Assisted human reproduction act* (S.C. 2004, c.2). Retrieved from https://laws-lois.justice.gc.ca/eng/acts/A-13.4/page-2.html#docCont.

Government of Canada. (2019a). *Make healthy meals with the eat well plate.* Retrieved from https://food-guide.canada.ca/en/tips-for-healthy-eating/make-healthy-meals-with-the-eat-well-plate/.

Government of Canada. (2019b). *Federal labour standards.* Retrieved from https://www.canada.ca/en/services/jobs/workplace/federal-labour-standards/leaves.html.

Green, J., Darbyshire, P., Adams, A., et al. (2015). Desperately seeking parenthood: Neonatal nurses reflect on parental anguish. *Journal of Clinical Nursing, 24*(13–14), 1885–1894. https://doi.org/10.1111/jocn.12811.

Hall, K. S., Kusunoki, Y., Gatny, H., et al. (2015). Social discrimination, stress, and risk of unintended pregnancy among young women. *Journal of Adolescent Health, 56*(3), 330–337. https://doi.org/10.1016/j.jadohealth.2014.11.008.

Halpern, S. H., & Garg, R. (2015). Evidence-informed medicine and labor analgesia. In *Epidural labor analgesia* (pp. 285–295). Cham, Switzerland: Springer.

Health Canada. (2009a). *Prenatal nutrition guidelines for health professionals—background on Canada's Food Guide.* Retrieved from https://www.canada.ca/en/health-canada/services/publications/

food-nutrition/prenatal-nutrition-guidelines-health-professionals-background-canada-food-guide-2009.html. [Seminal Reference].

Health Canada. (2009b). *Prenatal nutrition guidelines for health professionals—iron contributes to a healthy pregnancy.* Retrieved from https://www.canada.ca/en/health-canada/services/publications/food-nutrition/prenatal-nutrition-guidelines-health-professionals-iron-contributes-healthy-pregnancy-2009.html. [Seminal Reference].

Health Canada. (2011a). *Hepatitis B infection in Canada.* Retrieved from https://www.canada.ca/en/public-health/services/infectious-diseases/hepatitis-b-infection-canada.html. [Seminal Reference].

Health Canada. (2011b). *Pathogen safety data sheets: Infectious substances—Cytomegalovirus.* Retrieved from https://www.canada.ca/en/public-health/services/laboratory-biosafety-biosecurity/pathogen-safety-data-sheets-risk-assessment/cytomegalovirus.html. [Seminal Reference].

Health Canada. (2013a). *Canadian guidelines on sexually transmitted infections—management and treatment of specific infections: Genital herpes simplex (HSV) infections.* Retrieved from https://www.canada.ca/en/public-health/services/infectious-diseases/sexual-health-sexually-transmitted-infections/canadian-guidelines/sexually-transmitted-infections/canadian-guidelines-sexually-transmitted-infections-32.html. [Seminal Reference].

Health Canada. (2016a). *Public health notice—Zika virus.* Retrieved from https://www.canada.ca/en/public-health/services/public-health-notices/2016/public-health-notice-zika-virus.html.

Health Canada. (2016b). *Summary safety review: DICLECTIN (doxylamine and pyridoxine combination)—assessing safety in pregnancy.* Retrieved from https://www.canada.ca/en/health-canada/services/drugs-health-products/medeffect-canada/safety-reviews/summary-safety-review-assessing-diclectin-doxylamine-pyridoxine-combination-safety-pregnancy.html.

Health Canada. (2017a). *Canadian immunization guide—hepatitis B vaccine.* Retrieved from https://www.canada.ca/en/public-health/services/publications/healthy-living/canadian-immunization-guide-part-4-active-vaccines/page-7-hepatitis-b-vaccine.html.

Health Canada. (2017b). *Mercury in fish.* Retrieved from https://www.canada.ca/en/health-canada/services/food-nutrition/food-safety/chemical-contaminants/environmental-contaminants/mercury/mercury-fish.html.

Health Canada. (2018a). *Canadian guidelines on sexually transmitted infections—management and treatment of specific infections: Syphilis.* Retrieved from https://www.canada.ca/en/public-health/services/infectious-diseases/sexual-health-sexually-transmitted-infections/canadian-guidelines/sexually-transmitted-infections/canadian-guidelines-sexually-transmitted-infections-27.html.

Health Canada. (2018b). *Folic acid and neural tube defects.* Retrieved from https://www.canada.ca/en/public-health/services/pregnancy/folic-acid.html#wb-info.

Health Canada. (2019). *Canada's dietary guidelines.* Retrieved from https://food-guide.canada.ca/.

Health of Canada. (2013b). *Fertility.* Retrieved from https://www.canada.ca/en/public-health/services/fertility/fertility.html. [Seminal Reference].

Holley, S. R., & Pasch, L. A. (2015). Counseling lesbian, gay, bisexual, and transgender patients. In S. R. Covington (Ed.), *Fertility counseling* (pp. 180–196). Cambridge, UK: Cambridge University Press.

James, J. E. (2015). Review: Higher caffeine intake during pregnancy increases risk of low birth weight. *Evidence-informed Nursing, 18*(4), 111. https://doi.org/10.1136/eb-2014-102027.

Jarmasz, J. S., Basalah, D. A., Chudley, A. E., et al. (2017). Human brain abnormalities associated with prenatal alcohol exposure and fetal alcohol spectrum disorder. *Journal of Neuropathology & Experimental Neurology, 76*(9), 813–833. https://doi.org/10.1093/jnen/nlx064.

Jewkes, R., & Penn-Kekana, L. (2015). Mistreatment of women in childbirth: Time for action on this important dimension of violence against women. *PLoS Medicine, 12*(6), e1001849. https://doi.org/10.1371/journal.pmed.1001849.

Jhaveri, R. (2015). Prevention of hepatitis B virus vertical transmission: Time for the next step. *Pediatrics, 135*(5), e1286–e1287. https://doi.org/10.1542/peds.2015-0360.

Jyothi, N. (2015). Case study on post pregnancy related complication of pica. *International Journal of Nursing Care, 3*(1), 42–45. https://doi.org/10.5958/2320-8651.2015.0021.6.

King, T. L., & Brucker, M. C. (2016). *Pharmacology for women* (2nd ed.). Burlington, MA: Jones & Bartlett Learning.

King, T. L., Brucker, M., Fahey, J., et al. (Eds.). (2015). *Varney's midwifery* (5th ed.). Burlington, MA: Jones & Bartlett Learning.

Kovacs, G., & Briggs, P. (2015). Infections during pregnancy—varicella, herpes, cytomegalovirus, toxoplasma, Listeria, group B streptococcus. In *Lectures in obstetrics, gynecology and women's health* (pp. 133–137). Cham, Switzerland: Springer.

Kremer, M. E., & Arora, K. S. (2015). Clinical, ethical, and legal considerations in pregnant women with opioid abuse. *Obstetrics & Gynecology, 126*(3), 474–478. https://doi.org/10.1097/aog.0000000000000991.

Langer, O. (2015). *The diabetes in pregnancy dilemma: Leading the change with proven solutions* (2nd ed.). Shelton, CT: People's Medical Publishing House.

Lemyre, B., Jefferies, A. L., O'Flaherty, P., & Canadian Paediatric Society, Fetus and Newborn Committee. (2018). Facilitating discharge from hospital of the healthy term infant. *Paediatric Child Health, 23*(8), 515–522. Retrieved from https://www.cps.ca/en/documents/position/facilitating-discharge-from-hospital-of-the-healthy-term-infant.

Lewitt, M. (2015). Promoting normal physiologic birth through partnership with consumers, providers, and hospitals. *Journal of Obstetric, Gynecologic, and Neonatal Nursing, 44*, S21 10.111/1552-6909.12690.

Liat, S., Cabero, L., Hod, M., et al. (2015). Obesity in obstetrics. *Best Practice & Research Clinical Obstetrics & Gynaecology, 29*(1), 79–90. https://doi.org/10.1016/j.bpobgyn.2014.05.010.

Lissauer, T., Fanaroff, A. A., Miall, L., et al. (Eds.). (2015). *Neonatology at a glance* (3rd ed.). Somerset, NJ: Wiley-Blackwell.

Macones, G. (2015). *Management of labor and delivery* (2nd ed.). Somerset, NJ: Wiley-Blackwell.

Mader, S., & Windelspecht, M. (2015). *Human biology* (14th ed.). New York: McGraw-Hill Higher Education.

Malin, G. L., & Wallace, S. V. F. (2019). Cardiac disease in pregnancy. *Obstetrics, Gynaecology and Reproductive Medicine,* 1–5. https://doi.org/10.1016/j.ogrm.2018.12.008.

March of Dimes. (2015). *Birth defects.* Retrieved from http://www.marchofdimes.org/baby/birth-defects.aspx.

Mattson, S., & Smith, J. E. (2015). *Core curriculum for maternal-newborn nursing* (5th ed.). St. Louis, MO: Saunders.

McQueen, K., & Murphy-Oikonen, J. (2016). Neonatal abstinence syndrome. *New England Journal of Medicine, 375*(25), 2468–2479. https://doi.org/10.1056/NEJMra1600879.

Merriam-Webster. (2015). *Merriam-Webster's medical dictionary online.* Retrieved from https://www.merriam-webster.com/medical.

Michihata, N., Yamamoto, K. H., Mukaigawara, M., et al. (2015). Group B streptococcus immunization during pregnancy for improving outcomes. *Cochrane Database of Systematic Reviews,* (1), CD011496. https://doi.org/10.1002/1465185.

Moise, K. J. (2015). Overview of rhesus D alloimmunization in pregnancy. *UpToDate.* Retrieved from http://www.uptodate.com/contents/overview-of-rhesus-d-alloimmunization-in-pregnancy.

Money, D., Tulloch, K., Boucoiran, I., et al. (2014). Guidelines for the care of pregnant women living with HIV and interventions to reduce perinatal transmission: Executive summary. *Journal of Obstetrics and Gynaecology Canada, 36*(8), 721–734. https://doi.org/10.1016/S1701-2163(15)30515-6.

Mori, G. F. (2015). *From pregnancy to motherhood: Psychoanalytic aspects of the beginning of the mother-child relationship.* New York: Routledge.

National Aboriginal Council of Midwives (NACM). (2019). *What is an indigenous midwife.* Retrieved from https://indigenousmidwifery.ca/indigenous-midwifery-in-canada/.

National Collaborating Centre for Aboriginal Health (NCCAH). (2011). *Access to health services as a social determinant of First Nations, Inuit and Métis health.* Retrieved from https://www.nccah-ccnsa.ca/docs/fact%20sheets/social%20determinates/Access%20to%20Health%20Services_Eng%202010.pdf. [Seminal Reference].

Nicotine Dependence Clinic. (2019). *Prevention of gestational and neonatal exposure to tobacco smoke.* Retrieved from https://www.nicotinedependenceclinic.com/en/pregnets/home.

Norwitz, E. R., & Schorge, J. O. (2015). *Obstetrics and gynecology at a glance* (4th ed.). Malden, MA: Blackwell Publishing.

Ontario Council of Agencies Serving Immigrants. (2017). *Low cost healthcare.* Retrieved from https://settlement.org/ontario/health/ohip-and-health-insurance/low-cost-health-care/.

Ontario Ministry of Children, Community and Social Services. (2019). *Home page.* Retrieved from https://www.ontario.ca/page/ministry-children-community-and-social-services.

Ontario Ministry of Labour. (2019). *Pregnancy and parental leave.* Retrieved from https://www.ontario.ca/document/your-guide-employment-standards-act-0/pregnancy-and-parental-leave#section-2.

Oulman, E., Kim, T. H. M., Yunis, K., et al. (2015). Prevalence and predictors of unintended pregnancy among women: An analysis of the Canadian Maternity Experiences Survey. *BMC Pregnancy and Childbirth, 15*(260), 1–8. https://doi.org/10.1186/s1288-015-0663-4.

Pavord, S., & Maybury, H. (2015). How I treat postpartum hemorrhage. *Blood, 125*(18), 2759–2770. https://doi.org/10.1182/blood-2014-10-512608.

Pawluk, M. S., Campaña, H., Gili, J. A., et al. (2014). Adverse social determinants and risk for congenital anomalies. *Archivos Argentinos de Pediatria, 112*(3), 215–223. https://doi.org/10.1590/S0325-00752014000300004. [Seminal Reference].

Public Health Agency of Canada (PHAC). (2011a). *Maternal mortality in Canada.* Retrieved from http://publications.gc.ca/collections/collection_2012/aspc-phac/HP10-19-2011-eng.pdf.

Public Health Agency of Canada (PHAC). (2011b). *The sensible guide to a healthy pregnancy.* Retrieved from https://www.canada.ca/en/public-health/services/health-promotion/healthy-pregnancy/healthy-pregnancy-guide.html. [Seminal Reference].

Public Health Agency of Canada (PHAC). (2015). *About: Canadian prenatal nutrition program.* Retrieved from https://www.canada.ca/en/public-health/services/health-promotion/childhood-adolescence/programs-initiatives/canada-prenatal-nutrition-program-cpnp/about-cpnp.html.

Public Health Agency of Canada (PHAC). (2017a). Chapter 2: Preconception care. In *Family-centred maternity and newborn care: National guidelines.* Retrieved from https://www.canada.ca/en/public-health/services/maternity-newborn-care-guidelines.html.

Public Health Agency of Canada (PHAC). (2017b). *Section 6-4: Canadian guidelines on sexually transmitted infections—specific populations—pregnancy.* Retrieved from https://www.canada.ca/en/public-health/services/infectious-diseases/sexual-health-sexually-transmitted-infections/canadian-guidelines/sexually-transmitted-infections/canadian-guidelines-sexually-transmitted-infections-41.html.

Public Health Ontario. (2018). *Health effects of cannabis exposure in pregnancy and breastfeeding.* Retrieved from https://www.publichealthontario.ca/-/media/documents/eb-cannabis-pregnancy-breastfeeding.pdf?la=en.

Queenan, J. T., Spong, C. Y., & Lockwood, C. J. (2015). *Protocols for high-risk pregnancies: An evidence-informed approach* (6th ed.). Hoboken, NJ: John Wiley & Sons.

Raio, L., Bolla, D., & Baumann, M. (2015). Hypertension in pregnancy. *Current Opinion in Cardiology, 30*(4), 411–415. https://doi.org/10.1097/HCO.0000000000000190.

Rayburn, W. F., Jolley, J. A., & Simpson, L. L. (2015). Advances in ultrasound imaging for congenital malformations during early gestation. *Birth Defects Research Part A: Clinical and Molecular Teratology, 103,* 260–268. https://doi.org/10.1002/bdra.23353.

Reddy, B. S., Venkateswarlu, P., Umadevi, S., et al. (2015). Screening, pregnant women, seroprevalence, hepatitis B surface antigen among pregnant women attending antenatal clinics in Govt. General Hospital, Anantapuramu (A.P.). *Journal of Evolution of Medical and Dental Services, 4*(4), 555–558. https://doi.org/10.14260/jmeds/2015.82.

Rode, J. L., & Kiel, E. J. (2016). The mediated effects of maternal depression and infant temperament on maternal role. *Archives of Women's Mental Health, 19*(1), 133–144. https://doi.org/10.1007/s00737-015-1.

Rubin, R. (1967). Attainment of the maternal role. Part I. Processes. *Nursing Research, 16*(3), 237–245. https://doi.org/10.1097/00006199-196701630-00006. [Seminal Reference].

Rubin, R. (1984). *Maternal identity and the maternal experience.* New York: Springer. [Seminal Reference].

Sangkomkamhang, U. S., Lumbiganon, P., Prasertcharoensuk, W., et al. (2015). Antenatal lower genital tract infection screening and treatment programs for preventing preterm delivery. *Cochrane Database of Systematic Reviews* (2), CD006178. https://doi.org/10.1002/14651858.CD006178.pub3.

Sickle Cell Disease Association of Canada. (2016). *Bill S-211: Recognizing June 19 as the Canadian sickle cell awareness day.* Retrieved from http://www.sicklecelldisease.ca/pulsepro/pulsepro/data/files/Advocacy-Reception%20Book%202016-Final.pdf.

Silasi, M., Cardenas, I., Kwon, J., et al. (2015). Viral infections during pregnancy. *American Journal of Reproductive Immunology, 73*(3), 199–213. https://doi.org/10.1111/aji.12355.

Singh, A. E., Levett, P. N., Fonseca, K., et al. (2015). Canadian Public Health Laboratory Network laboratory guidelines for congenital syphilis and syphilis screening in pregnant women in Canada. *The Canadian Journal of Infectious Diseases & Medical Microbiology, 26*(Suppl. A), 23A–28A. Retrieved from https://www.ncbi.nlm.nih.gov/pmc/articles/PMC4353984/.

Slep, A. M. S., Foran, H. M., Heyman, R. E., et al. (2015). Identifying unique and shared risk factors for physical intimate partner violence and clinically-significant physical intimate partner violence. *Aggressive Behavior, 41,* 227–241. https://doi.org/10.1002/ab.21565.

Society of Obstetricians and Gynaecologists of Canada (SOGC). (2019a). *Group B streptococcus screening.* Retrieved from https://www.pregnancyinfo.ca/your-pregnancy/routine-tests/group-b-streptococcus-screening/.

Society of Obstetricians and Gynaecologists of Canada (SOGC). (2019b). *HIV screening*. Retrieved from https://www.pregnancyinfo.ca/your-pregnancy/routine-tests/hiv-screening/.

Society of Obstetricians and Gynaecologists of Canada (SOGC). (2019c). *Prenatal classes and preparing for delivery*. Retrieved from https://www.pregnancyinfo.ca/your-pregnancy/preparing-for-birth/prenatal-classes-and-preparing-for-birth/.

Solchany, J. E. (2013). *Promoting maternal mental health during pregnancy*. Seattle, WA: NCAST Programs. [Seminal Reference].

Spencer, L., Rollo, M., Hauck, Y., et al. (2015). The effect of weight management interventions that include a diet component on weight-related outcomes in pregnant and postpartum women: A systematic review protocol. *JBI Database of Systematic Reviews and Implementation Reports, 13*(1), 88–98. https://doi.org/10.11124/jbisrir-2015-1812.

Spong, C. Y. (2015). Prevention of the first cesarean delivery. *Obstetrics & Gynecology Clinics of North America, 42*(2), 377–380. https://doi.org/10.1016/j.ogc.2015.01.010.

Starling, P., Charlton, K., McMahon, A., et al. (2015). Fish intake during pregnancy and fetal neurodevelopment—a systematic review of the evidence. *Nutrients, 7*(3), 2001–2014. https://doi.org/10.1016/j.jnim.2014.10.118.

Statistics Canada. (2019). *Deaths, 2018*. Retrieved from https://www150.statcan.gc.ca/n1/daily-quotidien/191126/dq191126c-eng.htm.

Stevenson, D. K., Cohen, R. S., & Sunshine, P. (2015). *Neonatology: Clinical practice and procedures*. Maidenhead, UK: McGraw-Hill Education.Stockwell, F. (2015). *Maternal-infant bonding*. Retrieved from http://www.felicitystockwell.com/the-overview.

Swanson, J. R., & Sinkin, R. A. (2015). Transition from fetus to newborn. *Pediatric Clinics of North America, 62*(2), 329–343. https://doi.org/10.1016/j.pcl.2014.11.002.

Tewfik, T. L., Karsan, N., & Kanaan, A. (2015). Cleft lip and palate and mouth and pharynx deformities. *Medscape*. Retrieved from http://emedicine.medscape.com/article/837347-overview.

Tharpe, N. L., Farley, C. L., & Jordan, R. (2016). *Clinical practice guidelines for midwifery & women's health* (5th ed.). Burlington, MA: Jones & Bartlett Learning.

Tomson, T., & Klein, P. (2015). Fine-tuning risk assessment with antiepileptic drug use in pregnancy. *Neurology, 84*(4), 339–340. https://doi.org/10.1212/WNL.0000000000001197.

Tucker, C. M., Arthur, T. M., Roncoroni, J., et al. (2015). Patient-centered, culturally sensitive health care. *American Journal of Lifestyle Medicine, 9*(1), 63–77. https://doi.org/10.1177/1559827613498065.

von Mohr, M., Mayes, L. C., & Rutherford, H. J. V. (2017). The transition to motherhood: Psychoanalysis and neuroscience perspectives. *Psychoanalytic Study of the Child, 70*(1), 154–173. https://doi.org/10.1080/00797308.2016.1277905.

Whitney, E. N., & Rolfes, S. R. (2015). *Understanding nutrition* (14th ed.). Boston: Cengage Learning.

World Health Organization (WHO). (2009). *Reaching optimal iodine nutrition in pregnant and lactating women and young children*. Retrieved from https://www.who.int/nutrition/publications/micronutrients/WHOStatement__IDD_pregnancy.pdf. [Seminal Reference].

World Health Organization (WHO). (2016a). *Companion choice during labour and childbirth for improved quality of care*. Retrieved from http://apps.who.int/iris/bitstream/handle/10665/250274/WHO-RHR-16.10-eng.pdf;jsessionid=02DE112A789B57F06F-C59D1325061B07?sequence=1.

World Health Organization (WHO). (2016b). *Zika virus*. Retrieved from http://www.who.int/mediacentre/factsheets/zika/en/.

Zakšek, T. Š. (2015). Sexual activity during pregnancy in childbirth and after childbirth. In A. P. Mivsek (Ed.), *Sexology in midwifery* (pp. 87–115). Rijeka, Croatia: InTech.

# 11

# Infant

*Ellen Buck-McFadyen, RN, MScN, PhD*

Originating US chapter by *Susan Scott Ricci, CNE, MEd, MSN, ARNP*

## INTENDED LEARNING OUTCOMES

*After completing this chapter, the reader will be able to:*

- Evaluate the infant's health status and give examples of basic growth and developmental principles.
- Analyze the developmental tasks for the infant and the behaviour, indicating that these tasks are being accomplished.
- Explain the immunization schedule and other safety and health-promotion measures to a parent.
- Detect common parental concerns about infants and describe key components and strategies for parent education to allay these concerns.

- Examine accidents that occur during infancy and recommend appropriate counselling for accident prevention and safety.
- Differentiate ways in which nurses can be active in promoting policies and influencing legislation concerning health.
- Outline government strategies to meet the goals of improving infant health.

## KEY TERMS

Active immunization
Birth defect
Corrected age
Infant/child abuse
Herd immunity
Oral stage of development
Passive immunization
Parental self-efficacy

Failure to thrive
Positional plagiocephaly
Reflexes
Sensorimotor period
Sudden infant death syndrome (SIDS)
Trust versus mistrust
Weaning

## THINK ABOUT IT

### Car Seat Safety

Infants are at particular risk in automobile accidents. The proper use of child restraint systems can reduce the risk of death and injury significantly. Although the law in Canada requires caregivers to use infant and child restraints, and many public service campaigns encourage their use, more than half of children are not properly restrained in car seats (Bruce, Cramm, Mundle, et al., 2015).

Nurses must have up-to-date knowledge of child restraint systems and their proper use to help parents find new products and obtain the most current information available. Parents may rely on the person selling the infant car seat for their information about protection systems and the proper use of car seats. And while informational brochures and media campaigns may increase awareness of the need for properly fitted and installed child restraints, they often fall short

because they fail to provide explanations or demonstrations. As a result, parents may misinterpret the information that they receive.

- What type of program might you develop to reach and inform parents about the importance of car seat safety?
- In what settings might such a program be implemented?
- How would you modify your teaching plan to meet the needs of parents with low literacy?
- How would you modify your program to ensure that parents who come from cultural backgrounds different from your own would respond well to the information?

Infants are recognized as the most vulnerable and dependent members of society, and their well-being is often used to measure the overall health of society. Health is shaped by a broad set of determinants, including socioeconomic status, physical and social environments, genetics and biological influences, and access to health care. Providing a safe and sound source of attachment and interaction is paramount to healthy infant development. Caregiving activities and the context in which these activities occur are the primary ingredients of an infant's preparation for life and ultimate independence. Nurses play a vital role in influencing this positive interaction and the broader parenting environment through health promotion, advocacy, and education.

This chapter focuses on the infant and the infant's family during the infant's developmental period of 1 to 18 months. Because the infant is completely dependent on others, this chapter addresses the infant's parents and significant others as sources of health-promotion activities. The relationship initiated at birth between parents and the infant is the basis for the interdependence that is required for proper psychological and physical infant development. Health care providers must focus on parent education as a means of fostering healthy, satisfying relationships within the family unit, and promoting the development of healthy future generations.

The principles of normal growth and development are used as a structural framework for this chapter. Understanding these principles helps the nurse identify deviations from the norm and institute appropriate health-promoting interventions.

# BIOLOGY AND GENETICS

Human development begins when a single sperm penetrates a mature ovum. The changes that follow are undeniable and wondrous. During this early period of growth and development the infant depends completely on others, primarily the parents, to meet all personal needs (Table 11.1). To assist the parents in their understanding of their infant's needs and progress, the nurse must know what behaviours to expect at certain ages. These developmental landmarks serve as a basis for anticipatory guidance (Table 11.2). When parents know what to expect from their growing child and feel confident in their ability to facilitate these milestones, it can also promote closer family relationships.

## Developmental Tasks

Infant development begins before birth. A healthy pregnancy and a positive early childhood environment are essential to normal infant physical and mental health. Every infant faces developmental tasks and must accomplish them individually. Canada's cultural diversity means that parents may hold varying philosophies, values, and beliefs about child-rearing; yet, there are universal tasks of child development across all cultures (learning to walk and talk) that lead to common expectations and behaviours surrounding infant development (Bornstein, 2015).

The infant's first and most basic task is survival, which includes the physical tasks of breathing, sucking, eating, digesting, eliminating, and sleeping. Because many of these tasks involve the infant's mouth, this stage of life often is referred to

as the oral stage of development, reflecting the primary importance of the mouth as the centre of pleasure. More developmental tasks that must be accomplished during infancy are listed in Table 11.3. In the first year, infants learn to focus their vision, reach out, explore, and seek out things around them. During this time, infants also develop bonds of love and trust with their caregivers and others as part of their social and emotional development. Nurses can provide the infant's caregivers with guidance to encourage their infant's development by their:

- Talking to their infant, especially in a calming fashion
- Repeating sounds that their infant makes to help the infant learn to use language
- Reading to their infant to help develop and understand language and sounds
- Singing and playing music to help the infant develop a love for music and to help with brain development
- Giving their infant a great deal of loving attention to make the infant feel secure
- Praising their infant when something has been accomplished or learned (Centers for Disease Control and Prevention [CDC], 2018a)

To assist the infant's parents in encouraging achievement of these tasks, the nurse discusses the importance of stimulation and environmental interactions. Many neurological structures are far from completely developed at birth, with a significant period of plasticity during the first years of life that creates both opportunities and vulnerabilities for the developing brain (Gao, Lin, Grewen, et al., 2017). The brain volume doubles in size from birth to 1 year of age due to the development of neural connections, long-range axons, and myelination (Gao et al., 2017). The complex network of neural circuits that connect regions of the brain and the epigenetic mechanisms that alter DNA expression are a product of interaction between the infant's genes and their environment (Burns, Szyszkowicz, Luheshi, et al., 2018; Gao et al., 2017). Critical periods of brain development, prominent during the first year of life, are points in time where regions of the brain are more sensitive to environmental factors that provide instructive and adaptive signals for neural development and functional brain pathways (Inguaggiato, Sgandurra, & Cioni, 2017). This highlights the important role of the infant's caregivers, who provide the external stimuli that set the stage for brain development. During the early postnatal period, the most important external stimuli relate to a caregiver's sensitivity and responsiveness to infant cues as they establish a trusting infant–caregiver relationship (Inguaggiato et al., 2017). As the infant's environment expands, brain development relies on cognitive stimulation in the home through exposure to language, toys, books, and educational opportunities (Johnson, Riis, & Noble, 2016). While we have only a partial understanding of brain science and epigenetics, there is sufficient evidence to show that early life experiences shape the brain in ways that impact physical and mental health decades down the road (Inguaggiato et al., 2017).

When counselling parents, the nurse stresses the importance of a variety of stimuli within the infant's environment. A variety of auditory and visual stimuli should be available, such as colourful mobiles, music, spoken voice, and toys, to assist the

TABLE 11.1 **Growth and Development**

*During Infancy*

## 1 Month

- Follows and fixes on bright object with eyes when it moves within field of vision
- Still has head lag when pulled to sitting position
- Displays tonic neck, grasp, and Moro reflexes
- Turns head when prone, but unable to support it
- Displays sucking and rooting reflexes
- Holds hands in fists
- Looks intently at caregiver when talked to
- Makes small, throaty sounds
- Gains 140 to 200 g (5 to 7 ounces) weekly for 6 months
- Grows 2.5 cm (1 inch) monthly for 6 months
- Cries when hungry or uncomfortable
- Lifts head momentarily when prone

## 2 Months

- Has closed posterior fontanelle
- Listens actively to sounds
- Lifts head almost 45 degrees off table when prone
- Follows moving object with eyes
- Grasp reflex decreases
- Recognizes familiar faces
- Pays attention to speaking voice
- Assumes less-flexed position when prone
- Vocalizes; distinct from crying
- Turns from side to back
- Begins to have social smile

## 3 Months

- Visually inspects object and stares at own hand with apparent fascination when either appears in field of vision
- Has longer periods of wakefulness without crying
- Laughs aloud and shows pleasure in vocalization
- Holds head erect and steady; raises chest, usually supported on forearms
- Smiles in response to caregiver's face
- Recognizes faces, voices, and familiar objects
- Opens and closes hands, shakes toys
- Begins pre-language vocalizations (coos, babbles, and chuckles)
- Carries hand or object to mouth at will
- Grasp reflex absent
- Follows objects for 180 degrees
- Actively holds rattle, but will not reach for it
- Turns eyes to object placed in field of vision

## 4 Months

- Begins drooling, indicated by appearance of saliva; does not know how to swallow it
- Holds head steady when in sitting position
- Recognizes familiar objects
- Shows almost no head lag when pulled to sitting position
- Rolls from back to side and from abdomen to back
- Inspects and plays with hands; pulls clothing or blanket over face in play
- Begins eye–hand coordination
- Chews and bites
- Enjoys social interaction
- Demands attention by fussing
- Reaches out to people
- Bears some weight on legs when held upright
- Is aware and interested in new environment
- Grasps object with two hands
- Squeals

## 5 Months

- Reaches persistently; grasps with entire hand
- Plays with toes
- Begins to discover parts of his/her body
- Smiles at mirror image
- Begins to postpone gratification
- Shows signs of tooth eruption
- Sleeps through night without food
- Weighs twice the birth weight
- Sits with slight support
- Vocalizes displeasure when desired object is taken away
- Is able to discriminate strangers from family members
- Makes cooing noises
- Squeals with delight
- Looks for object that has fallen
- Rolls from back to stomach or vice versa

## 6 Months

- Gains approximately 85 to 140 g (3 to 5 ounces) weekly during the second 6 months
- Is able to lift cup by handle
- Begins to shuffle in locomotion
- Sits in high chair with straight back
- Begins to imitate sounds
- Vocalizes to toys and mirror image
- Recognizes caregivers
- Babbles with one-syllable sounds: "ma, ma, da, da"
- Chewing and biting occur
- Has definite likes and dislikes
- Likes to be picked up
- Plays peek-a-boo
- Makes "guh" and "bah" sounds

## 7 Months

- Has eruption of upper central incisors
- Bears weight when held in standing position
- Sits, leaning forward on both hands
- Fixates on one very small object
- Produces vowel sounds: "ba-ba" and "da-da"
- Shows fear of strangers
- Displays emotional instability by easy and quick changes from crying to laughing
- Repeats activities that are enjoyed
- Bangs objects together
- Develops taste differences
- Transfers objects from one hand to another
- Approaches toy and grasps it with one hand
- Imitates simple acts

## 8 Months

- Feeds self with finger foods
- Sits well alone
- Stretches out arms to be picked up
- Greets strangers with bashful behaviour
- Begins to show regular patterns in bladder and bowel elimination
- Responds to "no" but does not obey it
- Makes consonant sounds: t, d, and w
- Dislikes dressing and diaper change
- Releases object at will
- Shows nervousness with strangers
- Pulls toy toward self

*Continued*

## TABLE 11.1   Growth and Development—cont'd

### *During Infancy*

**9 Months**

- Creeps and crawls (backward at first)
- Shows good coordination and sits alone
- Responds to adult anger; cries when scolded
- Explores object by sucking, chewing, and biting it
- Responds to simple verbal requests
- Drinks from cup or glass with assistance
- Pulls self to standing position
- Begins to show fears of going to bed and being left alone
- Imitates waving "bye-bye"
- Sits for prolonged periods—10 minutes
- Releases object with flexed wrist
- Repeats facial expressions of adults
- Uses thumb and index finger in pincer grasp

**10 Months**

- Sits by falling down
- Says "da-da" and "ma-ma" with meaning
- Understands "bye-bye"
- Looks at and follows pictures in book
- Object permanence begins to develop
- Plays interactive games such as pat-a-cake
- Crawls and cruises about well
- Pays attention to own name
- Picks up objects fairly well
- Extends toy to another person without releasing
- Pulls self to standing position and stands while holding onto solid object

**11 Months**

- Is able to push toys and place several objects in container
- Attempts to walk without assistance
- Begins to hold spoon
- Explores objects more thoroughly
- Stands erect with help of person's hand
- May have eruption of lower lateral incisors
- Holds crayon to mark on paper
- Acts frustrated when restricted
- Imitates definite speech sounds
- Reacts to restrictions with frustration

**12 Months**

- Loses Babinski sign
- Understands simple verbal commands

- Develops evident hand dominance
- Weighs triple the birth weight
- Has equal circumference of head and chest
- Walks with one hand held
- Knows own name
- Turns pages in book
- Has slow vocabulary growth because of increased interest in walking
- Develops lumbar curve
- Uses spoon in feeding, but often puts it upside down in mouth
- Drops object deliberately for it to be picked up
- Shakes head for "no"
- Plays pat-a-cake
- Recovers balance when falling over
- Tries to follow when being read to
- Does things to attract attention
- Imitates vocalization lead

**15 Months**

- Creeps up stairs
- Uses "da-da" and "ma-ma" labels for correct parents
- Tolerates some separation
- Drinks from cup well, but rotates spoon
- Asks for object by pointing
- Plays interactive games such as peek-a-boo and pat-a-cake
- Expresses emotions; has temper tantrums
- Walks without help

**18 Months**

- Has closed anterior fontanelle
- Has long trunk, short and bowed legs, and protruding abdomen
- Walks upstairs with help
- Turns pages of book
- Has short attention span
- Begins to test limits
- Gets into everything
- Fills and handles spoon without rotating it, but spills frequently
- Runs clumsily and falls often
- Is extremely curious
- Places object in hole or slot
- Becomes communicative, social being
- Imitates behaviour of parents, such as mimicking household chores

Sources: Beckett, C., & Taylor, H. (2016). *Human growth and development* (3rd ed.). Los Angeles: Sage Publications; Berk, L. E., & Meyers, A. B. (2015). *Infants, children, and adolescents* (8th ed.). New York: Pearson Education.

infant in achieving developmental tasks. The sense of touch is also an extremely important stimulus, impacting the social attachment between the infant and caregiver, as well as the infant's level of brain activity and connectivity (Brauer, Xiao, Poulain, et al., 2016). Ensuring that appropriate sensory stimuli are available is vital to the infant's growth and developmental progression.

## Concepts of Infant Development

As infants develop, they go through a series of developmental stages that are important for all aspects of their personhood,

including physical, intellectual, emotional, and social aspects. The role of their caretakers is to provide encouragement, support, and access to activities that enable them to master key developmental tasks. The study of how a helpless infant grows and develops into a fully functioning, independent adult has fascinated many researchers. Their theories describe the development of human behaviour as overlapping stages that occur in somewhat predictable patterns in an individual's life (Child Development Institute, 2015). Because these developmental theories are presented in Chapter 9, only their specific application to the infant is discussed here.

## TABLE 11.2   Parenting Tasks for Developmental Landmarks in Infancy

| Age (Months) | Landmarks | Parenting Tasks |
|---|---|---|
| 2 | Smiles, coos, and makes gurgling sounds<br>Holds head up and pushes up when lying on tummy | Cuddle, talk, sing, and play with baby<br>Lay baby on tummy with toys close by |
| 4 | Babbles and copies sounds<br>Reaches for, holds, and shakes toy<br>Recognizes familiar people | Encourage and copy baby's sounds<br>Give age-appropriate toys like rattles<br>Set routines for sleeping and feeding |
| 6 | Responds to others' emotions<br>Begins to say consonant sounds and responds to own name<br>Rolls in both directions | Read books to baby<br>Point and name objects in the environment<br>Play on the floor with baby and encourage rolling over for toys out of reach |
| 9 | Looks for items someone hides and watches path of object falling<br>Pulls self to standing position<br>Uses pincer grasp to feed self | Play games with turn-taking and cause- and-effect, like rolling balls back and forth<br>Provide safe space to move and explore<br>Make finger foods available |
| 12 | Bangs things together and puts things in and out of container<br>Responds to simple requests and says words like "mama" or "dada"<br>Pulls to stand, walks holding furniture, may stand or walk alone | Encourage and praise good behaviour<br>Explain what's happening around child and ask them to label body parts or objects<br>Read, sing songs, and play with child<br>Provide safe environment |
| 18 | Plays pretend, knows what common objects are for, and hands things to others<br>Says several single words<br>Walks alone and pulls objects while walking<br>Eats with spoon and drinks from cup | Describe emotions and encourage empathy<br>Encourage pretend play<br>Provide balls, puzzles, blocks, push/pull toys<br>Encourage drinking and eating independently and do not scold for messiness |

Source: Centers for Disease Control and Prevention. (2018). *Developmental milestones.* Retrieved from http://www.cdc.gov/ncbddd/actearly/milestones/index.html.

## TABLE 11.3   Growth and Development

### Developmental Tasks Accomplished in Infancy

- Achieves physiological equilibrium after birth
- Establishes self as a dependent person, but separate from others
- Becomes aware of animate versus inanimate objects and familiar versus unfamiliar objects, and develops rudimentary social interaction
- Develops a feeling of affection for others and the desire for affection from others
- Manages the changing body and learns new motor skills, develops equilibrium, begins eye–hand coordination, and establishes rest–activity rhythm
- Learns to understand and control the physical world through exploration
- Develops a beginning symbol system, conceptual abilities, and preverbal communication
- Directs emotional expression to indicate needs and wishes

Sources: Centers for Disease Control and Prevention. (2018). *Developmental milestones.* Retrieved from http://www.cdc.gov/ncbddd/actearly/milestones/index.html; The Center for Parenting Education. (2016). *Tasks for infants through 18 months.* Retrieved from http://centerforparentingeducation.org/library-of-articles/child-development/developmental-tasks/#infants.

## Psychosocial Development

Erikson's psychosocial developmental theory is concerned primarily with a series of tasks or crises that each individual must resolve before encountering the next one. The central task during infancy is the development of a sense of trust versus mistrust. This occurs when adults meet an infant's basic needs for survival. The establishment of this basic trust or mistrust determines the manner in which the infant approaches all future stages of growth. The infant develops a sense of trust first in the mother (or other caregiver), and then in other significant people. Trust influences the infant's future relationships, allowing deeper commitment and intimacy. To develop trust the infant requires maximal gratification and minimal frustration to experience a healthy balance between inner needs and outer satisfaction. If the mother or caretaker is consistently responsive to the infant, meeting the physical and psychological needs, the infant will likely learn to trust his or her caretaker, view the world as a safe place, and grow up to be secure, self-reliant, trusting, cooperative, and helpful toward others.

A prompt, sensitive, and consistent response to the infant's needs helps foster security and trust because it enables the infant to predict what will happen within the environment. When unpredictability and disorganized routines exist, the infant will develop fear, anger, anxiety, and insecurity, which eventually lead to mistrust. The infant can demonstrate desire by crying but depends on the sensitivity and willingness of others to provide relief. If the most important people fail to do this, the infant has little foundation on which to build faith in others or self in adulthood. If the infant's needs are not met appropriately, the infant will grow up with a sense of mistrust and may view the world as unpredictable.

## Cognitive Development

Piaget's theory of cognitive development focuses on intellectual changes that occur in a sequential manner as a result of continual interaction between the infant and the environment. The theory is based on the idea that infants actively construct knowledge as they explore and manipulate the world around them (Carey, Zaitchik, & Bascandziez, 2015). Piaget's sensorimotor period (up to age 18 months) describes the time during which infants develop the coordination to master activities that allow them to interact with the environment. During this period the infant solves problems using sensory systems and motor activity rather than symbolic processes, which develop later.

Fetuses are able to distinguish light from dark, and sight is present at birth. Rod cells in the retina of the eyes, which are responsible for light perception, are functional at birth although the retina (the organ of visual perception) is not fully developed until approximately 4 months of age. The newborn infant can perceive colour and shape, and can focus on objects up to 25 cm (10 inches) from their face. Infants are startled by loud noises and are soothed by soft voices, indicating that their sense of hearing is functioning. Their hearing can also be tested with audio equipment at birth, a service that is routinely offered free of charge in several Canadian provinces and territories. Babies cry in response to painful stimuli and fuss when too hot or too cold; therefore, the senses of pain and temperature are also operative. Touching, stroking, and rocking typically comfort a fussing infant. Infants will also react to odours and tastes.

In addition to perceiving stimulation, the newborn is capable of reflexive behaviour. Reflexes are involuntary muscle responses that are normally exhibited after particular types of new stimulation (MedlinePlus, 2017a). These serve as important signs of nervous system development, and some infant reflexes, such as rooting and sucking, have survival value. The rooting reflex, activated by the angle of the lips or cheek being lightly stroked, helps the infant locate the food source. The infant will turn toward the side that is being stroked and will open the lips to suck. The sucking reflex is initiated when an object is placed in the infant's mouth. Together these reflexes ensure that the infant can obtain food. Infants also have reflexes that result in grasping, yawning, coughing, and sneezing. Armed with these reflexes and sensory capabilities, the infant is ready to begin interacting with the environment (seeing, hearing, touching, tasting, and smelling) to acquire valuable information.

The infant progresses in various ways between birth and age 18 months, with early capabilities changing and becoming intentional. Piaget outlines five stages within the sensorimotor period that describe the infant's development, from the early reflexive behaviour to differentiation between self and the environment (Table 11.4).

The infant in the sensorimotor period uses behavioural strategies to manipulate objects, to learn some of their properties, and to reach goals by combining several behaviours. The infant's behaviour is tied to the concrete and the immediate; schemes can be applied only to objects that can be perceived directly.

Knowledge of child developmental theories is extremely valuable to the nurse during interactions with infants. Understanding the infant's level of cognitive thought and emotional and social development helps the nurse decipher a child's communications more meaningfully and interpret behaviours and the processes that motivate the child more accurately.

## TABLE 11.4  Growth and Development
### Piaget's Five Stages of Infant Development

| Stage | Description |
|---|---|
| 1: birth to 1 month | Practice and modification of reflexes in response to new objects |
| 2: 1–4 months | Primary circular reactions: repeats reflexive actions that were previously enjoyed |
|  | Only the infant's own body is involved in activities |
|  | Begins to notice when objects disappear |
| 3: 4–8 months | Secondary circular reactions: repetitions involve objects in the external world |
|  | Appears to perform actions with a purpose |
| 4: 8–12 months | Engages in goal-directed actions |
|  | Combines two or more previously acquired strategies to obtain a goal |
| 5: 12–18 months | Uses active experimentation to achieve previously unattainable goals |
|  | Infant uses trial-and-error processes and observes results |

Source: Cherry, K. (2017). Piaget's stages of cognitive development. *Explore psychology.* Retrieved from https://www.explorepsychology.com/piagets-stages-cognitive-development/.

This knowledge can be incorporated in the anticipatory guidance offered to the parents. The nurse stresses that a variety of sensory and motor stimuli foster learning within the infant's environment.

To assist the nurse and parent in assessment of infant development, the Looksee Checklist (formerly the Nipissing District Developmental Screening [NDDS]), is an assessment tool that screens children from birth to 6 years of age (NDDS, 2019). A series of age-specific checklists track developmental skills in the areas of vision, hearing, communication, fine motor, gross motor, cognitive, social, emotional, and self-help. Parents complete a short list of yes/no questions and are advised to contact their health care provider if they answer "no" to any of the questions. Each checklist includes parenting tips to support the child's development.

The Rourke Baby Record is another common developmental screening tool used in primary care during well-baby/child visits (Rourke, Leduc, & Rourke, 2017). The Rourke Baby Record includes sections for the health care provider to monitor developmental milestones, growth and nutrition, physical examinations, immunizations, and provide anticipatory guidance for health promotion for children 1 month to 5 years of age.

The infant's growth trajectory is also important. Physical growth is a valid health status indicator that can provide early indication of health or nutritional problems. The nurse plots the infant's length, weight, and head circumference measurements on growth charts during each well-baby visit to observe for trends or disturbances in growth over time. The corrected age (actual age minus number of weeks the infant was preterm) is used to plot measurements for premature infants, and monitoring of body mass index (BMI) is recommended, beginning at 2 years old (Canadian Paediatric Society [CPS], 2018a). In 2006, the World Health Organization (WHO) released new international growth charts for children from birth to age 5 that represent the growth of children under economic conditions that support recommended health and nutritional practices, including infants who are primarily breastfed (CPS, 2018a). These charts were further adapted for use in Canada in 2014 and are recommended by the CPS as the tool of choice for monitoring child growth in primary care, community, and hospital settings. The nurse should have the skills and knowledge to accurately measure length/height, weight, and head circumference; plot anthropometric measurements on the growth chart; interpret trends in growth; and counsel parents, regarding their child's growth and development, with referral to a lactation consultant, dietitian, physician, or pediatrician if indicated.

## Sex

The infant's biological sex is determined at the moment of fertilization. Immediately after childbirth, the parents may ask, "Is it a girl or a boy?" The answer has far-reaching implications for many family units. Sex is one of the many important factors that influence parents' way of relating to the infant.

There are many biological and behavioural differences between male and female infants. Boys are, on average, larger and have proportionately more muscle mass at birth. Girls are generally smaller but physiologically more mature at birth and are less vulnerable to stress. Boys show more motor activity, whereas girls display a greater response to tactile stimulation and pain (Polan & Taylor, 2015). As the infant develops, further differences are noted. By 6 months, girls respond to visual stimulation with longer attention spans and are more socially responsive than are boys; girls also tend to sit up, walk, and crawl earlier than do boys. Girls also learn to communicate with language at an earlier age, whereas male infants use their whole bodies in communicating (Kail & Cavanaugh, 2015).

The sex of the infant, a major concern of many expectant parents, may well influence parental relationships and expectations. When stereotypes exist about fixed gender identities and expected gender roles, the infant's sex can evoke disappointment. In some cultures, having a male child is seen to be more socially and economically advantageous (Pulver, Ramraj, Ray, et al., 2016). Canada's population growth relies on immigration due to an aging population and declining fertility rates (El-Assal & Fields, 2018). Yet among some newcomers, a preference for sons and discrimination toward female children has persisted after immigration to Western countries (Pulver et al., 2016). At the same time, families of Western cultures tend to favour a "balanced family" in which they desire one child of each sex (Lowe, 2015). The importance and meaning of gender to parents should be explored by the nurse.

Health intervention focuses on the identification of high-risk families and the promotion of positive relationships between infants and parents. The nurse promotes the good health and developmental potential of the infant. Increasing the parents' feelings of adequacy and self-esteem will promote their acceptance and care of the infant. Most importantly, follow-up care for these families is a high priority to ensure that adequate support and help are available.

## Race and Ethnicity

Race and ethnicity are complex and dynamic concepts that have no consistent definition (Stevens, Ishizawa, & Grbic, 2015). Race generally refers to the classification of human beings into groups based on particular physical characteristics attributable to a common inheritance, such as skin colour, eye shape, and hair texture. Ethnicity is commonly associated with cultural characteristics such as language and religion (Stevens et al., 2015). While race has historically been used to explain patterns in health and illness, some consider this to be scientific racism and argue that "the classification of human beings into a small number of large population groups with defined biological and genetic differences is not warranted by any existing scientific data" (Perez-Rodriguez & de la Fuente, 2017, p. 38). Rather, race is considered to be a social construct and an important social determinant of health (Mikkonen & Raphael, 2010).

Race and ethnicity are primarily linked to health through social processes such as discrimination and social exclusion, and it is argued that social and economic conditions account for the health inequalities among minority populations rather than genetics (Ramraj, Shahidi, Darity, et al., 2016). When compared to White Canadians, Indigenous and Black Canadians have higher rates of chronic health conditions and poor self-rated health (Ramraj et al., 2016; Veenstra & Patterson, 2016). Infant mortality rates among Indigenous populations are more than two times higher than for non-Indigenous people, with higher rates of preterm birth, large-for-gestational age infants, stillbirths, and death from sudden infant death syndrome (SIDS) (Sheppard, Shapiro, Bushnik, et al., 2017). In addition to inequities in socioeconomic status, Indigenous peoples' health is affected by poor access to health care services and the long-term effects of colonization. Despite a growing awareness of the history of colonial practices such as residential schools and forced sterilization of Indigenous women, research suggests that racial stereotypes and stigma toward Indigenous peoples persists within health care institutions today (Goodman, Fleming, Markwick, et al., 2017). Providing culturally competent care requires nurses to be knowledgeable of families' broader social, cultural, economic, and historical context. Awareness of the context within which infants are born allows nurses to make referrals for community supports, advocate for resources, and seek upstream approaches to addressing health inequities in order to give children the best start in life.

## Genetics

In the past several decades, remarkable progress has been made in our understanding of the structure and function of genes and chromosomes. These advances have been aided by the complete sequencing of human DNA—our genome. This knowledge can now be applied to medical care. The desired and expected outcome of any pregnancy is the birth of a healthy baby. Parents experience disappointment when they discover that their baby has been born with a defect. A birth defect is an abnormality of structure, function, or metabolism as a result of a genetic or environmental influence on the fetus, often a combination of both. Couples may refrain from having another child because they have had one with a serious birth defect and do not want to risk another. In these situations, genetic counselling provides information that is needed to understand a hereditary disorder and its associated risks. The main goal of counselling is to explain birth defects to affected families and to allow prospective parents to make informed decisions about child-bearing.

Using the basic laws governing heredity and knowing the frequency of specific birth defects in the population, the genetic counsellor can often predict the probability of recurrence of a given abnormality in the same family. An important aspect of primary prevention is identifying families at increased risk and referring them for counselling (Nussbaum, McInnes, & Willard, 2016). The aspects to be reviewed in the initial interview include the following:

- *Maternal age.* The risk of having a child with Down syndrome increases significantly for the woman older than 35 years. In Down syndrome, there are three chromosomes in the 21 chromosome group (trisomy 21). Characteristic features of Down syndrome include almond-shaped eyes; small head, ears, and mouth; large, protruding tongue; broad, short hands and feet; low muscle tone; and some degree of developmental disability.
- *Ethnic background.* Several genetic disorders occur with higher frequency in certain groups due to a shared genetic inheritance. Anyone can be a carrier of Tay–Sachs disease, but the disease is most common among French-Canadians, Louisiana Cajuns, and the Ashkenazi Jewish population (National Tay-Sachs & Allied Diseases Association, 2016). People with African ancestry have a greater chance of carrying the sickle cell trait than the general population, and approximately 500 Canadians are currently living with a group of inherited red blood cell disorders called sickle cell disease (Sickle Cell Disease Association of Canada, 2018).
- *Family history.* Certain diseases, such as Huntington's disease and hemophilia, are hereditary. Huntington's disease is a neuro-degenerative disease characterized by emotional symptoms, deterioration of cognitive functions, and involuntary movements. Once symptoms have manifested themselves, a steady deterioration leads to death in approximately 10 to 30 years (National Institute of Neurological Disorders and Stroke, 2018). Approximately 7000 Canadians have Huntington's disease, and each of their children has a 50% chance of developing it (Huntington Society of Canada, 2017). Hemophilia is a coagulation disorder caused by a deficiency of a clotting factor; it leads to frequent and prolonged bleeding that can be life threatening. Approximately 3100 Canadians are presently living with hemophilia (Canadian Hemophilia Society, n.d.).
- *Reproductive history.* Spontaneous abortions, stillbirths, and previous live-born children with birth defects or slow development may indicate an increased risk.
- *Maternal disease.* Several maternal disorders are associated with a higher frequency of birth defects, including diabetes mellitus, seizure disorder, mental health disorder, and phenylketonuria. Prenatal diagnosis offers the couple the option of aborting a fetus that has certain genetic disorders. For many people, however, this option is unacceptable. Chapter 10 discusses the various tests used for prenatal diagnosis.

The nurse's role throughout the genetic counselling process is to provide the vital link between the counselling team and the high-risk couple. Nurses need to understand not only the foundations of genetics and genomics but also the implications of these sciences for those for whom they provide care. The nurse is involved in case finding, referral, and family education. As a result of the new and expanding technology devoted to genetic and genomic research, a growing number of genetic tests are available for the screening, diagnosis, and treatment of rare and common diseases. All nurses will need to become knowledgeable about the basics of genetics and genomics and their applications to clinical care so that they can provide quality health care that is appropriate to their setting, population, geographical location, access, and coverage. This knowledge will allow nurses to provide appropriate information to care recipients regarding genetic tests that are part of their own health care (Lopes, de Omena Bomfim, & Flória-Santos, 2015).

## ❖ GORDON'S FUNCTIONAL HEALTH PATTERNS

### ◆ Health Perception–Health Management Pattern

An important aspect of health promotion is aimed at assisting the infant and the infant's family to adopt behaviours to produce better physical and emotional health in adulthood. To reach this goal, the nurse encourages child-rearing practices that promote normal growth and development, and fosters attitudes and values compatible with health. Health promotion by nurses aims to prevent and minimize ill health of all individuals and their families. Nurses engage families in strategies to maintain health, support families in their decision making concerning their own health, and help families that need to negotiate the health care system (Arnold & Boggs, 2016). The nurse promotes the infant's health through the parents, who determine the care practices for the dependent infant.

Health is largely a subjective judgement. One's perception of health refers to physical, mental, and social well-being rather than the absence of disease (Public Health Agency of Canada [PHAC], 2016). The determinants of health include genetics and lifestyle, as well as a wide range of social, economic, and environmental factors (Government of Canada, 2018a). Promoting the health of an infant is additionally influenced by parental self-efficacy, which refers to parents' belief in their parenting competence and capacity to support their child's development (Amin, Tam, & Shorey, 2018). With this understanding, the nurse uses every opportunity to convey confidence in the parents' health perception–health management pattern and to improve their ability to implement behaviours that promote the infant's health. When parents learn and adopt behaviours that improve their own health, they are more likely to ensure that the health needs of their infant are met. Parental modelling of a healthy lifestyle increases the chances that good health practices will be retained throughout the child's life.

The goals of nursing practice with infants and their families are to promote individual motivation for health, to assist the family to identify health needs, and to develop problem-solving skills within the family unit using the family's own strengths and resources. To meet these goals, the nurse identifies the family's perception of good or poor health practices, which greatly influences participation in health-promoting activities. Age, gender, educational level, culture, income, and occupation combine to influence health perception. When parents believe that the infant is more susceptible to a health problem if promotional behaviour is not enacted, they become more motivated to adopt the behaviour.

The nurse helps the parents recognize their infant's susceptibility and the potential consequences when healthy practices are not instituted. The nurse works within the family's health perception framework to become acquainted with the characteristics that influence the infant's health. Unless caregivers meet their own personal needs, they will be unable to meet their infant's developmental needs. The empowerment and growth of parents is a key element to facilitate the successful development of their infants. The nurse supports the parents, strengthening their parental self-efficacy, providing information on meeting their infant's needs, and reinforcing their health perception–health management pattern.

While health management is influenced by the parents' knowledge, choices made, and behaviours adopted, other factors such as income, education, housing, and food security all play an important role in shaping the infant's opportunity for good health (PHAC, 2016). Health promotion, therefore, requires nurses to move beyond addressing lifestyle factors and consider how the social determinants of health can be addressed at the individual, community, and societal levels. By drawing the family's attention to the relationship between these social factors and health, the nurse can broaden their perception of what constitutes a healthy environment for raising a child and support health management by making referrals to appropriate supports and services, such as collective kitchens, housing and child care subsidies, employment services, and education or retraining opportunities.

## ◆ Nutritional-Metabolic Pattern

One of the most important aspects of health promotion in the infant is nutritional status. Many opinions have been expressed about the infant's nutritional needs. As research in this area continues, recommendations and opinions will change; however, some basic facts about nutrition remain fairly consistent. During the infancy period, it is all about milk—breast milk or formula. Milk will provide practically every nutrient the infant needs for the first year of life. Infant nutritional requirements are based on what is considered necessary to support life, provide for growth, and maintain health.

### Essential Nutrients

During infancy, a period of rapid growth, nutrient requirements per kilogram of body weight are proportionally higher than at any other time in the life cycle. Water, proteins, fats, carbohydrates, vitamins, and minerals are the essential nutrients in any diet. Because the first year of life is a period of rapid growth, nutritional needs during this period are especially important and always changing. Water is vital to survival. A person can live for several weeks without food but can survive only a few days without water. Because the infant's body weight is approximately 75% water, the baby must consume large amounts of fluid to maintain water balance. Under normal circumstances the water requirements of healthy infants who are fed adequate amounts of breast milk or properly

reconstituted infant formula are met by the breast milk or infant formula alone. Supplemental water is not necessary, even in hot, dry climates—in fact, breast milk composition adapts to the weather, with increasing water content during hot temperatures (La Leche League Canada, 2015).

The infant must also consume sufficient high-quality protein to facilitate growth and development. The recommended daily protein requirements are 9.1 g during the first 6 months and 11 g during the second 6 months (Government of Canada, 2006). No more than 20% of an infant's daily energy requirement should come from protein because infants are not able to process and excrete the excess nitrogen from higher-protein diets (US Department of Agriculture [USDA], 2015).

Carbohydrates should supply 30% to 60% of the energy intake during infancy. Approximately 37% of the calories in human milk and 40% to 50% of the calories in commercial formulas are derived from lactose or other carbohydrates. The recommended daily intake of carbohydrates is 60 g for infants up to 6 months of age and 95 g for infants 7 to 12 months old (Government of Canada, 2006).

For infants, 31 g of fats per day for the first 6 months of life and 30 g of fats per day during the second 6 months of life (approximately 40%–50% of the calories) are recommended (Government of Canada, 2006). These quantities are present in human milk and in all formulas prepared for infants. Significantly lower intakes, such as in cow and goat milk or plant-based milks, can result in an inadequate energy intake and are inappropriate substitutes for breast milk or formula (Health Canada, CPS, Dietitians of Canada, et al., 2015a).

Vitamins are essential nutrients in the infant's diet that regulate metabolism and allow more efficient use of carbohydrates, fats, and proteins within the body. Although most infants receive adequate vitamin intake through formula, breast milk, and food, recent research has raised a concern about a vitamin D deficiency in infants who receive only breast milk. Vitamin D deficiency causes rickets, a disorder involving poor mineralization and formation of bones. Since sunlight is the primary source of vitamin D, and infants are supposed to avoid direct sunlight for the first year of life, a vitamin D supplement of 400 IU is recommended for all breastfed infants from birth to 1 year old (Health Canada et al., 2015a).

Minerals are found in relatively small amounts in the infant's body but are vital elements in body structure and control of certain body functions. Mineral intake for infants appears to be adequate, except for iron. The full-term infant is born with stores of iron adequate to meet the needs for hemoglobin production for approximately 6 months. After this time, body stores need to be replenished to avoid iron-deficiency anemia. Although iron in human milk is bioavailable, both breastfed and formula-fed infants should receive an additional source of iron by 6 months of age. Meat, meat alternatives, and iron-fortified cereals are good sources of iron and therefore recommended as the infant's first foods. These can be paired with foods high in vitamin C to help with iron absorption (CPS, 2019a).

## RESEARCH FOR EVIDENCE-INFORMED PRACTICE

### Creating Exclusive Breastfeeding Knowledge Translation Tools With First Nations Mothers in Northwest Territories, Canada

*Background.* Breastfeeding is an ideal method of infant feeding that affects life-long health, and yet the uptake of breastfeeding in some Indigenous communities in Canada's north is low.

*Objective.* To determine the rate and determinants of exclusive breastfeeding in a remote community in the Northwest Territories (NWT) and to create knowledge translation tools to enhance breastfeeding locally.

*Methods.* First, a series of retrospective chart audits were conducted from hospital birth records and the local community health centre of women ($n = 198$) who gave birth from January 1, 2010, to December 31, 2012. Data collected included demographics and rate of exclusive breastfeeding. Second, semi-structured interviews with a purposive sample of mothers ($n = 8$) and one Elder were conducted to identify breastfeeding practices, beliefs, and the most appropriate medium to use to deliver health messages. Based on this information, two knowledge translation tools were developed in collaboration with a local community advisory committee.

*Results.* The rate of exclusive breastfeeding initiation in this remote region of the NWT was less than 30%. Thematic analysis revealed two overarching themes from the data: namely, "the pull to formula" (lifestyle preferences, drug and alcohol use, supplementation practices, and limited role models) and "the pull to breastfeeding" (traditional feeding method, spiritual practice, and increased bonding with infant).

*Conclusion.* There are a myriad of influences on breastfeeding for women who live in remote locations. Ultimately, society informs the choice of infant feeding for the new mother, since mothers' feeding choices are based on contextual realities and circumstances in their lives that are out of their control. As health care providers, it is imperative that we recognize the realities of women's lives and the overlapping social determinants of health that may limit a mother's ability or choice to breastfeed. Further health-promotion efforts—grounded in community-based research and a social determinants framework—are needed to improve prenatal and postnatal care of Indigenous women and children in Canada.

Source: Modified from Moffit, P., & Dickinson, R. (2016). Creating exclusive breastfeeding knowledge translation tools with First Nations mothers in Northwest Territories, Canada. *International Journal of Circumpolar Health, 75*(1). https://doi.org/10.3402/ijch.v75.32989.

A review of these requirements shows that breast milk or formula plus a vitamin D supplement meets most of the infant's nutritional needs. No data support the theory that solid foods are needed to meet these nutritional needs during the first 6 months of life.

### Breastfeeding

An infant's first and preferred source of nutrition should be breast milk. Ongoing evidence-informed practice findings strongly indicate that the lifelong health from breastfeeding that is bestowed on the infant also greatly contributes to the health status of the mother, the family, and society at large (Best Start Resource Centre, 2017a). Research throughout the years has demonstrated unequivocally that exclusive breastfeeding is the preferred method of infant feeding for the first 6 months of life, and should be encouraged for 2 years and beyond with appropriate complementary feeding (Health Canada et al., 2015a). Breast milk is often called the perfect food for the infant and for the mother, because of its composition and because it does not have to be purchased, cooked, or stored. The composition of breast milk changes during feedings and over time to accommodate the needs of the infant, and includes immunoglobulins and white blood cells to help prevent infections. Breastfeeding has been shown to improve children's cognitive development and reduce the risk of gastrointestinal illness, otitis media, respiratory infections, SIDS, and obesity (Health Canada et al., 2015a). Most women in Canada intend to breastfeed, and 90% of women initiate breastfeeding shortly after birth (PHAC, 2018a). Women in their 30s and with higher levels of education are more likely to breastfeed and for a longer duration, while the social determinants of health can limit some women's ability and choice to breastfeed (Research for Evidence-Informed Practice). Only

26% of women breastfeed exclusively to 6 months, with many citing an inadequate supply of breast milk (a rare condition) as their reason for stopping (Statistics Canada, 2015a). These statistics demonstrate that breastfeeding mothers need support from skilled and knowledgeable nurses in the immediate postpartum period and throughout the first years of an infant's life. Breastfeeding supports should provide a seamless transition between the hospital and community, and should include partners and families, offer peer-support programs, and provide help or advice 24/7 to improve breastfeeding outcomes in Canada (PHAC, 2018a).

WHO and the United Nations Children's Fund (UNICEF) developed the Baby-Friendly Hospital Initiative in 1991 in a global effort to increase breastfeeding (Breastfeeding Committee for Canada, 2017). Canada has adapted the international standards for the Canadian context and renamed it the Baby-Friendly Initiative to reflect the continuum of care. To become a baby-friendly facility in Canada, the 10 steps to successful breastfeeding must be implemented, as outlined in Box 11.1.

Women's decisions of whether to breastfeed are influenced in part by information they receive from their health care providers. Breastfeeding guidance given in the postpartum period that is congruent, sensitive, and effective increases the mother's knowledge and opportunity for breastfeeding success, whereas low levels of actual or perceived professional support are associated with higher use of formula (Radzyminski & Callister, 2015; Santos, Franca, Fernandes, et al., 2015). Because of their important role in the mother's choice of infant feeding, nurses can be instrumental in working toward increased breastfeeding rates by educating all women about the advantages of the practice (Box 11.2). In addition to professional support, breastfeeding initiation and

## BOX 11.1 Baby-Friendly Initiative: 10 Steps

- Have a written infant feeding policy that is communicated routinely to all staff, health care providers, and volunteers.
- Ensure that all staff, health care providers, and volunteers have the knowledge and skills necessary to implement the infant feeding policy.
- Inform pregnant women and their families about the importance and process of breastfeeding.
- Place babies in uninterrupted skin-to-skin contact with their mothers immediately following birth for at least 1 hour or until completion of the first feeding, or for as long as the mother wishes. Encourage mothers to recognize when their babies are ready to feed, offering help as needed.
- Assist mothers to breastfeed and maintain lactation should they face challenges, including separation from their infants.
- Support mothers to exclusively breastfeed for the first 6 months, unless supplements are medically indicated.
- Facilitate 24-hour rooming-in for all mother–infant dyads: mothers and infants remain together.
- Encourage responsive, cue-based feeding. Encourage sustained breastfeeding beyond 6 months with appropriate introduction of complementary foods.
- Support mothers to feed and care for their breastfeeding babies without the use of artificial teats or pacifiers (dummies or soothers).
- Provide a seamless transition between the services provided by the hospital, community health services, and peer-support programs. Apply principles of primary health care and population health to support the continuum of care, and implement strategies that affect the broad determinants that will improve breastfeeding outcomes.

Source: Breastfeeding Committee for Canada. (2017). *The BFI 10 steps and WHO code outcome indicators for hospitals and community health services*. Retrieved from http://breastfeedingcanada.ca/documents/Indicators.pdf.

## BOX 11.2 Advantages of Breastfeeding

**Breast Milk**
- Has the correct balance of all essential nutrients for infants
- Is full of immunological agents to protect against disease
- Is easier to digest than is formula
- Contains anti-inflammatory properties
- Promotes growth of *Lactobacillus bifidus*
- Reduces risk of childhood obesity, ear infections, and diabetes
- Reduces risk of allergies, asthma, and respiratory viruses
- Reduces risk of SIDS
- Reduces risk of overweight and obesity into adulthood

**Breastfeeding**
- Is cheaper and more convenient than formula
- Provides a unique bonding experience for both the infant and the mother
- Assists in the process of uterine involution and decreases postpartum vaginal bleeding
- Reduces mother's risk of some cancers, heart disease, diabetes, and osteoporosis
- Decreases environmental burden for disposal of formula cans and bottles
- Promotes weight reduction for new mother
- Delays return of mother's period and helps space pregnancies

*SIDS*, Sudden infant death syndrome.
Sources: Lauwers, J., & Swisher, A. (2016). *Counseling the nursing mother: A lactation consultant's guide* (6th ed.). Burlington, MA: Jones & Bartlett Learning; La Leche League. (2015). *Amazing milk: Made exclusively for babies*. Retrieved from https://www.lllc.ca/sites/lllc.ca/files/410_Amazing-MilkCMYK.pdf.

duration are influenced by societal attitudes toward breastfeeding, body image, conflicting responsibilities, and lack of familial support (Brown, 2017). These factors relate to social and cultural norms, and therefore individualized support and education that places breastfeeding responsibility solely on the mother can miss the opportunity to influence breastfeeding success by focusing on the wider environment and support system. This should include government enforcement of the International Code of Marketing of Breast Milk Substitutes that prohibits promotion of breast milk substitutes for children less than 6 months old, broad public health campaigns to promote acceptance of breastfeeding, increasing community supports for new mothers, and health care systems that support breastfeeding or become accredited as Baby Friendly (Brown, 2017). Policies that protect breastfeeding women from discrimination and require employers to accommodate women to breastfeed or express milk in the workplace (Canadian Human Rights Commission, n.d.) should also be broadly communicated as a strategy to ensure that women feel supported to continue breastfeeding beyond infancy.

Community nurses who are caring for breastfeeding mothers can support them by providing the following advice (and by providing the information presented in the Quality and Safety Scenario):
- You may be very thirsty, so have some water, milk, or juice when baby feeds.
- Watch the infant, not the clock. Look for early signs of wanting-to-feed behaviours.
- Provide your breastfeeding infant a vitamin D supplement of 400 IU.
- Try to rest when the infant sleeps, so you do not become overtired.
- There is no need to change your diet or restrict which foods you eat while you breastfeed; however, alcohol and medications pass into breast milk, so check with your doctor, nurse, midwife, or lactation consultant if you have questions.
- Sore nipples may mean baby is not latched on well; seek assistance regarding your technique.
- Expose nipples to air after each feeding and allow some breast milk to dry on nipples for their lubricating and anti-infective properties.
- You and your baby have the right to breastfeed anywhere, anytime.
- Learn about the use of breast pumps and milk storage, which can allow you to go back to work or school and continue breastfeeding.
- Join breastfeeding support groups for continued help within the community.
- Breastfeeding is more than just supplying nutrients for growth—it contributes to an intimate and special relationship between you and your infant (PHAC, 2015).

### Bottle Feeding

If the mother makes an informed choice to formula-feed rather than breastfeed her infant, it is important that the nurse provide nonjudgemental care and education in a way that supports the mother's autonomy and the therapeutic nurse–patient relationship (Wood, 2018). Mothers who formula-feed have been shown to experience feelings of guilt and stigma associated with their feeding choice and, given the large portion of Canadian women who are using at least some formula by the time their infant is 6 months of age, the risk to maternal well-being can be considered a widespread public health issue (Fallon, Komninou, Bennett, et al., 2017).

The nurse should provide information and resources about safe formula preparation and sterilization, how much and how often the infant should be fed, and how to hold the infant during feeding (Wood, 2018). Instruct the mother about safe preparation of infant formula as follows (Healthy Babies BC, 2018):

- Powdered and liquid concentrate formulas require mixing with boiled water; read and follow instructions carefully.
- Check the expiration date and condition of each container of formula.

- Bring water for mixing with formula to a rolling boil for 2 minutes.
- Wash hands thoroughly before preparing infant formula.
- Prepare the bottles, nipples, and other items by washing them with soap and water. Rinse well. Put all items in a large pot and boil for 2 minutes. Remove with tongs and air dry.
- Store the prepared formula in the refrigerator for no more than 24 hours.
- Warm the formula by placing it in warm water, never in a microwave oven.
- Shake the bottle well and feed the formula to the infant.
- Discard any formula the infant did not drink within 2 hours.

## ⚡ QUALITY AND SAFETY SCENARIO

### How to Hold Your Infant for Breastfeeding

- Have a bib or cloth ready to clean up spit-up.
- Sit comfortably and cradle the infant closely against your body.
- Keep the infant's head slightly higher than the body.
- Watch the infant drink; look for cues of being finished.
- Burp the infant half-way through the feed to help reduce spit-up.

#### How to Hold Your Infant for Breastfeeding
- Sit or lie down comfortably with your back supported.
- Make sure the infant has one arm on either side of your breast as you pull him/her close.
- Use firm pillows or folded blankets under the infant as a means of support during the feeding.
  As the infant gets older, the extra support will likely be unnecessary.
- Support the infant's back and shoulders firmly.
- Do not push on the back of the infant's head.
- The infant's face and body should be turned toward you, with the hip, shoulder, and ear all aligned.
- Touch the infant's top lip to your nipple; after the infant's mouth is open wide, pull him/her to your breast.

#### Three Common Breastfeeding Positions (Fig. 11.1)
*Football Hold*
- Hold the infant's back and shoulders in the palm of your hand.
- Tuck the infant up under your arm, keeping the infant's ear, shoulder, and hip in a straight line.
- Support the breast. After the infant's mouth is open wide, pull him/her quickly to you.
- Continue to hold your breast until the baby feeds easily.

*Lying Down*
- Lie on your side with a pillow at your back and lay the infant such that you are facing each other.
- To begin, prop yourself up on your elbow and support your breast with that hand.
- Pull the infant close to you, lining up his/her mouth with your nipple.
- After the infant is feeding well, lie back down. Hold your breast with the opposite hand.

- Cradle the infant in the arm closest to the breast with his/her head in the crook of your arm.
- Have the infant's body facing you, tummy to tummy.
- Use your opposite hand to support the breast.

*Across the Lap (Modified Cradle Hold)*
- Lay your infant on firm pillows across your lap.
- Turn the infant, facing you.
- Reach across your lap to support the infant's back and shoulders with the palm of your hand.
- Support your breast from underneath to guide it into his/her mouth.

**Breastfeeding Is Going Well When …**
- Your infant is feeding at least eight times in 24 hours. Some infants need to eat more frequently until they learn to breastfeed efficiently. Other infants gain weight although they feed less often.
- At least one breast softens well at each feeding.
- You feel a tug, but not pain, when the infant sucks.
- The infant's arms and shoulders are relaxed during the feeding.
- The infant has bursts of 10 or more sucks and swallows at the beginning of each feeding.
- As your breast softens, the infant slows down to two to three sucks and swallows at a time.
- Your infant is content when you finish breastfeeding.
- You see at least one wet diaper for each day of your infant's age (e.g., three wet diapers on day 3), up until day 5, and at least six wet diapers daily thereafter.
- Baby loses weight for the first 3 days, but regains birth weight by 10 to 14 days
- Signs that a good attachment has been made are:
  - The infant's nose is free from the breast.
  - The infant's chin is firmly pressed against the breast.
  - The infant has round cheeks.
- If any areola is visible, it should be more above the top lip versus the bottom lip.

Sources: Best Start Resource Centre. (2017). *Breastfeeding guidelines for consultants.* Retrieved from https://www.beststart.org/resources/breastfeeding/pdf/breastfdeskref09.pdf; Lauwers, J., & Swisher, A. (2016). *Counseling the nursing mother: A lactation consultant's guide* (6th ed.). Burlington, MA: Jones & Bartlett Learning.

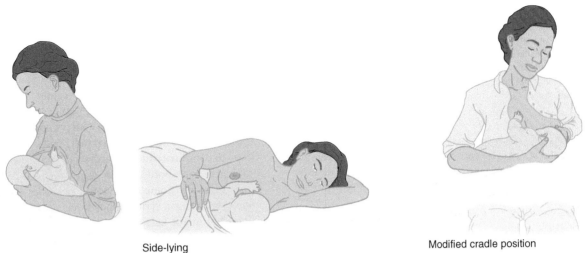

Football hold               Side-lying               Modified cradle position

**Fig. 11.1** Breastfeeding positions: (A) Football hold. (B) Side-lying. (C) Across the lap (modified cradle hold). (From HealthyFamilies BC. [2013]. *Breastfeeding positions*. Retrieved from https://www.healthyfamiliesbc. ca/home/articles/breastfeeding-positions.)

## Introduction of Solid Foods

The timing of the first introduction of solid food during infancy may have potential effects on lifelong health. Most children are physiologically and developmentally ready for their first foods at about 6 months of age (CPS, 2019b). The infant should be able to do the following developmental tasks before solid foods are introduced: sit with support, have good head and neck control, keep food in their mouth without pushing it out with their tongue, lean forward and open mouth when interested in food, and turn away when not hungry (CPS, 2019b). The risks of introducing complementary foods too early include eczema, diabetes, and overweight status at a later age, yet research finds that most mothers are introducing solids before 6 months (Fegan, Bassett, Peng, et al., 2017). Therefore support within the community and awareness campaigns about the timing of introduction to solid foods are needed to promote adherence to Health Canada's Nutrition for Healthy Term Infant recommendations.

The addition of foods should be governed by an infant's nutritional needs and readiness to handle different forms of foods (Brown & Rowan, 2016). Since an infant's stores of iron will be depleted around 6 months of age, it is important that a source of iron be added to the diet to prevent the development of iron-deficiency anemia. It is recommended that iron-rich foods be among the first solids introduced to the infant, and that they are served daily (Health Canada et al., 2015a). Meats, meat alternatives (such as eggs, tofu, legumes), and iron-fortified cereals are all good choices. Other foods, such as pureed fruits and vegetables, dairy products like yogurt and cheese, and grains like toast or rice, can be introduced according to culture and family preferences. It is recommended that salt, sugar, and spices be avoided, as well as choking hazards in the form of round-shaped foods like whole grapes or hotdogs (CPS, 2019b). Infants should also avoid honey until they are older than 1 year of age, due to the risk of botulism.

Parents should expose their children to a variety of tastes, colours, and textures. To support the developing neuro-muscular system, textures should be soft at 6 months (minced, pureed, mashed, or ground), progressing to lumpy textures by 8 months as the biting motion is developing, and to the texture of a range of typical family foods of tender consistency by 12 to 18 months when children acquire full chewing movements (Health Canada et al., 2015b). Finger foods should be offered all along to support infants' oral and motor development. Begin with safe textures, including pieces of soft-cooked vegetables, ripe fruit such as banana, grated cheese, and pieces of bread or toast (Health Canada et al., 2015b). Children can eat soft food from a spoon between 6 and 9 months of age, and try to use a spoon independently between 9 and 12 months of age (CPS, 2019b). Breast milk or formula will remain the most important drink until the child is at least 12 months of age, supplying approximately half of the energy needs of the infant, while food provides the other half (Health Canada et al., 2015b). However, older infants may be offered water from an open cup. Juice is not necessary, nor is it recommended, due to its association with diarrhea, dental caries, and the potential that it will reduce the infant's appetite for more nutritious foods (CPS, 2019b).

When teaching parents about the introduction of foods to their infants, it is important to emphasize their role in creating a positive and supportive environment that fosters healthy eating skills (Health Canada et al., 2015b). Parents should be encouraged to be sensitive to their infant's cues indicating hunger and satiety, allow their child to guide feeding by trusting their ability to decide when and how much to eat, and adjust expectations for eating behaviours based on the child's developmental stage. A few tips to assist parents in making the introduction of solid foods a smooth transition are listed in Box 11.3.

## Food Additives

In addition to their questionable nutritional value, additives in commercial baby food can negatively influence an infant's health status. The purposes of food additives differ, including adding nutritional value; preserving or extending shelf life; facilitating preparation; improving flavour, colour, and texture; and keeping flavours and textures consistent (WHO, 2015).

## BOX 11.3   Tips for Introducing Solid Foods

- The order of giving breast milk/formula or foods first does not seem to matter—decide which to offer first according to preference and the infant's cues.
- The infant's first foods can be many of the same foods that the rest of the family is eating. Buying commercially prepared infant foods is not necessary.
- It may take up to 10 times for a new food to be accepted—keep offering it over time and don't get discouraged.
- When introducing foods that are common allergens, introduce no more than one new food that day, and wait for 2 days to identify if it caused a reaction.
- As the infant learns how to handle solid foods, they may reflexively gag. This is normal.
- Reduce distractions in the environment. Look at, smile at, and talk to the infant during feeding.
- Never try to coerce the infant into eating—respect their hunger and satiety cues.

Sources: Canadian Paediatric Society. (2019b). *Feeding your baby in the first year*. Retrieved from https://www.caringforkids.cps.ca/handouts/feeding_your_baby_in_the_first_year; Health Canada, Canadian Paediatric Society, Dietitians of Canada, & Breastfeeding Committee for Canada. (2015b). *Nutrition for health term infants: Recommendations from six to 24 months*. Retrieved from https://www.canada.ca/en/health-canada/services/canada-food-guide/resources/infant-feeding/nutrition-healthy-term-infants-recommendations-birth-six-months/6-24-months.html.

Commercially prepared baby foods are generally safe, nutritious, and high quality. In response to consumer demand, baby food manufacturers have removed much of the added salt and sugar that their products once contained, and have eliminated most food additives. However, parents should be encouraged to read baby food labels carefully. A parent who wants the infant to have family foods rather than commercial baby food can puree a small portion of the table food at each meal, provided it has been cooked without the addition of salt or sugar. Making baby food is easy and economical. Written resources are available for parents who are interested in more details about home food preparation of food for infants.

### Weaning

Weaning is a gradual, caring process that introduces the infant to a cup, which replaces the bottle or breast. The biological norm and desired method for weaning is to allow the infant to self-wean. Weaning should be started when the infant and mother are ready. Developmentally, the infant can usually learn to use a cup beginning at 6 months; however, since breastfeeding is recommended to 2 years of age and beyond, this developmental milestone can be accomplished by offering small sips of water from an open cup between breastfeedings. For infants who are bottle-fed, the transition to a cup should take place by about 12 months of age and be complete by 18 months of age. This reduces prolonged bottle-feeding, which is associated with risk for dental caries and displacement of nutrient-rich foods (Health Canada et al., 2015b). Cow's milk can be introduced between 9 and 12 months of age, once the infant is eating a wide variety of iron-rich foods, and should not total more than 750 mL per day. Since cow's milk is low in iron, excess cow's milk consumption is a risk factor for iron-deficiency anemia because it displaces other iron-rich foods. Drinking milk from an open cup rather than from a bottle can help prevent excessive consumption (Health Canada et al., 2015b).

Some infants accept the cup readily; other infants are extremely reluctant to give up the bottle, especially the bedtime bottle. Allowing infants to sleep with propped bottles can lead to aspiration if the milk flows too rapidly or the infant becomes too sleepy to coordinate sucking and swallowing. Another potential problem is baby-bottle tooth decay, which involves decay of all upper teeth and some of the lower posterior teeth from direct contact with sugar, syrup, honey-sweetened water, or fruit juice. When the infant falls asleep and stops sucking on the bottle, the sugary solution pools around the infant's teeth and remains there for long periods. The carbohydrate in the solution is fermented into organic acids that demineralize the teeth until they decay. By not using the bottle as a pacifier, parents can prevent this condition.

Some additional tips for counselling parents are as follows:
- Keep a calm, relaxed attitude throughout the weaning process.
- Let the child lead the way; it could take days, weeks, or months.
- Anticipate the previous feeding times and offer a cup or snack instead.
- Do not force an infant to use a cup; it is more detrimental to wean an infant sooner than later.
- Introduce the cup for one feeding per day and progress until the breast or bottle is surrendered.
- Drop a feeding out every few days until the evening feeding is the last one left.
- Be sure the infant is getting enough nutrition from other sources.
- Remember that infants enjoy the accomplishment of using a cup; it is one of their first steps toward independence.
- Make sure to make up the bonding time with your infant by holding and cuddling the infant throughout the day (Williamson & Beatty, 2015).

### Anticipatory Guidance

The infant progresses from a diet of breast milk or formula alone to a diet of milk and solid foods within a short period. Understanding the infant's nutritional needs and developmental capabilities, the nurse can guide the parents in meeting them and, in the process, foster healthy family–infant relationships. The health-promotion activity used in meeting proper infant nutrition focuses on parent education and positive reinforcement of parenting abilities.

### ◆ Elimination Pattern

The infant develops an elimination pattern by the second week of life, usually associated with the frequency, amount, and type of feedings. Both breastfed and formula-fed infants progress from a pattern of having multiple stools per day in the early weeks to fewer stools per day after the first few months of life.

A breastfed infant's stools have a mushy golden-yellow colour and a seedy consistency, with a slightly sour but clean smell, dissimilar to stools passed later in life. A formula-fed infant's stools are firm, pasty, and smellier and resemble those of an infant eating solid food. The breastfed infant has many daily stools during the first and second months of life, progressing to one stool per day or even one stool every 4 to 5 days in the later months before solid foods are introduced. The bottle-fed infant has two to four stools per day during the first month, tapering to one a day or even fewer at the end of infancy (Polan & Taylor, 2015).

For the first year of life an infant cannot control the bowels. Bowel evacuation remains under involuntary, reflexive control until myelination of the spinal cord is complete, usually by 14 to 18 months of age (Kliegman, Stanton, St. Geme, et al., 2015). Nurses advise parents to delay toilet training until the infant is developmentally ready, most often between 2 and 4 years of age. The nurse also reassures breastfeeding parents who may become concerned if their infant goes for several days without having a bowel movement. When the infant's behaviour, feeding, and sleeping patterns are normal, no elimination problem exists. A breastfed infant rarely becomes constipated when consuming adequate amounts of breast milk. Urination increases as fluid intake increases. An infant who voids 6 to 12 times a day during the first few months of life is usually healthy and well hydrated. Voiding is involuntary until sometime during the second year of life, when bladder sensation develops. Irregular patterns of voiding characterize the remaining period of infancy.

### Anticipatory Guidance

Anticipatory guidance and health promotion concerning elimination patterns of the infant consist of parental teaching and reassurance, with special emphasis on good hygienic practices. For breastfeeding mothers, the infant's output is an important way of knowing whether the baby is feeding well and getting an adequate amount of breast milk. This requires the nurse to be aware of the early elimination pattern for effective teaching (see https://www.beststart.org/resources/breastfeeding/pdf/breastfdeskref09.pdf). Reassuring the parents about the infant's inability to control elimination is also important, so that their expectations are realistic.

### ◆ Activity-Exercise Pattern

Physical activity and exercise contribute to development and coordination throughout the life span; infants receive their exercise through play. Initially, infants engage in play with themselves, with their hands or feet, by responding to various sounds, and by rolling and getting into various positions. By manipulating objects and achieving pleasurable sensations, infants learn about themselves and the objects in the environment.

### Activity Through Play

Play is crucial for an infant's social, emotional, physical, and cognitive growth. Exploration is the heart of play, as it is how infants learn about their body and the world around them.

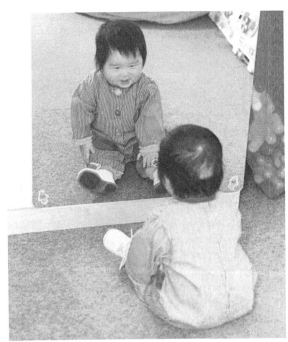

**Fig. 11.2** The Infant Enjoys Looking at Himself in the Mirror (From Hockenberry, M. J., & Wilson, D. [Eds.]. [2013]. *Wong's essentials of pediatric nursing* [9th ed.]. St. Louis: Mosby.)

Although the word *play* suggests physical activity, the infant's first play is actually an exercise of the senses. The infant's first toys are visual. Through play, infants learn to hone their senses, to exercise their physical abilities, and to relate to other people. Most of the infant's play is solitary and repetitious. As each discovery is made, self-confidence and pride in the achievement are reinforced (as is the skill) through repetition.

As the infant enters the second half of the first year and becomes mobile, the family should provide the infant with increasing opportunities for spontaneous play and exploration. A planned play period in a safe environment should be established. The infant should have unrestrictive clothing so that movement can be free and unhampered. The caregiver should not interfere directly with the play but should be attentive to the infant's needs.

An important nursing role is assisting parents to promote play, stressing the importance of providing opportunities that are appropriate for the infant's age. Buying expensive toys is unnecessary; common household items, such as pots, pans, lids, and spoons, provide excellent objects for play purposes.

### Activity Through Stimulation

Parental stimulation of the infant is an important developmental technique; the infant needs stimulation to learn about the world. This activity does not require expensive objects, but rather involves experiences in sight, sound, and touch that are free and can be provided by any parent (Fig. 11.2). Stimulation should include face-to-face interactions rather than screen time (TV, smart phones, computers, etc.), which does not support children's development at a young age and instead has been associated with lower cognitive ability, including language delays (CPS, 2017a). The CPS does not recommend any screen time for children younger than age 2. Examples of stimulating experiences for infants include the following:

- Having lullabies sung to them
- Listening to audio recordings of a heartbeat
- Seeing colourful mobiles in the crib
- Being rocked in a rocking chair
- Having a familiar face smiling close by
- Having space to wander when developmentally ready
- Looking at themselves in mirrors
- Listening to music

### Anticipatory Guidance

Knowledge of developmental milestones and early brain development allows the nurse to guide parents in proper play and stimulation for infants. Handing a 15-month-old child a ball and placing the child in a fenced-in back yard to play is not enough. These activities must provide interpersonal contact, activity, and exercise. Activity and exercise through stimulation and play are extremely important for healthy development (Johnson, Eberle, Henricks, et al., 2015).

### ◆ Sleep-Rest Pattern

The amount of sleep that infants need is closely related to their rate of growth. Initially, infants sleep approximately 80% of the time, as demanded by their rapid growth. As growth begins to slow toward the middle of the first year of life, less sleep is needed. The 12-month-old infant sleeps for only 12 of 24 hours, a pattern that remains essentially unchanged through the second year. Many new mothers think that there is a link between the amount of food fed to their infant and sleep duration. Studies indicate that infants who received more milk or solid feedings during the day were less likely to feed at night, but not less likely to wake (Brown & Harries, 2015). The findings have important implications for nurses who support new mothers with infant sleep and diet in the first year. Increasing infant calories during the day may reduce the likelihood of night feeding but will not reduce the need for mothers to attend to the infant in the night. To assist parents in understanding normal sleep and rest patterns, the nurse stresses that no set schedule exists (Table 11.5).

### Anticipatory Guidance

Infant sleep patterns are a common concern for new parents. Health-promotion activities can also help parents determine the individual needs of their infant. The nurse stresses that longer sleep patterns are signs of maturation and that sleep and rest are recognized as having a significant influence on the infant's growth and development. Sleep problems are highly prevalent in early childhood. Frequently, parents seek professional help when they suspect their child has a sleep problem. The nurse may offer the parents helpful comments for promoting infant sleep patterns, such as the following:

- Learn behavioural clues that signal that the infant is getting tired.
- Keep the environment well-lit during the day and quiet, with lights dimmed, at night.

**TABLE 11.5** **Growth and Development**
*Normal Sleep Patterns for Infants*

| Age (Months) | Hours in 24-Hour Period |
|---|---|
| 2–3 | Low: 10<br>Average: 16.5<br>High: 23 |
| 3–4 | Low: 8–10 nightly<br>High: 11–12 nightly (two or three naps daily) |
| 6–12 | 11–12 nightly (two or three naps daily) |
| 12–18 | 8–12 nightly (one or two naps daily) |

Sources: Baby Center. (2017). *Establishing good sleep habits: Newborn to three months.* Retrieved from http://www.babycentre.co.uk/a7654/establishing-good-sleep-habits-newborn-to-three-months; Stevens, M. S. (2015). Normal sleep, sleep physiology, and sleep deprivation. *Medscape.* Retrieved from http://emedicine.medscape.com/article/1188226-overview.

- Encourage the establishment of a bedtime routine (e.g., bath, pyjamas, feeding, and singing a song) and a consistent sleep schedule.
- Put the infant down in the crib or bassinet when they are drowsy but before they fall asleep.
- Comforting a crying infant will help them feel secure—you cannot spoil an infant!
- Daytime naps are important, and an overtired infant may have more trouble sleeping.
- Discuss normal development of infants' sleep and napping patterns.
- Review safe sleep practices (sleeping position, surface, environment) (Best Start Resource Centre, 2017b).

If parents express a sleep concern, the nurse assesses their reactions, considers their definition of the concern, assesses the sleep environment, and observes the infant's own unique sleep patterns. Only then can the nurse's health-promotion approach be individualized to assist the family in caring for the infant.

### Sudden Infant Death Syndrome

Sudden infant death syndrome (SIDS) is defined as the sudden death of an infant younger than 1 year old during sleep that is unexpected and unexplained after a thorough postmortem examination, including autopsy, a thorough history, and scene evaluation. SIDS is the only cause of death derived by exclusion of other causes. The incidence of SIDS in Canada decreased by over 300% from 2000 to 2013, likely due to fewer women smoking during pregnancy, more women breastfeeding, and the Back to Sleep campaign that encouraged caregivers to lay infants on their backs to sleep (Canadian Institute of Child Health, 2019). Despite its declining prevalence, SIDS continues to be the second leading cause of death for healthy infants under 1 year old in Canada (PHAC, 2018b). The exact cause of SIDS is unknown; however, it is believed to be related to a convergence of extrinsic stressors, a critical period of infant development, and dysfunctional or immature cardiorespiratory and arousal systems (Moon & Task Force on SIDS, 2017). Extrinsic stressors include prone sleeping position, being overheated, and airway obstruction. Exposure to prenatal and postnatal tobacco smoke can increase an infant's intrinsic vulnerability through several mechanisms,

## BOX 11.4 Safe Sleep for Your Baby Educational Campaign

- Provide a *smoke-free* environment before and after your baby is born.
- *Breastfeeding* can protect your baby.
- Always place your baby on his or her *back to sleep*, at naptime and night time.
- Provide your baby with a *safe sleep* environment that has a firm surface and no pillows, comforters, quilts, or bumper pads.
- Place your baby to sleep in a crib, cradle, or bassinet next to your bed.

Source: Public Health Agency of Canada. (2014). *Safe sleep for your baby* (p. 3). Ottawa: Minister of Health. Retrieved from https://www.canada.ca/content/dam/phac/aspc/migration/phac/aspc/hp-ps/dca-dea/stages-etapes/childhood/enfance/0-2/sids/pdf/sleep/sommeil-eng.pdf. © All rights reserved. Public Health Agency of Canada. Adapted and reproduced with permission from the Minister of Health, 2019.

including affecting the infant's arousal response. Other intrinsic risk factors include preterm birth, low birth weight, and being a twin. The risk of dying from SIDS is highest between 1 and 4 months of age, and is uncommon after 8 months of age (Moon & Task Force on SIDS, 2017). Families experiencing poverty and discrimination are more likely to have an infant affected by SIDS (Bartick & Tomori, 2019), and First Nations and Inuit populations have rates of SIDS that are seven times higher than non-Indigenous people in Canada (Sheppard et al., 2017).

The Public Health Agency of Canada (2018b) recommends several measures to reduce the risk of SIDS (Box 11.4). These include having a smoke-free environment before and after birth; placing the infant on his or her back to sleep for all naps and at bedtime; ensuring that there are no pillows, comforters, bumper pads, or other soft objects in the sleep environment; using a crib, cradle, or bassinet that has a firm mattress and meets Canadian safety regulations; breastfeeding; and room-sharing for the first 6 months. Research suggests that up to one-third of SIDS deaths could be prevented if pregnant women did not smoke, and up to half of SIDS deaths could be prevented by exclusive breastfeeding for 6 months (PHAC, 2018b).

One consequence of the Safe Sleep for Your Baby campaign is a significant increase in occipital flattening or cranial asymmetry, called positional plagiocephaly. This can impact caregivers' adherence to following the recommendations for placing infants in a supine sleeping position, due to concerns about the potential permanent impact on the infant's appearance (Martiniuk, Jacob, Faruqui, et al., 2016). In order to prevent a flat spot from developing, infants can be placed for sleep with their head at different ends of the crib on alternate days (CPS, 2016). They are likely to look away from the wall and toward the centre of the room, so changing their position in the crib encourages varied head positions for sleeping. Parents should be instructed to allow supervised tummy time when the infant is awake and should be cautioned about the amount of time their infant spends in a car seat, swings, or other infant carriers. Tummy time is a key intervention in preventing positional plagiocephaly and gross motor delays in infants. This prone position provides infants with increased physical challenges and gives them a chance to begin developing head

control by strengthening neck muscles. Nurses should educate the parents to introduce prone positioning in short periods several times a day, aiming for 10–15 minutes three times per day (CPS, 2016).

When an infant dies suddenly, unexpectedly, and for no apparent reason, a family crisis occurs. The parents are devastated and completely unprepared for the shock, reacting with intense guilt, blaming themselves and each other, and agonizing over the part they may have played in the infant's death. Because many unanswered questions remain, these feelings are universal. Parents think there is something they could have done to prevent the tragedy. In most cases, nothing could have been done. Too frequently, the first sign that something was wrong is death. The nurse is in an excellent position to help the family through this crisis. Dealing with the family's grief is very difficult. Many families find strength in their faith to help them through this difficult time. Other family members and close friends can assist the family in their grieving process. Many receive solace and support from talking to other parents who have lost an infant to SIDS. Parent support groups are available and the nurse can refer families to groups in their local area.

The nurse's main supportive role for families coping with SIDS is listening and offering compassionate guidance through the weeks and months that follow. The nurse encourages parents to talk about their infant. Too soon, family and friends expect the surviving family to "get over it." A parent, however, is never able to "get over it"; it is only put in perspective and not so near the surface. Nurses need to actively participate in helping parents through their grieving process and remember a standard time frame for grieving is not applicable (Andreotta, Hill, Eley, et al., 2015).

Nursing assessment of the infant at risk of SIDS includes observing the infant for apneic episodes. Usually, however, nursing assessment occurs after death and consists of support and providing appropriate resources for the family. Nursing diagnoses for sudden infant death might include the following:

- Spiritual distress, resulting from the loss of an infant
- Inadequate family coping, resulting from the loss of an infant
- Dysfunctional grieving, due to the parents' inability to cope

Nurses also discuss with the family feelings about caring for future children. Life can appear out of control, and parents may believe that they cannot care for another infant. These feelings must be resolved before another pregnancy is contemplated. When dealing with the families of SIDS infants, nurses can feel uncomfortable and helpless. As health professionals, they might speak in terms of easing the pain or alleviating the guilt of these families, but many times simple nonverbal human contact is sufficient to express concern and understanding.

## ◆ Cognitive-Perceptual Pattern

Cognition is the process by which an individual recognizes, accumulates, and organizes the knowledge of the environment, beginning with the perception or recognition of an event within that environment. Cognitive development is concurrent with biological, adaptive, and psychosocial achievement. The infant's biological and cognitive developmental patterns (Piaget's sensorimotor period) were discussed earlier in this chapter. The focus of this section is on the infant's sensory and language development and the importance of stimulation of both developmental areas. From birth, infants possess sensory capabilities; all sensory organs are well developed and functioning. As the infant is cared for and handled, the special senses become organized neurologically into a pattern of behaviour that will greatly influence subsequent development.

## Vision

Sight is the least developed sense at birth. The infant's initial visual impressions are unfocused and unfamiliar. The visual system of the newborn infant takes several months to develop. Because everything is new and only somewhat significant, visual stimuli must be moving, bright, contrasting, or flashing to capture the infant's attention. While their vision starts out at 20/400, by 1-week-old infants can focus on objects about 20 to 30 cm away, the distance to their caregiver's face while being fed or held. At 3 months, their vision is 20/40 and reaches 20/20 at 6 months (LoFrumento, 2018). To help stimulate the infant's vision, encourage parents to interact with their infant at a short distance so that they can see their face. Parents can also decorate their room with bright, cheerful colours or contrasting patterns and hang a brightly coloured mobile above the crib that has a variety of shapes. The infant's eyes are well developed at birth, but the muscles that attach the eyes to their sockets are weak. This weakness may be stressful to parents because the infant's eyes do not appear to function simultaneously. Parents can be assured that most infants coordinate their eye movements by the age of 3 months; by 6 months, this function is mature.

## Hearing

After the amniotic fluid has drained from the middle ear several days after birth, the infant's hearing becomes acute. Hearing is one of the better-developed senses in the infant; the fetus can even hear in utero and responds to loud sounds. The newborn can distinguish sound frequencies and turns toward a voice or another sound. The infant may be familiar with the mother's voice early in life. Sounds gradually gain significance and meaning when they are associated with caregivers, food, and pleasure.

The ability to listen and discriminate among sounds is an important task during infancy. Caretakers should talk to their infants, sing nursery songs, and make faces so the infants develop language and social skills. The use of baby rattles and musical mobiles is also a good way to stimulate the infant's hearing. The closer the infant is to the sound, the more easily the sound can be discriminated. The groundwork for verbal ability begins to develop long before words appear, and many believe that infants whose mothers talk to them tend to speak earlier than infants who are not exposed to these sounds (Burnham, Wieland, Kondaurova, et al., 2015). It is important that any hearing loss be detected early in life because of its impact on language development and opportunity for early intervention. Table 11.6 summarizes the infant's auditory development.

## TABLE 11.6    Growth and Development
### Normal Development of Hearing

| Age (Months) | Behaviour That Indicates Hearing |
|---|---|
| 1–3 | Is startled by loud noises |
| | Calms or smiles when spoken to |
| 4–6 | Turns eyes and head toward sound |
| | Pays attention to music |
| | Makes sounds that begin with p, b, and m |
| 6–9 | Responds to own name |
| | Understands simple words like "no" |
| | Recognizes familiar sounds |
| 9–12 | Points to familiar objects or people |
| | Imitates simple words and sounds |
| | Locates a sound in any direction |
| 12–18 | Follows simple spoken directions |
| | Distinguishes between sounds |
| | Spoken words are well on their way (at least 20 words by 18 months) |

Sources: Ontario Ministry of Children, Community and Social Services. (2016). *Your baby's speech and language skills from birth to 30 months.* Retrieved from http://www.children.gov.on.ca/htdocs/English/earlychildhood/speechlanguage/brochure_speech.aspx; National Institute on Deafness and Other Communication Disorders. (2017). *Your baby's hearing and communicative development checklist.* Retrieved from https://www.nidcd.nih.gov/health/your-babys-hearing-and-communicative-development-checklist.

## Smell

The ability to smell is fully developed at birth. The infant has many receptors in the nose but lacks the cilia that line the inside of the adult's nose. As a result, the infant has a keen sense of smell because odours reach the receptor cells easily. Within 2 weeks after birth, an infant can differentiate the odour of the mother's milk from other sources of milk, an ability developed when the infant is held closely (Berk & Meyers, 2015). At this time the infant begins associating the parents with their body odours, a perception that is important for infant–parent bonding.

## Taste

Taste buds in newborns can be found on the tonsils and the back of the throat, as well on the tongue. Infants use their sense of smell from the start and can localize odours by turning their heads in the direction of the odour. The sense of taste is present at birth, and salivation begins at approximately 3 months of age. The four primary sensations are sour, salty, sweet, and bitter. The taste buds for sweet tastes are more abundant during early life than they are in later life, which may account for the preference for sweets that is characteristic of infants and children. An infant's reaction to salty foods does not come until approximately 4 to 5 months of age.

## Touch and Motion

Touch is by far the most developed of all of the infant's senses, as it is the main way in which infants learn about their environment and bond with other people. The skin is the sensory organ for touch. Tactile sensation is well developed at birth, particularly on the lips and tongue. Perceptions of motion and touch are perhaps the most important of all senses. Rocking and other motions are sensations of equilibrium picked up by the middle ear. Skin-to-skin touching should be performed regularly; evidence shows that touch helps relieve infant stress and accelerates neuro-muscular development (Berk & Meyers, 2015). Infants respond with pleasure to rocking and other motions and to tactile sensations of warmth, closeness, and cuddling.

## Language Development

Language development, an important aspect of the infant's cognitive and perceptual pattern, is affected by development of the intellect, maturation of the central nervous system, development of the organs of speech, and exposure to human verbalization.

As in other areas of development, language acquisition follows a definite sequence. During the first 2 months, most of the infant's sounds are vowels and are made primarily in the front part of the mouth (Fogel, 2015). Crying is the major means of communication during this period. Cooing sounds are heard at approximately 2 to 3 months, usually in response to an adult's voice. By 6 months, babbling sounds are heard, and by 9 to 10 months, the infant forms two-syllable sounds. By 12 months, words such as "ma-ma," "bye-bye," and "da-da" are emerging. From 15 to 18 months, an expressive jargon with rhythmical intonations develops, but words are recognized only rarely. The infant uses jargon along with pointing to express wishes.

## Anticipatory Guidance

The nurse's knowledge and understanding of an infant's cognitive and perceptual behaviour facilitates interaction with infants and serves as a guide in parental counselling. The main focus centres on stimulation, because each of the infant's senses is receptive to environmental stimulation. This activity helps the infant learn from the environment. When an infant is exposed to appropriate sensory stimulation, greater curiosity, improved mental capabilities, accelerated neuro-muscular growth, enhanced gastro-intestinal functioning, quicker weight gain, more rapid language development, and pleasing mother–infant interactions are likely to occur (O'Connor, 2015).

Parents are the primary providers of pleasurable and stimulating experiences for the infant. The nurse assists them by offering suggestions about suitable stimuli for each sensory modality.

## ◆ Self-Perception–Self-Concept Pattern

Self-perception has a pervasive influence on all aspects of life. Self-concept consists of a set of attitudes regarding what each person thinks, believes, and feels about the self. These attitudes form a personal self-belief that is an abstraction referred to as "me." Many researchers believe that the infant determines self-existence by first noting that actions such as crying or smiling have an effect on others, which depends on receiving feedback (Berk & Meyers, 2015). Studies confirm that infants can identify themselves and, therefore, form a self-concept. Infants at 4 months of age were found to be particularly fascinated with their images in mirrors and smiled more at themselves than they did at pictures of other infants (Fivush & Waters, 2015).

As the infant continues to grow and mature, many circumstances combine to influence self-concept. How others relate to the infant's body and the messages that the infant receives from the body lead to knowledge of a physical self. The ability to use the body to influence others can lead the psychological self to conclude that someone cares about the infant (Feldman, 2015).

The infant's development of body image is gradual. At birth the infant has diffuse feelings of hunger, pain, anger, and comfort, but no body image. Initially, the infant knows only the self and regards the external world as an extension of the self. Only when infants begin to experience the environment through sensory modalities are they able to distinguish their bodies from animate and inanimate objects.

### Nursing Suggestions

The nurse plays a vital role in assisting parents to foster the development of a positive self-concept and a good body image in their infant. Socialization is unique and begins in infancy. Parenting skills and style have a strong influence on outcomes of integrated socialization as infants develop. The nurse first identifies personal self-concept and how it influences individuals (Reed, 2015). The nurse stresses that the way in which parents treat the infant influences the infant's self-concept. Basically, infants and young children incorporate their parents' interactions with them (good or bad) into their own view of self. Parents must understand that their infant's self-concept is an important, continuing event. What the infant knows and later believes about the self will affect all interactions with others, and by influencing what the infant will later attempt, the self-concept may have broad effects on the development of new skills. The mental state or the idea of "me" is that part of the self that makes reference to itself. This mental state develops over the first 2 years of life and is a function of both brain maturation processes and socialization (Reed, 2015).

## ◆ Roles-Relationships Pattern

What happens during the first few months of an infant's life matters a great deal because this period of life provides a blueprint for adult well-being and sets the foundation for what follows. Researchers have explored extensively the effect of early bonding between parents and their infants, emphasizing that this initial attraction sets the stage for the later development of love and affiliation. The bonding process has many other implications for the infant's future development as well (Polan & Taylor, 2015).

### Attachment and Bonding

The attachment relationship is a vital bond between the infant and the caregiver that, when secure, facilitates physical and psychological well-being. Various theories have attempted to explain the basis for attachment behaviour. Freudian psychoanalytical theory emphasizes that the bond between the child and the mother develops as a result of the mother's fulfillment of the infant's innate desire to socialize and the physical requirements for survival. Social learning theory contributes the principles of reinforcement to the attachment process; as the mother meets the infant's needs, discomfort is reduced or removed. The infant associates the pleasurable feeling of being satisfied with the mother, who becomes a significant other in the infant's life. The bonding process is the basis for the mother–infant relationship, which, in turn, forms the basis for the interdependence that is necessary for the infant's psychological and physical development. All infants are born with the building blocks that develop into attachment behaviours, and thus all infants have the ability to form an attachment relationship with their primary caregiver (Fivush & Waters, 2015).

Becoming a parent can be a transformational process for a person, and the process of bonding is also important for fathers. A review of the literature shows that fathers have a desire to nurture, love, and bond with their infants as equals in the parenting dyad (Scism & Cobb, 2017). While their bonding experience is often overlooked, nurses can help facilitate this father–infant relationship by engaging fathers in the immediate labour and birth process and subsequent physical care of the newborn. This is the initiation of an important long-term relationship; when fathers are involved in the lives of their children over time, it has an impact on child outcomes, such as improved academic achievement and reduced behavioural problems (Scism & Cobb, 2017). Social norms regarding the role of fathers have been changing in recent decades, including caregiving arrangements. As women have increasingly taken up higher education and careers outside of the home, there are more dual-income families, and women are less likely to become stay-at-home mothers, while the proportion of stay-at-home fathers is growing (Statistics Canada, 2016a). In addition, 1 in 8 of same-sex couples (who make up 0.9% of all couples in Canada) have children living with them (Statistics Canada, 2017a). While children tend to form a stronger attachment to one caregiver, there is no reason that this primary attachment figure must be the biological mother.

The impact of the parent–child relationship can reveal itself early in a child's life. Studies have shown that if the process of attachment is encumbered, problems are more likely to occur, such as child abuse, failure to thrive, and behavioural problems. Failure to thrive refers to a pattern of poor weight gain over time, and is a physical sign that an infant is receiving inadequate nutrition for optimal growth and development. This can be caused by a range of medical conditions and psychosocial issues, including poor parenting skills and lack of secure attachment (Homan, 2016).

Many factors are present when a relationship is being established and maintained. Most people enter a relationship with unrealistic expectations. Parents are no exception—they are going to be wise, patient, and devoted, and they will nurture their infant. Because the parents' self-esteem is associated closely with their infant's interactions and accomplishments, when parents' self-esteem is low, disappointment, anger, and a disturbance in the relationship with their infant can occur. In some instances, this disturbed parent–infant relationship is short-lived and nothing harmful develops. When a disturbed parent–infant relationship continues, however, the infant is at risk of abuse and behaviour problems (Innovative Practice).

## INNOVATIVE PRACTICE

### Ontario's Healthy Babies Healthy Children Program

Healthy Babies Healthy Children is a free home-visiting program that supports families with:
- having a healthy pregnancy
- developing a positive relationship with their child
- promoting their child's growth and development
- connecting them to resources and programs within their community
- working together to give their child the best start in life

Families are eligible if they are:
- a newcomer to Canada, here less than 3 years, and having their first baby in Canada
- concerned about or have questions about their child's growth and development and behaviours
- feeling alone with very few or no supports from family or friends
- experiencing or have a history of a physical and/or mental health illness (e.g., depression, anxiety) that is making pregnancy or parenting challenging
- a first-time or experienced parent with questions about parenting and building a healthy relationship with their child
- facing challenging life situations such as homelessness, domestic violence, or no OHIP (provincial health insurance)

Those eligible for the program can receive long-term home visiting from a public health nurse and family home visitor.

Source: City of Toronto. (n.d.). *Healthy Babies Healthy Children*. Retrieved from https://www.toronto.ca/community/people/children/parenting/pregnancy-and-parenting/pregnancy/during-pregnancy/prenatal-programs/healthy-babies-healthy-children/.

Infant/child abuse has occurred throughout history, yet its prevalence is difficult to estimate, partly because, like an iceberg, it is mostly hidden. Acceptable behaviour toward infants is largely a learned phenomenon; the art of parenting is not instinctively acquired, as many people believe. Abusing parents are seldom "monsters"; they are merely individuals ineffectively coping with the demands of parenthood, for which there is little or no preparation, at the same time that they experience significant other life stressors.

The scope of child abuse is extensive: approximately 33% of Canadians aged 15 and older experienced maltreatment as a child (Statistics Canada, 2017b). Child maltreatment refers to physical and/or sexual abuse experienced before the age of 15, and witnessing violence by their caregiver against another adult. Women were more likely to have been sexually abused, while men were more likely to have experienced physical abuse, and 93% of the abuse victims did not report it to police or child protection services. Children less than 4 years of age and those with special needs are the most vulnerable to abuse and neglect (CDC, 2018b). Risk factors for perpetrating abuse toward children include parents' own history of experiencing abuse, substance use and/or mental illness, having many dependent children, being a young parent, experiencing low socioeconomic status, community violence and deprivation, and poor social connections (CDC, 2018b).

Child abuse is an important cause of pediatric morbidity and death and is associated with major physical and mental health problems that can extend into adulthood. This means nurses may be the first point of contact when an infant or child experiences an abuse-related traumatic injury or seeks mental health care, and they must be prepared to recognize it and intervene. While physical trauma is not the only facet, it is the most overt indicator of a dysfunctional family unit and a disturbed parent–infant relationship (Fanetti, O'Donohue, Happel, et al., 2015).

Indications of physical abuse may include the following:

- Malnutrition, extensive dental caries, untreated diaper dermatitis, or neglected wounds
- Any injuries (fractures, bruises, mouth trauma, head or abdominal injuries) in a pre-ambulatory infant
- Multiple injuries at different stages of healing
- Explanation for an injury that is inconsistent with its pattern, age, and severity
- Notable delay in seeking medical attention
- Markedly different explanations for an injury from different people (Christian & Committee on Child Abuse and Neglect, 2015)

Signs of sexual abuse may include genital tissue injury and sexually transmitted infections (STIs); however, young children more often complain of gastro-intestinal symptoms or demonstrate behavioural signs of sexual abuse during a physical examination, such as anxiety or withdrawal, even when no anogenital abnormalities are present (Vrolijk-Bosschaart, Brilleslijper-Kater, Widdershoven, et al., 2017).

Abusing parents often have common patterns of behaviour. As children, their own parents may have abused them. In this way, child abuse is cycled from generation to generation. The development of the maternal role on which the infant depends for health, progress, and survival begins during the mother's early childhood. Unless she received love and proper mothering, she will have difficulty with a relationship that entails the complete dependency of another person. The residential school system is a well-documented example of how this cycle can occur. In Canada throughout the twentieth century, Indigenous children were separated from their parents and communities and forced to attend church-run residential schools in an attempt to assimilate them into Canadian society. Separation of families diminished parenting skills and interfered with the development of secure attachment between parents and children, while the oppression and abuse experienced by Indigenous people led to chronic stress, depression, anxiety, and low self-esteem. When these survivors of residential schools had their own families, their experiences left many caregivers unable to be emotionally present for their children, and some adopted negative coping strategies such as substance abuse and violence. This exposes the next generation of Indigenous children to adverse childhood experiences, and the intergenerational transmission of trauma continues (Aguiar & Halseth, 2015).

The abused infant or child is frequently singled out as someone who is different. This infant may be chronically ill, may have been born prematurely, may be hyperactive, may have been the product of a difficult and complicated pregnancy, or may have an obvious anomaly. Early bonding disturbances (inadequacies in feeding, holding, and caring for the infant) are characteristic signals.

The long-term effects of child abuse are profound. The Adverse Childhood Experiences (ACE) study during the 1990s was instrumental in revealing the impact of childhood abuse on adult health (Felitti et al., 1998, as cited in Hoft & Haddad, 2017). Cancer and diseases of the heart, lungs, and liver are all associated with having experienced childhood abuse, as are many of the behaviours that negatively impact health, such as smoking, alcohol and drug use, and risky sexual activity.

Nurses play a critical role in recognizing infants who have been intentionally harmed, because they are often the first to begin taking a history of the infant. The role of the nurse may include identifying abused infants with suspicious injuries who present for care, reporting suspected abuse to the Children's Aid Society for investigation, supporting families who are affected by infant abuse, coordinating with community agencies to provide immediate and long-term care to the victimized infant, providing court testimony when necessary, providing preventive care and anticipatory guidance in the health care setting, and advocating for policies that support and protect vulnerable infants (Christian & Committee on Child Abuse and Neglect, 2015). Nurses work collaboratively with community agencies to provide follow-up care for the infant in danger of continued abuse. Nurses take appropriate action if they suspect an infant is at risk. Some of the biggest challenges of child protection come from our own internal reluctance to act, but doing nothing is not an option and all nurses in Canada have a legal obligation to report suspected child abuse or neglect. The following measures may help with early identification of families who are at risk of abusing or neglecting their child:

- Questionnaires and offers of referrals for community support given to parents on postpartum units
- Recognition of parents who have difficulty relating to their infants through body language clues or verbalizations
- Follow-up home visits during the postpartum period by the public health nurse
- Crisis hotlines made available to parents in distress

Before focusing on nursing interventions, the nurse makes several observations to assist in identifying a high-risk infant by answering the following questions:

- Does the caregiver hold the infant close and establish eye contact?
- Does the caregiver speak negatively about the infant?
- Does the caregiver intensely dislike the duties of motherhood, such as diapering, feeding, and so on?
- Does the caregiver expect too much of the infant at a particular stage of development?
- Does the caregiver have a good support system available?
- Does the caregiver act overly concerned about the infant's sex?

Many communities are seeking ways in which child abuse can be prevented through educational efforts, improved agency coordination, and development of new collaborative efforts and services for parents and infants. It takes a community effort to address the problem.

## ◆ Sexuality–Reproductive Pattern

An infant's identity begins at birth, when the gendered child is identified and caretakers behave in a certain way toward the infant because of its sex. The infant's sexuality gives direction to its physical, emotional, social, and intellectual responses throughout life. Infants have a great oral sensitivity, enjoy skin-to-skin contact, and explore their own bodies for pleasure during the first year of life. A healthy, accepting attitude by caretakers is important in an infant's evolving sexual development.

## ◆ Coping–Stress Tolerance Pattern

The term *stress* implies intense reaction to an experience and changes in usual behaviour. Stress is a normal phenomenon that occurs throughout the life span, as, for example, when an individual experiences a developmental or situational crisis.

### Developmental Crisis

Developmental crises are turning points or periods of great change. Most stressors that an infant experiences are a necessary part of growth and development. For example, learning new skills creates stress. The infant who is unable to move forward while learning to crawl experiences stress. The infant expresses this stress by crying for help. Other stressors are more psychosocial in nature, such as being left with a babysitter or in an unfamiliar place.

### Situational Crisis

Situational crises are not anticipated easily and do not occur necessarily as part of the normal growth and development process. One major situational crisis during infancy is separation from the significant other. The following three distinct phases are evident in the reaction to separation (Coch, Dawson, & Fischer, 2015):

- *Protest.* Infant cries loudly, screams for the mother, and refuses attention of the substitute caregiver.
- *Despair.* Infant stops crying and becomes less active, withdraws, and becomes apathetic.
- *Withdrawal.* Infant takes an interest in the surroundings but tends to ignore or reject the mother when she returns, because she failed to meet the infant's needs.

Initially, with no time framework and no understanding of waiting, the infant has little ability to cope with stress. As maturity and a sense of security provided by the caregiver increase, the infant begins to wait a short time to have its needs met without protest. An infant who experiences stress reacts by crying, the main tool of communication. The infant gradually learns to tolerate greater stress with time.

### Nursing Interventions

Every family needs good information, concrete resources, and consistent support to thrive. Nursing interventions that assist the infant and the infant's family in stressful situations are listed in Box 11.5. By allaying anxiety in the infant's caregiver, the nurse facilitates coping behaviours in the infant. The stressful situation and the problem-solving activities can be turned into growth-producing experiences for the family, with coping capacities strengthened for the future.

---

**BOX 11.5** **Nursing Interventions to Assist in Stressful Situations During Infancy**

- Attempt to meet the infant's needs promptly.
- Allow favourite toy or item of security to be present during stressful experiences.
- Allow familiar caregiver to be present to calm the infant.
- Attempt to keep the number of strangers interacting with the infant to a minimum.
- Attempt to provide a warm and accepting environment for the infant.
- Allow freedom of expression (crying) to reduce tension in the infant.
- Identify the infant's established daily routine and try to follow through with it.
- Reinforce the infant's need for expression.
- Establish a trusting relationship with the infant.
- Provide opportunity for play so the infant can vent fears.
- Provide emotional support for the parents so they can, in turn, give support to their infant.
- Try the five "S" system to soothe a crying infant:
  - Swaddling
  - Side/stomach position (but not for sleeping)
  - Shushing sounds
  - Swinging
  - Sucking

Source: National Fatherhood Initiative. (2015). *Preventing child abuse: The crying baby.* Retrieved from https://www.fatherhood.org/fatherhood/preventing/child/abuse/the/crying/baby.

## ◆ Values–Beliefs Pattern

A value is a standard or principle that reflects a person's judgement on what is important in life. When people communicate, they send both the content message of the spoken words and the unspoken message of who they are and what they believe. Values are pervasive and important and give a focus to both individuals and groups within a particular culture. Because values are attitudes learned especially from significant others within the environment, the parents' values-beliefs pattern greatly influences the care and development of the infant. Values associated with a family's culture will also influence how they understand health and illness, what kinds of health-promotion activities are practiced and accepted, how they express themselves, and how family members support one another (CPS, 2018b).

### Nursing Interventions

By understanding and respecting the parents' value system, nurses works within their framework of values in the counselling situation. Nurses have an ethical responsibility to respect and value each patient's culture and beliefs, and to practice based on the principles of cultural competence and cultural safety (Canadian Nurses Association [CNA], 2018). This may be accomplished by the following:

- Consider how one's own cultural beliefs, values, and behaviours influence interactions with families.
- Assess and respect families' health-related values, attitudes, and beliefs, and incorporate these into the care plan.
- Be adaptable and flexible in working with diverse families.

Recognize your own position of power in the nurse–client relationship and seek to move away from a paternalistic model of care to one where families share power and responsibility.

The nurse collaborates with the parents to promote attitudes and behaviours that are consistent with healthy child development. Nurses accomplish this task by modelling, acting as a consultant by sharing pertinent information with parents, and modifying their own values. Nurses can anticipate a family crisis of values and can help to promote positive coping and effective use of social supports (Harkness & DeMarco, 2015).

First, modelling can be a potent influence on another individual's behaviour. In the counselling situation, the family looks to the nurse for guidance and assistance in promoting healthy child-rearing practices. The methods by which the nurse interacts with the infant, listens to the parents' concerns, and demonstrates respect for the family unit are influencing factors in changing behaviour.

Second, the nurse acts as a consultant to influence behaviour. Advice on child-rearing practices is overwhelming to parents; everyone has opinions. The nurse listens before giving advice to determine whether parents will accept the advice and to allow parents to decide whether the advice can be useful. Repeated attempts to convert parents to the nurse's value system can make them defensive and resistant to the advice.

Third, by expressing values and attitudes about healthy child-rearing practices, but remaining open to other approaches, the nurse influences the values-beliefs pattern. Parents can realize that they are free to change and are not bound to values that others outside their value system express (Gardner, Carter, Enzman-Hines, et al., 2016). Good communication can more effectively promote the health of the infant and the family.

## ❖ ENVIRONMENTAL PROCESSES

### ◆ Physical Agents

This section discusses various factors within the environment that can affect the infant's health status. The entire realm of accident prevention and safety promotion is applicable here. Adults take for granted that they are living in a world designed by adults for adults. They must constantly remind themselves that infants also live in this complex world and that they learn at a remarkable rate, primarily by exploring and playing in the environment. These experiences render them extremely vulnerable to accidents, a major problem and a challenging field for preventive measures.

Accidents occur in many situations: in the home, outdoors, on the playground, and in automobiles. Most accidents, however, occur in the home. Their number and seriousness is closely linked to the infant's developmental stage. Accidents tend to increase with the mobility of the infant, but even a 2-month-old infant can wiggle or fall from a high place. Keeping the environment free from hazards and ensuring caregiver supervision are crucial for this age group. Nurses have the opportunity to help parents and caregivers anticipate and understand the common hazards of early life and provide specific guidance for accident prevention.

Unintentional injuries are a significant cause of childhood morbidity and mortality in Canada, with transport-related injuries, drowning, and suffocation or choking the three leading causes of death for children aged 0–14 (Parachute, 2016). It is believed that 90% of unintentional childhood injuries are preventable (Richmond, D'Cruz, Lokku, et al., 2016). For children less than 4 years of age, suffocation or choking is the number one cause of death and falls are the leading cause of hospitalization, demonstrating where injury prevention efforts should be directed for this age group (Parachute, 2016).

The rate of mortality from childhood injuries has declined significantly over the past 60 years, with the timing of introduction of legislation and safety campaigns suggesting that public prevention efforts were at least partly responsible (Richmond et al., 2016). Some areas of success in promoting safety for infants include the development of flame-retardant sleepwear, car seats, and crib safety standards. It is important that nurses are aware of how to provide education to caregivers regarding how to select and properly use this equipment.

In the 1970s, legislation was developed to protect children from burns by instituting flammability requirements for children's sleepwear and bedding (Richmond et al., 2016). Sleepwear made for infants can be either made from a pure synthetic fibre, such as polyester or nylon, or from cotton or a cotton blend. Synthetic fibres will not burn as easily and are labelled as flame retardant. Parents should be advised to select flame-retardant sleepwear for their infant and to follow the laundry instructions carefully to maintain this properly. However, if the parents choose to dress their child in cotton that does not meet flammability requirements, they should choose tight-fitting clothing that is less likely to catch fire when exposed to a flame.

All cribs are required to meet strict safety standards, which were instituted in 1986 to prevent entrapment and suffocation deaths (Richmond et al., 2016). Any crib manufactured after this date should meet these standards, including those sold at second-hand stores. However, if parents accept a second-hand crib, they should be encouraged to look for recalls and safety alerts on the Government of Canada website (http://www.healthy-canadians.gc.ca/recall-alert-rappel-avis/index-eng.php?cat=4) and to check the following:

- The slats should be no farther than 6 cm apart. Wider slats could allow an infant's head to become trapped between them.
- There should be no decorations or projections that could snag an infant's clothes. Avoid cribs with decorative cutouts in the headboard or footboard.
- Some older cribs were painted with lead-based paint, which could poison an infant who mouths or chews the wood. If unsure, strip the old paint and repaint it with new lead-free enamel.
- No screws and bolts that hold the crib together should be missing, and all should be tight. Avoid cribs with drop side rails. If a drop side rail detaches or becomes loose, an infant may become trapped between the mattress and the railing.
- The crib mattress should be firm and should fit very snugly, with no room for the baby to become trapped between the mattress and the crib. Do not cover the mattress with plastic or a quilt, which can suffocate a baby.

## BOX 11.6    Safety Tips to Prevent Falls

- Keep sides up and firmly secured when the infant is in the crib.
- Place the infant seat on a stable surface, preferably the floor. The infant should be strapped in securely.
- Check high chairs, strollers, and carriages for safety, and restrain the infant who is active.
- All windows above the first floor should be locked and have operable window guards.
- Clean up food or liquid spills immediately from the floor.
- Close off stairways with doors or properly installed gates, at the top and bottom.
- To prevent falls, set the crib mattress at the lowest adjustment level after the infant can pull himself/herself up and stand.
- Place furniture away from windows and anchor pieces to the wall.
- Avoid the use of baby walkers.
- Never leave an infant alone on a bed, changing table, or piece of furniture.
- Avoid bringing strollers onto escalators.
- Best fall prevention is to watch, listen, and stay near the infant at all times.

Source: Remedy's Health Communities. (2015). *Preventing falls in babies*. Retrieved from http://www.healthcommunities.com/infant-safety/children/fall/prevention.shtml.

Encourage caregivers to never put an infant to sleep on a waterbed, pillow, quilt, beanbag chair, or sofa. All these surfaces increase the chance that a baby could suffocate or get the head or another part of the body trapped in the furniture. There should be no pillows or stuffed animals in an infant's crib, because they can cause suffocation. Crib quilt bumpers also pose a risk for suffocation and should not be used. When the infant learns to sit, the mattress should be lowered so the infant cannot fall out of the crib. Mobiles should be removed, and draperies and window blind cords must be well out of the infant's reach.

### Unintentional Injuries

*Falls.* Falls are most common after 4 months of age, when the infant has learned to roll over, but they can occur at any age. Falls involving infants happen more often in the home environment, on stairs, from furniture, and out of windows. The best advice is never to place an infant unattended on a raised surface that has no type of guard rails. When in doubt, the safest place is the floor. Safety tips to assist parents in preventing falls are listed in Box 11.6.

*Burns.* While burns are not one of the three leading causes of death or hospitalizations for Canadian children (Parachute, 2016), there are likely many burn or scald injuries that are not accounted for in reported statistics because most people seek medical attention outside of the hospital setting. Scalds are the most common type of burn-related injury for young children, often resulting from hot drinks or hot tap water (MacDougall, 2018). Improved residential hot water tanks with thermostat control has contributed to a decline in burn injuries (Richmond et al., 2016), and parents should be encouraged to set their hot water tank to no higher than 49°C. Contact burns from fireplaces and stoves are also common, and gates can be installed around fireplaces to prevent burns. In addition to creating a burn-proof environment, parents need to be within arm's reach of a child

who is near a burn hazard (MacDougall, 2018). Because nearly all burns are preventable, the attendant caregiver can experience severe guilt, and education about prevention is the best strategy beginning in infancy.

*Swallowing/choking on foreign objects.* Choking occurs when a foreign object becomes lodged in the throat, blocking air flow (National Safety Council, 2016). Choking is the leading cause of unintentional death in children aged 0 to 4 (Parachute, 2016). Any small object that an infant puts in the mouth has the potential to be swallowed and choked on. Liquids are the most common cause of choking in infants, whereas balloons, small objects, and foods are the most common causes of foreign-body airway obstruction in children (American Public Health Association, 2015). Parents should be advised that objects such as safety pins, peanuts, beads, coins, hot dogs, paper clips, nuts, corn, buttons, popcorn, chips, apple with peel, and parts of broken toys are frequently swallowed. Many objects can fit into this category and into the infant's mouth. The carelessness of a caregiver, relative, friend, or babysitter in leaving small objects available and within reach, or giving toys unsuited to the infant's stage of development, frequently causes these accidents.

When choking occurs, the adult should place the infant across the adult's knees and deliver five back blows with the palm of the hand followed by turning the infant face up and giving five chest thrusts with two fingers on the breastbone (MedlinePlus, 2017b). Repeat until the object is expelled or the infant becomes unresponsive. Cardiopulmonary resuscitation should be performed if the infant becomes unresponsive. The American Heart Association (2015) does not recommend use of under-the-diaphragm abdominal thrusts for choking infants younger than 1 year. Prevention of swallowing foreign objects is the best treatment.

The entire balance of safety for infants depends on allowing them plenty of opportunity to explore and play within the environment while protecting them from harmful agents. The nurse informs the infant's parents, babysitters, family friends, and day care workers about the need to childproof their environments when an infant is present. The nurse can explain ways to promote the safety of these varied environments (Box 11.7).

### Motor Vehicles

This section considers the effects of motion or action of forces on the infant; the focus here is on motor vehicle accidents.

Automobiles present a danger to people of all ages, but especially to infants. Usually an infant is injured because of improper restraint inside the automobile. Approximately 2000 children aged 1–4 are killed or injured in car collisions each year in Canada, and many of these outcomes could have been prevented with a proper restraint system (CPS, 2017b). Infants should be transported in a rear-facing car seat until they are at least 1 year of age and weigh 10 kg (22 lbs). Many car seats can be used in a rear-facing position until the child is 23 kg (50 lbs), and this is considered to be the safest position for the infant and toddler. The rear-facing car seat should be secured using a universal anchor system (UAS) in newer vehicles or with the seat-belt in older vehicles. It is important to read the instructions for the car seat and vehicle owner's manual to ensure it is installed

## BOX 11.7  Home Childproofing Tips

- Remove any heavy, sharp, or breakable objects from tables and low shelves.
- Bolt bookcases to the wall and remove heavy books to prevent falls.
- Test floor and table lamps to make sure they cannot be pulled over.
- Avoid placing toys, blankets, pillows, or bumper pads in the crib.
- Disconnect unused appliances and wrap up cords.
- Secure all other cords to prevent appliances from being pulled down.
- Safely discard unused and unneeded medicines.
- Avoid referring to medicines as candy.
- Post the Poison Control Centre phone number nearby.
- Store potentially toxic substances out of sight and reach.
- Close reachable outlets with safety covers.
- Avoid leaving an infant unattended in the bathtub, even for a moment.
- Avoid using tablecloths that can be pulled down by a crawling infant.
- Tie drapery and blind cords out of the infant's reach.
- Choose stair gates with openings too small for an infant's head and child-resistant fasteners such as pressure bars.
- Avoid accordion or expandable gates with openings that can trap an infant's head.
- Install smoke detectors and check the batteries at least once a month.
- Use sturdy screens in front of fireplaces.
- Place crib, playpen, and high chair well away from heaters, fans, and electrical outlets.
- Install childproof latches on drawers and cupboards. Store all cleaning compounds and detergents in a high, locked cupboard.
- Keep plants out of an infant's reach, as some are poisonous.
- Buy all medicines in bottles with childproof lids and keep them in their original labelled containers for identification in case of accidental ingestion.
- Install lids on garbage pails and never leave any harmful materials in them, such as sharp can lids or spoiled food.
- Place furniture away from windows and anchor pieces to the wall, such as TVs.
- Check the floor regularly for objects small enough to be swallowed.
- Cut blind cords into two pieces.

Source: Centers for Disease Control and Prevention. (2018). *Safety in the home and community*. Retrieved from http://www.cdc.gov/parents/infants/safety.html.

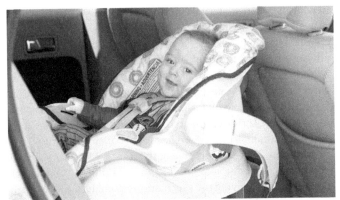

**Fig. 11.3** A Properly Secured Rear-Facing Infant Car Seat (iStockphoto/jenjen42)

properly. Once installed, it should sit at a 45-degree angle (Fig. 11.3) and should be secured tightly enough in the seat of the car that it cannot be moved from side to side or front to back more than 2.5 cm (1 inch). Once the infant has outgrown the rear-facing car seat and is over 1 year of age and 10 kg (22 lbs), they

may be turned facing forward and should stay in a forward-facing car seat until they are at least 4 years old and weigh 18 kg (40 lbs) (CPS, 2017b).

As many as 80–90% of car seats are used incorrectly (CPS, 2017b), which has significant implications for infant safety. It is important that nurses provide parents with guidance and education about the proper use of car seats. Nurses can also refer parents to local car seat clinics where they can have the installation checked by someone trained in car seat inspection. The following are tips for safe transportation of infants:

- The safest place for the infant's car seat is the middle of the back seat of the car.
- Fasten the harness snuggly—only one finger should fit between the strap and the baby's collarbone.
- The harness should be level with or slightly below the shoulders.
- The chest clip should sit at armpit level.
- Avoid thick or puffy clothing or snow suits which could compress during a crash, making the harness too loose, and allowing the infant to slide out of the car seat.
- Don't use bunting bags or sleeping bags, as these don't allow the crotch strap to fit snugly.
- Used car seats should be strongly discouraged because they may have been in an accident or could be expired or recalled.
- Car seats should be replaced if they are in a crash, even a minor one (CPS, 2017b).

Each year, some infants die of heat stroke after being left unattended in motor vehicles. More than half the deaths are of children younger than 2 years. On days when ambient temperatures exceed 30°C (86°F), the internal temperature of a vehicle quickly reaches 49°C (120°F) to 60°C (140°F) (Sims, 2015). At those temperatures, children are at great risk of significant health problems that can develop from a fever and dehydration to seizures, stroke, and death.

Even at relatively cool ambient temperatures, the temperature can rise inside the vehicle to more than 37.8°C (100°F), which places the infant at risk of hyperthermia. Vehicles heat up rapidly, with most of the temperature rise occurring within the first 10 minutes. Leaving the windows opened slightly does not significantly slow the heating process or decrease the maximal temperature attained (Kids & Cars, 2018).

Nurses can take the lead in increasing public awareness and improving parental education regarding heat rise in motor vehicles. The take-home message here is to never leave an infant alone in a motor vehicle. Make "look before you lock" a routine whenever you get out of the car. The nurse can also suggest the automobile safety precautions listed in Box 11.8. Much of automobile safety is common sense, but the nurse must cover all areas in anticipatory preventive teaching. The importance of automobile safety cannot be overemphasized.

### ◆ Biological Agents

The fetus is partially protected from some biological agents in the environment by the placental barrier and the mother's defence system. After birth, however, the infant is thrust into an environment that is filled with various bacteria, viruses, and potentially disease-causing agents. These organisms can be found everywhere in the infant's immediate environment,

## BOX 11.8   Automobile Safety Precautions

- Be a good role model. Make sure you always wear your seatbelt.
- Never leave a child unattended in a parked car or around cars.
- Never hold a child in the lap in the front seat.
- *Look before you lock* the car to make sure no child is left behind.
- Always use an infant car seat that is properly installed by following the manufacturer's instructions.
- Keep car doors and windows locked, even in driveways or garages.
- Use safety restraints for passengers and the driver.
- Do not be distracted by an infant while driving.
- Continue to use car seats as directed by the manufacturer; then use seatbelts.
- Never place an infant in a rear-facing car safety seat in the front seat of a vehicle that has a passenger air bag.
- Always lock your car and secure the keys so that children cannot access keys.
- Install a trunk-release mechanism so that children will not be trapped in the trunk.
- Take the child out of the car seat first, and then worry about getting other items (e.g., groceries) out of the car.
- If you see a child alone in a car, get involved. Call 911 immediately and get the child out of car immediately. It may save the child's life.

Source: American Academy of Pediatrics. (2018). *Car seats: Information for families*. Retrieved from https://www.healthychildren.org/English/safety-prevention/on-the-go-Pages/Car-Safety-Seats-Information-for-Families.aspx.

including on the skin of the caregiver. However, we are learning that these germs are not always harmful—in fact, infants exposed to bacteria from large animals, breastfeeding, and vaginal birth have lower rates of asthma, allergies, gastroenteritis, and type 1 diabetes via the impact of these early exposures on their gut microbiome (Johnson & Ownby, 2017). As we learn more about which environmental exposures are helpful versus harmful, we do have a vast amount of research demonstrating that the best way to protect infants from some of the most harmful disease-causing pathogens is with immunization.

### Immunization

Disease prevention by immunization is a public health priority and one of the world's greatest public health achievements (Government of Canada, 2018b). Currently, the recommended vaccine schedule protects children from 14 serious diseases. By exposing infants to either a killed or weakened version of the pathogen, these immunizations boost their immune response and are over 90% effective at preventing these diseases if they are encountered in the future. However, infants are too young to be fully vaccinated and individuals with a weak immune system may not respond adequately to be protected from infection. Therefore, herd immunity is important to protect these vulnerable individuals. Herd immunity refers to when a large portion of the population is vaccinated and therefore the opportunity for spread of vaccine-preventable disease throughout the community is reduced (Government of Canada, 2018b).

There is a small segment of the population that refuses to vaccinate their children, often called "anti-vaxxers" in the media. In order to increase families' acceptance of vaccination, it is important that health care providers listen and validate the parents' concerns, correct misconceptions in a nonjudgemental manner, and provide accurate information about the risks of vaccine-preventable diseases and safety of vaccines (CPS, 2018c). They can consider telling compelling stories to make the case for vaccination, and emphasizing that not vaccinating puts other vulnerable people at risk in addition to their own child. Finally, if the family is not convinced with one visit, health care providers should consider every encounter an opportunity for further discussion on the topic (CPS, 2018c).

The two types of immunization are active and passive immunization. In active immunization, all or part of a disease-causing microorganism or a modified product of that microorganism is injected into the body to make the immune system react defensively. This substance is generally a toxin of the disease organism; depending on the virulence and certain other characteristics of the organism, it is used in the vaccine in a live, killed, or attenuated form (American Academy of Pediatrics [AAP], 2015). The attenuated form is alive, but its virulence has been reduced significantly by treatment with laboratory procedures that use, for example, heat or chemicals, which reduces the potency of microorganisms. Examples of active immunization include diphtheria, tetanus, and acellular pertussis vaccine; inactivated polio vaccine; and measles, mumps, and rubella vaccine. Active immunity is relatively long lasting, waning over several years if at all.

Passive immunization is accomplished by injection of pre-formed antibodies from an actively immunized person or animal. After an individual has been exposed to a disease, a passive immunization as post-exposure prophylaxis is given to prevent the disease from developing. Passive immunizations provide a short immunity, usually 1 to 6 weeks, which will protect the person until the danger of contracting the disease has passed. Passive immunization also helps reduce the severity of the disease when it is contracted. Because of the short duration, active immunization is still needed for a person to remain permanently immune. Passive immunity also occurs naturally in newborns when maternal antibodies are passed through the placenta or in breast milk.

The National Advisory Committee on Immunization, an advisory body to the Public Health Agency of Canada, makes recommendations regarding current and newly available vaccines in Canada. Table 11.7 lists the current recommendations for healthy infants in Ontario; schedules are similar across provinces and territories, although they may differ in their timing of administration.

Immunization provides one of the most cost-effective means of preventing infection in infants. Immunizations not only help protect those receiving the vaccinations from developing potentially serious diseases but also help protect entire communities by preventing and reducing the spread of infectious agents. Immunization is additionally important because antibiotics cannot destroy viruses; therefore, immunization offers the most effective means of control. Nurses have a special responsibility to keep informed of the recommendations and document all vaccinations given. Emphasis must be placed on educating parents about the importance of immunization. Children need a series of vaccinations, starting shortly after birth, to be fully protected

## TABLE 11.7   Recommended Immunization Schedule for Infants in Ontario

| Age (Months) | Immunization |
| --- | --- |
| 2 | Diphtheria, Tetanus, Pertussis, Polio, Haemophilus influenzae type b (DTaP-IPV-Hib) + Pneumococcal Conjugate 13 (Pneu-C-13) + Rotavirus (Rot-1) |
| 4 | Diphtheria, Tetanus, Pertussis, Polio, Haemophilus influenzae type b (DTaP-IPV-Hib) |
| 6 | Diphtheria, Tetanus, Pertussis, Polio, Haemophilus influenzae type b (DTaP-IPV-Hib) |
| 12 | Pneumococcal Conjugate 13 (Pneu-C-13) + Meningicoccal Conjugate C (Men-C-C) + Measles, Mumps, Rubella (MMR) |
| 15 | Varicella (Var) |
| 18 | Diphtheria, Tetanus, Pertussis, Polio, Haemophilus influenzae type b (DTaP-IPV-Hib) |

Source: Ontario Ministry of Health and Long-Term Care. (2016). *Publicly funded immunization schedules for Ontario: December 2016.* Retrieved from http://www.health.gov.on.ca/en/pro/programs/immunization/docs/immunization_schedule.pdf.

against potentially serious diseases. To promote childhood immunization, the nurse can work toward increasing health education at the individual and community levels, be knowledgeable of the policies about immunization requirements for entry into the public school system and inform parents of these policies, send reminders for upcoming visits and needed immunizations, provide health services that make immunizations feasible and available, develop a close relationship with the family, and continue surveillance of the immunization status of every infant in the health care system.

## ◆ Chemical Agents

### Drugs and Medications

Despite advances such as childproof caps on medications, childproof packaging, increased educational efforts, and increased awareness of commonly ingested substances, deaths attributable to unintentional poisonings still occur. Unintentional poisonings are an unfortunate and usually preventable cause of death and disability in infants and children. The very nature of a young child predisposes the child to explore the surrounding environment. As children grow and learn to become independent, they are compelled to investigate new and interesting items, places, and objects, such as medications.

Among children younger than 5 years of age in Ontario, the top 10 exposures managed by the poison control centre are pain relievers (ibuprofen and acetaminophen), cleaning substances, cosmetics and personal care products, vitamins, foreign bodies, skin cream, plants, cough and cold medicines, pesticides, and antihistamines (Ontario Poison Centre, 2015). With the legalization of marijuana in 2018, a recent development in Canada is that children are having greater access to cannabis and may find edibles particularly appealing since they are often eaten in the form of candy. This has led to an increase in cannabis poisoning across Canada among children of all ages, including those younger than 4 years of age (Smith, 2018). It is important that safeguards be put in place when edible cannabis products

become legal (anticipated to occur in 2019), to prevent them from getting into the hands of children.

Recent changes in medication packaging and limits on the number of tablets contained in each bottle have reduced deaths resulting from overdose. Drug manufacturers are using childproof caps increasingly as a safety measure. Despite a concerted effort by manufacturers, childproof bottle caps differ in effectiveness (Ferguson, Osterthaler, Kaminski, et al., 2015). Frequently, the safety caps are adult proof, although children can readily open bottles with them.

This accessibility points to the dangers of medications, regardless of the bottle. All medications must still be secured in a safe place when infants are in the home or visiting other homes. Some additional guidelines to help prevent accidents involving medications include the following:

- Use a prescription medication only for the purpose and the person for whom it is intended. Do not use medication prescribed for someone else for a similar condition in the infant.
- Discard unused medications by taking them to dump into the garbage on toxic dump days; many infants have been poisoned by eating tablets found in the garbage at home.
- Request safety caps on all prescription medications.
- Keep all medicines under lock and key.
- Use the dosing device that comes with the medicine.
- Consider products not thought about as medicine, such as diaper rash remedies and eye drops.
- Have the telephone number of the nearest poison control centre readily available.

The main points to be emphasized in giving parents guidance in accident prevention are to eliminate specific environmental hazards from exploring infants, and to supervise infants while they play, gradually replacing supervision with safety training (Ferguson et al., 2015).

### Toxins

Colourful, interesting-looking houseplants add beauty to our homes, but they are often an irresistible attraction to a young infant or child. Infants and small children have a curious nature and have difficulty keeping their hands out of dirt-filled plant pots or resisting the temptation of eating leaves from the plant. Houseplants are another source of poison if ingested. Most people fail to think of houseplants as potentially poisonous because people do not consider eating them. However, infants test almost everything by putting things in their mouths, and a number of plants can be deadly when eaten. As a result, plants are one of the leading sources of poisoning of infants, and amateur foragers frequently learn the hard way that not everything that looks good can be eaten. Most plants, however, have an unpleasant taste and therefore are consumed only in small amounts. The effects of unintentional poisonings are typically dose dependent; therefore, as children age and their sense of taste becomes more defined, the risk of large-dose unintentional poisonings decreases because they are better able to discriminate the unpleasant taste.

Household plants are frequently placed on the floor, where the leaves or flowers are easy to pull off and taste. The best intervention for plant poisoning is prevention, which, in this case,

## TABLE 11.8   List of Poisonous Plants

### Any Part of the Following Plants

| | | |
|---|---|---|
| Amaryllis | English Ivy | Morning Glory |
| Angel's Trumpet | Eucalyptus | Mother-in-law's Tongue |
| Arrowhead vine | Euonymus | Narcissus |
| Autumn Crocus | Foxglove | Nightshade |
| Azalea | Gladiola | Oleander |
| Bittersweet | Holly | Potato (all green parts) |
| Black Locust | Horse Chestnut | Pothos |
| Boston Ivy | Hyacinth | Rhododendron |
| Caladium | Hydrangea | Rhubarb Leaves |
| Calla Lily | Iris | Rosary Bean |
| Castor Bean | Jack-in-the-Pulpit | Snake Berry |
| Chinese Lantern Plant | Jequirity Bean | Snow on the Mountain |
| Clematis | Jerusalem Cherry | Star of Bethlehem |
| Cotoneaster | Jimson Weed | St. John's Wort |
| Croton | Larkspur | Tobacco |
| Cyclamen | Lily-of-the-Valley | Tomato Plant (unripe) |
| Daffodil | Lobelia | Virginia Creeper |
| Daisy (Chrysanthemum) | Lupine | Water Hemlock |
| Delphinium | Marijuana | Wisteria |
| Dieffenbachia | Milkweed | Yew |
| Elephant's Ear | Mistletoe | |

### Seeds or Pits of the Following Fruit

| | | |
|---|---|---|
| Apple | Cherry | Nectarine |
| Apricot | Crab apple | Peach |

Source: Ontario Poison Centre. (2015). *Plants*. Retrieved from http://www.ontariopoisoncentre.ca/common-poisons/poisonous-plants/plants.aspx.

## BOX 11.9   Nursing Interventions to Prevent Plant Poisoning in Infants

- Keep plants, seeds, and bulbs out of reach of infants and young children.
- Know each plant in and around your home.
- Label each household plant.
- Never eat wild mushrooms or unfamiliar berries.
- Teach children not to put leaves, flowers, seeds, nuts, or berries in their mouths without checking with an adult first.
- Keep pesticides in their original containers and out of reach of children.
- Seek help whenever anyone chews or swallows a poisonous plant.
- Keep the local poison control centre telephone number handy.

Source: Parachute. (2019). *Poison prevention: Unintentional poisoning.* Retrieved from http://www.parachutecanada.org/injury-topics/item/poison-prevention-lt.

means previous knowledge. Table 11.8 identifies several common household and garden plants that are poisonous. The nurse should know which plants are harmful when ingested or how to readily access this information, and must inform parents of the potential dangers to infants.

Safety education is stressed at all well-baby visits, beginning in the first 6 months of life. Prevention of plant poisoning and other accidents depends on a reciprocal relationship between protection and education that must be related to age. Encourage parents to keep all poisonous substances, medicines, cleaning agents, health and beauty aids, paints, and plants locked in a safe place out of an infant's sight and reach. This might include purses, if medications are kept in them. Cannabis products should be treated and stored like all other medications. Parents should find out the names of all the plants in and around the house because if someone ingests one of them, the poison control centre will need to know this specific information. Never store poisonous substances in containers other than original ones (e.g., empty jars or soda bottles). Anticipatory guidance should also include the phone number for the local poison control centre, early recognition of common signs and symptoms of poisoning, and the importance of never giving remedies before the poison control centre has been contacted. When parents are provided with anticipatory guidance, particular emphasis must be placed on the prevention of unintentional poisonings. Guidance should be given on the basis of developmental age rather than chronological age (Parachute, 2019).

As nurses, part of our role is that of education. Talking with parents outside the health care arena would be a great start. Girl or Boy Scout meetings, meetings of parent–teacher associations, church gatherings, day care centres, and other community-based activities can provide a forum for teaching and learning, and such training sessions could also provide an opportunity for questions to be answered.

Box 11.9 lists specific safety measures for parents to prevent plant poisoning of infants.

Susceptibility to environmental toxicants depends on the child's developmental stage and interactions within the physical, biological, and social environment. Infants are at particular risk of exposure to toxic factors in the environment; as dependent, developing organisms, they are inherently vulnerable. Generally, the exposure of infants to potential toxins is quite different from that of adults because of differences in physical environment, activities, and diet. Daily activities of infants, such as proximity to the floor or carpet inside the home and the lawn or soil outside, hand-to-mouth behaviours, and smaller body size and composition, place them at great risk of exposure to environmental toxins. The floor inside the home is an important microenvironment for infants because their breathing zones are low and many chemicals are concentrated near the floor. Ingestion, inhalation, and dermal exposure can occur. Infants are exposed to a host of environmental pollutants on a regular basis. These exposures occur through all possible environmental media: air, water, soil, and food. Infants have a unique exposure pattern and unique vulnerabilities. For example, some studies identify that the infant's oral habits and unique diet (ingesting more fruits, vegetables, and water than do adults) magnify their exposure to certain agents. Finally, because infants have a longer life span, toxins that have a long latency or cumulative toxicity (such as certain carcinogens) pose a greater risk to them than to adults (Falck, Mooney, Kapoor, et al., 2015).

Pesticides are internationally used harmful chemicals that are used to control pest attack on crops. In general, pesticides are used to kill insects (insecticides), weeds (herbicides), fungi (fungicides), and rodents (rodenticides). Some pesticides that are used to control insects that feed on cereal grains, fruits, and vegetables are notorious for their slow accumulation in human tissue. Over sufficient time, exposure to relatively small amounts of pesticides can result in the buildup of toxic quantities and lead to chronic disease in humans. Pesticides pollute water sources and agricultural products, and consumption of their residues by drinking water or the eating of foods may lead to serious health risks (Hashim, 2015). All pesticides have the ability to harm infants if they are exposed to them. The essence to decreasing the health hazards of pesticides is to limit exposure to them by use of precautionary measures and to have knowledge of their chemistry to decrease their hazards.

Lead is another environmental toxin that has no known physiological role in the human body. Lead exposure is a public health concern, especially in early childhood because young children are more prone to practice hand-to-mouth activity, play on the floor where dust with lead may settle, and they absorb lead more easily than adults. Even low amounts of lead exposure can affect cognitive development, leading to lower IQ scores and attention-related problems (Government of Canada, 2018c). However, lead poisoning in Canada has declined over time and young children have been shown to have the lowest blood lead concentrations of all Canadians (Statistics Canada, 2015b). While lead can still be found in water, soil, dust, and air, it was more common in our environment when it was still used in paint and gasoline. In houses built before 1960, lead-based paint was probably used on the inside and outside of the home (Government of Canada, 2017). For homes built between 1960 and 1990, the exterior paint would likely contain lead and the interior would have smaller amounts. If this paint is chipping or flaking, it can be a hazard to young children. Numerous toys made in China have been recalled and deemed unsafe because they contain lead-based paint. Lead in the air, water, dust and soil comes primarily from industrial processes, transportation (particularly air), and mining (Government of Canada, 2016a).

Human potential and development are clearly important natural resources, and a growing body of evidence links increased lead exposure to impaired intellectual performance and potential. Clinical lead poisoning is preventable; excess lead in the infant's environment is made by, and should be eliminated by, human beings. Lead has now been removed from gasoline, paint, and pipes that supply water in Canada. Recently, the Government of Canada (2018c) also tightened their consumer product safety regulations regarding the amount of lead allowed in children's toys. However, some people are more at risk of being exposed to lead and inadvertently exposing their children—for example, parents who work at a smelter, refinery, or other industry where they are exposed to lead, and parents with a hobby like making stained glass, lead shot, or lead fishing weights—and must, therefore, take extra precautions. Nurses can recommend the following measures to reduce infants' exposure to lead:

- Keep areas in which the infant plays as dust-free and clean as possible.
- Do not remove lead paint yourself.
- Do not keep drinks in lead crystal containers for a long time, and do not serve drinks from crystal glassware to pregnant women or young children.

- If lead solder is used for a hobby in the home, keep children away from the area and wash hands well after handling lead.
- If work involves lead, change clothes and bathe before entering the home or environment of infants (e.g., day care centres).
- Do not burn waste oil, coloured newsprint, battery casings, or painted wood in a fireplace (Government of Canada, 2016b).

Air pollution is another risk to infants' health, and young children are more at risk for breathing in air contaminants than are other age groups. This is because infants' lungs are less developed and able to handle toxic damage, and their higher ventilation rates and mouth breathing increase their intake of air pollutants. This can impact infants' lung development, and lead to respiratory illnesses and premature mortality (Gouveia & Junger, 2018). Families can check the Air Quality Health Index levels for their local area on a daily basis and engage in outdoor activities that are as far away as possible from roadways and other sources of pollution to reduce the risks associated with air pollution (Government of Canada, 2016c).

Infants do not necessarily escape noxious chemicals when they are indoors. The levels of contaminants that cause air pollution are approximately the same indoors as they are outdoors, with perhaps higher indoor concentrations of carbon monoxide, nitrogen dioxide, and various hydrocarbons from tobacco smoke; poorly ventilated heating and cooking equipment; and aerosol sprays. There are radon checks and carbon dioxide detectors that can be used to assess the presence of these contaminants. Many consequences of exposure to air pollution may not be observed during infancy but can surface in problems that affect both physical and mental well-being over a lifetime.

Toxicants are widely dispersed throughout the environment of infants. It is essential for nurses to understand the potential routes of exposure, toxic effects, and strategies for prevention of exposure so as to provide anticipatory guidance to parents and family members.

## ❖ DETERMINANTS OF HEALTH

### ◆ Social Factors and Environment

#### Community and Work

As infants grow and develop, their boundaries extend beyond the home environment. Many mothers and fathers of infants return to the workforce, placing the infants in community day care centres. *Day care* refers to the care provided for infants in a centre-based facility. It involves the caring for and supervising of infants by someone other than the parent or guardian.

Today, few young families can escape financial burdens. The two-income and single-mother families are ways of life, and the trend will continue; 69% of families who have children living at home are dual-earner couples in Canada (Uppal, 2015), demonstrating why the need for child care service is growing. This situation is usually an emotional issue for families when they return to work and still have a young child at home, and the separation process can be traumatic for both the infant and the parent.

Findings from social science research regarding the effects of day care on an infant's development and health can be summarized as follows: little evidence suggests that day care permanently enhances or slows intellectual development, although high-quality day care can support the cognitive and language development of children from impoverished homes; the home and family are still more influential for child development, even for children who spend significant time in nonparental care; the quality of day care is important, and generally formal centres have higher quality of care than informal home-based options; day care can be used without damaging the parent–child attachment relationship; and day care can lead to an increase in communicable diseases, ear infections, and the flu, without evidence of long-term effects (Shpancer, 2017).

Canada offers maternity and parental leave benefits that provide some financial support and job security until the infant is 1 year of age. While most parents take advantage of this important social benefit, approximately 26% of infants under 1 year of age use child care (Sinha, 2015). The question of how old an infant should be before being placed in day care is frequently asked of health professionals. Many experts believe that a mother and infant should have 4 to 6 months together before the mother returns to work. Brazelton and Sparrow (2015) make a good case for the mother and infant transitioning through four stages of attachment together before the mother returns to work:

- In the first stage, which takes 10 to 14 days, the infant learns to be attentive to the mother, and the mother learns cues from the infant about being both ready for and tired of attentiveness.
- The second stage, which lasts 8 weeks, is a stage of playful interaction, when the mother learns how to recognize the infant's nonverbal cues and helps the infant maintain the alert state.
- The third stage, from the 10th week to the fourth month, is when the mother and infant learn to play games together.
- During the fourth stage, which occurs in the fourth month, infants rapidly learn about themselves and their world. A mother, when possible, should spend the first 4 months with her new infant.

Parents in Canada rely on three types of child care situations, in fairly equal proportions: formal day care centres; home day cares; and private arrangements such as relatives or nannies (Sinha, 2015). The nurse has a vital role in assisting families with infants who need day care to help them sort through the many options available in the local area. Many factors are reviewed when a family is looking for an appropriate day care program; the nurse can counsel and guide the family in its search. The means by which the nurse counsels and guides the family in selecting a day care centre are as follows:

- Promote awareness of the three types of day care available in their local communities.
- Counsel parents on questions to ask employees of a prospective day care facility (Box 11.10).
- Help parents learn ways to cope with the separation behaviours manifested by their infant:
  - Remain calm in the situation.
  - Attempt to reduce the number of adults who interact with the infant and always introduce them.

---

### BOX 11.10    Prospective Day Care Facility Questions

- How much does it cost? Are there additional fees?
- Are there subsidized spots available at the centre?
- How flexible are the drop-off/pick-up times?
- How do parents communicate with caregivers?
- Are you licensed?
- How many children do you care for?
- How do you ensure the health of children?
- What happens when a child is sick?
- What safety measures are in place?
- What kinds of snacks and meals do you provide?
- Is food prepared on-site or catered in?
- Can you accommodate our family's dietary/allergy needs?
- Is a fridge available for breast milk and is there a schedule for feeding?
- What will my child do throughout the day?
- How do play materials support learning, creativity, and social interaction?
- How much time is spent outside?
- How are different cultural traditions integrated into the program?
- How are family members integrated into the program?
- What happens if a child is angry or upset?
- What qualifications do staff and providers have?
- Does someone on staff have CPR and first aid training?
- What happens when the staff or provider is sick or away?

*CPR,* Cardiopulmonary resuscitation.
Source: Ontario Ministry of Education. (2018). *Questions to ask a child care provider.* Retrieved from https://www.ontario.ca/page/questions-ask-child-care-provider. © Queen's Printer for Ontario, 2016. Reproduced with permission.

---

- Instruct parents to ask the question: Where do the infants sleep and are they separate from older children? Exposure to older children increases the risk of infection.
- Encourage the parents to bring an infant's special cuddly toy from home to the day care facility to promote security.
- Listen to the parent's understanding of the separation and expected behaviours.
- Reassure parents that it takes time for the infant to make the transition from the parent to another caregiver and vice versa.
- Emphasize that at certain developmental stages stranger anxiety may be heightened (8 months), and separation behaviours of crying and clinging may be repeated.
- Work toward promoting a good relationship among parents, the infant, and the caregiver by providing opportunities for open discussions of concerns.

## Culture and Ethnicity

Culture is defined as a set of learned values, beliefs, attitudes, and practices that are passed from generation to generation (Polan & Taylor, 2015). Culture plays an important role in influencing an infant's development, and what is considered "normal" development differs greatly from one culture to the next. Culture defines how health care information is received, how rights and protections are exercised, what is considered to be a health problem, how symptoms and concerns about the problem are expressed, who should provide treatment for the problem, and what type of treatment should be given. In short, culture is the lens through which one views the world, affecting everything that an individual and that individual's family perceives and does.

The developing infant is subject to the influences of culture from the moment of conception. Partly because of the long dependency period, the family environment is the setting within which the infant experiences overall cultural attitudes. The lives of infants tend to be more under the direct control of parents or other caregivers than the lives of older children, who are often actively involved in selecting their own environments through contacts with peers, teachers, and other adults. The special demands of infancy require extensive and specific caregiving routines across cultures. Effective parenting styles also vary as a function of culture. The parents' perceptions of illness, wellness, roles, child-rearing practices, religious values, language, and health practices are all modelled for the infant. In short, culture helps form the infant's view of the world (Bornstein, 2015; CPS, 2018b).

The family's ethnicity includes ideas about health, illness, food preferences, moral codes, and family life that persist across generations and survive even the upheaval of coming to a new country. All cultural groups confront repeated challenges as they transfer their families from familiar to unfamiliar surroundings. Infants are exposed to an appropriate mode of behaviour that is in accordance with their family's cultural standards. By observing and imitating family members, infants take cues for behaviour. These perceptions are then incorporated into their own self-concepts (Calkins, 2015).

Cultural competence is grounded in humility, involving self-reflection and self-critique of personal biases and an emphasis on building respectful partnerships that are based on mutual trust (CNA, 2018). In attempting to foster trust with diverse populations, nurses need to help women and their families feel comfortable enough to engage in a dialogue and share information. One approach is being careful not to prejudge as foolish or ill-conceived specific cultural practices and beliefs about health care. For example, among families from Mexico, Guatemala, and Central American countries, when an infant develops a sunken fontanelle it is considered a symptom of trauma caused by experiences such as driving on a bumpy road, sucking on an empty body, or improperly holding an infant (Killion, 2017). The remedy for this might include slapping the soles of the feet, pushing up on the palate of the mouth, or nonviolently shaking an infant in an upside-down position. Instead of deeming such practices foolish, the nurse should let the families know that an effective practice is to ensure the infant gets lots of breast milk or formula to drink, and then support them with infant feeding. This ensures the infant's hydration and safety are prioritized, yet it does not demean their cultural practices. With such an approach, families are not embarrassed to let nurses know about their traditional cultural practices. This will help bridge the gap and build trust in their relationship.

> ### BOX 11.11 Factors That Facilitate Multicultural Health Care by Nurses
>
> - Self-exploration of values and beliefs concerning other cultures and their beliefs
> - Knowledge of the historical experience, recent and long term, of ethnic groups that live in the community
> - Knowledge of demographic data that include family size, socioeconomic status, and future expectations that are characteristic of diverse ethnic groups
> - Understanding and sensitivity to cultural health care practices different from their own
> - Recognition of traditional beliefs and cultural attitudes toward health and illness
> - Awareness of the nature of problems encountered by ethnic group members when they enter the health care system, including fear and distrust of health care providers, language barriers, and discrimination by caregivers

To assess and plan appropriate interventions for different ethnic groups, nurses must be aware of their own cultural backgrounds. An important consideration is to examine all customs and values in relative terms, seeing none as either good or bad (Box 11.11). Change is inevitable in family life, whether it is resisted or welcomed. An important function of the nurse is to help families monitor the rate of change that is acceptable to various members and reach a consensus.

Culturally competent nursing improves outcomes for nurses, organizations, and those seeking care. Providing safe and high-quality care to families of different cultural backgrounds should be considered an entry-level competency for nurses, and part of our social justice mandate (CNA, 2018). Research has identified several strategies that nurses can use that improve communication and reduce stress for culturally diverse populations: answering questions carefully, teaching by demonstration, and taking time to explain in simple English. In addition, when women feel that nurses truly care for their infant, it facilitates communication across multiple barriers because mothers feel safe to ask questions or express needs (Lee & Brann, 2015). Thus, nurses who are mindful of the specific views of a culture respect the boundaries of the particular cultural perceptions, beliefs, and practices. Culturally competent nurses have achieved efficacy in communication skills and incorporate health care practices and beliefs of a particular culture into health care plans. Furthermore, respect for the individual's cultural values is viewed as essential if the nurse is to successfully help the family achieve a state of health and wellness.

The nurse identifies the power structure within a given cultural group. This knowledge may help dictate which family member to approach with the health teaching. Although the nurse might assume it would be the infant's mother, this may not necessarily be the case, because in some cultures the primary decision maker regarding matters of child welfare is the father or grandmother (Andrews & Boyle, 2015). The nurse assesses the cultural groups' practices and beliefs before planning interventions, as approaches to infant care differ among cultural groups (Diversity Awareness).

## ⊕ DIVERSITY AWARENESS

### *Quick Guide for Cross-Cultural Nursing Care*

The dominant North American attitudes about infants and approaches to infant care have undergone many changes in the past several years. With the increased numbers of women in the workforce, fathers are becoming more involved in infant care, and day care for infants is increasing. Although children are valued, and raising children within the nuclear family remains a priority, an increasing number of women are focusing on careers, delaying childbirth, and limiting family size.

Members of some cultures view child-bearing and child-rearing differently. The birth of a child is crucial for women of some cultures, whose social role and status are attained through reproduction within the marital relationship. Preference for a male child exists among families of many cultures, particularly Middle Eastern and Asian cultures (Roudsari, Zakerihamidi, & Khoei, 2015).

In the dominant Western culture, an infant is frequently wrapped warmly in blankets, placed in an infant seat or stroller, and put to sleep in a crib in a room separate from the parents. Mothers from other cultures may choose to carry or wrap their infants differently, such as carrying their infants with them at all times and sleeping with them. Inuit infants may be carried in the Amauti, a warm parka with a built-in pouch to allow the infant to be carried on either the woman's front or back (Ontario Association of Children's Aid Societies [OACAS], 2015). Indigenous families may also rely more heavily on an extended community to participate in child-rearing, and their children are given more respect, freedom, and autonomy than is common within a Western parenting philosophy (OACAS, 2015).

Cultural beliefs and practices are continually evolving and changing. Nurses acknowledge and explore their meanings with all the families they meet. Nurses work actively to reduce the experience of culture shock for ethnic minority families, remembering that Western medical beliefs and practices may appear strange to others. All behaviour must be evaluated from within the context of the family and the family's cultural background and experience.

Nurses must facilitate health-promoting attitudes and practices and show empathic concern and respect for individuals of all cultural backgrounds. By incorporating the assessment of cultural beliefs and practices into the individual's plan of care, nurses can demonstrate respect and take a step forward in developing culturally appropriate patterns of caring.

The family is the primary health care provider for the infant. The family determines health promotion for the family, including when an infant is ill. Many cultural groups choose between the traditional beliefs that they believe to be appropriate and Western medical treatment, whereas others may implement both. Nurses are cautious in imposing their own values, beliefs, and attitudes on others. Rather than judging people, the nurse ascertains how each family's values and beliefs influence health outcomes.

The nurse remembers that all behaviours must be evaluated from within the context of the family's cultural background and experiences. Nurses who strive to foster health-promoting attitudes and behaviours begin at the most basic level: empathic concern and respect for the individual. By incorporating the assessment of cultural beliefs and practices into the infant's plan of care, nurses demonstrate respect, reduce alienation, and take a step toward developing culturally appropriate patterns of health promotion. Respecting another's language and religion is extremely important.

#### Reflective Questions

Think about the attitudes and beliefs that you were raised with in your home as a child. Consider gender roles, who made decisions, what kinds of remedies were used when you were sick, what kinds of foods you ate, whether you were breastfed or bottle fed, and how you were cared for.

- How does this influence your understanding of health, health promotion, and health care?
- How will this impact your work with families that are different from your own?

Sources: Andrews, M. M., & Boyle, J. S. (2015). *Transcultural concepts in nursing care* (7th ed.). Philadelphia: Lippincott Williams & Wilkins; Roudsari, R. L., Zakerihamidi, M., & Khoei, E. M. (2015). Socio-cultural beliefs, values and traditions regarding women's preferred mode of birth in the north of Iran. *International Journal of Community Based Nursing and Midwifery, 3*(3), 165.

## Language

Language is an important medium for understanding and working together. The nurse may avoid or tend to mumble a person's name when it is foreign; people hesitate to express themselves when the material is unfamiliar. The nurse must consider how the individual who speaks a different language feels about being unable to express thoughts and feelings or to understand what is being said. Both parties may play the avoidance game.

The nurse takes steps to remove communication barriers, including the following:

- Using a professional interpreter to help in the communication process
- Using pictorial flash cards in the individual's native language to assist in explaining instructions
- Sending a health care worker to an educational centre or school to learn the basics of the language to help in the interpreting process in the health care facility

Even a person who speaks the nurse's language may not understand and comprehend instructions given by the nurse. The negative impact of poor communication is huge, resulting in poor health outcomes, health inequities, and high health care

costs. The importance of good health communication is relevant to all populations seeking care, including those from culturally and linguistically diverse backgrounds (Andrews & Boyle, 2015).

## Religion

Some health care providers believe that religion plays no role in individuals' health care practices; therefore, they eschew people's religious, spiritual, or ethical concerns and deal mainly with the physical or psychological problems at hand. However, the individual's religious, spiritual, and ethical concerns are generally the major source for human values when health care services are being evaluated.

Religious beliefs can become risk factors when they affect decisions concerning treatment. An example may be the parents who refuse a blood transfusion, surgery, or other medically indicated treatment required to save their infant's life. A court order is needed in many instances to treat these infants. Decisions regarding an infant's health care are the parents' responsibility, based on their customs and beliefs, and when the life of the child is not in imminent danger, this should be respected. Deciding not to offer an opinion may be extremely difficult, but usually the opinion is unwanted. Religion is often a powerful force, and when the nurse causes conflict and interferes, a gap can be formed. This gap may force the parents to seek nonprofessional health care to help them with their health-related and religious ideas about birth, death, stress, birth control, and other matters. To work successfully with an individual, the person's religious background should be explored and understood thoroughly. Most nurses recognize that attending to the spiritual needs of families enhances the overall quality of their nursing care and the satisfaction of their care recipients.

## ◆ Levels of Policy Making and Health

### Legislation

Enormous strides have been made in infant health in the past decade: many common, lethal infections have been eradicated (smallpox), malnutrition is seldom seen in Canada, and perinatal and infant mortality rates continue to decline. Health and well-being are accepted rights of every Canadian, without regard to race, gender, age, sexuality, economic or social status, or creed. The *Canada Health Act* is the piece of federal legislation that enshrines this right, which "aims to protect, promote and restore the physical and mental well-being of residents of Canada and to facilitate reasonable access to health services without financial or other barriers" (Government of Canada, 2018d, para 1).

Despite the universal health benefits and positive trends in the health of Canadian women and children, infant mortality rates among some groups, such as Indigenous populations, remain high (Sheppard et al., 2017). Additionally, rates of low birth weight have risen between 2000 and 2013 from 5.6% to 6.3% of all births (Statistics Canada, 2016b). This has a significant impact on the infants' long-term health, as low birth weight increases the risk of SIDS, diabetes, hypertension, heart disease, asthma, blindness, and hearing problems (Statistics Canada, 2016b). To address these problems, factors that increase the risks of poor child outcomes must be identified.

Many of the risk factors for low birth weight are preventable, with up to half of such births being attributed to modifiable risk factors (Johnson, Jones, & Paranjothy, 2017). Smoking is the single most influential risk factor, and other modifiable risk factors include substance use (both alcohol and illicit drugs), low maternal BMI, and maternal infections including STIs. Young mothers who experience material deprivation tend to experience more than one risk factor, which suggests that addressing individual risk factors may not be effective and that the broader context for the family must be considered (Johnson, Eberle, Henricks, et al., 2015). Many of the modifiable risk factors for low birth weight will continue to influence the child's health and development after birth, and it is important that nurses work at the family, community, and societal levels to help address the social and economic context.

Legislation is an upstream intervention to address the social determinants of health and increase families' access to secure income, employment, housing, education, and food security. The federal government has recently increased the Canada Child Benefit, a monthly tax-free payment that is adjusted to income, in order to help with the costs of raising children and to reduce childhood poverty. In 2018, the federal government introduced the first ever National Housing Strategy, including an investment of $40 billion over 10 years to reduce housing need and cut chronic homelessness by half (Government of Canada, 2018e). Subsidies for housing, education, employment retraining, and child care are managed at the provincial or municipal level. An example of legislation that has helped support many families with young children is Quebec's universal subsidized child care program, in which parents pay a fee ranging from only $7 to $21 per day (Fortin, 2017). These broad macroeconomic policies act on the distribution of socioeconomic factors to increase equity and "level up" the social positions of the most vulnerable families (Mantoura & Morrison, 2016).

*Nursing's role.* Nurses have important roles in promoting change in response to a continually expanding knowledge base, health care needs, and government legislation. By actively participating in groups involved with health and social service planning, the nurse helps make governmental policy more responsive to infants' and families health care needs. Health promotion essentially relates to collective or population well-being, which is wholly compatible with all the nurse's roles. Nurses need to work together with other professionals, agencies, and local people to improve the health and well-being of infants and all people (Christie, Parkes, & Price, 2015).

The nurse may engage in the development of health care policies at the following three stages: identifying resources for the community to meet its specific needs; planning for resources not available to the community; and coordinating the resources available to the community to promote better use of them.

Additionally, the nurse can advocate for policies that impact the social determinants of health by becoming a member of a professional nursing organization, a health planning council, a community coalition or concerned citizen's group, or an advisory group that makes recommendations to any of the three levels of government (federal, provincial/territorial, or municipal). In this capacity, nurses' responsibility is to share their expertise with the other committee members, collaborate in identifying needs and priorities, and advocate for upstream strategies and legislation that address the various factors that lead to health inequities. Because nurses have first-hand experience with many community needs and marginalized groups, they are in a good position to speak out and inform others.

### Economics

Virtually every major health problem is found more frequently in segments of the population with low income than in high-income groups. The infant mortality rates are highest among the lowest-income Canadians, and also higher in Indigenous and materially disadvantaged communities (PHAC, 2018c).

In Canada, roughly 17% of children are living in a low-income household (Statistics Canada, 2017c). Income determines the quality of other social determinants of health, such as housing and food security; impacts stress and psychological functioning; and contributes to social exclusion (Mikkonen & Raphael, 2010). Parents with low incomes are often unaware of their infant's developmental needs; they are frequently faced with many environmental and social stresses that demand their time, energy, and other resources (Rapaport, 2015). Many parents have so many unfulfilled needs of their own that they cannot meet their infants' needs. In many cases, infants from families in poverty have delayed language development. With limited educational and life experiences, their parents are often unable to be ideal models for language development. Infants learn early language sounds from their parents, but their attempts at language must be reinforced.

Armed with the knowledge of how economics can affect the infant's growth, development, and health status, the nurse, before deciding on interventions, assesses the family situation by performing the following tasks:

- Establish a relationship with the family to obtain pertinent information.
- Evaluate the home environment in which the infant interacts.
- Elicit the parents' health perceptions about their own health and that of the infant, and consider their strengths and resources.
- Offer assistance for the family to navigate the health care system for their infant.
- Complete a thorough physical examination, including developmental assessment, of the infant to identify any areas requiring early intervention.
- Identify community resources and income supports that are available to the low-income family.

The take-home message is that poverty is like any other epidemiological exposure in infants that has health consequences. To the extent that nurses can reach out to these families, they may have a real positive impact on those infants' lives going forward.

### ◆ Health Services/Delivery System

The health care delivery system is diverse and large; many different sectors merge to provide infant care. Within this enormous, multidisciplinary system, the nurse is an advocate who facilitates the family's passage through the many facets of care. Table 11.9 lists a suggested schedule for health-promotion infant care.

The value of health promotion and preventive health care has been validated; it is cost-effective and is here to stay. As nurses' roles continue to expand within the various parts of the health care system, their duty is to keep pace with the needs, concerns, resources, and available strategies for health promotion. Because many conditions that cause morbidity or death in infants are preventable when health-promotion practices are used, nurses have an opportunity to impact the health of infants, families, and society at large by intervening early and using a range of health-promotion strategies that include education, advocacy, and policy development.

## ❖ NURSING APPLICATION

Nurses can do more to ensure the health of our youngest and most vulnerable population. It is the responsibility of all nurses to make health-education and health-promotion activities an integral part of their professional role. The primary role of the nurse in promoting the health of an infant is to provide the family with education during the most critical developmental period. Initial health-promotion efforts should focus on the nutritional needs of the infant during the first 18 months of life. Basic principles of biological growth and development set the stage for appropriate developmental tasks and psychological growth in the coming months. Nurses can make a difference in the lives of infants and their families by encouraging early and adequate prenatal care for the mother, supporting the transition from the hospital to the home, providing increased access to infant care services, and supporting childhood health surveillance.

The nurse promotes the health of infants through their interactions with their parents as infants are dependent on them for care. The nurse is in a position to encourage practices in the home that create the optimal conditions for normal growth and development. An important starting point for the nurse is to teach new parents about the nutritional value of breastfeeding and to encourage those efforts. Professional support and education play a vital role in increasing the rates of breastfeeding women.

Following a routine immunization and well-child health visit schedule is another aspect of health promotion for the infant. Nurses play a role in this task by educating parents about the importance of immunization. In addition, nurses should remain informed about the immunization recommendations and assist the family in maintaining documentation of vaccines administered, as well as removing barriers to accessing health care.

Injuries and accidents are a major concern for the infant population. Accident prevention and safety are topics that should be addressed by the nurse when working with families. Although it is difficult to address the many ways in which an infant can be injured, nurses should be prepared to educate parents about the most common hazards. Some of the educational topics that can be addressed include fall and burn prevention, choking hazards, unintentional poisonings, environmental hazards, and automobile safety. In addition, a significant source of illness in infants and children is associated with infectious diseases from either a bacterial or a viral source. Particularly in younger infants, parents should be taught about the importance of frequent handwashing, avoidance of sick contacts, and signs and symptoms of illness that require immediate medical attention.

Essentially, health promotion should be viewed as an umbrella concept that encompasses all health-related activities that contribute to the formation of a state of health in that individual or community. It should include education, disease prevention, and environmental health-promotion measures. The health-promotion goals of the nurse working with infants are met through the family. The nurse must ascertain the health perceptions and motivation of the family, including the use of positive or negative health practices. The family must be motivated to provide good health practices for the infant. As the nurse plans health-promotion activities for families of infants, it is imperative that factors influencing health

## TABLE 11.9  Suggested Schedule for Health-Promotion Infant Care

| Age (Months) | Promotional Activity | Age (Months) | Promotional Activity |
|---|---|---|---|
| 1 | Complete physical assessment | 9 | Infant's need for space to crawl about |
|  | **Parent discussion includes:** |  | Playing games with infant: pat-a-cake, peek-a-boo, waving bye-bye, and shaking hands |
|  | Basic infant needs: to be touched, held, rocked, and talked to |  | Appropriate toys: blocks, stack toys, and jack-in-the-box |
|  | Supervised tummy time while awake |  | Nutrition: finger foods, variety of textures, introducing cup |
|  | Healthy sleep habits | 12 | Complete physical assessment |
|  | Appropriate toy: colourful mobile |  | Immunizations: pneumococcal conjugate 13 (Pneu-C-13) + meningococcal conjugate C (Men-C-C) + measles, mumps, rubella (MMR) |
|  | Nutrition: breast milk and vitamin D or formula |  | **Parent discussion includes:** |
| 2 | Complete physical assessment |  | Accident prevention |
|  | Immunizations: diphtheria, tetanus, pertussis, polio, *Haemophilus influenzae* type b (DTaP/IPV/Hib) + pneumococcal conjugate 13 (Pneu-C-13) + rotavirus (Rot-1) |  | Infant's need to touch and investigate environment, with supervision |
|  | **Parent discussion includes:** |  | Parent's need to read, show pictures, and repeat body parts to infant |
|  | Need of infant to be exposed to a variety of stimuli within environment |  | Child care/return to work |
|  | Need of infant for change of scenery |  | Sleeping patterns |
|  | Colic and other common problems |  | Appropriate toys: sets of measuring cups, nesting toys, pots and pans, and wooden spoons |
| 4 | Complete physical assessment |  | Nutrition: breast milk or homogenized milk |
|  | Immunizations: diphtheria, tetanus, pertussis, polio, *Haemophilus influenzae* type b (DTaP/IPV/Hib) | 15 | Complete physical assessment |
|  | **Parent discussion includes:** |  | Immunization: varicella (Var) |
|  | Stimulation of infant |  | **Parent discussion includes:** |
|  | Providing a mirror in which the infant can see reflection |  | Age of curiosity in infant |
|  | Being talked to and played with |  | Toys appropriate for age: push-pull toys and ball |
|  | Appropriate toy: rattle |  | Accident prevention |
|  | Nutrition: delaying introduction of solid foods |  | Elimination patterns |
| 6 | Complete physical assessment |  | Discipline: stress positive aspects of behaviour when possible |
|  | Immunizations: diphtheria, tetanus, pertussis, polio, *Haemophilus influenzae* type b (DTaP/IPV/Hib) | 18 | Complete physical assessment |
|  | **Parent discussion includes:** |  | Immunization: diphtheria, tetanus, pertussis, polio, *Haemophilus influenzae* type b (DTaP/IPV/Hib) |
|  | Accident prevention |  | **Parent discussion includes:** |
|  | Teething |  | Accident prevention |
|  | Allowing infant to crawl to explore environment |  | Encouragement of vocalization |
|  | Stranger anxiety |  | Socialization with other small children |
|  | Nutrition: introduction of iron-containing foods |  | Importance of reading to child |
| 9 | Complete physical assessment |  | Setting limits on behaviour |
|  | **Parent discussion includes:** |  | Coping mechanisms of parents |
|  | Accident prevention |  |  |
|  | Dental caries prevention: cleaning teeth daily |  |  |

Sources: American Academy of Pediatrics. (2018). *AAP schedule of well-child care visits*. Retrieved from https://www.healthychildren.org/English/family-life/health-management/Pages/Well-Child-Care-A-Check-Up-for-Success.aspx; Rourke, L., Leduc, D., & Rourke, J. (2017). *Rourke Baby Record*. Retrieved from http://www.rourkebabyrecord.ca/default.

perception are identified. The ability of the nurse to provide a supportive relationship with the parents is a key element in facilitating successful infant development. The nurse working with this population has a unique opportunity to influence the health status of both the infant and the family for years to come.

The leadership of nurses in collaboration with other health care providers will be key to improving the health of future generations. While progress is being made on the social determinants of health, nurses still have an important role to play in advocating for resources and policies that support the health of all infants, especially the most vulnerable.

## CASE STUDY

### Homelessness: Families With Infants

As a community health nurse in an inner-city health centre, you are increasingly aware that the homeless population in your city appears to be the forgotten aggregate. Your community health centre provides primary care to a culturally diverse and Indigenous population. As a nurse, you believe that the population who are homeless within your city has numerous health needs. Beyond the basic requirements, many individuals who are homeless have mental and substance abuse problems, a deficiency in life skills, and poor family support, and most of all lack access to child health services.

The homeless population has all the usual health problems you would expect in the general population, in addition to other problems resulting from being without a home. Although there are several glaring concerns, you plan to focus your attention first on securing immunizations for the homeless infants and, second, on obtaining formula for them.

#### Reflective Questions

- In planning health services for this special population, what facts do you need to know?
- What barriers to accessing health care confront these families?
- How can you overcome some of the barriers in developing your plan for health care?

#### Discussion

- In planning health services for this special population, what facts do you need to know? The following are some of the first questions that should be asked:
  - How many homeless infants are in this aggregate?

- Where are they?
- How can they access health care in the city?

To answer these questions, it might be prudent to collaborate and partner with other health and social service agencies, local hospitals, and the public health department. Collaboration and partnering can bring in additional resources and reduce duplication and gaps in services.

- What barriers to accessing health care for infants confront these families?
  - Lack of transportation
  - Lack of trust in the medical establishment
  - Judgemental care on the part of health care providers and nurses
  - No health insurance card or permanent address to order one
  - Preventive care, such as immunizations, not a priority when you are hungry
  - No money to get prescriptions filled or transportation to get there
  - Waiting until the condition is serious before seeking treatment
- How can you overcome some of the barriers in developing your plan for health care?
  - Provide health care in the city shelters for use by homeless families.
  - Set up a mobile health care team and visit the shelters to provide care.
  - Offer immunizations for all family members.
  - Establish educational sessions within the shelters to provide information.
  - Stress the importance of preventive measures to reduce illness in infants.
  - Offer breastfeeding education and support in the shelter system.
  - Obtain free formula to give to homeless bottle-fed infants.
  - Work closely with other health and social service providers within the community.

## CARE PLAN

### Homelessness: Families With Infants

Homelessness is a community dilemma and an example of an economic problem that places infants at risk. Family homelessness disproportionately affects people who are Indigenous, racialized, newcomers to Canada, parents with a disability, and single mothers (Canadian Observatory on Homelessness, 2018). Homeless infants within these families are more likely to lack immunizations, proper nutrition, a safe environment, and a stable family situation. The community health nurse in this chapter's case study wants to address two aspects of homeless infants: immunizations and nutrition.

#### Nursing Issue

Inadequate health maintenance related to nonadherence to appropriate immunization schedule as manifested by increased incidence of communicable diseases

#### Defining Characteristics

- History of lack of health-seeking behaviour by caregiver
- Lack of financial or other resources
- Reported or observed impairment of personal support systems
- Lack of knowledge regarding health-promotion practices
- Difficulty accessing routine health care
- Limited basic personal resources

#### Related Factors

- Ineffective family coping
- Perceptual-cognitive impairment
- Lack of material resources
- Ineffective individual coping

#### Expected Outcomes

The caretaker of the infant will:
- Begin health-seeking behaviour on behalf of the infant
- Increase health-promotion and health-maintenance knowledge
- Gain access to available health care resources
- Participate in life change to improve health status; meet goals for health care maintenance

#### Nursing Interventions

- Assess caretaker's feelings, values, and personal situation.
- Assess for family patterns, economic issues, and cultural patterns that influence adherence.
- Support the caretaker and family to apply for health card if they have not got one.

## ⦿ CARE PLAN—cont'd

### *Homelessness: Families With Infants*

- Assist the caretaker and family to access health care resources available to them.
- Refer the caretaker and family to community agencies to address social and economic issues.
- Educate the caretaker and family on the importance of immunizations and disease prevention.
- Provide follow-up care to increase the chance of health status change occurring.

#### Nursing Issue

Potential for imbalanced nutrition—less than body requirement due to nutritional and socioeconomic factors as manifested by low height and weight measurements for chronological age on growth chart

#### Defining Characteristics

- Pale conjunctival and mucous membranes
- Poor muscle development
- Inadequate food intake to maintain body weight
- Weight loss, fatigue, frequent irritable, fussy, crying behaviour
- Growth and development milestones not met
- Frequent illnesses, suggesting depressed immunity

#### Related Factors

- Inability to obtain adequate food or fluid or both to nourish body because of socioeconomic factors

#### Expected Outcomes

The infant will demonstrate the following:

- Progressive weight gains toward desired goal
- Weight within normal range for height and weight
- Infant consuming adequate nourishment
- Free of signs of malnutrition

#### Nursing Interventions

- Assess healthy body weight for age and height.
- Observe infant's ability to consume food and fluids.
- Monitor food and fluid intake weekly.
- Access nutritional resources for the caretaker or family.
- Refer family to appropriate community agencies to meet needs.
- Assist the caretaker or family to identify area needing change that will make the greatest contribution to improve nutrition.
- Implement instructional dialogue that is appropriate for their level.
- Provide follow-up care to assist them in changing their health status.

---

### BOX 11.12  Newborn Screening and Genomics

Infants in Canada are offered newborn screening shortly after birth to allow for early detection, diagnosis, and treatment of conditions that might otherwise not be identified until symptoms appear and irreversible damage has occurred. Genomic sequencing can identify genetically based conditions that routine blood tests used to screen newborn babies cannot detect. The standard newborn screening blood tests look for chemical changes and, typically, screen newborns for metabolic and endocrine diseases, sickle cell disease, cystic fibrosis, severe combined immune deficiency, and critical congenital heart disease that are caused by a gene mutation. Researchers have tallied more than 6000 such inherited disorders caused by a single mutated gene and other genes are associated with higher risks of certain conditions, such as heart disease. Imagine being able to anticipate a child's health all the way to adulthood.

In the next few decades, every infant's genome can be sequenced and used to shape a lifetime of personalized strategies for disease prevention, detection, and treatment.

But this brave new world is fraught with technical and ethical issues that have some scientists questioning whether it is appropriate for infants to have their genome sequenced and what information children and parents should receive about the results.

Every individual's genome is loaded with "variant" genes, and harmful mutations make up just a small fraction of them. Researchers have only begun to catalogue which variants cause problems. Questions arise about the wisdom of telling parents and children about conditions for which there is no effective treatment or of letting them know about disorders that will not affect a child until adulthood. Families will need to decide this, as this latest technology moves forward.

Sources: Bavley, A. (2016). Genome sequencing holds tremendous promise for infants, but issues abound. *The Kansas City Star*. Retrieved from http://www.kansascity.com/news/business/health-care/article21973176.html; Ontario Ministry of Health and Long-Term Care. (2018). *Newborn screening*. Retrieved from http://www.health.gov.on.ca/en/pro/programs/newborn/; National Human Genome Research Institute. (2016). *Newborn screening*. Retrieved from https://www.genome.gov/27556918.

# SUMMARY

Never before has health promotion been more important than it is today. Nurses must have evidence-informed understanding of the significant effect that can be made through health-promotion interventions and communicate this understanding to families they care for. Society is changing, as are people's needs and ideas. Families today want more information and knowledge, and they demand that health care providers be more responsive to their needs. Their demand has been a catalyst for the nurse's expanded health care role and responsibility for health promotion. Nurses have been "touted" as potential major contributors to society's health promotion and illness prevention. Nurses are in the forefront of the health-promotion movement through their practice. Health promotion by nurses is associated with common universal principles of health education. Nurses should be able to plan, implement, and evaluate health-promotion interventions for infants and their families to improve their health outcomes.

Health-promotion and disease-prevention practices that are applicable during infancy can be used in the nurse's expanded role. A four-pronged approach is stressed:

- Giving anticipatory guidance to the family unit as the infant grows and develops
- Teaching and counselling to ensure the infant's optimal development
- Being a family advocate to ensure the safety and development of the family unit
- Screening infants to identify infants at risk of developing a condition, via history gathering, physical examination, and observation of parent–child interaction

Anticipating potential health problems during infancy and effectively intervening to avert these problems are nursing processes that promote health. Early detection and reduction of risk factors avoid many health problems, such as abuse. By anticipating problems and helping families to avoid them, the nurse promotes health maintenance.

Using the infant's normal growth and development, psychosocial tasks, common health problems, and health maintenance strategies, the nurse assesses the infant, the family, and the infant's developmental status to provide anticipatory guidance.

By teaching (Box 11.12), an essential component of the nursing process, the nurse transmits knowledge to families to ensure continuity of care and long-term health maintenance. By counselling, the nurse listens to the identified problem, helps the family to recognize the real issues, and allows the family to make its own decisions regarding health care.

Because the infant is in no position to advocate for itself effectively, the nurse assumes the role of advocate. The ultimate goal of nursing intervention in maintaining the infant's health is future self-care. As the infant grows and matures, well-established family health maintenance habits can only enhance the lives of healthy future generations. The nurse is challenged to join this effort of investment in the future.

## Evolve Chapter Features

http://evolve.elsevier.com/Canada/Edelman/healthpromotion/
- Review Questions

# REFERENCES

Aguiar, W., & Halseth, R. (2015). *Aboriginal peoples and historic trauma: The processes of intergenerational transmission*. Prince George, BC: National Collaborating Centre for Aboriginal Health.

American Academy of Pediatrics (AAP). (2015). *Red book 2015: Committee on infectious diseases*. Retrieved from http://redbook.solutions.aap.org/book.aspx?bookid=1484.

American Heart Association. (2015). *Infant CPR*. Retrieved from http://www.heart.org/HEARTORG/CPRAndECC/CommunityCPRandFirstAid/CommunityProducts/Infant-CPR-Anytime_UCM_428979_Article.jsp.

American Public Health Association. (2015). *Injury and violence prevention*. Retrieved from https://www.apha.org/topics-and-issues/injury-and-violence-prevention.

Amin, N. A. L., Tam, W. W. S., & Shorey, S. (2018). Enhancing first-time parents' self-efficacy: A systematic review and meta-analysis of universal parent education interventions' efficacy. *International Journal of Nursing Studies, 82*, 149–162. https://doi.org/10.1016/j.ijnurstu.2018.03.021.

Andreotta, J., Hill, C., Eley, S., et al. (2015). Safe sleep practices and discharge planning. *Journal of Neonatal Nursing, 21*(5), 195–199.

Andrews, M. M., & Boyle, J. S. (2015). *Transcultural concepts in nursing care* (7th ed.). Philadelphia: Lippincott Williams & Wilkins.

Arnold, E. C., & Boggs, K. U. (2016). *Interpersonal relationships: Professional communication skills for nurses* (7th ed.). Philadelphia, PA: Elsevier.

Bartick, M., & Tomori, C. (2019). Sudden infant death and social justice: A syndemics approach. *Maternal and Child Nutrition, 15*,e12652. https://doi.org/10.1111/mcn.12652.

Berk, L. E., & Meyers, A. B. (2015). *Infants, children, and adolescents* (8th ed.). New York: Pearson Education.

Best Start Resource Centre. (2017a). *Breastfeeding matters: An important guide to breastfeeding for women and their families*. Retrieved from https://www.beststart.org/resources/breastfeeding/breastfeeding_matters_EN_LR.pdf.

Best Start Resource Centre. (2017b). *Sleep well, sleep safe*. Retrieved from https://www.beststart.org/resources/hlthy_chld_dev/pdf/BSRC_Sleep_Well_resource_FNL_LR.pdf.

Bornstein, M. H. (2015). Culture, parenting, and zero-to-threes. *Zero to Three, 35*(4), 2–9.

Brauer, J., Xiao, Y., Poulain, T., et al. (2016). Frequency of maternal touch predicts resting activity and connectivity of the developing social brain. *Cerebral Cortex, 26*, 3544–3552. https://doi.org/10.1093/cercor/bhw137.

Brazelton, T. B., & Sparrow, J. A. (2015). *Discipline: The Brazelton way* (2nd ed.). Old Saybrook, CN: Tantor Media.

Breastfeeding Committee for Canada. (2017). *The BFI 10 steps and WHO code outcome indicators for hospitals and community health services*. Retrieved from http://breastfeedingcanada.ca/documents/Indicators.pdf.

Brown, A. (2017). Breastfeeding as a public health responsibility: A review of the evidence. *Journal of Human Nutrition and Dietetics, 30*, 759–770. https://doi.org/10.1111/jhn.12496.

Brown, A., & Harries, V. (2015). Infant sleep and night feeding patterns during later infancy: Association with breastfeeding frequency, daytime complementary food intake, and infant weight. *Breastfeeding Medicine: The Official Journal of the Academy of Breastfeeding Medicine, 10*(5), 246–252.

Brown, A., & Rowan, H. (2016). Maternal and infant factors associated with reasons for introducing solid foods. *Maternal and Child Nutrition, 12*(3), 500–515.

Bruce, B., Cramm, C., Mundle, K., et al. (2015). Roadside observation of child passenger restraint use. *Advances in Pediatric Research, 2*(24). https://doi.org/10.12715/apr.2015.2.24.

Burnham, E. B., Wieland, E. A., Kondaurova, M. V., et al. (2015). Phonetic modification of vowel space in storybook speech to infants up to 2 years of age. *Journal of Speech, Language, and Hearing Research: Journal of Speech Language Hearing Research, 58*(2), 241–253.

Burns, S. B., Szyszkowicz, J. K., Luheshi, G. N., et al. (2018). Plasticity of the epigenome during early life stress. *Seminars in Cell & Developmental Biology, 77*, 115–132. https://doi.org/10.1016/j.semcdb.2017.09.033.

Calkins, S. D. (2015). *Handbook of infant biopsychosocial development*. New York: Guilford Publications, Inc.

Canadian Hemophilia Society (n.d.). *What is hemophilia?* Retrieved from https://www.hemophilia.ca/what-is-hemophilia/.

Canadian Human Rights Commission (n.d.). *Pregnancy and human rights in the workplace: Policy and best practices*. Retrieved from https://www.chrc-ccdp.gc.ca/eng/content/policy-and-best-practices-page-2.

Canadian Institute of Child Health. (2019). *The health of Canada's children and youth: A CICH profile*. Retrieved from https://cichprofile.ca/module/8/section/7/page/rate-of-infant-deaths-due-to-sudden-infant-death-syndrome-sids-canada-2000-to-2013/.

Canadian Nurses Association (CNA). (2018). *Position statement: Promoting cultural competence in nursing*. Retrieved from https://www.cna-aiic.ca/-/media/cna/page-content/pdf-en/position_statement_promoting_cultural_competence_in_nursing.pdf?la=en&hash=4B394DAE5C2138E7F6134D59E505DCB059754BA9.

Canadian Observatory on Homelessness. (2018). *Families with children*. Retrieved from https://www.homelesshub.ca/about-homelessness/population-specific/families-children.

Canadian Paediatric Society (CPS). (2016). *Preventing flat heads in babies who sleep on their backs*. Retrieved from https://www.caringforkids.cps.ca/handouts/preventing_flat_heads.

Canadian Paediatric Society (CPS). (2017a). Screen time and young children: Promoting health and development in a digital world. *Paediatrics and Child Health, 22*(8), 461–468. Retrieved from https://www.cps.ca/en/documents/position/screen-time-and-young-children.

Canadian Paediatric Society (CPS). (2017b). *Car seat safety*. Retrieved from https://www.caringforkids.cps.ca/handouts/car_seat_safety.

Canadian Paediatric Society (CPS). (2018a). *Promoting optimal monitoring of child growth in Canada: Using the new World Health Organization growth charts*. Retrieved from https://www.cps.ca/en/documents/position/child-growth-charts.

Canadian Paediatric Society (CPS). (2018b). *How culture influences health*. Retrieved from https://www.kidsnewtocanada.ca/culture/influence.

Canadian Paediatric Society (CPS). (2018c). *Working with vaccine-hesitant parents: An update*. Retrieved from https://www.cps.ca/en/documents/position/working-with-vaccine-hesitant-parents.

Canadian Paediatric Society (CPS). (2019a). *Iron needs of babies and children*. Retrieved from https://www.caringforkids.cps.ca/handouts/iron_needs_of_babies_and_children.

Canadian Paediatric Society (CPS). (2019b). *Feeding your baby in the first year*. Retrieved from https://www.caringforkids.cps.ca/handouts/iron_needs_of_babies_and_children.

Carey, S., Zaitchik, D., & Bascandziez, I. (2015). Theories of development: In dialog with jean Piaget. *Developmental Review, 38*, 36–54.

Centers for Disease Control and Prevention (CDC). (2018a). *Child development: Infants (0–1 year of age)*. Retrieved from http://www.cdc.gov/ncbddd/childdevelopment/positiveparenting/infants.html.

Centers for Disease Control and Prevention (CDC). (2018b). *Child abuse and neglect: Risk and protective factors*. Retrieved from https://www.cdc.gov/violenceprevention/childabuseandneglect/riskprotectivefactors.html.

Child Development Institute. (2015). *Ages and stages*. Retrieved from http://childdevelopmentinfo.com/ages-stages/.

Christian, C. W., & Committee on Child Abuse and Neglect. (2015). The evaluation of suspected child physical abuse. *Pediatrics, 135*(5), e1337–e1354.

Christie, J., Parkes, J., & Price, J. (2015). The public health practitioner. In J. Hughes, & G. Lyte (Eds.), *Developing nursing practice with children and young people* (pp. 87–102). Ames, IA: Blackwell.

Coch, D., Dawson, G., & Fischer, K. W. (2015). *Human behavior, learning, and the developing brain: Typical development*. New York: Guilford Publications.

El-Assal, K., & Fields, D. (2018). *Canada 2040: No immigration versus more immigration*. Ottawa: The Conference Board of Canada. Retrieved from https://www.conferenceboard.ca/temp/ba5cd24d-bdb0-437c-937b-df5b229a20b0/9678_Canada2040_NIC-RPT.pdf.

Falck, A. J., Mooney, S., Kapoor, S. S., et al. (2015). Developmental exposure to environmental toxicants. *Pediatric Clinics of North America, 62*(5), 1173–1197. https://doi.org/10.1016/j.pcl.2015.05.005.

Fallon, V., Komninou, S., Bennett, K. M., et al. (2017). The emotional and practical experiences of formula-feeding mothers. *Maternal and Child Nutrition, 13*, e12392. https://doi.org/10.1111/mcn.12392.

Fanetti, M., O'Donohue, W., Happel, R. F., et al. (2015). Child abuse and neglect. In *Forensic child psychology* (pp. 105–124). Hoboken, NJ: John Wiley & Sons.

Fegan, S., Bassett, E., Peng, Y., et al. (2017). Adherence to complementary feeding recommendations and implications for public health. *Public Health Nutrition, 19*(4), 638–649. https://doi.org/10.1017/S1368980015001433.

Feldman, R. S. (2015). *Child development* (7th ed.). New York: Pearson Education.

Ferguson, R. W., Osterthaler, K., Kaminski, S., et al. (2015). *Medicine safety for children: An in-depth look at calls to poison centers*. Washington: Safe Kids Worldwide. Retrieved from https://www.safekids.org/sites/default/files/research_reports/medicine_safety_study_2015_v7-lr.pdf.

Fivush, R., & Waters, T. E. A. (2015). Patterns of attachments across the lifespan. In R. A. Scot, & S. M. Kosslyn (Eds.), *Emerging trends in the behavioral and social sciences: An inter-*

disciplinary, searchable, and linkable resource (pp. 1–10). San Francisco: Wiley.

Fogel, A. (2015). *Infant development: A topical approach* (2nd ed.). Cornwell-on-Hudson, NY: Sloan Educational Publishing.

Fortin, P. (2017). *Quebec daycare: A success that must now focus on equity. The Globe and Mail.* April 27. Retrieved from https://www.theglobeandmail.com/opinion/quebec-daycare-a-success-that-must-now-focus-on-equity/article34823036/.

Gao, W., Lin, W., Grewen, K., et al. (2017). Functional connectivity of the infant human brain: Plastic and modifiable. *The Neuroscientist, 23*(2), 169–184. https://doi.org/10.1177/1073858416635986.

Gardner, S. L., Carter, B. S., Enzman-Hines, M. I., et al. (2016). *Merenstein & Gardner's handbook of neonatal intensive care* (8th ed.). St. Louis: Mosby.

Goodman, A., Fleming, K., Markwick, N., & Western Aboriginal Harm Reduction Society, et al. (2017). "They treated me like crap and I know it was because I was Native": The healthcare experiences of Aboriginal peoples living in Vancouver's inner city. *Social Science & Medicine, 178*, 87–94. https://doi.org/10.1016/j.socscimed.2017.01.053.

Gouveia, N., & Junger, W. L. (2018). Effects of air pollution on infant and children respiratory mortality in four large Latin-American cities. *Environmental Pollution, 232*, 385–391. https://doi.org/10.1016/j.envpol.2017.08.125.

Government of Canada. (2006). *Dietary reference intakes.* Retrieved from https://www.canada.ca/en/health-canada/services/food-nutrition/healthy-eating/dietary-reference-intakes/tables/reference-values-macronutrients-dietary-reference-intakes-tables-2005.html. [Seminal Reference].

Government of Canada. (2016a). *Releases of lead to the environment.* Retrieved from https://www.ec.gc.ca/indicateurs-indicators/default.asp?lang=En&n=4F1AE114-1&pedisable=true.

Government of Canada. (2016b). *Reduce your exposure to lead.* Retrieved from https://www.canada.ca/en/health-canada/services/home-garden-safety/reduce-your-exposure-lead.html.

Government of Canada. (2016c). *Air quality and children's health.* Retrieved from https://www.canada.ca/en/environment-climate-change/services/air-quality-health-index/children-health.html.

Government of Canada. (2017). *Lead-based paint.* Retrieved from https://www.canada.ca/en/health-canada/services/home-safety/lead-based-paint.html.

Government of Canada. (2018a). *Social determinants of health and health inequalities.* Retrieved from https://www.canada.ca/en/public-health/services/health-promotion/population-health/what-determines-health.html.

Government of Canada. (2018b). *Vaccines for children: Deciding to vaccinate.* Retrieved from https://www.canada.ca/en/public-health/services/vaccination-children.html.

Government of Canada. (2018c). *Consumer products containing lead regulations: SOR/2018-83. Canada Gazette, Part II, 152*(9). Retrieved from http://www.gazette.gc.ca/rp-pr/p2/2018/2018-05-02/html/sor-dors83-eng.html.

Government of Canada. (2018d). *Canada health act.* Retrieved from https://www.canada.ca/en/health-canada/services/health-care-system/canada-health-care-system-medicare/canada-health-act.html.

Government of Canada. (2018e). *National housing strategy: A place to call home.* Retrieved from https://www.placetocallhome.ca/.

Harkness, G. A., & DeMarco, R. (2015). *Community health and public health nursing: Evidence for practice* (2nd ed.). Philadelphia: Lippincott Williams & Wilkins.

Hashim, M. (2015). Pesticides and drinking water. *Journal of Advanced Botany and Zoology, 3*(1). https://doi.org/10.15297/JABZ.V3I1.05.

Health Canada, Canadian Paediatric Society (CPS), Dietitians of Canada, & Breastfeeding Committee for Canada. (2015a). *Nutrition for healthy term infants: Recommendations from birth to six months.* Retrieved from https://www.canada.ca/en/health-canada/services/canada-food-guide/resources/infant-feeding/nutrition-healthy-term-infants-recommendations-birth-six-months.html#a9.

Health Canada, Canadian Paediatric Society (CPS), Dietitians of Canada, & Breastfeeding Committee for Canada. (2015b). *Nutrition for healthy term infants: Recommendations from six to 24 months.* Retrieved from https://www.canada.ca/en/health-canada/services/canada-food-guide/resources/infant-feeding/nutrition-healthy-term-infants-recommendations-birth-six-months/6-24-months.html.

Healthy Babies, B. C. (2018). *How to choose, prepare and store infant formula.* Retrieved from https://www.healthyfamiliesbc.ca/home/articles/how-choose-prepare-and-store-infant-formula.

Hoft, M., & Haddad, L. (2017). Screening children for abuse and neglect: A review of the literature. *Journal of Forensic Nursing, 13*(1), 26–34. https://doi.org/10.1097/JFN.0000000000000136.

Homan, G. J. (2016). Failure to thrive: A practical guide. *American Family Physician, 94*(4), 295–300.

Huntington Society of Canada. (2017). *Living at-risk for Huntington disease.* Retrieved from https://www.huntingtonsociety.ca/wp-content/uploads/2017/03/Living-At-Risk-Mar-2017.pdf.

Inguaggiato, E., Sgandurra, G., & Cioni, G. (2017). Brain plasticity and early development: Implications for early intervention in neurodevelopmental disorders. *Neuropsychiatrie de l'Enfance et de l'Adolescence, 65*, 299–306. https://doi.org/10.1016/j.neurenf.2017.03.009.

Johnson, J. E., Eberle, S. G., Henricks, T. S., et al. (2015). *The handbook of the study of play.* Lanham, MD: Rowman & Littlefield Publishing Group.

Johnson, C. D., Jones, S., & Paranjothy, S. (2017). Reducing low birth weight: Prioritizing action to address modifiable risk factors. *Journal of Public Health, 39*(1), 122–131. https://doi.org/10.1093/pubmed/fdv212.

Johnson, C. C., & Ownby, D. R. (2017). The infant gut bacterial microbiota and risk of pediatric asthma and allergic diseases. *Translational Research, 179*, 60–70. https://doi.org/10.1016/j.trsl.2016.06.010.

Johnson, S. B., Riis, J. L., & Noble, K. G. (2016). State of the art review: Poverty and the developing brain. *Pediatrics, 137*(4), e20153075. https://doi.org/10.1542/peds.2015-3075.

Kail, R. V., & Cavanaugh, J. C. (2015). *Human development: A life-span view* (7th ed.). Boston, MA: Cengage Learning.

Kids & Cars. (2018). *Look before you lock.* Retrieved from http://www.kidsandcars.org/wp-content/uploads/2018/10/Heatstroke-fact-sheet-2018-1.pdf.

Killion, C. M. (2017). Cultural healing practices that mimic abuse. *Annals of Forensic Research and Analysis, 4*(2), 1042.

Kliegman, R. M., Stanton, B., St Geme, J., et al. (2015). *Nelson textbook of pediatrics* (20th ed.). St. Louis: Elsevier.

La Leche League Canada. (2015). *Thursday's tip: Breastfeeding in a heat wave.* Retrieved from https://www.lllc.ca/thursdays-tip-breastfeeding-heat-wave.

Lee, A., & Brann, L. (2015). Influence of cultural beliefs on infant feeding, postpartum and childcare practices among Chinese-American mothers in New York City. *Journal of Community Health, 40*(3), 476–483.

LoFrumento, M. A. (2018). Your guide to baby's vision and hearing. *Parents.* Retrieved from https://www150.statcan.gc.ca/n1/en/pub/82-003-x/2017011/article/54886-eng.pdf?st=625p9mdH.

Lopes, L. C., de Omena Bomfim, E., & Flória-Santos, M. (2015). Genomics-based health care: Implications for nursing. *International Journal of Nursing Didactics, 5*(2), 11–15.

Lowe, P. (2015). Milk for a girl and bananas for a boy: Recipes and reasons for sex-preference practices in a British internet forum. *Women's Reproductive Health, 2*(2), 111–123. https://doi.org/10.1080/23293691.2015.1089150.

MacDougall, F. (2018). Preventing burn injuries to children in the home. *Canadian Nurse.* Retrieved from https://www.canadian-nurse.com/articles/issues/2018/january-february-2018/preventing-burn-injuries-to-children-in-the-home.

Mantoura, P., & Morrison, V. (2016). *Policy approaches to reducing health inequalities.* Montréal, Québec: National Collaborating Centre for Healthy Public Policy.

Martiniuk, A., Jacob, J., Faruqui, N., et al. (2016). Positional plagiocephaly reduces parental adherence to SIDS guidelines and inundates the health system. *Child: Care, Health and Development, 42*(6), 941–950.

MedlinePlus. (2017a). *Infant reflexes.* Retrieved from https://medlineplus.gov/ency/article/003292.htm.

MedlinePlus. (2017b). *Choking: Infant under 1 year.* Retrieved from https://medlineplus.gov/ency/article/000048.htm.

Mikkonen, J., & Raphael, D. (2010). *Social determinants of health: The Canadian facts.* Toronto, ON: York University School of Health Policy and Management. [Seminal Reference].

Moon, R. Y., & Task Force on SIDS (2017). SIDS and other sleep-related infant deaths: Evidence base for 2016 updated recommendations for a safe infant sleeping environment. *Pediatrics, 138*(5), e20162940. https://doi.org/10.1542/peds.2016-2940.

National Institute of Neurological Disorders and Stroke. (2018). *Huntington's disease information page.* Retrieved from https://www.ninds.nih.gov/Disorders/All-Disorders/Huntingtons-Disease-Information-Page.

National Safety Council. (2016). *Choking prevention and rescue tips.* Retrieved from http://www.nsc.org/learn/safety-knowledge/Pages/safety-at-home-choking.aspx.

National Tay-Sachs & Allied Diseases Association. (2016). *Tay-Sachs disease.* Retrieved from https://www.ntsad.org/index.php/the-diseases/tay-sachs.

Nipissing District Developmental Screening (NDDS). (2019). *Looksee checklist by NDDS.* Retrieved from https://www.lookseechecklist.com/en/.

Nussbaum, R., McInnes, R. R., & Willard, H. F. (2016). *Thompson & Thompson genetics in medicine* (8th ed.). Philadelphia, PA: Elsevier Health Sciences.

O'Connor, A. (2015). All about sensory development. *Nursery World,* 22–26. Retrieved from https://www.nurseryworld.co.uk/nursery-world/feature/1149541/eyfs-practice-about-sensory-development.

Ontario Association of Children's Aid Societies (OACAS). (2015). *Working with First Nations, Inuit, and Metis families who have experienced family violence.* Retrieved from http://www.oacas.org/wp-content/uploads/2015/08/fn_eng_guide.pdf.

Ontario Poison Centre. (2015). *Current top 10.* Retrieved from http://www.ontariopoisoncentre.ca/common-poisons/Current-Top-10/Top-10-Lists.aspx.

Parachute. (2016). *Unintentional injury trends for Canadian children, June 2016.* Toronto: Author. Retrieved from http://horizon.parachutecanada.org/en/article/unintentional-injury-trends-for-canadian-children-june-2016-report/.

Parachute. (2019). *Poison prevention: Unintentional poisoning.* Toronto: Author. Retrieved from http://www.parachutecanada.org/injury-topics/topic/C16.

Perez-Rodriguez, J., & de la Fuente, A. (2017). Now is the time for postracial medicine: Biomedical research, the national institutes of health, and the perpetuation of scientific racism. *The American Journal of Bioethics, 17*(9), 36–47. https://doi.org/10.1080/15265161.2017.1353165.

Polan, E., & Taylor, D. (2015). *Journey across the lifespan: Human development and health promotion* (5th ed.). Philadelphia: F.A. Davis.

Public Health Agency of Canada (PHAC). (2015). *Ten valuable tips for successful breastfeeding.* Retrieved from https://www.canada.ca/en/public-health/services/health-promotion/childhood-adolescence/stages-childhood/infancy-birth-two-years/breastfeeding-infant-nutrition/valuable-tips-successful-breastfeeding.html.

Public Health Agency of Canada (PHAC). (2016). *Health status of Canadians 2016.* Ottawa, ON: Public Health Agency of Canada (Cat. No. 978-0-660-05480-3). Retrieved from http://healthycanadians.gc.ca/publications/department-ministere/state-public-health-status-2016-etat-sante-publique-statut/alt/pdf-eng.pdf.

Public Health Agency of Canada (PHAC). (2018a). *Family-centred maternity and newborn care: National guidelines. Chapter 6.* Retrieved from https://www.canada.ca/en/public-health/services/publications/healthy-living/maternity-newborn-care-guidelines-chapter-6.html#a10.

Public Health Agency of Canada (PHAC). (2018b). *Safe sleep.* Retrieved from https://www.canada.ca/en/public-health/services/health-promotion/childhood-adolescence/stages-childhood/infancy-birth-two-years/safe-sleep.html.

Public Health Agency of Canada (PHAC). (2018c). *Key health inequalities in Canada: A national portrait.* Catalogue No. HP35-109/2018E-PDF.

Pulver, A., Ramraj, C., Ray, J. G., et al. (2016). A scoping review of female disadvantage in health care use among very young children of immigrant families. *Social Science & Medicine, 152,* 50–60. https://doi.org/10.1016/j.socscimed.2016.01.027.

Radzyminski, S., & Callister, L. C. (2015). Health professionals' attitudes and beliefs about breastfeeding. *The Journal of Perinatal Education, 24*(2), 102–109.

Ramraj, C., Shahidi, F. V., Darity, W., Jr., et al. (2016). Equally inequitable? A cross-national comparative study of racial health inequalities in the United States and Canada. *Social Science & Medicine, 161,* 19–26. https://doi.org/10.1016/j.socscimed.2016.05.028.

Rapaport, L. (2015). *More poor babies get checkups when parents get extra help.* Reuters Health. Retrieved from http://www.reuters.com/article/2015/06/03/us-healthcare-poverty-infant-care-idUSKBN0OJ2MP20150603.

Reed, L. (2015). Early socialization. *International Journal of Childbirth Education, 30*(2), 31–34.

Richmond, S. A., D'Cruz, J., Lokku, A., et al. (2016). Trends in unintentional injury mortality in Canadian children 1950–2009 and association with selected population-level interventions. *Canadian Journal of Public Health, 107*(4–5), e431–e437.

Roudsari, R. L., Zakerihamidi, M., & Khoei, E. M. (2015). Socio-cultural beliefs, values and traditions regarding women's preferred mode of birth in the north of Iran. *International Journal of Community Based Nursing and Midwifery, 3*(3), 165.

Rourke, L., Leduc, D., & Rourke, J. (2017). *Rourke baby record.* Retrieved from http://www.rourkebabyrecord.ca/default.

Santos, M., Franca, A. P., Fernandes, O., et al. (2015). Parental knowledge on breastfeeding: Contributions to a clinical supervision model in nursing. *International Journal of Information and Education Technology, 5*(1), 10–13.

Scism, A. R., & Cobb, R. L. (2017). Integrative review of factors and interventions that influence early father-infant bonding. *Journal of Obstetric, Gynecologic, and Neonatal Nursing, 46*, 163–170.

Sheppard, A. J., Shapiro, G. D., Bushnik, T., et al. (2017). Birth outcomes among first Nations, Inuit and Metis populations. (Cat. No. 82-003-X). *Health Reports, 28*(11), 11–16. Ottawa: Statistics Canada. Retrieved from https://www150.statcan.gc.ca/n1/en/pub/82-003-x/2017011/article/54886-eng.pdf?st=625p9mdH.

Shpancer, N. (2017). Nonparental daycare: What the research tells us. *Psychology Today*. Retrieved from https://www.psychologytoday.com/us/blog/insight-therapy/201710/nonparental-daycare-what-the-research-tells-us.

Sickle Cell Disease Association of Canada. (2018). *General knowledge*. Retrieved from https://www.sicklecelldisease.ca/eng/2018/09/28/general-knowledge/.

Sims, J. D. (2015). *The no-nonsense guide to heat wave, drought, & hot weather safety* (2nd ed.). North Carolina: Lulu Books & Beyond the Spectrum Books.

Sinha, M. (2015). *Child care in Canada*. (Cat. No. 89-652-X). Ottawa: Statistics Canada. Retrieved from https://www150.statcan.gc.ca/n1/pub/89-652-x/89-652-x2014005-eng.htm.

Smith, K. (2018). Spike in cannabis poisoning in kids a concern for doctors: 'It's candy and it tastes great'. *Global News*. October 11. Retrieved from https://globalnews.ca/news/4534284/cannabis-poisoning-edibles-doctors/.

Statistics Canada. (2015a). *Breastfeeding trends in Canada*. (Cat. no. 82-624-X). Ottawa: Statistics Canada. Retrieved from https://www150.statcan.gc.ca/n1/pub/82-624-x/2013001/article/11879-eng.htm.

Statistics Canada. (2015b). *Lead, mercury, and cadmium concentrations in Canadians, 2012 and 2013*. Retrieved from https://www150.statcan.gc.ca/n1/pub/82-625-x/2015001/article/14209-eng.htm.

Statistics Canada. (2016a). *Changing profile of stay-at-home parents*. Retrieved from https://www150.statcan.gc.ca/n1/pub/11-630-x/11-630-x2016007-eng.htm.

Statistics Canada. (2016b). *Low birth weight newborns in Canada, 2000 to 2013*. Retrieved from https://www150.statcan.gc.ca/n1/pub/82-625-x/2016001/article/14674-eng.htm.

Statistics Canada. (2017a). *Census in brief: Same-sex couples in Canada in 2016*. Retrieved from https://www12.statcan.gc.ca/census-recensement/2016/as-sa/98-200-x/2016007/98-200-x2016007-eng.cfm.

Statistics Canada. (2017b). *Family violence in Canada: A statistical profile, 2015*. Retrieved from https://www150.statcan.gc.ca/n1/daily-quotidien/170216/dq170216b-eng.htm.

Statistics Canada. (2017c). *Children living in low income households*. Retrieved from https://www12.statcan.gc.ca/census-recensement/2016/as-sa/98-200-x/2016012/98-200-x2016012-eng.cfm.

Stevens, G., Ishizawa, H., & Grbic, D. (2015). Measuring race and ethnicity in the censuses of Australia, Canada, and the United States: Parallels and paradoxes. *Canadian Studies in Population, 42*(1–2), 13–34.

Uppal, S. (2015). *Employment patterns of families with children*. (Cat. No. 75-006-X.) Ottawa: Statistics Canada. Retrieved from https://www150.statcan.gc.ca/n1/en/pub/75-006-x/2015001/article/14202-eng.pdf?st=UIEr7xh1.

US Department of Agriculture (USDA). (2015). *Nutritional needs of infants*. Retrieved from http://www.nal.usda.gov/wicworks/Topics/FG/Chapter1_NutritionalNeeds.pdf.

Veenstra, G., & Patterson, A. C. (2016). Black-White inequalities in Canada. *Journal of Immigrant and Minority Health, 18*(1), 51–57. https://doi.org/10.1007/s10903-014-0140-6.

Vrolijk-Bosschaart, T. F., Brilleslijper-Kater, S. N., Widdershoven, G. A., et al. (2017). Physical symptoms in very young children assessed for sexual abuse: A mixed method analysis from the ASAC study. *European Journal of Pediatrics, 176*, 1365–1374. https://doi.org/10.1007/s00431-017-2996-7.

Williamson, C., & Beatty, C. (2015). Weaning and childhood nutrition. *Education and Inspiration for General Practice, 8*(3), 141–145.

Wood, R. B. (2018). Effective communication strategies for nurses to discuss infant feeding with new mothers during hospitalization. *Maternal Child Nursing, 43*(4), 218–224.

World Health Organization (WHO). (2015). *Food additives*. Retrieved from http://www.who.int/topics/food_additives/en/.

# 12

# Toddler

*Bahareh Singla, RN, MN*

Originating US chapter by *Diane Marie Welsh, CNE, RN, MSN, ARNP*

## INTENDED LEARNING OUTCOMES

*After completing this chapter, the reader will be able to:*

- Describe the physical growth, developmental, and maturational changes that occur during the toddler period.
- Examine the recommended health-promotion and disease-prevention visits for the toddler with the appropriate topics for anticipatory guidance for the parents.

- Compare and contrast developmentally appropriate approaches to toddlers at different ages.
- Analyze the factors that contribute to the heightened vulnerability of toddlers to injury and abuse.

## KEY TERMS

Amblyopia
Autism spectrum disorders (ASD)
Autonomy
Child abuse
Conditioned-play audiometry
Doubt
Egocentrism
Lumbar lordosis
Masturbation
Night terrors
Object permanence
Otitis media

Parallel play
Preoperational stage
Rituals
Sensorimotor stage
Shame
Strabismus
Styes
Temperament
Toilet training
Visual-reinforcement audiometry
World Health Organization (WHO) growth charts

### ? THINK ABOUT IT

#### Reframing the Terrible Twos

A young mother tells the nurse that she is convinced her 22-month-old child, who used to be the sweetest child around, has entered what must be the terrible twos. She reports that her child's favourite words include "mine" and "no," with "no" being the response to every request the mother makes. In addition, the child is becoming increasingly stubborn and just threw her first public temper tantrum. The mother says that she is tired of saying and hearing "no" and turns to the nurse for help.

- How does the nurse explain the relationship between the child's stage of psychosocial development and meaning behind the child's behaviours?
- What suggestions can the nurse give the mother to respond sensitively to her child's evolving need for independence while balancing her own need to provide for and protect her child?

Having spent their first year of life getting to know and trust their parents and other child care providers and their immediate environments, toddlers' increasing mobility now allows

them to begin to expand their worlds, bringing excitement and challenges to both themselves and their parents. Toddlers are ready to develop a sense of self and separate from their parents; understanding and respecting this evolving independence is a common parental challenge. Their behaviours can be frustrating, but the toddlers' delight in their own emerging competence and achievements can bring a sense of joy and accomplishment to everyone around them (Kochanska, Kim, Boldt, et al., 2013).

Nurses explain to parents and other primary care providers the many physical and developmental changes that occur in toddlers and describe how these changes contribute to their vulnerability to injury and overall health, as well as to the health and vulnerability of the family unit (Centers for Disease Control and Prevention [CDC], 2015c). Unfortunately, the recommended schedule for health-promotion and disease-prevention visits for this age group advocates fewer contacts than during infancy. Parents may begin to fall into a pattern of illness care, missing opportunities to receive anticipatory guidance and health-promotion information until they are required by preschool or school prerequisites. The nurse plays an integral role in encouraging health-promotion efforts and behaviours (Hockenberry & Wilson, 2015; Levickis, McKean, Walls, et al., 2019).

## BIOLOGY AND GENETICS

The toddler period begins at 12 to 18 months and extends to 3 years of age. The overall growth rate slows significantly, and the increasingly active toddler begins the process of shedding baby fat and straightening his or her posture. Toddlers have a protuberant abdomen, accentuated by a lumbar lordosis, and a characteristic gait, in which their feet are planted wide apart and appear flat due to an extra fat pad in the instep for stability.

A slow, steady growth in height of 5 to 10 centimetres per year and in weight of 1.5 to 2.5 kilograms per year occurs during toddlerhood, and growth remains steady until puberty. Birth weight usually quadruples by [f × 2] years of age, and the toddler's height at age 2 years is approximately 50% of the final adult height (Hockenberry & Wilson, 2015). Growth charts are used to determine the parameters within which an individual toddler's growth lies for head circumference, height, and weight. The Canadian Paediatric Society (CPS) recommends using the World Health Organization (WHO) growth charts, adapted for Canada, to monitor growth for infants and children up to 2 years of age. The toddler's height may be measured with the toddler in a recumbent position for length, as in infancy, or in a standing position for stature.

The nurse continues to measure head circumference throughout the toddler period. The anterior fontanelle usually closes by 18 months, the skull begins to thicken, and by 24 months it is 80% of its adult size (Hockenberry & Wilson, 2015).

The kidneys are well differentiated by the toddler years, and urine specific gravity and other urine findings are similar to those of adults. The daily excretion of urine for the 2-year-old child is 500 to 600 mL, increasing to 750 mL for the 3-year-old child. Toddlers empty their bladders less frequently than infants and begin to develop voluntary control of urination. However, full bladder control comes later and begins after 18 to 24 months, when the toddler first becomes physiologically able to control the bladder.

The toddler's gastro-intestinal tract also reaches functional maturity, although it continues to grow into adulthood. The toddler tends to need meals and snacks more frequently than an older child or adult. Most toddlers develop sufficient voluntary control of internal and external anal sphincters to accomplish successful bowel training. Bowel control usually occurs before urinary control.

Lung capacity continues to increase as the toddler grows, and the respiratory rate decreases from a mean of 30 breaths per minute at 1 year of age to 25 breaths per minute at 3 years. The diameter of the toddler's upper respiratory tract is small compared with that of an older child or adult. This may lead to mouth breathing when the nose is obstructed with mucus (Fig. 12.1). This small diameter, coupled with the toddler's exploratory nature and lack of judgement in deciding what to place in the mouth, can result in accidental airway obstruction, which demands emergency action.

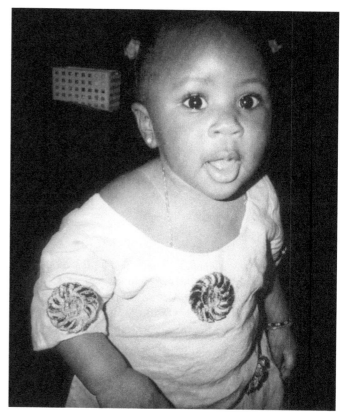

**Fig. 12.1** Toddler Demonstrates Mouth Breathing

The proximal anatomy of the ear, eustachian tube, and nasal pharynx continue to resemble those of the infant more closely than those of the adult, continuing the risk of otitis media. The tonsils and adenoids remain proportionately large during the toddler years (Ball, Dains, Flynn, et al., 2015).

With the exception of reproductive functions, most endocrine organs become functionally mature during the toddler and preschool years, although function continues at a minimum. The production of glucagon and insulin can be limited or labile, producing variations in blood glucose levels throughout early childhood. The production of cortisol, aldosterone, and deoxycorticosterone by the adrenal cortex remains somewhat limited, but they appear to function effectively in protecting the young child from the hazards of fluid and electrolyte imbalance well known in infancy. Secretion of epinephrine and norepinephrine from the adrenal medulla increases sufficiently to perform homeostatic functions of the autonomic nervous system and to mediate certain aspects of increased emotional components of behaviour. Regulation of growth during early childhood remains one of the most important functions of the endocrine system.

Changes in the circulatory system include a decrease in heart rate, an increase in blood pressure, and a change in vascular resistance in response to growth in the size of various blood vessel lumens. The toddler's heart rate ranges from 80 to 120 beats per minute, and the mean blood pressure is 90/56 mmHg. Getting the toddler to sit still for a blood pressure reading can be difficult, but it is worth the effort to obtain several baseline readings for future reference.

The capillary beds gradually increase their capacity to respond to heat and cold in the environment, providing the toddler with more effective thermoregulation. Toddlers can also begin to take voluntary measures to relieve the discomfort of heat or cold. For example, the older toddler can put on clothing or move to warmer or cooler areas, assisting physiological efforts to maintain a constant internal thermal environment.

The immune response continues to mature. As toddlers expand their worlds through playgroups and day care centres, exposure to new and different organisms is greatly increased. They may experience a period during which they appear to succumb to many minor respiratory tract and gastro-intestinal tract infections. As immunity begins to develop against the organisms in their new environments, their resistance similarly increases.

Passive immunity to communicable disease acquired through transfer of maternal antibodies during fetal life has disappeared, and active immunity through the initial immunization series is usually completed by the age of 18 months. The next scheduled immunizations do not occur until age 4 to 6 years, before the toddler enters kindergarten. If a toddler is behind in the initial immunization series, the child's care provider should be notified so that appropriate adjustments can be made to the child's catch-up immunization schedule (Public Health Agency of Canada [PHAC], 2019). Canada's immunization schedules vary by province and territory. For updated immunization schedules and the latest guidance refer to the provincial and territorial immunization information at https://www.canada.ca/en/public-health/services/canadian-immunization-guide.html.

All 20 primary or deciduous teeth erupt by the end of toddlerhood (Fig. 12.2). The timing of these eruptions can differ widely, but a variation in the sequence alerts the nurse to inquire about early trauma to the mouth or familial traits for non-sequential tooth eruption. Application of fluoride varnish to primary teeth is recommended shortly after the teeth erupt through the gum. Important aspects of dental care at this age are included in health teaching and are listed in Box 12.1.

A mature swallowing pattern, using the tongue rather than the cheeks, has not yet developed, and toddlers continue to be at risk of choking. Toddlers who are mouth, rather than nose, breathers because of ongoing respiratory illness or allergies may have an underdeveloped palatal arch. With normal breathing, the tongue rests on and naturally widens the palate; however, when the child is forced to breathe through the mouth, the tongue rests in the lower jaw, not on the palate. This resultant narrowing of the palatal arch predisposes these toddlers to dental crowding when the permanent teeth erupt (Guilleminault, Abad, Chiu, et al., 2015).

An increase in the size and strength of muscle fibres continues. During this period, as during infancy, the use of muscle tissues is the primary stimulus for increased size and strength for gross and later fine motor movement. Myelination of the corticospinal tract is functionally sufficient to support most movement, but achievement of full control does not occur until much later in life. Throughout early childhood, voluntary motor movement is often accompanied by involuntary movements on the opposite side of the body. This mirroring of action is more pronounced in children who have some damage to the central nervous system, but the mechanisms by which this occurs are unknown. The toddler generally does not show complete dominance of one side of the body and may still switch hands when eating, throwing a ball, or engaging in other-handed activities.

Genes are passed from each parent to the child, and great similarities may show between the generations. Most genetic syndromes and disease entities are diagnosed either during the prenatal period or during infancy. However, some genetic

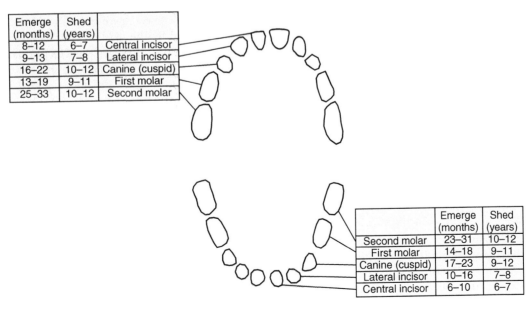

Maxillary (upper) teeth

| Emerge (months) | Shed (years) | |
| --- | --- | --- |
| 8–12 | 6–7 | Central incisor |
| 9–13 | 7–8 | Lateral incisor |
| 16–22 | 10–12 | Canine (cuspid) |
| 13–19 | 9–11 | First molar |
| 25–33 | 10–12 | Second molar |

| | Emerge (months) | Shed (years) |
| --- | --- | --- |
| Second molar | 23–31 | 10–12 |
| First molar | 14–18 | 9–11 |
| Canine (cuspid) | 17–23 | 9–12 |
| Lateral incisor | 10–16 | 7–8 |
| Central incisor | 6–10 | 6–7 |

Mandibular (lower) teeth

Fig. 12.2 Eruption (and Shedding) of Primary Teeth

---

### BOX 12.1   Nursing Interventions
#### To Promote Dental Health Care for Toddlers

**Brushing**

- When teeth are present, begin to use a soft-bristled brush.
- Brush teeth daily using non-fluoridated toothpaste for toddlers aged 1 to 2 years. Fluoride toothpaste may be introduced between 3 and 4 years of age.
- Introduce only a moist toothbrush at first. After the toddler has accepted the toothbrush, begin using toothpaste. Only a pea-sized amount of fluorinated toothpaste is recommended. If the child does not like the taste of the toothpaste, use plain water.
- Toothpaste should contain supplemental fluoride if not in the water supply. Use oral fluoride supplementation before tooth eruption and only for high-risk populations. When used, the total daily fluoride intake from all sources should not exceed 0.05–0.07 mg F/kg body weight in order to minimize the risk of dental fluorosis.
- Toddlers do not have the motor coordination to brush their own teeth. They may enjoy imitating parents and put the toothbrush in their mouths, but an adult should be responsible for the actual brushing.
- Brush daily; for many toddlers, this practice becomes part of the bedtime routine. When the child appears too tired to cooperate in the evening, the parent should choose some other time of day when this important task will not be so difficult.

**Foods**

- Limit intake of foods high in sugar because they contribute to dental caries.
- Avoid juice, because it is unnecessary; if you do offer it, limit to 125 mL daily.
- When the young toddler still drinks from a bottle, only plain water should be given. Milk and juices should be offered by cup. If milk or juice is given in a bottle, it should never be done at naptime or bedtime.

**Visits to the Dentist**

- The first visit to the dentist should occur at 12 months of age.

Sources: Canadian Dental Association. (2012). *Canadian Dental Association position on the use of fluorides in caries prevention*. Retrieved from https://www.cda-adc.ca/en/about/position_statements/fluoride/; Canadian Paediatric Society. (2018). *Healthy teeth for children*. Retrieved from https://www.caringforkids.cps.ca/handouts/healthy_teeth_for_children.

---

syndromes and diseases are not detected until the toddler years or even later. The most common initial sign is a change in growth pattern or developmental delays.

Developmental delays are often not diagnosed during infancy because the subtle language, motor, or cognitive deficiencies do not interfere with the expected performance and behaviour of the infant as they do with those of the more actively developing toddler.

## ❖ GORDON'S FUNCTIONAL HEALTH PATTERNS

### ◆ Health Perception–Health Management Pattern

Toddlers may eventually learn that being sick means feeling bad or having to stay in bed, but they have little, if any, understanding of the meaning of health. They may perform requested health-promotion activities, such as brushing teeth, but they may simply brush their teeth as part of their bedtime ritual and not because they know that this activity will prevent dental caries. Toddlers depend on their parents for health management; thus their overall health is significantly influenced by their parents' health perceptions and health-management priorities.

Toddlers identify with parents, caregivers, and other important role models, internalizing a wide range of lifestyle attributes. Parents' and caregivers' health perceptions and health behaviours should model the perceptions and behaviours desired for health promotion. Toddlers whose parents eat a variety of foods are more likely to try new foods. Such modelling increases the chances that good practices are retained throughout the toddler's life. The nurse's task is to help parents strengthen their confidence and self-esteem as parents and provide them with the information needed to anticipate and meet the developmental needs of their toddler as they develop as a family.

### ◆ Nutritional-Metabolic Pattern

The Canadian Paediatric Society (CPS, 2018a) supports the following nutritional recommendations regarding breastfeeding:

- Breast milk from birth to 6 months. Exclusive breastfeeding provides all of the nutrients needs during the first few months of life.
- Breastfeeding may continue for as long as the mother and child are comfortable.
- After 12 months of age, toddlers should not consume more than 500 mL to 720 mL (16 to 24 ounces) of milk each day, as any more would cause the child to feel full from the milk and refuse solid foods. There is an increased risk that a toddler may develop iron-deficiency anemia if more than the recommended daily amounts of milk are consumed.
- The introduction of solid foods should begin at approximately 6 months of age.
- The use of a bottle with milk or juice, especially at bedtime, has also been associated with dental caries (baby-bottle tooth decay) because of the high sugar content. If parents want to give a bottle at bedtime, it should contain only water.

Fruit juice and other drinks are often over-consumed because they taste good, are conveniently packaged and easily carried around by the toddler, and because they are viewed as being nutritious. However, the CPS (2019a) advises serving fresh fruit instead of juice, because this adds healthy fibre to the child's diet. Toddlers should be offered water instead of juice for thirst and between meals and snacks. Juice (if served) should be limited to 125 mL daily. A decrease in the growth rate during toddlerhood results in a decrease in appetite. Parental health teaching should include maintaining a daily record kept over a 3- to 5-day period, as it presents a better picture of a child's intake and is a useful teaching tool for this age group.

Toddlers often use mealtime as an occasion to assert individuality and control as well as exploration. Families will differ in their expectations of eating behaviour and mealtime routines. The nurse's best guide for parents of toddlers is to remind them that parents are in charge of what food is offered, when it is offered, and where it is offered (Research for Evidence-Informed Practice). Box 12.2 lists some nursing interventions to promote healthy eating in toddlers. However, it is up to the toddler to decide the amount of food to consume. Periodically,

## BOX 12.2   Nursing Interventions

### Promoting Healthy Eating in Toddlers

- Routines are important to toddlers. Serve scheduled meals and snacks. Parents are responsible for what, when, and where the toddler eats. The toddler decides whether to eat and how much.
- Schedule meals and sleep periods such that the child is awake and alert during mealtime.
- Turn off the television. Mealtime should be a relaxed and pleasant time, free of distractions.
- Serve small portions and let your toddler ask for more.
- Offer simple, single foods, because mixtures of foods are often rejected.
- Serve your toddler's favourite foods along with new ones. Several introductions may be necessary before the toddler accepts a new food. Make sure you eat it too.
- Encourage the use of utensils, but accept that toddlers still often need to use their fingers.
- Do not use food to bribe, reward, or punish your toddler.
- Avoid foods that may cause choking, such as hard candy, mini marshmallows, popcorn, pretzels, chips, and spoonfuls of peanut butter, nuts, and seeds, large chunks of meat, hot dogs, raw carrots, dried fruits, and whole grapes.
- Drinking more than 700 mL of milk per day can reduce your child's appetite for other healthy foods. For those younger than 2 years, do not use reduced-fat, low-fat, or fat-free (skim) milk because children younger than 2 years need the extra fat for their developing nervous systems.

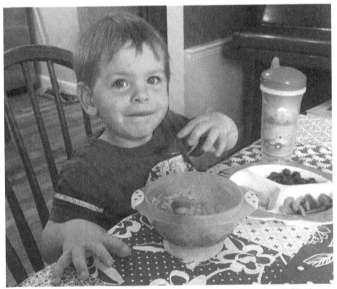

**Fig. 12.3** Toddlers Need Healthy, Age-Appropriate Food Choices

a toddler may even refuse a meal altogether. Parents need to be encouraged to offer healthy, age-appropriate food choices (CPS, 2019b; Fig. 12.3). Ensure that toddlers do not consume empty calorie juices and high-carbohydrate snacks that are often given to children prior to mealtime. Furthermore, parents should not focus too much attention on food intake or punish children for refusing food. Toddlers may learn how easily parents can be controlled by their behaviour around food intake and may then continue the behaviour for the attention alone.

## RESEARCH FOR EVIDENCE-INFORMED PRACTICE

### Asthma, Diet, and Toddlers—A Cure?

The toddler diet can be challenging, as toddlers often prefer non-nutritious and highly sweetened food. Imagine that same toddler with asthma or wheezes and that the possibility of following a Mediterranean diet might eliminate asthma symptoms. A meta-analysis evaluating the relationship between adherence to the Mediterranean diet during pregnancy and childhood and the risk of asthma and wheeze in children was conducted by Zhang, Lin, Fu, and colleagues in 2019. The meta-analysis included 18 observational studies of moderate to high quality. Participants who consumed a Mediterranean diet consumed foods low in saturated fatty acids, rich in carbohydrates, fibre, and antioxidants, with a high content of monounsaturated fatty acids and *n*-3 polyunsaturated fatty acids. High adherence to a Mediterranean diet during pregnancy and childhood revealed a short-term benefit on wheeze. There was a short-term benefit of this diet for those with current wheezes and those with diagnosed asthma; however, there did not appear to be a benefit for those with current severe wheezes. The researchers note that the Mediterranean diet might be beneficial in asthma development because it might have the ability to counteract oxidative stress that occurs in the respiratory tract.

Previous research indicated that the Mediterranean diet could potentially reduce the risk of asthma and wheeze (Simopoulos, 2008). Results from this study indicated that while there was some short-term benefit of diet adherence during pregnancy and childhood on risk of wheeze, no empirical evidence supported a long-term effect on severe asthma. However, a limitation of this study included a lack of randomized controlled trials, which would provide evidence that is more accurate.

Source: Zhang, Y., Lin, J. Fu, W., et al. (2019). Mediterranean diet during pregnancy and childhood for asthma in children: A systematic review and meta-analysis of observational studies. *Pediatric Pulmonology, 54,* 949–961. https://doi.org/10.1002/ppul.24338.

Maintaining a record of food intake over time, the nurse can demonstrate the adequacy of the nutrients that the toddler is already receiving during mealtimes and help parents develop a plan to offer more of the essential foods during meals (Government of Canada, 2019a). Children with inadequate nutrition are predisposed to impaired immune systems, leading to infections and delayed healing and recovery. They are also predisposed to depletion of muscle mass, leading to diminished functional capacity. In addition, although inadequately understood, nutrients and gut microbiota interact with one another for brain and behavioural development (Oriach, Robertson, Stanton, et al., 2016).

The family who has a vegetarian or vegan diet may need some assistance from the nurse or a dietitian. Vegetarian and vegan diets differ widely, so it is important to assess the foods that are eaten, which foods or food groups that have been eliminated from the diet, and any supplements that are used.

### ◆ Elimination Pattern

**Toilet training** is often a major parental concern during toddlerhood. The nurse anticipates this developmental stressor and initiates discussion with the parents to determine their understanding of the child's signs of developmental readiness and their attitude and commitment to establishing a toileting pattern for their toddler. Emotional and physiological readiness for toilet training rarely develops before 18 months of age.

## BOX 12.3 Nursing Interventions

### *Initiating a Toileting Program for Toddlers*

Interest in and awareness of bowel and urinary elimination usually begin by 18 months of age.

- Before beginning toilet training, parents should check their toddlers for the prerequisite skills, which include being able to walk well, stoop and recover, stay dry for at least 2 hours during the day, and communicate sensation before elimination, as well as the discomfort of wet or messy pants and the need for assistance.
- When these prerequisites are present, introduce the child to a potty seat or chair. The potty chair should provide secure seating with the child's feet touching the floor. The potty seat should be used with a small step stool to create the same effect.
- Because of the gastro-colic reflex, bowel elimination is more likely after a meal, so this is a good time to place the toddler on the potty. When a pattern of bowel or urinary elimination is identified, use this pattern as a guide for placing the child on the potty.
- Encourage the toddler to stay on the chair for 2 to 3 minutes and always explain what to do ("Go potty") rather than what not to do ("Don't wet your pants"). Do not refer to elimination as dirty or yucky. Remember this is your child's first creation.
- Praise the child for desired behaviour. Introduce underwear as a badge of success. Ignore undesired behaviour and never punish the child by scolding the child, spanking the child, or other punitive measures.

  Remember that daytime dryness is usually achieved by 3 years of age and ahead of night-time dryness, where the need to wear a diaper remains.

Parents who begin before their child is ready usually experience frustration.

### Nursing Interventions

By suggesting the sequence in Box 12.3, the nurse assists parents with toilet training. The parent, who can approach toilet training with a relaxed attitude, accepting some delays and frustrations, will have a better chance of success and a more positive outcome for the toddler.

### ◆ Activity-Exercise Pattern

Toddlers are always busy—emptying garbage cans and drawers; building and destroying towers; throwing, kicking, and chasing after balls; or dressing and undressing. Many of their activities are repeated, providing practice opportunities for their newly realized skills. The various toys designed for toddlers capitalize on this ability to explore and imagine with laptop trainers, electronic colouring tablets, musical instruments, and books with accompanying audiovisual disks.

During the toddler period, children will advance from taking their first step to running, climbing stairs, and even pedalling a tricycle. They enjoy pushing and pulling, whether it is an unsuspecting laundry basket or a push-pull toy made for the job. They scribble spontaneously, usually with vigour, and will emerge from toddlerhood capable of copying a circle and creating tadpole-like figures. They learn to use a spoon and a fork with some dexterity and to wash their hands. They also advance from being dressed by others to dressing themselves with assistance, although at times they resist it.

The CPS recommends 180 minutes of physical activity throughout the day for children aged 1 to 2 years (CPS, 2018b). This activity can be planned and organized or unstructured, and can include free play (CPS, 2018b). For children aged 3 to 4 years, 60 minutes of energetic play is recommended (CPS, 2018b). Toddlers spend most of their waking hours at play—exploring their expanding environment, imitating others' actions, and creating a safety net of rituals around the routines of eating, sleeping, and everything in between. In their enthusiasm to try many activities, toddlers invariably take on tasks that are beyond their abilities, which can result in frustration and an occasional well-known temper tantrum. Their exploratory nature and limited, but advancing, skills also make them vulnerable to injury.

Most toddlers are interested in other children. However, this interest is limited because toddlers, although ready to be with other children, are not ready to share. Successful social encounters with toddlers are best described as parallel play, where children play side by side, doing similar things with similar toys, but each working independently (Charlop, Lang, & Rispoli, 2018). Sharing and cooperative play will not develop until well into the preschool age.

The Canadian Paediatric Society's Active Kids Healthy Kids program endeavours to engage health professionals in promoting an active lifestyle to patients. For more information on encouraging activity in toddlers, please refer to *Your Busy Toddler: Games, Toys and Play in the Second Year of Life* on the CPS website at https://www.caringforkids.cps.ca/handouts/your_busy_toddler.

### Nursing Interventions

When parents inquire about what toys and activities to provide for their toddler, the following are suggested:

- Provide toys that challenge the child to develop new skills: toys that require skills slightly above the child's present level, but not so advanced that the child cannot achieve some success.
- Provide opportunities for new learning. This may be as basic as a book with pictures of new animals or a walk through the produce section of the grocery store to point out fruits and vegetables.
- Provide opportunities for social encounters with other children, but do not force playing together. Creating separate yet parallel space, with the use of small mats or hula hoops as boundaries, is recommended.
- Follow the child's lead. Let the toddler choose and explore new toys or objects, within safe limits.
- Make sure the toy is safe for the toddler and does not have any parts that can be removed and swallowed, have lead paint, or can cause harm to the curious toddler.

The heightened expectations of some parents to raise the high-achieving child often begins in the toddler period. Consistent quality interactions with parents and others in their environment provides the advantage with cognitive development in childhood. The CPS recommends no screen time, including television, videos, tablets (iPads), and computers, for children younger than 2 years; and for children aged 2 to 5 years, recommends less than 1 hour daily (CPS, 2017b). For interactive computer games that may include touch screens (on smartphones and tablets), the parent needs to be there with the toddler so that two-way conversation occurs. Ideally, children should be encouraged to explore their interests, with parents responding to their cues. Past research associated television watching by toddlers with interference at a critical time when language development occurs and suggested that this can cause a delay in that process. The more time children view television increases the probability of delayed cognitive, language, and motor development, and increased exposure is associated with greater risk (Lin, Cherng, Chen, et al., 2015). Additionally, the more television shows with advertising watched, the more likely the child will become obese (Lobstein, Jackson-Leach, Moodie, et al., 2015). For more information on helping parents support their toddler's activity, use of technology, and exploration in a safe and educational way, visit the Childcare Canada—Technology in Early Childhood website at https://www.childcarecanada.org/resources/issue-files/technology-early-childhood, or the Zero to Three website at http://www.zerotothree.org.

### ◆ Sleep-Rest Pattern

Toddlers' need for sleep decreases to 12 hours a day, including one or two naps of shorter duration. Naps can be replaced by quiet time, allowing a brief period to unwind from a busy or noisy activity. Sitting together in a rocking chair for a soothing song or quiet music or reading side by side or together can be suggested by the nurse.

The toddler may be involved in an activity and not be aware of fatigue, especially when visitors are in the home or some interesting new toys have been discovered. All parents are familiar with the child who is overtired but unable to relax enough to sleep. Parents can potentially avoid this dilemma by scheduling nap and quiet time even when there are houseguests or holidays that pre-empt the toddler's routine.

Rituals are characteristic of this age, and most toddlers have a nap and bedtime ritual. The following might be a typical pattern: eating a nutritious snack, followed by bathing, brushing teeth, listening to a story, getting a kiss, and having overhead lights turned off and the night light turned on. Following this ritual is important because the toddler gets a sense of security when ending the day. Changing this ritual can be upsetting. The nurse encourages parents to establish and follow the bedtime ritual as closely as possible, even when visitors, family illness, or travel makes the routine more difficult. In addition, incorporate rituals as much as possible when the toddler stays outside the home; for instance, staying overnight at their grandparent's house or during a hospitalization.

Many toddlers will try to delay sleep by calling for water, another story, or another kiss, or by making other requests. Parents should be certain that the toddler has opportunities for adequate interaction with them during the day, follow the usual bedtime ritual, and be firm and consistent in resisting any requests for attention once settled into bed. Encouraging toddlers to use transition or security objects, such as stuffed animals or blankets, helps them to self-quiet and console themselves both at bedtime and during new situations (Fig. 12.4).

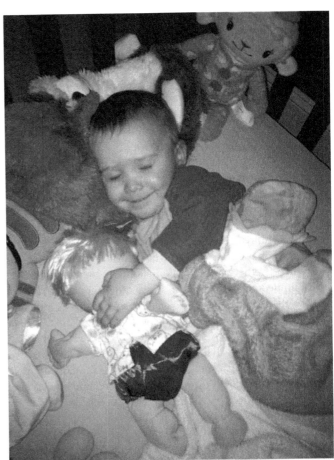

Fig. 12.4 Toddlers need adequate sleep for healthy growth, and their stuffed toys can help them feel more secure.

Night terrors may begin in toddlerhood, typically occurring in children aged 3 to 12 years. Night terrors are different from nightmares, which generally begin at a later age and result in the child awakening and being able to recall the frightening dream. Typically, these do not occur in isolation; night terrors usually occur 2 to 3 hours after falling asleep when sleep moves from the deepest stage of non-REM (non–rapid eye movement) sleep to light REM sleep. The child who experiences night terrors does not waken completely, but cries out, appears terrified, and is difficult to arouse. Eventually, usually after 5 to 10 minutes, the child falls back into quiet sleep. Parents need to be reassured that these episodes will become less frequent as the child develops. The parents should talk in a soothing voice but should not try to awaken the child. If the child does waken, the parents should then provide comfort and tuck the child back in bed.

### ◆ Cognitive-Perceptual Pattern

Toddlers who have experienced the security of a nurturing and reliable source of protection and attachment during infancy have a strong base from which to begin to explore and learn about their expanding world. They begin toddlerhood in Piaget's sensorimotor stage of cognitive development and start moving to the preoperational stage. Their advancing thought-processing skills and abilities to use the language precede the development of egocentrism, an inability to put oneself in another's shoes. Toddlers who come running into a room asking their parents

"Where is it?" are confused when parents respond, "Where is what?" They assume their parents and all others share their same thoughts and cannot understand why they do not.

Toddlers interpret and learn about objects and events, not in terms of general properties but in terms of their relationship with them or their use to them. Their thoughts are dominated by what they see, hear, or otherwise experience, and they want to experience everything. Two- to three-word phrases are most often related to present events, describing an action, a desire, or a possession (e.g., "Mommy, me up!").

Both receptive and expressive language skills are developing rapidly in toddlers; however, their receptive language skills far outweigh their expressive language ability, and toddlers often use gestures until words are found to represent the meanings already acquired. Toddlers also learn the use of inflection. "Mommy" may mean "Pick me up" on one occasion and "I'm scared" or "Where are you?" on another. Often frustrated by their limited repertoire of expressive language (approximately 400 words), young toddlers default to using "no" as a method of gaining control over a situation or expressing themselves (see the Think About It box at the beginning of this chapter).

By age 3 years, children have mastered the basics of language function, form, and content, and these fundamentals will continue to be refined throughout childhood and adolescence. Table 12.1 outlines the landmarks of speech, language, and hearing ability for this age group.

Toddlers have a solid understanding of object permanence and are no longer easily distracted when a desired toy, blanket, or parent is missing. Many toddlers will sit patiently in front of the washing machine while a favourite blanket is laundered or stare out of a front window awaiting a parent's return. They can inadvertently put themselves in harm's way as they pursue an object or person they sense is just out of view.

The toddler period is dominated by play, which is repetitive and ritualistic. When bouncing a ball, toddlers are trying to learn various aspects of the object, and repetition is the best teacher. Toddlers' ritualistic behaviours help them to master skills and decrease anxiety, and the addition of a seemingly endless string of questions to these behaviours can test the limits of the most patient parents. These queries, however, must be acknowledged and answered in a manner that not only provides solutions but also validates and reinforces the toddler's burgeoning curiosity. The nurse explains the "terrible twos" by teaching parents and caregivers that this is a normal stage of child development where a toddler alternates between reliance on adults and a new desire for independence. Frustration becomes heightened as the toddler is trying to express independence without the emotional vocabulary to do so. This is often expressed using anger or aggression.

Autism spectrum disorders (ASD) are defined as pervasive neuro-developmental disorders with onset in infancy or childhood and characterized by impaired social interactions, language, and communications, combined with restricted and repetitive behaviours, interests, or activities (American Psychiatric Association [APA], 2013). Signs of ASD typically appear in early childhood, with Canadian prevalence rates of 1 in 66 (15.2 per 1000) in 2015 (Ofner, Coles, Decou, et al., 2018).

Boys are diagnosed with ASD four to five time more frequently than girls (CDC, 2014; Ofner et al., 2018). There is no single treatment that works for all children with autism; however, there are many options available, including applied behaviour analysis. This involves the principle that positive reinforcement increases the frequency of the desired behaviour. It is best to implement treatment early in the child's development. See https://autismcanada.org/ for more information.

## Hearing

The ability to hear and listen to others is critical for speech and language development. Listening includes attending to what is heard, discriminating among the various qualities of sound, cognitively associating what is heard with previously learned experiences, and remembering what is heard. Children who are exposed to and hear large amounts of varied speech tend to learn language more quickly than children who do not (Jones & Rowland, 2017). The quantity and quality of language to which the toddler is exposed is thought to be more important for the development of listening ability, and therefore receptive language skills, than it is for the development of expressive language skills (Perryman, Carter, Messinger, et al., 2013). Toddlers often seek repetition of auditory input, as observed in their seemingly endless repetition of sounds, words, and combinations of words. This repetition is their way of practising and organizing new language (Clark, 2018) (see Table 12.1).

Hearing loss is one of the most common conditions present at birth. If undetected during early infancy, even mild hearing loss can impede speech, language, cognitive, and emotional development (Cupples, Ching, Button, et al., 2018). Health care providers need to continue to monitor, screen, and refer children for formal audiological evaluation if they develop signs of identified risk factors for hearing loss. The timing and number of hearing re-evaluations for children with risk factors should be individualized. The Canadian Paediatric Society recommends that all newborns receive hearing screening to ensure early diagnosis and intervention, with reassessment for all children who experience developmental or learning difficulties (Patel & Feldman, 2018).

Younger toddlers are screened using visual-reinforcement audiometry, in which stimulus tones and visually animated reinforcers (e.g., a lighted toy) are paired and presented together. After the toddler has been conditioned to expect this relationship, the visual reinforcer is withheld, and the sound is presented alone. The toddler looks for the visual reinforcer in response to the sound, and the visual reinforcer is then presented as a reward. Conditioned-play audiometry is used for older toddlers and preschool children. The child is first taught to play listening games, using blocks or rings. The child learns to wait and listen for a sound and then perform a motor task (e.g., places a block, a bucket, or a ring on a stacking stick) in response. The motor task is followed by social reinforcement. Non-calibrated toys or noisemakers and signals that lack frequency specificity are inappropriate screening methods and should be used only as gross indicators for monitoring.

Otitis media, or middle ear infection, is one of the leading causes of visits to health care providers during the toddler years and the primary reason for which antibiotics are

## TABLE 12.1   Growth and Development
### Landmarks of Speech, Language, and Hearing Ability During the Toddler Period

| Age (Months) | Receptive Language | Expressive Language | Related Hearing Ability |
|---|---|---|---|
| 18 | Up to 50 words; recognizes between 6 and 12 objects by name, such as *dog, cat, bottle, ball*; identifies three body parts, such as *eyes, nose, mouth*; understands simple, one-step commands such as *give me the doll, open your mouth, stick out your tongue* | Up to 20 words; jargon and echolalia are present; uses names of familiar objects and one-word sentences, such as *go* or *eat*; uses gestures; uses words such as *no, mine, eat, good, bad, hot, cold*, and expressions such as *oh-oh, what's that, all gone*; use of words can be quite inconsistent; 25% of speech intelligible | Has begun to develop gross discrimination by learning to distinguish between highly dissimilar noises, such as doorbell and train, barking dog and automobile horn, or mother's and father's voices |
| 24 | Up to 1200 words; knows *in, on, under*; identifies *dog, ball, engine, bed, doll, scissors, hair, mouth, feet, nose, cup, spoon, car, key*; distinguishes between one and many and formulates a negative judgement (a knife is not a fork); understands simple stories; follows simple, two-step directions; is beginning to make distinctions between *you* and *me* | Up to 270 words; jargon and echolalia almost gone; average 75 words per hour during free play; talks in words, phrases, and two-word to three-word sentences; averages two words per response; first pronouns appear, such as *I, me, mine, it, who, that*; adjectives and adverbs are only beginning to appear; names objects and common pictures; refers to self by name, such as *Katrina go bye-bye*; uses phrases such as *I want, go bye-bye, want cookie, ball all gone*; 60% of speech intelligible | Refinement of gross discriminative skills |
| 30 | Up to 2400 words; identifies action in pictures and objects by use; carries out one-part and two-part commands, such as *pick up your shoe and give it to mommy*; knows what is used to drink liquids, what goes on the feet, what is used to buy candy; understands plurals, questions, difference between boy and girl, the concepts *one, up, down, run, walk, throw, fast, more, my* | Uses up to 425 words; jargon and echolalia — no longer exist; averages 140 words per hour; names words such as *chair, can, box, key, door*; repeats two digits from memory; average sentence length is approximately 2.5 words; uses more adjectives and adverbs; demands repetition from others, such as *do it again*; nearly always announces intentions before actions; begins to ask questions of adults; 75% of speech intelligible | |
| 36 | Up to 3600 words; understands *both, two, not today*, what to do when thirsty (hungry, sleepy), why people have stoves; understands *wait, later, big, new, different, strong, today, another*, and taking turns at play; carries out two-item and some three-item commands, such as *give me the ball, pick up the doll*, and *sit down*; identifies several colours; is aware of past and future | Up to 900 words in simple sentences, averaging three to four words per sentence; averages 170 words per hour; uses words such as *when, time, today, not today, new, different, big, strong, surprise, secret*; can repeat three digits, name one colour, say name, give simple account of experiences, and tell stories that can be understood; begins to use more pronouns, adjectives, and adverbs; describes at least one element of a picture; is aware of past and future; uses commands such as *you make it* and expressions such as *I can't, I don't want to*; verbalizes toilet needs; expresses desire to take turns; communication includes criticisms, commands, requests, threats, questions, answers; 85% of speech intelligible | Starts to distinguish dissimilar speech sounds, such as the difference between *ee* and *er*, although there may be some difficulty with the concepts of *same* and *different* |

Sources: Modified from Hockenberry, M. J., & Wilson, D. (Eds.). (2015). *Wong's nursing care of infants and children* (10th ed.). St. Louis, MO: Mosby; Ports, N. L., & Mandleco, B. L. (2011). *Pediatric nursing: Caring for children and their families* (3rd ed.). Clifton Park, NY: Thomson Delmar Learning; Quevedo, L. A., Silva, R., Godoy, K., et al. (2011). The impact of maternal post-partum depression on the language development of children at 12 months. *Child: Care, Health and Development, 38*(3), 420–424.

prescribed for these children. Discussing the current literature and evidence-informed reports and recommendations often helps parents understand the proper use of antibiotics, which is also imperative in preventing antibiotic resistance. When it is deemed necessary to use an antibiotic, nurses teach how to administer the medication safely and stress the importance of taking the medication at the prescribed time and for the full duration of the course, which is indicated by an empty container of medication, not by the absence of initial symptoms.

## Vision

Toddlers' visual acuity is usually approximately 20/40, although gaining their cooperation for screening is often difficult and not recommended unless parents, caregivers, or health care providers identify a concern. Depth perception is still immature, although more developed than in infancy.

Amblyopia is one of the major health care concerns for this age group, occurring in two to four of every 100 children (Canadian Association of Optometrists, n.d.-a). It is defined as diminished, or loss of, vision in an eye that has not received adequate use. The eye looks normal, but it is not being used normally. Because the brain favours the other eye, the term "lazy eye" is often used. The most common cause of amblyopia is strabismus, but it may also occur when one eye is more nearsighted, farsighted, or astigmatic than the other. Occasionally, amblyopia is caused by other eye conditions such as a cataract.

Amblyopia is preventable and treatable, especially if detected early. The earlier detection of amblyopia will contribute to the greater chance for a complete recovery. It is strongly recommended that children have their eyes examined at the following times: between 6 and 9 months, between 2 and 5 years, and yearly after starting school (Canadian Association of Optometrists, n.d.-b; CPS, 2018c). Management of amblyopia depends on the cause and may include surgery or paralytic, autonomic, and centrally acting pharmacological agents. However, no matter what the cause, management will involve making the child use the lazy eye, the eye with reduced vision. There are two ways to accomplish this: use of atropine eye drops or patching of the stronger eye (Canadian Ophthalmological Society, n.d.). If glasses are worn with the patch, the nurse will help the parents secure them with the active toddler.

Strabismus is a deviation of the line of vision from the midline that results from extraocular muscle weakness or imbalance and is commonly referred to as crossed eye. One or both eyes may turn in, out, up, or down, and this can be constant or intermittent. Marked or continuous strabismus is usually noticed early by the parents and health care providers and is therefore treated early; the subtler deviations are often unnoticed until older toddlerhood or the preschool years (Pritchard & Ellis, 2016). Every toddler should be screened for strabismus as part of the routine eye examination that is performed by the health care provider or nurse practitioner during well-child visits.

Other signs of vision problems that the nurse observes or that parents report in their toddlers include the following red flags:
- Rubs eyes excessively
- Shuts or covers one eye, tilts head, or looks sideways to view an object
- Has difficulty or is irritable when doing close work
- Blinks, squints, or frowns when viewing objects
- Holds books close to eyes
- Has red, encrusted, or swollen eyelids
- Has red, inflamed, or watery eyes
- Develops recurring styes (swelling at the edge of the eyelid)

### Taste and Smell

Toddlers are beginning to take control of their world and have the capacity to taste and smell, new skills that are rapidly used. Toddlers often refuse to even taste something that looks or smells displeasing to them or eat something that they recall as tasting terrible. They are able to react accurately to a sensation that a taste or smell arouses in them, and they begin to learn conditioned association between certain smells and culturally acceptable values. Foods and smells found in one family or culture become palatable and accepted, and those that are unacceptable become displeasing. Many of our adult eating habits, food likes and dislikes, and visceral responses to odours have their roots in this period.

## ◆ Self-Perception–Self-Concept Pattern

According to Erikson (1995, 1998), the developmental task of toddlers is to acquire a sense of autonomy while overcoming a sense of doubt and shame. To exert autonomy, toddlers must relinquish the dependence on others that was enjoyed during infancy. Continued dependency has the potential to create a sense of doubt in toddlers about their ability to take control of, and ultimately take responsibility for, their own actions. Toddlers seem to thrive when parents can accommodate their increasing autonomy yet maintain a strong parenting presence that includes a full measure of patience, enough parental self-confidence to set appropriate limits, and the ability to realize that their toddler's negative behaviour is not directed at them and their egocentrism is not a reflection on them.

The toddler must explore the world, not only the physical aspects but also the interpersonal aspects of relationships, to develop a true sense of autonomy. Exploring the physical world involves poking into, climbing onto, crawling under, tasting, smelling, and taking apart the objects encountered. Children explore relationships with others by searching for the limits of the their power: If a no or a temper tantrum means control of another person's behaviour, the child learns that one's own self is more powerful than the other person's self. The toddler continually practises separateness to develop a sense of autonomy.

This process can be frustrating and confusing for parents. The toddler may say a vehement "no" when offered a drink and then scream and cry when the drink is taken away; the parents may wonder whether the toddler wants the drink. Probably the answer is yes, but the toddler may also need to express autonomy by refusing it. Occasionally, the same toddler who displays a strong need for autonomy spontaneously cuddles or even clings to a parent. These conflicting desires can be confusing to both the parent and the toddler. The toddler's need for more autonomy may conflict with parental expectations, safety limits, or the rights of other children or adults. Any of these conflicts result in feelings of frustration. A typical toddler response to frustration is the well-known temper tantrum.

Conversely, the concept of child autonomy, where children are allowed the freedom to explore their environment, promoting independence, is a value that is openly recognized and respected by Indigenous people in Canada (Muir & Bohr, 2014). The Inuit in Canada also view autonomy and independence as being intrinsic to the child–parent relationship, because parents look for indications from their children to guide their own response (McShane, Hastings, Smylie, et al., 2009).

### Nursing Interventions

The nurse assesses the toddler–parent relationship to determine the following:

- How is the toddler expressing the need for autonomy?
- How do the parents perceive these actions?
- How does the toddler respond to frustration in exploring the environment or controlling personal and others' actions?
- How do the parents respond to the toddler's display of frustration?
- What provisions are the parents making to allow safe choices for the toddler?

The nurse's teaching focuses on the aspects that are troublesome for the toddler–parent relationship. The following examples are some general concepts to include:

- Match the environment to the child's needs and abilities. Childproof the home such that the child can explore safely. Provide toys that the child can master. Give opportunities to play with more challenging toys, but do not make these toys the rule.
- Give advance notice of a change in activity, such as lunch or nap time. Use transition rituals and objects.
- Do not offer a choice if there is not one. For example, rather than ask if the toddler wants to take a bath, say "It is time to take a bath. Do you want to take it upstairs or downstairs, or do you want to start at the face and move down to the toes or start with the toes and wash the face last?" This allows the toddler to be in charge and the task of bathing to be achieved.
- Set and enforce consistent limits such that the toddler will come to develop control within these limits.
- To prevent temper tantrums, keep routines simple and consistent, set reasonable limits and give rationales, avoid "head-on clashes," and provide choices.
- If temper tantrums occur, provide a safe environment for the toddler, identify the tantrum's cause, and help the toddler regain control. Do not reason, threaten, promise, hit, or concede. Respond consistently and follow through on discipline free of anger. Over-criticizing and restricting the toddler may dampen enthusiasm and increase feelings of shame and doubt.
- Praise the toddler's skills and abilities. Never miss an opportunity to catch your toddler being good. Be positive. Remember to say "yes" occasionally.

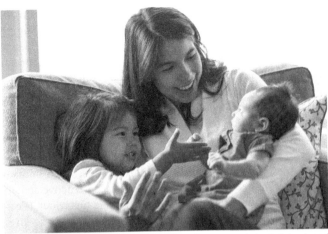

**Fig. 12.5** It is a big change for a toddler when a new baby is introduced to the family. (iStockphoto/FatCamera)

### ◆ Roles-Relationships Pattern

By toddlerhood, children typically know their mother, father, and older siblings and have established some form of reciprocal relationship with them (Perry, Hockenberry, Lowdermilk, et al., 2017). Toddlers' capability for relationships is limited and usually reflects their egocentric approach to everything else. Parents' and siblings' roles are understood, just like everything else in their lives, in terms of how those roles relate to the toddler. One family member may be the fixer of toys or the comforter of bruises, another the troublemaker who takes away toys.

Toddlers are interested in everything, and parent, caregiver, and siblings' activities or possessions are often imitated and preferred. Frequently the desire to be like or have something that belongs to a sibling creates sibling rivalry. This happens between toddlers and their older siblings, but even more when a new, younger sibling is introduced (Fig. 12.5). A new baby who is often loud, unable to play, unable to be touched or explored too vigorously, and demands and gets too much parental attention quickly becomes a nuisance to toddlers, who have been known to inform their parents that they can "take the new baby back where it came from now." Realizing the new sibling is here to stay, toddlers often regress, reverting to earlier, previously abandoned infantile behaviour such as losing toileting skills, wanting to be fed or dressed, or even communicating by "baby talk." They are usually trying to retain or regain a sense of mastery and, once reassured, will progress through this stage. This process is not the end of sibling rivalry but only the beginning of what will assume many forms and require ongoing negotiation from all family members. Parents cannot stop sibling fighting by forbidding it, but reasonable limits can be established. One way to deescalate fighting is to remove the reward of the fight. Generally, the desired outcome in the toddler's mind is to see the self is rewarded and the sibling is punished. When parents do not reward the toddler or punish the sibling, or when they do not take sides, the gain is missing and fighting becomes less satisfactory. This approach does not mean that all fighting will stop, but the child will look for other ways of getting approval.

Sibling relationships and parent–child relationships can be difficult subjects for parents to discuss. Parents may think that any hint of discord indicates an unhealthy family (Wulff, St. George, & Tomm, 2015). The nurse includes normal family development and role relationships as part of the anticipatory guidance given during the toddler years. Toddler behaviours are frustrating for all parents, and discipline can often be influenced as much by parental emotions as by parenting knowledge and skill (Gravener, Rogosch, Oshri, et al., 2012). Discipline and limit settings refers to action taken to enforce established rules of acceptable behaviour (Perry et al., 2017). Nurses can support parents to establish realistic and concrete rules. When limit setting and discipline are positive, children can test their limits of control, channel undesirable feelings into constructive activity, and learn boundaries of socially acceptable behaviour (Perry et al., 2017). When parents experience high levels of stress related to challenging child behaviour, dysfunctional parent–child interactions and low levels of available resources, physical abuse, and emotional abuse can occur (Beckerman, van Berkel, Mesman, et al., 2017).

## Child Abuse

Child abuse and maltreatment is not limited to a particular age or particular families. However, it is more likely to occur with a major change or turmoil (Bartlett, Kotake, Fauth, et al., 2017; CDC, 2015b) in the family or when parental role models were abusive. Toddlerhood is a trying time for the most patient of parents, and nurses are alert to family changes and stresses as well as to warning signs of abuse (Box 12.4). Many injuries are difficult to differentiate from accidental injury and, at times, may even be confused with culturally appropriate healing practices (Diversity Awareness). Statistics reveal that 32% of Canadians have experienced some form of abuse before the age of 16 (26% physical abuse, 10% sexual abuse, and 8% exposure to intimate partner violence) (PHAC, 2018; Statistics Canada, 2017b). Of significance, rates of childhood abuse among Indigenous people have now reached 40%. According to the Canadian Incidence Study of Reported Child Abuse and Neglect, types of childhood trauma include exposure to intimate partner violence (34%), neglect (20%), physical abuse (20%), emotional abuse (9%), and sexual abuse (3%) (PHAC, 2010).

The toddler years have the greatest incidence of child maltreatment with at least 1 in 7 children experiencing child abuse and/or neglect each year (CDC, 2019), with 27% of nonfatal cases reported for children aged 3 years or younger and 70% of deaths from child maltreatment occurring in children younger than 3 years (CDC, 2015b). Nonfatal cases appearing in emergency departments, pediatrician offices, and day care centres may be the only opportunity for health care providers to prevent later death from continued child maltreatment.

Laws in Newfoundland, Saskatchewan, Prince Edward Island, and the Northwest Territories allow for professionals who work with children to report suspected child maltreatment to the Royal Canadian Mounted Police (RCMP), which is in turn obligated to report these to the local child welfare authorities. In most other provinces and territories, suspected maltreatment should be reported directly to the local child protection society.

---

### BOX 12.4   Warning Signs of Child Abuse

- Parental delay in seeking help
- Inconsistencies in the history of how the injury occurred
- Recurrent unexplained illnesses
- Injury inconsistent with the history or the child's developmental capability
- Old, unexplained fractures evident on radiographs
- Bruises confined to back surface of the body—neck to knees
- Bare spots and broken hair
- Pattern of injury or bruising descriptive of object used to inflict injury (belt or belt buckle, hand, cigarette, hot water)
- Burns with sharply demarcated edges or circumferential patterns
- Perineal injuries of any kind

For more information about recognizing signs of child abuse, visit the Child Welfare Information Gateway at https://www.childwelfare.gov/pubs/user-manuals/childcare/.

---

### 🌐 DIVERSITY AWARENESS

#### Evaluating a Child for Child Abuse With Cultural Sensitivity

Nurses are required by law to report cases of suspected child abuse to their local child protective agency. The nurse who takes a careful health history may discover that what might appear to be characteristic burns or bruises associated with child abuse may instead be the product of a traditional culturally appropriate healing practice. The following are three examples of healing practices found in the Pacific Islander and Asian populations that might create such confusion.

**Coining (Cao Gio)**
Coining is a common healing practice used among Pacific Island and Asian families within North America. Traditionally, coining is used for conditions associated with "wind" illnesses, as well as a wide variety of febrile illnesses. The lesions seen from coining are produced by rubbing a warm oil or balm on the skin and firmly abrading the skin with a coin or special instrument. The practice produces linear petechiae and ecchymosis on the chest and back that often resemble strap or belt marks. The appearance of the deep red-purple skin colour is confirmation that the person had bad wind in the body.

**Cupping (Ventouse)**
Cupping involves the creation of a vacuum inside a special cup or glass by burning the oxygen out of it and then promptly placing it on a person's skin surface. Cupping draws blood and lymph to the body surface that is under the cup or glass, increasing local circulation. The purpose for doing this is to remove cold and damp "evils" from the body or to assist blood circulation, or both. The procedure is frequently used to treat lung congestion. The resulting circular ecchymotic marks are approximately 5 cm in diameter and resemble nonaccidental trauma.

**Moxibustion**
Moxibustion involves burning moxa (the dried leaves of *Artemisia vulgaris*), wormwood, or another slow-burning material on or as close to the skin as possible. This practice is most commonly used in Chinese and Japanese culture to improve a body function or for pain relief. It can leave skin burns and scarring.

**Reflective Questions**
- Do you believe that employing any of these cultural practices constitutes child abuse? Why?
- How would you ask careful, sensitive, and respectful questions regarding diverse cultural health beliefs and healing practices?

Child abuse and maltreatment in First Nations communities has been delegated to First Nations Child and Family Service Agencies (FNCFSAs), and any reporting should be made to the appropriate FNCFSA (Government of Canada, 2019b). British Columbia and Ontario have both partially and fully delegated FNCFSAs; partially delegated FNCFSAs are not authorized to receive or assess reports of child abuse and maltreatment; therefore reports must be made to the local child protection society. In the Northwest Territories and Prince Edward Island, there are no FNCFSAs, thus all abuse reports must be made to the local child protection society.

Typically, parental responses to childhood injuries include a spontaneous reporting of the details of the illness or injury accompanied by concern, questions about progress and discharge, difficulty in leaving the child, and an attempt to identify with the child's feelings. These parents may also experience guilt for not protecting the child from the accident and may offer gifts to compensate for these feelings of guilt. In contrast, neglectful or abusive parents are often hesitant to provide information about the illness or injury; they may be evasive or even contradict themselves, appearing irritated by the inconvenience of being questioned. Abusive parents may not exhibit guilt feelings and often contend that the toddler was solely responsible for the injury.

Although these signs of potential abuse are certainly not present in all abusive parents, their presence alerts the nurse to assess and observe further. The nurse also remembers that some of these signs may be found in nonabusive parents, and that the presence of these signs serves only as a cue for further assessment. All nurses are required by law to report any and all suspected child abuse to the local child protective authorities.

### Sexuality-Reproductive Pattern

The toileting process, during which attention is focused on the genital area, may precipitate the toddler's curiosity about genital organs. The nurse includes this aspect when teaching about toilet training, giving parents time to consider their feelings and decide on their approach to genital exploratory behaviour and masturbation. Some parents accept the child's curiosity, whereas others see this as an opportunity to introduce their own sexual values and taboos (Healthy Children, 2015).

The nurse encourages parents to approach this curiosity and exploration, as well as masturbation, as a normal developmental process. These behaviours provide toddlers with an opportunity to become better acquainted with their bodies. Many parents are uncertain about the vocabulary they should use and often create cute, unrelated words rather than provide the correct anatomical terms. The use of cute alternative words is often a reflection of parental discomfort or embarrassment. Using correct terms will help toddlers develop accurate knowledge about sexuality and communicate more effectively if inappropriate touching by others occurs. For example, a young boy was initially ignored by day care providers because he said an older boy ate his "pickle." After repeated episodes, the parents were contacted because the child seemed so upset (even though day care workers gave him

a new pickle to eat). The parents shared that "pickle" was their name for penis.

### Coping–Stress Tolerance Pattern

Perceptions of events and reactions to them are filtered through children's developing cognitive, emotional, and social capacities. The relevance of life events and the child's vulnerability to their impact depend on the given developmental period (see the case study and care plan at the end of this chapter). A child's temperament refers to the emotional and behavioural responses to their environment and others across situations, especially those involving change or stress (Perry et al., 2017). Chess and Thomas (1986) originally described three common temperament patterns that they believe are innate: the easy child; the difficult child; and the slow-to-warm-up child. The easy child is cuddly, affectionate, and easy to manage. Children with a difficult temperament, however, are less adaptable, are more intense and active, and have more negative moods.

Although temperament has generally been accepted as inborn, it can be influenced by environmental characteristics and exerts an influence on psychosocial adjustment by way of its effect on parent–child interactions. Nurses assist parents in recognizing their toddler's innate behavioural qualities as expressions of temperament and in developing management strategies. According to the goodness-of-fit interactive model of temperament, adults can accommodate their demands and expectations in ways that match the child's behaviours, including learning strategies to help toddlers adapt positively to social expectations.

Toddlers are developing new ways to cope with the myriad of new stresses that come with being a toddler. As is typical of their stage of development, coping is egocentric and reflective of their need for autonomy. Typical stressors include new siblings, babysitters, day care, toilet training, parental limit setting, and an endless string of tasks involving skills they have yet to develop.

Toddlers often imitate their parents' behaviour, and this includes their methods of dealing with stress. They also regress, at times, to earlier infantile behaviour when overwhelmed, until they regain some sense of mastery. Parents can help to anticipate and prepare toddlers for stressful experiences before they happen. However, they need to remember that toddlers' sense of time and ability to recall are limited. Preparations should be honest, simple, and focused on what the toddler will experience. Enough time should be provided for the toddler to rehearse the coping behaviour with the parent, but not so early before the event that the toddler forgets.

The nurse helps the parents anticipate developmental stressors and suggests age- and temperament-appropriate coping behaviours for toddlers. Early efforts at dealing with stress are an essential step to more mature coping responses as the child grows (Lieberman, 2017).

### Values-Beliefs Pattern

Healthy behaviours are expressions of positive values and beliefs. These values and beliefs are learned, and their recognition and acceptance are fundamental to the integrity of every child. Toddlers believe rules are absolute and behave, according to Kohlberg, out of a fear of punishment. However, toddlers' environments should not only help them become aware of right and wrong but also contribute to their sense of security, belonging, and autonomy. Moral development forms throughout childhood as children acquire greater capacities for processing, self-control, and understanding of their own feelings (Barner & Baron, 2016).

Because most of toddlers' developing values and beliefs depend on their interactions with parents, the nurse's assessment questions are often directed to or focused on the parent or caregiver. The following are some examples of questions asked by the nurse:

- What are the family's values and beliefs about what is right and wrong?
- How does the parental approach to limit setting reflect these values and beliefs?
- What religious, spiritual, or cultural traditions and activities do the family have?
- How is the toddler included in these traditions and activities?

Children are exposed to and begin to participate in and imitate their family's religious rituals and practices during toddlerhood. They are often taught prayers and songs with a religious theme that are tied into what the family believes are right and wrong. Toddlers may be able to learn the words to these simple prayers and songs, but parents should be cautioned that knowing the words does not mean that toddlers understand the full meaning of what is said. This early introduction into the family's religious beliefs is important as a socialization factor but should not be assumed to produce a good child.

The creation of values and beliefs in young children is related to their developmental stage and is reflected in their behaviours. An important aspect of teaching young children what is right and wrong involves stating what acceptable behaviour is and then reinforcing the behaviour when it occurs. Parents often attend to toddlers only when they are misbehaving, leaving them alone when they are being good. In this scenario, toddlers receive no attention for acceptable behaviour but gain their parents' attention when they misbehave. The nurse can remind parents to catch their toddlers being good and give them the same or more attention.

## ❖ ENVIRONMENTAL PROCESSES

### ◆ Physical Agents

#### Accidents

Toddlers are at high risk of accidental injury because they lack judgement and experience and have only rudimentary problem-solving skills, limited physical coordination, and a heightened level of curiosity about their environment. There are also behavioural and environmental factors that increase toddlers' risk of injury, such as being in new situations (Kuhn & Damashek, 2015). Most parents think that it is natural for children to get hurt and that childhood injuries are just a part of growing up. However, most injuries are predictable and preventable and can cause disabilities requiring long-term care.

Furthermore, they can cause more deaths than all childhood diseases combined.

Childhood injuries are a significant public health issue, as unintentional injury is the leading cause of death and morbidity among Canadian children, and can have consequences that can last throughout the child's lifetime (PHAC, 2009). One in every 10 toddlers who come to the emergency department is treated for accidental injury. Male toddlers tend to have more injuries than their female counterparts, but the overall numbers of accidental injuries peak during toddlerhood for both male and females. A second peak occurs for males during adolescence. Major causes of accidental injury in toddlers involve falls, drownings, and threats to breathing; these are the three leading causes of injury-related deaths in children (CPS, 2012). Other causes of unintentional injury involve motor vehicle and non-motor vehicle land transportation, fire, and poisoning.

In comparison to the non-Indigenous population, children living in First Nations, Métis, and Inuit areas of Canada are twice as likely to experience unintentional injuries (Oliver & Kohen, 2015). The young children in these groups have higher injury and death risk due to land transportation, fire, and drowning/suffocation. These findings possibly reflect limited resources, exposure, living conditions, and activities specific to living in northern areas, suggesting that new strategies and approaches are needed to narrow the disparities that continue to exist.

### Structural Hazards

Houses and other buildings can be hazardous for toddlers. Their desire to explore lures them to locations that older children or adults would not consider. The toddler will climb onto furniture or fixtures, out of windows, or into small spaces. Injuries that result from these explorations can range from minor scrapes and bruises to fatal head injuries. Ideally, homes are "baby-proofed" before the infant begins scooting and crawling (i.e., before they become increasingly mobile). Parents should reassess the safety of their home as their child acquires new skills. Injuries to toddlers occur most often when they fall from furniture, high chairs, changing tables, stairs, windows, and playground equipment. When the child or family visit the home of a friend or relative, it must be inspected for hazards, or the toddler must be confined to one safe room. Many injuries occur in unfamiliar environments.

Preventive measures for structural hazards include the following:

- Do not leave a toddler unattended.
- Use gates at the top and bottom of stairways, and at doors.
- Keep chairs away from countertops and tables to prevent toddlers from climbing.
- Securely anchor large television screens and other electronic equipment that can fall onto toddlers.
- Lock doors to dangerous areas and use gates and window guards.
- Store guns in a locked, safe area out of reach.

### Toys

Toys commonly found in homes are another source of injury. Parents should inspect not only the toys that are in their own homes but also the toys given to the toddler outside the home by relatives, friends, babysitters, or day care personnel (see the Case Study and Care Plan at the end of this chapter). Many toys that are likely to be safe for older children are extremely hazardous for the toddler. Of concern are small, removable parts, magnets and batteries, toxic paint or stuffing, sharp edges, and flammable material.

### Sports

Although sporting and recreational equipment is a major source of accidents in older children and adolescents, parents and health care personnel occasionally forget that such equipment can also be dangerous to toddlers. Improper storage of this equipment is a primary danger. Accessible firearms that are loaded and unlocked are deadly hazards, and bodybuilding weights and other heavy equipment easily overwhelm toddlers, who may pull these objects down on themselves. Toddlers should always be supervised closely, especially in new environments or on playground equipment.

As toddlers become more mobile, they are introduced to riding toys, tricycles, and bicycles. Nurses remind parents about the need for bicycle helmets, and most provinces require bicycle helmets that are fitted properly and worn every time the toddler rides or is a passenger on a bicycle.

### Drowning

Children between the ages of 1 and 3 years are at the highest risk of drowning because most of them do not know how to swim and do not have the skills to keep their heads above water or to get out of the water. Toddlers can drown in water just deep enough to cover their noses and mouths. Although swimming pools and other natural bodies of water are a big part of the problem, even pails of water, toilets, bathtubs, and wading pools are dangerous. When toddlers fall into a pail of water or a toilet, it is hard for them to straighten up because all their weight is forward. Toddlers should never be left unattended—even for a few seconds—near a bathtub, hot tub, wading or swimming pool, toilet, pail of water, or small creek. All swimming pools should be fenced and have self-closing gates and latches. Toddlers must be constantly supervised whenever they are near any body of water, regardless of its size or depth. When swimming or boating, they should be fitted properly with government-approved age-appropriate personal flotation devices.

### Burns

Approximately 1.8 million children visit emergency departments every year in Canada (Klassen & Crockett, 2019). Hot tap water, boiling water, coffee, tea, and food are the most common sources of injury, resulting in scalds from hot liquids. These very painful and often debilitating injuries often occur as toddlers begin to gain mobility and explore their environments, inadvertently touching hot surfaces or spilling hot liquids on themselves. They may also put their mouths on live electrical cords or their fingers into electrical sockets and become seriously burned, as well as tip their walkers or themselves into fireplaces or woodstoves.

The nurses' role is to educate parents regarding the following:

- Never eat, drink, or carry anything hot while holding a child.
- Lower the water heater temperature to 49°C.
- Never leave hot beverages or foods within a child's reach.
- Put children in a playpen while cooking.
- Never leave a toddler unattended in the bathtub. It takes only a moment to turn on the hot water.
- Put screens around fireplaces or woodstoves.
- Do not let children handle food directly from the microwave oven.
- Use burners at the back of the stove and turn pot handles in toward the stove.
- Install and maintain smoke detectors, replacing batteries annually.

### Motor Vehicles

Motor vehicle–related injuries, which include both passenger and pedestrian injuries, are the primary injury in children from 1 to 4 years of age. For the toddler, passenger injury is more frequent and often involves the lack of use or misuse of child safety seats. Child safety seats, when properly installed and used, have reduced the risk of death and serious injury to children. Unfortunately, improper installation and use of child safety seats are widespread problems, with some experts reporting that more than 72% of them are misused in some way (CDC, 2015a). Canada does not have a national network of car seat clinics; there are, however, several organizations related to child and road safety (Transport Canada, 2018). Provinces and territories regulate the use (e.g., age, height, and weight restrictions) of child car seats.

The rear-facing child safety seat supports a young child's head, neck, and spine, helping to reduce stress to the neck and spinal cord in a crash. When children outgrow their re-facing seat and weigh at least 10 kg, the nurse confirms with the parents that they can switch to forward-facing child safety seats. These seats have a built-in harness for enhanced protection during sudden stops or collisions. Booster seats are recommended for children who weigh at least 18 kg. All children younger than 12 years should be seated in the rear seat. Rear-seat position is safer than the front seat for all child safety seats, and no child should be seated in the front passenger seat due to serious injury or death that can occur if car air bags are deployed (Transport Canada, 2018). During the toddler years, it is safest to keep children in a forward-facing rear seat with a harness until they reach the seat's maximum height or weight 18–30 kg. The nurse can provide a list of approved car seats and local retail outlets or agencies that sell, lend, or rent car seats.

Parents should be warned that toddlers may be injured or killed when they are hit by drivers backing up in their own driveways and often by members of their family or nearby neighbours. They are too small to be visible by a driver backing up and are quick to run out after a departing parent or relative who thinks they are still safely inside.

## ◆ Biological Agents

### Bioterrorism

Threats about bioterrorism, and concerns about agents such as *Escherichia coli* (*E. coli*) continue to evolve. Other bioterrorism risks that are of concern for children include botulism, salmonellosis, and typhus. Children are especially at risk of these bacterial hazards because of their physiology. Compared with adults, they have a faster respiratory rate, increased skin permeability, higher skin to body mass ratio, and less body fluids (Jarvis, Browne, MacDonald-Jenkins, et al., 2019). Nurses provide information that can assist parents in dealing with their toddler's and their own fears. Nurses encourage parents to:

- Talk about their fears and worries.
- Stick to family diet routines that help toddlers maintain a varied and nutritious diet.
- Supervise toddlers' television viewing.
- Educate themselves, the best protection against unnecessary fear. Toddlers will be less fearful if they see that their parents are not afraid.

Many parents feel that toddlers, because of their immature immune systems and varied diet, are especially vulnerable to certain agents such as *E. coli*. Fearful parents might request antibiotics when they hear of an *E. coli* outbreak, just to be certain their child does not get sick, despite confirmation the child was never exposed to contaminated food. The nurse should reassure parents and explain that administration of antibiotics when they are not indicated leads to adverse conditions that have global implications. Many antibiotics, especially those identified for *E. coli* management, can have significant side effects. Overuse of antibiotics when they are not necessary can lead to the development of medication-resistant forms of bacteria. If this happens, the antibiotics will not be able to kill the resistant bacteria the next time the child needs the same antibiotic to treat common ear, sinus, or other infections.

The Canadian Paediatric Society does not have a position statement on bioterrorism; however, the American Academy of Pediatrics website addresses numerous issues related to bioterrorism and children (http://www.aap.org), including the development of a teaching toolkit for parents to use with their children.

◆ **Chemical Agents**

**Poisoning**

Poisoning happens 10 times more often among young children aged 1 to 4 years than in their older counterparts. The Public Health Agency of Canada estimates an average of three deaths each year from unintentional poisoning, with an additional 900 children hospitalized with serious injuries (Parachute, 2019). Toddlers aged 1 to 2 years are at the greatest risk. They are becoming more mobile, enabling them to explore and discover poisonous substances in the home. These include prescription and over-the-counter medications, alcohol, household products, plants, cosmetics, lead-based paint, and cigarettes (Quality and Safety Scenario). They are also at risk because they still use their mouths as a way of exploring. Although many parents take precautions against poisoning in their own homes, some forget that toddlers can be poisoned away from the home, while visiting grandparents or other relatives (e.g., see the case study and care plan at the end of this chapter). Further information

**⚡ QUALITY AND SAFETY SCENARIO**

*Preventing Accidental Poisonings in the Home*

- All household, garden, and car products should be kept out of reach.
- Keep medications out of reach in locked cabinets.
- Use childproof caps on medication.
- Keep all products and medication in their original containers for easy identification.
- No poisonous plants should be kept in the house. A list, which includes poinsettia, amaryllis, *Aloe vera*, English ivy, mistletoe, chrysanthemums, and spider plants, is available from local poison control centres.
- Avoid outdoor plants and shrubs that are poisonous, including azaleas and chrysanthemums.
- Supervise the toddler's activity at all times.
- Post the local poison centre telephone number next to every telephone, including your cell phone.

can be found at the Canadian Association of Poison Control Centre website (http://www.capcc.ca/).

The toddler, because of limited experience and cognitive level, is unaware that these items are harmful. Many emergency department (ED) calls and visits are precipitated by a toddler's ingestion of a potentially or actually harmful substance. These incidents are likely to occur in the kitchen, bathroom, bedroom, or work area, and are usually discovered by the parent or caretaker who finds an open or empty container or a half-eaten leaf or other substance.

When parents or caregivers suspect that a toddler has ingested a poisonous substance, they should call the poison control centre, even if the child appears perfectly healthy. Each centre is part of a nationwide effort to provide immediate information about poisonings. Parents should not attempt to induce vomiting without specific instructions from the centre. Vomiting can cause further harm if the child is drowsy, unconscious, or convulsing; or if the substance ingested is corrosive, such as lye or a strong acid. The administration of vomit-inducing agents (e.g., ipecac) should be avoided because there is no evidence from clinical studies to support improved outcomes for poisoned patients, and it may delay the administration or reduce the effectiveness of oral antidotes (Benzoni & Gibson, 2019).

Chronic poisonings, such as lead poisoning, are often undetected until irreversible damage has occurred. Primary prevention involves teaching parents about risk factors and dangers of lead poisoning and the importance of a diet that encourages decreasing fat intake, because lead is retained in fat. Vitamin C, calcium, and iron intake reduce lead levels in the body. Secondary prevention involves performing periodic screening of blood lead levels in all young children identified as at risk. Health Canada, under the Government of Canada's *Hazardous Products Act* and regulations, requires that all toys, furniture, and products manufactured for small children be free of lead-based paint products. However, imported toys and furniture or antique and older family furniture or paint in older houses may have been painted with a lead-based product.

## ❖ DETERMINANTS OF HEALTH

### ◆ Social Factors and Environment

#### Day Care

During the toddler years, many parents return to work, requiring the introduction of the toddler to an alternative care environment. The nurse can provide counselling about the decision to place a child in day care and the resulting emotions, as well as guidelines for selecting a safe child care or day care provider.

The Ontario Ministry of Education recommends a four-step approach as a guideline for selecting a child care provider or day care centre: (1) consider the type of care child needs; (2) identify at least three programs to review; (3) interview potential child care providers; and (4) observe the program or setting. During the interview, it is important to obtain a comprehensive overview of the care provider's program to determine whether it is a good fit for your family.

- Ask about cost; enrollment; ages served; daily activities; accreditation and licensing regulations; caretaker credentials and experience; and policies about visiting, illness, and nutrition.
- Look at provider–child interactions, safety, and the quality of the learning material and toys.
- Check references.
- Talk to parents with children attending the centre or being cared for by the provider about discipline and responsiveness to parents, and talk to local child care resource or referral agencies and licensing offices.
- Make a decision based on specific criteria.
- Think about safety, values, fit for you and your toddler, and affordability.
- Get and stay involved.
- Talk to the provider regularly about how your child is doing, to your child about what the children are doing each day, and to other parents.
- Visit often, announced and unannounced, and at various times of the day. (CPS, 2017a; Ontario Ministry of Education, 2019)

Regardless of the reasons for the parents wanting or needing day care for their child, the traditional expectation of caring for the young child at home continues to influence the parents' concept of what they should do for their child. Parents must be reassured that a day care environment congruent with the family environment is not detrimental to the child. If a child is placed in a setting that is detrimental to physical or emotional development, the parent may need assistance in selecting an alternative setting. Changes in caregivers are difficult for toddlers, and regressive behaviours may surface during transition periods.

#### Culture and Ethnicity

Culture influences everything we do, know, and believe. Each culture possesses its own values, attitudes, and practices with regard to family and child-rearing. Toddlers continue to be shaped by the cultural values and beliefs of their parents and families, the first of many socializing forces they will encounter. As their world expands, other forces and subcultures, including peers, the media, and their schools, will also be encountered.

Unlike older children, toddlers do not question the cultural practices of the family. The toddler who refuses to do certain expected things usually does so out of a need for autonomy and control rather than a questioning of beliefs. However, nurses remind parents of this, because parents may be feeling the pressure of cultural norms and expectations. This is especially true for families who have emigrated recently.

Guided by the *Calls To Action* from the Truth and Reconciliation Commission of Canada (TRC, 2015), it is important to consider the cultural, social, and historical aspects of Indigenous communities when assessing Indigenous children, as differences in parenting norms may be apparent. It is imperative that comprehensive evaluation of child development occurs, to inform patient-centred and culturally relevant health decisions. When nurses have a clear understanding of the cultural differences in parenting and health practices that occur in Indigenous communities, they are better able to ensure the health and well-being of the toddler and address the cultural needs of children, their families, and the community.

Nurses are prepared to provide culturally sensitive and competent care. Knowledge and respect for various cultural worldviews, customs, values, and traditions are needed to negotiate different approaches in developing a health-promotion plan with families. Health care practices are often culturally influenced. For example, if a culture views immunizations as being dangerous or unnecessary, the toddler may be unprotected from certain communicable diseases. Collaboration with communities is important to help facilitate a better understanding of the child's cultural context and how that influences health practice. Incorporation of knowledge, respect, and negotiation facilitates the development of respectful and reciprocal relationships, which are grounded in trust, and promote effective, high-quality health outcomes (Verdon, Wong, & McLeod, 2016).

### ◆ Levels of Policymaking and Health

A lack or paucity of economic resources is capable of affecting the toddler's health and well-being. In 2015, approximately 17% of children in Canada were living in low-income households—approximately 1.2 million children out of 6.8 million in total (Statistics Canada, 2017a). Toddlers who live in poverty experience poor child outcomes, particularly cognitive and educational outcomes (Chaudry & Wimer, 2016).

#### Legislation

Local, provincial, territorial, and federal legislation specific to the toddler is directed primarily toward safety and injury prevention. Many provinces have passed legislation requiring the use of child safety seats, bicycle helmets, and temperature limits for household hot water heaters.

Child maltreatment-reporting laws, under the jurisdiction of provincial and territorial governments, provide protection for a child or developmentally disabled adult, define abuse and neglect, require that a report be made to a designated agency in the case of actual or suspected abuse or neglect, and define the responsibility of the protecting agency. These laws also provide for a central registry of reported cases of abuse. Nurses are aware that they are required by law to report suspected child abuse, and should familiarize themselves with the child abuse and neglect laws in their province or territory.

Children's rights have earned increased attention both nationally and internationally. In 1991, Canada signed the Convention on the Rights of the Child (CRC) human rights treaty to protect children. Protection includes:

- *Non-discrimination.* Children should not be discriminated against based on race, religion or abilities.
- *Best interest of the child.* All decisions are made in the best interest of the child (e.g., budgets, policy, law).
- *Right to life, survival, and development.* Children have the right to develop, live, and survive in healthy ways.
- *Respect for the views of the child.* Children have the right to provide input into decisions that affect them. Adults are encouraged to listen to and consider the opinions of children. (United Nations [UN] Human Rights: Office of the High Commissioner, 1991)

*In 2019, the federal government introduced Bill C-92, An Act Respecting First Nations, Inuit and Métis Children, Youth and Families* that is consistent with the TRC's *Calls to Action.* This legislation was created in collaboration with Indigenous, provincial, and territorial stakeholders with the goal of ensuring that Indigenous children and youth remain connected to their families, communities, and culture. It recognizes their unique culture and supports Indigenous communities and groups to develop policies and laws based on their history, cultures, and circumstances. Guided by national principles such as best interests of the child, cultural continuity, and equality, the Act also enables Indigenous groups and communities to establish partial or full jurisdiction over child and family services (Parliament of Canada, 2019).

### ◆ Health Services/Delivery System

The health of toddlers is significantly affected by the health care delivery system in the place where they live (Waterston, Grueger, Samson, et al., 2015). Canada has a publicly funded universal health care model that provides accessible health care to all. The *Canada Health Act* does not include general oral health care, although governmental dental programs do exist. For example, in Ontario, dental care is covered for children 18 years of age and younger through the Ontario Disability Support Program.

Toddlers need to explore their environment in order to attain a basic mastery. This is also true during encounters with health care providers. They may need to observe and listen as their parents interact with the health care providers, be introduced to and allowed to manipulate examination equipment, and be given simple explanations and choices so that they can maintain some degree of control. Taking the time to enlist the cooperation of a toddler will make the health care visit more productive and conducive to information exchange and health care teaching.

### ❖ NURSING APPLICATION

Educating parents about health promotion and disease prevention in the toddler age group is similar to that for the infant. The nurse involved with the family provides education, focusing on expected physical and developmental changes that occur during the toddler stage. This is the period of life from approximately 18 months to 3 years of age.

In addition to educating the parents, the nurse is able to begin to teach some health-promotion activities to the toddler. Examples of this type of toddler education are nutrition and oral hygiene. At this stage of development, it is crucial that caregivers model healthy behaviours and eating patterns. Parents may need education from the nurse on providing age-appropriate food choices while discouraging the intake of empty calories.

The nurse dealing with the toddler and the family can engage in screening activities. Assessments should be performed to evaluate the toddler for hearing loss and vision disturbances. Some conditions associated with vision or hearing can be treated if detected early.

As toddlers begin to explore their autonomy, they become at risk of accidental injury. Parents should be educated about objects on which the child may climb, possibly creating a crush or entrapment injury. They should also be aware of hazardous toys, sports equipment, drowning, burns, poisoning, and motor vehicle safety. In addition to this, medical personnel must remain alert to the potential for child abuse and report any suspicious injuries.

Another important element of health promotion with the toddler age group is educating the parents about routine health examinations and the childhood immunization schedule. Vaccination is one of the most successful public health interventions and has led to the elimination and control of diseases that were once common. In Canada, scheduled vaccines prevent illnesses such as diphtheria, tetanus, pertussis (whooping cough), polio, *Haemophilus influenzae* type B (Hib), rotavirus, hepatitis B, measles, mumps, rubella, chickenpox, pneumococcal and meningococcal diseases, and human papillomavirus virus (HPV). The timing for each vaccination varies among provinces and territories. Despite their effectiveness in controlling infectious diseases, parental hesitancy about vaccines is emerging due to misinformation regarding disease, safety, and effectiveness (Dubé, Gagnon, Ouakki, et al., 2016). Providing accurate information, reassurance, and support in a nonjudgemental manner from nurses and other health care providers is important for vaccine acceptance (Dubé et al., 2016). Nurses need to work with parents to remain informed about changes in immunization recommendations and educate families as the changes occur. Nurses working with families need to remain knowledgeable about the resources available in the community that may provide free or low-cost injections.

## CASE STUDY

### Grandparents Provide Care: Jean-Luc

Maria and François are the parents of 18-month-old Jean-Luc. They plan to take a week-long vacation while leaving Jean-Luc with his grandparents at their house. Because Jean-Luc is the first grandchild, the older couple is eager to spend time with him, but they have expressed concern about caring for a toddler.

**Reflective Questions**

- What do the parents need to discuss with the grandparents concerning safety issues?
- What psychosocial issues of a toddler are important for both the parents and the grandparents to consider?
- What resources are available for today's grandparents?

## CARE PLAN

### Grandparents Provide Care: Jean-Luc

**Nursing Issue**

At risk of injury related to change in environment and change in primary caregiver(s)

**Defining Characteristics**

At risk of injury as a result of environmental conditions interacting with the individual's adaptive and defensive resources.

**Related Factors**

- Heightened level of curiosity about environment
- Lack of more mature judgement and experience
- Limited height and physical coordination

**Risk Factors**

- Change in living environment to grandparents' home
- Grandparents' home not "childproofed"
- Change in primary caregiver(s) from parents to grandparents
- Grandparents not up to date with caregiver/safety knowledge for toddlers

**Expected Outcomes**

- Grandparents will receive instruction regarding toddler care/safety.
- Grandparents will take necessary precautions to childproof their home.
- Grandparents will identify available resources to assist in toddler care/safety.
- Toddler will remain free of injury while in grandparents' care.

**Interventions**

- Surveillance: safety.
  - Conduct a safety check in grandparents' home/community.
  - Provide a safety checklist for grandparents.
- Assist grandparents in identifying resources/support.
  - Contact community groups to emphasize community safety concerns.
- Risk identification.
  - Identify potential risk factors in grandparents' home/community.
- Teaching: toddler care/safety.
  - Teach grandparents about toddler care/safety issues.

## SUMMARY

This period can be an exciting and challenging time for both toddlers and their parents. Parents who have encouraged their toddlers' desire to explore can now delight in their developing sense of adventure as they enter their preschool years. The world is a wonderful place for the toddler who has known and experienced support, affection, and protection.

**Evolve Chapter Features**

http://evolve.elsevier.com/Canada/Edelman/healthpromotion/
- Review Questions

## REFERENCES

American Psychiatric Association (APA). (2013). *Diagnostic and statistical manual of mental disorders: DSM-5* (5th ed.). Arlington, VA: American Psychiatric Association. [Seminal Reference].

Ball, J. W., Dains, J. E., Flynn, J. A., et al. (2015). *Seidel's guide to physical examination* (8th ed.). St. Louis: Mosby.

Barner, D., & Baron, A. S. (2016). *Core knowledge and conceptual change*. New York: Oxford University Press.

Bartlett, J. D., Kotake, C., Fauth, R., et al. (2017). Intergenerational transmission of child abuse and neglect: Do maltreatment type, perpetrator, and substantiation status matter? *Child Abuse & Neglect, 63*, 84–94. https://doi.org/10.1016/j.chiabu.2016.11.021.

Beckerman, M., van Berkel, S. R., Mesman, J., et al. (2017). The role of negative parental attributions in the associations between daily stressors, maltreatment history, and harsh and abusive discipline. *Child Abuse & Neglect, 64*, 109–116. https://doi.org/10.1016/j.chiabu.2016.12.015.

Benzoni, T., & Gibson, J. (2019). *Ipecac.* In StatPearls (Internet). Treasure Island, FL: StatPearlsPublishing. 2020 Jan. Retrieved from https://www.ncbi.nlm.nih.gov/books/NBK448075/.

Canadian Association of Optometrists. n.d.-a, Canadian Association of Optometrists (n.d.-a). *Amblyopia (lazy eye)*. Retrieved from https://opto.ca/health-library/amblyopia-lazy-eye.

Canadian Association of Optometrists (n.d.-b). *The eye exam*. Retrieved from https://opto.ca/health-library/the-eye-exam.

Canadian Ophthalmological Society (n.d.). *Amblyopia ("Lazy eye")*. Retrieved from https://www.cos-sco.ca/vision-health-information/conditions-disorders-treatments/pediatric-eye-conditions/lazy-eye/.

Canadian Paediatric Society (CPS). (2012). *Child and youth injury prevention: A public health approach*. Retrieved from https://www.cps.ca/en/documents/position/child-and-youth-injury-prevention. [Seminal Reference].

Canadian Paediatric Society (CPS). (2017a). *Child care: Making the best choice for your family*. Retrieved from https://www.caringforkids.cps.ca/handouts/child_care.

Canadian Paediatric Society (CPS). (2017b). *Screen time and young children*. Retrieved from https://www.caringforkids.cps.ca/handouts/screen-time-and-young-children.

Canadian Paediatric Society (CPS). (2018a). *Breastfeeding*. Retrieved from https://www.caringforkids.cps.ca/handouts/breastfeeding.

Canadian Paediatric Society (CPS). (2018b). *Physical activity for children and youth*. Retrieved from https://www.caringforkids.cps.ca/handouts/physical_activity.

Canadian Paediatric Society (CPS). (2018c). *Vision screening in infants, children and youth*. Retrieved from https://www.cps.ca/en/documents/position/children-vision-screening#ref14.

Canadian Paediatric Society (CPS). (2019a). *Healthy eating for children*. Retrieved from https://www.caringforkids.cps.ca/handouts/healthy_eating_for_children.

Canadian Paediatric Society (CPS). (2019b). *When your child is a picky eater*. Retrieved from https://www.caringforkids.cps.ca/handouts/when_your_child_is_a_picky_eater.

Centers for Disease Control and Prevention (CDC). (2014). *CDC estimates 1 in 63 children has been identified with autism spectrum disorder*. Retrieved from http://www.cdc.gov/media/releases/2014/p0327-autism-spectrum-disorder.html. [Seminal Reference].

Centers for Disease Control and Prevention (CDC). (2015a). *Child passenger safety: Get the facts*. Retrieved from http://www.cdc.gov/motorvehiclesafety/child_passenger_safety/cps-factsheet.html.

Centers for Disease Control and Prevention (CDC). (2015b). *Child maltreatment: Risk and protective factors*.

Centers for Disease Control and Prevention (CDC). (2015c). *Learning the signs, act early: Developmental milestones*. Retrieved from http://www.cdc.gov/ncbddd/actearly/milestones/index.html.

Centers for Disease Control and Prevention (CDC). (2019). *Child abuse & neglect*. Retrieved from https://www.cdc.gov/violenceprevention/pdf/CAN-factsheet.pdf.

Charlop, M. H., Lang, R., & Rispoli, M. (2018). More than just fun and games: Definition, development, and intervention for children's play and social skills. In *Play and social skills for children with autism spectrum disorder* (pp. 1–16). New York: Springer.

Chaudry, A., & Wimer, C. (2016). Poverty is not just an indicator: The relationship between income, poverty, and child well-being. *Academic Pediatrics, 16*(3), S23–S29. https://doi.org/10.1016/j.acap.2015.12.010.

Chess, S., & Thomas, A. (1986). The New York longitudinal study: From infancy to early adult life. In R. Plomin, & J. Dunn (Eds.), *The study of temperament changes, continuities and challenges* (pp. 39–52). Hillsdale, NJ: Lawrence Erlbaum. [Seminal Reference].

Clark, E. V. (2018). Conversation and language acquisition: A pragmatic approach. *Language Learning and Development, 14*(3), 170–185. https://doi.org/10.1080/15475441.2017.1340843.

Cupples, L., Ching, T. Y., Button, L., et al. (2018). Language and speech outcomes of children with hearing loss and additional disabilities: Identifying the variables that influence performance at five years of age. *International Journal of Audiology, 57*(Suppl. 2), S93–S104. https://doi.org/10.1080/14992027.2016.1228127.

Dubé, E., Gagnon, D., Ouakki, M., et al. (2016). Understanding vaccine hesitancy in Canada: Results of a consultation study by the Canadian immunization research network. *PloS One, 11*(6), e0156118. https://doi.org/10.1371/journal.pone.0156118.

Erikson, E. H. (1995). *Childhood & society* (35th anniversary ed.). New York: Norton. [Seminal Reference].

Erikson, E. H. (1998). *The life cycle completed*. New York, NY: Norton. [Seminal Reference].

Government of Canada. (2019a). *Make healthy meals with the eat well plate*. Retrieved from https://food-guide.canada.ca/en/tips-for-healthy-eating/make-healthy-meals-with-the-eat-well-plate/.

Government of Canada. (2019b). *First Nations child and family services*. Ottawa: Author. Retrieved from https://www.sac-isc.gc.ca/eng/1100100035204/1533307858805.

Gravener, J. A., Rogosch, F. A., Oshri, A., et al. (2012). The relations among maternal depressive disorder, maternal expressed emotion, and toddler behavior problems and attachment. *Journal of Abnormal Child Psychology, 40*(5), 803–813. https://doi.org/10.1007/s10802-011-9598-z. [Seminal Reference].

Guilleminault, C., Abad, V. C., Chiu, H. Y., et al. (2015). Missing teeth and obstructive pediatric sleep apnea. *International Journal of the Science and Practice of Sleep Medicine, 19*(73), 1–8. https://doi.org/10.1007/s11325-015-1238-3.

Healthy Children. (2015). *Common childhood habits*. Retrieved from https://www.healthychildren.org/English/family-life/family-dynamics/communication-discipline/Pages/Common-Childhood-Habits.aspx.

Hockenberry, M. J., & Wilson, D. (Eds.). (2015). *Wong's nursing care of infants and children* (10th ed.) St. Louis, MO: Mosby.

Jarvis, C., Browne, A., MacDonald-Jenkins, J., et al. (2019). *Physical examination and health assessment* (3rd Canadian ed.). Toronto: Elsevier Canada.

Jones, G., & Rowland, C. F. (2017). Diversity not quantity in caregiver speech: Using computational modeling to isolate the effects of the quantity and the diversity of the input on vocabulary growth. *Cognitive Psychology, 98*, 1–21. https://doi.org/10.1016/j.cogpsych.2017.07.002.

Klassen, T., & Crockett, L. (2019). *Why Canada should invest in emergency care for children*. Evidence Network. Retrieved from https://evidencenetwork.ca/why-canada-should-invest-in-emergency-care-for-children/.

Kochanska, G., Kim, S., Boldt, L. J., et al. (2013). Promoting toddlers' positive social-emotional outcomes in low-income families: A play-based experimental study. *Journal of Clinical Child and Adolescent Psychology, 42*(5), 700–712. https://doi.org/10.1080/15374416.2013.782815. [Seminal Reference].

Kuhn, J., & Damashek, A. (2015). The role of proximal circumstances and child behaviour in toddlers' risk for minor unintentional injuries. *Injury Prevention, 21*(1), 30–34. https://doi.org/10.1136/injuryprev-2014-041247.

Levickis, P., McKean, C., Walls, E., et al. (2019). Training community health nurses to measure parent–child interaction: A mixed-methods study. *The European Journal of Public Health, 0*(0), 1–6. https://doi.org/10.1093/eurpub/ckz155.

Lieberman, A. F. (2017). *The emotional life of the toddler*. New York: Simon & Schuster.

Lin, L. Y., Cherng, R. J., Chen, Y. J., et al. (2015). Effects of television exposure on developmental skills among young children. *Infant Behavior and Development, 38*, 20–26. https://doi.org/10.1016/j.infbeh.2014.12.005.

Lobstein, T., Jackson-Leach, R., Moodie, M. L., et al. (2015). Child and adolescent obesity: Part of a bigger picture. *Lancet, 385*(9986), 2510–2520. https://doi.org/10.1016/S0140-6736(14)61746-3.

McShane, K. E., Hastings, P. D., Smylie, J. K., & The Tungasuvvin-gat Inuit Resource Centre, et al. (2009). Examining evidence for autonomy and relatedness in urban Inuit parenting. *Culture & Psychology, 15,* 411–431. https://doi.org/10.1177/1354067X09344880. [Seminal Reference].

Muir, N., & Bohr, Y. (2014). Contemporary practice of traditional Aboriginal child rearing: A review. *First Peoples Child and Family Review, 9*(1), 66–79. [Seminal Reference].

Ofner, M., Coles, A., Decou, M. L., et al. (2018). *Autism spectrum disorder among children and youth in Canada 2018.* Ottawa: Public Health Agency of Canada.

Oliver, L. N., & Kohen, D. E. (2015). *Unintentional injury hospitalizations among children and youth in areas with a high percentage of Aboriginal identity residents: 2001/2002 to 2005/2006.* Ottawa: Statistics Canada. Retrieved from https://www150.statcan.gc.ca/n1/pub/82-003-x/2012003/article/11699-eng.htm.

Ontario Ministry of Education. (2019). *Choosing child care.* Retrieved from http://www.edu.gov.on.ca/childcare/choosing.html.

Oriach, C. S., Robertson, R. C., Stanton, C., et al. (2016). Food for thought: The role of nutrition in the microbiota-gut-brain axis. *Clinical Nutrition Experimental, 6,* 25–38. https://doi.org/10.1016/j.yclnex.2016.01.003.

Parachute. (2019). *Policy: Poison prevention policy.* Retrieved from https://parachute.ca/en/professional-resource/policy/poison-prevention/.

Parliament of Canada. (2019). *Bill C-92, an act representing first Nations, Inuit and Métis children, youth and families.* Retrieved from https://www.parl.ca/DocumentViewer/en/42-1/bill/C-92/royal-assent.

Patel, H., & Feldman, H. (2018). The Canadian Paediatric Society position statement: Universal newborn screening. *Paediatric Child Health, 16*(5), 301–305.

Perry, S. E., Hockenberry, M. J., Lowdermilk, D. L., et al. (Eds.). (2017). *Maternal child nursing care in Canada* (2nd ed.). Milton, ON: Elsevier Canada.

Perryman, T. Y., Carter, A. S., Messinger, D. S., et al. (2013). Brief report: Parental child-directed speech as a predictor of receptive language in children with autism symptomatology. *Journal of Autism and Developmental Disorders, 43*(8), 1983–1987.

Pritchard, C., & Ellis, G. S. (2016). *Approach to visual acuity assessment and strabismus evaluation of the pediatric patient. Practical management of pediatric ocular disorders and strabismus.* New York: Springer, 3–23.

Public Health Agency of Canada (PHAC). (2009). *Leading causes of death, Canada, 2004, males and females combined: Counts (crude death rate per 100,000).* Ottawa: Author. [Seminal Reference].

Public Health Agency of Canada (PHAC). (2010). *Canadian incidence study of reported child abuse and neglect—2008: Major findings.* Ottawa: Author. [Seminal Reference].

Public Health Agency of Canada (PHAC). (2018). *Family violence: How big is the problem in Canada?* Ottawa: Author. Retrieved from https://www.canada.ca/en/public-health/services/health-promotion/stop-family-violence/problem-canada.html.

Public Health Agency of Canada (PHAC). (2019). *Canada's provincial and territorial routine (and catch-up) vaccination routine schedule programs for infants and children.* Ottawa: Author. Retrieved from https://www.canada.ca/en/public-health/services/provincial-territorial-immunization-information/provincial-territorial-routine-vaccination-programs-infants-children.html.

Simopoulos, A. P. (2008). The importance of the omega-6/omega-3 fatty acid ratio in cardiovascular disease and other chronic diseases. *Experimental Biology and Medicine, 233*(6), 674–688. https://doi.org/10.3181/0711-MR-311. [Seminal Reference].

Statistics Canada. (2017a). *Children living in low-income households.* Retrieved from https://www12.statcan.gc.ca/census-recensement/2016/as-sa/98-200-x/2016012/98-200-x2016012-eng.cfm.

Statistics Canada. (2017b). *Family violence in Canada: A statistical profile, 2015.* Retrieved from https://www150.statcan.gc.ca/n1/daily-quotidien/170216/dq170216b-eng.htm.

Transport Canada. (2018). *Car seat safety.* Ottawa: Author. Retrieved from https://www.tc.gc.ca/en/services/road/child-car-seat-safety.html.

Truth & Reconciliation Commission of Canada (TRC). (2015). *Calls to action.* Retrieved from http://trc.ca/assets/pdf/Calls_to_Action_English2.pdf.

United Nations Human Rights: Office of the High Commissioner. (1991). *Convention on the rights of the child.* Retrieved from https://www.ohchr.org/Documents/ProfessionalInterest/crc.pdf. [Seminal Reference].

Verdon, S., Wong, S., & McLeod, S. (2016). Shared knowledge and mutual respect: Enhancing culturally competent practice through collaboration with families and communities. *Child Language Teaching and Therapy, 32*(2), 205–221. https://doi.org/10.1177/0265659015620254.

Waterston, S., Grueger, B., Samson, L., & Canadian Paediatric Society (CPS), & Community Paediatrics Committee (2015). Housing need in Canada: Healthy lives start at home. *Paediatrics and Child Health, 20*(7), 403–407. https://doi.org/10.1093/pch/20.7.403.

Wulff, D., St George, S., & Tomm, K. (2015). Societal discourses that help in family therapy: A modified situational analysis of the relationships between societal expectations and healing patterns in parent-child conflict. *Journal of Systemic Therapies, 34*(2), 31–44.

Zhang, Y., Lin, J., Fu, W., et al. (2019). Mediterranean diet during pregnancy and childhood for asthma in children: A systematic review and meta-analysis of observational studies. *Pediatric Pulmonology, 54,* 949–961. https://doi.org/10.1002/ppul.24338.

# 13

# Preschool Child

*Erin Ziegler, RN(EC), MN, PhD, PHC-NP*

Originating US chapter by *Susan Ann Denninger, PT, DPT, PCS, Kristi Coker, RN, PhD, Kevin K. Chui, PT, DPT, PhD, GCS, OCS, CEAA, FAAOMPT*

## INTENDED LEARNING OUTCOMES

*After completing this chapter, the reader will be able to:*

- Explain the physical and psychosocial changes occurring during the preschool years that influence child and family health needs.
- Discuss the concepts of cognitive development of preschoolers using Piaget's theory.
- Review the Public Health Agency of Canada concepts that pertain to preschool children and their families.
- Describe family teaching and nursing support for the typical sleep disturbances of the preschool years.

- Differentiate the nursing roles regarding vision and hearing screening for preschoolers.
- Compare coping skills of preschoolers with those of younger children.
- Outline the primary prevention immunization requirements for preschoolers.
- Identify warning signs of cancer in preschoolers.
- Recognize signs, symptoms, and clinical features of and risk factors for asthma in preschoolers.
- Identify the major causes of injuries during the preschool years.

## KEY TERMS

Acute lymphocytic leukemia (ALL)
Amblyopia
Asthma
Centring
Chloroma
Deduction
Doll or puppet play
Eccrine sweat gland function
Egocentrism
Expressive language
Gender independent
Heterophoria
Heterotropia

Homeostasis
Induction explanation
Initiative
Irreversibility
Ishihara test
Lactose intolerance
Looksee Checklist
Mnemonic techniques
Mutual storytelling
Myopic vision
Neuroblastoma
Nightmares
Night terrors

Otitis media
Parental divorce
Preoperational stage
Receptive language
Refractive errors
Retinoblastoma
Rourke Baby Record
Strabismus
Transductive reasoning
Vaccine hesitancy
Vineland Social Maturity Scale
Wilms' tumour

## ? THINK ABOUT IT

### Aggressive Behaviour

Phillip, age 4 years, started preschool 2 weeks ago after spending his early years at home with his mother and his 18-month-old sister. His mother recently returned to her job as an accountant, works 9 hours a day, and is fatigued when she picks up Phillip at 5:00 p.m. Phillip's father travels for his job but is home on weekends to spend time with his family. Although Phillip's mother always believed that Phillip was shy because he was quiet, during the last week at child care he started hitting his peers and becoming loudly vocal at story time. His mother, believing that Phillip's behaviour is related to her return to work, feels embarrassed and frustrated by his behaviour, especially because she enjoys her new job and the extra income.

- What factors might be contributing to Phillip's changed behaviour?
- How might you define Phillip's temperament? Why?
- What discussions might you have with Phillip's parents to help them understand, respond to, and change their son's behaviour for the better?

The preschool child (age 3–6 years) has a more developed body structure, an ability to control and use the body, and a facility with language that more closely resembles that of the adult than that of the toddler. The major psychological thrust of this period of development is mastery of self as an independent human being, with a willingness to extend experiences beyond those of the family. Although historically the end of early childhood in the Western world was marked by entrance into the formalized educational system, increasing numbers of children in Canada begin formalized schooling during their preschool years.

## BIOLOGY AND GENETICS

The protuberant abdomen of the toddler disappears during the preschool years as the pelvis begins to straighten and the abdominal muscles develop. The hips gradually rotate inward, replacing out-toeing with straight or slight in-toeing. Mild in-toeing (metatarsus adductus) may remain during the preschool years, but anything beyond a mild level should be investigated and treated.

Growth rates remain steady from age 3 to 6 years. Average preschoolers gain approximately 2 kg (4 pounds) of body weight and 7 cm (2 inches) of height each year, whereas head circumference increases by less than 2 cm during the entire preschool period. During early childhood, skin matures in its ability to protect the child from outer invasion and loss of fluids. The skin's capacity to localize infection increases but remains less than that of a mature person. Negligible secretion of sebum makes the skin fairly dry. Eccrine sweat gland function, part of the body's heat-regulation mechanism, gradually matures, but the quantity of eccrine sweat produced in response to heat or emotion remains minimal. Apocrine sweat glands, located primarily in the axillae, areolas of the breast, and the anal area, remain nonsecretory during this period.

The kidneys reach full functional maturity by the end of infancy and early toddlerhood, with only their size changing during the preschool years. By the end of the preschool years, urine excretion ranges from 650 to 1000 mL (19–30 ounces). Under normal homeostatic conditions, the preschooler's renal system conserves water and concentrates urine on a level that approximates adult abilities. Under conditions of stress, however, the kidneys lack the ability to respond fully and to maintain homeostasis when compared with the more rapid response of the adult renal system.

Growth of gastro-intestinal organs continues through the preschool years without functional changes. Children achieve full voluntary control of elimination. Lactose intolerance, intolerance to milk products manifested by diarrhea, often appears during the preschool years. This condition, more common in children of East Asian or African descent, can be managed successfully by elimination of lactose from the diet.

Lung capacity continues to increase, with a gradual decrease in respiratory rate. Preschoolers make better decisions than toddlers about objects they place in their mouths, resulting in fewer instances of choking and obstruction. A gradual increase in the size and shape of the ears coincides with decreases in the incidence of otitis media (middle ear infection). Tonsils and adenoids are large compared with their throat, which may contribute to noisy breathing and upper respiratory tract infection in preschoolers.

The cardiovascular system enlarges in proportion to general body growth. Heart rate for preschoolers ranges from 40 to 70 beats per minute, with a mean blood pressure of 100/60 mm Hg. Early hypertension develops in some children during the preschool years; therefore routine measurement of blood pressure is indicated, particularly in children with a strong family history of hypertension (see Chapter 14). Preschool children maintain adequate hemoglobin levels when dietary intake is sufficient. Bone marrow of the ribs, the sternum, and the vertebrae become fully established as primary sites for red blood cell formation. The liver and spleen continue to form erythrocytes and granulocytes.

The immune system continues to develop. Preschoolers boost their immune response to common pathogens as exposure occurs. Group activities, such as joining preschool or play groups, increase exposure and, subsequently, escalate the incidence of common contagious illnesses during the time of exposure, regardless of the child's age. Initial encounters with such group activities usually result in increases in illness. Later, these children may be less prone to common contagious diseases because of their early exposure to infectious illnesses and their consequent immunity.

Primary teeth finish erupting by late toddler or early preschool years. Initial permanent teeth generally erupt toward the end of the preschool period. Permanent teeth tend to erupt approximately 6 months earlier in girls than in boys. Older preschoolers usually take responsibility for dental hygiene, although all children need gentle guidance about proper brushing and appropriate nutritional intake for healthy teeth. Parents should continue to assist with brushing and supervise flossing and fluoride intake. Risk of fluorosis exists in children younger than 8 years and is influenced by both the dose and the frequency of exposure to fluoride during tooth development (Wright, Hanson, Ristic, et al., 2014). Balancing this risk of opacity against the prevention of caries involves assessment of the amounts of fluoride the child receives from various sources. Fluoride sources include public water supply in some regions, foods, drinks, fluoride supplements, and accidentally swallowed toothpaste (Carey, 2014). Because the preschool period is an age of caries formation, regular dental checkups are essential. The Canadian Paediatric Society (CPS) recommends use of a smear (the size of a grain of rice) of non-fluoridated toothpaste up to age 3 years. After the third birthday, a pea-sized amount of fluoride toothpaste may be used. Children should have regular dental visits every 6 months. Fluoride varnish is recommended in the primary care setting every 3 to 6 months, starting at tooth emergence. Over-the-counter fluoride rinse is not recommended for children younger than 6 years because of the risk of their swallowing higher-than-recommended levels of fluoride (Clark & Slayton, 2014). Nurses assess whether the child is receiving preventive dental care. Parents should be encouraged to begin or maintain this care. Suggestions for promoting good oral hygiene as part of general health-promotion teaching can be found in Chapter 14.

Musculo-skeletal and neurological development reaches a level that allows seemingly effortless walking, running, and climbing. Older preschoolers' ability to copy figures and draw recognizable pictures indicates their advancing fine motor abilities, and they are eager to demonstrate these skills to others. Practice, increases in muscle size, continuing associations among existing neural pathways, and the establishment of new pathways for already accomplished tasks are a few of the many complex factors that contribute to the advances in neurological function observed during early childhood. These advances in fine motor, gross motor, cognitive, communicative, and social-emotional skills are outlined in Table 13.1.

## Biological Sex and Gender

Biological sex refers to the genetically assigned sex of male or female based on chromosomes, XX for females and XY for males. Boys tend to experience more childhood illnesses than do girls from 3 to 6 years of age (see Chapter 12). Traditionally, boys have been encouraged to take more risks than girls and they have more accidents than do preschool girls, who may have been encouraged to choose more sedentary activities. For example, in their study of 476 preschool children (50% male), Brown, Pfeiffer, McIver, and colleagues (2009) found that 3-year-old boys were more active than 3-year-old girls. In today's society, boys and girls have more opportunities to choose the same activities, but preschool activities can also be geared to be gender neutral to encourage more female participation. Gender-neutral activities such as tag, hide-and-seek, kick ball, duck, duck, goose, red rover, and obstacle courses may encourage physical activity for both boys and girls. It will be interesting to observe whether societal changes or preschool policy changes will reflect accident or obesity statistics in the future.

Preschoolers are more aware of their gender than are toddlers and may imitate societal stereotypes more closely. Additionally, at this age, children may begin to express their personal gender identity, a personal sense of self as male or female which may not be related to their sex assigned at birth. Gender independent children are those with a gender expression or identity which differs from their biological sex. Some children may strongly express a gender role different from their biological sex or express fluidity in their gender. Gender independence is a natural expression diversity. Support for gender independent children should concentrate on an affirmative model focused on parents learning to support their child. Goals include strengthening the parent–child bond, promoting the child's self-worth, and advocating for safe spaces in schools and social interactions (Payne, 2012).

## Ethnicity

Ethnicity, with its related economic and cultural issues, can influence health care practices at this age, as is the case at all ages. Cultural preferences and economic issues, therefore, influence the environments and other health-promoting behaviours, such as nutrition and recreation (Brown et al., 2009; Division of Adolescent and School Health, National Center for Chronic Disease Prevention and Health Promotion, 2011; Dogra, Meisner, & Ardern, 2010; Lee & Im, 2010).

## Genetics

The signs and symptoms of most genetic problems appear during infancy or the toddler years, whereas other genetic problems will be noted during adolescence. Those most likely to appear during the preschool years are cystic fibrosis, Duchenne muscular dystrophy, fragile X syndrome, Williams syndrome, and autism, which is generally considered a genetic disorder with a high degree (90%) of heritability (Freitag, Staal, Klauck, et al., 2010). These disorders, characterized by aberrant social interaction, communication, and stereotyped patterns of behaviour, affect 0.5% to

### GENOMICS

#### Cystic Fibrosis

The field of cystic fibrosis (CF) has benefited from developments and advancements in genomics in terms of detection, understanding, and monitoring of the disease state. Infants with CF are structurally normal at birth; however, they have an inability to control bacterial infection, which plays a key role in early CF lung disease pathogenesis. Research and application of novel molecular techniques to explore the human microbiome has helped develop an understanding of CF airway microbiology and how it differs from that of those without the disease. CF is caused by one of several defects in cystic fibrosis transmembrane conductance regulator, which regulates fluid flow within cells and affects the components of sweat, digestive fluids, and mucus. The G551D mutation, in particular, is characterized by a dysfunctional cystic fibrosis transmembrane conductance regulator that cannot transport chloride through the ion channel. In 2012, Health Canada approved Kalydeco (ivacaftor) for use in Canada for patients with the G551D mutation and since further approved for ten additional disease mutations. Ivacaftor increases the transport of chloride through the ion channel by binding, and thus for the first time is able to treat the underlying cause of CF instead of its symptoms.

Sources: Cystic Fibrosis Canada. (2019). *Kalydeco®*. Retrieved from https://www.cysticfibrosis.ca/our-programs/advocacy/access-to-medicines/kalydeco; Milla, C. E. (2013). Cystic fibrosis in the era of genomic medicine. *Current Opinion in Pediatrics, 25*(3), 323–328.

1.0% of the population and are often diagnosed or suspected in the preschool years, when social interaction plays a larger role in development (Boyd, Odom, Humphreys, et al., 2010; Freitag et al., 2010).

Genetic conditions (Genomics) diagnosed early in life affect the child's health, and nursing strategies focus on continuing parent education, assessing the child's development (including complications), and providing interventions to support family coping (Boyd et al., 2010).

## ❖ GORDON'S FUNCTIONAL HEALTH PATTERNS

### ◆ Health Perception–Health Management Pattern

Preschoolers have a fairly accurate perception of the external parts of their own bodies based on what they can see and do; they may be extremely curious about the body of a member of the opposite gender. Their concepts of what is inside the body and how its internal functions operate are vague and inaccurate. Preschoolers view the internal part of the body as hollow. Most preschoolers can name one or two items inside the body (blood, bones). Many of their questions involve body functions. Anxiety surrounding the body and fear of mutilation and death pervade the children's concerns. Their size as compared with that of adults produces a sense of vulnerability and fear of loss of control (Price & Gwinn, 2012).

By age 4 or 5 years, children have amassed their beliefs about health from the family. They begin to understand that they play a role in their own health. The preschooler often becomes upset over minor injuries. Pain or illness may be viewed as a punishment. The preschooler's declaration, "If you don't put your seat belt on you will get in an accident," is a statement that reflects

## TABLE 13.1 Growth and Development

### Developmental and Behavioural Milestones for Preschool Children

| Age (year) | Expectations |
| --- | --- |
| 3 | At this age, the typical child: <br>• Understands two- and three-step directions; throws ball forward at least 1 metre; walks upstairs; can stand on one foot <br>• Has self-care skills (self-feeding, self-dressing) <br>• Knows own name, age, and gender <br>• Engages in imaginative play that becomes more elaborate with specific themes or story lines demonstrated; enjoys interactive play; plays with others comfortably <br>• Speech understood by family all the time; speaks in sentences of five or more words |
| 4 | At this age, the typical child: <br>• Alternates feet when descending stairs; jumps forward; hops on one foot, and can stand on one foot for up to 3 seconds <br>• Holds and uses a pencil with good control <br>• Cuts paper into two pieces <br>• Brushes own teeth <br>• Dresses self, including buttons and zippers <br>• Gives first and last name <br>• Is toilet trained during the daytime for both bowel and bladder <br>• Sings songs or says rhymes; understands three-part directional sentences <br>• Knows what to do if cold, tired, or hungry <br>• Tells stories with clear beginning, middle, and end <br>• Talks about daily experiences and things that are used at home (food, appliances) <br>• Can name four colours <br>• Takes turns and shares when in group play <br>• Draws a person with three or more body parts <br>• Tells you what he/she thinks is going to happen next in a book |
| 5 | At this age, the typical child: <br>• May be able to skip; can walk on tiptoes; stop, start and change direction when running <br>• Draw lines, simple shapes, and some letters <br>• Holds pencil correctly <br>• Tells long stories about past experiences <br>• Dresses and undresses without supervision <br>• Knows common shapes and most of the alphabet <br>• Begins to understand right and wrong, fair and unfair <br>• Engages in dramatic make-believe and dress-up play <br>• Enjoys the companionship of other children; usually plays well in groups; talks about having a best friend <br>• Has good articulation, uses appropriate tenses and pronouns <br>• Can count to 10 |
| 6 | At this age, the typical child: <br>• Can catch a small ball; can hop on one foot for 3 metres; can walk on a beam/curb without falling; can skip across a room <br>• Cuts out simple shapes following an outline <br>• Listens while others are speaking <br>• Shows understanding of right from wrong <br>• Counts up to 10; prints own first name; prints numbers up to 10 <br>• Understands right from left <br>• Pays attention and follows instructions in a group |

Modified from Nipissing District Developmental Screening (NDDS). (2019). *Looksee Checklist*. Retrieved from https://www.lookseechecklist.com.

the idea of expected immediate and absolute cause and effect. The preschooler cannot conceive that the purpose of the seat belt is to prevent injury in the event of an accident, not prevention of the accident itself.

Although preschoolers are not completely responsible for their own health management, they certainly contribute by brushing their teeth, taking medication, wearing appropriate clothing for inclement weather, and performing other actions. Preschoolers' memory of these activities can be sporadic, but they are at least beginning to be their own health care agents (Yoo, Slack, & Holl, 2010).

Reinforcement of health-promotion activities, which occurs in the home and child care environments, helps to instill behaviours that affect self-esteem, safety, and an individual's overall balance with life. For example, family support for active lifestyles provides one way for parents to be a positive role model and children are 6.3 times more likely to be active with parentally influenced behaviour (Zecevic, Tremblay, Lovsin, et al., 2010).

In addition, the preschool environment influences health-promotion activities for many children in this age group. For example, when Brown and colleagues (2009) directly observed children in 20 preschool settings, they demonstrated that aspects of the preschool environment affected children's activity levels. Preschool settings with more resources also offered a greater variety of activities. Even these preschools with more resources were well below the physical activity time recommended (180 minutes per day) by the Canadian Society for Exercise Physiology (CSEP, 2017). Their findings provide further support for those of Bower, Hales, Tate, and colleagues (2008), who demonstrated that in preschool settings, children participated in physical activity for approximately 80 minutes more in settings with more resources than children in settings with fewer resources. These findings indicate a need for health-promotion advocacy and policy development focused on the environment. Many community bookstores carry health-promotion-focused books appropriate to the preschool population; these references provide information for discussion among parents, caregivers, and children on the importance of healthy behaviours for success in life.

## ◆ Nutritional-Metabolic Pattern

Establishing healthful nutritional and physical activity behaviours begins during childhood. Children should eat a variety of foods, with at least five servings of fruits and vegetables per day. Children aged 3 to 5 years old should receive 1100 to 1650 calories per day, depending on their activity level and gender (Government of Canada, 2019a). *Canada's Dietary Guidelines* recommend choosing whole-grain foods and eating plenty of fruits and vegetables and protein-rich foods. Preschool children need to eat small amounts of food more often throughout the day. Servings can be divided up into smaller amounts and served throughout the day (Government of Canada, 2019a). Fat requirements in preschool children are higher than those for older children, but fat consumption should consist primarily of unsaturated fat, with saturated fat, *trans*-fatty acids, and cholesterol intake as low as possible.

Specific issues that impact the preschool age include bone growth, iron-deficiency anemia, milk intake, salt intake, sugar intake, and dentition. For bone growth, children aged 1 to 8 years require a calcium intake of approximately 700 to 1000 mg (Government of Canada, 2012c). To prevent iron-deficiency anemia, preschool children should consume 7–10 mg of iron a day. Deficiencies in iron can cause behavioural and intellectual deficiencies (Canadian Paediatric Surveillance Program, 2011). Salt and sugar intake should be moderate. The contribution of sugar intake to caries development is well established. For example, Warren, Weber-Gasparoni, Marshall, and colleagues (2009) examined factors associated with carcinogenicity in 128 children. Their study suggests that sweetened beverages, in particular, are associated with the development of caries.

Nutrition and dentition impact health at all ages. Pain from dental caries, infection, and poorly maintained teeth affects appetite and chewing ability, with a subsequent impact on future nutritional status. The frequency of dental caries in children has declined dramatically in recent years because of preventive measures, such as use of fluoride toothpaste, fluoridation of community water supplies, implementation of sound dietary practices, and use of dental sealants. Oral health promotion involves self-care and population-based initiatives, along with professional care (CPS, 2018). Nurses interface with families in a variety of these settings and are therefore in an ideal position to impact dental health promotion.

As early childhood progresses, intense food preferences emerge. This behaviour is a natural outgrowth of the increased physical capacity to react to the taste and textures of foods and the realization that expressing an opinion about food is a way to control the environment. Older preschoolers frequently refuse to try new foods. The favourite foods for this age are meat, cereal grains, baked products, fruits, and sweets. Selecting finger foods that facilitate independence helps the preschooler learn to eat without assistance. Examples of appropriate nutritional foods include cheese, crackers, small pieces of meat, and celery stuffed with cheese or peanut butter. Parents' support for food choices has been demonstrated to be an effective strategy to promote healthy food choices in this age group (Marshall, Golley, & Hendrie, 2011). Parents should provide nutritious foods, avoiding salty and sweet foods. Parents should encourage good nutritional habits to help establish healthy eating behaviours. Increased consumption of fats and processed foods along with diminished physical activity has contributed to a significant increase in the frequency of obesity and type 2 diabetes in children and adolescents (Government of Canada, 2016; Liou, Liou, & Chang, 2010). Family tolerance for individual food preferences differs, and children differ in their tendency to develop strong likes and dislikes. When families reach extreme differences over food preferences, major conflicts may arise, requiring insightful counselling to achieve a mutually satisfying solution. For example, some families may institute a "take a little taste before your refuse" standard for foods at the preschool age. Nurses collaborate with families to discover comfortable approaches to maintain nutritional adequacy of foods that children prefer. Community nurses use a variety of approaches and recognize the wide range of possibilities that exist for families of differing cultures.

Preschoolers begin to eat meals away from home more often than toddlers. Minimal standards require licensed child care centres and preschools to serve foods using recommended dietary allowances of basic nutrients. Parents should communicate regularly with preschool personnel about foods eaten at home and away from home to provide healthy food variety. Preschoolers in group settings learn both positive and negative eating habits and food preferences from care providers and other children. School settings are ideal for community health nurses to impact the nutritional patterns of the preschool child (Water, 2011). Communication about nutritional intake habits reinforces positive behaviours and discourages negative habits at home.

Preschoolers struggle with the intricacies of using utensils. In the later years of the preschool period, children attain skill with spoons, demonstrate fair proficiency with forks, and manage knives for spreading soft foods on bread or crackers. Most preschool children, however, need help cutting meat and pouring liquids from large, heavy containers. Preschoolers enjoy helping to prepare family meals and may be capable of simple tasks, such as washing fruits and vegetables. Involving young children in meal preparation teaches them about healthy nutrition. Sharing important family functions nurtures self-esteem and a sense of value.

The prevalence of food allergy in children in Canada continues to increase, affecting up to 7% of children (AllerGen, 2015). Most allergies develop before the age of 2 years. The foods most likely to cause allergic reactions in the preschool age group include milk, eggs, and peanuts (Fleischer, Perry, Atkins, et al., 2012). Reactions to peanuts tend to decrease over time; however, children who experience peanut allergy should avoid allergens, and their parents should receive written emergency plans along with instructions for epinephrine injection (Fleischer et al., 2012). Clear food labelling and education are essential for prevention of allergic reactions. Many preschools have banned foods such as peanut products as a precautionary measure. Parents may need help identifying potential hazardous situations and communicating their child's needs to preschool personnel. A food allergy action plan that includes a written emergency plan should be developed for parents to use to facilitate communication regarding the child's allergies. Educational resources are available at http://www.cofargroup.org/.

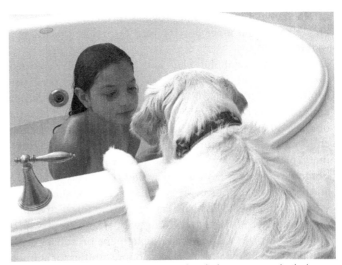

Fig. 13.1 Preschool children can enjoy their pet even at bath time.

### ◆ Elimination Pattern

Toilet training is an important milestone in child development (Kaerts, Van Hal, Vermandel, et al., 2012). Older preschool children are capable of and responsible for independent toileting. Their verbal skills have developed to better communicate their needs, they begin to insist on performing independently, and they are proud of their accomplishments (Kaerts et al., 2012). These developmental achievements provide additional signs for independence with elimination patterns. They may forget to flush the toilet or wash their hands when they are rushed, but they have the physical ability to perform the skills. Preschoolers should not be teased or punished when they are unable to perform independently. If their clothing becomes soiled, they should be responsible for changing their clothes and reminded gently and encouragingly of ways to avoid problems in the future. (Enuresis and encopresis are discussed in Chapter 14.)

### ◆ Activity-Exercise Pattern

Play continues to be the primary activity for preschoolers as well as for toddlers; however, preschoolers explore intently and demonstrate increased coordination and confidence with motor activities. They venture farther from home than toddlers. Many activities involve other children (Fig. 13.1) and involve

modelling behaviour. Particularly in group care settings, children should be monitored for safe activities that enhance gross and fine motor skills while creating fun in movement.

Most 4-year-old children separate easily from their parents, play simple interactive games, dress themselves, copy a number of basic geometrical figures well, and draw recognizable people. Preschoolers enjoy using language skills to tell stories and ask questions. Their physical abilities include balancing on one foot, jumping, and running (Driscoll & Nagel, 2008). Generally, preschoolers appreciate an audience, enjoy practicing new skills, and demonstrate mastered skills to others. Play constitutes an important role in preschoolers' social and psychological development. Play offers a vehicle that allows them to explore while experimenting with who they are, who they might become, and how they relate to others socially. The drama of play allows preschoolers to view themselves from another perspective. Play often reveals the child's reality and complex perception of the world.

Children mimic the behaviour of people familiar to them, expanding their representation beyond self and rehearsing what has been demonstrated to them as appropriate behaviour (Driscoll & Nagel, 2008). Young children seldom assume the role of a younger child or infant while playing. They usually assume adult roles and use a doll for the younger child. Through play, preschoolers learn to exert control over their own behaviour. Assuming an adult role in play allows children to consciously adopt more mature behaviours. Patterns of behaviour used in play can be transferred to actual situations. For example, children who express their anger in a play situation aggressively by vocalizing their distress, scolding the offending party, or using withdrawal of attention are likely to respond with aggression or tantrum behaviour when facing frustration or anger in real-life situations. Observing children at play, as seen by the study group Brown and colleagues (2009) used in their research, reveals natural physical capacities of children better than observation in an examination or testing environment, and provides further evidence of the child's social and inner development for use by practitioners in the field.

Observing symbolic play and imitation play in peer groups helps nurses assess social competency as their perceptions unfold (Driscoll & Nagel, 2008). At first the new child in a peer group may be expected to stand back and observe other children before manipulating a toy. Preschool children engage in more interactive play, particularly dramatic play, than at any other age. Two or more children may become involved in an imaginary plot, especially when toys and equipment support a particular scenario, such as toy kitchen equipment. Patterns emerge in the interactive processes of play: initiating, deciding with whom to play, play themes/roles/rules, and finally enactment or collaborative pretending. These patterns provide opportunities for support to facilitate play initiation and collaborative play (Driscoll & Nagel, 2008). Much of the preschooler's play involves fantasy. The young child frequently invents an imaginary companion who plays, eats, and sleeps with the child. The section entitled Cognitive-Perceptual Pattern addresses more fully the aspects of fantasy during the preschool stage; however, the goal of symbolic or pretend play is to derive meaning from their play experience using their knowledge and skills acquired. The play is a way to integrate previously learned ideas and skills (Driscoll & Nagel, 2008).

Most preschoolers spend some time in a group setting each week. Ground rules at these facilities govern sharing, *quiet* times, and group activities. Although time orientation remains incompletely developed in preschoolers, they have an idea about past and future. They enjoy planning activities with their parents for the future. Visiting the library to review books about wild animals, packing lunches, and choosing what clothes to wear may preface a trip to the zoo.

The preschooler regulates body activities with more purpose and copes with limit setting better than the toddler, but has much energy and requires outlets for this energy during the day. The young child requires physical activity for energy expenditure. Physical activity for the developing child may be more appropriately described as either locomotor play or active play (Pellegrini & Smith, 1998). Active play increases from the toddler to the preschool period, and then declines by approximately 10% for each advancing year of age (Hinkley, Salmon, Okely, et al., 2012). Hinkley and colleagues (2012) concluded that efforts to promote children's physical activity should seek to influence children's preference for physical activity, parent rules, and gender-specific strategies. Becker, McClelland, Loprinzi, and colleagues (2014) investigated whether active play during recess was associated with self-regulation and academic achievement in prekindergarten children. The results revealed that higher active play was associated with better self-regulation and higher scores on early reading and math assessments. Nurses should encourage parents to engage the preschool child in active, locomotor, and rough-and-tumble play. Parents and child care directors/school administrators should also encourage physical activity and work together to overcome perceived barriers that

might limit the young child's ability to access physical activity (Gagne & Harnois, 2014).

Although this age group needs physical activity, many preschoolers spend long periods each day watching television, watching videos, and playing electronic games. Occasionally, parents use the electronic diversions inappropriately to entertain the child. Although some excellent television, video, and electronic game programming is available for preschoolers, many electronic entertainment options focus on adult themes and violence. Many experts agree that television, videos, and electronic games disengage the child's mind and support less learning (Frost, Wortham, & Reifel, 2008) (see Chapter 14). Parents should remember that preschoolers who rely on television, videos, and electronic games do not have enough life experiences to interpret many of the issues presented in adult shows (violence, interpersonal relationships, moral decisions); might be missing opportunities for interacting with other children or adults and other opportunities for active learning; and cannot judge which shows are appropriate for them. In addition, these electronic activities usually offer sedentary recreation, hindering the development of an active healthy lifestyle. Parents should choose which electronic devices and activities are appropriate for their child, limiting time and promoting physical activity in lieu of sedentary play. Furthermore, taking time to share activities provides the child with an opportunity for discussion and for the child to ask questions (Frost et al., 2008). Nurses should explain to parents and preschoolers the relationship between watching television/screen time and lack of physical activity that leads to health problems such as obesity (Frost et al., 2008). Family support for engaging in physical activity has been shown to affect children's health-promoting behaviours. In a study of 93 children and their parents, Marshall and colleagues (2011) demonstrated that parental influence shaped children's physical activity and nutritional health-promoting behaviours.

The latest *Canadian 24-Hour Movement Guidelines for the Early Years*, released in 2017, recommended that preschoolers should accumulate at least 180 minutes of physical activity (including at least 60 minutes of moderate-to-vigorous physical activity), obtain between 10 and 13 hours of sleep, and engage in no more than 1 hour of screen time (CSEP, 2017). Very few preschool-aged children in Canada met all three recommendations (13%); however, 61.8% met the physical activity recommendations, and no associations were found between meeting individual or combined recommendations and indicators of adiposity (Chaput, Colley, Aubert, et al., 2017).

Gordon's health promotion–health maintenance, nutritional-metabolic, and activity-exercise patterns clearly overlap and should be considered together during the assessment phase so as to plan and intervene successfully (Marshall et al., 2011). Resources for these patterns may be used together to provide optimal health promotion. Physical activity in the preschool child is not typically structured exercises. Children do not usually need formal muscle-strengthening programs, such as lifting weights. Younger children usually strengthen their muscles through play activities such as climbing on a jungle gym or trees, riding a tricycle, playing ball, and running/jumping with parents and peers.

## Sleep-Rest Pattern

According to the *Canadian 24-Hour Movement Guidelines,* preschoolers should sleep from 10 to 13 hours a day including naps, with consistent bedtimes and wake-up times (CSEP, 2017). A recent study found that a high proportion of preschool children (83.9%) met the sleep duration recommendations (Chaput et al., 2017). For many older preschoolers, a nap is not necessary. Quiet time provides a welcome respite for the parent, along with a chance for the active preschooler to relax before afternoon activities. Many child care/preschool environments routinely provide rest periods, enhancing rest and relaxation with soft music and a story. An afternoon rest also gives the young child energy for the evening routine, when family members have other duties beyond work and school.

Sleep-time habits, falling asleep, and waking up during the night present challenges for families with preschool children (National Sleep Foundation, 2011). The preschooler's expanded imaginative play and increased physical activity during the day may provoke night-time fears, nightmares, sleepwalking, and sleep terrors, which are at a peak during this stage of development (National Sleep Foundation, 2011).

### Bedtime Ritual

Preschoolers usually require a ritual of activities at bedtime to move from playing and being with others to being alone and falling asleep. These children prolong bedtime routines more often than the toddler. They insist on sleeping with the light on, take a treasured object to bed, request parental attention after being told good night, and experience delays falling asleep. The bedtime ritual generally lasts 30 minutes or longer. Parents honour reasonable rituals, but repeated requests for attention afterward are handled firmly and consistently. Consistency with the routine helps to ameliorate bedtime battles (Hoban, 2010). Vigorous resistance to bedtime challenges parents more during the preschool period than at any other developmental stage. Behavioural insomnia in children occurs when this resistance is associated with a negative association with sleep (Vriend & Corkum, 2011). Preschoolers learn to use the behaviours that meet their needs and control the family regardless of the disruption created.

### Nursing Interventions

When a demanding bedtime behaviour extends beyond 1 year or an episode persists longer than 1 hour, the nurse explores the family situation. A comprehensive assessment in this case includes the following elements:  -
- Description of early episodes
- The manner in which these early episodes were managed and the progression of events since then
- Current bedtime behaviours of the child and siblings
- Identification of parental temperament and the resulting responses of the parents and family members
- Feelings of the parents and child about each other and about the bedtime situation
- Stressful events and changes that have occurred in the past several years
- Behaviour of the child at other times of the day
- Parents' thoughts about the reasons why these episodes continue
- Parents' ideas about strategies to use now

The nurse observes interactions within the family. A home visit at mealtime provides an excellent method to observe active interaction. In the office or clinic setting the nurse can ask a parent to teach the child a task or give directions. The nurse remains as unobtrusive as possible while observing the interaction. The first-hand observation of parent–child interaction, along with the detailed history, usually provides the nurse with adequate baseline information to decide whether to manage the situation in the primary care setting or refer the family to a child behaviour specialist. Sharing recent literature about management techniques for children with differing temperaments helps families understand more about the behaviours. For example, the findings from a study of more than 1500 children by Prior, Cini, Bavin, and colleagues (2011) support that temperament in children may be somewhat modifiable and that parents may consider strategies to influence their preschooler's behaviour that focus on their temperament. Research-based strategies should be used to help parents reach their goals related to managing bedtime concerns.

### Sleep Disturbances

Night terrors and nightmares characterize the night-time wakening problems that generally occur during the preschool years. Night terrors manifest themselves as frightening dreams that cause the child to sit up in bed, scream, stare at an imaginary object, breathe heavily, perspire, and appear in obvious distress (see Chapter 12). Children, not fully awake, may be inconsolable for 10 minutes or more, before they relax and return to a deep sleep. In most cases the child does not recall the dream and in the morning does not remember the incident (Hoban, 2010). These night terrors can start at approximately age 2 years but are more common during the preschool years. Night terrors rarely occur in older children and adults, and only approximately 6% of preschool children have them. Night terrors and nightmares trigger apprehension for the parents (Hoban, 2010).

Nightmares (anxiety dreams) are a more common cause of night wakening. Although infants and toddlers probably have nightmares, their limited verbal skills hinder their relating details of the incidents. After age 3 years, nightmares occur frequently. Approximately 20% of the night is spent dreaming. Dreams frighten preschoolers as they connect to the larger world with their active imaginations and fantastic ideas. These children can waken fully and feel fearful and helpless. Usually they provide vivid descriptions at the time, and they frequently remember the event the following morning. Consolation can be given by a parent who sits with the child, listens to descriptions and fears about the dream, and reminds the child that dreaming is natural and sleep will soon return (Hoban, 2010).

Helping children appreciate the meaning of the words *pretend* and *real* facilitates growth during this phase of childhood. When the parent reads a story to the child or the child tells a make-believe tale, the parents can specify that these are "pretend" and did not really happen. The parent relating a true event can say, "This is real." Children differentiate between the two concepts as they develop cognitively.

## Recommendations

Parents of a preschooler can benefit from knowing the following facts:

- Bedtime rituals of 30 to 45 minutes are common for pre-schoolers. These rituals, because of their importance to children, are respected within reasonable limits. Maintaining a regular consistent and relaxing routine facilitates sleep (National Sleep Foundation, 2011).
- Night-wakening events are common during the preschool years. A consistent sleep environment with the same bed in a room that is cool, quiet, and dark without a television promotes sleep (National Sleep Foundation, 2011). Children who waken at night are reassured and encouraged to return to sleep.
- Parents have clear rules about children sleeping with them if the children will not stay in their own beds.
- Restricting the watching of frightening television shows and the reading of frightening stories and discussing "real" versus "pretend" ideas and stories can help lessen the incidence of nightmares.

## ◆ Cognitive-Perceptual Pattern

During the preschool years, children cultivate their conceptual and cognitive capacities. The quality of the child's care environment enhances these gains. Family and cultural values influence preschoolers' perceptions and their reaction to events (Gonzalez-Mena, 2012). Internalization of family rules has been associated with social competency in this age group (Kochanska, Koenig, Barry, et al., 2010). Preschoolers gradually differentiate today from yesterday and define tomorrow and the future more clearly as concepts of time emerge. The child becomes more oriented in space and develops an awareness of the location of the home within the neighbourhood. The child also begins to structure daily activities and to value certain activities, objects, and people above others.

### Piaget's Theory

The older toddler enters the first substage of the preoperational stage described by Jean Piaget (see Chapter 12). The hallmark of this preconceptual substage includes the ability to function symbolically using language. The preschool child demonstrates increased symbolic functioning during the intuitive substage, from 4 to 7 years of age. The predominant feature of this and the following period is the concrete thought process, as compared with adult abstract thinking. As they experience symbolic mental representations, preschoolers process mental symbols as though they were actually participating in the event. Adults analyze and synthesize symbolic information without concrete connections between the mental process and the actual event. At this stage, mental abstraction, such as skipping from one part of an operation to another, reversing the operation mentally, or thinking of the whole in relation to the parts, is not feasible.

The egocentrism that is characteristic of the preschool years exemplifies this concept of concrete thinking. At this stage, children concentrate solely on their own perspective. They consider only their own personal meanings for symbols. The preschooler wonders why another person fails to follow these idiosyncratic communications.

Furthermore, attention focuses solely on one part of an object without shifting. This behaviour, termed centring by Piaget, illustrates the child's inability to consider more than one factor at a time when solving simple problems. For example, a child can be given two identical cups containing equal amounts of water and asked which cup contains the greater amount of water. During the preoperational stage, the child responds that they contain the same amount of water. The child is then asked to pour the water from each cup into two different containers (one flat and wide, the other tall and narrow). When asked which container has more water, the child always identifies one. The child usually selects the taller, narrower container with water at the higher height. When the water is again transferred to the identical cups and the experiment is repeated, the child returns to the original conclusion that the amounts are equal.

This experiment also illustrates the trait of irreversibility. The child is unable to connect the reversible operation, the transfer of the water back into the original cup, to reach the logical conclusion that the differently shaped containers may hold the same amount of water. The child cannot mentally associate that the transformation from one state to another relates to the shape of the container, not the amount of the water.

Finally, Piaget describes the preoperative stage of thinking as transductive reasoning. The child cannot proceed from general to particular (deduction) or from particular to general (induction); rather, the child moves only from particular to particular in making associations and solving problems. For example, Piaget relates an association made by one of his children between being hunchbacked and being ill. When a hunchbacked neighbour was unable to visit one day because he had a communicable illness, the child understood that the neighbour was ill. However, when the child was told later that the neighbour was better and that she could go see him, her conclusion was that now his hunched back was straight and well. She thought in terms of the man being well or ill, but she placed the man in one or the other category and assumed that he possessed all the attributes and meanings that she linked symbolically with either trait.

The cognitive development of preschoolers is reflected in their symbolic games, which become significantly more orderly and representative of reality (Box 13.1). They begin to incorporate the reality of the world, as it exists outside the self. They increasingly seek play objects that represent models of authentic objects in their environment (Langevin, Packman, & Onslow, 2009). Preschoolers progressively imitate more social rules in their play. Social interactive play predominates as the young child develops a more secure sense of self.

Preschoolers may have one or more imaginary companions who exist for differing periods. These fantasy companions assume the form of another child, an animal, or some other friendly or fearsome creature. Preschoolers may save special chairs, insist that an extra place be set at the table, and talk at length to this companion. Imaginary companions serve an important function; they are controlled totally by

## BOX 13.1 Play as a Method of Learning: Preschool Child

Throughout life, play develops cognitive, affective, and psychomotor skills that are important for the effective performance of life skills. For the preschool child, the following play activities provide the foundation for later competency and socialization-skill refinement:

- Arts and crafts (jewellery making, painting, drawing, ceramics, printmaking)
- Group sports (softball, volleyball, hockey, soccer, swimming)
- Skating, skateboarding
- Bicycling
- Puzzles
- Gymnastics
- Games (board, card, knock-knock jokes, computer)
- Secret clubs
- Imaginary play (being in playhouse productions)
- Horseback riding

the child and are not a threat. In this way the preschooler practices social interactions, controls a fearsome beast, or blames someone for naughty behaviour without fear of being scolded, shame, or attack. Imaginary companions do and say only what the child wills.

### Vision

Vision capabilities, which are well developed by 2 years of age, continue to undergo refinement during the early childhood period. By approximately age 6 years, the child should approach a 20/20 visual acuity level. The possibility of developing amblyopia decreases; it appears most frequently during infancy through approximately the fourth year (see Chapter 12). Depth perception and colour vision become fully established, and the child recognizes subtle differences in colour shading by the sixth year. Maximal visual capability is usually achieved by the end of the preschool years.

Visual capacity throughout the rest of life deteriorates rather than improves. This phenomenon relates partly to changes in the refractive power of the lens and developmental changes that occur in the shape of the eyeball. In the normal sequence of growth, the eyeball becomes increasingly spherical, losing the short shape typical of infancy and progressing to the point at which light converges accurately on the surface of the retina. This change occurs at approximately 6 years of age. When this change occurs before the sixth year, growth continues past the point of ideal light conversion, the eyeball lengthens, and the child may develop early myopic vision, which will progress with age. Glasses are always indicated for the child who develops myopia before approximately age 8 years.

Early detection requires regular screening with standardized tests such the Snellen screening test, which, when administered under standardized procedures, has the advantage of rendering a reliable estimate of actual visual acuity (Hockenberry & Wilson, 2015). The child must be able to understand the test requirements of either pointing in the direction of the *E* or naming the letters.

The Canadian Paediatric Society recommends regular vision screening of children starting at age 3 years (CPS, 2009). Children who do not pass a vision screen should be taken to an optometrist or ophthalmologist for further examination. Refractive errors (inability of the eye to focus on an object) can be significant in the preschool child. The prevalence of refractive errors (5–7%) and amblyopia (2–4%) in preschool children places vision loss as an important public health concern; however, some screening tests reveal only refractive errors (O'Donoghue, Rudnicka, McClelland, et al., 2012). Children younger than 7 years with amblyopia demonstrate significant improvement in vision when treated, providing a rationale for screening and early recognition programs. The pupillary light reflex provides a screening approach for heterotropia, a condition in which the child's eyes do not focus together to transmit effective, coordinated binocular vision. When the child has heterotropia, the light from a penlight held approximately 50 cm (20 inches) from the eyes reflects off the pupil slightly off-centre. Consistent and observable strabismus (crossing of the eye) may be noted. The cover test provides further evidence of a tendency for the child's eyes to cross, known as heterophoria. The child focuses on a spot 36 cm (14 inches) away, then 6 m (20 feet) away. As the child gazes at the designated spot, one eye is covered completely for several seconds (the eye and eyelashes must not be touched), and then the cover is removed abruptly. If the covered eye moves from the line of vision of the uncovered eye, that eye has a tendency toward muscle imbalance and must be evaluated further.

Colour blindness presents a particular problem for younger children because many cues encountered at school depend on the child's ability to distinguish colours. With early detection the child is able to receive assistance to interpret visual cues, thus minimizing the disadvantage of being colour blind. The nurse screens the child for certain types of colour discrimination difficulties by asking the child to respond to various colours in the environment; however, accurate testing for all types of colour blindness requires a specialized tool, such as the Ishihara test, which uses a series of cards with colour-tinted letters and figures.

Preschoolers may be aware of some discomfort or limitations with vision. The nurse gathers the history from the parents, including the questions listed in the Vision section in Chapter 12, about signs of eye problems.

The preschooler is asked questions to elicit information about the following symptoms:

- Itching, burning, or "scratchy" eyes
- Poor vision
- Dizziness, headaches, or nausea after close eye work
- Blurred or double vision

### Hearing

During the preschool years, hearing develops to the level of an adult, when the ability to attend to and interpret what is heard becomes more refined. The 4-year-old preschooler begins to discriminate among remarkably similar speech sounds, such as the difference between sounds made with "f" and "th" or "f" and "s." It is generally accepted that the hearing ability of preschoolers can be hindered by repeated middle ear infections (otitis media). Otitis media with effusion can occasionally result in temporary hearing loss. Parents who notice language delays because of ear infections should be referred to their health care provider for appropriate follow-up care for their children (Hockenberry & Wilson, 2015). Parental reports of difficulty should be taken seriously. Clear evidence supports that effective newborn hearing screening programs correct problems early and often correct developmental delay (Houston, Mufioz, Bradham, et al., 2011). The most effective programs have rigorous evaluation of their policies, procedures, processes, and outcomes (Houston et al., 2011; Yoshinaga-Itano, 2011).

Audiometric methods most accurately measure the child's ability to hear. Preschool children possess the developmental capability to have standard audiometric tests performed on them. The child can follow directions by this age, and most preschoolers enjoy demonstrating their abilities and cooperate easily during vision and hearing screening examinations (Hockenberry & Wilson, 2015).

To ensure success, the nurse encourages a positive experience by adhering to the following points:

- Use equipment skillfully.
- Use age-appropriate language. Avoid the word test to limit anxiety or fear of failure.
- Encourage the child to ask questions and scrutinize the equipment.
- Perform screening before other intrusive or painful procedures.
- Perform screening in a quiet, private area without distractions.
- Praise the child for cooperating.
- Allow rest periods when the child becomes distracted or tired.
- Discuss results with the child in age-appropriate language.

## Sensory Perception

Sensory abilities contribute to preschoolers' skill to perceive and interact with the world. Both sensory acuity and sensory perceptual abilities mature during the preschool years. The nature of the visual stimulus determines the response. Preschoolers respond powerfully to visual illusions and have difficulty discriminating right and left mirror images. Confusion commonly occurs with the letters "b," "d," "p," and "q."

## Language

Cognitive and sensory abilities contribute to preschool language development. Toward the end of the preschool period, expressive language rivals that of an adult except for minor deficiencies in refinement, vocabulary, and structure. Language ability depends on aptitude, opportunities to use language, the quality and quantity of language used at home, and the range of experiences. Regardless of expressive capacity, the child develops receptive language during the preschool years that provides a vital foundation for later communication. Throughout early childhood, receptive capacity exceeds expressive capacity. Children comprehend meanings of words and phrases not contained in their expressive vocabulary. Associations between concepts materialize, although the child lacks the ability to explain these concepts. Table 13.2 outlines the receptive and expressive language skills of preschoolers.

During the early childhood years, rhythm develops as an important dimension in speech capacity. Between 3 and 5 years of age, children practice speaking by mimicking adult language patterns. Practice expands neuromotor capacities, and verbal interaction develops vocabulary and sense of grammatical structure. Hesitations, repetitions, and frequent revisions in speech reflect attempts to expand language capacity. Adults may label such preparation as stuttering, but these inaccuracies actually represent normal speech maturation. Stuttering originates during this developmental period, associated with response and reaction from adults and other children to the normal preschool broken speech pattern (Langevin et al., 2009). Reactions of impatience while waiting for the child to express thoughts and negative social interactions decrease the child's opportunities to use language. Insisting children use correct speech before capacity for fluent speech develops may hinder normal speech development. As many as 60% of expressive language delays resolve during the preschool years (Conti-Ramsden & Durkin, 2012). As nurses help parents provide anticipatory guidance for language development, they should maintain vigilance to identify those children who are not outgrowing their language difficulties. These children encounter lifelong obstacles with learning and socialization. Suggestions for nurses to assist parents and to facilitate preschoolers' language development are listed in Box 13.2.

## Memory

Memory plays an important role in language development and learning in general (Archibald, Joanisse, & Edmunds, 2011). Archibald and colleagues (2011) examined 12 preschool students and demonstrated an association between memory and verbal ability. At the preschool level, children label pictures, group objects, and mimic others as ways to aid memory, performing these tasks with less precision than the older child. Younger children benefit from suggestions about how to group items using characteristics to remember. Preschoolers remember pictures better by saying names of pictures rather than simply hearing the name of a picture when it is first shown. Preschoolers do not spontaneously use rehearsal or other mnemonic techniques for remembering, but they do use and benefit from rehearsal when it is suggested. The nurse tests memory by asking the child to repeat an arbitrary sequence of numbers. By approximately age 5 years, children are able to repeat four consecutively named numbers easily.

## Testing of Developmental Level

Parents of preschool children determine their child's readiness for school programs. The child's skill level, the child's and the family's psychosocial status, and the characteristics of the school program under consideration contribute to readiness determination. Early identification of developmental and emotional disorders is critical to the well-being of children and is an integral function and an appropriate responsibility of all pediatric health care professionals.

## TABLE 13.2 Growth and Development
### Landmarks of Speech, Language, and Hearing Ability During the Preschool Period

| Age (Months) | Receptive Language | Expressive Language | Related Hearing Ability |
|---|---|---|---|
| 42 | Up to 4200 words; knows words such as *what, where, how, funny, we, surprise, secret*; knows number concepts to two; knows how to answer some questions accurately, such as: Do you have a dog? Which is the girl? What toys do you have? | Up to 1200 words in mostly complete sentences averaging four to five words per sentence; uses all 50 phonemes; 7% of sentences are compound or complex; averages 203 words per hour; rate of speech is accelerating; relates experiences and tells about activities in sequential order; uses words such as *what, where, how, see, little, funny, they, we, he, she, several*; can recite a nursery rhyme; asks permission; 95% of speech is intelligible | |
| 48 | Up to 5600 words; carries out three-item commands consistently; knows why people have houses, books, umbrella, key; knows nearly all colours; knows words such as *somebody, anybody, even, almost, now, something, like, bigger, too*, full name, one or two songs, number concepts to four; understands most preschool stories; can complete opposite analogies such as brother is a boy, sister is a girl, and in daytime it is light and at night it is dark | Up to 1500 words in sentences averaging five to six words per sentence; averages 400 words per hour; counts up to three, repeats four digits, names three objects, repeats nine-word sentences from memory; names the primary colours, some coins; relates fanciful tales; enjoys rhyming nonsense words and using exaggerations; demands reasons why and how; questioning is at a peak, up to 500 questions a day; passes judgement on own activity; can recite a poem from memory or sing a song; uses words such as *even, almost, something, like, but*; typical expressions might include "I's so tired," "You almost hit me," "Now I's make something else" | Begins to make fine discriminations among similar speech sounds, such as the difference between *f* and *th* or *f* and *s*; has matured enough to be tested with an audiometer; at this age, formal hearing testing can usually be done; not only has hearing developed to its optimal level but also listening has become considerably refined |
| 54 | Up to 6500 words; knows what materials a house, window, chair, and dress are made of and what people do with eyes and ears; understands differences in texture and composition, such as hard, soft, rough, smooth; begins to name or point to penny, nickel, dime; understands *if, because, why, when* | Up to 1800 words in sentences averaging five to six words; now averages only 230 words per hour—is satisfied with less verbalization; does little commanding or demanding; likes surprises; approximately one in 10 sentences are compound or complex, and only 8% of sentences are incomplete; can define 10 common words and counts up to 20; common expressions are "I don't know," "I said," "tiny," "funny," "because"; asks questions for information and learns to manipulate and control people and situations with language | |
| 60 | Up to 9600 words; knows number concepts to five; knows and names colours; defines words in terms of use, such as a bike is to ride; defines wind, ball, hat, stove; understands qualifiers such as *if, because, when*; knows purpose of horse, fork, and legs; begins to understand *left* and *right* | Up to 2200 words in sentences averaging six words; can define ball, hat, stove, policeman, wind, horse, fork; can count five objects and repeat four or five digits; definitions are in terms of use; can single out a word and ask its meaning; makes serious inquiries—"What is this for?" "How does this work?" "Who made those?" "What does it mean?"; language is now essentially complete in structure and form; uses all types of sentences, clauses, and parts of speech; reads by way of pictures, and prints simple words | |

Modified from Hockenberry, M. J., & Wilson, D. (Eds). (2015). *Wong's nursing care of infants and children* (10th ed.). St. Louis, MO: Mosby.

To obtain a more specific measure of developmental age, the nurse uses one of several screening tools designed for use with the preschool child. These validated instruments help to identify children at risk of developmental delay or disorder. Screening instruments are not diagnostic tools. In the primary care setting, screening for developmental age can be performed using the Rourke Baby Record (Rourke, Leduc, & Rourke, 2017) or the Looksee Checklist (NDDS, 2019), formerly called the Nipissing District Developmental Screen. The Rourke Baby Record, used by practitioners, is an evidence-informed tool for children up to age 5. It addresses growth and nutrition monitoring, developmental screening, physical examination parameters, vaccinations, and a guide for safety and health promotion. The Looksee Checklist is a parent report tool to monitor development from 1 month to 6 years.

When a screening tool result is positive/concerning, the nurse should take additional steps to meet the needs of the parent and child. An early return visit should be made to provide additional developmental surveillance as well as anticipatory guidance for the family. Most importantly, the child should be referred for developmental and/or medical evaluations. Early developmental intervention/early childhood services should also be initiated if necessary.

Children who are ready for school demonstrate competencies in areas other than measurable skill performance. Complex home environments with stable caring adults or safe, predictable physical environments with regular, stimulating activities, peers, and materials contribute to readiness. Social norms define expectations; therefore, home values that align with school values are more likely to result in children characterized as ready for school. Conversely, when

---

**BOX 13.2** **Nursing Suggestions to Encourage Language Development in Preschoolers**

- Read to the child. Encourage the child to be an active listener. Pause during the story to ask questions, such as "What do you think will happen next?" and "Why do you think the boy said that?" and "What would you do now?" Praise the child's storytelling and creativity with stories.
- Always respond to the child's questions. Occasionally a response must be delayed; for example, when the parent is driving in heavy traffic and the child asks a question that requires a complex answer, the parent might say "That's a very good question; let's talk about that as soon as we get home." The parent should remind the child of the question later and respond if the child still expresses interest.
- Never tease or criticize a child about speaking style. If the child speaks so fast as to be fumbling over words, then the parent might say "I can't listen that fast. Slow down a little for me." This is much more encouraging than is the statement "You talk too fast. No one can understand you."
- Play language-focused games, such as naming the colours of houses or kinds of flowers as parent and child walk to the store.

---

school expectations differ from those at home, children are less likely to be considered ready for school (Conti-Ramsden & Durkin, 2012).

### Autism Spectrum Disorders

Statistics from the Public Health Agency of Canada (PHAC, 2018) identify that approximately one in 66 Canadian children are diagnosed with autism spectrum disorders (ASD). ASD is four times more common among boys than girls, and has been diagnosed in an estimated one in 42 boys and one in 165 girls in the Canada. ASD is the umbrella diagnosis for all subtypes (autistic disorder, childhood disintegrative disorder, pervasive developmental disorder—not otherwise specified, and Asperger's syndrome).

These conditions are considered genetically determined disorders and are only rarely associated with nongenetic risk factors, such as advanced maternal age (Sandin, Hultman, Kolevzon, et al., 2012), maternal valproic acid use during pregnancy, congenital rubella, and cerebral palsy (Freitag et al., 2010). Although the genetic foundation is well recognized, no single gene or gene family is linked to the disorders (LeBlanc & Fagiolini, 2011; Mefford, Batshaw, & Hoffman, 2012). Chromosome microarray analysis is a promising area for assessment of ASD and currently provides diagnosis 15% to 20% of the time (Mefford et al., 2012).

Multiple studies have linked ASDs with atypical birth weight (high or low), low Apgar scores, hemolytic disease, hyperbilirubinemia (jaundice), respiratory distress, advanced parental age, length of gestation, and environmental factors (viruses), all of which may be subtle and complicated by the genetic influence (May-Benson, Koomar, & Teasdale, 2009). In their study of 467 children with ASD, May-Benson and colleagues (2009) provided support for the idea that there is no unique combination of characteristics, but rather a composite of risk factors that provide suspicion for the disorders.

More recently, there has been a question on whether an association between assisted reproductive technology (ART) conception

and autism exists. Fountain, Zhang, Kissin, and colleagues (2015) found in a population-based sample in California that the incidence of autism was twice as high for ART births as for non-ART births. However, they also explain that the association between ART and autism can be primarily explained by adverse prenatal and perinatal outcomes and multiple births. Research is also being performed to look at potential differences in ART procedures and parental infertility diagnoses as they might factor into the incidence of autism in ART-conceived infants. For example, there is a higher incidence of autism during the first 5 years of life when intracytoplasmic sperm injection was used compared with in vitro fertilization and a lower incidence when parents had unexplained infertility (among singletons) or tubal factor infertility (among multiples) compared with other types of infertility (Kissin, Zhang, Boulet, et al., 2015).

Careful observation is vital during this time of language and communication development to assess children for ASD because most cases of ASD are diagnosed in children (LeBlanc & Fagiolini, 2011). Most children have symptoms in the first year of life (Shumway, Thurm, Swedo, et al., 2011); however, a formal diagnosis of autism is typically not made until a child is 2 years old. This assessment includes the family history, clinical history, and physical assessment with a focused neurological examination. Various screening tools exist for the nurse to use to identify children at risk of autism. The Modified Checklist for Autism in Toddlers is a widely used, two-stage parent-completed screening tool for children aged 16 to 30 months (Robins, Fein, & Barton, 2018). For higher functioning older children, the Childhood Asperger Syndrome Test and the Social Communication Questionnaire are well-developed and validated screening tools.

Manifestations differ considerably (Freitag et al., 2010; May-Benson et al., 2009). Assessment of cognitive and behavioural symptoms is the cornerstone of diagnosis, and early detection may help families address advancing behavioural aberrations sooner (LeBlanc & Fagiolini, 2011). The families of these children manage multiple behavioural and physical challenges early in the child's life; therefore, health providers need to remain apprised of current trends in pediatric development connected to the disorders (May-Benson et al., 2009). Providers should consider the prenatal events mentioned earlier in this section along with childhood stressors (e.g., chronic ear infections, sleeping/eating problems, absent/brief crawling phase, language delays, atypical responses to sensory stimulation, lack of separation anxiety, and failure to attain motor skill developmental milestones) as warning signs that warrant further assessment (LeBlanc & Fagiolini, 2011; May-Benson et al., 2009).

In 2016 a population-based ASD surveillance study was published that looked at the characteristics and prevalence of ASD in 4-year-old children (Christensen, Bilder, Zahorodny, et al., 2016). The study authors concluded that when compared with diagnosis in 8-year-old children, ASD were diagnosed in the 4-year-olds approximately 5 months earlier (27 months compared with 32 months, respectively), demonstrating improved methods of early identification. They also found that 4-year-old children with ASD were more likely to have intellectual disability than 8-year-old children in the same communities. Lastly, they concluded that among 4-year-old children, girls and White children were more likely to receive their first comprehensive, developmental evaluation by age

### Health Promotion With Preschoolers: Environmental Accountability

*Rationale for Teaching Preschoolers About Environmental Protection*
- Environmental education at an early age will produce environmental practitioners of the future.
- Preschoolers can learn basic concepts of environmental accountability and gain a sense of empowerment when they perceive that they make a difference to the future world.
- Health care providers, in consultation with child care providers, can promote environmental education that is based on their knowledge of child growth and development and concerns about overall health.

*Basic Ways for Preschoolers to Help the Environment and Promote Overall Societal Health*
- Use water wisely.
- Use electricity only when necessary.
- Recycle.
- Avoid using balloons.
- Plant trees, protect plants, and grow a garden.
- Create a compost pile.
- Care for birds.
- Clean up the neighbourhood.
- Decrease the amount of garbage; say "no" to Styrofoam and plastic garbage bags, and use paper cups and reusable cloth bags for groceries.
- Recycle old toys by giving them to others.
- Buy and use only Earth-friendly school supplies.
- Walk rather than ride in the car.
- Use live Christmas trees and replant them.

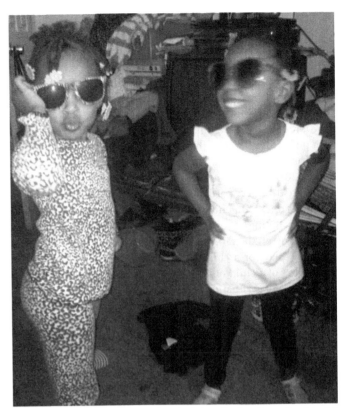

Fig. 13.2 Two preschoolers using their imagination to pretend to be movie stars.

3 years compared with boys and Black children, demonstrating that although there have been improvements in early diagnosis, at-risk populations still exist for later diagnosis/identification.

It is critical that autism and developmental delay be detected early in an effort to minimize delay and reduce educational costs. Neural circuits, which create the foundation for learning, behaviour, and health, have increased plasticity within the first 3 years and become increasingly difficult to change over time. Diagnosis in the preschool child or earlier is imperative. The brain in strengthened by positive early experiences, stable relationships, appropriate nutrition, and supportive environments. High-quality early intervention can change the child's developmental trajectory and improve outcomes for families, children, and communities (Center on the Developing Child at Harvard University, 2010).

## ◆ Self-Perception–Self-Concept Pattern

During the preschool years, basic self-concept emerges from the child's personal struggle for autonomy. As children develop beyond the toddler years, they refine their sense of self through both task-oriented and socially oriented experiences. By reinforcing skills and successfully accomplishing tasks, preschoolers build self-esteem, enhancing overall health. Social acceptance helps children feel successful in their role as a child, sibling, and friend. Preschoolers investigate roles through rich imagination. Pretending to be the parent or baby allows preschoolers to imagine experiences and feelings of others (i.e., empathy) and safely experiment with new ideas (Price & Gwinn, 2012).

Preschool children learn about their roles in their child care environments and learn that being dependable within their world is important. When children perceive their value in improving the world in which they live, they experience good feelings about themselves, and, ultimately, demonstrate improved mental and physical health. Many simple ways to improve the environment are available, and when children learn ways to contribute to environmental health, they often reinforce these behaviours in their parents (Quality and Safety Scenario).

### Erikson's Theory

Preschoolers develop a sense of initiative through their vigorous motor activity and active imagination (Fig. 13.2). Erikson views this growth as the most central developmental task in the emerging self-concept of the preschool years. By praising preschoolers' efforts and providing opportunities for new experiences, parents promote development of initiative. Rather than requiring a particular behaviour, parents should provide avenues for experimentation. Preschoolers then feel mastery, thus encouraging repetition. With mastery, preschoolers become more confident about trying new actions.

## ◆ Roles-Relationships Pattern

Family members continue to play a vital role in the preschooler's life, but peers become increasingly significant as development progresses. Preschoolers receive ideas and information from peers. They may subsequently question rules or expectations at home, comparing them with their friends' situations.

Discussion about family values and behaviours that are acceptable in one place but not in another helps them understand differences.

Preschoolers understand gender expectations regarding jobs, activities, and competencies of people in their lives. Ideas about gender differences in work roles or activities are based on models in the home, at child care or preschool centres, and on television. Parents and caregivers should be aware of the powerful influence that the environment has on role perceptions (Bower et al., 2008; Brown et al., 2009; Kochanska et al., 2010). When inaccurate portrayals of male and female roles are depicted, parents and caregivers should discuss more accurate ones with children. Preschoolers experiment through play, including adopting family roles. These roles differ depending on the family structure and function. For example, the role-play for a child of gay or lesbian parents may differ from that of a child of heterosexual parents. As the mother or father in a play situation, the preschooler sets limits, punishes, praises, and makes outlandish demands on the invented child. Play represents an important strategy for preschoolers to use for stress reduction and experimentation with new roles. By playing different roles, children safely experience the effects of their behaviour and understand others' roles more clearly. Parents also better understand the effects of their own actions when they observe the behaviours of their child. Nurses help parents use their observations to improve interactions with their child.

Compared with toddlers, preschoolers relate to older children in the family on a more equal basis. Although their cognitive, motor, and language skills are less refined, preschoolers participate in some activities with their older siblings. Younger children may admire and imitate an older sibling. This behaviour flatters the older child initially, but with continued persistence may develop into a source of frustration for the sibling. The older sibling, in a more powerful position, may resort to violence (Phillips, Phillips, Grupp, et al., 2009).

Social interaction during the preschool period prepares the child for school. Through experience within the family, with peers, and with other adults, the child acquires readiness to interact in group situations, follow directions, take turns, recognize others' rights, channel energy toward an assigned activity, and demonstrate increasing independence. School readiness can be assessed by use of several relevant tests, as discussed in this chapter. The nurse who sees the child repeatedly in an office, clinic, or group care or preschool setting assesses progress as the child develops social competencies. Comparing the preschooler's current, more mature behaviour with previous behaviour provides insight into that child's readiness for school. This method of evaluation, however, prevents comparison with other children of the same age. For example, school personnel may view a child who reflects a quiet temperament and is introverted or subdued as overly attached to the mother in comparison with other children the same age. However, if the child's earlier social behaviour is known, the behaviour may be interpreted as a progression toward independence.

Evidence of social competency can be obtained by discussion and evaluation of the child's family drawings. Children can be given the opportunity to draw pictures while they are waiting for outpatient visits, and the drawings can be used to begin the assessment process. The nurse observes the drawing and responds to any comments or questions volunteered by the child. When asked for advice or assistance, the nurse encourages the child to proceed with drawing. Positive encouragement for the child's efforts may be used, particularly with reluctant children. After the drawing is finished, the nurse discusses the sketch with the child to identify the people and describe individual characteristics. The nurse writes the names of each family member on the picture and documents the perceptions the child describes. Open-ended questions such as "What do you like best about your brother?" or "When do you get angry with your sister?" can be posed to encourage the child to describe the family interaction patterns. When an adult family member is present, the nurse explains the purpose of the drawing and interview and requests that the adult withhold comments or questions until the activity is completed. Any areas of concern or questions should be discussed, assuring the parent that confidentiality will be maintained. The child's perceptions can be verified with the adult at the conclusion of the interview, or further information can be sought to clarify them.

The Vineland Social Maturity Scale provides an objective, standardized estimate of social functioning and social maturity (Scattone, Raggio, & May, 2011). This tool profiles the child's self-help skills, self-direction, locomotion, communication, and social relations. The scoring system seems to be culturally and socioeconomically neutral. The investigator collects data by observing the child's behaviour and interviewing the mother or primary caregiver. Designed to measure progression toward independence, this instrument uses direct observation of the child's behaviour whenever possible, with the interview data being used only if needed to complete the assessment (Scattone et al., 2011).

These kinds of tools elicit cues indicative of family stress and strain. Parental divorce commonly creates disruption in family relationships. Discussion of the results of the assessment offers the opportunity to discuss family situations that otherwise might have remained unmentioned. Children's responses to changes in family circumstances depend on their developmental stages and their relationships before the change. Divorce represents a final decision, usually culminating from a period of conflict, stress, and changing relationships. Although preschoolers definitely sense stress in the home, they cannot articulate their feelings or determine their origin. Children react to changes in various ways, including regression, confusion, or irritability. Asking the same questions repeatedly—such as "Is Daddy coming home for supper tonight?" or "Why doesn't Daddy stay here anymore?"—can be a child's way of expressing difficulty in coping with or comprehending the situation.

Parents in the midst of marital problems or divorce frequently lack the psychological energy or patience to deal with questions and altered behaviour. Nonetheless, their children desperately need closeness, patience, and consistent responses from their parents. Nurses act as advocates for children by helping parents explore ways to address regression and irritability. As parents develop skills to explain situations, they realize children are deeply affected during times of family disruption, regardless of their behaviour (Kaakinen, Gedaly-Duff, & Hanson, 2010).

Parents need to connect emotionally with their children to demonstrate that love will continue for the child despite dissolution of the marriage. Books appropriate to the preschooler's cognitive and emotional level can help parents address children's feelings and needs during divorce.

### Child Abuse

The social processes within families and communities that create child abuse are multifaceted and complex. Research focuses on the complexity of the abuse cycle and the challenges involved in resolution. Parents and caregivers who experience workplace stress, financial worries, and other frustrations may project their anger and abuse toward their children physically, emotionally, or sexually. Effective primary and secondary prevention interventions involve promoting awareness of violence as a social problem, opposing violence to women, and offering community or school programs to teach nonviolent conflict resolution skills to people of all ages. Prevention of child neglect and abuse is the focus of many health-promotion programs. Recognition of signs of child abuse is important, and health care providers are mandated to report suspected abuse (Government of Canada, 2012a). Although it is important for families to begin to teach children about how to respond to strangers, child abuse in general and sexual abuse in particular occur more often within a family than with a stranger as the perpetrator. Most children suffer the abuse from someone who is familiar to them. The Government of Canada (2012b) provides helpful information about child abuse and maltreatment at https://www.canada.ca/en/public-health/services/health-promotion/stop-family-violence/prevention-resource-centre/children/child-maltreatment-canada.html.

## ◆ Gender and Sexuality-Reproductive Pattern

Preschoolers recognize there are two genders and identify with their own gender. Appropriate and positive representations of both genders on television and in role models, such as working mothers, allow preschoolers to interpret gender roles broadly and define their own roles more realistically (Hockenberry & Wilson, 2015). Body image, a part of gender identity, also includes perception of sex organs. Preschoolers develop curiosity at this age, including inquisitiveness about bodies and sexual functions of others. Questions should be answered simply and factually. Teasing preschoolers about this interest or implying that sexual information is unacceptable or naughty promotes negativity. Positive feelings about all aspects of the self (including gender role) create positive self-esteem. Many children's books address self-esteem in young children and provide interesting and informative approaches to nurturing overall health promotion in this age group.

## ◆ Coping–Stress Tolerance Pattern

### Play Approaches

Assessing self-concept in preschool children who struggle to articulate their feelings presents a challenge for the nurse. Play can elicit behaviours that indicate sense of self and self-esteem, future success or failure, sense of acceptance, and competence. Doll or puppet play provides valuable insight into a child's sense of self. Dolls or puppets, including those representing a young child of the same gender, race, and cultural background

as the preschooler, should be available (Hockenberry & Wilson, 2015). If the child spontaneously begins to engage the dolls or puppets in imaginary activity, no further guidance should be given. With a reluctant child, the nurse begins to pretend, using examples for the child, such as going to the store, moving the dolls through the related activities, and then involving the child. Frequently, preschoolers continue the scenario to tell their personal stories.

A related technique is mutual storytelling. The nurse begins a story for the child to finish. The nurse might begin with a standard line, such as "Once upon a time there lived a [girl, boy, cow, monkey, etc.] who …" The nurse then pauses for the child to continue. If the child hesitates, the nurse resumes the story for another sentence or two and asks what the figure in the story is doing. As the child supplies details, the nurse offers encouragement to continue, asking questions such as "And then what happened?" or "How did the child feel?"

The child's inner nature can be explored along several dimensions. The emotional theme of the story is noted and should be congruent with the child's tone and expression. For example, a child who centres on a theme of aggression and destruction but describes the character's anger in a monotone is demonstrating incongruence between content and expression. The child's emotionless response suggests difficulty with expressing feelings. At the conclusion of the story, possible meanings can be revealed by the nurse asking whether the child feels similar to any of the characters or would like to be any of the characters.

Although these dimensions may be explored for meaning, interpretation of a child's behaviour in these play situations remains highly speculative. Determining possible themes or estimating the child's self-esteem requires several encounters. Additionally, the nurse's personality and approach influence the child's spontaneity and ability to tell a story. Observed behaviour and responses without associated interpretation should be recorded for future reference. Interpretations of the behaviour and responses are avoided until validated by a specialist.

### Coping Mechanisms

Preschoolers use coping mechanisms similar to those of the toddler (separation anxiety, regression, denial, repression, and projection). Protest behaviour in the form of temper tantrums normally disappears as a stress response in the older preschooler. Temper tantrums that persist through the fifth year indicate a lack of matured coping responses. The child uses tantrums and continues to gain the desired result.

Preschoolers lack the cognitive awareness, social abilities, and motives for communication of adults and older children. They display temperaments and tantrums that appear oppositional to older individuals. Through positive interactions with parents and caregivers, preschoolers frequently learn how to organize their bodies, abilities, and environment to move successfully to the next stage of development (Brown et al., 2009; Luby, Belden, Sullivan, et al., 2009). A positive relationship between the child's temperament and the demands of the environment (also known as goodness of fit) can be attained by social interaction, which, in turn, prevents the development of problem behaviours later (Box 13.3).

Preschoolers possess a considerable range of experiences and memories; therefore, they respond more maturely to stress than do toddlers. Positive coping resources are determined by some of the following variables:

- Availability of emotional comfort and the child's inner resilience
- Ability to work on task
- Availability of play materials and toys
- Opportunity to engage in activities (Kalpidou, Power, Cherry, et al., 2004)

Preschoolers use many of the coping mechanisms developed during their toddler years, but they generally show greater ability to verbalize frustration, have fewer temper tantrums, and display more patience in experimentation to resolve difficulty than the typical toddler. Preschoolers refine their problem-solving skills. Through fantasy play, they investigate solutions or responses to stressful events and find inner control for challenging situations.

Occasionally, projection and fantasy lead parents to consider their child dishonest. When faced with the question "Did you break this dish?" the preschooler might respond, "No, Teddy did it." The child might even relate a detailed story of the toy bear mishap. Preschoolers tend to project blame. Active fantasies help tell the story. Parents should not accuse the preschooler of lying, but rather the adult should help the child decide whether the story is pretend or real. The concepts of pretend and real help encourage children to discuss nightmares, television shows, stories, and their own active imaginations (Garrison, Liekweg, & Christakis, 2011).

Compared with toddlers, preschoolers better perceive their ability to control and manage situations. Strict adherence to rituals or game rules controls situations. As discussed, preschoolers have longer and more rigid bedtime rituals than those of toddlers. Preschoolers also dislike losing games and may structure the rules to ensure they win. Older children and adults may be able to accept these structures, but these controlling behaviours frustrate other preschoolers because they also need to win. Gentle, consistent direction by parents and caregivers about how to play games fairly and how to move toward positive group outcomes helps preschoolers develop a sense of morality, which is important for later life success and happiness. See the Case Study and Care Plan at the end of this chapter for an example of ineffective coping in a preschool child.

## ◆ Values-Beliefs Pattern

Preschoolers, like toddlers, lack fully developed consciences; however, at age 4 to 5 years these children do demonstrate some internal controls on their actions. Immaturity limits the consistency and effectiveness of these internal controls. With the child's concrete perspective, the internal controls may be rigid; therefore, a preschooler may feel overwhelming guilt when behaviour and internal controls conflict. Cognitive developmental level determines, for the most part, preschoolers' maturity and their feelings about their behavioural fluctuations. Cognitive development continues with dramatic transformation during these years, explaining the differences not only among children

---

**BOX 13.3    The Challenge of Temperament and Preschoolers**

Temperament, which describes the way in which an individual behaves or responds to new situations and to life occurrences, has consistently been associated with psychopathology and family function since the early work of Terry Brazelton with maternal attachment in 1978 (Healey, Flory, Miller, et al., 2011; Joosen, Mesman, Bakermans-Kranenburg, et al., 2012). Most children can be defined as *easy, difficult,* or *slow to warm up to* on the basis of how they react to their surroundings and to people. Temperament and parental stress are linked; however, multiple other factors influence interactions between the parent and the child, including the child's own temperament (Healey et al., 2011; Prior et al., 2011). For many adults, the challenge in parenting is to learn how to work with a child's temperament, which can differ from the parents' or other children's temperaments, in efforts to attain family happiness. Coping skills and stress management for families, particularly those with children defined as difficult, may improve family function (Healey et al., 2011).

Sources: Healey, D. M., Flory, J. D., Miller, C. J., & Halperin, J. M. (2011). Maternal positive parenting style is associated with better functioning in hyperactive/inattentive preschool children. *Infant & Child Development, 20*(2), 148–161, https://doi.org/10.1002/icd.682; Joosen, K. J., Mesman, J., Bakermans-Kranenburg, M. J., et al. (2012). Maternal sensitivity to infants in various settings predicts harsh discipline in toddlerhood. *Attachment & Human Development, 14*(2), 101–117; Prior, M., Bavin, E., Cini, E., et al. (2011). Relationships between language impairment, temperament, behavioural adjustment and maternal factors in a community sample of preschool children. *International Journal of Language & Communication Disorders, 46*(4), 489–494.

---

but also for different times in the same child. Modelling and induction explanation, moving from specific to general, influence moral behaviours appreciably. Modelling stems from many sources, not all of which leave positive impressions. Parents affect the availability of models by screening television shows, carefully selecting child care situations, and monitoring play sessions. Responsible parents verify the suitability of the models. More detailed inductive explanations, based on the child's cognitive level, are generally comprehended by the preschool population.

Preschoolers control their behaviour to retain parental love and approval. From their perspective, parental disapproval represents a decrease in the child's importance from the parent's viewpoint. The child therefore suffers a decline in self-esteem, which motivates a change in behaviour. Guilt results from perceived reduction of self-esteem, a critical step in the development of conscience. Moral actions are demonstrated in simple activities, such as taking turns and sharing. These actions stem from the assumption that other people have rights and desires that are as important as the rights and desires of preschoolers.

Preschoolers frequently express their values by stating who or what they like or what they want to be when they become adults. These values change frequently, even within a few minutes. Preschoolers occasionally use statements of value as punishment for playmates or family members and display insensitivity to the effect of their remarks on others. Preschoolers ask endless questions. When they ask these questions about moral actions or feelings, they may simply be asking "How does this work?" and not questioning the underlying parental value. The same intent exists when the child asks about the spiritual values that the parent may be teaching.

## RESEARCH FOR EVIDENCE-INFORMED PRACTICE

### Effectiveness of Parents' Language Interventions for Preschool Children

Roberts and Kaiser (2011) conducted a systematic meta-analysis of 18 studies with participants aged 18 to 60 months that met the following criteria: used a comparison group; used a parental intervention; and included a child communication component with at least one language outcome measure. Almost half of the studies evaluated used the Hanen Program for Parents and focused stimulation. Effect sizes were determined for each study, as well as seven language outcome variables. Intellectual disabilities and parent report versus direct observation measures were also compared. This meta-analysis indicated that parent-implemented language interventions have significant positive influence on both receptive and expressive language skills in preschool children, regardless of whether they have intellectual impairment. The findings from this analysis provide evidence to support the use of parent-implemented interventions for preschool children with language impairments.

Source: Roberts, M. Y., & Kaiser, A. P. (2011). The effectiveness of parent-implemented language interventions. A meta-analysis. *American Journal of Speech-Language Pathology, 20*(3), 180–199.

Parents may enroll their child in Sunday school or other faith-oriented classes or activities. The preschool child generally enjoys the social aspects of these activities and receives some important modelling of values from the involved adults and from working with peers as they struggle to develop morality (Kochanska et al., 2010).

Life beginnings and death concepts fascinate preschoolers. Because of their limited emotional experiences with death, some ask about dead insects and the process of death with great interest, occasionally with insensitivity. Others become upset with the idea of dying, assuming that when someone becomes angry and wishes them dead, they will cease to exist. Many children worry about who will care for them if their caregivers die, whether pain comes with death, what causes death, and what happens after someone dies. Children who actually lose a loved one to death can experience sleep disturbances and other behavioural changes as part of the grieving process. Parents, on the basis of their own religious and cultural values, should respond to children in a supportive and open manner to provide an accurate interpretation of death. In some cases, counselling may be needed if the parents are unable to cope with their duties or if the child has significant behavioural problems as a result of the family disruption. Assessment using the preschooler's drawings in such situations provides an accepted method to explore their perceptions about family relationships, death, and the afterlife (Selwyn, Boraschi, & Ozkula, 2009).

## ❖ ENVIRONMENTAL PROCESSES

### ◆ Physical Agents

For many children, physiological, psychosocial, and environmental factors create health problems that interfere with physical, social, and educational activities of normal development (Hockenberry & Wilson, 2015). Major disruptions limit fulfillment of the child's potential in adulthood. The environmental processes that affect toddlers also affect preschoolers. Preschoolers have more refined problem-solving skills, are more coordinated, and have more experience with a variety of situations than do toddlers. Although preschoolers recognize and avoid some environmental hazards, they remain impulsive and immature. Population-based programs ensure that screening occurs at the most developmentally appropriate time (Research for Evidence-Informed Practice).

Because many preschoolers attend child care programs, many have been trained to use 911 and can access help in emergencies when this phone code exists. At this age a child needs to know his or her name, address, and how to say "no" to strangers.

### Injuries

Accidents and injuries are often predictable and preventable (CPS, 2012; Ingram, Deave, Towner, et al., 2011). As preschoolers become more independent, causes of injury change; they may chase a ball into a busy street or suffer from sports-related injuries. Preschoolers continue to need supervision to prevent injury related to their developmental age. Nurses guide families to provide a safe environment for preschoolers with opportunities to explore without negative consequences (Box 13.4).

Of all injuries, two-thirds occur in children and adolescents. Although preschoolers have fewer accidents than toddlers, accidental injury continues to be a predominant cause of morbidity in this age group. Preschoolers are most likely to sustain injuries related to falls, poisonings, and thermal injuries than any other accidental injuries; however, as the child's age increases toward school age, these injuries begin to decline in number (CPS, 2012; Ingram et al., 2011; Orton, Kendrick, West, et al., 2012).

Motor vehicle accidents consistently remain the top-ranked reason for death attributable to injury in the preschool age group (CPS, 2012). In Canada, all jurisdictions have seatbelt and child restraint laws. The Canadian National Survey on Child Restraint Use 2010 found that, unfortunately, children younger than 8 years old are not using the recommended child passenger restraints (Snowdon, Hussein, & Ahmed, 2011). The overall critical misuse for child restraints is approximately 73% (Decina & Lococo, 2005). To promote correct car seat use, Weaver, Brixey, Williams, and colleagues (2013) recommend conducting meaningful formative research, developing and evaluating injury prevention message strategies, evaluating existing programs and recommendations, conducting transdisciplinary work, and supporting partnerships between manufacturers, retailers, and injury prevention specialists.

Each province and territory has its own height, weight, and age restrictions for child restraints. As children outgrow a rear-facing car seat at approximately age 2 years old and weigh at least 10 kg, they should move to a forward-facing car seat with a five-point harness. Children should remain in a forward-facing car seat with a harness for as long as possible, up to the highest weight and height allowed by the car seat manufacturer. School-aged children should transition to a booster seat when the weight and/or height are above the forward-facing limit. Children younger than 13 years old should ride in the back seat of a motor vehicle, particularly

## BOX 13.4    Injury Prevention for Preschoolers

A safe and developmental-stimulating environment allows children of all ages to explore without negative consequences. When teaching parents how to modify their homes for preschoolers, the nurse should consider the following requirements for child safety.

### Safe Sleep Environment

Provide beds with guardrails (as needed), soft corners, and appropriate bedding to prevent suffocation.

### Well-Ventilated but Optimal Temperature Environment for Play

Provide safe play areas by using electrical outlet covers, handrails in stairwells, toy boxes with lids that lock securely, nonslip floor materials, well-anchored furniture, and appropriate soft ground coverings and padding for outdoor play equipment.

### Burn Prevention

Use only a cool mist humidifier for management of upper respiratory tract infections; dress a child only in flame-retardant clothing, particularly at bedtime.

### Appropriate Installation and Use of Emergency Home Equipment

Discuss the importance of properly operating smoke detectors and fire extinguishers, and practice a plan for escape from the home in case of emergency.

### Connection to Emergency Services

Post 911 on all phones; teach the child how to use 911 and how to report the child's name and address over the phone; parents should be trained in cardiopulmonary resuscitation and the use of abdominal thrusts.

### Prevention of Aspiration

Monitor use of balloons and eating habits of preschoolers.

### Safe Daily Home Environment

Close doors of the dishwasher, oven, washer, and dryer; mark all glass doors with decals to delineate doors; use gates at the top and bottom of stairs for the younger child; set water heater temperature at a maximum of 48.9°C (120°F) to avoid burns; store all poisonous substances out of the reach of children; discourage running in the house; avoid using throw rugs on bare floors.

### Prevention, Recognition, and Management of Poison Ingestion or Exposure

Know how to use syrup of ipecac, and have the nearest poison control centre phone number within easy access; learn how to evaluate burns or blisters around the mouth, odour of poisons, empty containers around the child, stomach distress, or changes in normal activity level that might indicate poison ingestion.

### Water Safety

Monitor bathtub and pool activity; teach preschooler swimming skills (usually by age 4 years); ensure that all pools are fenced.

### Bicycle Safety

Ensure that the child is riding a developmentally appropriate bicycle with a federally approved safety helmet and is schooled in the rules of riding in the street and interacting with strangers.

### Lead Concerns

Avoid exposure to items with a high lead content in the home (paint, wrapping paper, earthenware, coloured newspaper); ensure that children are monitored when lead exposure is a concern.

### Environmental Contaminants Hazardous to the Child's Health

Avoid exposure to tobacco smoke, nitrous oxide from wood-burning stoves, asbestos, pesticides, radiation, and factory-produced irritants.

Source: Hockenberry, M. J., & Wilson, D. (Eds). (2015). *Wong's nursing care of infants and children* (10th ed.) St. Louis: Mosby.

---

because of potential injury or death from a passenger seat air bag that could inflate in a severe car accident. In 2013, changes were made by car manufacturers regarding the use of LATCH (*Lower Anchors and Tethers for Children*) for older children using child restraints. This is important in the preschooler because, per the new guidelines, in general, if the combined weight of the car seat and child is more than 29 kg (65 pounds), LATCH should not be used. Instead of LATCH, the seat belt should be used. Each car seat and car manufacturer has slightly differing regulations, so parents are encouraged to have a certified car seat technician install their child's seat to ensure proper and safe installation. It is important to note that each province has differing laws regarding child safety restraints. However, these laws are often minimum requirements, are not updated often, and are not always reflective of best practice.

Nurses actively participate in health-promotion programs in communities and emergency departments that help families use car restraints correctly. Unfortunately, in one study, despite comprehensive nursing education and training programs during the postpartum period, car safety seat misuse was frequent (Rogers, Gallo, Saleheen, et al., 2013). When families have to consider financial constraints to comply with the requirements to restrain their children, nurses are often

the first line of information. Nurses provide information about resources available locally through agencies such as hospitals, health care provider's offices, United Way, Safe Kids Worldwide (2018), the fire department, and other community organizations.

Household furniture and fixtures also remain a hazard for preschoolers, as do structural features such as stairs and windows. A meta-analysis found that home safety interventions were effective in significantly increasing the proportion of families with fitted stair gates (Kendrick, Young, Mason-Jones, et al., 2013). Nursery and toy injuries decrease during the preschool years. Sports and recreational injuries increase in preschool children. This elevated incidence occurs because many preschoolers are involved in group sports, riding bicycles, and using playground equipment. Preschoolers need a broad range of play areas and experiences. Conscientious parents supply age-appropriate limits and supervision (Ingram et al., 2011; Price & Gwinn, 2012). Preschoolers lack the skill or judgement to ride bicycles in the street. They need instruction about safe use of playground equipment. Adult supervision of most preschooler activities, group sports in particular, is required to prevent injury.

Preschoolers begin to safely handle basic tools, kitchen equipment, and cleaning supplies. Children at this age take pride in participating in household projects with a supervising parent. They spend much of their time in the home and in the preschool or child care centre. The facilities pose the same potentially harmful environmental conditions as the home, as well as some additional threats to safety.

## Burns

Scalds and direct flame burns are major hazards for preschoolers. For many young children, thermal injury results in an emergency department visit or hospital admission (Ingram et al., 2011). Thermal injury (unintentional fire/burn) ranks among the top five causes of death from injuries in Canadian children from birth to 14 years of age (Safe Kids Canada, 2007). The number of deaths of preschool children in house fires is nearly double that of children of other ages. Children of this age experiment with matches and fire, and they may be unable to escape from a fire once it starts. The measures discussed in Chapter 12 to reduce scald burns in the home apply to this age group as well. Preschoolers should be taught about the dangers of matches, open flames, and hot objects. Parents and caregivers should model appropriate use of active and potentially dangerous burning devices. In a study of five emergency departments, the majority (58%) of thermal injuries were scalds from beverages (49.6%), domestic water (37.6%), and food (12.7%), most frequently caused by pull-down (48%) and spill (32%) mechanisms (Kemp, Jones, Lawson, et al., 2014). A meta-analysis found that home safety interventions were effective in significantly increasing the proportion of families with safe hot tap water temperatures, functional smoke alarms, and a fire escape plan (Kendrick et al., 2013).

## Drowning

Children older than 3 years are at lower risk of drowning in the bathtub, but at greater risk of drowning in a swimming pool, than the toddler. Drowning ranks among the top five causes of death from injuries in children up to 14 years of age (Safe Kids Canada, 2007). Preschool children aged 1 to 4 years are at highest risk of drowning, with two near-drowning episodes for every fatality. Most children are close to safety when drowning occurs. With this in mind, it is important to supervise young children when they are near a body of water, to install fencing to isolate a residential pool from the house, for young children to use personal floatation devices while bathing or playing near a natural body of water, and to teach children how to swim and that swimming alone is unsafe. Preschoolers should receive instruction in water safety and swimming, and should always be supervised by a trained adult or older person. The Canadian Paediatric Society suggests that at by 4 years of age and older, children should start swimming lessons (CPS, 2017). Because a good outcome depends on early resuscitation, it is reasonable to encourage parents and pool owners to learn cardiopulmonary resuscitation.

Preschoolers have the cognitive ability to learn water survival. They should always wear a personal flotation device or PFD (i.e., life jacket) when they are on boats, even when they know how to swim, and they must be supervised when near water, even shallow water. The CPS recommends the following strategies to prevent drownings: adult supervisor (one adult for every two young children), pool fencing, pool alarms, lifeguards, cardiopulmonary resuscitation training, swimming instructions, and PFDs (CPS, 2017; Weiss, 2010).

## Mechanical Forces

Bicycle accidents become a greater source of injury during the preschool years. Many bicycle accidents involve automobiles, and most of these accidents result from the child's errors. Parents should set reasonable and age-appropriate limits on bicycle use. An epidemiological study of nonfatal bicycle injuries seen by emergency departments (Chen, Dunn, Chen, et al., 2013) reported that 5.6% of patients were aged 0 to 4 years (110 injuries per 10,000) and 20.5% were aged 5 to 9 years (389 injuries per 10,000). In children aged 0 to 4 years and children aged 5 to 9 years, 17% and 39% of injuries involved a motor vehicle collision, respectively. For both age groups, in order of incidence, the three most common injured body parts were the face, head, and hands. The two most common locations of the injury were in the street (55.5%) and in the home (28.4%). Most injuries occurred during the summer months (in order of incidence, July, August, June). The transition from tricycle to bicycle provides an excellent time for a child to begin using a helmet. Federally approved bicycle helmets are effective in reducing head trauma, a major cause of death among young children. A study implemented an educational bicycle safety program for kindergarten-aged children and found that they were able to improve their knowledge of appropriate helmet-wearing technique (Cusimano, Faress, Luong, et al., 2013).

Preschoolers, as passengers or pedestrians, are at great risk of an automobile-related accident. At this age, pedestrian injury is more likely to occur than is passenger injury. Preschoolers should be taught proper street-crossing techniques and, generally, should be supervised when crossing streets. Schwebel, Davis, and O'Neal (2012) discussed risk factors for child pedestrian injuries, which include developmental factors (cognitive and perceptual), distraction, temperament and personality, social influences (parents and peers), environmental risks, attention-deficit/hyperactivity disorder, and sleep and fatigue. The prevention strategies reviewed include parental instruction, school-based instruction (including crossing guards), street-side training, technology-based training, and community-based training.

## ◆ Biological Agents

Preschoolers seem healthier than toddlers, with fewer illnesses of the respiratory and gastrointestinal tracts. They have developed antibodies to many common organisms through exposure. Children usually become ill more often when they enter their first group situation, where they may be exposed to new organisms. This concerns parents and should be discussed by the nurse before the child begins attending a group setting. Increasingly, child care settings provide instruction to children about appropriate handwashing techniques to decrease disease transmission and provide relevant health-promotion teaching (Rosen, Zucker, Brody, et al., 2011).

Immunization recommendations are reviewed annually by the National Advisory Committee on Immunizations (NACI) and updated with professional educational tools and parent-friendly resources. These resources for professionals and families can be found in a variety of formats, in both English and French, at https://www.canada.ca/en/public-health/services/immunization/national-advisory-committee-on-immunization-naci.html. NACI publishes the *Canadian Immunization Guide* with the most current recommendations, with a particular focus on the immunization needs of children. The 2018 recommendations can be found at https://www.canada.ca/en/public-health/services/canadian-immunization-guide.html. The child with a full course of immunizations as an infant receives repeated doses of diphtheria, tetanus, and acellular pertussis; measles, mumps, and rubella; and varicella vaccines between the fourth year and the sixth year (Government of Canada, 2018a). Most provinces require that all children in a school setting be fully immunized. In Canada, only 1.5% of children have not been vaccinated (PHAC, 2016). However, despite this high rate of vaccination, recently, there have been multiple outbreaks of measles, mumps, and rubella in Canada. Vaccine hesitancy is defined by the World Health Organization (2019) as a refusal or reluctance to vaccinate despite vaccines being available. Parents who choose not to immunize their children usually make this choice based on lack of confidence in the effectiveness or safety of the vaccines, a perceived low risk of their child acquiring the disease, and a lack of convenience and accessibility in obtaining the vaccines (Shen & Dubey, 2019).

Although vaccines provide an extremely safe way to combat communicable disease, issues about safety do arise. Because autism is often diagnosed around the same time a child is vaccinated, some parents have connected the onset of their child's autism with the vaccine. The CPS (2016) refutes this association and cites numerous studies that report no link between various vaccinations and autism (for more information see https://www.caringforkids.cps.ca/handouts/vaccines-common-concerns). The risk of consequences of the disease itself far outweighs any vaccine risk, but without first-hand experience with vaccine-preventable diseases such as measles, *Haemophilus influenzae* type b, or polio, families today may minimize their severity (Diekema, 2012). Nurses must remain informed about recommended vaccines, their schedule, and their risks and benefits, to provide accurate evidence-informed information to families.

Nurses who remain informed about the reasons for avoidance of immunization will be better able to increase parents' understanding of the possible consequences of omitting a dose. Incomplete immunization may also occur as a result of parental forgetfulness or procrastination. Mandatory immunization for school entry provides an effective incentive for these parents. Advances on the horizon include more combination vaccines to decrease the cost of administration. Noninjectable vaccines that could be inhaled or eaten would greatly enhance pediatric immunization programs with ease of administration and simplified storage.

Continued efforts to vaccinate all children are needed, especially children living in poverty, particularly in large cities, where they are traditionally undervaccinated (Diekema, 2012; Gilmour, Harrison, Asadi, et al., 2011). Nurses use immunization registry programs to consolidate records, to remind parents, to evaluate the person's scheduled program, and to analyze issues for a particular population. Registry programs avoid duplication and are of particular value for the preschool age group that may not be involved in day care or preschool with mandated immunization. The *Canadian Immunization Guide* publishes recommendations for individuals who have omitted doses for some reason. Routine and catch-up immunization schedules are provincially regulated and available through provincial public health units or the Government of Canada website (https://www.canada.ca/en/public-health/services/provincial-territorial-immunization-information/provincial-territorial-routine-vaccination-programs-infants-children.html). When immunizations have been omitted or delayed, the immunization schedule continues from the dose of the last vaccine. Parents should be fully informed about the potential side effects of immunizations.

## ◆ Chemical Agents

Preschoolers face exposure to environmental pollutants. The young child's skin area relative to body mass is twice that of an adult's, which increases the risk of toxicity. Environmental exposure has been implicated in the increased prevalence of learning disabilities because of the unique vulnerability of a child's brain to chemicals (Landrigan & Goldman, 2011; Trasande & Liu, 2011; Tucker, 2012). Disparities exist among populations with regard to their risk. Ethnicity, socioeconomic status, and geographical location all have an impact on the risk of exposure (Landrigan & Goldman, 2011).

Chemical agents of concern for toddlers, such as pesticides, lead, and passive smoke, continue to merit consideration in the preschool population. Preschoolers, however, become more independent and understand the concepts of safe and poisonous.

In Canada, poisoning is the fifth leading cause of injury deaths, hospitalizations, and emergency department visits, with approximately half of all poison exposures occurring in children younger than 6 years of age (Parachute Canada, 2019). Even though manufacturers enclose many children's medications in childproof packaging, the product may be administered incorrectly by the caregiver, or the child may experiment with another family member's colourful pills. For example, the medication used to treat attention-deficit/hyperactivity disorder, methylphenidate, poisons many children.

Many household products, medications, carbon monoxide, pesticides, lead, mercury, polychlorinated biphenyls, ethers, and poisonous plants pose hazards to preschoolers. Secondary smoke and lead exposure represent negative chemical influences on the growing child.

Preschoolers should receive verbal explanations about poisonous or dangerous substances, but parents cannot rely on preschoolers to remember instructions. Preschools and child care facilities often incorporate topics about environmental pollutants and dangerous substances into their curricula to promote the health of preschoolers. Information about poison control is widely available online through the Canadian Association of Poison Control Centres (http://www.capcc.ca/en). The toll-free Canadian Poison Centre number is 1-800-268-9017; however, it is recommended that individuals call their local poison control centre first. Information about provincial centres can be found at http://www.ontariopoisoncentre.ca/get-help-now/Canadian%20Poison%20Centres/-canadian-poison-centres.aspx.

Parents should teach children about the four forms of poison, which are *solids* (air fresheners, pills, vitamins, aspirin, lipstick), *liquids* (cleaning products, fuel, alcohol), *sprays* (furniture polish, oven cleaner, room deodorizer), and *invisibles* (carbon monoxide, space heater fumes). Communication with parents about environmental dangers remains a major role of the child care provider.

## Cancer

Childhood cancers are uncommon; however, they remain the most common disease-related cause of death (Canadian Cancer Society, 2019). Even though mortality has decreased, the incidence of brain and other central nervous system tumours has increased (Landrigan & Goldman, 2011). Acute lymphocytic leukemia (ALL), the most common childhood cancer, accounts for approximately 32% of the cases of cancer in children (Canadian Cancer Society, 2019). Although less common than other solid tumours, retinoblastoma merits attention because of the possible loss of vision. Remarkable advances in long-term survival of children with cancer have occurred. Early detection remains the key to successful treatment; therefore, early, aggressive efforts have been invested in detection programs. Some of the increases in the rates of diagnosis may be attributed to improved imaging techniques and early detection.

### Leukemia

The incidence of ALL rises from age 2 years, peaks at age 5 years, and diminishes through later childhood and adolescence. The dominant signs and symptoms of ALL appear suddenly, but often the child demonstrates a prodromal period of weakness, malaise, anorexia, fever, and tachycardia. Bone pain, petechiae, and hemorrhages after minor procedures such as dental extractions are encountered frequently. When an unexplained infection does not respond to management, suspicion should arise. Early detection and treatment of ALL has resulted in a marked increase in 5-year survival rates. Survival depends on the age at diagnosis, with the best survival rates occurring when diagnosis occurs during the preschool years (Hockenberry & Wilson, 2015).

With suspected leukemia, the nurse institutes secondary prevention strategies with an assessment that includes the following parameters:
- Examination of the cervical and peripheral lymph nodes
- Palpation and percussion of the liver and spleen
- Inspection of the skin for systemic signs of leukemia, such as pallor, purpura, petechiae, and chloroma, which is a localized tumour mass that has a greenish appearance and may be found in the skin, orbits, or other tissues in granulocytic forms of leukemia

- Inspection of the mouth for enlarged tonsils; hyperplasia of the gums; and red, friable gingivae
- Palpation of the sternum, bones, and joints for tenderness and pain

The rate of leukemia is higher in children with Down syndrome; therefore school nurses and public health nurses should monitor these children for early signs of the disease.

### Wilms' Tumour

Most cases of Wilms' tumour occur in children younger than 5 years. A strong correlation exists between Wilms' tumour and several congenital malformations. Genetic links may contribute to its occurrence in children with bilateral tumours and those who have family members with the disorder. When Wilms' tumour, aniridia (a congenital malformation of the iris of the eye), genitourinary malformations, and mental developmental delay occur together, the genetic association strengthens. However, survivors of Wilms' tumour that is unilateral at diagnosis possess a low risk of producing a child who will develop the disease. Information about the risk factors for Wilms' tumour is not definitive. The 5-year survival rates for children with this disease are excellent (Hockenberry & Wilson, 2015).

### Retinoblastoma

Even as the most common intraocular tumour in younger children, in Canada approximately 20 children are diagnosed with retinoblastoma each year (Canadian Cancer Society, 2019). Most of these children are younger than 5 years. Genetic mutations contribute to the incidence of retinoblastoma, usually causing the bilateral form of the disease. Even though the tumour is uncommon, the scientific work surrounding its diagnosis and management has resulted in many of the methods used for treatment of other cancers. Survival rates are excellent (Hockenberry & Wilson, 2015).

The history usually reveals a slow symptom progression. To determine risk factors, the following questions should be asked:
- Do tumours of the eye run in your family?
- If tumours of the eye run in your family, which relatives were affected and how were they treated?
- Have you noticed that your child has eye problems (crossed or lazy eyes or difficulty seeing)?
- Have you noticed any changes in your child's eyes?

Screening eye examinations for high-risk children include the following:
- Visual acuity
- Red reflex, which appears whitish with retinoblastoma (cat's eye reflex)
- Ophthalmoscopic findings
- Lid lag, which is found with exophthalmos
- Strabismus, by doing the cover-uncover test

The cat's eye reflex and strabismus are the most common signs of retinoblastoma. Any suspicious findings indicate referral for further evaluation.

### Neuroblastoma

Neuroblastoma, a cancer of the sympathetic nervous system, begins in the abdomen, primarily in the adrenal gland, approximately 70% of the time. The remaining 30% of cases originate in cervical, thoracic, or pelvic areas. Parodi, Merlo, Ranucci, and colleagues (2014) reported a connection between maternal characteristics and perinatal factors in patients with neuroblastoma. More than 90% of diagnoses occur by age 5 years. Unfortunately, many of the children have metastases when the cancer is identified. Frequently, symptoms of secondary distribution bring the child to the health professional. The survival rate for children in whom neuroblastoma is diagnosed during the preschool years is increasing, but in other age groups it has remained static. There is little convincing evidence of specific risk factors. Prenatal exposure to pesticides and hormones and use of certain medications suggest an increased risk (Landrigan & Goldman, 2011).

Cancer in a child can be frightening to parents, particularly if there is a strong family history of cancers of any kind. Early detection continues to be associated with increased survival rates. Secondary prevention programs should include the warning signs of cancer in children. Routine procedures, such as a bath, provide opportunities for parents to examine the child for physical symptoms of disease that are outlined in Box 13.5.

## Asthma

The incidence of asthma, a chronic inflammatory disorder of the airways, affects more children and youth than adults (Government of Canada, 2018b). The inflammation in this disorder contributes to a hyper-responsive airway, limited airflow, and respiratory symptoms that include breathlessness, wheezing, cough, and chest tightness. The causes include genetic predisposition, allergens such as animal dander or dust mites, exposure to tobacco smoke, low birth weight, and frequent respiratory infections early in life. Multiple factors contribute to exacerbation of asthma symptoms and can include high levels of exposure to tobacco smoke, pollutants, allergens, cold air, exercise, and chest infections. In addition to the generally known allergens of house mite dust and pet and rodent dander, cockroach particles have been implicated (Government of Canada, 2015).

## ❖ DETERMINANTS OF HEALTH

Many factors can have an influence on health. Determinants of health can include personal, environmental, economic, and social factors. They can influence the health of individuals in positive and negative ways. One example is income, individuals living in poverty have more negative health outcomes compared with those who are not affected by low income and poverty. Thus, when collecting health assessment data using a framework such as Gordon's Functional Health Patterns, it is important to include data related to the preschooler's social, economic, and physical home environment.

## ◆ Social Factors and Environment

Some preschoolers become involved with groups outside their families, such as group child care settings, church groups, or family involvement in other activities, by age 3 years. Other children of the same age experience little outside contact. A preschool setting introduces the child to a

wider social arena. Parents learn to release their child to encourage independent activity in a safe, supervised setting. Preschoolers test their independence, interactive skills, and self-discipline as they learn to function in a group. Preschool provides a transition to kindergarten and Grade 1, where group interaction skills are expected. Parents often select a preschool on the basis of geographical closeness to their home or a friend's recommendation, using the most practical

---

### BOX 13.5   Warning Signs That May Indicate Childhood Cancer

Cancer remains a leading cause of death in children younger than 15 years, second only to injuries.

**General**
- Sudden unexplained weight loss
- Persistent poor appetite
- Unexplained lack of energy
- Tires constantly
- Noticeably pale

**Leukemia or Lymphomas: "Liquid Tumours" (Cancer of the Blood, Blood-Making System, Lymph Nodes)**
- Anemia (fatigue, feeling cold, lightheaded, shortness of breath, pale)
- Persistent infections
- Fever
- Bruising without injury and purple or red patches appearing on the skin
- Loss of appetite
- Swollen glands (lymph nodes) unrelated to infection
- Persistent bone pain or limping
- Paleness of the lips, skin, nails, or lining of the eyes

**Brain Tumour**
- Headaches, frequently with early morning vomiting
- Vision changes (blurred or double vision)
- Dizziness
- Seizures
- Unexplained, persistent changes in behaviour
- Changes in mobility

**Kidney Tumours (Wilms, Tumor)**
- Lump in the abdomen or abdominal enlargement
- Blood in the urine
- Bulging of the eyes
- Unexplained, persistent cough or chest pain
- A firm mass in the muscles

**Make Bath Time Examination Time**
- These complaints or physical findings should be interpreted only as warnings of possible serious disease. When these warnings are present, you should consult your physician at once.
- Do not forget that your children must be examined by a health care provider every year. The earlier cancer is detected, the better the chances are for a cure. With current treatment methods of surgery, radiation therapy, and chemotherapy (administration of anticancer medications), the survival rate of children with certain forms of cancer has increased dramatically.

Source: American Cancer Society. (2019) *Types of Cancer that Develop in Children.* Retrieved from https://www.cancer.org/cancer/cancer-in-children/types-of-childhood-cancers.htmlchildcancersymptoms.

## BOX 13.6    Evaluating a Child Care Setting

Child care that meets the needs and expectations of parents will most likely ensure a happy preschooler as well. The questions that parents should consider in evaluating and choosing a child care setting include the following:

- Will my needs and those of my child be best met with a caregiver in a family home, commercial centre, or preschool, or by having a person come to my home to care for my child?
- What kinds of backup plans will I need or will be available if the provider becomes ill?
- What are my standards for nutrition, safety, sanitation, and health, and can these standards be met at the chosen child care facility?
- How important is it to my child to be with other children? How many children would be ideal for my child's socialization needs?
- What personality attributes and educational preparation do I desire in my child's caregivers? What attributes do I dislike, and how will I deal with these attributes to maximize the care given to my child? How important is caregiver stability to me? Can I comfortably communicate with the staff to collaborate with my child's learning?
- What educational philosophy do I want in the setting? What involvement do I wish to have in the educational mission of the facility?
- Do the hours of the facility meet my personal and professional needs? Is close access to my job or home important to me?
- How are the children grouped, and what is the caregiver-to-child ratio?
- Does the cost of the service meet my financial needs? Can I pay part-time fees during vacation or when my child is ill for a lengthy period?
- Is accreditation of the facility mandatory for me to use it?
- What is my internal response or my general feelings about the setting when I visit it before my child's enrollment? Are the caregivers interacting with and responsive to the children? Are the children happy and interactive? Are the children's individual needs addressed appropriately? Is the environment supportive of my child's care? Is discipline appropriate?

## DIVERSITY AWARENESS

### Preschool

Three groups of 36 Chinese children (each with a mean age of 61 months) were studied to identify cognitive abilities that might distinguish children at risk of dyslexia: teacher- or parent-reported (and health care professional–confirmed) language delay; family history of dyslexia; and not at risk.

The cognitive skills studied included syllable awareness, tone detection, rapid automated naming, visual skill, and morphological awareness. Compared with the control group, the language-delayed group of children scored significantly lower on all measures. Children in the familial risk group performed significantly worse only on tone detection, morphological awareness, and word recognition.

Testing these skills may be important assessment tools for diagnosing the risks of reading problems and may be associated with broader cognitive impairment as found previously in various Indo-European languages.

#### Reflective Question
- How would your own personal cultural values affect how you interpret the results of this study? Would it change the care that you provide to this population?

Source: McBride-Chang, C., Lam, E., Doo, S., et al. (2008). Word recognition and cognitive profiles of Chinese pre-school children at risk for dyslexia through language delay or familial history of dyslexia. *Journal of Child Psychology and Psychiatry, 49*(2), 211–218.

approach (Box 13.6). With many child care facilities and options now available, parents frequently visit and evaluate a number of settings to determine the most appropriate for their needs (Bower et al., 2008).

### Culture and Ethnicity

Family cultural heritage continues to shape preschoolers. Health-promotion assessment should adapt to cultural differences (Diversity Awareness). For example, a child who has never seen snow may not be able to know that it is cold. Unlike toddlers, preschoolers frequently ask why the family follows certain practices. These young children notice differences from one family to another. Their playmates may celebrate different holidays or practice family rituals different from their own. As preschoolers experience more activities outside their home, differences become more apparent. Discussion about the strength of cultural differences provides an excellent learning opportunity (Andrews & Boyle, 2015).

Preschoolers also notice ethnic differences in appearance and pronounce skin colours, eyes, and hairstyles as "pretty" or "ugly." The socialization process forms presumptions similar to those of their family or playmates. Parents and caregivers who teach and role model positive behaviours allow children to see differences in others as being positive rather than negative. Mass media influences on physical attractiveness also contribute and become more significant to the adolescent.

Certain cultures apply more pressure for children to assume responsibility for younger siblings or household tasks. Confusion develops in preschoolers when the family's culture differs from that of most playmates. Disciplinary approaches differ from culture to culture. Uncertainty also results when parents integrate their cultural background into the community standards but the grandparents adhere to traditional cultural practices, rituals, and child-rearing ideas.

### ◆ Levels of Policymaking and Health

Many safety-focused legislative bills have affected preschoolers: for example, the Canada Consumer Product Safety Act (CCPSA) includes safety requirements for children's toys and related products that pose risks for suffocation, strangulation, and other injuries (Government of Canada, 2019b). School issues, as discussed in Chapter 15, also affect this age group. The *Campaign 2000 Report Card on Child Poverty* (Campaign 2000 Report Card, 2016) reports that in Canada, 1 in 5 children live in poverty; furthermore, this rate increases to 40% of Indigenous children living in poverty. Family homelessness, homelessness amongst dependent children and youth, is a significant and unrecognized issue in Canada.

In Canada approximately 35,000 people are homeless every night. For every person who is absolutely homeless, there are at least three more who fall into the "hidden homelessness" category, which often includes families and children (Gaetz, Gulliver-Garcia, & Richter, 2014; Gaetz, O'Grady, Kidd, et al., 2016).

## Economics

Poverty influences preschoolers as it does any child. Unlike toddlers, preschoolers become more aware of family economic status. A preschooler may know that the family lacks money for toys but recognizes less the comprehensive limits to resources that influence the family lifestyle. In some cases, the family's financial history prevents attendance at preschool or influences exposure to expanded learning activities. Preschoolers realize money acquires food, toys, and clothes, but they do not yet have a concept of economic values. The child might trade an expensive item for a trinket that looks more interesting. A child who uses the earnings to buy something realizes that more must be earned to buy more things. The child thus begins to learn the concepts of earning and spending.

## ❖ NURSING APPLICATION

Preschoolers show much interest in the tools and procedures of a health screening examination (Price & Gwinn, 2012) (Box 13.7). These inquisitive children may play with the stethoscope, otoscope, and other diagnostic instruments. The nurse explains the tests in age-appropriate terminology and expects the child to cooperate for most of the visit. Preschoolers may show self-control during injections but definitely need a parent close by to offer support and encouragement. The nurse includes the preschooler in the history by directing questions about dietary intake and health practices, such as tooth brushing, favourite activities, and friends. At this age, children begin taking some interest in health, developing the cognitive maturity to learn many health-promotion skills that they will use for the rest of their lives.

---

### BOX 13.7 Health Promotion and Primary Prevention for Preschool Children

**Annually**
- Health history
- Height and weight
- Vision screening (age 3–4 years)
- Hearing screening
- Oral health screening
- Obesity prevention
- Developmental and behavioural assessment
- Physical examination

**Periodically**
- Immunizations based on recommended schedule
- Ensure currency of immunizations
- Diphtheria, tetanus, acellular pertussis
- Inactivated poliomyelitis vaccine
- Pneumococcal
- Measles, mumps, rubella
- *Haemophilus influenzae* type b
- Varicella
- Assess health inequalities and living conditions
- Screen for abuse and neglect

**Screenings for High-Risk Children**
- Lead
- Tuberculosis
- Cholesterol

**Anticipatory Guidance**
- Injury prevention
- Child safety car seat (age less than 5 years) or seat belt
- Lap and shoulder belt (age 5 years or older)
- Use helmet and avoid traffic when bicycling
- Smoke detectors, flame-retardant sleepwear
- Hot water temperature less than 49°C
- Window and stair guards, pool fence
- Safe storage of medications, toxic substances, firearms, matches
- Close availability of syrup of ipecac, poison control phone number
- Parents and caretakers trained in cardiopulmonary resuscitation
- Violence prevention
- Nutrition and exercise
- Limit saturated fats; maintain caloric balance; and emphasize grain, fruit, vegetable intake
- Regular fun physical activity
- Tobacco
- Effects of passive smoking
- Anti-tobacco messages

---

## CASE STUDY

### *Preschool Child: Ricky*

Ricky, age 4 years, arrives in the clinic with his mother. Ricky lives with his mother and father, who both work full-time, and his infant sister. Their extended family lives in a different city more than 200 km away. Both parents are of average height and in good health. Ricky's mother mentions that Ricky often expresses frustration, particularly in regard to food. Conflict over food occurs every day. Mealtime is a battle to get him to eat, unless his mother feeds him. Ricky's baby sister seems to tolerate all baby foods, but requires her mother to spoon-feed. Ricky's mother is quite frustrated and concerned that he will become malnourished.

**Reflective Questions**
- What additional assessment information would you collect?
- What questions would you ask, and how would you further explore this issue with the mother?
- In what ways does the distance of the extended family influence this family's approach to health promotion?
- What factors would you consider to determine whether malnourishment is a factor in this family?

## ◎ CARE PLAN

### Ineffective Coping in Preschool Child: Ricky

**Nursing Issue**

Inadequate coping resulting from parental feedback for regressive behaviours and lack of consistent limits and fulfillment of appropriate responsibilities

**Defining Characteristics**

- Parent verbalization of need for help
- Changes in the usual behaviour patterns of the child

**Related Factors**

- Inconsistent methods of parental discipline
- Inadequate impulse control
- Lack of social skills

**Expected Outcomes**

- The child will separate from his parents without incident (tantrum, crying).
- The child will join a community or church peer group activity.
- The child will perform one household task (picking up his toys) before bedtime every evening.
- The child will demonstrate independent self-care behaviours (feed himself).
- The parents will have clear, consistent, and age-appropriate expectations for behaviour.
- The parents will explain the rationale for limiting a socially unacceptable or unsafe behaviour as soon as it is displayed.

**Interventions**

- Discuss with the parents the process of growth and development and the child's need to learn how to compromise, take turns, and channel energy appropriately.
- Use a prescreening developmental questionnaire to validate general assessment data.
- Encourage the parents to leave the child in someone else's care while they go shopping or to see a movie.

- Encourage the mother to formulate a bedtime ritual with the child that does not include her sitting in his room until he falls asleep.
- Discuss with the parents and the child what "jobs" he can do at home and the expectation that they be performed daily.
- Suggest laying out the child's clothes so that he can dress himself. Set a time to be dressed, such as before or after a certain television program.
- Explore with the parents the availability of playgroups or community activities for the child.
- Encourage the parents to take the child to the neighbourhood playground so that he can meet and play with other children.
- Have the child help around the house alongside his parents. Specify "work" and "play" times.
- Encourage the parents to praise the child for age-appropriate behaviours, being careful not to bribe him to perform.
- Discuss the principles of discipline consistency, immediacy, realistic expectations, and clear explanations.
- Recognize the parents' frustration and encourage them to try different approaches, such as limited choices, diversion, and incentives ("when you finish your meat, we'll play a game").
- Suggest that the parents keep a diary of how long an approach was tried and how consistently the child responded.
- Discuss the decrease in appetite and reliance of food fads that typify the child's age. Review the principles of nutrition, timing of snacks, and ways of making food attractive to children.
- Refer the parents and the child to a dietitian for nutrition counselling.

**Evaluation**

- Parents make appropriate verbal, nonverbal, and eye contact.
- Parents demonstrate correct caregiver techniques.
- Parents verbalize intent to maintain relationships.
- Parents attend routine well-child care appointments.
- Parents provide developmentally appropriate play activities.
- Parents describe healthy ways to express frustration.

## ▮ SUMMARY

Schedules for preventive health care during the preschool years include visits at 4 and 5 years of age. Each visit includes an ongoing history; growth, physical, and developmental assessment; and discussion of age-appropriate developmental concerns.

In addition to the office or clinic contact, the nurse may consult with a preschool nurse or a nurse for a primary school and preschool. Early exposure to and reinforcement of health care information as part of preschool education lays a foundation for later healthy lifestyle habits, which influence overall societal health. Health as a curricular subject during the school-age years continues this focus. The school nurse's role in health promotion and prevention of illness is discussed in Chapter 14.

**Evolve Chapter Features**

http://evolve.elsevier.com/Canada/Edelman/healthpromotion/

- Review Questions

## REFERENCES

AllerGen. (2015). *New estimates of food allergy prevalence in Canada.* Retrieved from http://allergen-nce.ca/new-estimates-of-food-allergy-prevalence-in-canada/.

American Cancer Society. (2019). *Types of cancer that develop in children.* Retrieved from https://www.cancer.org/cancer/cancer-in-children/types-of-childhood-cancers.htmlchildcancer symptoms.

Andrews, M. M., & Boyle, J. S. (2015). *Transcultural concepts in nursing care* (7th ed.). Philadelphia: Lippincott.

Archibald, L., Joanisse, M., & Edmunds, A. (2011). Specific language or working memory impairments: A small scale observational study. *Child Language Teaching and Therapy, 27*(3), 294–312.

Becker, D. R., McClelland, M. M., Loprinzi, P. D., et al. (2014). Physical activity, self-regulation, and early academic achievement in preschool children. *Early Education & Development, 25*(1), 56–70. https://doi.org/10.1080/10409289.2013.780505.

Bower, J. K., Hales, D. P., Tate, D. R., et al. (2008). The childcare environment and children's physical activity. *American Journal of Preventive Medicine, 34*(1), 23–29. https://doi.org/10.1016/j.amepre.2007.09.022. [Seminal Reference].

Boyd, B. A., Odom, S. L., Humphreys, B. P., et al. (2010). Infants and toddlers with autism spectrum disorder: Early identification and early intervention. *Journal of Early Intervention, 32*(2), 75–98. https://doi.org/10.1177/1053815110362690.

Brown, W. H., Pfeiffer, K. A., McIver, K. L., et al. (2009). Social and environmental factors associated with preschoolers' non-sedentary physical activity. *Child Development, 80*(1), 45–58. https://doi.org/10.1111/j.1467-8624.2008.01245.x. [Seminal Reference].

Campaign 2000 Report Card. (2016). *A road map to eradicate child and family poverty.* Retrieved from http://campaign2000.ca/wp-content/uploads/2016/11/Campaign2000NationalReportCard2016Eng.pdf.

Canadian Cancer Society. (2019). *Childhood cancer statistics.* Retrieved from http://www.cancer.ca/en/cancer-information/cancer-101/childhood-cancer-statistics/?region=qc.

Canadian Paediatric Society (CPS). (2009). *Vision screening in infants, children and youth.* Retrieved from https://www.cps.ca/en/documents/position/children-vision-screening.

Canadian Paediatric Society (CPS). (2012). *Child and youth injury prevention: A public health approach.* Retrieved from https://www.cps.ca/en/documents/position/child-and-youth-injury-prevention.

Canadian Paediatric Society (CPS). (2016). *Vaccines: Common concerns.* Retrieved from https://www.caringforkids.cps.ca/handouts/vaccines-common-concerns.

Canadian Paediatric Society (CPS). (2017). *Water safety for young children.* Retrieved from https://www.caringforkids.cps.ca/handouts/water_safety.

Canadian Paediatric Society (CPS). (2018). *Healthy teeth for children.* Retrieved from https://www.caringforkids.cps.ca/handouts/healthy_teeth_for_children.

Canadian Paediatric Surveillance Program (CSEP). (2011). *Iron-deficiency anemia in children.* Retrieved from https://www.cpsp.cps.ca/uploads/publications/RA-iron-deficiency-anemia.pdf.

Canadian Society for Exercise Physiology (CSEP). (2017). *Canadian 24-hour movement guideline.* Retrieved from https://csepguidelines.ca/.

Carey, C. M. (2014). Focus on fluorides: Update on the use of fluoride for the prevention of dental caries. *Journal of Evidenced-Based Dental Practices, 14,* 95–102. https://doi.org/10.1016/j.jebdp.2014.02.004.

Center on the Developing Child at Harvard University. (2010). *The foundations of lifelong health are built in early childhood.* Retrieved from http://developingchild.harvard.edu/resources/the-foundations-of-lifelong-health-are-built-in-early-childhood/.

Chaput, J. P., Colley, R. C., Aubert, S., et al. (2017). Proportion of preschool-aged children meeting the Canadian 24-hour movement guidelines and associations with adiposity: Results from the Canadian health measures survey. *BMC Public Health, 17*(Suppl. 5), 829. https://doi.org/10.1186/s12889-017-4854-y.

Chen, W. S., Dunn, R. Y., Chen, A. J., et al. (2013). Epidemiology of nonfatal bicycle injuries presenting to United States emergency departments, 2001–2008. *Academic Emergency Medicine: Official Journal of the Society for Academic Emergency Medicine, 20*(6), 570–575. https://doi.org/10.1111/acem.12146.

Christensen, D. L., Bilder, D. A., Zahorodny, W., et al. (2016). Prevalence and characteristics of autism spectrum disorder among 4-year-old children in the Autism and Developmental Disabilities Monitoring Network. *Journal of Developmental and Behavioral Pediatrics: Journal of Developmental and Behavioral Pediatrics, 37*(1), 1–8. https://doi.org/10.1097/DBP.0000000000000235.

Clark, M. B., & Slayton, R. L. (2014). Fluoride use in caries prevention in the primary care setting. *Pediatrics, 134,* 626–633. https://doi.org/10.1542/peds.2014-1699.

Conti-Ramsden, G., & Durkin, K. (2012). Language development and assessment in the preschool period. *Neuropsychology Review, 22*(7), 1–18. https://doi.org/10.1007/s11065-012-9208-z.

Cusimano, M. D., Faress, A., Luong, W. P., et al. (2013). Evaluation of a bicycle helmet safety program for children. *The Canadian Journal of Neurological Sciences, 40,* 710–716.

Decina, L. E., & Lococo, K. H. (2005). Child restraint system use and misuse in six states. *Accident Analysis & Prevention, 37,* 583–590. https://doi.org/10.1016/j.aap.2005.01.006. [Seminal Reference].

Diekema, D. S. (2012). Improving childhood vaccination rates. *New England Journal of Medicine, 366*(5), 391–393. https://doi.org/10.1056/NEJMp1113008.

Division of Adolescent and School Health, & National Center for Chronic Disease Prevention and Health Promotion. (2011). School health guidelines to promote healthy eating and physical activity. *MMWR Recommendations & Reports, 60*(5), 1–78.

Dogra, S., Meisner, B. A., & Ardern, C. I. (2010). Variation in mode of physical activity by ethnicity and time since immigration: A cross-sectional analysis. *International Journal of Behavioral Nutrition and Physical Activity, 7*(10), 1–11. Retrieved from http://www.ijbnpa.org/content/7/1/75.

Driscoll, A., & Nagel, N. G. (2008). *Early childhood education: Birth–8: The world of children, families, and educators* (4th ed.). Upper Saddle River, NJ: Allyn and Bacon. [Seminal Reference].

Fleischer, D. M., Perry, T. T., Atkins, D., et al. (2012). Allergic reactions to foods in preschool-aged children in a prospective observational food allergy study. *Pediatrics, 130*(1), e25–e32. https://doi.org/10.1542/peds.2011-1762.

Fountain, C., Zhang, Y., Kissin, D. M., et al. (2015). Association between assisted reproductive technology conception and autism in California, 1997–2007. *American Journal of Public Health, 105*(5), 963–971. https://doi.org/10.2105/AJPH.2014.302383.

Freitag, C. M., Staal, W., Klauck, S. M., et al. (2010). Genetics of autistic disorders: Review and clinical implications. *European Child & Adolescent Psychiatry, 19*(3), 169–178. https://doi.org/10.1007/s00787-009-0076-x.

Frost, J. L., Wortham, S. C., & Reifel, S. C. (2008). *Play and child development* (3rd ed.). Upper Saddle River, NJ: Prentice-Hall. [Seminal Reference].

Gaetz, S., Gulliver-Garcia, T., & Richter, T. (2014). *The state of homelessness in Canada 2014.* Toronto: The Homeless Hub Press. Retrieved from https://www.homelesshub.ca/sites/default/files/attachments/SOHC2014.pdf.

Gaetz, S., O'Grady, B., Kidd, S., et al. (2016). *Without a home: The National Youth Homelessness Survey.* Toronto, ON: Canadian Observatory on Homelessness Press. Retrieved from https://www.homelesshub.ca/YouthWithoutHome.

Gagne, C., & Harnois, I. (2014). How to motivate childcare workers to engage preschoolers in physical activity. *Journal of Physical Activity and Health, 11,* 364–375.

Garrison, M. M., Liekweg, K., & Christakis, D. A. (2011). Media use and child sleep: The impact of content, timing, and environment. *Pediatrics, 128*(1), 29–35. https://doi.org/10.1542/peds.2010-3304.

Gilmour, J., Harrison, C., Asadi, L., et al. (2011). Childhood immunization: When physicians and parents disagree. *Pediatrics, 128* (Suppl. 4), S167–S174. https://doi.org/10.1542/peds.2010-2720E.

Gonzalez-Mena, J. (2012). *Child, family and community, family centered early care and education* (6th ed.). Upper Saddle River, NJ: Prentice-Hall.

Government of Canada. (2012a). *Child maltreatment: A "what to do" guide for professionals who work with children.* Retrieved from https://www.canada.ca/en/public-health/services/health-promotion/stop-family-violence/prevention-resource-centre/children/child-maltreatment-what-guide-professionals-who-work-children.html.

Government of Canada. (2012b). *Child maltreatment in Canada.* Retrieved from https://www.canada.ca/en/public-health/services/health-promotion/stop-family-violence/prevention-resource-centre/children/child-maltreatment-canada.html.

Government of Canada. (2012c). *Vitamin D and calcium—updated dietary reference intakes.* Retrieved from https://www.canada.ca/en/health-canada/services/food-nutrition/healthy-eating/vitamins-minerals/vitamin-calcium-updated-dietary-reference-intakes-nutrition.html#a7.

Government of Canada. (2015). *Asthma.* Retrieved from https://www.canada.ca/en/public-health/services/chronic-diseases/chronic-respiratory-diseases/asthma.html.

Government of Canada. (2016). *Childhood obesity.* Retrieved from health/services/childhood-obesity/childhood-obesity.html#a11.

Government of Canada. (2018a). *Canadian immunization guide.* Retrieved from https://www.canada.ca/en/public-health/services/canadian-immunization-guide.html.

Government of Canada. (2018b). *Asthma in Canada.* Retrieved from https://infobase.phac-aspc.gc.ca/datalab/asthma-blog-en.html.

Government of Canada. (2019a). *Canada's dietary guidelines.* Retrieved from https://food-guide.canada.ca/en/.

Government of Canada. (2019b). *Industry guide to Health Canada's safety requirements for children's toys and related products.* Retrieved from https://www.canada.ca/en/health-canada/services/consumer-product-safety/reports-publications/industry-professionals/industry-guide-safety-requirements-children-toys-related-products-summary/guidance-document.html#a2.

Healey, D. M., Flory, J. D., Miller, C. J., et al. (2011). Maternal positive parenting style is associated with better functioning in hyperactive/inattentive preschool children. *Infant and Child Development, 20*(2), 148–161. https://doi.org/10.1002/icd.682.

Hinkley, T., Salmon, J., Okely, A. D., et al. (2012). Correlates of preschool children's physical activity. *American Journal of Preventative Medicine, 43*(2), 159–167. https://doi.org/10.1016/j.amepre.2012.04.020.

Hoban, T. F. (2010). Sleep disorders in children. *Annals of the New York Academy of Sciences, 1184*(1), 1–14. https://doi.org/10.1111/j.1749-6632.2009.05112.x.

Hockenberry, M. J., & Wilson, D. (Eds.). (2015). *Wong's nursing care of infants and children* (10th ed.) St. Louis, MO: Mosby.

Houston, K. T., Mufioz, K. F., Bradham, T., et al. (2011). Newborn hearing screening: An analysis of current practices. *Volta Review, 111*(2), 109–120.

Ingram, J. C., Deave, T., Towner, E., et al. (2011). Identifying facilitators and barriers for home injury prevention interventions for preschool children: A systematic review of the quantitative literature. *Health Education Research, 27*(2), 258–268.

Joosen, K. J., Mesman, J., Bakermans-Kranenburg, M. J., et al. (2012). Maternal sensitivity to infants in various settings predicts harsh discipline in toddlerhood. *Attachment & Human Development, 14*(2), 101–117.

Kaakinen, J., Gedaly-Duff, V., & Hanson, S. (2010). *Family health care nursing: Theory, practice and research* (4th ed.). Philadelphia: F. A. Davis.

Kaerts, N., Van Hal, G., Vermandel, A., et al. (2012). Readiness signs used to define the proper moment to start toilet training: A review of the literature. *Neurology and Urodynamics, 31*(4), 437–440.

Kalpidou, M. D., Power, T. G., Cherry, K. E., et al. (2004). Regulation of emotion and behavior among 3- and 5-year-olds. *The Journal of General Psychology, 131*(2), 159–178. [Seminal Reference].

Kemp, A. ,M., Jones, S., Lawson, Z., et al. (2014). Patterns of burns and scalds in children. *Archives of Disease in Childhood, 99*(4), 316–321.

Kendrick, D., Young, B., Mason-Jones, A. J., et al. (2013). Home safety education and provision of safety equipment for injury prevention (review). *Evidence-Based Child Health: A Cochrane Review Journal, 8*(3), 761–939.

Kissin, D. M., Zhang, Y., Boulet, S. L., et al. (2015). Association of assisted reproductive technology (ART) treatment and parental infertility diagnosis with autism in ART-conceived children. *Human Reproduction, 30*(2), 454–465. https://doi.org/10.1093/humrep/deu338.

Kochanska, G., Koenig, J. L., Barry, R. A., et al. (2010). Children's conscience during toddler and preschool years, moral self, and a competent, adaptive developmental trajectory. *Developmental Psychology, 46*(5), 1320–1332. https://doi.org/10.1037/a0020381.

Landrigan, P. J., & Goldman, L. R. (2011). Children's vulnerability to chemicals: A challenge and opportunity to strengthen health and environmental policy. *Health Affairs, 30*(5), 842–850. https://doi.org/10.1377/hlthaff.2011.0151.

Langevin, M., Packman, A., & Onslow, M. (2009). Peer responses to stuttering in the preschool setting. *American Journal of Speech-Language Pathology, 18*(3), 264–276. [Seminal Reference].

LeBlanc, J. J., & Fagiolini, M. (2011). Autism: A "critical period" disorder? *Neural Plasticity, 2011*, 921680.

Lee, S. H., & Im, E. (2010). Ethnic differences in exercise and leisure time physical activity among midlife women. *Journal of Advanced Nursing, 66*(4), 814–827. https://doi.org/10.1111/j.1365-2648.2009.05242.x.

Liou, Y. M., Liou, T., & Chang, L. (2010). Obesity among adolescents: Sedentary leisure time and sleeping as determinants. *Journal of Advanced Nursing, 66*(6), 1246–1256. https://doi.org/10.1111/j.1365-2648.2010.05293.x.

Luby, J. B., Belden, A., Sullivan, J., et al. (2009). Shame and guilt in preschool depression: Evidence for elevations in self-conscious emotions in depression as early as age 3. *Journal of Child Psychology and Psychiatry, 50*(9), 1156–1166. https://doi.org/10.1111/j.1469-7610.2009.02077.x. [Seminal Reference].

Marshall, S., Golley, R., & Hendrie, G. (2011). Expanding the understanding of how parenting influences the dietary intake and weight status of children: A cross-sectional study. *Nutrition and Dietetics, 68*(2), 127–133.

May-Benson, T. A., Koomar, J. A., & Teasdale, A. (2009). Incidence of pre-, peri-, and post-natal birth and developmental problems of children with sensory processing disorder and children with autism spectrum disorder. *Frontiers in Integrative Neuroscience, 3*, 31. [Seminal Reference].

Mefford, H. C., Batshaw, M. L., & Hoffman, E. P. (2012). Genomics, intellectual disability, and autism. *New England Journal of Medicine, 366*(8), 733–743. https://doi.org/10.1056/NEJMra1114194.

National Sleep Foundation. (2011). *Children and sleep.* Retrieved from https://www.sleepfoundation.org/.

Nipissing District Developmental Screening (NDDS). (2019). *Looksee checklist.* Retrieved from https://lookseechecklist.com/en/.

O'Donoghue, L., Rudnicka, A. R., McClelland, J. F., et al. (2012). Visual acuity measures do not reliably detect childhood refractive error—an epidemiological study. *PLoS ONE, 7*(3):e34441.

Orton, E., Kendrick, D., West, J., et al. (2012). Independent risk factors for injury in pre-school children: Three population-based nested case-control studies using routine primary care data. *PLoS ONE, 7*(4):e35193. https://doi.org/10.1371/journal.pone.0035193.

Parachute Canada. (2019). *Poison prevention.* Retrieved from http://www.parachutecanada.org/policy/item/261.

Parodi, S., Merlo, D. F., Ranucci, A., et al. (2014). Risk of neuroblastoma, maternal characteristics and perinatal exposures: The SETIL study. *Cancer Epidemiology, 38*(6), 686–694. https://doi.org/10.1016/j.canep.2014.09.007.

Payne, J. (2012). *Supporting gender independent children and their families.* Retrieved from https://www.researchgate.net/publication/284552073_Supporting_Gender_Independent_Children_and_their_Families.

Pellegrini, A. D., & Smith, P. K. (1998). The development of play during childhood: Forms and possible functions. *Child and Adolescent Mental Health, 3*(2), 51–57. [Seminal Reference].

Phillips, D. A., Phillips, K. H., Grupp, K., et al. (2009). Sibling violence silenced: Rivalry, competition, wrestling, playing, roughhousing, benign. *Advances in Nursing Science, 32*(2), E1–E16. https://doi.org/10.1097/ANS.0b013e3181a3b2cb. [Seminal Reference].

Price, D. L., & Gwinn, J. F. (2012). *Pediatric nursing* (11th ed.). St. Louis, MO: Saunders.

Prior, M., Cini, E., Bavin, E. L., et al. (2011). Relationships between language impairment, temperament, behavioural adjustment and maternal factors in a community sample of preschool children. *International Journal of Language & Communication Disorders, 46*(4), 489–494.

Public Health Agency of Canada. (2016). *Vaccine coverage in Canadian children: Results from the 2013 Childhood National Immunization Coverage Survey (CNICS).* Ottawa: Public Health Agency of Canada. Retrieved from https://www.canada.ca/en/public-health/services/publications/healthy-living/vaccine-coverage-canadian-children-highlights-2013-childhood-national-immunization-coverage-survey.html.

Public Health Agency of Canada (PHAC). (2018). *Autism spectrum disorder among children and youth in Canada 2018.* Retrieved from https://www.canada.ca/content/dam/phac-aspc/documents/services/publications/diseases-conditions/autism-spectrum-disorder-children-youth-canada-2018/autism-spectrum-disorder-children-youth-canada-2018.pdf.

Roberts, M. Y., & Kaiser, A. P. (2011). The effectiveness of parent-implemented language interventions. A meta-analysis. *American Journal of Speech-Language Pathology, 20*(3), 180–199.

Robins, D., Fein, D., & Barton, M. (2018). *Modified checklist for autism in toddlers. Revised with follow up.* Retrieved from https://mchatscreen.com/wp-content/uploads/2015/09/M-CHAT-R_F_Rev_Aug2018.pdf.

Rogers, S. C., Gallo, K., Saleheen, H., et al. (2013). Can nurse education in the postpartum period reduce car seat misuse among newborns? *Journal of Trauma and Acute Care Surgery, 75*(4 Suppl. 3), S319–S323. https://doi.org/10.1097/TA.0b013e31829cba75.

Rosen, L., Zucker, D., Brody, D., et al. (2011). Enabling hygienic behavior among preschoolers: Improving environmental conditions through a multifaceted intervention. *American Journal of Health Promotion, 25*(4), 248–256. https://doi.org/10.4278/ajhp.081104-QUAN-265.

Rourke, L., Leduc, D., & Rourke, J. (2017). *Rourke baby record.* Retrieved from http://www.rourkebabyrecord.ca/pdf/RBR%202017%20National%20English%20-%20Black%20170926.pdf.

Safe Kids Canada. (2007). *Child and youth unintentional injury.* Retrieved from https://www.cssd.gov.nl.ca/publications/pdf/healthyliving/unintentional_injuries_child.pdf.

Safe Kids Worldwide. (2018). *Car seat safety tips.* Retrieved from http://www.safekids.org/car-seat.

Sandin, S., Hultman, C., Kolevzon, A., et al. (2012). Advancing maternal age is associated with increasing risk for autism: A review and meta-analysis. *Journal of the American Academy of Child & Adolescent Psychiatry, 51*(5), 477–486.

Scattone, D., Raggio, D. J., & May, W. (2011). Comparison of the Vineland adaptive behavior scales, second edition, and the Bayley scales of infant and toddler development, third edition. *Psychological Reports, 109*(2), 626–634. https://doi.org/10.2466/03.10.PR0.109.5.626-634.

Schwebel, D. C., Davis, A. L., & O'Neal, E. E. (2012). Child pedestrian injury: A review of behavioral risks and preventative strategies. *American Journal of Lifestyle Medicine, 6*(4), 292–302.

Selwyn, N., Boraschi, D., & Ozkula, S. M. (2009). Drawing digital pictures: An investigation of primary pupils' representations of ICT and schools. *British Educational Research Journal, 35*(6), 909–928. [Seminal Reference].

Shen, S., & Dubey, V. (2019). Addressing vaccine hesitancy: Clinical guidance for primary care physicians working with parents. *Canadian Family Physician, 65*(30), 175–181.

Shumway, S., Thurm, A., Swedo, S. E., et al. (2011). Brief report: Symptom onset patterns and functional outcomes in young children with autism spectrum disorders. *Journal of Autism and Developmental Disorders, 41*(12), 1727–1732. https://doi.org/10.1007/s10803-011-1203-3.

Snowdon, A., Hussein, A., & Ahmed, E. (2011). *Canadian National Survey on Child Restraint Use.* Retrieved from https://www.tc.gc.ca/media/documents/roadsafety/Child_Restraint_Survey_2010.pdf.

Trasande, L., & Liu, Y. (2011). Reducing the staggering costs of environmental disease in children, estimated at $76.6 billion in 2008. *Health Affairs, 30*(5), 863–870. https://doi.org/10.1377/hlthaff.2010.1239.

Tucker, P. G. (2012). *Principals of pediatric environmental health—course WB2089.* Washington, DC: US Department of Health and Human Services, Agency for Toxic Substances and Disease Registry. Retrieved from http://www.atsdr.cdc.gov/csem/csem.html.

Vriend, J., & Corkum, P. (2011). Clinical management of behavioral insomnia of childhood. *Psychology Research and Behavior Management, 4*(1), 69–79. https://doi.org/10.2147/PRBM.S14057.

Warren, J. J., Weber-Gasparoni, K., Marshall, T. A., et al. (2009). A longitudinal study of dental caries risk among very young low SES children. *Community Dentistry and Oral Epidemiology, 37*(2), 116–122. https://doi.org/10.1111/j.1600-0528.2008.00447.x. [Seminal Reference].

Water, T. (2011). Critical moments in preschool obesity: The call for nurses and communities to assess and intervene. *Contemporary Nurse: A Journal for the Australian Nursing Profession, 40*(1), 60–70. https://doi.org/10.5172/conu.2011.40.1.60.

Weaver, N. L., Brixey, S. N., Williams, J., et al. (2013). Promoting correct car seat use in parents of young children: Challenges, recommendations, and implications for health communication. *Health Promotion Practice, 14*(2), 301–307. https://doi.org/10.1177/1524839912457567.

Weiss, J. (2010). Prevention of drowning. *Pediatrics, 126*(1), e253–e262. https://doi.org/10.1542/peds.2010-1265.

World Health Organization. (2019). *Ten threats to global health in 2019.* Retrieved from https://www.who.int/emergencies/ten-threats-to-global-health-in-2019.

Wright, J. T., Hanson, N., Ristic, H., et al. (2014). Fluoride toothpaste efficacy and safety in children younger than 6 years. *Journal of the American Dental Association, 145*(2), 182–189. https://doi.org/10.14219/jada.2013.37.

Yoo, J., Slack, K. S., & Holl, J. L. (2010). The impact of health-promoting behaviors on low-income children's health: A risk and resilience perspective. *Health & Social Work, 35*(2), 133–143. https://doi.org/10.1093/hsw/35.2.133.

Yoshinaga-Itano, C. (2011). Achieving optimal outcomes from EHDI. *ASHA Leader, 16*(11), 14–17. https://doi.org/10.1044/leader.FTR2.16112011.14.

Zecevic, C., Tremblay, L., Lovsin, T., et al. (2010). Parental influence on young children's physical activity. *International Journal of Pediatrics, 2010,* 468526. https://doi.org/10.1155/2010/468526.

# 14

# School-Aged Child

*Tanya Spence, RN, MN, CNCCP(c)*

Originating US chapter by *Leslie Kennard Scott, MLDE, CDE, PPCNP-BC, APRN, PhD*

## INTENDED LEARNING OUTCOMES

*After completing this chapter, the reader will be able to:*

- Identify expected physical and developmental changes occurring in the school-age child.
- Explore stages of cognitive development of the school-age child, particularly its relation to academic skills and performance.
- Appraise relevant health-promotion needs and common health risk factors found in the school-age child.
- Analyze cultural, societal, peer influence, and stress on development in the school-age child.
- Describe common developmental problems that occur in the school-age child, including ways to assist parents in the management of these common problems.
- Determine strategies for family (parents) to improve self-concept, socialization abilities, and reduce stress in the school-age child.

## KEY TERMS

Astigmatism
Asthma
Attention-deficit/hyperactivity disorder (ADHD)
Auditory acuity
Auditory learners
Bullying
Child abuse
Chronic serous otitis media
Classifying and ordering
Concrete operation
Conservation
Coping strategies
Dental caries
Depression
Discipline
Disorders of arousal
Dyslexia
Encopresis
Enuresis
Gastroenteritis
Genomics
Human papilloma virus

Hyperopic (farsighted)
Hypertension
Individualized educational plan
Industry versus inferiority
Intelligence
Intelligence quotient (IQ)
Kinesthetic learners
Latchkey children
Learning disability
Lice
Limit setting
Malocclusion
Menarche
Meningococcal vaccination
Moral development
Myopia (nearsightedness)
Obesity
Orthodontic care
Ossification
Overweight
Pediculosis
Peer groups
Phonics

Preconventional
Puberty
Punishment
Scabies
Screen time
Self-concept
Self-discovery
Self-esteem
Sexual abuse
Sleep apnea
Sleep talking
Sleepwalking
Snellen chart
Socialization
Somatization
Standardized growth charts
Tooth eruption
Tympanograms
Visual acuity
Visual learners
Vision screening programs

### School-Age Bullying

Liam is 9 years old and has recently started demonstrating withdrawn behaviour. His mother reports "he used to enjoy school." Recently, he has mentioned wanting to stay home from school and has become apathetic regarding participating in school-related activities. Two weeks ago, his mother reports she began driving him to school. "He hasn't wanted to walk to school with his friends lately. I don't understand what is going on; he tells me 'it's nothing.'" He was performing well in school until this most recent grading period. His teacher has voiced concern that Liam seems "distracted" and is not participating in group work conducted in class. Liam's father has voiced frustration that he seems to be "losing" things too. "Earlier this week he lost his backpack. Last week it was a jacket."

- Is Liam's behaviour typical for a 9-year-old male child?
- How might a 9-year-old female child's behaviour differ from Liam's in this situation?
- As a health care provider, how might you guide this family in finding ways to address Liam's behaviour?
- How might you assist/counsel Liam on developing skills associated with resilience?
- Are there any further underlying issues that may be contributing to Liam's behaviour?

"The school-age years" is a span of time between a child's entrance to kindergarten and the beginning of adolescence, a range from 6 to 10 years of age. During this period observable differences in growth, development, and cognitive ability are prominent. Consider how different the child entering kindergarten is from the preadolescent, particularly the differences in size as well as mental ability. Children grow (physically) much more slowly during this period as compared with growth during infancy and adolescence. Fine and gross motor skills are being perfected, and mental abilities grow tremendously as the child learns to read, write, and compute mathematics, in addition to other topics of interest (Table 14.1). Relationships outside the family, including peer groups, are also developing during this phase of growth and development.

Most children are relatively healthy during this period. Health-promotion and health-maintenance strategies are important. During this period of development, children learn to accept personal responsibility and participate in the management of self-care tasks in the areas of personal hygiene, nutrition, physical activity, sleep, and safety. Nurses fill a significant role in the facilitation of parental roles and child roles in meeting growth, developmental, and self-care aspects of the school-age child (SickKids Staff, 2011).

## BIOLOGY AND GENETICS

A child's growth and development is influenced by genetic inheritance, nutrition, and the physical-sociocultural environments in which the child lives. School-age children have an overall slimmer appearance as compared with preschool children. Their legs are longer as compared with the rest of the body, allowing greater strength, balance, coordination, and fluidity of motion in running, jumping, climbing, throwing, and riding a bicycle (SickKids Staff, 2011).

### TABLE 14.1 Growth and Development
**Motor Development of the School-Age Child**

| Age (years) | Gross Motor | Fine Motor |
|---|---|---|
| 5 | Dresses independently<br>Runs well and jumps | Prints letters<br>Ties shoes, buttons<br>Draws triangle, square |
| 6–8 | Balances on one foot for 10 seconds<br>Can perform tandem gait<br>Pedals a bicycle<br>Is skilled in physical activities, running, skipping | Spreads with knife<br>Holds pencil with fingertip<br>Draws a person with three to six parts<br>Cuts and pastes<br>Aligns letters horizontally<br>Knows right from left |
| 8–10 | Has good body balance<br>Enjoys vigorous activities<br>Has increased coordination | Spaces words and letters with writing<br>Draws a diamond<br>Has good eye–hand coordination<br>Bathes self<br>Sews and builds models |
| 10–12 | Balances on one foot for 15 seconds<br>Catches a fly ball<br>May experience clumsiness from prepubertal growth spurt<br>Possesses all basic motor skills similar to adult | Writes well<br>Has skills similar to those of an adult |

Source: Ball, J. W., Bindler, R. C., & Cowan, K. J. (2013). *Child health nursing: Partnering with children & families.* Upper Saddle River, NJ: Prentice Hall.

Most body systems reach an adult level of function during the school-age years. Before 6 years of age, children use the diaphragm as the primary breathing muscle. After 6 years of age, thoracic muscles develop, and the respiratory rate slows to 14 to 24 breaths per minute (Moses, 2015). The school-age child's head circumference continues to grow. However, after age 5 years, head growth slows until puberty, at which time the head and brain reach adult circumference measurements (53–54 cm; 21 inches) (SickKids Staff, 2011). The heart slowly grows in size, and the heart rate slows to an average rate of 60 to 160 beats per minute, approaching that of an adult. Mean blood pressure is lower in this age group and is dependent on age, height, weight, and sex (Dionne, Harris, Benoit, et al., 2017). The gastro-intestinal system is maturing with increased stomach capacity, resulting in less need for snacks and decreased calorie needs as compared with the preschooler. Bladder capacity increases. The immune system is better able to produce an antibody–antigen response (Durani, 2015). By puberty, the endocrine system (with the exception of reproductive function) approaches adult capacity and function.

### Elevated Blood Pressure

The long-term effects of elevated blood pressure, hypertension, in adults are well known and documented. The realization that adult hypertension often begins in childhood has encouraged efforts to screen young children for elevated blood pressure. The Canadian Paediatric Society (CPS, 2016) recommends that children have their blood pressure measured every 1–2 years between the ages of 6 and 13 years old. In Canada, the prevalence of hypertension in children is 1–2% and is associated with obesity and sedentary activity patterns (CPS, 2016). There are data suggesting that the incidence of elevated blood pressure in children is decreasing and that obesity rates are stabilizing. Blood pressure among school-age children may vary and therefore should be compared with norms for age, height, and sex (Dionne et al., 2017).

Hypertension in children is defined as a systolic or diastolic blood pressure at the 95th percentile for age, height, and sex, measured on at least three separate occasions. A family history of hypertension or identification of an elevated blood pressure in a child mandates additional evaluation by the primary care physician. The strongest effect on blood pressure in obese children was found to be the body mass index (BMI). Height, weight, and BMI should be measured and calculated for all children during routine health visits (Dionne et al., 2017).

## Physical Growth

Although many children have "spurts" of growth alternating with periods of minimal growth, height and weight growth velocities assume a slower and steadier pace as compared with earlier years of growth. The school-age child gains approximately 5 cm (2 inches) in height per year and 2 to 3 kg (4.4–6.6 lbs) in weight per year until puberty, at which time growth rates increase. (Lourenco, Villamor, Augusto, et al., 2012). BMI correlates with body fat and has been linked to future obesity and poor health in children. Physical and emotional health problems can arise that include high blood pressure, type 2 diabetes, sleep apnea, bone and joint problems, low self-esteem, depression, and being teased or bullied by peers (Government of Canada, 2019a). BMI continues to increase through childhood and adolescence. BMI for age is recommended for screening children greater than 2 years of age to identify individuals who are potentially underweight, overweight, or obese (CPS, 2014). Indigenous children tend to be slightly larger and Asian Canadian children tend to be somewhat smaller than their counterparts of European descent, as plotted on growth charts that are believed to be standardized for various ethnic groups (World Health Organization [WHO], 2015a). Children with intellectual, developmental, genetic, or other disorders often have growth patterns that are different from healthy children. Before the onset of puberty there is little difference in size between boys and girls. However, toward the latter part of this developmental stage, girls tend to grow more rapidly in height and weight (Harding, 2015). A pre-adolescent increase in height and weight tends to occur at approximately 10 years of age in girls and 12 years of age in boys. However, maturation rates differ, resulting in a wide range of sizes in both boys and girls, particularly among those aged 10 to 12 years (Harding, 2015; Lourenco et al., 2012).

Girls tend to mature, enter puberty, and stop growing earlier than boys. From birth, girls tend to have more fat than boys, and after puberty girls have a greater percentage of body weight derived from fat. Adiposity has a direct correlation to puberty onset in girls, yet conversely relates to a delayed pubertal onset in boys (Bordini & Rosenfield, 2011).

School-age children tend to be concerned about their rate of growth, weight, time of menarche, and final height. These children need to understand that the timing and extent of their physical changes usually reflect their genetic inheritance. When one is assessing a child's height, weight, and BMI, and before referring to standardized growth charts, the height of the child's family must be taken into consideration. For more information, see https://www.cps.ca/en/tools-outils/who-growth-charts. For example, the child whose height is in the third percentile may have parents who are shorter than average. Shorter height can be expected because of the family's genetic composition. Likewise, although the average age of menarche is at approximately 12.7 years in Canadian girls, one study in 2010 shows that there is variation in the age of menarche depending on the province of residence, household income, and family type. (Al-Sahab, Ardern, Hamadeh, et al., 2010). With sufficient body fat to stimulate hormones needed for menses, girls can have their first menstrual period between age 11 years and age 15 years and still be considered normal. As a result of better nutrition and differences in lifestyle, girls appear to experience menarche earlier than did girls of 30 years ago (Harding, 2015). Although the school-age child experiences numerous physical changes before adolescence, changes in three physical areas are of particular interest: oral development, lymphoid tissue, and motor skills development.

## Oral Development

Teeth enable a person to speak, chew, and smile. They also help give the face shape and form. The school-age child appears to be constantly losing or gaining a tooth. Deciduous, or baby, teeth are usually lost in the same order in which they initially erupted. School-age children begin shedding their first teeth when they are approximately 6 to 7 years of age, and the process is complete with the loss of the second molars at 11 to 13 years of age. The first permanent teeth, the 6-year molars, erupt at 6 to 7 years of age and continue to erupt until the third molars (wisdom teeth) appear at approximately 17 to 22 years of age. The child aged between 6 and 13 years loses and gains approximately four teeth per year. A 13-year-old child should have 28 teeth, having lost 20 deciduous teeth (Peristein, 2013). When deciduous teeth erupt, only the crown is lost; the root has been reabsorbed in the developing permanent tooth. As the child's mouth becomes filled with the larger, permanent teeth, the shape of the jaw and the facial appearance normally change. Girls tend to experience earlier permanent tooth eruption than do boys (Canadian Dental Association, 2018).

The rapid change in the number and type of teeth and the uneven growth in the child's jaw may cause malocclusion, an unacceptable relationship of the teeth in one jaw to those in the other. Dentists evaluate children to determine if the cleaning happening at home is sufficient and if there are any identified problems that need to be addressed right away (Canadian Dental Association, 2018). Some children will grow out of any identified problems, but others may need orthodontic care and appliances (braces) to correct problems or improve their appearance. Peer reaction to braces is addressed as part of the teaching about body changes; this teaching may decrease problems with the child's self-concept or body image as a result of looking different. School dental programs include education about conscientious tooth care for the child who wears braces, because these frequently make brushing and flossing more difficult, especially for the school-age child who lacks manual dexterity.

Dental problems can have a devastating effect on children, and poor dental health can affect the psychological, functional, and social areas of a child's well-being (CPS, 2018a). A 2010 Canadian Health Measures Survey reported that 57% of Canadian children aged 6 to 11 years have had a cavity, and rates of dental cavities among children 2 to 4 years of age is increasing. In some Indigenous communities in Canada the prevalence of dental decay in children exceeds 90% (CPS, 2018a). In contrast to the publicly funded health care system in Canada, Canadians are largely responsible for financing their children's dental care. Up to 32% of Canadians have no third-party dental insurance and do not qualify for government subsidized programs that are available. Dental health has been identified as one of the most costly diseases in Canada and much of the burden of dental disease occurs in low-income families, Indigenous children, new immigrants, and children with special health care needs (CPS, 2018a).

### Lymph Tissue

Lymph tissue grows rapidly throughout childhood, reaching maximal size before puberty, after which it begins to decrease in size, most likely as a result of changes in the concentrations of sex hormones. The amount of lymphoid tissue of a child up to 10 years of age often exceeds that of an adult (Kanwar, 2015). This is most often reflected in the size of the tonsils. As a result, tonsils that appear pathologically enlarged to a parent can be normal for the child's age. Additional lymphoid tissue during the school-age period generally helps this group to have a stronger immune response than do younger and older children. This is a result of the immune system being activated by environmental antigens and exposure to common organisms (Kanwar, 2015).

### Motor Skills Development

Neurological, skeletal, and muscular changes combine to increase the child's overall motor abilities. With maturation of the nervous system by age 7 or 8 years, the brain's two hemispheres articulate to allow the child more control over and coordination with motor tasks.

The child grows taller because of lengthening of the long bones that continues into adolescence. Ossification, replacement of cartilage with bone, occurs throughout childhood but is not complete until adulthood (Jarvis & Luctkar-Flude,

2019). Therefore special attention must be paid to well-fitting shoes that protect the child's feet, ensure comfortable walking on different surfaces, and offer grip on smooth surfaces (Caring for Kids, 2018). Children at this age also need protective sports equipment and conditioning exercises before sports to prevent fractures and other injuries (HealthlinkBC, 2017.) However, the child builds new bony tissue during the entire period of childhood, which generally allows rapid healing of fractures. Overweight children typically have greater bone density as compared with their normal-weight peers. Although they have greater bone density, this does not translate into reduced risk of fractures and joint pain. Overweight children have more joint and muscle pain than their normal weight counterparts and are more likely to experience bone fractures, possibly due to greater fall forces or a greater tendency to fall (Nielson, Srikanth, & Orwoll, 2012).

Muscle mass also increases with muscle strength. During the school-age years, physically active boys are slightly stronger than girls, but this difference is not significant until adolescence. With these changes the child has the potential to perform more complex fine motor and gross motor functions but must practise to perfect these skills. Children willingly exercise their new-found skills and feel pride when others see their improved skill level when bike riding, tying shoes, and engaging in team sports, for example.

## ❖ GORDON'S FUNCTIONAL HEALTH PATTERNS

A public health nurse assigned to a school can be an integral and influential person for the school-age child. The nurse in the school enables children to attain optimal health, development, and learning potential. Gordon's functional health patterns can be used to comprehensively assess the school-age child.

### ◆ Health Perception–Health Management Pattern

The school-age child understands an abstract definition of health and sometimes the factors causing illness, but this understanding differs from that of an adult. Most school-age children perceive symptoms and show an ability to participate in health-promoting behaviours. Health-promoting behaviours taught at school and home must meet the school-age child's cognitive level (concrete operation) and moral level (external rules and forces) to be effective. Teaching strategies using cognitive, psychomotor, and affective senses can help children learn responsibility for their own health (Shroff, 2015). This knowledge provides an excellent foundation for health-promotion behaviours during the school years.

School-age children's understanding of illness is directly correlated with their cognitive development and follows a direct sequence of developmental stages. It is important for nurses to integrate the child's developmental views on illness because this has direct implications for plans related to health education. When specifically asked about their ideas on causes of illness, school-age children usually state the germ theory, the punishment theory, or the external forces theory. Although many younger school-age children know that germs play a role in illness, they have limited understanding of how germs work (Brogan, 2015). They may believe that a misdeed or misbehaviour caused their illnesses.

Various cultural influences may also contribute to a child's understanding of illness. Health care providers need to recognize that culture, ethnicity, and religion will influence the child's beliefs about health and illness. Sensitivity to differences between the child's cultural background and your own is important; you need to be aware of your own bias and values. Difference in both verbal and nonverbal communication will influence the care of the child (CPS, 2018b).

Parents, caregivers, nurses working in schools, and teachers teach health-promotion concepts, and they spend time monitoring and reinforcing preventive health practices, such as personal hygiene, dental care, and good nutrition. Role-playing, reading age-appropriate books, and modelling of health-promotion behaviours (e.g., washing hands) may also help children make the link between behaviour and improved health. Unfortunately, by imitating some caregivers, children can become passive, asking few questions, doing as they are told, and perpetuating poor choices. These responses may also be caused by children's developmental and cultural obligation to obey authority figures. Parents, caregivers, nurses in the schools, and teachers need to make commitments to demonstrate and teach healthy behaviours at home and in school; this helps children develop health values as part of their educational process toward reaching a healthy adulthood.

Counselling the child and the child's family on a broad definition of health, one that includes personal and environmental health and safety, requires an awareness of the school-age child's normal perceptions of health (Inman, van Bakergern, Larosa, et al., 2011). Public health nurses working in schools, in consultation with teachers, are in a prime position to use such information to present content in a manner beneficial to the school-age child's level of understanding. Topics may include some of the following content areas: cultural difference of causes and management of illnesses; causes of personal and environmental health problems; and critical issues affecting the school-age child's general health and self-esteem. A holistic and comprehensive approach with other public health, education, and community partners is required to address the health concerns of students. Health is viewed in the broad sense of physical, mental, emotional, and social health. According to a report published by the Community Health Nurses Initiatives Group in Ontario in 2015, nurses maximize their contributions in the school setting through promoting health with individual students, promoting health within the classroom, school-wide health promotion, and community-level health promotion. The Registered Nurses Association of Ontario (RNAO) has developed some Best Practice Guidelines to support and inform public health nurse practice within schools. Some of these guidelines include prevention of childhood obesity, establishing therapeutic relationships, crisis intervention, promoting asthma control, and enhancing healthy adolescent development.

## ◆ Nutritional-Metabolic Pattern

School-age children, like all people, need a well-balanced diet. Since children spend a large portion of their day at school, making healthy food choices is essential. Healthy school lunches and snacks provide children with the energy and nutrients they need to get through their day. *Canada's Dietary Guidelines* (Government of Canada, 2019a) recommends creating a healthy food environment for children. This includes limiting their exposure to highly processed foods and drinks and increasing their access to healthy food choices, including fresh fruits and vegetables. Involving children in planning and packing healthy lunches and snacks teaches them how to make good choices, improves their food skills, and makes children feel a part of the process.

School-age children often eat foods low in iron, calcium, and vitamin C, and foods that have a higher fat and sodium content than foods their parents ate when they were this age. There is a disjuncture between current dietary practices and recommended dietary intake of children. These behaviours place children at risk of poor nutritional habits, obesity, iron-deficiency anemia, and chronic illnesses such as diabetes and hypertension (Klish, 2015). The rates of unhealthy weights among children have risen steadily in recent decades, with 30% of children aged 5–17 years in Canada being overweight or obese today. If childhood obesity trends do not reverse, children today may have a shorter life expectancy than their parents (Canadian Medical Association, 2015). The public health nurse in the school can be an integral component and assume a leadership role in the education of school-age children on the health and cognitive benefits of consuming nutritional sound foods.

### Factors Influencing Food Intake

Access to food, the influence of mass media, and contemporary busy lifestyles play a role in poor food choices. A multitude of television and billboard messages pressure children to eat certain foods, many of which contain large amounts of salt, sugar, and calories. In 2018, the House of Commons passed the *Child Health Protection Act* (Bill S-228), which bans the advertising of certain foods and drinks to children under the age of 13 years, in an effort to reduce obesity rates (Government of Canada, 2019b). Marketing of food and drinks will become restricted, starting in 2021, and Health Canada will develop the regulatory guidelines to oversee this change.

Children are more sedentary than ever with the widespread use of television, video games, and electronic devices. In 2017, the CPS released guidelines on screen time, recommending that children over the age of 5 years of age have a 2 hour daily maximum of exposure (CPS, 2017a). Screen time refers to time spent with any screen, including television, video games, computers, smart phones, and tablets. A 2012 Canadian study found that children who watched an hour of television per day were 50% more likely to be overweight than those who watched less (Shenouda & Timmons, 2012). Watching television and online content exposes children to advertisements for unhealthy foods and can encourage snacking, which increases overall caloric intake. Screen time also reinforces sedentary behaviour, which, combined with increased food intake or unhealthy food choices, places children at increased risk for health problems (Hingle & Kunkel, 2012).

Although some school-age children willingly try new foods, many continue to dislike vegetables, fruits, casseroles, spicy foods, and iron-rich foods, and prefer a small range of foods. Some children may eat only raw vegetables and fruits and go through a phase of eating only one food at lunch, such as a peanut butter sandwich. These practices seldom hurt the child nutritionally.

Children frequently make their own after-school snacks and need supervision regarding the content. Daily consumption of foods high in vitamins A and C, fruits, and vegetables should be encouraged. With parental, caregiver, or teacher help and positive reinforcement, school-age children can learn to calculate nutrition needs, plan family meals, and eat better for their overall health. These activities also assist school-age children in developing wise decision-making practices, feelings of empowerment about health, and healthy food habits for the rest of their lives.

Healthy choices must be an available and an easily recognizable option. Some communities in Canada—specifically, northern, rural, and remote communities—may not have the same access to nutritious foods and are further challenged to adopt healthy eating practices. Social determinants of health, including income, also limit some families' abilities to effectively make healthy food choices (Government of Canada, 2011, p. 4).

Canadian families have such busy lives that they may eat few meals together. A positive environment for nutrition and socialization during a shared mealtime is important. Parents encourage positive food habits for each family member, and pressure to eat certain foods is avoided to prevent power struggles between the parent or caregiver and the child. A child's nutritional pattern usually reflects family patterns (Robson, Couch, Peugh, et al., 2016). For example, parents who skip breakfast tend to have trouble convincing their children to eat breakfast. Educating children as a group to eat healthy foods can be successful because of the powerful influence of a peer group (people of the same age, experience, and, usually, sex). The child whose friend is eating a chocolate bar usually prefers the same rather than an apple for a snack.

### Nutrition Education

Nutrition education incorporated into the general curriculum of school-age children throughout their educational experience is important. Despite evidence that the school can serve as an environment for nutritional health-promotion education, not all schools require nutrition education from kindergarten through Grade 12 (Cardoso da Silveria, Taddei, Guerra, et al., 2013). The World Health Organization stated that school policies and programs should support the adoption of healthy diets and physical activity. Public health nurses that work in schools, teachers, parents, and families need to be involved in achieving the objective of developing healthy habits in our children (WHO, 2008). Teachers and school personnel also serve as role models for optimal eating and exercise habits for children in their charge

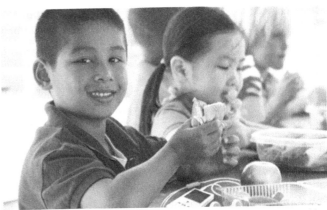

**Fig. 14.1** Children should be encouraged to eat plenty of vegetables and fruit daily.

The Government of Canada has established *Canada's Dietary Guidelines* (Government of Canada, 2019a), which are applicable for all ages. The daily nutritional needs include the following (Fig. 14.1):

- Eat plenty of vegetables and fruits, whole grain foods, and protein foods. Choose protein foods that come from plants more often. Choose foods with healthy fats instead of saturated fats.
- Limit highly processed foods. If you choose these foods, eat them less often, and in small amounts.
- Make water your drink of choice. Replace sugary drinks with water.
- Use food labels.
- Be aware that food marketing can influence choices.

Indigenous cultures in Canada sometimes have different food choices because of values and traditions of their culture. The Government of Canada has created a tailored food guide that reflects the importance of traditional food and how to incorporate these with store-bought foods. This food guide can be found at https://www.canada.ca/en/health-canada/services/food-nutrition/canada-food-guide/eating-well-with-canada-food-guide-first-nations-inuit-metis.html.

### Overweight and Obesity

Overweight and obesity are major nutritional problems that have reached alarming proportions among adults and children in Canada and the United States. The Expert Committee on the Assessment, Prevention, and Treatment of Child & Adolescent Overweight and Obesity lists the following definitions for use in children and adolescents (Barlow, 2017):

- Individuals 2 to 18 years of age with a body mass index (BMI) greater than the 95th percentile for age and sex or a BMI exceeding 30 kg/m$^2$ (whichever is smaller) should be considered obese.
- Individuals with a BMI greater than the 85th percentile, but less than the 95th percentile, should be considered overweight.

The problem of overweight and obesity in children and adolescents has increased significantly in the last 50 years. Childhood obesity is a major concern for parents, along with substance abuse and smoking. In Canada, obesity rates for children aged 2 to 17 years of age decreased slightly from 35% in 2004 to 30% in 2015 (PHAC, 2018). The percentage of boys who are considered obese (defined by a BMI over 30) is currently 14.5%, and for girls it is 9.5%. Evidence suggests that adult obesity begins in infancy or childhood and results from both genetic and environmental factors. For example, a child whose overweight parents constantly use food as a reward faces a greater risk of obesity than does a child of thin parents who do not reward the child with food. Excessive food intake and lack of physical activity also lead to obesity, and, once overweight, these children tend to exercise even less. Obesity occurs more frequently in Indigenous populations in Canada. There is no one data source in Canada for obesity among Indigenous populations, but the Government of Canada reports that obesity rates remain higher in indigenous populations compared with non-Indigenous populations: obesity among children and youth is high, varying from 16.9% among Métis to 20% among off-reserve First Nations, to 25.6% among Inuit (Government of Canada, 2006).

Being overweight increases the risk of hypertension, diabetes, sleep apnea, orthopedic problems, and heart disease. Experts believe that overweight and sedentary behaviours are the primary risk factors for the development of insulin resistance, hyperlipidemia, hypertension, type 2 diabetes, and heart disease (American Heart Association [AHA], 2015b; Nielson, Danielson, & Sorenson, 2011). There is also evidence that postprandial hyperinsulinemia may result in excessive weight gain (Klish, 2015). In addition, hormones released during the pubertal years make the situation worse in that these hormones cause the body to use insulin less effectively, leading to insulin resistance and thus increasing the risk of development of type 2 diabetes.

Current evidence suggests that being overweight is associated with obstructive sleep apnea. Whether each disease state increases the expression of the other is unclear (CDC, 2015a). The potential association between short sleep duration and childhood overweight has been described in the literature (Bonuck, Chervin, & Howe, 2015; Research for Evidence-Informed Practice). Longer sleep durations are associated with higher degrees of activity, which may assist with weight loss. Recent findings support the proactive approach of ensuring adequate sleep in the prevention of overweight in children.

The overweight and obese child faces ridicule by peers and discrimination later in life. These responses reinforce an already low self-esteem and poor body image and cause a cycle of personal isolation that influences a child's success, current and future (Griffiths, Parsons, & Hill, 2010; Klish, 2015). Helping the overweight and obese child change lifestyle patterns requires intensive intervention, including the support of parents. Even with these interventions, few overweight children achieve or maintain significant weight loss because of the complexity of factors (environmental, cultural, economic, and psychological) involved. In addition, there are reports that failure to maintain weight loss may be associated with impulsivity behaviours (Van den Berg, Pieterse, Malik, et al., 2011). Some success has been achieved by programs that include implementation of reasonable

## RESEARCH FOR EVIDENCE-INFORMED PRACTICE

### Sleep Duration Relation to Overweight in Children

The purpose of this study was to better describe the association between short sleep duration or sleep problems with childhood overweight. Emerging research has introduced the association between sleep and the regulation of many physiological functions, including energy balance, appetite, and weight maintenance. The researchers sought to determine if the association of short sleep duration and overweight in children existed while controlling the data for measures such as quality of the home environment, parenting, and child behaviour problems.

A longitudinal study of 785 children and their parents who were enrolled in the US National Institute of Child Health and Human Development Study of Early Childcare and Youth Development was conducted. Data were collected regarding BMI, sex, and socioeconomic status in Grade 3 and Grade 6 students. Questionnaires regarding sleep and home environment were completed by the participant's mother at the same time intervals.

The findings revealed an association between short sleep duration in Grade 6 and overweight in Grade 6. Shorter sleep duration in Grade 3 was independently associated with overweight in Grade 6, regardless of the child's weight in Grade 3. For every additional hour of sleep in Grade 6, the child was 20% less likely to be overweight in Grade 6. For every additional hour of sleep in Grade 3, the child was 40% less likely to be overweight in Grade 6. Sleep problems were not associated with overweight in children.

Adequate sleep duration in childhood may offer a protective effect on weight maintenance and overweight risk in children. One preventive approach to overweight in children may simply be to ensure adequate sleep in childhood.

Source: Lumeng, J., Somashekar, D., Appugliese, D., et al. (2007). Shorter sleep duration is associated with increased risk for being overweight at ages 9 to 12 years. *Pediatrics, 120*(5), 1020–1029.

caloric restriction; eating a variety of low-fat and low-cholesterol foods; and use of diet support groups, physical exercise, peer counselling groups, and habit changes (AHA, 2015a,b). However, intervention sometimes fails because some school-age children do not show concern about being overweight. Nursing suggestions for parents who are interested in preventing obesity in their school-age children are given in Box 14.1.

## ◆ Elimination Pattern

Most children have full bowel and bladder control by 5 years of age. Control involves the ability to undress and dress, to wipe and flush, and to clean hands. The child's elimination patterns are similar to the adult's, with urination occurring six to eight times a day and bowel movements averaging one or two times a day. For some school-age children, however, elimination continues to be a problem.

### Enuresis

Involuntary urination at an age when control should be present is called enuresis (Kaneshiro, 2016; National Health Service, 2015). Children with primary enuresis have never achieved bladder control, and those with secondary enuresis have periods of dryness and recurrent enuresis. Involuntary nocturnal urination (bedwetting) that occurs at least once a month is defined as nocturnal enuresis, and wetting during the day has been termed

## BOX 14.1 Nursing Interventions to Prevent Overweight/Obesity During the School-Age Years

- Make social and physical environments where children learn and play more supportive of physical activity and healthy eating.
- Encourage parents to be a role model for their child—be active; plan physically active family outings.
- Limit the amount of time spent watching television, playing video games, and using the computer/Internet.
- Look at ways to increase the availability and accessibility of nutritious foods and decrease the availability and accessibility of foods and beverages high in fat, sugar, and/or sodium.
- Encourage the family to assess "fast food" consumption and explore/ develop eating habits that support a healthier diet as defined by *Canada's Dietary Guidelines*.
- Encourage the child to participate in food/meal selection and preparation.
- Support lunch choices that meet overall healthy nutrition intake.
- Identify the risk of overweight and obesity on children and address it early.

Source: Government of Canada. (2011). *Curbing childhood obesity: A federal, provincial and territorial framework for action to promote healthy weights*. Retrieved from https://www.canada.ca/content/dam/phac-aspc/migration/phac-aspc/hp-ps/hl-mvs/framework-cadre/pdf/ccofw-eng.pdf.

diurnal enuresis. Enuresis should be considered not a disease but a variation of normal development. Enuresis affects 7% of boys and 3% of girls at 5 years of age (Goldberg, 2014).

Nocturnal enuresis causes disruption for both the child and the family. The child may frequently experience teasing from classmates and siblings. It can have profound effects on life socially, emotionally, and behaviourally. Although many forms of enuresis do not pose any significant health risk, there are social stressors. A night away from home appears impossible because of fear of wetting. Parents may be angry about the frequent bed changes and laundering and may try punishments, thinking that the child should be able to control the problem. Parental stress places additional pressure on the child, who may already have low self-esteem and lack self-confidence as a result of a perceived inability to control the problem (Pillinger, 2015).

Often because they lack information, frustrated families seek help. Many therapies exist, yet require a high degree of motivation from the child and parents. Their views must be taken into consideration when one is considering various treatment options. In addition to providing information, the nurse provides active support to facilitate coping. If a child does not have a urinary tract infection, various forms of management may be considered. These include wet alarm systems, bladder training and retention control, waking schedules, medication therapy, and hormone therapy. Each method has advantages, disadvantages, and cost considerations, but all require consistency and time from the child and parents, as well as positive reinforcement by the parents, to reach a successful outcome (Pillinger, 2015).

Diurnal enuresis is often called intermittent incontinence. This term describes a urinary pattern most often seen in school-age girls. These children may demonstrate "holding on" behaviours resulting in daytime incontinence, intermittent voiding, and straining before voiding (Austin et al., 2016). It is not clear why children delay urination or empty their bladders only partially, thus promoting overflow incontinence. Evaluation of these children begins with a urine culture to rule out urinary tract infection. If no infection exists or symptoms persist after treatment, then the intervention is focused on increasing fluid intake to prevent "holding" and establishing a voiding routine of every 2 hours, with a conscious effort to empty the bladder completely. The nurse can be instrumental in helping the child and parents understand the problem and its management.

### Encopresis

Another elimination problem that may occur in children is encopresis, defined as the persistent voluntary or involuntary passing of stool into the child's underpants after age 4 years. In most cases the problem has no discernible physiological cause and is not related to laxative use. There may be a history of inconsistent toilet training or early life stress in affected children. Encopresis is a common complication of chronic constipation. More than 90% of children with encopresis have a history of recent constipation and/or painful bowel movements (Barron, 2015). Once children become constipated or have hard and painful stools, they begin to hold their bowel movements to prevent further pain. This creates a cycle that leads to fecal impaction and rectal distension. Stool then begins to leak around the impaction and leaks through the child's rectum, often without the child's knowledge. In most cases, soiling occurs during the day when the child is awake and active. Soiling at night is uncommon.

Encopresis is often associated with recurrent abdominal pain and, for many, enuresis as well. Often these children have emotional difficulties that began before or resulted from encopresis. They experience poor peer relationships and self-esteem, perhaps attributable to their offensive odour. Awareness of this childhood problem is necessary to appropriately identify the affected child, refer the child for treatment, and support the child and the family during a bowel management program and counselling.

### ◆ Activity-Exercise Pattern

Physical activity in children is an important aspect of health and an integral component of health promotion. Childhood is considered to be a critical time in which regular physical activity behaviours are acquired and fostered (Fig. 14.2). Generally, the school-age child is naturally active, although many do not meet current activity recommendations (CDC, 2015b; Craggs, Corder, van Sluijs, et al., 2011). Boys are typically more active than girls (Fig. 14.3). In addition, those who perceive their neighbourhood as unsafe or do not have at least one parent who exercises are less likely to exercise themselves. Physical activity and participation in sport activities tends to decrease with age, particularly among girls. The CPS (2018c) recommends that children aged 5–11 years accumulate at least 60 minutes of exercise daily, including vigorous-intensity activities and activities that strengthen muscle and bone at least 3 days per week.

As previously discussed, impressive changes in motor skills occur between the age of 6 years and the age of 12 years, allowing the child to engage in many activities that develop strength,

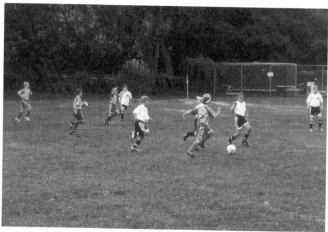

**Fig. 14.2** Peer play is important during the school-age years.

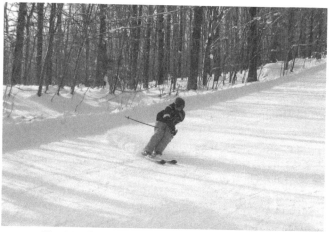

**Fig. 14.3** Boys are typically more active than girls.

balance, and coordination (see Table 14.1). Exercise typically occurs through group activities and organized sports such as hockey and soccer, through individual activities such as gymnastics and ballet, and through unorganized play such as bike riding, sledding, rollerblading, and imaginary play. Play provides important learning and health promotion, and for this reason should be encouraged consistently during the school-age years. For many children, involvement in physical activities is fun and connects them to their peers, family members, and other important people in their lives (Milteer, Ginsburg, & Mulligan, 2012).

Play activities also promote social, personal, and cognitive development. School-age children frequently prefer interacting with peers rather than with the family. This desire for peer interaction, usually with one of the same sex, extends beyond school and carries over to play and outside activities. A child's skill in motor tasks wins the respect of other children and provides a feeling of self-accomplishment (CDC, 2015c). Organized sports, such as hockey, teach team cooperation, competition, and other social skills. Concerns exist that young children have experienced too much physical and psychological pressure to perform in sports. This has generated a renewed commitment by many parents to focus more on the fun of sports than on the winning of games (Craggs et al., 2011). Organized activities such as

Scouts and 4-H clubs teach children about group functioning, processes involved in performing a task, and the power of social relationships to create change. These lessons can prepare them for the discipline needed for a job later in life. Overall, children who perform well in these activities feel good about themselves and their competence, and enhance a sense of industry. Parents and teachers who compliment children when they perform well enhance self-esteem as well.

As part of play, school-age children incorporate new cognitive skills, including the ability to count and sort objects. Children of this age express pleasure in their collections of stamps, rocks, or other objects. Understanding the concepts of fair and consistent rules found in games requires cognitive skills of memory, logical reasoning, and the desire to work with others. Many children like to read, which provides ideas about life and cultures that differ from their own, thereby enhancing their acceptance of human diversity. The nurse helps parents promote healthy play activities for children by encouraging the following (CDC, 2015c):

- Family activities that focus on physical activity and togetherness between parents or caregivers and children
- Use of a library card to encourage reading on a variety of topics and to teach responsibilities involved with borrowing
- Monitoring of daily television and computer use that detracts from physical activity and more active mental activities
- Encouragement of both group and solitary activities to support the child's overall development

## ◆ Sleep-Rest Pattern

### Sleep Patterns

Most school-age children have no difficulties with sleep. Generally, their sleep requirements and patterns are more similar to those of an adult than those of a younger child. Individual needs vary on the basis of activity, age, and state of health, but most school-age children sleep between 10 and 12 hours a night without naps during the day (American Academy of Sleep Medicine, 2014; Gupta, 2014). Unlike younger children, school-age children experience few difficulties with going to bed. Most children and parents can agree on a bedtime with some flexibility on non-school nights and adhere to that agreement. When problems arise regarding bedtime, children may be testing parents who have not been clear and firm about their expectations for their children going to bed or have not been willing to discuss the arrangement with their children (Boyse, 2010). Although many Canadians accept the idea that school-age children should sleep in their own beds, some other cultures encourage the family or siblings to sleep together (Martin, 2013; Queensland Health, 2014). In the school-age child, bed-sharing does not have any impact on sleep patterns, nor does it show any long-term effects toward health, positive or negative (Boyse, 2010).

### Sleep Disturbances

The most common sleep problems that occur during the preschool and early school-age years are night terrors (see Chapter 13), sleepwalking, sleep talking, and enuresis. As a group, these disturbances have been called disorders of arousal (Boyse, 2010) and share the following characteristics:

- They occur immediately before a rapid eye movement state of sleep.
- Most occur 1 to 2 hours after going to sleep.
- There is a family history of sleep problems; boys experience more sleep problems than girls.
- Problems reflect normal central nervous system immaturity of the child.
- Problems may be influenced by fatigue and stress within the child.
- Problems do not involve the respiratory system.

Approximately one in six children (15%) aged 5 to 12 years has sleepwalked at least once, but far fewer children walk in their sleep persistently. Sleepwalking is most likely due to the brain's inability to regulate sleep–wake cycles because of immaturity of the central nervous system. It occurs more often in boys and often occurs with enuresis (Gupta, 2014). Shortly after going to sleep, the child may suddenly sit up in bed, make repetitive finger and hand movements, or walk, usually for a short time. In most cases, however, the child stays in bed. The child may mumble when talking to a parent or other person (sleep talking). The words tend to be simple but unclear to the listener. Often the child falls back to sleep quickly after talking or walking (Boyse, 2010; Robinson, 2014).

Parents who are concerned about sleepwalking or sleep talking need to know that most children outgrow these episodes with central nervous system maturation. However, parents should protect their child from injury by placing gates at the top of stairs and removing sharp objects from the child's path. Most parents find that the easiest solution is to direct the sleepwalker back to bed, where the child returns to a normal sleep. Occasionally, parents can intervene effectively by implementing relaxation techniques for their child before bedtime, avoiding stressful and fatiguing situations, and providing consistency with sleep preparation patterns (American Academy of Sleep Medicine, 2014; Boyse, 2010). If children have many episodes of sleepwalking or sleep talking, or if parents express particular concern, they may need further evaluation and treatment by health care providers.

## ◆ Cognitive-Perceptual Pattern

The school-age child spends extensive time in settings that require mastery of new ideas and concepts. The child's basic intelligence, heredity, and environment encourage or discourage learning. Mastery of ideas and learning requires intact senses, such as vision, hearing, language, and memory capabilities that allow cognitive development and acquisition of skills needed for later life success (Goswami, 2015). Unfortunately, many children in society lack these capabilities and will have learning problems if these are not identified early through parental awareness, school observations, or routine health care assessments. For further information about school-age tests or procedural preparations, see http://www.nlm.nih.gov/medlineplus/ency/article/002058.htm (Kaneshiro, 2014).

## Piaget's Theory

Piaget (2001) refers to the age span of 7 to 11 years as the period of concrete operations, a stage when children learn by manipulating concrete objects and lack the ability to perform thinking operations that require abstraction. During this time the child moves from egocentric interactions to more cooperative interactions and increased understanding of many concepts gained through environmental connections (Hanfstingl, Benke, & Zhang, 2019). Children increasingly change their reasoning from intuitive to logical or rational operations (rule-governed actions) and engage in serial ordering, addition, subtraction, and other basic mathematical skills. The operations of this period are termed concrete because the child's mental operations or actions still depend on the ability to perceive specific examples of what has happened. Older school-age children use both concrete and recently acquired abstract operations, which add flexibility and control to their thinking and meet developmental needs of adolescence. Unlike the egocentric preschooler, a school-age child begins to take the other person's point of view into account. This trait does not emerge suddenly. The new skill appears occasionally and then more frequently as the child's mental capacity and experience grow.

During the school-age period, the child understands a number of expanding concepts regarding objects, including the concept of conservation of substance (Hanfstingl, Benke, & Zhang, 2019). When asked if a difference exists in the amount of liquid poured into two glasses of different shapes, the preschool, preoperational child focuses on the different shapes and says "yes." The concrete operational school-age child realizes that no change has occurred in the amount of the liquid despite the change in shape. Conservation of numbers, weight, volume, and quantity, required to understand basic mathematics, sequentially develops as the school-age child gains chronological age and experience.

The concept of time also develops during this period. Children begin to learn to tell time and understand the passage of time. By age 8 years, most children understand the difference between past and present, and history becomes meaningful. The concept of human aging becomes increasingly understandable, and the child can comprehend the difference between an 18-year-old person and an 80-year-old person.

Two major operations of the school-age period are classifying and ordering. The child classifies or groups objects by their common elements and understands the relationship between groups or classes. For example, when given 12 wooden beads, some brown and some white, the child understands that the beads may be grouped by their colour and by their material. Conversely, the preschool child focuses only on one property of the beads, such as colour. The newfound ability to classify objects shows in the school-age child's interest in collections, such as stamps or coins (Hanfstingl, Benke, & Zhang, 2019). Children in school frequently "order" their world; they line up in school according to height, they repeat numbers and letters in their classic order, and they receive numbers in school to reflect an alphabetized surname. These two operations (classifying and ordering) must exist to learn to read, understand the concepts of numbers, and learn subjects based on relations, such as history (the relation of events in time) and geography (the relation of places in space).

## Vision

The child's sensory abilities continue to develop during the school-age years. Visual capacity should reach optimal function by the sixth or seventh year (Heiting, 2015). Peripheral vision and the ability to discriminate fine colour distinctions should be fully developed as well. Although many 4 year olds have 20/20 vision, a school-age child should have a visual acuity of at least 20/30 in each eye, as measured by the Snellen chart, an assessment tool for children who can read some letters (Segre, 2015).

Physiological changes occur in the eye during the school-age years. Eyes in the preschool years are normally hyperopic (farsighted), a condition in which the visual image of an object falls behind the retina. However, unlike older individuals, preschool children do not need glasses because their eyes normally accommodate by adjusting their lenses. For most children, vision becomes normal as the shape of the eye changes and lengthens with maturation. However, many school-age children need visual correction to prevent academic difficulties and headaches and dizziness when reading or doing close work. The peak incidence of hyperopia diagnosis in school-age children is at approximately 6 years of age (Castagno, Fassa, Carret, et al., 2014).

Twenty-five percent of school-age children have visual problems. In Canada, most provinces provide coverage for regular eye exams for children. Vision screening programs for school children are intended to help identify those children who have or may potentially have a vision problem that may affect physiological or perceptual processes of vision or that could interfere with school performance. Vision screenings are not diagnostic, nor do they lead to treatment, but rather only indicate a potential need for further care. The nurse in the school is in an optimal position to ensure eye screenings are performed, and encourages parents of children with deficits to seek further optometric care to correct these defects so that these children can learn more effectively.

Two visual problems are common in the age group of the school-age child. Many school-age children inherit myopia (nearsightedness), a condition in which the visual image of an object falls in front of the retina, causing the child to have difficulty seeing distant objects. The other condition, astigmatism, causes blurred vision because the image is focused poorly on the retina because of changes in the surface of the cornea or lens. Eyeglasses correct the defects, but the problem must be identified before it can be solved. For example, a child with myopia may not realize that their visual images are impaired. Children with corrective lenses often express delight and surprise when they first see the fully focused and rich detail of the world after experiencing less-refined visual acuity for some time.

## Hearing

The child's hearing ability (auditory acuity) is nearly complete by 7 years of age, although some maturation continues into adolescence. Hearing deficits occur less frequently than visual deficits, but hearing loss affects up to 8% of youth aged 6 to 19 in Canada (Statistics Canada, 2016). This deficit compromises learning in school and important socialization with peers. Chronic serous otitis media, or long-term fluid in the middle ear, remains a common cause of hearing deficit in both the preschool years and the early school-age years (American Academy of Otolaryngology, 2015). New concerns about the potential for long-term hearing loss in children who listen to loud music have been raised.

All school-age children, especially those with a history of recurrent ear infections or fluid behind the eardrum, should have periodic hearing evaluations (National Institute on Deafness and Other Communication Disorders, 2012). Various treatments exist for acute otitis media, including antibiotics and the recent discovery that xylitol gum may be of some preventive benefit (Azarpazhooh, Lawrence, & Shah, 2011). Work continues on a vaccination for prevention of otitis media infections. Tympanograms, used to measure the sensitivity of the tympanic membrane to vibrations induced by pressure and sound waves, help detect and monitor this problem as part of well-child and ill-child care (American Academy of Audiology, 2011). By providing education on hearing protection for school-age children, the school nurse plays an important role in the maintenance of this important sense for the future.

## Sensory Perception

Children learn simultaneously through many senses, and most teaching approaches incorporate this concept. For example, young school-age children see a letter, hear its sound, and feel its shape. With this approach, children learn in a number of ways to interpret an event (Willingham, Hughes, & Doboly, 2015). For example, some children learn best by listening (auditory learners), others by doing (kinesthetic learners), and others by engaging all sensory modalities (auditory, kinesthetic, and visual learners). Because no two children have exactly the same sensory acuity, sensitivity, or discrimination, all children build slightly different perceptions and conceptions of the world around them and do not follow the same timetable to grasp concepts. Therefore, teaching approaches must be individualized to meet the learning needs of most children.

Of all the senses, visual perception has been studied the most, primarily because of its role in helping children learn to read. Studies have examined children's abilities to discriminate parts of a picture (to see a figure within a picture). Children usually progress from the preschool stage, during which they perceive visual stimuli more as a whole, to the school-age stage, during which they perceive more details, and finally to the point at which they perceive and integrate both. This process helps children recognize letters; the first step needed for reading. Children may first be able to differentiate between obviously different letters, such as "h" and "o," but may have difficulty with letters similar in appearance, such as "b" and "d," until they can distinguish details more effectively.

## Language

Language develops rapidly during the school years. Most school-age children enter this period with an ability to understand and speak a language, but with only a basic knowledge of reading and writing. By the end of the school-age period, most children have acquired at least a functional ability in both areas. Language development mandates that a child has visual perception for reading, auditory acuity and perception for understanding spoken language, and fine motor skills for both articulation and handwriting.

The full capacity to imitate sounds develops during the childhood years. Between 6 and 7 years of age, the child shows the ability to produce proper articulation for most vowel and consonant sounds. However, some have difficulty expressing sounds for "s," "l," "z," "sh," "ch," and "r." By 7 years of age the child should be able to articulate all sounds for speaking, and by age 12 years has a vocabulary of approximately 4000 words. Understanding of the syntax (grammar) and semantics (meaning) of language continues to develop. The child uses more complex sentences and understands multiple meanings for the same word and metaphors. The child should be able to recognize and correct spelling and grammatical errors by 8 or 9 years of age. The capacity to learn foreign languages is at an optimal level at this stage and provides the rationale for foreign language instruction during the school-age years. Foreign language instruction also provides children with information about other cultures and an opportunity to understand people who are different from themselves.

Much of the child's time in school focuses on learning to read and write. Learning to read is a complex process, beginning with letter and sound recognition (American Academy of Pediatrics [AAP], 2015a). Letters combine to form words that the child must learn to decode. Words combine to form sentences, and so on. Most children need help from teachers, peers, parents, or older children to learn to read effectively. Some researchers believe that children learn best by sounding out the individual letters of a word (phonics), whereas others think that learning the word as a whole unit is better. Both processes have value, and likely a combination of both is most effective (AAP, 2014). Considering the wide range of processes that support development of reading skills (conceptual, perceptual, verbal, and motor), it is not surprising that most children experience some difficulty in learning to read (AAP, 2014).

Handwriting requires eye–hand coordination, motor control, and perceptual abilities (Harron, 2014). Primarily a motor skill, handwriting does not reflect mental capacity. Many bright children and adults have poor handwriting, and vice versa. Boys tend to have more problems with legible handwriting than do girls. Writing style does not approach adult-level maturity until the end of late childhood, but the handwriting should reflect the child's handedness. No reversal of letter outlines should occur by age 7 or 8 years, and the relative size of letters should be uniform. By age 8 or 9 years, letter strokes should be firm, even, and flow with ease. The individual who has difficulty with handwriting may use a typewriter, computer, or graphics to produce a satisfactory written product. Tutoring by a handwriting specialist can help children with dyslexia, a term defining the tendency to reverse the normal appearance of letters and numbers in writing.

## Memory

Memory abilities, both short term and long term, improve for school-age children. Strategies such as organizing, classifying, and labelling information help them retain information. Rehearsal, repeating an item to be learned, is also a helpful memorization strategy. At age 5 years, children use rehearsal when someone suggests or models it; at age 10 years, they rehearse spontaneously. Memory abilities improve with practice and through various strategies, such as placing the words that need to be remembered in a song or by rhyming words (Raghubar, Barnes, & Hecht, 2010).

## Intelligence

Intelligence tests assess a person's mental abilities and compare them with the abilities of other people through the use of numerical scores. Although the term "intelligence" is used as if there is agreement on what it means, in reality there is much debate as to how this term should be and has been defined. For example, debate has surrounded whether intelligence should be considered an inherent cognitive capacity, an achieved level of performance, or a qualitative construct that cannot be measured. Psychologists have debated whether intelligence is learned or inherited, culturally specific or universal, or one or several abilities (Kendler, Ohlsson, Turkheimer, et al., 2015). Although these debates are ongoing, evidence is increasing that traditional intelligence tests measure specific forms of cognitive ability that are predictive of school functioning but do not measure the many forms of intelligence that are beyond these more specific skills, such as music, art, and interpersonal and intrapersonal abilities.

The concept of intelligence usually conveys an ability to think and process information learned earlier in life. Scores on an intelligence test should measure the child's basic abilities as compared with those of others of the same age and experience level and, ideally, should predict performance in school or society. However, this is not always the case. Intelligence test scores tend to differ because each test, or each form of the same test, measures slightly different samples of abilities and reflects the test author's philosophy on intelligence. It is important to note that some intelligence tests may be culturally insensitive (123test, 2012). For example, the words on the test may not be part of an ethnic group's usual vocabulary, causing children to miss these items on an intelligence test.

Canada does not routinely use intelligence testing for children; however, children may take achievement tests that measure the amount of information learned in a specific area and offer insight into a child's overall intelligence. Although intelligence and achievement tests should measure different issues (basic ability versus learned achievement), their results correlate well. Some researchers believe this correlation exists because both tests actually measure the same thing (achievement, notability).

Reports from intelligence and achievement testing differ. Intelligence tests usually provide a number that represents intelligence quotient (IQ). An IQ of 90 to 110 is considered average (BMJ Best Practice, 2015). Achievement tests compare the child's performance with that of other children and report scores as percentiles. For example, a score in the 20th percentile of a test means the child scored better than only 20% of other children of the same age in that skill. The Wechsler Intelligence Scale for Children (WISC), which assesses cognitive functioning in verbal comprehension, visual-spatial ability, working memory, processing speed, and fluid reasoning in children aged 6–16 years, can be used to identify giftedness, learning disabilities, or general cognitive strengths and weaknesses (Hrabok et al., 2014). Scores on the five WISC subscales can be combined and converted into a Full Scale Intelligence Quotient (FSIQ), which is designed to measure overall intelligence.

Current beliefs accept that people inherit some of their intelligence but that environmental factors also influence opportunities for learning and overall intelligence. Most likely, the greatest environmental influence is socioeconomic, reflected in the correlation in scores: children from low-income families tend to score lower on intelligence tests than do children from middle-income or high-income families. The reason for this probably relates to many subfactors, such as nutrition, language, parental reinforcement and encouragement, and sociocultural environmental stimuli.

### Learning Disabilities

According to Statistics Canada, 3.2% of Canadian children have a learning disability, and the years when children transition for home to school are a key time to assess children and provide accommodations to support their learning needs (Learning Disabilities Association of Canada, 2017). Many terms and definitions have been used to describe the impairments of children who have normal or above-normal intelligence and usually do not have visual, hearing, or motor handicaps or emotional problems, yet have difficulties in school learning (Disabled World, 2015). Some children have minor, almost unnoticeable difficulties, whereas other children are so impaired that they appear to be mentally delayed until their impairment has been diagnosed and they have been helped. An individual child may have more than one developmental disorder. Some children will develop behaviour and self-esteem problems as a response to their inability to function satisfactorily (BMJ Best Practice, 2015).

One well-known condition that causes difficulty in the child's adjustment to the school setting is attention-deficit/hyperactivity disorder (ADHD), a disorder that reflects developmentally inappropriate degrees of inattention, impulsiveness, and hyperactivity (AAP, 2011a). ADHD is the most common neuro-behavioural disorder of childhood and among the most prevalent chronic health conditions affecting school-age children. Frequently, these children have high energy, intuitiveness, and creativity, personal characteristics that help them succeed in some facets of their lives. Despite diagnostic criteria for ADHD developed by the American Psychiatric Association (2013), the problem has been difficult to assess, primarily because the child manifests symptoms in varying degrees in different settings and with different people (Box 14.2). Some symptoms associated with ADHD have been identified as changes to the *DRD4* gene (Dadds, Schollar-Root, Lenroot, et al., 2016). Current ADHD guidelines recommend using nonpharmacological interventions as part of

---

### BOX 14.2 Diagnostic Criteria for Attention-Deficit/Hyperactivity Disorder

Diagnosing a child with attention-deficit/hyperactivity disorder (ADHD) is a process with several steps and can be difficult. The first step for families is to speak with a health care provider. Diagnosis can be made by a primary care provider, like a pediatrician or nurse practitioner, or a psychologist or psychiatrist (CDC, 2018). A diagnosis of ADHD uses the criteria outlined in the *Diagnostic and Statistical Manual of Mental Disorders (DSM-5)* that outlines essential behaviours over a broad age range. The CPS has questionnaires, rating scales, and screening tools that are completed by the health care provider, family, and educators. A diagnostic evaluation consists of several visits to a physician or nurse practitioner, a detailed history, in-depth evaluation of the family and child, and the engagement of schools to ensure appropriate diagnosis (CPS, 2018d). To ensure adequate diagnosis, the DSM-5 outlines core symptoms and characteristics of ADHD. In addition, the child must demonstrate that:

- Symptoms are severe, persistent (present before 12 years of age and >6 months), and inappropriate for the child's age and developmental level.
- Symptoms are associated with impairment in academic achievement, peer, and family relations and adaptive skills.
- If there is a discrepancy of symptoms across settings, it is important to identify why the discrepancy exists.
- Specify the type of ADHD presentation as either combined presentation (criteria are met for inattention, hyperactivity-impulsivity), predominantly inattentive presentation (criteria are met for inattention), or predominantly hyperactive-impulsive presentation (criteria are met for hyperactivity-impulsivity).
- Specify current severity (mild, moderate, or severe), based on the symptoms and degree of functional impairment.

Source: Canadian Paediatric Society. (2018). *ADHD in children and youth: Part 1—etiology, diagnosis and comorbidity*. Retrieved from https://www.cps.ca/en/documents/position/adhd-etiology-diagnosis-and-comorbidity.

---

### GENOMICS

#### *Medicine in Children*

Clinical genome sequencing and exome sequencing technologies are becoming promising tools for determining genetic causality of numerous diseases in children, including cystic fibrosis, asthma, autism spectrum disorders, and childhood cancers. Genomic medicine is looking to find genetic mutations that drive various disease states so as to yield new targets against which novel therapies may be developed (Downing, Wilson, Zhang, et al., 2012). The next generation of medical treatments and therapies are being designed to better improve outcomes for many childhood conditions. Nurses are well positioned to incorporate genetic and genomic information across all aspects of health care. This translation of clinical, medical research technologies into practice is not without challenges (Thiffault & Lantos, 2016). However, nurses have an opportunity to close the gap between research and therapeutic developments.

Sources: Downing, J. R., Wilson, R. K., Zhang, J., et al. (2012). Pediatric Cancer Genome Project. *National Genetics, 44*(6), 619–622; Thiffault, I., & Lantos, J. (2016). The challenge of analyzing the results of next-generation sequencing in children. *Pediatrics, 137*(Suppl), 83–87.

---

the treatment plan for children and adolescents (CPS, 2018d). The *Canadian ADHD Practice Guidelines* (Canadian ADHD Resource Alliance [CADDRA], 2018) recommend medication treatment in only the more severe cases, with a more holistic approach taken in Canada, individualized to the child. ADHD is a chronic medical condition and requires long-term planning by health care providers. There are five tiers for intervention outlined by the CADDRA: adequate education of children and their families; behavioural interventions; psychological treatment; educational accommodations; and medical management. One novel therapy that has demonstrated a sustained treatment effect when treatment is completed and withdrawn is neurofeedback (Van Doren, Arns, Heinrich, et al., 2019). Neurofeedback is a noninvasive and safe non-pharmacological complementary and alternative therapy that uses a brain–computer interface to promote self-regulation of brainwave activity, which leads to improved attention and focus. Screening is completed by caregivers, teachers, and health care providers to compare results, confirm diagnosis, and develop the appropriate course of treatment for the child. ADHD and learning disorders often coexist and can mimic one another. ADHD can also exist with other conditions such as depression, anxiety, and aggression. Appropriate assessment of the child is crucial to help target treatment correctly (CADDRA, 2018). These interventions may also be successful in management of ADHD-affected adults. However, with the use of genomics, new treatments and therapies may be developed to better match the needs of the individual with ADHD (Dadds et al., 2016; Genomics).

The nurse's role with the child who has a learning disability is varied. The nurse may participate in detection of the problem and consultation during evaluations, collaborate with the school administration on implementation of a treatment plan and referral to resources, assist as a liaison between school and home environments, and be a source of instruction for both the child and the family to improve overall development and the family's adaptation to meet the needs of this unique child.

In Canada, the Canadian *Charter of Rights and Freedoms* makes it clear that every individual in Canada, regardless of physical or mental health disorder, is to be considered equal and must have the same access to all government programs (Government of Canada, 2018a). This means that students are to be instructed among those who are not disabled and to the maximal extent appropriate for the student's needs.

The nurse plays a vital role in promoting the school-age child's overall cognitive and perceptual health, helping to prevent problems in these areas. The nurse must talk to parents and school administration personnel about any child who has language articulation problems beyond 6 or 7 years, because this child should be evaluated by a professional. The nurse helps parents understand their child's level of cognitive and sensory abilities so that learning expectations are realistic. Through educational materials sent to the child's home or provided during school meetings, the nurse may address the socialization needs and development of school-age children. The nurse also needs to help parents understand common tests used for child intelligence and achievement screening (Atherton, 2013). In addition, the nurse helps evaluate a child believed to have a learning disability when the child may actually have a health problem, general immaturity, or an environmental deficit (poverty or divorce; Krause-Parello & Samms, 2010).

## ◆ Self-Perception–Self-Concept Pattern

Through each of the developmental processes of physiological growth, cognitive development, and social development, children progressively engage in an important process of self-discovery. Through these processes, children actively build and create their own personalities, develop relationships with others, and expose themselves to a wide range of experiences that influence their behaviour, attitudes, and values.

### Erikson's Theory

The stage of personality development described by Erikson for the school-age child is industry versus inferiority. The major task to be accomplished is full mastery of whatever the child is doing (sense of industry). The child focuses on success in personal and social tasks and avoidance of a sense of inferiority. Inferiority occurs with repeated failures at attempted tasks and with little encouragement or trust from people important to the child. With mastery of the tools of the culture in relation to those of the peer group, a sense of worth and understanding of the self develops (Erikson, 1993, 1994).

### Self-Concept

Self-concept develops over time and through a variety of experiences and relationships. For example, by being responsible for a pet's care and by showing love to this animal, the older school-age child nurtures a positive self-concept. The way in which others, especially peers, view the child influences the sense of self (Ferrer & Fugate, 2014; Sturaro, van Lier, Cuijpers, et al., 2011). Increasing cognitive abilities facilitate better understanding of the identifying factors of others (ethnicity, disability, or gender) and how those others compare with the child. Self-concept includes self-esteem, sense of control, and body concept.

***Self-esteem.*** Self-esteem has been defined as the extent to which an individual believes oneself to be capable, significant, successful, and worthy (AAP, 2015b). The younger school-age child has a limited self-concept, but one that develops with successful completion of the tasks of this period (Erikson's sense of industry). Although engaged in more activities outside the home, the child still depends on the family, as defined by one's culture, to develop high self-esteem. In school, teachers or group leaders frequently reward those who have succeeded in a task with badges, stars, or privileges (tangible objects that validate success).

The peer group's influence on the school-age child's self-esteem is unquestionable. Acceptance by a peer group contributes to feelings of self-worth and a sense of belonging to a desired group. Competition or collaboration with peers in school, clubs, and activities also influences feelings of adequacy and feelings of success (Women's & Children's Health Network, 2013). Parents must be encouraged to expose their school-age children to interesting activities of their choice, involving peers, to nurture their self-esteem and sense of uniqueness.

Concern has been voiced about school-age girls suffering a decline in self-esteem that affects their school achievements. Some research indicates that boys receive more praise in school than do girls, and girls receive criticism on the content of their work, whereas boys receive more criticism on the appearance of their work (Garey, 2015). Girls experience greater competition now than in earlier times, and they face pressures about personal appearance. Various authors report that girls need strong adults to support their ways of thinking and behaving in a world often built on "male values." Girls tend to have high self-esteem if they perceive parental harmony that supports perceptions of balance within themselves and promotes their emotional health (Garey, 2015).

In encouraging development of self-esteem in all school-age children, the nurse remembers that a child needs to experience success with tasks, and completely structured activities may not provide this opportunity for some children. A child who succeeds in some things and receives acceptance by peers gains a sense of competence and worth, is self-confident, and has high self-esteem, which are important qualities for life survival.

*Sense of control.* As the school-age child matures and makes choices, a sense of control develops about the self and the environment. Children with an internal locus of control believe they are responsible for their behaviour and accomplishments and tend to have higher levels of achievement than do children who believe in an external locus of control. The latter think that fewer reasons exist for them to try hard at a task, because others or fate determines life results. Older children and girls tend to have a more internalized locus of control than do younger children and boys.

*Body concept.* The school-age child's concept of the body and its functioning also changes from the preschool period and adds to overall self-concept. By age 8 to 11 years, children know that parts of the body constitute a related whole. The 11-year-old child can name twice the number and functions of internal body structures that a 6-year-old child can and frequently understands the functions of the cardiovascular, musculo-skeletal, and nervous systems. For example, the 7-year-old child knows that the heart is important and that it beats, whereas the 13-year-old child knows that the heart pumps blood. Changes or differences in the body may frighten the school-age child until the child understands normal developmental processes, such as losing deciduous teeth. Physical differences, such as freckles, can provoke ridicule and isolation. Children in this age group frequently feel threatened by others with deformities. Children with chronic illness worry that their peer relationships will be negatively influenced if others know about their illness. Children who learn about body differences, by meeting people with chronic health problems as well as by reading and discussion of anxiety about differences, increase their knowledge of the body and ways to maintain health. They also gain an understanding of the value of each person, despite their differences.

### ◆ Roles-Relationships Pattern

The family environment provides a sense of security that allows the school-age child to cope with uncertainties in the external environment. Although many live in single, divorced, or same-sex parenting households, the family structure generally encourages a child's cognitive growth through exposure to a variety of experiences that bolster the desire to achieve and develop positive self-esteem.

Parents, caregivers, and children interact in a variety of ways to show love and companionship for each other. Caregivers, such as grandparents or extended family members, protect the dependent child and teach the learning child. The caregiver–child relationship is not equal, primarily because caregivers and parents serve as authority figures that establish the rules needed for the functioning of the family and safe growth of the child. During the school-age years, the child's increasing maturity, independence, and responsibility begin to reduce the amount of parental authority and structure needed. In some cultures, parents set higher standards for child independence than parents of other diverse populations (Women & Children's Health Network, 2013). With increasing independence, the child prioritizes school and peer group relationships to develop socialization skills and understand group social mores (Sturaro et al., 2011). These connections will help prepare the child for future relationships.

School-age children also begin to broaden their interests outside the home, often encouraged by parents. Unfortunately, some older children may become involved in gangs, behaviour that causes much stress for both children and their parents. The child's changing world frequently alters family schedules and patterns, supporting studies that have found that parents express the least amount of parental satisfaction when their oldest child is between 6 and 13 years of age. The relationships between siblings differ, depending on birth order, culture, sex, and age differences and perceived power of siblings. Siblings interact with one another in a number of roles, such as playmates, teacher–learner, protector–dependant, and adversaries, based on feelings of jealousy and rivalry that often occur in families. School-age children cope with these feelings better than do preschool children because they have outlets outside the family, including school and friends. Parents can minimize conflicts by recognizing each child's needs and level of maturity and by providing guidance and support.

As children mature, they assume more responsibilities within the family and the community. School-age children learn responsibility for allowance, household chores, self-care, and pets and acquire a sense of empowerment as an integral part of the family. This is the period during which families often give allowances or children earn money through chores or small jobs, such as paper routes. The amount of an allowance may relate to cultural values. In one study, Asian children earned higher allowances than did other children from diverse population groups for completing fewer chores and for meeting higher standards of academic performance (Goldstein & Brooks, 2012). School-age children learn valuable life lessons by earning and spending their allowances.

Children learn socially accepted behaviours when their parents engage in limit setting (defining expected behaviour and consequences when limits are not honoured). Violent behaviour must be discouraged, and nonviolent methods to reach resolutions for personal problems should be encouraged (Box 14.3). Parents who express their feelings, explain why things happen, and listen to their children while setting limits encourage the development of self-control and positive self-esteem. Some families with school-age children find it helpful to have periodic

## BOX 14.3 The School-Age Child: Points for Effective Discipline

Effective discipline is essential to family harmony and individual child growth and reflects cultural beliefs. The goal of discipline is to encourage and reinforce positive child behaviours, eliminate inappropriate child behaviours, improve parent–child communication, and meet parental needs. It is about changing behaviour, not punishing children. Trust between caregiver and child should be maintained and constantly built upon. Disciplining children is one of the most important, yet difficult, parenting responsibilities. The goal of effective discipline is to foster appropriate and acceptable behaviour in children and raise emotionally mature adults (Nieman & Shea & CPS Community Paediatrics Committee, 2004).

The foundation of effective discipline is respect and consistency. Specifics of discipline strategies for school-aged children include the following:

- Praise and approval should be used liberally; reinforce desirable behaviour
- Use of appropriate motivators
- Withdrawal or delay of privileges, consequences, and time out
- Avoid nagging and making threats without consequences
- Apply rules consistently
- Set reasonable and consistent limits
- Know and accept age-appropriate behaviour
- Allow for the child's temperament and individuality
- Prioritize rules

Source: Modified from Nieman, P., & Shea, S., & Canadian Paediatric Society Community Paediatrics Committee. (2004). Effective discipline for children. *Paediatric Child Health, 9*(1), 37–41. Retrieved from https://www.uottawa.ca/health/sites/www.uottawa.ca.health/files/ped-_behavior_effective_discipline_for_children.pdf.

## BOX 14.4 Warning Signs of Child Maltreatment

- Physical evidence of abuse or neglect, including previous injuries
- Conflicting stories about the "accident" or injury from the parents or others
- Injury or complaint inconsistent with the child's history or developmental level (e.g., the child received a concussion and broken arm from falling off a bed)
- Signs and symptoms consistent with signs of abuse and inconsistent with history, vague recall of event (e.g., chief complaint is a cold when there is evidence of first-degree and second-degree burns)
- Inappropriate response of caregiver, such as an exaggerated or absent emotional response, refusal to give consent for additional tests or agree to necessary treatment, excessive delay in seeking treatment, or absence of the parents
- Inappropriate response of child, such as little or no response to pain, fear of being touched, excessive or lack of separation anxiety, or indiscriminate friendliness to strangers
- Child's report of physical or sexual abuse
- Previous reports of abuse in the family
- Repeated visits to emergency facilities with injuries

Source: Smith, M., & Segal, J. (2016). *Child abuse and neglect.* Retrieved from http://www.helpguide.org/articles/abuse/child-abuse-and-neglect.htm.

family meetings during which everyone discusses family issues, rules, and responsibilities. Behaviour contracts between the parent and the child provide direction and may also encourage improved behaviour by delineating favourable consequences when the terms of the contract are followed.

### Child Maltreatment

Child maltreatment refers to the harm, or risk of harm, that a child may experience while in the care of a trusted caregiver. The harm may occur through the person's direct actions or through the neglect of a component of care necessary for a child to grow and develop in a healthy way. In 2012 the Government of Canada defined five types of child maltreatment. These include: physical abuse, sexual abuse, neglect, emotional harm, and exposure to family violence. According to the Canadian Child Welfare Research Portal, a 2008 national study estimated that almost a 250,000 child-maltreatment–related investigations were conducted in Canada that year; 22% of those cases involved indigenous children (Public Health Agency of Canada [PHAC], 2008). The impact of child maltreatment on children can be minor or short-lived, but can also have severe and/or long-lasting effects on a child's physical, emotional, and social health and development (Government of Canada, 2012).

Abused children have an increased likelihood of becoming violent adults and of abusing their own children. The factors that increase the risk of abuse include family poverty, culture, limited maternal education, needy child syndrome, presence of a stepfather, lone-parent status, parental substance use, and teenage parenthood (AAP, 2011b). However, child abuse also occurs in families that do not have these risk factors. Cultural factors must be considered in detecting abuse. For example, coin rubbing of the chest (used in the Asian ethnic group for treatment of respiratory tract infections) leaves abrasions that may be perceived as abuse by a nurse assessing an ill child. National governmental agencies and professional organizations require that health care providers report suspected abuse and participate in preventing, assessing, and treating victims. Provincial/territorial nurse practice acts require nurses to report suspected cases of abuse. Ultimately, nurses help interrupt the vicious cycle of abuse by becoming involved in community coalitions and innovative evidence-informed programs that prevent and intervene in child and family abuse.

Unfortunately, relationships between children and adults are not always positive. Sexual abuse, use of a child for sexual exploitative purposes, has become a more common but often hidden problem for a variety of reasons (AAP, 2011b; US Department of Health and Human Services [USDHHS], 2011): the child may be too frightened to talk about the situation, families and society do not want to admit its existence, Internet traffic has supported pornography and pedophilia, and fewer agencies exist to respond to these cases. Many victims know their abusers (many are parents), and people in positions of authority (e.g., teachers, coaches, or clergy members) may be abusers. The child may comply for a variety of reasons, such as a need to be good or a need to keep the family together. Emotions are complex and change as the child grows, but they often lead to adult anxiety, depression, and physical symptoms and illnesses. Males less often report sexual abuse but are more likely than girls to suffer negative emotional effects from incest, a form of sexual abuse.

As in any type of suspected abuse, nurses assist these children by recognizing those at risk and those experiencing abuse and referring them to relevant resources. All people who work with young children must acknowledge the warning signs of abuse (Box 14.4). When sexual abuse is suspected, an in-depth interview and examination must be conducted by a specially trained, multidisciplinary team that is sensitive to the needs of the child and can validate the abuse. Most authorities believe that children who describe sexual abuse are telling the truth because the details are usually specific and trauma is evident. Therefore, a child's story should be believed unless it is disproved.

### ◆ Sexuality-Reproductive Pattern

The preschool child learns about sex differences and begins to model the general societal behaviours expected of a female or male child. The child enters the school-age years with a strong identification with the parent of the same sex. The child continues to learn the concepts and behaviour of the gender role and incorporate these into the self-concept. This challenge is significant for all children, but more so for gender-diverse children. Societal stereotypes related to gender roles continue to influence the school-age child's ideas of male and female roles. Fortunately, most children receive early teaching about gender roles that emphasizes that sex does not determine one's choices, personality, or behaviour. As a result of this teaching, children increasingly choose occupations based on their skills and interests, rather than on what appears appropriate because of their sex.

The school-age child's increasing awareness of the body, its functioning, and a need for sexual identity combine to foster a desire for knowledge about the biological aspects of sexual function. Late in the school-age period, when the physical changes of puberty have begun, concern and curiosity about sexual issues frequently develop. A child may become extremely attached to another of the same sex, and they may explore one another's sexual organs. This is common exploratory behaviour and may not reflect true gender diversity. With the advent of physical changes of puberty, the school-age child desires more privacy in a bedroom shared with no one. As noted earlier, the physical changes of puberty appear gradually over several years.

Children frequently share questions about sexual matters with their peer group. Parents are often uncomfortable or unsure of what sexual information to give to their children and when to give it. Many health care agencies sponsor short programs to educate parents and older school-age children, in a supportive environment, about body and mental changes during preadolescence and puberty. An increasing number of age-appropriate books that focus on emotional and body changes can be used at home and in school to increase children's understanding. Particularly because menstrual cycles start earlier now than they did 50 years ago, education about body changes and puberty appears appropriate as part of later school-age education.

The nurse plays an important role in sex education in health care and education settings. This professional should be receptive to answering questions in this area and at each health care visit. The nurse employed in the school is in an ideal position to teach group, sex education programs using literature and games. Children at this age appear to respond most favourably with sex-segregated classes because of their general discomfort with sexual topics and unique needs and questions. Some schools appropriately incorporate these classes into school curricula as part of a health-promotion curriculum.

Other schools have special programs focused only on sex education based on parental desires or school board policies. Most school-age children have the cognitive skills to respond to programs on responsible sexuality, including discussions on abstinence and condom use, pregnancy, sexually transmitted infections, and the human immunodeficiency virus (Krause-Parello & Samms, 2010). The nurse also wants to include program content specific to disabled children, who face unique body changes and concerns and need to understand ways others can express affection to them without causing accusations of abuse.

### ◆ Coping–Stress Tolerance Pattern

The school-age child must learn to cope with stress as part of the developmental process. Through a health-promotion program, children can learn to identify symptoms of stress (pounding heart, stomach "butterflies," and sweaty hands) and ways to cope with these perceived stresses (e.g., deep breathing and walking) before they cause illness. The child actually faces many stressful experiences in life, including competition, homework deadlines, failure at home or school, and decisions whether to cheat, steal, or even join an unpopular peer group. The young school-age child may never have shared his or her life with other children the same age, and cultural values learned earlier in life may not be reflected in school or in peer relationships. Threats to the child's security (e.g., bullying) cause feelings of helplessness and anxiety that may affect the ability to function successfully. Grief over the death of a loved one, parental divorce, loss of a favourite activity because of misbehaviour, or expulsion from a favourite peer group may cause negative behaviour. Parents need to provide appropriate discipline in responding to this behaviour, but should also listen and analyze factors related to the problem so as to increase the child's feelings of control and decrease stress for the family.

Children use a variety of coping strategies, healthy behaviours intended to buffer perceived stressful events. However, in a very stressful situation or many stressful situations, a child may be unable to move beyond the coping behaviours. In conversations with teachers and parents, the nurse may offer a variety of strategies for coping with a school-age child's problems, enabling the child to cope and learn from others (Table 14.2). These strategies may involve role-playing or referral to literature on the problem topic to interrupt the child's negative behaviour cycle and improve family health (see Table 14.2). The nurse may also refer a child to relevant religious and spiritual leaders, on the basis of school-age children's belief that prayer will help them cope with an otherwise uncontrollable situation.

#### Parental Divorce

More than half of all marriages end in divorce, leaving many school-age children to face stress related to their parents' separation. Often children experience a feeling of loss, although they may hope that their parents will reunite at some point. Box 14.5 discusses the effects of divorce on a school-age child. Children's responses vary with their level of development (Kim, 2011). Factors such as economic security; availability of both of their parents, other family, church,

## TABLE 14.2  The School-Age Child's Coping Strategies and Nursing Interventions to Promote Coping

| Coping Strategies | Nursing Interventions |
| --- | --- |
| Use of defence mechanisms (regression, denial, repression, projection, displacement, sublimation) | Accept child's use of defence mechanisms as temporary, healthy coping responses; provide child with options for moving to more age-appropriate ways of responding to stressors. |
| Cognitive mastery (problem solving, communication) | Ask children what they know of the situation and how they might handle it; encourage questions; use diagrams and models to help explain; encourage child to verbalize feelings and use past successful strategies that might help deal with present stressors; try personalized approaches, such as books, puppets, and manipulation of equipment, to increase feelings of control when faced with a stressful situation; encourage praying and other communications to a chosen deity as appropriate |
| Controlling, holding behaviours | Encourage child to participate and to make decisions; accept child's need to direct as appropriate; set consistent age-appropriate limits; respond to signals for help; let child be responsible for self-care |
| Use of repetition | Use books, games, and other communication media to work through feelings; emphasize "OK" for child to continue to ask questions and to receive answers that assist in coping |
| Use of humour | Be a good listener and participate in riddles and jokes used by child; be a good sport with school-age children's desire to play jokes on each other; share stories and cartoons with child |
| Motor activity, aggression, protest behaviour | Encourage physical activity to deal with stress; accept appropriate behaviour; establish limits on behaviour for group safety |
| Withdrawal (resurgence of separation anxiety) | When child is separated from the family, child may have separation anxiety; encourage close emotional contacts between child and significant others (friends, family, church members); allow favourite objects from home to be brought to the hospital or a new environment for child |

## BOX 14.5  Effects of Divorce on the School-Age Child

School-age children tend to view life in black and white and are likely to blame one parent for the breakup. Boys, especially, mourn the loss of their fathers and frequently express anger at their mothers. Both boys and girls have great difficulty accepting their parents' new dates. Crying, daydreaming, and problems with friends and school are common divorce-related behaviours in children of this age.

Here are some suggestions that might help the school-age child cope with divorce of parents:

- *Discourage reconciliation fantasies.*
  Have parents avoid dinners, outings, or holiday celebrations with the ex-spouse. This only fuels the child's fantasies. Instead, emphasize the finality of divorce.
- *Make sure the child has the phone number of the absent parent.*
  Both parents should encourage easy access and frequent conversations with the noncustodial parent.
- *Do not allow the child to manipulate the parents into buying more possessions.*
  School-age children are likely to feel deprived. Although they may intensify requests for playthings or other possessions, do not try to retain child's affection through material objects. Even children of divorce need to be told "No!"
- *Talk to the child's teachers or school counsellors about the divorce.*
  School personnel may better understand possible learning or behavioural problems and will likely offer extra support.

Source: Pickhardt, C. (2011). *Impact of divorce on young children and adolescents.* Retrieved from http://www.psychologytoday.com/blog/surviving-your-childs-adolescence/201112/the-impact-divorce-young-children-and-adolescents.

and school supports; and quality of interactions with their parents can influence the child's ability to cope with divorce. Unfortunately, many parents become so immersed in their own feelings that they fail to support their children (Pickhardt, 2011). Conflicts over custody, child support, and visitation rights add to the child's difficulty in coping. Sometimes the school system becomes the child's advocate to encourage the parents to provide a supportive environment during divorce proceedings. Despite this intervention, some children do not cope well with the divorce and have emotional consequences that result in juvenile behaviour problems or require long-term counselling (see the Case Study and Care Plan at the end of this chapter).

### Somatization and Depression

Children, like adults, use defence mechanisms to cope, with various degrees of success. Two strategies used by the school-age child to respond to uncontrollable situations are somatization and depression.

Some children respond to a stressful situation by transferring their feelings to a physical problem (somatization). In this phenomenon, school-age children, unable to discuss their concerns, complain of stomach aches or headaches, symptoms reflective of functional or psychogenic pain. These children may also develop discrete, repetitive movement habits called tics. In many cases the child with these problems must be evaluated to determine whether an underlying physiological cause exists. The child and the family will then need assistance in understanding the child's concerns to define successful ways to cope with the behaviour.

Depression occurs in up to 2% of school-age children (CPS, 2018e) and more often in boys than in girls during the school-age period. Depression reflects a disturbance of mood, when a child displays sadness, guilt, or worthlessness, and other unusual behaviours that disengage the child from peers and the family. In defining depression in children, most authors emphasize that they are referring to a more long-term syndrome in which the child's normal development and functioning become impaired, not a periodic sadness that all children occasionally experience. The factors that place a child at risk of depression include homelessness, death of a parent or significant other, divorce, long-term hospitalization, chronic illness, learning problems, and emotional turmoil at home. Parents and teachers look for symptoms of depression, including anorexia, sleeplessness, lethargy, changed affect, aggressive behaviour, frequent crying, and withdrawal from previously enjoyed activities.

Although it has been concluded that there is insufficient evidence to routinely screen all school-age children for depression, the nurse can serve an important role in identifying any child who appears to be depressed and in notifying parents about the need for further assessment. Depending on the child and the situation, differing amounts of counselling and individual child guidance may be required. Nurses in schools and outpatient settings are often the ideal helpers because they have the skills and time needed to help a child cope with a helpless feeling and its cause.

Healthy social and emotional development in the early years lay the foundation for resilience and mental health throughout life. In Canada, an estimated 1.2 million children and youth are affected by mental illness, and less than 20% of those will receive treatment. The Mental Health Commission of Canada's (MHCC) Youth Council has created a youth version of the Mental Health Strategy for Canada. This strategy is a recommendation for action and a blueprint for change to ensure the well-being of all young Canadians (MHCC, 2018). A priority goal involves implementing comprehensive school health initiatives that promote mental health for all students. Strategies include targeted prevention efforts for those at risk, reducing the stigma associated with mental health issues, and removing financial barriers that inhibit access to clinical resources.

## ◆ Values-Beliefs Pattern

Children make decisions related to moral and ethical issues every day. Should they tell the teacher which classmate broke the rule? Should they share their candy with a younger sibling? For these situations, the child makes a decision on the basis of the level of moral development. Moral development involves choosing the most appropriate behaviour on the basis of one's values and feelings related to the situation. Environmental factors and culture strongly influence a child's moral development, as do the type of family discipline, role models, people with whom the child identifies, and the child's rehearsal and practice of moral behaviour.

### Kohlberg's Theory

Most researchers agree that the younger school-age child is at the preconventional level, a level of moral development characterized by self-interest only. The child continues to do many things simply to avoid getting in trouble and does not understand the reason for rules, but also performs actions that will benefit the self (Kohlberg, 1981). During later childhood (10–13 years) most children progress to the conventional level, a stage of moral development defined by concern about group interests and values. The conventional level of moral judgement involves the child looking to others for approval and to societal authority for a definition of rules. Children aged 10 to 12 years judge a behaviour in terms of the intention of the offender, understand the "golden rule" concept, and engage in behaviour that

maintains a valued relationship. The conventional level coincides with Piaget's cognitive level of concrete operations and the child's increased social involvement with people outside the home (Kohlberg, 1981).

### Moral Behaviour Problems

Some moral behaviour problems, such as lying, stealing, or cheating, are common during the school-age years. Cultural, religious, and parental values influence a child's moral development, concept of right and wrong, and consequences of not demonstrating moral behaviour. Preschool and younger school-age children frequently lie as a result of fantasy, exaggerations, or inaccurate understanding. As children mature, they may use the defence mechanism of denial to block upsetting situations and maintain self-esteem. The lie then becomes an unconscious act. Older children often lie because they fear punishment or ridicule. Children may cheat because of a desire to win, do well in competitive society, or "look good" for their peers. Children usually steal when they think they will not be caught and they think that there is no other way to get what they want (McLeod, 2015). Although these actions can be quite upsetting for parents, they are common developmental behaviours. Parents frequently need reassurance that the child is normal and will probably outgrow the behaviour with parental assistance. They may need help in developing fair rules for behaviour and communicating their expectations for a child's behaviour to meet parental and cultural values. Therefore, the nurse encourages the parents to warn the child clearly not to steal, lie, or cheat; offer other, more socially acceptable, ways to cope with the stressor causing the behaviour; and then apply appropriate punishment congruent with an understanding of the event.

## ❖ ENVIRONMENTAL PROCESSES

### ◆ Physical Agents

School-age children, similar to those of all other age groups, face daily exposure to environmental agents and factors that may cause injury, illness, or death. Many of these agents and factors are harmless if appropriately used or if there is minimal exposure. Examples include physical agents such as fires; mechanical agents such as bicycles, skateboards, and cars; biological agents such as bacteria; chemical agents such as asbestos; and radiological agents such as X-rays. Death rates from these agents differ among ethnic groups because of access to health care and environmental issues. According to the WHO's 2008 World Report on Child Injury Prevention, approximately 950,000 children aged 17 and under were killed by an injury in 2004, and 87% of these deaths were due to unintentional and potentially preventable causes (CPS, 2012). Injury is also the leading cause of death among Indigenous children and youth.

### Unintentional Injuries

Unintentional injuries are the leading cause of death and disability for children and youth in Canada. They accounted for 15% of the hospitalizations of children under the age of 12 in 2005. Twenty percent of injuries involving serious trauma result in serious head injuries and lifelong disability. The main causes of head injuries include motor vehicle collisions, falls, and sports injuries (PHAC, 2009). Unintentional injuries in Indigenous children in Canada occur at a rate of three to four times the national average (CPS, 2017b). The nurse has a significant role in educating parents and school personnel on ways to prevent dangers to school-age children and to become involved in public initiatives to create a safer society for them (Safe Kids, 2013).

The agent, host, and environment must be considered when one is developing solutions to decrease the number of unintentional injuries. The type of agent varies with the child's age. Most fatal injuries during the school-age period occur from motor vehicle collisions when the child (host) is a passenger or pedestrian (walking or riding a bike). Other fatal injuries occur from fires and burns, riding bicycles, drowning, and use of firearms. Most common nonfatal injuries tend to be caused by simple agents that produce simple injuries. Despite helmet laws, many school-age children continue to experience head injuries related to recreational equipment, such as bicycles, swings, skateboards, and trampolines (CDC, 2014). Slightly older children have an increased number of injuries from contact sports and cuts, falls, and burns.

Specific unintentional injury factors relate to the host—the school-age child (Quality and Safety Scenario). Children in this age group tend to become hurt because of their carefree attitude, curiosity, love of mimicking older people, and intense oral tendencies. Among children in Canada aged 14 and under the proportion of unintentional injury deaths and hospitalization by gender is 63% boys and 37% girls (CPS, 2012). Boys have more unintentional injuries than girls, perhaps attributable to differences in personalities, societal expectations, child-rearing practices, and increased propensity for risk-taking behaviours.

## ⚡ QUALITY AND SAFETY SCENARIO

### *Safety Concerns Specific to School-Age Children*

Because of increased independence, school-age children face significant exposure to situations threatening their health. Consequently, the parents of these children must be involved in community and legislative activities that provide safe play environments. Additionally, at appropriate health visits, health care workers should provide anticipatory guidance to parents in the following areas:

**Bicycle Safety**
Each child should have a well-maintained bicycle, ride only in safe areas approved by the parents, observe rules for vehicle traffic, ride on the side of the road with traffic, "bike defensively," and use an approved riding helmet.

**Street Safety**
Children should look right, left, then right again to check the safety of crossing a street; children should cross only at safe and well-monitored intersections, preferably with an adult present; ensure parental supervision when children play close to streets and heavy traffic areas.

**Motor Vehicle Safety**
Children should wear a seat belt or be in an age-appropriate booster seat as needed; older children should ride with a restraint system and in the back seat until age 12 years.

**Pool Safety**
All children should have swimming lessons and swim with a buddy or adult who swims well; all pools should have drain covers; children should avoid swimming after a heavy meal and avoid "roughhousing" behaviour around the pool; children should be monitored by the parents during swimming.

**Firearm Safety**
Adults need to lock away guns and ensure gun safety locks are intact; parents need to educate children *never* to touch guns.

**Playground Safety**
All playground equipment should meet federally approved standards; children should be trained on how to use equipment safely; equipment should be evaluated for safety and repaired before children use it.

**Fire Safety**
Working smoke detectors should be in place in the home and school; the family needs to have a fire evacuation plan and practice it; children need to wear fire-retardant clothing at night; children should not play with matches, open fires, fireworks, or open wires that can cause injury and fire.

**Toxin Safety**
Children should avoid insecticides, radiation sources, inappropriate use of medications, and pollution sources; parents need to store all known toxins, chemicals, and household cleaning agents in an adequately ventilated location that is inaccessible to children.

**Stranger Safety**
Children should play with friends, have a plan for returning home, know the home phone number and address, play in a safe and known area, and report any suspicious activity threatening their safety to an appropriate adult; children should know how to say "no" and how to locate assistance when in an unsafe situation.

**Sports Safety**
Children need to engage in age-appropriate activities and wear protective equipment relevant to the sport; parents need to ensure safety and maintenance of all sports equipment; parents need to caution children against hazardous sports, such as tramlining.

**Animal Safety**
Parents should teach children to avoid strange animals, especially sick or injured ones, and ensure that personal pets receive vaccinations; parents need to teach children not to mistreat pets and not to place their faces close to any animal.

Although nurses offer suggestions to parents to improve their children's play safety, studies have shown that few parents follow these suggestions. The reasons for this behaviour include parental difficulty in assessing the safety of and age appropriateness of play equipment, the amount of effort involved, and a lack of money to create a safe play area. The nurse helps parents respond to these perceived barriers. With more children using skateboards and rollerblades, the nurse also encourages the use of child safety helmets and knee, elbow, and wrist guards to prevent muscle sprains and bone fractures. The school offers an on-site opportunity for teaching children, teachers, and parents about accident prevention. In addition to providing this guidance, nurses can participate in legislative and educational actions to increase community consciousness about child safety.

The physical environment of the child dictates the type or frequency of unintentional injuries, which occur in the home, neighbourhood, and school. Most happen outdoors, which means that school-age children face a greater risk of automobile or bicycle injuries than of poisoning or falls, indoor accidents that occur predominantly in younger children. More injuries (drowning and pedestrian–vehicle accidents) occur in the summer than in the winter because of children's outside play. Socioeconomic level affects children's physical environments and access to dangers. For example, space heaters place children of low-income families at risk of burns, whereas skiing places wealthier children at risk of injury.

The social environment, which includes the family, school, and playmates, also plays a role in accidents. Although little research has focused on the physical trauma caused by heavy backpacks that many school-age children use, these bags exert significant pressure against functionally immature muscles of the back and torso. Daily carrying of bulging backpacks causes muscle strain, headaches, improper posture, shoulder slouch, and other physical problems. Additionally, teachers' expectations that all textbooks be available both in the classroom and at home must be considered. At least one study has shown that children will change their backpack-carrying behaviours if they are involved in a school-based program focused on this topic (AAP, 2012).

## Drowning

Drowning accounts for 15% of all injury-related deaths of children in Canada (CPS, 2012). Between 2001 and 2010, two-thirds of children who drowned in Canada were younger than 15 years. Sixty percent of child drownings occur during the months of June, July, and August. Children drown in private pools five times more frequently than they do in public pools. Among drowned children under 19, only 35% had intended to be in the water (e.g., swimming or wading); 33% of children drowned after entering the water unintentionally by falling or accidental submersion (Canadian Red Cross, 2013). Water safety measures can help reduce drowning, along with the many other injuries that occur around water, such as falls in slippery areas. Environment and safety teaching can influence the number of school-age children dying of drowning.

## Burns

Each year many children become victims of house fires, many of which occur during the winter months from Christmas trees, space heaters, and fireplace malfunctions. Many homes lack working smoke detectors because of incorrect installation or inadequate testing. If a fire occurs in a home with a smoke detector, the risk of death is decreased by 40–50% (CDC, 2012). Most burned children survive, frequently with various degrees of physical and psychological scars. Children need to learn about fire safety, including the importance of avoiding situations involving fire and practicing fire drills routinely at school and home. The nurse encourages parents to understand other practices to prevent fire-related problems, including parental purchase of flame-retardant sleepwear for children.

## Firearms

From 2008 to 2012 there were 15 suicides, 10 homicides, 7 unintentional deaths, and 2 undetermined types of firearm deaths among children under 15 years of age (CPS, 2018f). Children are at increased risk for firearm injury due to their immature cognitive development. The CPS recommends that health care providers routinely screen for the presence of a firearm in the home. Families with firearms in the home should store them in a locked area apart from ammunition. All family members should be knowledgeable about gun safety. Much debate has been raised recently regarding the use of toy guns by children. Unlike video game use, the use of toy guns during childhood does not increase the likelihood of violent or aggressive behaviour later in life. Additionally, nonpowder firearms (e.g., air guns and BB guns) are dangerous weapons that should never be used by children unless supervised closely by an adult. Paintball and airsoft guns must be used in supervised arenas with proper safety gear (CPS, 2018f).

## Sports and Recreation

Accidents from sports and other recreational activities increase during the school-age years and include lacerations, contusions, hematomas, concussions, sprains, and fractures. Some evidence exists that adolescents now have more musculo-skeletal injuries because of involvement in repetitive team sports earlier in their lives. This suggests that society needs to examine the current emphasis on initiating young children with musculo-skeletal immaturity into team sports such as football, hockey, soccer, and basketball. Intense social pressure for children to participate in these sports means that parents and school systems must ensure that each child has protective body devices to prevent injuries, as well as psychological support to allow a child to benefit from the team sport. There is a further need to increase safety by ensuring that each child fits the sport, has adequate hydration during the game, and engages in conditioning exercises before and after the game for prevention of injuries. Furthermore, the literature supports societal need to focus more on the collaborative skills children learn by being part of a team, rather than the intense focus on winning philosophy found in many school-age team sports.

Playgrounds help children to stay active and healthy. They are a place where children can play with their peers, run, jump, and have fun. Caregivers need to ensure that children stay safe on playgrounds. Most injuries that occur are the result of falling off equipment, although children can also be get caught in equipment or get otherwise injured on a playground (Caring for Kids, 2017). The Canadian Standards Association sets playground equipment standards in Canada. If playgrounds are poorly maintained or fail to meet these standards, they can be a hazard for children. There are things caregivers can do to ensure safety of children on playgrounds. Ensuring a proper surface area like rubber, wood chips, or sand can help prevent serious injury in the case of a fall. The area should be free from hazards such as broken glass or garbage. The equipment should have strong barriers and handrails to prevent falls, and all equipment should be firmly attached to the ground (Caring for Kids, 2017). Caregivers should stay close to children at all times, appropriately supervise activity on playgrounds, and teach children about safety when playing.

## Mechanical Forces

Motor vehicles and bicycles are the two most common mechanical agents that cause injury to school-age children.

*Motor vehicles.* The leading cause of death in Canada in children and youth is motor vehicle accidents, which account for 17% of all injuries (Yanchar, Warda, & Fuselli, 2012). Children die as passengers in cars, as pedestrians, and as bicycle riders. In Canada, over 20,000 children were injured or killed in motor vehicle accidents in 2017 (Government of Canada, 2019c). Bicycle-related injuries account for approximately 4% of all youth injuries seen in Canadian Emergency Departments and account for 5% of all deaths due to accidental injury for children younger than 15 years of age. Helmet use in children can reduce the risk of head and brain injury by approximately 60% (Hagel, Yanchar, CPS, et al., 2013). Each province/territory in Canada has its own laws regarding helmet use on bicycles, with eight provinces having laws requiring helmet use for minors.

Automobile passenger injuries can be prevented, or the significantly reduced. For example, proper and consistent use of approved belt-positioned booster seats for children that have outgrown their forward-facing seat and weigh at least 18 kg (40 lbs). Each province/territory in Canada may have its own age, height, and weight restrictions, so it is important that caregivers refer to the laws in their home province or territory (Government of Canada, 2018b). Transition to a seat belt should only occur when the child has outgrown the booster seat and the caregiver has ensured that the seat belt fits the child. The minimum age, weight, and height for seat belts varies from one province to another. All child car seats must meet Canadian Motor Vehicle Safety standards, and caregivers should look for the maple leaf and the word "Transport" on the seat to ensure it meets those standards.

The reasons given by parents and children for their not using seat belts or booster seats include forgetting to use the device, having difficulty reaching and fastening belts, feeling discomfort from wearing the belt or using the seat, and receiving misinformation about the need for the belt or seat for short trips. Clearly, consistent use of booster seats by young children and seat belts by older children and adults, who model seat-belt behaviour to their children, will occur only when legal enforcement occurs.

Urban children younger than 15 years old experience more than half of all pedestrian–automobile accidents. These occur when they are using rollerblades, skateboards, and skate scooters and tend to be more severe (head injuries) than passenger injuries. Many factors cause pedestrian accidents: children often have difficulty interpreting traffic signs and judging the speed of cars, and they forget to look carefully before crossing the street. Although overcrowding, poverty, high volume of traffic, stress, and unsafe play areas influence children's street safety, various principles can direct interventions to decrease the number of street dangers.

*Bicycles and motorized vehicles.* Many accidents occur each year with young children on bicycles, motorized skateboards, and all-terrain vehicles (ATVs). Most of these are not serious, but deaths occur among young children who have suffered head trauma or significant body injury from inappropriate use of

this equipment. Caring for Kids recommends that only people at least 16 years old ride ATVs. These vehicles can weigh over 300 kg (661 lbs) and can reach high speeds. In Canada, 34% pf ATV-related deaths are among youth less than 16 years old, and children under age 16 years are more likely to suffer a head injury or bone fracture in an ATV accident (Caring for Kids, 2019). Bicycle accidents occur most frequently near the child's home and during the day, and commonly involve injuries from the spokes when children ride behind the bike seat. More boys than girls experience these injuries from bicycles, motorized skateboards, and ATVs, perhaps because of their greater risk-taking behaviour (Daly, Kallan, Arbogast, et al., 2010).

In response to children's developmental behaviour related to bicycles, motorized skateboards, and ATVs, the nurse addresses safety issues. Additionally, nurses encourage parents to teach and reinforce safe bicycling habits to their children and should sponsor helmet and bike programs within the school (Box 14.6).

## ◆ Biological Agents

School-age children face constant exposure to bacterial, viral, and other biological agents that pose threats to or improve their overall health (e.g., immunizations). Compared with the pre-school child, the school-age child has fewer illnesses. The most

---

**BOX 14.6  Nursing Interventions to Prevent Accidents During the School-Age Period**

### Strategies for Counselling

- Discuss accident prevention at optimal times, such as during prenatal visits or well-child visits, after the arrival of a new sibling, or after an accident.
- Rather than discussing all topics at once, pick the main concerns for the developmental level of the child at each well-child visit. For the school-age child, these topics include motor vehicle, water, fire, and bicycle safety.
- Repeat information at other visits to emphasize its importance.

### Community Actions

- Use supplemental materials, such as pamphlets, to reinforce the verbal information.
- Support local and national legislation that sets standards for potentially harmful agents.
- Encourage children to wear a bicycle helmet and other protective gear when appropriate. Many nurses have been active in lobbying for bicycle helmet requirements in their province/territory.
- Consult with manufacturers on safe designs of materials used by children.
- Report objects that are potentially hazardous.
- Participate in local activities that promote accident prevention.
- Educate groups, such as schoolchildren and parent organizations.

Recommended national resources for injury prevention (Yanchar, Warda, & Fuselli, 2012):
- Canadian Paediatric Society: https://www.cps.ca
- Canadian Paediatric Surveillance Program: https://www.cpsp.cps.ca
- Safe Kids Canada: http://www.parachutecanada.org/safekidscanada
- ThinkFirst Foundation of Canada: http://www.thinkfirst.ca
- Safe Communities Canada: http://www.safecommunities.ca
- SMARTRISK: http://www.parachutecanada.org/smartrisk
- Canadian Red Cross: https://www.redcross.ca
- Health Canada: https://www.hc-sc.gc.ca
- Public Health Agency of Canada (PHAC): https://www.phac-aspc.gc.ca
- Transport Canada: https://www.tc.gc.ca

frequent illness continues to be upper respiratory tract infections (URIs), illnesses shared among schoolchildren who fail to practice good handwashing techniques and avoidance of ill peers. These illnesses cause children to lose school days and learning opportunities. Most URIs result from viruses, but bacteria can play either a primary or a secondary role. Two problems associated with URIs are streptococcal infection ("strep throat") and otitis media.

Strep throat occurs frequently among school-age children. A child with an infection from group A streptococcus may have a severe sore throat, fever, and malaise, or may have only a minor sore throat. A throat culture confirms the diagnosis, and antibiotic treatment typically cures the infection. Children are noninfectious after 24 hours of treatment and may return to school (Wald, 2015). If not treated, the affected child may develop rheumatic fever or acute glomerulonephritis as a secondary infection following the sore throat. Greater transmission of streptococcal infection occurs in areas where there is close personal contact during colder weather. The school nurse's preventive efforts focus on teaching the children good handwashing techniques and identifying children who complain of sore throats. Children with throat infections caused by other streptococci, such as group B, do not usually require treatment, because these infections generally do not cause the same serious complications.

Otitis media rates have subsided with the integration of the pneumococcal and influenza vaccines into the immunization schedule. Acute otitis media is often self-limiting and can often be regarded as a complication of a preceding or concomitant URI. Most cases of otitis media will resolve spontaneously. Without specific treatment, symptoms abate within 24 hours in 60% of children and settle within 3 days in 80% of children (Toll & Nunez, 2012). The nurse is in an integral position to help support the family and educate them on risk factors associated with otitis media and nonpharmacological therapies that may alleviate symptoms and discomfort during the course of illness.

The school-age child may experience other illnesses. The frequency of gastro-intestinal tract infection (gastroenteritis) decreases during the school-age years but is still the second most common acute condition of childhood. Usually caused by a virus, gastro-intestinal tract infections cause vomiting and diarrhea. Older and larger school-age children have little chance of rapid dehydration; they basically react to the illness the same as do adults and need to be treated similarly. Gastroenteritis is contagious, and therefore the nurse should monitor schoolchildren for symptoms of illness and encourage proper handwashing to prevent transmission of the virus from one child to another.

Scabies and pediculosis are common skin disorders among school-age children, involving extreme itchiness of either the body (scabies) or the head (pediculosis), and are easily spread to other children (Gupta, 2015). The nurse educates parents to visualize the mites and lice or use a lice comb to check their children for mites and lice when they complain of itchiness or seem to be constantly scratching their heads. Previously, children with lice could not come to school until they were lice-free,

which isolated students from their peers and influenced school funding based on student attendance.

The objectives of immunization programs are to prevent, control, or eliminate vaccine-preventable diseases, and in Canada the responsibility for immunizations is shared between the federal and provincial governments (Government of Canada, 2016). National guidelines for immunization practices including recommended immunization schedules are listed on the Government of Canada public health website. There are a growing number of Canadians who have vaccine hesitancy, whether refusing the vaccine or delaying the schedule because of concerns about immunization. Loss of public confidence can reduce the number of people who are immunized and result in a resurfacing of vaccine-preventable diseases. The decision to immunize a child should be done in partnership with the health care worker, and candidly communicating information about the safety of vaccines and their benefit–risk ratio is necessary (Government of Canada, 2016).

## ◆ Chemical Agents

A number of potentially toxic chemical agents exist in the environment, and the child is exposed to these through inhalation, ingestion, or direct contact. Children are particularly susceptible to chemical hazards. Food and medications are two sources of chemicals ingested by children on a regular basis, and some older school-age children ingest tobacco as a result of cigarette smoking. Although normally safe, some foods and medications can be harmful when used inappropriately. Other environmental hazards include pollution, heavy metals (lead and mercury), and pesticides.

The nutritional needs of the school-age child were discussed earlier in this chapter. As stated, children frequently eat foods with large quantities of sugar, salt, and fat, and with chemical additives. The effects of some of these additives have been questioned, and concern has been expressed about the effect of biochemically altered food on children and future generations. On a short-term basis, some foods may cause allergic reactions; on a long-term basis, some may contribute to the development of coronary disease, hypertension, and cancer. Nurses are aware that the child's diet may contribute to future health problems, and therefore assess intake and counsel the child and parents accordingly about ways to improve it.

The incidence of poisoning decreases during the school-age years as children become more aware of the appropriate uses of medications and other agents. Childproof containers have decreased exposure of children to dangerous poisons and chemicals in the home. However, children continue to face exposure to medications, alcohol, and glue inhalants because of less monitoring by working parents, and older school-age children face exposure to recreational drugs, primarily through their peers and older children. In the school environment, the nurse and school personnel need to encourage students to engage in wise decision making about recreational drug use that will affect their future and overall health.

With pressure on older school-age children to smoke cigarettes, attention must be paid to effective strategies to prevent this behaviour. In Ontario, more children in

Grades 7–12 are using electronic cigarettes than tobacco cigarettes. In 2017, approximately 11% of children in this age group used electronic cigarettes, and 19% used cannabis (Ontario Student Drug Use and Health Survey, 2017). Attention to smoking as part of a health-promotion program seems merited because so many children begin smoking at a young age; in addition, many believe that this habit leads people to experiment with riskier substances (cocaine and methamphetamines).

In 2018 Canada enacted the *Tobacco and Vaping Products Act*, which regulates the sale, labelling, and promotion of tobacco and vaping products sold in the country. The act aims to protect young people and non-users of tobacco and vaping products from exposure to and dependence on nicotine from the use of electronic and tobacco cigarettes. The act also aims to enhance public awareness of the health hazards of using these products (Government of Canada, 2018c). The federal *Non-smokers Health Act* restricts smoking in federally regulated workplaces and public place under federal jurisdiction. Most provinces and territories have laws restricting the exposure to second-hand smoke in public places (Government of Canada, 2015).

Pollution and air quality can be a concern for some Canadian children. Air pollution irritates the eyes and the respiratory tract, causing URIs, ear infections, and allergies. More children now experience asthma, and many inner-city children face higher rates of this disease because of poor air quality, including secondary and tertiary smoke. Knowing the negative effects of air pollution and smoking on their health, many school-age children participate in school projects to improve their environmental health.

Children also face exposure to various toxic materials in their environment. Progress has been made in the past decades to reduce children's exposure to chemical hazards. Lead, for example, has been removed from gasoline and paint. This, in turn, has resulted in significant reductions in children's blood lead levels. Lead exposure continues to exist. Children are exposed to lead through parents' clothes, shoes contacting lead-infused soil, lead in older residential water pipes, traditional medications in some cultures, and in school building structures. Children living in poverty receive high exposure from lead-based paint used on older and less expensive homes. The long-term effects of lead on children remain unclear, but some evidence indicates children suffer neurotoxic effects from this type of exposure. High lead levels in children contribute to dental caries and hearing loss.

Routine use of chemicals to control insects and undesirable weeds in landscaping has led to increasing concerns about children's exposure to these agents. With increased interest in more natural substances to control insects and gardening problems, perhaps less reliance will be placed on chemicals for these problems in the future. Knowing the primary source of exposure to the most hazardous materials and avoiding these materials are often sufficient to accomplish real risk reduction and offer substantial protection within the child's environment (WHO, 2015b). Various behaviours can be implemented to create a safe environment and minimize health risks associated with hazardous chemical exposure. Nurses are instrumental in the assistance and support of parents, schools, and community agencies in the implementation of these behaviours, such as the use of nonhazardous cleaners and pesticide-free foods, and further monitoring of the environment for hazardous materials.

### X-ray Exposure

The child receives exposure from both naturally occurring radiation and human-made ionizing radiation. Exposure occurs in various degrees with radiographic examinations of teeth and bone, from nuclear power plants and explosions, and in the management of many childhood cancers. Children exposed to high levels of radiation risk developing breast or thyroid cancer or leukemia and compromised growth. With little advocacy in this area, nurses and other professionals improve children's health by becoming active in initiatives that focus on prevention of chemical and radiation hazards.

## Cancer

Childhood cancer is relatively uncommon in Canada, although it is the most common cause of disease-related deaths, and is second only to injury-related deaths among Canadian children. Cancer behaves differently in children and is found in different parts of the body than it is for adults. Generally, tumours grow more quickly in children as compared to adults, and children are more likely to develop leukemia and lymphoma (Canadian Cancer Society, 2019). In children 0–14 years of age, leukemia is the most common cancer, and it accounts for 32% of all new cancer diagnoses. Among the 12 major types of childhood cancers, leukemia and cancers of the brain and central nervous system (second most common forms of childhood cancers) account for more than 50% of all cancer deaths in children (Canadian Cancer Society, 2019). Lymphomas (Hodgkin's disease and non-Hodgkin's lymphoma) also affect school-age children and adolescents as the third most common group of malignancies. Non-Hodgkin's lymphoma is more common during the school-age years, and boys experience this malignancy three times more often than do girls. The most common symptom is abdominal pain caused by intestinal obstruction or organ compression. With effective treatment regimens, children with limited disease may be cured but may experience side effects of treatment later in life (e.g., development of cataracts, dental problems, learning difficulties). Advances are being made with the use of genomic sequencing and the use of genomic medicine to explore novel treatments with the goal of improving childhood cancer outcomes (Downing, Wilson, Zhang, et al., 2012). Children with cancer present a challenge to the nurse because they are in various stages of recovery, may be developmentally delayed as a result of prolonged periods of absence from peer groups during therapy, and may fear a recurrence of their disease. The nurse provides psychological and emotional support to affected children and their families to help children develop peer relationships and meet developmental goals important to them during the school-age years.

# ❖DETERMINANTS OF HEALTH

The school-age child interacts daily with other children and adults to become more independent by age 12 years. Mutual problem solving by the child and the parents or friends frequently occurs at this age related to a higher level of maturity in social relationships and concerns. Exposure to a variety of social roles and expectations of others strengthens the process of socialization so that the child develops social competence—the ability and skills to participate effectively in the social interactions of society. Social competence includes both the obvious social behaviours and an inner understanding of the appropriateness of behaviours.

Several elements play a role in the development of the child's social competence. The child's desire for a sense of industry encourages interactions, positive relationships, and accomplishments within society. Cognitive development supports understanding of relationships and effective problem solving. Moral judgement helps the child understand consequences and fairness in relationships. Understanding and obeying authority help to maintain order in society. Social sensitivity is a result of social interactions and requires the child's ability to perceive the social cues of others, understand the roles of others, and communicate verbally with them. Social behaviours are also a part of social competence; these are learned most frequently through imitation, role modelling, and reinforcement of others' behaviours. The interaction of all these elements produces a level of social competence and simultaneously plays a role in the child's self-perception. Individuals frequently see themselves as others see them.

## ◆ Social Factors and Environment

### Peers

The strongest relationships that school-age children develop outside their families are with their peers (other children encountered in the neighbourhood and school). The peer group acts as a new social system, becoming increasingly influential in the child's life. All children continue to be influenced significantly by the family, the culture of the family, and many other environmental factors, but the peer group begins to influence lifestyle, habits, and speech patterns and formulate standards of behaviour and performance. The standards of the peer group become vitally important, and children attempt to conform to its rules. Being accepted by the peer group becomes more important than being accepted by anyone else (Ferrer & Fugate, 2014). Conforming to the pressures of peers becomes an issue, especially when it interferes with the parents' expectations. When children realize that their own goals, desires, and aspirations might be quite different from those held by the peer group or the school, they must find ways to cope and perform according to the new standards if they are to succeed. The degree to which children fit in socially, learn to cope, and receive satisfaction from the group is a powerful determinant of healthy socialization.

A child may have one best friend or several important friends and a mutual understanding and willingness to help each other. Friendship groups that form during this age may change and become goal directed, such as groups composing a sports team. These groups frequently have set rules or rituals that connect the members. During the middle school years, friendships often revolve around same-sex relationships, videos, songs, books, and media shared by the group. Later in the school-age years, the development of sexual relationships with members of the opposite sex occurs during dating and mixed parties.

School-age children also become increasingly involved with adults outside the family, including teachers, coaches, and others who become role models, all of whom influence the child's view of the world and self. Although this influence may not be as significant as that of a child's peers, long-term ideas and beliefs frequently develop from these relationships. Children usually perceive some similarity between themselves and their models, those of the same sex with similar physical or behaviour traits. During these years, children may not maintain a strong identification with the parent of the same sex, but they tend to adopt other adult models with whom they can identify.

### Working Parents

Both dual-career couples and lone-parent families influence their children's safety when no adult is present to monitor the environment after school. Many latchkey children who are left alone until their parents return from work follow directions given by their parents. These directions may include beginning dinner in anticipation of their parents' return or completing homework while remaining inside the home with the doors locked.

Parents and school-age children often disagree about how old is "old enough" to be left at home alone or with an older sibling. Although the school-age child might consider being at home alone to be a real mark of maturity, children who look after themselves after school can become more isolated and miss peer relationships important to their development. Nurses give guidance to families who must cope with the issue of after-school care for school-age children to ensure that relevant and safe decisions are made.

### Culture and Ethnicity

School-age children focus more on the influences of their culture on their lives than do younger children. Aspects of North American culture that the child must confront include poverty and affluence, ethnic differences, acceptance of these differences, and the power of media as a cultural phenomenon in North American society. Preschool children may notice ethnic differences, but school-age children increasingly show evidence of being aware of these differences. This is a time during which attitudes toward others develop on the basis of family and community attitudes. Although prejudice exists among some school-age children, they may be encouraged to view people from different cultures and ethnic backgrounds in a positive light. Many schools appropriately focus on the importance of other cultures by having multicultural awareness weeks. During these times, children dress, eat, and live as other cultures do, allowing them to recognize the uniqueness of individual cultural beliefs and values (Diversity Awareness).

## 🌐 DIVERSITY AWARENESS

### How Culture Influences the Health of Children New to Canada

- Culture is a pattern of ideas, customs, and behaviours shared by a particular people or society. It is constantly evolving.
- The speed of cultural evolution varies. It increases when a group migrates to and incorporates components of a new culture into their culture of origin.
- Children often struggle with being "between cultures"—balancing the "old" and the "new." They essentially belong to both, whereas their parents often belong predominantly to the 'old' culture.
- One way of thinking about cultures is whether they are primarily "collectivist" or "individualist." Knowing the difference can help health care providers with diagnosis and with tailoring a treatment plan that includes a larger or smaller group.
- The influence of culture on health is vast. It affects perceptions of health, illness, and death, beliefs about causes of disease, approaches to health promotion, how illness and pain are experienced and expressed, where patients seek help, and the types of treatment patients prefer.
- Both health care providers and patients are influenced by their respective cultures. Canada's health system has been shaped by the mainstream beliefs of historically dominant cultures.
- Cultural bias may result in very different health-related preferences and perceptions. Being aware of and negotiating such differences are skills known as *cultural competence*. This perspective allows care providers to ask about various beliefs or sources of care specifically, and to incorporate new awareness into diagnosis and treatment planning.
- Demonstrating awareness of a patient's culture can promote trust, better health care, lead to higher rates of acceptance of diagnoses, and improve treatment adherence.

#### Reflective Questions

Reflect on your own cultural background:

- How might your values and beliefs impact the care that you give to children with the same cultural background?
- How might they impact the care that you give to children with a different cultural background?

Source: Canadian Paediatric Society. (2019). *How culture influences health.* Retrieved from https://www.kidsnewtocanada.ca/culture/influence.

## Screen Time

Television, video games, and electronic handheld devices exert a major influence on ideas and behaviour in North American culture. Unfortunately, many television programs and video games pose harm to children because of their messages and because such activities prevent children from engaging in physical activity. Advances in gaming offer an option for increased activity during gaming activities. Video games and gaming systems have been developed that encourage movement during gaming. Energy expenditure more than doubled when sedentary screen times were converted to active screen time.

Computers connected to the Internet pose a danger unless locking devices have been installed to prevent school-age children from accessing inappropriate websites. Additional concerns have focused on the violent themes of programming, persuasive television commercials, unrealistic depiction of the world, unhealthy food intake, and the passivity of television viewing.

Many times, certain ethnic or racial groups implement the violence in these media sources, leading children to stereotype these groups as the perpetrators of violence. Violence viewed through media sources, such as television and online, have been linked to aggressive thoughts and behaviours, desensitization, and a pessimistic world-view (Scharrer, 2019). One positive note is that adults who discuss violence with children by pointing out that these acts are unacceptable and cause pain to others can help inhibit some childhood aggression. Discussion of recent acts of violence committed by young people in such a context also helps. Anger-control programs, as part of school health-promotion programs, also help decrease societal violence and produce more collaborative workers needed for the future.

The average child views an overwhelming number of television commercials by age 18 years, and these commercials influence daily and future choices and behaviours. Many television commercials focus on sugary foods that cause damage to teeth, diminish overall healthy habits, and lead to increased rates of obesity. Young children cannot always separate the program from the commercials and believe that they must purchase products the television says to buy. Many childhood authorities question the ethics of exposing children to any type of advertising. Although concern about the effect of advertising has led to programming changes during children's watching time, more work is needed to send more socially responsible messages.

The world as presented on many television shows does not accurately reflect the real world. Despite an increasingly diverse and aging population, stereotypes of women and minority groups and a predominance of younger actors continue to make money for the media industry. Parents and health care providers should monitor television viewing to ensure the age appropriateness of the material, respond to television stations about inaccuracies in the content, and write letters to their newspaper or television networks to express concerns about the material presented. Parents may also participate with their children in responding to media presentations on learning and moral themes.

Exposure to digital devices such as tablets and smart phones is increasing in Canada. The CPS (2017a) recommends no more than 2 hours per day of recreational screen time for school-aged children. Screen time is defined as time spent on any screen, including computers, smart phones, tablets, video games, and television. Parents can positively influence their children's behaviours by setting limits on screen time and modelling this themselves. Some recent studies confirm a strong correlation between parents' screen time and that of their children.

There is concern that face-to-face parent–child interactions and family time are being displaced by time spent on screens. There is evidence that screen time can also influence less time spent reading. To mitigate risks associated with screen time, parents can be present and engaged when screens are used, be aware of content and prioritize educational and age-appropriate programming, and use parenting strategies that teach self-regulation and limit setting of devices. Parents and caregivers should model healthy screen use by engaging in reading, outdoor play, and hands-on activities with their children and turn off their own devices during family time at home (CPS, 2017a).

## Children with Disabilities

Throughout this chapter, policies and laws that support the health and well-being of the school-age child have been discussed. These include guidelines for safety, nutrition, physical activity, and social environments. In Canada, there are 10 different types of disabilities identified. These include: seeing, hearing, mobility, flexibility, dexterity, pain, learning, developmental, mental, and memory. Over 200,000 Canadian children live with some form of disability that affects their quality of life (Easter Seals, 2016).

Children with disabilities in Canada have the right to equality in all aspects of life, including health care and education. Regardless of whether the disability is behavioural, emotional, intellectual, speech, hearing, or visual, children have the right to free public education in Canada. Provinces and territories differ across the country in regards to their policies and regulations for education of children with disabilities. Even though the majority of support is managed by each province, there are many similarities between approaches to education across the country (Angloinfo Canada, 2019).

## Poverty

The low income rate in Canada is approximately 8.8% (Government of Canada, 2014). In 2014, over half a million children were living in low-income families in Canada. Children under the age of 18 who live with a single parent are more likely to live in low-income circumstances. Some groups in Canada have significantly higher rates of low income, such as single parents, recent immigrants, Indigenous people, and people with disabilities; 40% of Indigenous children in Canada live in poverty and approximately one-third of food bank users across Canada in 2016 were children (Canada Without Poverty, 2018).

Many homeless children face poor living conditions and high rates of depression related to few friends and poor health status. Migrant children face more disease (e.g., tuberculosis, scabies, and ear infections), injury, and dental caries, and pose treatment challenges because of their transient status. Indigenous populations are over-represented among the homeless population in virtually all urban centres in Canada (Canada Without Poverty, 2018). The effects of limited financial resources on children include higher mortality rates at all ages than in those who are not poor or migrant and more school days lost because of illnesses. Numerous problems exist for children in poverty, including greater developmental delay as a result of poor nutrition; increased peer rejection; poorer self-concept; increased risk of accidents, substance use and abuse or neglect by parents; and greater overall poor coping abilities.

Nurses interacting with poor families and their children should be aware of federal, provincial, and local resources to assist families financially. Local resources often include food banks, assistance with costs of a child's education, childcare, and housing support. Public health nurses in schools can advocate for children who are in need and help identify programs that may benefit a school's population, such as breakfast and/or lunch programs. The nurse improves the overall health of children by encouraging relationships with appropriate role models and by reinforcing strong family relationships that help children develop resilient and positive self-images.

Family wealth may have a negative influence on the school-age child if there is frequent substitute caregiving of varying quality attributable to parental absence, extremely high or unreasonable parental expectations, availability of material possessions but little child awareness of relevant responsibilities, and easy access to medications and alcohol and similar dangers. The nurse reinforces the need in wealthy families for consistent demonstration of parental love and support, firm limits on appropriate behaviour, and the value of recognizing the child's unique abilities. The nurse also offers ideas that will help decrease risk-taking behaviour (e.g., substance use) and increase parent–child connection until a parent is in the home.

When discussing children raised in poverty or affluence, the nurse remembers at least two points. First, many variables affect each child, often in different ways, to influence overall development. Second, although personality and support networks help a child in a socially poor environment to excel later in life, most authorities believe that problems of affluence are easier to overcome than are the all-pervasive problems of poverty.

## ◆ Health Services/Delivery System
### Well-Child Care

The CPS (2016) recommends that at every 1 to 2 years, children 6 years of age or older have a well-child examination by either a physician or a nurse practitioner. In the ideal situation, the child has a primary health care provider, one person or practice from which the child receives wellness and illness care coordinated by members of a health care team. Unfortunately, many North American children still do not have this quality of care (see the Poverty section earlier). Parents may find it challenging to find primary care providers they can see regularly. There are various online resources available in many areas of the country to help families find a doctor accepting new patients. Community health centres and various organizations for low-income or immigrant families may be able to assist in finding a health care provider for children.

The nurse encourages the school-age child and the parents to be active members of any health evaluation. Children may give some of their own history, answer questions, and discuss their health concerns. During the history, the child's privacy should be respected. Some children in this age group want a parent present during the examination; others do not. When possible, the nurse spends at least some time alone with the child to allow discussions that the child may not feel comfortable with when the parents are present. The examinations can also be a time for education on how the body works and ways to keep it healthy. Preventive information on diet and exercise can be offered relevant to prevention of obesity, cardiovascular disease, and diabetes. Information can also be obtained on school adjustment and performance, particularly because this is a major portion of the child's life. School performance can reflect the child's cognitive and general development. If there are any concerns, the nurse obtains more information through separate testing or discussion with school officials. Health education is directed to both the child and the parents for the best results. Activities that the child performs alone and with the family can give a picture of relationships and adjustments that relate to the child's health (see the Care Plan at the end of this chapter).

A challenge for nurses who work with school-age children is to maintain their normal healthy status and prevent illness. This task is accomplished through a variety of health-promotion mechanisms, such as examination, guidance, education, and legislation. The success of this health-promotion approach has been illustrated in at least one study in which Black American children improved lifestyle choices when engaged in an intervention focused on cardiovascular health. Many professionals have noted that school-age children guided by the nurse generally seek health and use various resources to attain, maintain, or regain optimal health for their future productivity. Aspects of the nursing process are implemented when one is structuring a program to maintain the child's health (such as seen with an assessment of immunization status), promote health habits (seen with teaching bicycle safety), and prevent illness (seen by obtaining throat cultures to detect streptococcal infection).

Nurses have many opportunities and settings to help them implement their interventions as consultants, board members, and active providers of care. For example, nurses and school-age children interact during well-child evaluations and at school. Nurses in other roles, such as in public health positions and in hospitals, also play a role in health promotion, although these nurses must often focus more on helping the child and the family respond to an illness or a crisis. Local and national groups influence the health of children through their activities and regulations. These include organizations such as Boy Scouts and Girl Scouts, Big Brothers and Big Sisters, charities such as the Red Cross, and various federal and provincial government agencies.

As an integral part of the community, the school system has the responsibility to provide a healthy school environment and a comprehensive health-education program. In some areas, nurses, physicians, and other health care personnel work as a team in the school health program, which includes health care and maintenance and education. The nurse advocates and searches for resources so that each child has a source of health care, or the nurse is a nurse practitioner who delivers care. School health programs range from an occasional mention of body care and the changes of puberty to a full program that integrates physical and mental health principles into all aspects of the educational experience.

Comprehensive school health services require an interdisciplinary, coordinated effort between health care providers and educators. However, when available, public health nurses offer educational and interpersonal skills to initiate health-promotion teaching that improves the overall health of consumers (students, parents, teachers, and community). Nurses have a wide scope of practice, including that of referring parents to relevant resources aimed toward activities that improve the school environment and its inhabitants.

The nurse's role in planning health maintenance for children of a school varies, depending on the type of health-maintenance program. In one system, the school nurse may refer children to resources available to provide a source of health care, whereas in another system, the school nurse functions as a nurse practitioner. On the basis of the scope of practice

## INNOVATIVE PRACTICE

### School Emergency Preparedness

Because children spend a significant portion of their day in school, pediatric emergencies such as exacerbation of a medical condition, behavioural crisis, and accidental/intentional injuries are likely to happen. As a result of the likelihood of such risks, many school districts have emergency response plans (ERPs). The purpose of an ERP is to establish procedures within the school for the administration of emergency first aid services, emergency treatments, and administration of emergency medications for students. A plan helps schools prepare to respond to life-threatening medical emergencies in the first minutes before the arrival of emergency medical service (EMS) personnel. All procedures established in the ERP are to be followed during school hours, at school-sponsored activities, and on school buses and other school property.

Because injuries are the most common life-threatening emergency encountered, teachers, trainers, nurses, and other school personnel should be trained and know the general principles of first aid. Schools now employ fewer nurses, who often rotate between schools, resulting in many schools being without medical coverage for several hours/days each week. As a result, much of the emergency care is the responsibility of teachers and other school personnel.

An ERP should have the following core elements so as to save the greatest number of lives with the most efficient use of school equipment and personnel:

- Establish an efficient and effective campus-wide communication system for each school.
- Develop a coordinated and practiced ERP with the nurses in schools, educators, families, and the EMS system, with appropriate evaluation and quality improvement.
- Reduce the risk of life-threatening emergencies by identifying students at risk and ensuring that each has an individual emergency care plan and by reducing the risk of injury and disease triggers at the school.
- Train and equip teachers, staff, and students to provide cardiopulmonary resuscitation and first aid.
- Establish an automated external defibrillator program in schools.

Many schools across Canada have emergency plans in place, although the regulation of this happens at the level of the school boards. The Pan-Canadian Joint Consortium for School Health (2019) discusses partnerships between schools and health care at a provincial level, outlining the various initiatives all Canadian provinces and territories have in place for school health promotion and emergency plans. Preparedness of schools to manage life-threatening emergencies requires the commitment of the entire community. The nurse is in a prime position to facilitate these community efforts and orchestrate partnerships between school officials, local EMS, school personnel, and local pediatricians to ensure the planning and implementation of a disaster plan.

and provincial/territorial legal requirements, the school nurse monitors and updates children's immunizations and identifies and intervenes with children who have acute or chronic health care problems, such as scoliosis, strep throat, common cold, or child abuse. Increasingly, school nurses provide sophisticated care according to evidence-informed protocols for chronically ill school-age children who have been integrated into the regular academic environment. On the basis of provincial/territorial regulations, the nurse also engages in completing vision, hearing, and scoliosis screening at regular intervals. In most schools the nurse works with the school's physician, community physicians, and parents in meeting children's and community health needs.

For all school-age children, the community health or public health nurses plays a role in developing a healthy educational environment through promoting a comprehensive and age-appropriate health-education program focused on children becoming responsible for their own health. A program aimed at accident prevention in and around the school is part of the nurse's role. The program includes assessing the school for pedestrian and automobile traffic patterns, broken playground and classroom equipment, ice and snow dangers, poorly maintained toilet facilities, and inappropriately prepared food. Regular practice drills are held to acquaint teachers and students with emergency procedures (i.e., fire, bomb, or intruder threats or actual events; Innovative Practice). All people in the school are prepared to respond to chemical hazards. The nurse implements existing school-based programs on substance and alcohol use.

It is also important to consider the role of the nurse in fostering a healthy social environment in the school. The nurse examines the social interactions of the children and interacts with them to promote positive relationships. However, social problems continue to constitute a major concern for many children during this time. Children may experience difficulty in making the initial transition away from the family and gaining satisfaction from a group of peers. Children may make the initial adjustment but then have difficulties interacting with others (e.g., bullying). When problems such as these arise, the nurse, parents, and school system determine the reasons for this behaviour and intervene appropriately.

## ❖ NURSING APPLICATION

The nurse working with the school-age child has a unique and exciting opportunity to engage the child in health-promoting behaviours. Most school-age children are able to participate in the teaching strategies if the strategies are geared toward the child's appropriate cognitive ability. As the age range of the school-age child is from 5 to 12 years, the nurse must consider the mental ability and comprehension of each developmental stage.

Nurses can teach health-promotion behaviours directly to the child through spending time demonstrating, monitoring, and reinforcing preventive health practices such as handwashing, dental hygiene, nutrition, and physical activity. These activities can be taught through age-appropriate reading materials, modelling, and role-playing. Engaging the child in these practices may also help the child conceptualize the link between the behaviour and disease prevention. The nurse must partner with parents to model healthy behaviours at home, at school, and in the community settings.

A variety of methods can be used to educate children on health and nutrition. Keeping culture, socioeconomics, and media influences in mind, the nurse should teach children concepts about food choices, exercise habits, and the ways overall health is impacted by those choices. Nutrition education can be individualized to the age of the child through use of games, activities, colourful food guides, and simple cooking activities.

Physical activity in childhood is crucial in promoting healthy behaviours that continue into adulthood. Exercise for this age group is generally provided in group activities and sports. Physical activity provides the school-age child with peer interaction and social relationships. This aspect of health promotion should be encouraged by the nurse as well as the family.

As with younger age groups, health promotion of the school-age child focuses on education about routine health examination and the childhood immunization schedule. The nurse provides the families with immunization recommendations and must remain updated on current guidelines. The nurse also focuses on prevention of childhood injuries by educating children about seat-belt and bicycle safety, as well as other things with a potential for causing injury.

Screening for health problems is another aspect of caring for the school-age child. Screenings are generally conducted for problems with vision, hearing, height, weight, and oral health. The nurse may be the first person to identify a potential issue with regard to an acute or chronic condition. At that time the nurse gathers assessment data to determine if the child needs immediate treatment or a referral to another provider. For the nurse working with school-age children and their families, the role is often one of providing education, case management, consulting, counselling, and community outreach.

## CASE STUDY

### Change in Usual Communication Pattern in School: Joey

Joey is an 8-year-old boy in elementary school. His teacher has voiced a growing concern regarding his classroom behaviour. In the past 2 months Joey has become more withdrawn from his classmates and rarely participates in class discussion. This is a new behaviour in that he "used to talk all the time, and raise his hand to answer questions in class." His teacher reports that they were discussing family and family roles in class this week. Joey became very aggressive and yelled, "My dad isn't at home anymore 'cause of my mom." He went on to say, "I really miss dad. My mom's new boyfriend isn't nice and won't buy me stuff, like my dad does." His teacher determines Joey's parents are divorced. A parent–teacher conference has been scheduled to discuss Joey's behaviour because it is now affecting his grades in school.

**Reflective Questions**

- Is Joey's behaviour appropriate for his age?
- Joey's parents do not understand his change in behaviour. His father yells, "If she would let me spend more time with *my* son, Joey wouldn't be having trouble with school. She doesn't care about *my* son now that *she* has *her* new boyfriend." How might the nurse respond to this situation?
- What interventions might be effective for Joey's parents and teacher in improving his classroom behaviour and school performance?

## ◎ CARE PLAN

### Change in Usual Communication Pattern in School: Joey

**Nursing Issue**
Inadequate coping resulting from disruption of home environment

**Defining Characteristics**
- Frequent absences from school (1 day per week in the past 2 months)
- Change in quality of schoolwork: grades have deteriorated in the past month
- Verbal outbursts in class

**Related Factors**
- Parents separated 9 months ago
- Lives with mother; her boyfriend moved into home 2 months ago
- Mom reports, "He frequently complains of headaches and stomach aches, but his doctor can't find anything wrong." Results in frequent absence
- Visits father every other weekend
- No siblings

**Expected Outcomes**
- Child will decrease number of absences from school related to "headache/stomach ache" complaints.
- Child's grades will improve during the 9-week period.
- Parents will become more involved with the school, so as to establish a relationship with the school that addresses the needs of the child related to home and school.

**Interventions**
- Assess level of family problems within the home regarding communication between parents and visitation with the child.
- Assess somatic complaints by the child. Have the child complete a "headache diary"/"stomach ache diary" to determine aggravating/alleviating factors. Document the frequency of complaints and discuss/review them with the parents.
- Meet the child to assess academic and emotional needs as they relate to home and school. Discuss the findings with the child's parents.
- Meet the parents to develop a plan to help the child meet academic goals and address the emotional needs of the child. Involve the child's teacher in plan development.
- Offer community resources to address emotional needs of the child such as support groups for children of divorced parents, Boys and Girls Clubs of Canada, and peer play groups. Include information for parent support resources as well.
- Offer after-school tutoring to facilitate the meeting of academic goals as desired.
- For further information on developing care plans, see Carpenito-Moyet (2016).

## ▊ SUMMARY

Many changes occur in children during the exciting period of the school-age years. The child's development progresses from the immaturity of the preschooler to the beginning of adolescence and eventual adulthood. Cognitive abilities increase dramatically, adding to the desire to master tasks and the ability to develop moral judgement. The child's world expands beyond the family unit, as school and peers begin to exert a major influence. Opportunities for nurses during this period occur primarily in ambulatory settings, with the school nurse frequently the most effective and influential health care provider for children of this age group and their families.

### Evolve Chapter Features
http://evolve.elsevier.com/Canada/Edelman/healthpromotion/
- Review Questions

## REFERENCES

123 test. (2012). *Culture fair intelligence tests.* Retrieved from http://www.123test.com/culture-fair-intelligence-tests/.

Al-Sahab, B., Ardern, C., Hamadeh, M. J., et al. (2010). Age at menarche in Canada: Results from the national longitudinal survey of children & youth. *BMC Public Health, 10,* 736.

American Academy of Audiology. (2011). *Childhood hearing screening guidelines.* Retrieved from http://www.cdc.gov/ncbddd/hearingloss/documents/AAA_Childhood%20Hearing%20Guidelines_2011.pdf.

American Academy of Otolaryngology. (2015). *What is otitis media and ear infection?* Retrieved from http://www.entnet.org/HealthInformation/childrensEaraches.cfm.

American Academy of Pediatrics (AAP). (2011a). Clinical practice guideline ADHD: Clinical practice guidelines for the diagnosis, evaluation, and treatment of attention-deficit, hyperactivity disorder in children and adolescents. *Pediatrics, 128*(5), 1007–1022.

American Academy of Pediatrics (AAP). (2011b). *Child abuse and neglect.* Retrieved from http://www2.aap.org/sections/childabuseneglect/.

American Academy of Pediatrics (AAP). (2012). *Injuries, manufacturer warnings do not deter ATV use by children under age 16.* Retrieved from https://www.aap.org/en-us/about-the-aap/aap-press-room/pages/Injuries-Manufacturer-Warnings-Do-Not-Deter-ATV-Use-by-Children-under-Age-16.aspx.

American Academy of Pediatrics (AAP). (2014). Literacy promotion: An essential component of primary care. *Pediatric Practice, 134*(2). Retrieved from http://pediatrics.aappublications.org/content/pediatrics/early/2014/06/19/peds.2014-1384.full.pdf.

American Academy of Pediatrics (AAP). (2015a). *Helping your child learn to read.* Retrieved from https://www.healthychildren.org/english/ages-stages/preschool/Pages/Helping-Your-Child-Learn-to-Read.aspx?nfstatus=401&nftoken=00000000-0000-0000-0000-000000000000&nfstatusdescription=ERROR%3a+No+local+token.

American Academy of Pediatrics (AAP). (2015b). *Helping your child develop a healthy sense of self-esteem.* Retrieved from https://www.healthychildren.org/English/ages-stages/gradeschool/Pages/Helping-Your-Child-Develop-A-Healthy-Sense-of-Self-Esteem.aspx.

American Academy of Sleep Medicine. (2014). *Sleep & children*. Retrieved from http://yoursleep.aasmnet.org/topic.aspx?id=8.

American Heart Association (AHA). (2015a). *Healthy eating habits start at home*. Retrieved from http://www.heart.org/HEARTORG/GettingHealthy/NutritionCenter/HealthyEating/Healthy-Eating-Habits-Start-at-Home_UCM_461862_Article.jsp#.VlsKCNKrTIU.

American Heart Association (AHA). (2015b). *Overweight in children*. Retrieved from http://www.heart.org/HEARTORG/Getting-Healthy/Overweight-in-Children_UCM_304054_Article.jsp.

American Psychiatric Association. (2013). *Diagnostic and statistical manual of mental disorders* (5th ed.). Washington: American Psychiatric Association.

Angloinfo Canada. (2019). *Special needs education in Canada*. Retrieved from https://www.angloinfo.com/how-to/canada/family/schooling-education/special-needs-education.

Austin, P. F., Bauer, S. B., Bower, W., Chase, J., Franco, I., Hoebeke, P., et al. (2016). The standardization of terminology of lower urinary tract function in children and adolescents: Update report from the standardization committee of the International Children's Continence Society. *Neurourology and Urodynamics*, 35(4), 471–481.

Azarpazhooh, A., Lawrence, H. P., & Shah, P. S. (2011). Xylitol prevents acute otitis media in children up to 12 years of age. *Cochrane Database of Systematic Reviews*, 11, CD007095.

Barlow, S. E. (2007). Expert committee recommendations regarding the prevention, assessment, and treatment of child and adolescent overweight and obesity: Summary report. *Pediatrics*, 120(Suppl. 4), S164–S192.

Barron, S. A. (2015). *Encopresis (soiling)*. Retrieved from http://kidshealth.org/parent/emotions/behavior/encopresis.html#.

BMJ Best Practice. (2015). *Assessment of learning difficulties and cognitive delay*. Retrieved from http://bestpractice.bmj.com/best-practice/monograph/884.html.

Bonuck, K., Chervin, R. D., & Howe, L. D. (2015). Sleep disordered breathing, sleep duration, and childhood overweight: A longitudinal study. *The Journal of Pediatrics*, 166(3), 632–639. https://doi.org/10.1016/j.jpeds.2014.11.001.

Bordini, B., & Rosenfield, R. L. (2011). Normal pubertal development: Part II: Clinical aspects of puberty. *Pediatrics in Review*, 32(7), 281–292.

Boyse, K. (2010). *Sleep problems*. Retrieved from http://www.med.umich.edu/yourchild/topics/sleep.htm.

Brogan, R. J. (2015). *What is a germ?* Retrieved from http://kidshealth.org/kid/talk/qa/germs.html#.

Canada Without Poverty. (2018). Retrieved from http://www.cwp-csp.ca/poverty/just-the-facts/.

Canadian ADHD Resource Alliance (CADDRA) (2018). *Canadian ADHD practice guidelines* (4th ed.). Retrieved from https://www.caddra.ca/wp-content/uploads/CADDRA-Guidelines-4th-Edition_-Feb2018.pdf.

Canadian Cancer Society. (2019). *Childhood cancer statistics*. Retrieved from http://www.cancer.ca/en/cancer-information/cancer-101/childhood-cancer-statistics/?region=on.

Canadian Dental Association. (2018). *Dental development*. Retrieved from http://www.cda-adc.ca/en/oral_health/cfyt/dental_care_children/development.asp.

Canadian Medical Association. (2015). *Obesity in Canada: Causes, consequences and the way forward*. Retrieved from https://sencanada.ca/content/sen/committee/412/SOCI/Briefs/2015-06-10CanadianMedicalAssocWrittenObesityBrief_e.pdf.

Canadian Paediatric Society. (2017a). *Screen time and young children: Promoting health and development in a digital world*. Retrieved from https://www.cps.ca/en/documents/position/screen-time-and-young-children.

Canadian Paediatric Society. (2018d). *ADHD in children and youth: Part 1—Etiology, diagnosis and comorbidity*. Retrieved from https://www.cps.ca/en/documents/position/adhd-etiology-diagnosis-and-comorbidity.

Canadian Paediatric Society (CPS). (2012). *Child and youth injury prevention: A public health approach*. Retrieved from https://www.cps.ca/en/documents/position/child-and-youth-injury-prevention.

Canadian Paediatric Society (CPS). (2014). *WHO growth charts for Canada*. Retrieved from https://www.cps.ca/en/tools-outils/who-growth-charts.

Canadian Paediatric Society (CPS). (2016). *Greig health record*. Retrieved from https://www.cps.ca/en/tools-outils/greig-health-record.

Canadian Paediatric Society (CPS). (2017b). *Preventing unintentional injuries in Indigenous children and youth in Canada*. Retrieved from https://www.cps.ca/en/documents/position/unintentional-injuries-indigenous-children-youth.

Canadian Paediatric Society (CPS). (2018a). *Oral health for children—a call for action*. Retrieved from https://www.cps.ca/en/documents/position/oral-health-care-for-children.

Canadian Paediatric Society (CPS). (2018b). *Cultural competence for child and youth health professionals*. Retrieved from https://www.kidsnewtocanada.ca/culture/competence.

Canadian Paediatric Society (CPS). (2018c). *How much for school-age children? (5–11 years)*. Retrieved from https://www.cps.ca/en/active-actifs/how-much-for-school-age-children.

Canadian Paediatric Society (CPS). (2018e). *Depression in children and youth*. Retrieved from https://www.kidsnewtocanada.ca/mental-health/depression.

Canadian Paediatric Society (CPS). (2018f). *The prevention of firearm injuries in Canadian youth*. Retrieved from https://www.cps.ca/en/documents/position/the-prevention-of-firearm-injuries-in-canadian-youth.

Canadian Red Cross. (2013). *Facts and figures: Child drownings in Canada*. Retrieved from https://www.redcross.ca/crc/documents/What-We-Do/Swimming-Water-Safety/facts-and-figures-water-safety-week-2013.pdf.

Cardoso da Silveria, J. A., Taddei, J. A., Guerra, P. H., et al. (2013). The effect of participation in school-based nutrition education interventions on body mass index: A meta-analysis of randomized, controlled community trials. *Preventive Medicine*, 56(3–4), 237–243.

Caring for Kids. (2017). *Playground safety*. Retrieved from https://www.caringforkids.cps.ca/handouts/playground-safety.

Caring for Kids. (2018). *Footwear for children*. Retrieved from https://www.caringforkids.cps.ca/handouts/footwear_for_children.

Caring for Kids. (2019). *Are ATVs safe for children and youth?* Retrieved from https://www.caringforkids.cps.ca/handouts/all_terrain_vehicles.

Carpenito-Moyet, L. J. (2016). *Nursing diagnosis: Application to clinical practice* (15th ed.). Philadelphia: Lippincott Williams & Wilkins.

Castagno, V. D., Fassa, A. G., Carret, M. L., et al. (2014). Hyperopia: A meta-analysis of prevalence and a review of associated factors among school-age children. *BMC Ophthalmology*, 14, 163. https://doi.org/10.1186/1471-2415-14-163.

Centers for Disease Control and Prevention (CDC). (2012). *Protect the ones you love: Child injuries are preventable*. Retrieved from http://www.cdc.gov/safechild/burns/index.html.

Centers for Disease Control and Prevention (CDC). (2014). *Pedestrian safety*. Retrieved from http://www.cdc.gov/Motorvehiclesafety/Pedestrian_safety/index.html.

Centers for Disease Control and Prevention (CDC). (2015a). *Overweight and obesity: Basics about childhood obesity.* Retrieved from https://www.cdc.gov/obesity/childhood/index.html.

Centers for Disease Control and Prevention (CDC). (2015b). *How much physical activity do children need?* Retrieved from http://www.cdc.gov/physicalactivity/basics/children/.

Centers for Disease Control and Prevention (CDC). (2015c). *Youth activity guideline toolkit.* Retrieved from http://www.cdc.gov/healthyschools/physicalactivity/guidelines.htm.

Centers for Disease Control and Prevention (CDC). (2018). *Attention-deficit/hyperactivity disorder.* Retrieved from https://www.cdc.gov/ncbddd/adhd/diagnosis.html.

Craggs, C., Corder, K., van Sluijs, E. M., et al. (2011). Determinants of change in physical activity in children and adolescents. *American Journal of Preventive Medicine, 40*(6), 645–658.

Dadds, M. R., Schollar-Root, O., Lenroot, R., et al. (2016). Epigenetic regulation of the DRD4 gene and dimensions of attention-deficit disorder in children. *European Child & Adolescent Psychiatry, 25*(10), 1081–1089.

Daly, L., Kallan, M. J., Arbogast, K. B., et al. (2010). Risk of injury to child passengers in sport utility vehicles. *Pediatrics, 117*(1), 9–14.

Dionne, J. M., Harris, K. C., Benoit, G., et al. (2017). Hypertension Canada's 2017 guidelines for the diagnosis, assessment, prevention and treatment of pediatric hypertension. *Canadian Journal of Cardiology, 33*(2017), 577–585. https://doi.org/10.1016/j.cjca.2017.03.007.

Disabled World. (2015). *Cognitive disabilities: Information on intellectual disabilities.* Retrieved from http://www.disabled-world.com/disability/types/cognitive/.

Downing, J. R., Wilson, R. K., Zhang, J., et al. (2012). Pediatric cancer genome project. *National Genetics, 44*(6), 619–622. https://doi.org/10.1038/ng.2287.

Durani, Y. (2015). *Body basics: The immune system.* Retrieved from http://kidshealth.org/en/parents/immune.html#.

Erikson, E. H. (1993). *Childhood and society* (2nd ed., reissued). New York: W. W. Norton. [Seminal Reference].

Erikson, E. H. (1994). *Identity, youth and crisis* (35th ed., reissued). New York: W. W. Norton. [Seminal Reference].

Ferrer, M., & Fugate, A. (2014). *The importance of friendship for school-age children.* Retrieved from https://www.frontierdistrict.k-state.edu/family/child-development/docs/school-age/ImportanceFriendship.pdf.

Garey, J. (2015). *13 ways to boost your daughter's self-esteem.* Retrieved from http://www.childmind.org/en/posts/articles/2012-9-25-13-ways-help-build-your-daughters-self-esteem.

Goldberg, J. (2014). *Enuresis in children.* Retrieved from http://www.webmd.com/mental-health/enuresis.

Goldstein, S., & Brooks, R. (2012). *Raising resilient children.* Retrieved from https://www.psychologytoday.com/blog/raising-resilient-children/201211/giving-children-allowance-nurturing-resilience.

Goswami, U. (2015). *Children's cognitive development and learning.* Retrieved from http://cprtrust.org.uk/wp-content/uploads/2015/02/COMPLETE-REPORT-Goswami-Childrens-Cognitive-Development-and-Learning.pdf.

Government of Canada. (2006). *Aboriginal peoples survey.* Retrieved from https://www.canada.ca/en/public-health/services/health-promotion/healthy-living/obesity-canada/prevalence-among-aboriginal-populations.html. [Seminal Reference].

Government of Canada. (2011). *Curbing childhood obesity: An overview of the federal, provincial and territorial framework for action to promote healthy weights.* Retrieved from https://www.canada.ca/en/public-health/services/health-promotion/healthy-living/curbing-childhood-obesity-federal-provincial-territorial-framework/curbing-childhood-obesity-overview-federal-provincial-territorial-framework-action-promote-healthy-weights.html.

Government of Canada. (2012). *Child maltreatment in Canada.* Retrieved from https://www.canada.ca/en/public-health/services/health-promotion/stop-family-violence/prevention-resource-centre/children/child-maltreatment-canada.html#Typ.

Government of Canada. (2014). *Towards a poverty reduction strategy—A background on poverty in Canada.* Retrieved from https://www.canada.ca/en/employment-social-development/programs/poverty-reduction/backgrounder.html#h2.4-h3.1.

Government of Canada. (2015). *Federal laws.* Retrieved from https://www.canada.ca/en/health-canada/services/health-concerns/tobacco/legislation/federal-laws.html.

Government of Canada. (2016). *Canadian immunization guide: Key immunization information.* Retrieved from https://www.canada.ca/en/public-health/services/publications/healthy-living/canadian-immunization-guide-part-1-key-immunization-information.html.

Government of Canada. (2018a). *Rights of people with disabilities.* Retrieved from https://www.canada.ca/en/canadian-heritage/services/rights-people-disabilities.html.

Government of Canada. (2018b). *Choosing a child car seat or booster seat.* Retrieved from https://www.tc.gc.ca/en/services/road/child-car-seat-safety/choosing-child-car-seat-booster-seat.html#_The_four_stages.

Government of Canada. (2018c). *Tobacco and Vaping Products Act.* Retrieved from https://www.canada.ca/en/health-canada/services/health-concerns/tobacco/legislation/federal-laws/tobacco-act.html.

Government of Canada. (2019a). *Canada's dietary guidelines.* Retrieved from https://food-guide.canada.ca/en/guidelines/.

Government of Canada. (2019b). *Restricting advertising of certain foods to children under 13 years of age.* Retrieved from https://www.canada.ca/en/health-canada/services/marketing-health-claims/restricting-advertising-children.html.

Government of Canada. (2019c). *Canadian motor vehicle traffic collision statistics 2017.* Retrieved from https://www.tc.gc.ca/eng/motorvehiclesafety/canadian-motor-vehicle-traffic-collision-statistics-2017.html.

Griffiths, L. J., Parsons, T. J., & Hill, A. J. (2010). Self-esteem and quality of life in obese children: A systematic review. *International Journal of Pediatric Obesity, 5*(4), 282–304.

Gupta, R. C. (2014). *All about sleep.* Retrieved from http://kidshealth.org/parent/general/sleep/sleep.html#.

Gupta, R. C. (2015). *Head lice.* Retrieved from http://kidshealth.org/parent/infections/common/head_lice.html#.

Hagel, B. E., Yanchar, N. L., & Canadian Paediatric Society, & Injury Prevention Committee. (2013). Bicycle helmet use in Canada: The need for legislation to reduce the risk of head injury. *Paediatrics and Child Health, 18*(9), 475–480. https://doi.org/10.1093/pch/18.9.475.

Hanfstingl, B., Benke, G., & Zhang, Y. (2019). Comparing variation theory with piaget's theory of cognitive development: More similarities than differences? *Educational Action Research, 27*(4), 511–526.

Harding, M. (2015). *Normal and abnormal puberty.* Retrieved from http://patient.info/doctor/normal-and-abnormal-puberty.

Harron, W. (2014). *Your child's handwriting—Signs of handwriting problems.* Retrieved from http://kidshealth.org/parent/positive/learning/handwriting.html#.

HealthlinkBC. (2017). *Preventing children's injuries from sports and other activities.* Retrieved from https://www.healthlinkbc.ca/health-topics/abo6102.

Heiting, G. (2015). *Eye exams for children.* Retrieved from http://www.allaboutvision.com/eye-exam/children.htm.

Hingle, M., & Kunkel, D. (2012). Childhood obesity and media. *Paediatric Clinics of North America, 59*(3), 677–692. https://doi.org/10.1016/j.pcl.2012.03.021.

Hrabok, M., Brooks, B. L., Fay-McClymont, T. B., & Sherman, E. M. (2014). Wechsler intelligence scale for children-(WISC-IV) short-form validity: A comparison study in pediatric epilepsy. *Child Neuropsychology, 20*(1), 49–59. https://doi.org/10.1080/09297049.2012.741225.

Inman, D. D., van Bakergern, K. M., Larosa, A. C., et al. (2011). Evidence-based health promotion programs for schools and communities. *American Journal of Preventive Medicine, 40*(2), 207–219. https://doi.org/10.1016/j.amepre.2010.10.031.

Jarvis, C., & Luctkar-Flude, M. (2019). Musculo-skeletal system. In C. Jarvis, A. J. Browne, J. MacDonald-Jenkins, et al. (Eds.), *Physical examination & health assessment* (3rd Canadian ed.) (pp. 625–686). Toronto: Elsevier Canada.

Kaneshiro, N. K. (2014). *School-age test or procedure preparation.* Retrieved from http://www.nlm.nih.gov/medlineplus/ency/article/002058.htm.

Kaneshiro, N. K. (2016). *Bedwetting.* Retrieved from https://medlineplus.gov/ency/patientinstructions/000703.htm.

Kanwar, V. S. (2015). *Lymphadenopathy.* Retrieved from http://emedicine.medscape.com/article/956340-overview#showall.

Kendler, K. S., Ohlsson, H., Turkheimer, R., et al. (2015). Family environment and the malleability of cognitive ability: A Swedish national home-reared and adopted-away cosibling control study. *Proceedings of the National Academy of Sciences of the United States of America, 112*(15), 4612–4617. https://doi.org/10.1073/pnas.1417106112.

Kids, S. (2013). *Injury trends fact sheet.* Retrieved from http://www.safekids.org/sites/default/files/documents/skw_overview_fact_sheet_oct_2013.pdf.

Kim, H. S. (2011). Consequences of parental divorce for child development. *American Sociological Review, 76*(3), 487–511. https://doi.org/10.1177/0003122411407748.

Klish, W. J. (2015). *Comorbidities and complications of obesity in children and adolescents.* Retrieved from http://www.uptodate.com/contents/comorbidities-and-complications-of-obesity-in-children-and-adolescents.

Kohlberg, L. (1981). *The philosophy of moral development.* San Francisco: Harper & Row. [Seminal Reference].

Krause-Parello, C. A., & Samms, K. (2010). School nurses in New Jersey: A quantitative inquiry on roles & responsibilities. *Journal for Specialists in Pediatric Nursing, 15*(3), 217–222.

Learning Disabilities Association of Canada. (2017). Prevalence of learning disabilities. Retrieved from https://www.ldac-acta.ca/prevalence-of-learning-disabilities/.

Lourenco, B. H., Villamor, E., Augusto, R. A., et al. (2012). Determinants of linear growth. *BMC Public Health, 12,* 265. http://www.biomedcentral.com/1471-2458/12/265.

Martin, L. (2013). *Sleep in different cultures.* Retrieved from http://www.howsleepworks.com/anthropology_cultures.html.

McLeod, S. (2015). *Piaget's theory of moral development.* Retrieved from http://www.simplypsychology.org/piaget-moral.html.

Mental Health Commission of Canada. (2018). *MHS: A youth perspective.* Retrieved from https://www.mentalhealthcommission.ca/English/initiatives/11849/mhs-youth-perspective.

Milteer, R. M., Ginsburg, K. R., & Mulligan, D. A. (2012). The importance of play in promoting healthy child development and maintaining strong parent-child bond: Focus on children in poverty. *Pediatrics, 129*(1), e204–e213. https://doi.org/10.1542/peds.2011-2953.

Moses, S. (2015). *Pediatric vital signs.* Retrieved from http://www.fpnotebook.com/cv/exam/pdtrcvtlsgns.htm.

National Health Service. (2015). *Bedwetting.* Retrieved from http://www.nhs.uk/Conditions/Bedwetting/Pages/Introduction.aspx.

National Institute on Deafness and Other Communication Disorders. (2012). *Office visits to U.S. physicians resulting in primary diagnosis of otitis media.* Retrieved from http://www.nidcd.nih.gov/health/statistics/Pages/officevisits.aspx.

Nielson, L. S., Danielson, K. V., & Sorenson, T. I. A. (2011). Short sleep duration as a possible cause of obesity: Critical review analysis of the epidemiological evidence. *Obesity Review, 12*(2), 78–92.

Nielson, C. M., Srikanth, P., & Orwoll, E. S. (2012). Obesity and fracture in men and women: An epidemiologic perspective. *Journal of Bone and Mineral Research, 27*(1), 1–10. https://doi.org/10.1002/jbmr.1486.

Nieman, P., Shea, S., & Canadian Paediatric Society Community Paediatrics Committee. (2004). Effective discipline for children. *Paediatric Child Health, 9*(1), 37–41. Retrieved from https://www.uottawa.ca/health/sites/www.uottawa.ca.health/files/ped-_behavior_effective_discipline_for_children.pdf. [Seminal Reference].

Ontario Student Drug Use and Health Survey. (2017). *Drug use among Ontario students.* Retrieved from http://www.camhx.ca/Publications/OSDUHS/2017/index.html.

Pan-Canadian Joint Consortium for School Health. (2019). Retrieved from http://www.jcsh-cces.ca/.

Peristein, D. (2013). *My child has a tooth, now what?* Retrieved from http://www.medicinenet.com/tooth_eruption_chart/views.htm.

Piaget, J. (2001). *Psychology of intelligence.* Florence, KY: Routledge. [Seminal reference].

Pickhardt, C. (2011). *Impact of divorce on young children and adolescents.* Retrieved from http://www.psychologytoday.com/blog/surviving-your-childs-adolescence/201112/the-impact-divorce-young-children-and-adolescents.

Pillinger, J. (2015). *Bedwetting (enuresis).* Retrieved from http://www.netdoctor.co.uk/diseases/facts/bedwetting.htm.

Public Health Agency of Canada (PHAC). (2008). *Canadian incidence study of reported child abuse and neglect.* Retrieved from http://cwrp.ca/sites/default/files/publications/en/CIS-2008-rprt-eng.pdf. [Seminal Reference].

Public Health Agency of Canada (PHAC). (2009). *The chief public health officer's report on the state of public health in Canada.* Retrieved from https://www.canada.ca/en/public-health/corporate/publications/chief-public-health-officer-reports-state-public-health-canada/report-on-state-public-health-canada-2009/chapter-3.html.

Public Health Agency of Canada (PHAC). (2018). *Tackling obesity in Canada: Canada obesity and excessive weights in Canada.* Retrieved from https://www.canada.ca/en/public-health/services/publications/healthy-living/obesity-excess-weight-rates-canadian-children.html.

Queensland Health. (2014). *Health care provider's handbook on Hindu patients.* Retrieved from https://www.health.qld.gov.au/multicultural/support_tools/hbook-hindu.pdf.

Raghubar, K. P., Barnes, M. A., & Hecht, S. A. (2010). Working memory and mathematics: A review of developmental individual differences and cognitive approach. *Learning and Individual Differences, 20*(2), 110–122. https://doi.org/10.1016/j.lindif.2009.10.005.

Robinson, J. (2014). *Overview of sleepwalking*. Retrieved from http://www.webmd.com/sleep-disorders/guide/sleepwalking-causes.

Robson, S. M., Couch, S. C., Peugh, J. L., et al. (2016). Parent diet and quality and energy intake are related to child diet quality and energy intake. *Journal of the Academy of Nutrition and Dietetics, 116*(6), 984–990. https://doi.org/10.1016/j.jand.2016.02.011.

Scharrer, E. (2019). Teaching about media violence. *The International Encyclopedia of media literacy*, 1–10. https://doi.org/10.1002/9781118978238.ieml0231.

Seals, E. (2016). *Disability in Canada: Facts and figures*. Retrieved from https://easterseals.ca/english/wp-content/uploads/2016/12/Disability-in-Canada-Facts-Figures.pdf.

Segre, L. (2015). *The eye chart and 20/20 vision*. Retrieved from http://www.allaboutvision.com/eye-test/.

Shenouda, N., & Timmons, B. W. (2012). *Preschool focus: Physical activity and screen time*. Child health and exercise medicine program (Issue 5). Hamilton, ON: McMaster University.

Shroff, A. (2015). *Piaget's levels of learning*. Retrieved from http://www.webmd.com/children/piaget-stages-of-development.

SickKids, Staff. (2011). *Physical development in school-age children*. Retrieved from https://www.aboutkidshealth.ca/Article?contentid=712&language=English.

Statistics, Canada. (2016). *Hearing loss of Canadians, 2012 to 2015*. Retrieved from https://www150.statcan.gc.ca/n1/pub/82-625-x/2016001/article/14658-eng.htm.

Sturaro, C., van Lier, P. A., Cuijpers, P., et al. (2011). The role of peer relationships in the development of early school-age externalizing problems. *Child Development, 82*(3), 758–765.

Thiffault, I., & Lantos, J. (2016). The challenge of analyzing the results of next-generation sequencing in children. *Pediatrics, 137*(Suppl. 1), 83–87.

Toll, E. C., & Nunez, D. A. (2012). Diagnosis and treatment of acute otitis media: Review. *Journal of Laryngology & Otology, 126*(10), 976–983. https://doi.org/10.1017/S0022215112001326.

US Department of Health and Human Services (USDHHS). (2011). *Child maltreatment 2010*. Retrieved from http://www.acf.hhs.gov/programs/cb/pubs/cm10/cm10.pdf#page=31.

Van Doren, J., Arns, M., Heinrich, H., et al. (2019). Sustained effects of neurofeedback in ADH: A systematic review and meta-analysis. *European Child & Adolescent Psychiatry, 28*, 293–305. https://doi.org/10.1007/s00787-018-1121-4.

Van den Berg, L., Pieterse, K., Malik, J. A., et al. (2011). Association between impulsivity, reward responsiveness and BMI in children. *International Journal of Obesity, 35*(10), 1301–1307.

Wald, E. R. (2015). *Sore throat overview*. Retrieved from http://www.uptodate.com/contents/sore-throat-in-children-beyond-the-basics.

Willingham, D. T., Hughes, E. M., & Doboly, D. G. (2015). Scientific status of learning styles theories. *Teaching of Psychology, 42*(3), 266–271. https://doi.org/10.1177/0098628315589505.

Women, & Children's Health Network. (2013). *Self-esteem*. Retrieved from http://www.cyh.com/HealthTopics/HealthTopicDetails.aspx?p=114&np=141&id=1702.

World Health Organization (WHO). (2008). *School policy framework: Implementation of the WHO global strategy on diet, physical activity and health*. Retrieved from https://www.who.int/dietphysicalactivity/SPF-en-2008.pdf?ua=1. [Seminal Reference].

World Health Organization (WHO). (2015a). *Growth reference data for 5–19 years*. Retrieved from http://www.who.int/growthref/en/.

World Health Organization (WHO). (2015b). *Environmental risks*. Retrieved from http://www.who.int/ceh/risks/en/.

Yanchar, N. L., Warda, L. J., & Fuselli, P. (2012). Child and youth injury prevention: A public health approach. *Paediatrics and Child Health, 17*(9), 511.

# 15

# Adolescent

*Barbara Wilson-Keates, RN, MS, PhD*

Originating US chapter by *Susan Rowen James, RN, PhD*

## INTENDED LEARNING OUTCOMES

*After completing this chapter, the reader will be able to:*

- Summarize the physical growth, developmental, and maturational changes that occur during adolescence.
- Discuss the recommended schedule of health-promotion and preventive health visits for adolescents and the appropriate topics for inclusion during each visit.

- Analyze factors that contribute to risk-taking behaviours and situations during adolescence.
- Develop a health teaching plan addressing some of the physical, emotional, social, and spiritual challenges facing adolescents.

## KEY TERMS

Acne
Adolescence
Body image
Cyberbullying
Eating disorders
Egocentrism
Idealism
Identity
Introspection

Obesity
Peer group
Precocious puberty
Puberty
Risky behaviours
Scoliosis
Sexually transmitted and blood-borne infections (STBBIs)
Social media
Tanner staging

## ❓ THINK ABOUT IT

### Risk Behaviours in Adolescents

The mortality rate for adolescents (age 15–19 years) is four times higher than it is for school-age children (age 5–14 years) (Statistics Canada, 2019a). Currently, suicide is the second leading cause of death in adolescents (Mental Health Commission of Canada, 2018). By the age of 17, more than half of Canadian youth are sexually active, and, of those who are sexually active, 25% report not consistently using any method of birth control (Canadian Paediatric Society [CPS], 2019).

- What growth and developmental factors make adolescents susceptible to engaging in risky behaviours?
- What anticipatory guidance and strategies might be offered to adolescents and their families to prevent this risky behaviour?

The term *adolescence* is frequently used to describe the transitional stage with significant physiological and psychological changes beginning with the onset of puberty, at approximately age 10 to 13 years, and lasting until adulthood,. Many Canadian researchers and developmental specialists use the age span from 13 to 19 years as a working definition of adolescence (Public Health Agency of Canada [PHAC], 2010). The term *adolescence* refers to the psychosocial, emotional, cognitive, and moral transition from childhood to young adulthood, whereas *puberty* refers to the development and maturation of the reproductive, endocrine, and structural processes that lead to fertility.

Rapid change in physical, psychosocial, spiritual, moral, and cognitive growth creates an extremely tenuous sense of balance. A pivotal developmental period, adolescence offers health care providers unique opportunities for providing health-promotion and preventive services to adolescents and their families. The PHAC (2019a) emphasizes that focusing on supportive relationships with family, school, peers, and community promotes adolescent health, in addition to enhancing protective factors against risk. Family support is the most critical factor in the promotion of positive health outcomes for youth, including adopting a healthy lifestyle and avoiding risk behaviours. School climate helps to prevent bullying and violence, while peer support protects positive health behaviours, but does not necessarily prevent risk behaviours. Community support also facilitates positive health outcome for adolescents.

## BIOLOGY AND GENETICS

### Sex and Puberty

In contrast to the slow, steady growth of childhood, adolescents experience accelerated physical growth that dramatically alters their body size and proportions. Additionally, adolescents experience the onset of puberty. Changes associated with the onset of puberty occur in a predictable sequence, but the onset and duration of the sequence differ among individuals. Females usually begin puberty 2 years earlier than males and experience their growth spurt earlier. White females are maturing earlier than in the past, and body mass index (BMI) is correlated with earlier onset of puberty for both males and females (Statistics Canada, 2016a). Adolescents who do not follow the normal sequence or who have not begun pubertal development by age 14 years, for males, and age 13 years, for females, should have an endocrine evaluation (Merck Manual, 2019).

The physical changes experienced during adolescence are mediated primarily by the hormonal regulatory systems in the hypothalamus, pituitary gland, gonads, and adrenal glands (Fig. 15.1). The hypothalamus releases gonadotropin-releasing hormone (GnRH), which stimulates the anterior pituitary to release the gonadotropin hormones luteinizing hormone (LH) and follicle-stimulating hormone (FSH) (Copstead & Banasik, 2013). In females, this stimulates development of the ovaries and estrogen production. Once sexual maturation is complete, the ongoing release of hormones controls menses, pregnancy, and lactation. In males, LH results in enlargement of the testes and the development of Leydig cells in the testes, which produce testosterone. FSH stimulates the development of the seminiferous tubules of the testes, leading to spermatogenesis and fertility.

During puberty, primary sexual characteristics begin to develop and secondary sexual characteristics emerge. Primary sexual characteristics involve the organs necessary for reproduction, such as the penis and testes in boys and the vagina and uterus in girls. Secondary sexual characteristics are external features that are not essential for reproduction. Breast development, facial and pubic hair growth, and lowering of the voice

are examples of secondary sexual characteristics (Table 15.1). Estrogen produces all secondary sexual characteristics except axillary and pubic hair, which are controlled by adrenal androgens. Sexual maturity rating, also referred to as *Tanner staging*, is used widely to assess and monitor the degree of maturation of an adolescent's primary and secondary sexual characteristics. Each of the characteristics—breast, pubic hair, and genitals—is staged separately (from 1 to 5) and compared with the expected sequencing (Fig. 15.2).

Breast development is usually confined to females; however, some degree of unilateral or bilateral breast enlargement, termed *gynecomastia*, may appear early in male puberty, just before the growth spurt. Gynecomastia is usually temporary and typically disappears. However, occasionally it persists and leads to body image problems and can be surgically reduced if psychological assessment warrants it.

The first sign of puberty in males is a thinning of the scrotal sac and enlargement of the testicles. Ejaculation is considered a milestone of male puberty and precedes fertility by several months. Nocturnal emissions, or wet dreams, can concern adolescent males because the events happen beyond their control.

For females, the first sign of puberty is the appearance of breast buds, followed by the growth spurt. The onset of menstruation, or menarche, occurs approximately 2 years after the appearance of the breast buds and near the end of the growth spurt (see Fig. 15.2).

Familiarity with the stages of development of sexual characteristics and their expected sequence helps the nurse monitor the adolescent's progression through puberty and detect any variations that might herald an alteration in normal growth and development.

Precocious puberty is the appearance of physical signs of puberty before the age of 9 in boys and before the ages of 7 or 8 years in girls. Children undergoing precocious puberty should have their growth and history reviewed, to help identify individuals in need for further evaluation (Canadian Paediatric Society, 2017a).

Before the growth spurt, many adolescents experience a transient increase in the amount of body fat or adipose tissue. As puberty progresses the proportion of total body weight composed of fat usually declines, particularly in boys. Body fat begins to accumulate again in both sexes after their growth spurt, but at a slightly higher rate in females.

## Other Physical Changes

The heart grows in size and strength. Blood volume and blood pressure increase, and the heart rate decreases to adult levels. These cardiovascular changes occur earlier in females, corresponding with puberty. Compared with adolescent males, adolescent females also generally have higher pulse rates and slightly lower systolic blood pressure. Adolescents are identified as hypertensive when their systolic or diastolic blood pressure is at or above the 95th percentile (based on age, sex, and height) on three separate occasions. Functional murmurs are common in adolescents (Government of Canada, 2013).

Respiratory rate decreases throughout childhood, reaching an average rate of 15 to 20 breaths per minute during

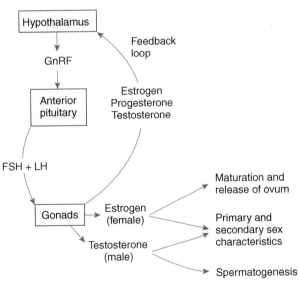

**Fig. 15.1** Hormonal interaction among hypothalamus, pituitary, and gonads.
*FSH*, Follicle-stimulating hormone; *GnRH*, gonadotropin-releasing hormone; *LH*, luteinizing hormone. (From Hockenberry, M. J., & Wilson, D. [2015]. *Wong's nursing care of infants and children* [10th ed.]. St. Louis: Mosby.)

adolescence. Respiratory volume and vital capacity increase, particularly in males. The larynx and vocal cords grow, producing the characteristic voice changes of puberty. Both male and female voices become deeper, and laryngeal cartilage enlarges, with both effects more pronounced in males.

The gastro-intestinal system reaches functional maturity during the school-age years. However, it continues to grow along with the growth spurt (Guyton & Hall, 2011).

Permanent teeth begin erupting at approximately 6 years of age, and all 32, except the third molars, or wisdom teeth, are in place by 13 to 14 years of age. Third molars are often pulled during adolescence to make space for the other permanent teeth. It is not uncommon for one or more of the third molars not to develop, and this lack of development (agenesis) is often familial. Dental decay and periodontal disease are not uncommon, particularly among Indigenous adolescents (Government of Canada, 2013).

The sweat and sebaceous glands both become more active during adolescence. The sweat glands are located primarily in the axillary, genital, and periumbilical areas and are the primary

## TABLE 15.1 Growth and Development

### Sexual Maturity Rating, Tanner Stages: Developmental Stages of Secondary Sexual Characteristics

| Stage | Male Genital Development | Pubic Hair Development | Female Breast Development | Other Changes |
|---|---|---|---|---|
| 1 | Prepubertal | No distinction between hair over pubic area and hair over abdomen | | |
| 2 | Initial enlargement of scrotum and testes; reddening and texture changes of scrotum | Sparse growth of long, straight, downy hair at base of penis or along labia | Enlargement of areolar diameter; small area of elevation around papillae (breast bud) | Usual time of peak height velocity for girls |
| 3 | Initial enlargement of penis, mainly in length; further growth of testes and scrotum | Hair becomes dark, coarse, and curly; spreads sparsely over entire pubic area | Further elevation and enlargement of breasts and areolas, with no separation of their contours | Usual time of menarche; facial hair begins to grow on upper lip and voice deepens in boys |
| 4 | Further enlargement of penile diameter, testes, scrotum, and glans | Further spread of hair distribution, not extending to thighs | Areolas and papillae project from breast to form secondary mound | Usual time of peak height velocity for boys; axillary hair begins to grow |
| 5 | Adult in size and contour | Adult in amount and type; spreads to inner surface of thighs | Adult, with projection of papillae only; recession of areolas into general breast contour | |

Modified from Hockenberry, M. J., & Wilson, D. (2015). *Wong's nursing care of infants and children* (10th ed.). St. Louis: Mosby.

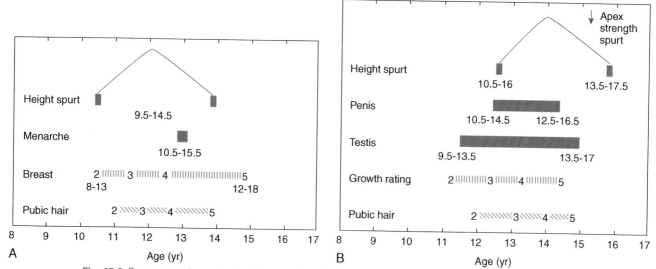

**Fig. 15.2** Sequences of events at adolescence in girls (A) and boys (B). Single numbers (*2, 3, 4, 5*) indicate stages of development. The average is represented. A range of ages when each event may begin and end is indicated by inclusive numbers listed below each event. (Modified from Herman-Giddens, M., Slora, E. J., Wasserman, R. C., et al. [1997]. Secondary sexual characteristics and menses in young girls seen in office practices: A study from the Pediatric Research in Office Settings Network. *Pediatrics, 99*[4], 505–512; Hockenberry, M. J., & Wilson, D. [2015]. *Wong's nursing care of infants and children* [10th ed.]. [Figs. 17-2 & 17-5]. St. Louis: Mosby; Marshall, W., & Tanner, J. [1970]. Variations in pattern of pubertal changes in boys. *Archives of Diseases in Childhood, 45*[239], 13–23.)

source of body odour. The sebaceous glands are located primarily on the face, neck, shoulders, upper back, chest, and genitals. They can become clogged and inflamed, leading to the common teenage condition called acne. Acne is seen in nearly 90% of adolescents, with a higher prevalence and severity in males than in females (Canadian Dermatology Association, 2019).

## Scoliosis

During the growth spurt, adolescents may manifest signs of a common skeletal deformity called scoliosis, which is a lateral S-shaped curvature of the spine (Fig. 15.3). The curve is typically convex to the right. Classifications of scoliosis include secondary or functional, congenital, neuromuscular, constitutional, and idiopathic, which has an infantile, juvenile, or adolescent onset. Approximately 10% of all adolescents have a mild truncal asymmetry; however, curves greater than 20 degrees are abnormal and can progress to significant curvature during the growth spurt (Scoliosis Research Society, 2019). Idiopathic scoliosis is the most common type and is significantly more prevalent in females.

Although early screening and early intervention may help reduce the impact of scoliosis, the *Canadian Guide to Clinical Preventative Health Care* (CPS, 2016a) does not recommend screening for idiopathic scoliosis in asymptomatic adolescents. There is evidence that asymptomatic individuals have a mild clinical course and that interventions such as braces and exercise may not improve back pain or quality of life. Potential harms include unnecessary medical evaluations and psychological side effects, especially related to wearing corrective braces. Referral for orthopedic evaluation occurs when the curvature measures more than 5 to 7 degrees, measured by a scoliometer when the adolescent is in the Adams position (see Fig. 15.3B).

## Genetics

Most genetic problems are discovered during infancy and early childhood. Some syndromes, however, may not be diagnosed until adolescence. Turner's syndrome in females and Klinefelter's syndrome in males result from alterations in the X chromosome. These genetic disorders, which affect both physical and cognitive development, are frequently discovered during the assessment of an adolescent who has delayed or irregular pubertal development, and require referral to an appropriate specialist.

Since the sequencing of the human genome, information on genetic predisposition to disease has expanded exponentially. For example, genomics research has demonstrated a genetic basis for conditions seen during adolescence, such as acne, scoliosis (Genomics), substance abuse, depression, eating disorders, and autoimmune conditions (e.g., lupus erythematosus and celiac disease) (CPS, 2017a). The risk of conditions of concern to adolescents, such as breast cancer, type 2 diabetes, and cardiovascular disease, can now be identified through genetic testing. A request for genetic testing by a competent, well-informed adolescent for the purpose of reproductive decision making should be considered and must be accompanied by appropriate counselling. The decision to include his or her family in the decision making should be made by the adolescent. Although newborn screening for genetic disease is routinely performed, predictive screening for adolescents should be postponed until the adolescent is competent to decide whether they want the information.

Family history, however, not only can help health care providers make a diagnosis if the adolescent shows signs of a disorder but can also help to reveal whether there is an increased risk of a disease for the adolescent.

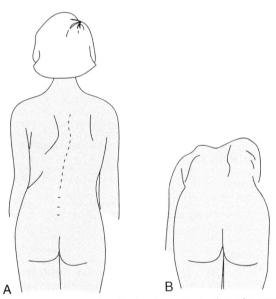

**Fig. 15.3 Scoliosis Screening** So that the entire back can be seen, the adolescent should remove all clothing from the upper body when being assessed for scoliosis. (A) While the adolescent stands up straight, check for any asymmetry; observe and palpate the body for differences in shoulder or scapular height, prominence of either scapula or hip, waist asymmetry, and misalignment of the spinous processes. Lateral curvature and thoracic convexity of the spine indicate scoliosis. (B) With feet together, legs straight, and arms hanging freely, the adolescent bends forward until the back is parallel with the floor. Check for prominence of the ribs, or rib hump, on one side only and hip and leg asymmetry. With scoliosis, the chest wall on the side of convexity is prominent, and the scapula on the side of convexity is elevated.

### GENOMICS

#### *Scoliosis*

For many years the cause of adolescent idiopathic scoliosis (AIS) has been elusive to determine. A body of research reveals that AIS is significantly more prevalent in girls than in boys (up to 10 times more prevalent), that AIS occurs in families, and that the condition is multifactorial. Multifactorial inheritance patterns suggest that a combination of genetics, hormonal and muscle imbalances, and environmental influences affects the occurrence of AIS. In the past several years, as genome sequencing has allowed more precise identification of genetic contributions to various diseases, multiple studies have tried to determine an exact genetic inheritance pattern for AIS. Researchers have identified multiple genes that possibly increase susceptibility and are associated with various aspects of spinal development and growth. Unfortunately, researchers have not identified evidence that would suggest a specific genetic pattern, but have concluded that AIS is caused by multiple genes that are modified by environmental influences.

Source: Haller, G., McCall, K., Jenkitkasemwong, S., et al. (2018). A missense variant in *SLC39A8* is associated with severe idiopathic scoliosis. *Nature Communications, 9*(1), 4171.

## ❖ GORDON'S FUNCTIONAL HEALTH PATTERNS

### ◆ Health Perception–Health Management Pattern

Teens have fewer acute illnesses than younger children and fewer chronic illnesses than adults. They are seen in health care facilities less frequently than younger children and adults, and they are rarely hospitalized. Yet they need to be monitored, because adolescence is a pivotal developmental period, with numerous physical, psychosocial, and spiritual changes. The CPS (2016a) recommends that the frequency of preventive visits for adolescents be every 1 to 2 years. Box 15.1 lists interventions for a periodic health examination. It is vital to remember that not all sections of the examination must be covered during each visit. Nurses may use personal discretion when choosing specific topics to discuss. At least part of the adolescent's visit should be conducted in private, with parents or guardians excused, as confidentiality is key to a successful nurse–adolescent relationship. While variations exist across Canada, minors may give informed consent to medical treatment provided they understand and appreciate the proposed treatment, inherent risks,

and possible outcomes and benefits. However, it is important to explain that the rules of confidentiality do not pertain to cases of homicidal or suicidal indication and emotional, physical, or sexual abuse.

A crucial component for understanding adolescent health is an adolescent's own perceptions of health, illness, and health care services. Too often, their sense of invincibility and "Peter Pan" ideology couples with typical adolescent experimentation and risky behaviours to produce deleterious health care choices and outcomes. Caught somewhere between childhood and adulthood, teens may no longer feel as if they are being attended to by pediatricians, pediatric nurse practitioners, and pediatric nurses, yet, at the same time, are often misunderstood by adult health care providers. Health care services for adolescents that are available, visible, confidential, and flexible need to be developed. Unmet health care needs during adolescence may result in poor health outcomes during adulthood (Landstedt, Hammarström, & Winefield, 2015). The reasons that contribute to unmet health care needs include lack of appropriate access, financial constraints, and adolescent attitudes that health is not

---

### BOX 15.1 Interventions Recommended for the Periodic Health Examination: 11 to 17 Years of Age

**Screening**
- Height, weight, and BMI, and BMI percentile
- Blood pressure
- Vision and hearing
- Tanner stage
- Anemia
- Hyperlipidemia
- Urinalysis
- Tuberculosis—if at risk
- Eating disorders
- Sports injuries
- Tattoos and piercings
- Substance use assessment
- Depression screening
- HIV screening (age 16–18 years)
- If sexually active, STI screening
- Counselling

**Injury and Violence Prevention**
- Lap and shoulder belts in car
- Bicycle, motorcycle, all-terrain vehicle helmets
- Protective gear for sports, work, and other physical activities
- Learn first aid and cardiopulmonary resuscitation
- Skin cancer, sun exposure (or exposure through tanning beds), sunscreen sun protection factor 15 or higher
- Safe storage and use of firearms

**Substance Use**
- Avoid tobacco, alcohol, and drug use

- Avoid alcohol or drug use while driving, swimming, boating, riding a bike or motorcycle, or operating farm equipment or other machinery
- Do not ride with a driver who has been using alcohol

**Sexual Behaviour**
- Abstinence, resisting sexual pressures, saying no
- STI prevention and protection
- Unintended pregnancy, contraception
- Date rape

**Diet and Exercise**
- Choose a variety of healthy foods
- Balance caloric intake and energy expenditure
- Limit fat and cholesterol; emphasize grains, fruits, and vegetables
- Adequate calcium, iron, and folic acid

**Dental Health**
- Regular (every 6 months) visits to dental care provider
- Brush teeth at least twice a day and floss daily
- Avoid tobacco products

**Immunization**[a]
- Tdap vaccine at age 11 to 12 years; Td vaccine every 10 years thereafter
- HPV vaccine: males and females between the ages of 9 and 13 years; ideally before they become sexually active
- Meningococcal vaccine: a booster dose of Men-C-C vaccine or of a quadrivalent (Men-C-ACYW) vaccine is routinely given at 12–14 years of age
- Influenza vaccine yearly
- Catch-up vaccines—HPV, hepatitis B; measles, mumps, rubella; varicella (two-dose schedule); hepatitis A (if indicated)

*BMI,* Body mass index; *HIV,* human immunodeficiency virus; *HPV,* human papillomavirus; *STI,* sexually transmitted infection; *Td,* tetanus, diphtheria; *Tdap,* tetanus, diphtheria, acellular pertussis.
[a]Public Health Agency of Canada. (2018). *Canadian immunization guide: Recommended immunization schedules.* Retrieved from https://www.canada.ca/en/public-health/services/publications/healthy-living/canadian-immunization-guide-part-1-key-immunization-information/page-13-recommended-immunization-schedules.html#p1c12a2.

important. Whereas adults search for health information using the Internet, adolescents are more likely to use social media (e.g., Facebook, Twitter, YouTube) to obtain health information (Bottorff, Struik, Bissell, et al., 2014). Because these sites are unmonitored for accuracy, nurses need to advise adolescents and their parents to verify information with their health providers. For information regarding health care services for adolescents, visit Health Canada youth health information website at https://www.canada.ca/en/services/health/youth-health.html.

Adolescents are in the process of developing health habits and patterns of problem solving that are likely to last a lifetime. The cognitive and psychological changes that they experience can affect their adherence to health-promotion and disease-prevention strategies. Teens do not always consider the health risks of their behaviour and have an overall sense of invulnerability to illness or injury. Peer influence is primary, and parental input is often rejected. Parents need, however, to be vigilant to recognize when their adolescent needs assistance with avoiding situations that could lead to irreparable harm (CPS, 2018a). Parental monitoring, which involves knowing where the adolescent is, knowing with whom he or she is communicating, setting clear behavioural expectations, and sensitivity to adolescent behaviour changes, has been shown to be protective against adolescent risk behaviour. Role modelling appropriate health behaviours is also a known protective factor against risk (CPS, 2018a). Parents, however, need to guard against overprotection, sometimes known as overparenting or helicopter parenting, because this behaviour can lead to overdependence and lack of confidence as the adolescent transitions to adulthood. Parents who are perceived by their children as being overcontrolling (e.g., give undue advice or assistance, are overly involved with the adolescent's activities, or fail to allow the adolescent to solve problems) can contribute to increased anxiety, stress or depression, low self-regulation, decreased self-confidence, and exaggerated egocentric behaviour (Moilanen & Manuel, 2019). Nurses can advise parents to strike a balance between the desire to overprotect their children and allowing them increasing autonomy as adolescents become increasingly capable of more independent decisions about their health behaviour.

Parents, teachers, and health care providers will be more successful in assisting teens to manage their health needs wisely if they treat them as joint partners in planning the care for which the adolescents themselves will assume responsibility. Key components of successful health supervision include gradually facilitating adolescent independence and decision making, involving parents and schools in a holistic approach to health promotion, and effective communication.

## ◆ Nutritional-Metabolic Pattern

Although many adolescents gravitate to low-nutrient, processed foods, it is essential that they consume a well-rounded diet that provides a variety of high-nutrient, low-sugar, and low-fat foods and beverages (Health Canada, 2019a). Adolescents are the age group with the highest daily consumption of total dietary sugars, mostly consumed through sweetened fruit drinks and soft drinks. Adolescents need to consume daily calorie amounts appropriate for their level of physical exercise (females,

1600–1800 calories; males, 1800–3200 calories) found primarily in vegetables, fruits, whole grains, fish, and nuts. Nurses need to assist teens with following a healthy diet and educate them about the appropriate nutrients, such as protein (especially for vegetarians), calcium, vitamin D, and iron and folic acid (for females) (O'Connor et al, 2018). Recommending regular consumption of milk to prevent later osteoporosis is essential, especially for adolescent girls, as is avoidance of high-sugar and diet beverages. The nurse can encourage adolescents to eat breakfast every day to improve academic performance, or to carry protein snacks. An excellent resource for nurses and adolescents regarding dietary considerations is the Healthy Eating for Teens website: https://food-guide.canada.ca/en/tips-for-healthy-eating/teens/. Regarding vegetarian diets, CPS (2018b) recommends that a well-balanced vegetarian diet can provide for the nutritional requirements of adolescents, but that evaluation of appropriate caloric intake is needed. Adequate protein intake and sources of essential fatty acids, iron, zinc, calcium, and vitamins $B_{12}$ and D should be ensured. Supplementation may be required in cases of strict vegetarian diets with no intake of any animal products.

Many teens have concerns about their body, proper nutrition, and exercise. The media not only portray the ideal body as thin, lean, or muscular but at the same time promote access to unhealthy high-fat, high-sugar, processed foods. Asserting their newfound autonomy, teens may choose dietary intake as a mechanism to gain control over their changing bodies, exert independence, or experiment with a new identity or cause, such as becoming a vegetarian. All of this occurs as their body's nutrient and energy demands increase in preparation for and in response to the adolescent growth spurt. Teen activities, including sports and other vigorous extracurricular physical activity, can further increase these demands. Gymnasts, runners, bodybuilders, rowers, wrestlers, dancers, and swimmers are particularly vulnerable to eating disorders because their sports necessitate weight restriction. Complicating matters are teens' overwhelming desire to "fit in" with their peers, which often prevails and can lead to unhealthy dietary practices

### Eating Disorders

The occurrence of eating disorders results from a combination of genetic and environmental factors, mediated as well by internal and external factors prevalent during puberty (e.g., family, peer, and media influences) (Kreipe, 2016). In Canada, the lifetime prevalence of eating disorders among adolescents is 3% (National Initiative for Eating Disorders [NIED], 2018). Major eating disorders include anorexia nervosa, bulimia nervosa, and binge eating disorder. In general, eating disorders have a higher prevalence in females, but they affect both sexes and people of all cultures. Most adolescents with an eating disorder experience comorbid mental health conditions, such as anxiety, depression, alcohol addiction, or obsessive-compulsive disorder, and suicide ideation is not uncommon (National Eating Disorder Information Centre [NEDIC], 2014). Adolescents who meet the criteria for eating disorders should be referred to an interprofessional team that is experienced and skilled in working with these disorders

At one end of the eating disorder spectrum is anorexia nervosa and bulimia nervosa. At the other end is binge eating disorder and obesity. Distorted body image is a hallmark of anorexia nervosa in both males and females. Body image specifically refers to the picture of and feelings about various characteristics of one's body. In females, particularly, and to a lesser extent in males, distorted body image may be related to self-objectification, or judging one's personality or character strictly by one's appearance (Tylka & Wood-Barclow, 2015). Media images and positive or negative comments about appearance from others can contribute to self-objectification.

The onset of anorexia nervosa is typically in response to low self-esteem and real or imagined obesity. Adolescents with anorexia nervosa are typically female, perfectionists, and high achievers. Symptoms or warning signs include a relentless pursuit of thinness, self-starving with significant weight loss, lack of menstruation (in females) and decreased sexual interests (in males), compulsive physical activity, preoccupation with food, portioning food carefully, and eating only small amounts of only certain foods. The adolescent may also have brittle hair and nails; dry, yellowish skin; growth of fine hair over the body; constipation; mild anemia and muscle weakness; and often complains of feeling cold. The severe restriction of food intake eventually contributes to dangerous malnourishment. It is estimated that 10% of individuals will die within 10 years of the onset of the disorder (NEDIC, 2014).

Pro-eating disorder websites and other social media sites may target adolescents in order to promote eating disorders, particularly anorexia nervosa, as a lifestyle choice rather than a deadly illness. Also known as ana or pro-ana, these communities may lead adolescents to falsely believe that they are okay and that an eating disorder is a choice. The sites make disordered eating seem normal and glamorous and may encourage adolescents to do harmful things (NEDIC, 2014).

Bulimia nervosa has symptoms or warning signs that are different from those of anorexia nervosa. Teens with bulimia nervosa typically binge on huge quantities of high-calorie foods and then purge by self-induced vomiting and/or use of laxatives. Binge episodes may alternate with diets, resulting in dramatic weight fluctuations. These teens often try to hide the signs of vomiting by running water as a sound cover. Purging poses serious threats to the teen's health, including dehydration, sometimes fatal electrolyte imbalances, and erosion of tooth enamel.

At the other end of the eating disorder spectrum is binge eating disorder, which can often contribute to obesity. Similar to the teen with bulimia nervosa, the teen with binge eating disorder frequently consumes large amounts of food while feeling a lack of control over eating. However, this disorder is different from bulimia nervosa because these teens usually do not purge their bodies of the excess food they consume during their binge episodes. Adolescents who are binge eaters experience lack of control over eating, the inability to stop eating when full, social difficulties, altered mood, and decreased self-esteem (NEDIC, 2014). Binge-eating disorder can increase the risk of type 2 diabetes, high blood pressure, or weight concerns.

Because of the multiple factors contributing to the occurrence of an eating disorder, there is no one method that can prevent its occurrence. However, when working with families of adolescents, nurses can recommend family members de-emphasize the adolescent's body proportions or shape, encourage healthy eating and participation in regular exercise, emphasize the adolescent's positive and unique aspects, and foster the adolescent's self-esteem (Canadian Mental Health Association [CMHA], 2019a). It may also be helpful to connect with support groups for individuals with an eating disorder, as well as support groups for their families and friends. In addition, a dietitian or nutritionist can teach eating strategies and eating habits to support recovery goals.

The obese adolescent consumes too many calories for the amount of energy expended. The prevalence of obesity has nearly tripled over the last 25 years, with up to 26% of young people being overweight or obese, and 41% of their Indigenous peers being overweight or obese (CPS, 2012a). The cause of obesity is multifactorial, but key factors include excessive caloric intake, sedentary behaviour patterns, inadequate physical activity, and lack of exercise. Other research has identified depression, chronic stress, and inadequate sleep as additional predictors of adolescent obesity. Obesity can be detrimental to adolescents' self-esteem and social development, because they often become trapped in a vicious cycle of social rejection, isolation, inactivity, and continued obesity. Adolescent obesity has a poor prognosis, with most obese adolescents becoming obese adults. Health consequences of adolescent obesity can include type 2 diabetes, hypertension, obstructive sleep apnea, nonalcoholic steatohepatitis, poor self-esteem, and a lower health-related quality of life (CPS, 2017b).

Indigenous populations, ethnic minorities, and adolescents who live in apartments or public housing, or in neighbourhoods where outdoor play is curtailed by weather or a lack of safe facilities, are also at higher risk for obesity (CPS, 2012a). Urban sprawl with limited access to recreational opportunities, parks, and neighbourhood playgrounds especially impacts low-income families and may also lead to obesity. Although quality daily physical education (PE) classes in schools have been eliminated in favour of academics, regular PE actually improves academic performance and reduces stress (Hobin, So, Rosella, et al., 2014).

To promote physical activity and reduce the incidence of obesity, nurses should encourage adolescents to complete at least 60 minutes of moderate to vigorous physical activity daily, including muscle and bone strengthening at least three times a week. Recreational screen time should be limited to 2 hours daily (Canadian Society for Exercise Physiology [CSEP], 2019). Clinicians are encouraged to screen for depression, anxiety, and low self-esteem and refer to a mental health professional if required. Strategies for good sleep habits should also be promoted. Advocating and promoting national policies for achieving health among teens and for removal of health disparities for Indigenous youth is also strongly recommended (CPS, 2016a). Teens can access information about physical activity, sedentary lifestyle, and sleep at *Canadian 24-Hour Movement Guidelines* (https://csepguidelines.ca/children-and-youth-5-17).

## Obesity, Type 2 Diabetes, and Teens

Diabetes is a group of diseases marked by high levels of glucose in the blood, which, if not attended to, lead to blindness, kidney failure, amputations, heart disease, and stroke. Type 2 diabetes, formerly called adult-onset diabetes, is the most common form. People can develop it at any age. Soaring obesity rates are making type 2 diabetes, a disease that used to be seen mostly in adults older than 45 years, more common among teens and young people. A recent study showed that 44% of Canadian youth with new-onset type 2 diabetes were Aboriginal (Diabetes Canada, 2018).

More than anything, adolescents need reassurance about their bodies. Parents, teachers, and health care providers will be more successful in helping teens assume responsibility and manage their ongoing health needs if they approach and treat them as partners in planning their care. Assessment is of particular importance. Nurses working with adolescents need to be aware of abnormal changes in weight, body image distortion, abnormal food behaviour, including thinking about food, and obsessive exercise. Nurses can engage adolescents and help them create an individualized wellness plan that addresses body image, diet, weight concerns, and physical activity.

## ◆ Elimination Pattern

The renal and gastro-intestinal systems are functionally mature by adolescence, and elimination patterns are consistent with those found in adults. Abnormal variation can occur in teens with eating disorders. It is important to remember that an adolescent's need for privacy or self-protection may inhibit normal elimination in public places, such as schools.

## ◆ Activity-Exercise Pattern

During adolescence the alterations in body composition and growth of lean muscle mass allow the teen to experience increased physical strength and endurance. All adolescents should be taught that regular exercise can increase their endurance and improve their appearance and general state of health and that these positive effects can extend into adulthood.

Many teens participate in organized sports, and the preparticipation sports examination is one of the most common reasons adolescents seek primary care (Fig. 15.4). This examination offers an opportunity for nurses to identify adolescents at risk, evaluate their general state of health, and promote healthy lifestyle behaviours (Box 15.2). Along with eating disorders related to maintaining or losing weight for sports participation, adolescent athletes are subject to overuse injuries. Often these injuries are related to the specific sport in which the adolescent engages. The sports environment can contribute to or prevent overuse. The factors contributing to injury include environmental temperature (too hot or too cold), type of playing surface, emotional pressure from parents or coaches, inappropriate equipment, and inadequate training of coaches (Canadian Safety Council, 2019). Nurses need to work closely with athletes and coaches to be sure the approach to sports participation is healthy and free of injury potential.

## ◆ Sleep-Rest Pattern

During adolescence the amount of time needed each night for sleep declines in comparison with earlier childhood needs. Although their sleep patterns differ greatly, adolescents need at least 8 to 10 hours of sleep per night (Tremblay, Carson, Chaput, et al., 2016). Adolescents who are employed, those involved in extracurricular sports, and those who have "too much on their plate" are at increased risk of sleep deprivation. They stay up late and are then forced to wake up before their sleep cycles have finished because the high school day has such an early start. Many adolescents send and receive text messages at bedtime after room lights have been turned off, which can interfere with a good night's sleep. Even a moderate level of night-time texting can greatly increase the likelihood of having long-term fatigue. Adolescents without sufficient sleep can find it difficult to concentrate and learn, or even stay awake in classes. Too little sleep might also contribute to mood disorders and behavioural problems. Adolescents who drive when they are sleep deprived can cause accidents, which could lead to death. Nurses can suggest that adolescents keep their cell phones, computers, and other electronic devices out of their bedrooms at night. Nurses can also suggest strategies for daily living that help adolescents cope with the challenge of balancing their varied responsibilities while preventing exhaustion or burnout. Adolescents can access more sleep information and recommendations at *Teens and Sleep: Why You Need It and How To Get Enough* (https://www.caringforkids.cps.ca/handouts/teens_and_sleep?).

## ◆ Cognitive-Perceptual Pattern

### Piaget's Theory of Cognitive Development

Adolescence is characterized by a shift in cognitive abilities to Piaget's stage of *formal operations* (Piaget, 1969). Piaget's theory used the term *formal* to represent the emergence of ability to focus on the "form" of thoughts, objects, and experiences rather than on the exact content, which in turn lays the groundwork for abstract thinking. These new cognitive abilities are reflected in adolescent behaviours in several ways.

The first change is that because of their new ability to "think about their thinking," adolescents become highly introspective. As introspection increases, they develop an internalized audience that provides them with a means to evaluate questions such as "Who am I?" "How do others see me?" and "Where am I going?" Introspection also combines with a re-emergence of egocentrism, leading to their sense of being the primary focus—special, unique, and exceptional (Piaget, 1969). Being exceptional adolescents means being the exception, thinking that nothing can happen to them, but only to others. This type of thought can contribute to the risk-taking behaviours for which adolescents are well known:

- I can get drunk on weekends and not develop a drinking problem.
- I won't get pregnant; I've had sex for 6 months and haven't gotten pregnant yet.
- I can take those turns at 100 km per hour and not lose control.

Another behavioural manifestation of adolescents' formal operations is an intolerance of things as they are. They are able to

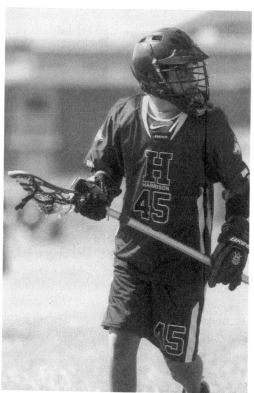

**Fig. 15.4** Adolescents frequently participate in organized activities, especially sports.

---

### BOX 15.2    Adolescent Preparticipation Sports Examination

#### *Areas for Special Concern*

- Previous trauma, including concussion
- Exertional symptoms
- Cardiovascular disease, including presence of a heart murmur and symptoms of Marfan syndrome
- Family history of premature cardiac conditions or sudden cardiac death
- Hypertension
- Asthma
- Seizure disorder
- Splenomegaly, or enlarged spleen, often seen with infectious mononucleosis
- Absence of paired organs: eye, kidney, testicle, or ovary

Source: Mirabelli, M. H., Devine, M. J., Singh, J., et al. (2015). The preparticipation sports evaluation. *American Family Physician, 92*(5), 371–376.

---

conceptualize things as they might or could be, rather than how they are, and can think of elaborate means for achieving these changes—now. With this new-found capability, they constantly challenge the ways things are and challenge themselves to consider the way things can or should be. Teens can be vehement in trying to convince others of their viewpoints and untiring in their support of causes that align with them. This idealism can lead to a rejection of family beliefs, religion, or social causes, which do not appear to the adolescent to be working fast enough to solve the problems of society. Although this idealism appears to most adults to be a flight from reality, it is a necessary stage in formal thinking. Reality is recognized, but only as a subset of

many other possibilities that need to be aligned with their own thinking. Eventually, their thinking becomes less egocentric and omnipotent, giving way to an appreciation of differences in judgement between themselves and others (Piaget, 1969).

### Erikson's Theory of Psychosocial Development

Erikson's theory of psychosocial development describes the central task of adolescence as being the establishment of identity, with the primary risk being *role confusion* (Erikson, 1968). Although it may appear that adolescents are involved in a final rather than a transient or initial stage of development, identity formation in adolescence provides a means of moving into and through what might be termed an identity crisis.

This crisis involves a restaging of each of the previous stages of psychosocial development (Erikson, 1968). Development of trust in self and others, as emphasized in infancy, is encountered again as the adolescent searches for people and ideologies in which to have faith. Toddlerhood, and its search for autonomy, is also revisited as adolescents search for independence from their primary family units. The preschooler's challenge, a sense of initiative rather than guilt, resurfaces as the adolescent searches for direction and purpose. The school-age child's developing sense of industry is carried into the adolescent period also, as teens make choices in social, recreational, volunteer, academic, familial, and occupational activities. The confusion and hesitation in making these choices arise from fears of participating in activities that will not afford them the opportunity to excel or win the approval of their peers.

Erikson (1968) says that the extent to which these earlier tasks were accomplished successfully predicts the success of the current developmental stage, therefore, influencing an adolescent's resourcefulness and success in experimenting with the new identity. When the threat of identity confusion is exceedingly great, delinquent behaviour and alterations in mental health can occur. This threat is enhanced by conditions of poverty, racism, and other social inequities (see Box 15.7).

The pursuit of a meaningful ideology and an individual identity frequently creates a puzzling combination of shifting interests and sudden extremes in action. Erikson views this behaviour as an attempt to try on various roles and to search for some stable principle that might last through the testing of extremes and be carried into adulthood. Reassuring parents that this behaviour is normal during adolescence and encouraging them to maintain positive communication with their adolescents is an important nursing function.

### Time Orientation

Adolescents look at time differently than they did as younger children. They realize that the response to a problem can, and sometimes should, be delayed to think through the possibilities for approaching the problem. Additionally, teens develop a future orientation and are able to delay immediate gratification to gain more satisfaction in the future.

### Language

Advances in cognitive skills are reflected in an increased understanding of language. Formal operations and more abstract

## TABLE 15.2 Deciphering and Conversing in the Latest Text Messaging Lingo

| Message | Meaning |
| --- | --- |
| ROFL | Rolling on the floor laughing |
| LOL | Laughing out loud |
| YOLO | You only live once |
| NVM | Never mind |
| POS/MOS/DOS | Parent over shoulder/Mom over shoulder/Dad over shoulder |
| 9 | Parent watching |
| 99 | Parent no longer watching |
| CD9 | Code 9: parent watching or in room |
| RUOK | Are you okay? |
| XLNT | Excellent |
| F2F | Face to face |
| Zzz | Sleeping, bored, tired |
| Y | Why |
| B4N | Bye for now |
| YYSSW | Yeah yeah sure sure whatever |
| JK | Just kidding |
| FOMO | Fear of missing out |

thought processes require expression in different words than did the more concrete thoughts of younger children. Adolescents give complex definitions, frequently including all possible meanings or uses. Interpretations of pictures or stories are intricate and abstract. Older teens are capable of using and understanding complex sentence structure, although they, like adults, may not use these complex sentences routinely in their speech.

Both receptive and expressive vocabularies increase during adolescence. As with all ages, receptive vocabulary far exceeds expressive vocabulary. The adolescent's vocabulary frequently includes slang. Slang may be centred on topics such as drug use, popular dress, music, and certain peer activities, or it may be more pervasive, in which case adults or "outsiders" may have difficulty following a conversation between two teens. The surge in cell phone use, instant and text messaging, and online social media has given rise to an entirely new set of communications to decipher (Table 15.2).

### ◆ Self-Perception–Self-Concept Pattern

The term *self-perception,* which is often used interchangeably with the terms *self-concept* and *self-esteem,* refers to both the description of the self and to the evaluation of, or feelings about, that description. Tied together and brought to the forefront in adolescence, both self-perception and body image dominate, influence, and are influenced by individual, peer, and societal norms and expectations.

Assessment, anticipatory guidance, education, and counselling are strategies the nurse can use to guide the adolescent in developing a self-perception that incorporates a healthy body image. It is important for parents, teachers, and health care providers to remember to praise adolescents for who they are rather than for what they do, value each of them as unique, demonstrate belief in their abilities to grow and develop, and delight in their discoveries of themselves and their unique means of expressing this.

### Acne

Teenage acne can influence self-perception, as it is a contributor to alterations in appearance. Most adolescents experience some degree of acne, especially during puberty, and they are typically concerned about their skin changes. The sebaceous glands increase production of sebum, a primary factor in the pathogenesis of acne. The sebaceous follicles become clogged with sebum and debris, forming open (blackheads) or closed (whiteheads) comedones. The incidence of acne within families suggests that hereditary factors are involved.

Thorough examination of the adolescent's skin and a discussion of its impact on the overall body image are necessary to determine appropriate management strategies. Intervention should include teaching the individual about the pathophysiological nature of acne. Knowledge allows the adolescent to become instrumental in its management and helps dispel common myths about acne and its care.

The approach to acne management is a stepwise approach according to the severity; all recommended management strategies take between 6 and 8 weeks to be effective (Canadian Dermatology Association, 2019). Washing the skin with mild soap and water two times a day is the best way to remove surface dirt and oil. Vigorous scrubbing should be discouraged because the skin can become irritated, leading to follicular rupture. The adolescent should not attempt to remove the pustules and papules that form. Squeezing the lesion can result in further irritation of the gland and permanent injury to the tissue. Adolescent females need to be careful when selecting makeup. Most preparations, when applied extensively over the face, prevent adequate exposure to air and light, especially those that have a fat base. Sunlight can have a beneficial effect on acne; however, prolonged exposure should be avoided. Stress can exacerbate acne in some adolescents. In these cases, stress-management techniques should be considered. The effect of diet on acne is a highly controversial issue. Evidence indicates that dietary restrictions specific to acne are unnecessary.

Recent guidelines from the Canadian Dermatology Association (2019) suggest that a combination of topical cleansers or creams (salicylic acids or benzoyl peroxide) can be used for mild acne. Should the condition worsen, or be more severe than mild acne, prescription-strength treatments can be added and may include topical formulations, such as antibiotics, retinoids (vitamin A derivatives), benzoyl peroxide, anti-inflammatory medications (e.g., dapsone and azelaic acid) and fixed dose combinations. Oral (systemic) medication can include antibiotics, retinoids, or hormonal agents (i.e., birth control pills, spironolactone).

Adolescents with acne need support and understanding. The nurse can help adolescents and their families understand that management does not result in immediate improvement. In fact, topical agents may make acne appear worse initially, with any improvement occurring slowly over several months.

## Body Art and Piercing

Adolescence is a developmental period full of identity experimentation and risk-taking behaviour. Body piercing and tattooing have become popular forms of expression of individuality and personal values, particularly among adolescents, and are intimately related to self-perception. Although body art and piercing have traditionally been associated with those outside the mainstream, such as gang members and incarcerated individuals, these activities have now become more of an accepted, mainstream phenomenon (Roggenkamp, Nicholls, & Pierre, 2017). However, adolescents need to realize that each carries health risks.

Metallic rings, rods, studs, and barbells have pierced many sites on adolescent bodies: ears, lips, cheek, tongue, nipples, navels, noses, eyebrows, genitalia, and eyebrows. Local infection is the most common complication of body art and piercing, with infection rates ranging from 9% to 35% (Duval Smith, 2016). Additional complications include hepatitis and human immunodeficiency virus (HIV) infections, keloid scar formation, tooth injury or cracking, and periodontal disease.

Nurses can explore with adolescents the reasons for acquiring body art and explain the potential short-term and long-term consequences to assist with their decision making. To prevent infection from body piercing, the nurse needs to advise the adolescent to use meticulous handwashing when cleaning piercing sites. The sites should be cleaned with sterile saline and sometimes antibacterial soap and protected from injury (Association of Professional Piercers [APP], 2019). Adolescents with new tattoos need to avoid sun exposure and apply a moisturizing lotion to the site (American Academy of Dermatology [AAD], 2016). With both types of body art, adolescents should notify the provider of any signs of infection.

## ◆ Roles-Relationships Pattern
### Families

Until adolescence, the younger child is highly dependent on the parents and other adults. Striving for identity and increased independence, the adolescent begins to spend increased time away from the family. Parents sense a narrowing of their influence as their teen not only begins to prefer the company of peers and other adults but also begins to question familial beliefs and values. Parents may respond by setting unreasonably strict limits and asking intrusive questions about their teen's activities, friends, and ideas or decide to drop all rules and limits and assume that the adolescent can now manage alone. Neither of these approaches works well.

Whereas adolescents strive for a sense of identity and independence, their parents try to learn how to let go. Each is temporarily unsure of the relationship with the other, and the family unit may experience more stress than at any previous time. Furthermore, this period is often prolonged because more teens remain financially dependent on their families as they move into young adulthood.

Some families experience better outcomes than do other families. Families in which parents maintain a willingness to listen and demonstrate an ongoing affection for and acceptance of their adolescent yet still maintain some consistent limits experience more constructive, positive outcomes during this period. This situation does not mean that parents necessarily agree with their teen's ideas or actions, but rather that they are willing to hear what the adolescent has to say and to negotiate some limits. Parents may need assistance in determining negotiable versus non-negotiable rules and in developing ways to voice their concerns in an honest, open way. Even when teens do not want to "discuss" a topic, they need to know why their parents are concerned.

### Peers

Faced with the need to become autonomous, achieve identity, and become productive, the adolescent often turns from the family to the peer group to find a safe psychosocial shelter in which to develop. Belonging to an informally organized clique, crowd, gang, or group is the primary means with which to make the transition from the young child's allegiance to the family to a member of a group. Identification with a group is proclaimed through conformity to standards of clothing, behaviour, language, and values. This feature of the adolescent subculture persists despite the strong inclination in society as a whole toward greater levels of individuality.

The peer group is a vehicle for disengaging from the family unit and, as such, provides a means of achieving the goals of independence and individualization. Adolescents talk a great deal with their peers. Whether on the phone, online, or in person, they can discuss a 10-minute situation for hours on end. This sharing of thoughts and impressions is important. The telephone or computer can provide a "safe" mechanism for the teen to interact with members of the opposite sex as they share intimate ideas and concerns and begin to experience the closeness and caring that develops into the capacity to form a future intimate relationship.

*Youth gangs.* Becoming increasingly independent, adolescents test the limits of authority, experiment with a variety of roles, question adult values and authority, and look to peers for affirmation. They may feel pressure to join gangs or feel threatened by them. Adolescents in both urban and rural areas can have exposure to, and participate in, gangs. Gangs function as a peer group for adolescents who may feel socially inadequate, feel alienated from mainstream Canadian society, or exhibit low self-esteem. There are more than 430 active gangs in Canada, with 7000 members. Almost half of youth gang members are males under the age of 18. Many members began their involvement as children (Royal Canadian Mounted Police [RCMP], 2018). The RCMP (2018) defines a *youth gang* as a group of people who participate in criminal behaviour with the purpose of gaining power, recognition, and control, and generally use intimidation and violence to achieve their goals. The top four reasons to join a gang were to get respect, money, protection, and to fit in (Grekul & LaBoucane-Benson, 2008). Youth at risk of joining a gang tend to be from societal groups with the greatest levels of inequality and social disadvantage. Although not all gangs exhibit delinquent behaviour, more than a third of individuals accused in a criminal incident were youth aged 12 to 17 and young adults aged 18 to 24 (Public Safety Canada, 2014). In 2016, police in Canada reported 141 gang-related homicides, an increase of 45 from 2015. The largest increases in the number of gang-related homicides committed with a firearm were reported in Ontario and British Columbia (RCMP, 2018).

Indigenous gangs make up about 20% of Canada's gang population, as membership may be seen as an escape from poverty in order to obtain the necessities of life. In addition, with a large number of incarcerated Indigenous people in Canada, gang membership is often a key to survival. Many Indigenous youth who join gangs have a parent who has been, or is a current gang member. Indigenous gangs can be traced to the residential schools and may be seen as a way to cope with past trauma (Goodwill & Ishiyama, 2015). The longer an individual is involved in gangs, the more problems the adolescent may incur, including dropping out of school, lack of employment opportunities, and increased exposure to drug and alcohol use. Important connections with family, friends, and their community may also weaken. Nurses can alert parents to the signs that their adolescent may be associating with a gang. These include new and extensive body art, secrecy about friends, wearing symbolic clothing or colours, worsening school performance and truancy, unwillingness to attend family gatherings, having large sums of money or new expensive items that cannot be explained, contact with law enforcement, and possible substance use (RCMP, 2018). Encouraging strong and positive relationships with friends during adolescence and increased vigilance by parents can be protective against gang membership.

## ◆ Sexuality-Reproductive Pattern

### Adolescent Sexual Issues

The emergence of secondary sexual characteristics increases adolescents' awareness of themselves as sexual human beings. They fantasize about relationships and sex and gradually experiment with dating and a myriad of coital and noncoital physical contacts. Adolescents become sexually active for a variety of reasons. They have sex for affection, because of peer pressure, as a symbol of maturity, as spontaneous experimentation, to feel close, or because it feels good or right. In 2015, approximately 28% of Grade 10 males and 29% of Grade 9 females had had sexual intercourse at least once (PHAC, 2016). In addition, 28% of males and 21% of females reported having their first intercourse prior to the age of 14. Condoms were the contraceptive method of choice for 70% of both males and females. Generally, 16 years is the age of consent to sexual activity, but there are exceptions, depending on partners who are close in age and who are not in a position of power or trust (Department of Justice, 2017).

Of all sexual assault incidents, nearly half (47%) were committed against women aged 15 to 24 (Statistics Canada, 2014). Indigenous women were three times as likely to report being a victim of violence than non-Indigenous women, presumably due to several factors which have been linked to victimization—a history of childhood maltreatment, mental health disorders, and substance abuse—which are more common among the Indigenous population (Statistics Canada, 2016a).

During adolescence, teens are discovering what it means to be emotionally, physically, or romantically attracted to people of the same gender (gay, lesbian), the other gender (heterosexual), or either gender (bisexual). Gender identity is an individual's internal and psychological sense of self as female, male, both, or other (Registered Nurses Association of Ontario [RNAO], 2007). Approximately 4% of Canadian youth self-identify as lesbian, gay, bisexual, transgender, intersex, queer, and two-spirit (LGBTQ2) (University of Toronto, 2019). Being gay or transgender is not something that a person can change or can select to change. Often teens recognize their sexual orientation and gender identity with little doubt from an early age, whether or not they reveal it to others. Some gay teens may comfortably accept their sexuality, while others may find it more difficult to accept.

In addition to the usual stresses among adolescents, such as school, developmental changes, and peer pressure, LGBTQ2 youth have higher rates of mood and anxiety disorders, poorer self-perceived health status, and suicide. They are also more likely to be victims of bullying, including social and cyberbullying and violence, and face a greater risk of social isolation.

When providing culturally appropriate care, nurses can create a supportive, nonjudgemental climate that enables disclosure and optimizes social support for both LGBTQ2 adolescents and their families. Rainbow Health Ontario offers several educational resources for health care providers that are available at https://www.rainbowhealthontario.ca/training/#about.

The technological revolution has opened up a limitless world of unmediated information to adolescents and has led to increased issues of online risky behaviours. The use of online social networks such as Facebook, Twitter, Instagram, and other messaging sites continues to increase rapidly among all age groups and segments of our society, presenting new opportunities for the exchange of sexual information, as well as for potentially unsafe encounters between predators and the vulnerable or young. Additionally, adolescents who use the Internet to seek sexual information often receive conflicting messages and inaccurate facts. Sexting has been recognized as an increasing occurrence for several years and is a global practice among teens and young adults. Sexting refers to sending a text message with sexually explicit content or a sexually explicit picture. This type of texting can cause emotional pain for the person in the picture, as well as the sender and receiver (Canadian Centre for Cybersecurity, 2018).

Knowing that adolescents are heavily invested in these and other sexual issues, nurses are capable and willing to discuss them with adolescents in a variety of settings, such as health care providers' offices and clinics. Nurses need to be comfortable with their own sexuality; able to discuss the subject of sex and sexual orientation, contraception, and protection against sexually transmitted and blood-borne infections (STBBIs); and be aware of their own limitations, beliefs, and biases. Anticipatory guidance about the decision to become sexually active, to use contraception, and to obtain protection from STBBIs needs to be provided before adolescents encounter a situation in which they need this information (see Tables 16.2 and 16.3). This is also a good time to introduce the adolescent to breast and testicular self-examinations (Quality and Safety Scenario).

## ⚡ QUALITY AND SAFETY SCENARIO

### Performing Breast and Testicular Self-Examination

Breast self-examination (BSE) or testicular self-examination (TSE) should be performed once a month so that teens become familiar with the usual appearance and feel of their breasts or testicles. This routine makes noticing any changes from one month to another easier. Finding a change from "normal" is the main idea behind regular self-examination. The best time for females to perform a BSE is 2 or 3 days after their period ends, when the breasts are least likely to be tender or swollen. For males, the best time for a TSE is during or immediately after a warm shower.

**Breast Self-Examination**

- Stand in front of a mirror. Inspect both breasts for anything unusual, such as any discharge from the nipples, puckering or dimpling of the skin, or marked asymmetry.
- While watching closely in the mirror, clasp your hands behind your head and press your hands forward, and inspect the breast again.
- Next, press your hands firmly on your hips and bow slightly toward the mirror as you pull your shoulders and elbows forward, and inspect the breast again.
- Next, raise one arm. Use three or four fingers to explore the breast firmly, carefully, and thoroughly. Beginning at the outer edge, press the flat part of your fingers in small circles, moving the circles slowly around the breast. Gradually work toward the nipple. Be sure to examine the entire breast. Pay special attention to the area between the breast and the armpit, including the armpit itself. Feel the breast for any unusual lump or mass under the skin.
- Gently squeeze the nipple and look for a discharge. Repeat the examination on the other breast.

The last two steps should be repeated lying down. This position flattens the breast and makes examination easier. Some women perform BSE in the shower. Fingers gliding over soapy skin make concentrating on the texture underneath easier.

**Testicular Self-Examination**

- Cup or support the testicles with one hand and feel them with the other.
- Gently roll each testicle between the thumb and fingers. There should not be any pain.
- Feel the testicles for any swelling or hard lumps on the surface of the testicles. Testicles are normally oval, firm, smooth, and rubbery. One may be slightly larger than the other.
- A natural tube-like structure, the epididymis, is along the back of the testicle. Learn what it feels like.

Sources: Lowdermilk, D. L., Perry, S. E., & Cashion, M. C. (2011). *Maternity nursing* (8th ed.). St. Louis: Mosby; Neinstein, L. S., Gordau, C. M., Katzman, D. K., et al. (2008). *Adolescent health care: A practical guide* (5th ed.). Philadelphia; Lippincott Williams & Wilkins.

## Adolescent Pregnancy

For health care providers, adolescent pregnancy is viewed as a high-risk situation because of the serious health risks and potential complications for both the mother and the infant. For politicians and governmental agencies, it is a social problem that makes overwhelming demands on social and economic resources. For adolescents and their families, it may be seen as positive and normal or the worst disaster imaginable. No matter what the perspective, adolescent pregnancy represents a myriad of concerns with far-reaching social, educational, financial, and emotional effects.

Nearly 13,000 infants are born to adolescent mothers (<20 years of age) each year in Canada (Statistics Canada, 2019b). There was an overall 47% decrease in adolescent births between 1990 and 2010, levelling with a birth rate of 13.5 per 1000. However, there are some geographic differences, with the Atlantic provinces showing an increase in birth rates during the same period. Indigenous females are more than three times as likely to be mothers before the age of 20 than non-Indigenous women (Statistics Canada, 2016b). Immigrant women (visible minority or not) in Canada have a lower likelihood of being teenage mothers than native-born women not in a visible minority.

Adolescent pregnancy has a myriad of negative outcomes for both the mother and the child. For the mother, these include a significant decline in her future prospects, especially educational and economic, reliance on government-sponsored assistance, and poverty (CPS, 2016b). For the child born to adolescent mothers there is a higher risk of prenatal death, preterm birth, and low birth weight. Low birth weight, which may result from disparities in access to prenatal care, is associated with infant death and other health and developmental problems. Furthermore, these children often fall victim to abuse and neglect and are more likely to struggle academically, which further limits their educational opportunities, vocational options, and financial security. Later, as adolescents, they are at higher risk for substance use, early sexual activity, and becoming adolescent parents themselves.

Most adolescent fathers are on average 5 years older than the adolescent mother. Over 80% of these fathers do not live with their child, although weekly visits are common (CPS, 2016b). Their financial contribution may be limited as they, too, are often living in poverty with limited education, tenuous employment, and potentially, a criminal history. Nurses need to ask about psychosocial stressors, offer resources and support, while keeping in mind that domestic violence and relationship problems may jeopardize family safety. However, it is vital to note that paternal involvement may benefit both maternal and child outcomes. Involving fathers may reduce maternal postpartum depression, promote breastfeeding and family functioning as well as strengthen psychosocial, cognitive, and behavioural well-being of the child.

The current practice point highlights the unique health needs of adolescent parents and their children, and recommends some basic strategies to optimize outcomes. When pregnancy occurs, adolescents and their families deserve honest and sensitive counselling about options available to them, as well as the support systems available for them throughout the pregnancy, birth, and subsequent parenting. Nurses not only need to encourage early paternal involvement and reinforce reproductive health-education efforts but also need to encourage adolescents to build on the strengths in their lives and opportunities available to them (see Chapter 16 for additional information about pregnancy and contraception).

## Coping–Stress Tolerance Pattern

When all the changes that occur in adolescents are aligned with their need to separate from their parents and gain a sense of their own independence, their ability to cope is put to the test over and over again. Common coping mechanisms, and the strategies the nurse can use to encourage teens to use them in adaptive ways, are listed in Box 15.3.

However, too often adolescents are unable to balance the stresses, lacking the appropriate skills and outlets, adequate support systems, or available mental health intervention. Depression, suicide, and substance abuse emerge as life becomes overwhelming and the future unimaginable.

### Depression

As with many other diseases, the rate of depression increases with age, and the incidence continues to increase during adolescence. In Canada, approximately 5% of male youth and 12% of female youth have experienced a major depressive episode (CMHA, 2019a). The total number of 12- to 19-year-olds in Canada at risk for developing depression is an astounding 3.2 million. While the exact cause of depression is unknown, many factors are likely to play a role, including family history, personality, life events, and developmental changes.

Depression is suspected when the adolescent uses words such as down, sad, low, blue, hopeless, worried, bored, or discouraged, and exhibits several of the following symptoms:

- Change in weight or appetite
- Insomnia or hypersomnia
- Decreased energy or fatigue
- Loss of interest and pleasure in usual activities
- Out-of-proportion feelings of self-reproach or guilt
- Difficulty concentrating; declining school performance
- Preoccupation with death or suicidal ideation

Evidence suggests that when health care providers complete a mental health screening questionnaire for adolescents during periodic health examinations, referrals to appropriate mental health management and resources increase (CPS, 2016a). Once depression is recognized, help can make a difference for 80% of youth who are affected and allow them to get back to their regular activities.

Nurses need to lead the way in screening and assessing teens for mental health problems, including depression. Moreover, nurses may encourage mental health promotion in teens by teaching them effective coping skills, self-care strategies, and stress-reduction techniques.

### Suicide

Adolescence is a period of considerable stress and, when coping mechanisms and social supports are inadequate, suicide may emerge as an outcome. In Canada, suicide has become the second leading cause of death among adolescents, aged 10 to 24 years, and Canada's youth suicide rate is the third highest in the industrialized world (Canadian Children's Rights Council, 2019). A national survey revealed that one in seven (14%) of Canadians aged 15–24 had experienced suicidal thoughts. Indigenous youth die by suicide 5 to 6 times more often than non-Indigenous youth (Mental Health Commission of Canada, 2019). In addition, suicide ideation and behaviour is higher among LGBTQ2 youth (Egale Canada Human Rights Trust, 2019). It is estimated that for every completed suicide, there are at least 20 suicide attempts. Males are more likely to die from suicide, while females are more likely to attempt suicide.

These figures might not even reflect the full scope of the problem because many suicides may be classified as accidental deaths. Along with well-known risk factors, such as bullying, depression, and exposure to self-harm on digital media, the risk factors for suicide may be related to physical and cognitive developmental changes. The physical and emotional changes during puberty in younger children evolve into older adolescents achieving a cognitive level that allows them to more carefully solve problems and look at consequences. Suicide during adolescence is not an impulsive or spontaneous act: it is selected carefully only after other problem-solving methods have failed and suicide is viewed as the only option (Canadian Children's

---

### BOX 15.3 Coping Mechanisms of Adolescents

**Cognitive Mastery**
The adolescent attempts to learn as much as possible about the situation or stressor. This strategy is common for the adolescent with a chronic illness. The nurse can assist by clarifying any misinformation, sharing research findings, and encouraging a discussion of feelings.

**Conformity**
The adolescent attempts to be a mirror image of peers, which includes dress, language, attitudes, and actions. The nurse must respect this need for sameness and can also encourage discussion of feelings about differences among teens.

**Controlling Behaviour**
Adolescents must be in charge of some aspects of life and can no longer accept family and school rules without question as they did in the past. This need for control extends to health care. The nurse cannot simply give directions or instructions, but rather should present the options and allow the adolescent to partner with the nurse to work out an acceptable plan.

**Fantasy**
The adolescent may use fantasy as a way to escape or experiment. The nurse can encourage the teen to use fantasy constructively to develop creative plans to deal with a stressful situation.

**Motor Activity**
Engaging in sports, dancing, running, or other physical activity can be an effective tension-releasing strategy, and can also provide an instant peer group. The nurse can encourage physical activity and offer information about protective gear and injury prevention.

Rights Council, 2019). Adolescent suicide can be prevented. Distressed adolescents tend to give clues, both verbally and nonverbally. Any single clue may mean nothing, but when several clues are noted, they should be recognized as important warning signs. Box 15.4 outlines vigilant warning signs for parents, teachers, health care providers, and peers to prevent adolescent suicide. Any signs of suicide or threat to commit suicide should be taken seriously and require immediate intervention and referral. An adult should remain with the adolescent until medical assistance becomes available. Nurses can teach adolescents to be sensitive to the signs that may indicate a friend is suicidal and to seek adult assistance immediately.

## Values-Beliefs Pattern

Values and beliefs are learned phenomena that serve as guides for decision making and actions. With the development of abstract thought, adolescents begin to expand their understanding of good and bad or right and wrong, to include autonomous moral principles that have validity apart from the authority of a parent or society and instead are based on the individual's beliefs. Their newly discovered maturity in moral reasoning is situational and relational and is often superseded by psychosocial developmental needs and influences. Adolescents may think or feel something is wrong or bad. yet may act contrary to that belief because of peer pressure or the need to declare their independence.

Adolescents often align their values and beliefs with a particular religion, philosophical school of thought, social movement or cause, or other formal system, using it to make decisions about what is right or wrong, best or worst, and important or trivial. During adolescence, these alignments can change drastically and often, causing strife and concern for parents, yet providing the teen with different ranges of experience from which to base eventual and lasting choices. Kohlberg's theory of moral development (Kohlberg, 1981) demonstrates that the adolescent begins to make the transition to the postconventional stage, equating what is right with the idea of justice and basing actions on the recognition of the universal principles underlying laws and social agreements.

As adolescents struggle with their journey to discover who they are, parents, teachers, and health care providers need to provide positive role modelling, reinforce positive behaviours, and remember the difficulty of their own journeys. It is often when we like them the least that they need us the most.

## Environmental Processes

Because adolescents are in developmental transition, their lifestyle choices may have a significant effect on their current and future health. These choices are particularly sensitive to the immediate physical and social environments. These environmental influences include their family members, friends, community, school, neighbourhood, and work environments. Several critical types of adolescent health behaviours—including alcohol and drug use, injury and violence, tobacco use, nutrition, physical activity, and sexual behaviours—have been identified as contributing to the leading causes of death and disability among adults and youth.

## Physical Agents
### Unintentional Injury

Unintentional injury, along with suicide and homicide, continues to be the leading cause of death, hospitalization, and disability among Canadian youth. Approximately 71% of all deaths from unintentional injury among adolescents, aged 15 to 19 years, are attributed to injuries caused by motor vehicle crashes (CPS, 2012b). For Indigenous teens, the death rate from unintentional injuries is on average three to four times higher than for non-Indigenous youth, particularly from motor vehicle crashes and drownings (Banerji, CPS, & First Nations, Inuit, and Métis Health Committee, 2012). Motor vehicle crashes are a significant cause of nonfatal injury as well. Whether drivers, passengers, pedestrians, or cyclists, few adolescents take measures to reduce their risk of injury, with 15% rarely or never using a safety belt and 90% rarely or never using a bicycle helmet. Evidence also suggests that distractions, such as talking or texting on cell phones, eating, or playing with the radio, increase teen drivers' risk of being involved in a crash.

Nurses talk to teens about the consequences of texting while driving and encourage teens to wear their safety belts and avoid driving, or riding with someone, under the influence of drugs or alcohol. The tendency to play loud music and change the tune or disc often, as well as the pressure to answer cell phones, can also be distracting, as can a car full of other teens. Recognizing this and that teens have a much higher night-time crash fatality rate, many provinces have enacted new driver restrictions and night-time curfews.

### Sports Injuries

Organized sports in and out of school provide adolescents with experiences in competition, teamwork and effort, and conflict resolution. They also provide a valuable means for adolescents

---

### BOX 15.4   Warning Signs of Suicide Risk in Adolescents

**Behavioural Changes**
- Increased risk taking
- Increased incidence of accidents
- Substance use and abuse
- Physical violence to self, others, or animals
- Decreased appetite
- Alienation from family or peer group
- Giving away personal items
- Writing letters or notes, essays, and poems with suicidal content

**Cognitive and Mood Changes**
- Expression of hopelessness
- Increasing rage or anger
- Dramatic swings in affect
- Sleep disorders
- Preoccupation with death
- Difficulty concentrating
- Hearing voices, seeing things or people
- New-found interest in religion or cult

to develop self-esteem. However, adolescents are particularly vulnerable to sports injuries. Their coordination skills are developing, their judgement is often immature and inadequate, their epiphyses have not yet closed, and their extremities are poorly protected by stabilizing musculature. They can also become obsessed or driven to perform beyond their capabilities or to the exclusion of all other activities. The use of performance-enhancing substances, such as steroids, which have been unfortunately modelled by many professional athletes, can create another potential extreme scenario that places the adolescent at risk of injury.

Although traumatic brain injury (concussion) is caused by falls or other mechanical injury, the most frequent contributing factor in Canadian adolescents is participation in sports and recreational activities (Canadian Safety Council, 2019). Hockey, rugby, and ringette are the sports with the highest proportion of brain injuries among youth. Among injured Canadian youth, 53% of head injuries in children 10 to 14 years of age and 43% of head injuries in adolescents 15 to 19 years of age were sport-related, while concussion accounted for 9% to 12% of injuries in high school athletes (CPS, 2014). Even a minor impact injury to the head or neck, with or without loss of consciousness, can result in long-term physical, emotional, and cognitive effects if it is not appropriately managed, including deficits in cognition, altered neurological status, problems concentrating in school, and fatigue. Traumatic brain injury should be managed by a provider who is experienced in recognizing the signs and symptoms and who is experienced in concussion management. Several reliable and valid assessment instruments are available to assist health care providers in diagnosis (CPS, 2014).

As a consequence of a body of evidence suggesting that traumatic brain injury effects can be severe in adolescents, the Government of Canada has developed a concussion "toolbox" that includes evidence-informed information, practical tools, and protocols for coaches, athletes, parents, schools, and health care providers for appropriate guidance in the prevention, recognition, and management of concussions (Health Canada, 2018). Both physical and cognitive rest are essential aspects for recovery. Cognitive rest includes limiting activities that require mental exertion, such as reading, texting, school work, electronic games, and watching television (CPS, 2014). As symptoms improve, teens may gradually increase cognitive tasks and social activities, provided that symptoms are not exacerbated.

The nurse advocates the proper use of protective gear during all activities and a thorough preparticipation sports examination, along with concussion training for coaches and parents. The nurse also monitors adolescents for overuse, overexertion, or overinvestment in a sport.

### Violence

Although the rate of adolescent victims of violence has decreased in the past two decades, adolescents still experience risk of injury and death from violence in their homes, schools, and communities. In Canada, 12% of victims of crime were youth aged 12 to 17 years, while one third of Indigenous youth have been victims of violent crimes compared to one quarter of non-Indigenous youth (Statistics Canada, 2016b). Although Canada's rate of firearm ownership is lower than that of the United States, adolescent males are disproportionately at risk of firearm injuries, particularly when weapons are kept in the home (Austin & Lane, 2018). Adolescents often report a fear of violence and try to avoid situations where they might be vulnerable to it, including the home or even the bathroom at school. Victims of violent crime can experience both short-term and long-term physical and psychological health problems. Fig. 15.5 outlines the inter-relationships of internal and external precipitating factors that increase an adolescent's vulnerability to and for violent behaviours.

Bullying occurs when there is an imbalance of power; when someone intentionally and repeatedly says or does harmful things to someone else. It may occur one-on-one or in a group(s) of people. Four types of bullying exist: (1) physical, where your body or objects are used to cause harm, such as hitting, punching, or kicking; (2) verbal, where words are used to hurt someone, such as teasing, insults, or threats; (3) social bullying, where your friends or relationships are used to hurt someone, such as gossiping or spreading rumours; and (4) cyberbullying (RCMP, 2019). Cyberbullying involves the use of electronic media, such as the Internet, social media sites, or text messages, to repeatedly intimidate or harass other teens. Examples include posting embarrassing photos of someone online, pretending to be another person, or sending threatening emails or text messages. Sextortion, a form of cyberbullying, involves the threat of releasing shared intimate videos, images, or explicit messages online in order to receive payments to prevent the public release of such videos, images, or messages. Cyberbullying is different from other forms of bullying as it can harm a victim 24 hours a day and 7 days a week, and can follow them into their home, which is usually a safe environment from traditional bullying.

In a Canadian survey, 16% of youths in Grades 7 to 9 had been bullied on more than 12 occasions during the previous year. Males are more likely to be a physical bully and to be a victim of physical bullying, while females are more likely to be a social bully and to be a victim of social bullying. Males and females were equally as likely to be a verbal bully as well as a victim of verbal bullying (RCMP, 2019). Being bullied in any form may lead to school absences, social isolation, and serious emotional distress, including depression and suicide (Public Safety Canada, 2018). In addition, adolescents who bully are 37% more likely than adolescents who do not bully to commit criminal offences as adults and have a higher risk of substance use, school absences, and may be bullied themselves. Public Safety Canada (2018) has created an informative website for many school and community programs to help prevent and reduce bullying at https://www.publicsafety.gc.ca/cnt/rsrcs/pblctns/bllng-prvntn/index-en.aspx#a05. In addition, there is also a national tip line to report online sexual exploitation of children and adolescents at https://www.cybertip.ca/app/en/projects-public_awareness.

Nurses engage adolescents to examine and discuss the messages in social media, videos, songs, movies, games, and

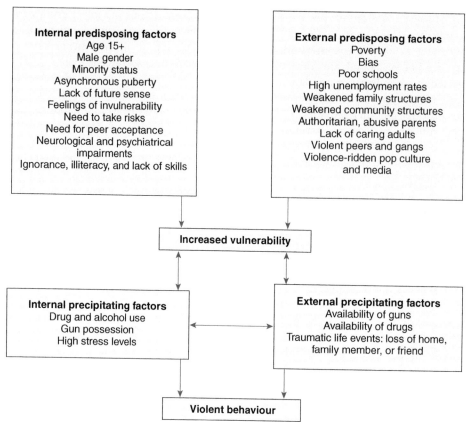

**Fig. 15.5** Factors contributing to adolescent violence.

television shows. Discussing their developing sense of self, their sense of belonging, and where that sense is found, and their fears, may help nurses to intercept an adolescent who might otherwise turn to violence. Discussing frightening news events with adolescents in a realistic, contextual way might also help nurses mitigate fear and anxiety. Teens who are valued and nurtured by caring adults have the best chance of emerging from adolescence unscathed. Nurses may also discuss cyberbullying with adolescents; encourage them to talk to a trusted adult if they receive harassing text messages and to consider options such as rejecting texts from unknown numbers; and tell them that it is inappropriate and possibly illegal to send harassing text messages to others.

Working with parents is essential. Nurses can encourage parents to be vigilant regarding their adolescent's use of electronic media, including restricting use or using parental controls, if necessary. Total screen time should be limited to no more than 2 hours a day for children of all ages and removing access to all electronic device at bedtime (CPS, 2017b). Parents need to be aware of websites accessed by their adolescent, including YouTube sites, gaming sites, text messaging programs, and social media. Adolescents may be resistant to parental monitoring because of the perception that it invades their privacy; however, nurses can suggest that parents discuss these issues with teens before providing them with electronic access so that adolescents know from the outset that spot checking will occur and the consequences of inappropriate use.

## ◆ Biological Agents

### Infection

Infectious mononucleosis is a self-limiting viral infection transmitted by direct contact with oropharyngeal secretions. It is prevalent among adolescents and is often referred to as the "kissing disease"; however, it can occur in younger children. It is caused by Epstein–Barr virus. Typically, adolescents complain of a sore throat, lymph node enlargement, and lethargy. Both splenomegaly and hepatomegaly can occur, creating a risk of injury. The condition is self-limiting and resolves with symptomatic care and appropriate rest.

Invasive meningococcal disease (IMD) is serious, often resulting in fulminant sepsis or meningitis. IMD in Canada is primarily attributable to serogroups B and C. There are routine programs for serogroup C vaccine (Men-C-C) at 12 months of age, with some provinces and territories routinely providing additional earlier doses. A booster dose of Men-C-C vaccine or of a quadrivalent (Men-C-ACYW) vaccine is routinely given at 12–14 years of age (CPS, 2018c). In Canada, there have no identified risks of meningococcal disease among university or college students who live in dormitories or residence halls.

Adolescents are at the period of life with high sexual energy that may lead to high levels of risky behaviours attributable to an increased sense of invulnerability. As adolescents experiment with and explore their sexual development and emerging independence, they engage in risky sexual behaviour and expose themselves to increased risk of acquiring **STBBIs**. STBBIs commonly include gonorrhea, syphilis, chlamydia, herpes simplex virus infection, human papillomavirus (HPV) infection, trichomoniasis, hepatitis B, and HIV infection. Chlamydia is the most frequently reported STBBI in Canada and predominately affects females aged 15–24 years. Rates of gonorrhea are increasing faster among adolescent females than adolescent males (CPS, 2018d). Indigenous people in Canada accounted for an estimated 10% all Canadians with HIV (Canadian AIDS Treatment Information Exchange [CATIE], 2016).

Many contributing factors have been identified and found to negatively impact this significant adolescent health problem. Factors such as inconsistent use of contraceptives and protective devices, increasingly earlier age of and more frequent sexual activity, lower self-esteem, depression, social and peer pressure, and an adolescent's sense of invincibility were related to higher risks of STBBIs (PHAC, 2019b).

The decision to screen is based on risk factors and symptoms, both genital and systemic, while recognizing that rectal and pharyngeal gonococcal infections are often asymptomatic. Ideally, all of a patient's sexual contacts should be identified, tested, and treated appropriately, although ensuring full disclosure and follow-up in individuals with multiple sexual partners may be challenging. Screening is recommended for high-risk adolescents, including those who are sexually active, have had a previous STBBI, are a victim of sexual abuse or assault, use injection drugs, practice unsafe sex, are homeless, or have spent time in a detention facility. Canadian guidelines for STBBI screening are available on the Public Health Agency of Canada website, including links to a mobile application (PHAC, 2019b). STBBIs are reportable diseases and nurses should be familiar and comply with a timely reporting process in their area. Public health authorities can assist in tracing contacts when needed.

The Pan-Canadian Sexually Transmitted and Blood-Borne Infection Framework for Action is based on four interconnected pillars that span the continuum of STBBI care: prevention; testing; initiating care and treatment; and ongoing care and support. It aims to reduce stigma and discrimination that create vulnerabilities to STBBI, improve access to testing, treatment, and ongoing care and support (PHAC, 2018).

Discussions about sexuality, sexual activity, contraception, and the prevention of STBBIs should start early with adolescents, ideally *before* they become sexually active (CPS, 2018d). Although parents may be involved in discussions on this sensitive topic, it is also essential that youth have opportunities to discuss sexual issues with care providers alone and in confidence. Confidentiality maximizes the likelihood of obtaining a complete sexual history and engaging on questions and concerns that youth might not be comfortable sharing with a parent. The law protects youths' right to receive confidential care for their sexual and reproductive health, including prescriptions for contraception and treatment of STBBIs, as long as they are mature enough to understand the nature and consequences of treatment. It is important to consider youth perspectives on sexually transmitted infections (STIs) and sexual health, including those from diverse Canadian populations and regions (Research for Evidence-Informed Practice).

## RESEARCH FOR EVIDENCE-INFORMED PRACTICE

### Youth Perspectives on Sexually Transmitted Infections and Sexual Health in Northern Canada

Little research has explored the perspectives of youth in Northern Canada regarding sexual health and sexually transmitted infections (STIs), despite high rates of STIs. A qualitative study was conducted with 17 youth (aged 14–19 years) in three Nunavut communities. The research was conducted within an Indigenous knowledge framework with a focus on Inuit ways of knowing to explore youth experiences of talking about sexual health and relationships with their family, peers, teachers, or other community members. The majority of youth participants described sexual health in terms of condom use and STIs and used terms they had learned in school. The preferred source of knowledge about sexual health and relationships was their parents or caregivers, and they did not report using the Internet to access sexual health information. The participants described sexual health in terms of both desire and love, and related their sexual decision making to broader community contexts and determinants of health, such as unemployment and poverty.

Nurses working in Northern Canada may employ these findings to tailor interventions to address the concerns of the youth related to promoting sexual health. The researcher suggests that these include parent–adolescent educational interventions using social determinants of health lens and a holistic approach that considers physical, emotional, mental, and spiritual health.

Source: Healey, G. (2016). Youth perspectives on sexually transmitted infections and sexual health in Northern Canada and implications for public health practice. *International Journal of Circumpolar Health, 75,* 30706. doi:10.3402/ijch.v75.30706

## Cancer

Adolescents are affected by many of the same cancers as are younger children, such as leukemia, osteogenic sarcoma, lymphomas, and central nervous system tumours. Older adolescents are entering the period of their lives during which cancer of the reproductive and related organs is more common. For females, the focus is on cervical and breast cancer; for males, testicular cancer is of concern.

The peak incidence of breast and cervical cancer is during middle age, and breast and cervical cancers are actually rare in the teenage years. Risks for later development of these cancers can occur during adolescence, so prevention and surveillance are essential. Breast self-examination, which has been highly recommended for many, has recently been questioned as a routine practice for most adolescents. The extremely small incidence of breast cancer in teens has caused some health care providers to de-emphasize this practice for them. However, most still feel that regular examination of the breasts is a life-long habit that should begin as soon as the female adolescent develops (see Quality and Safety Scenario box, earlier).

Cervical cancer is detected with a Papanicolaou (Pap) smear, obtained from the cervix during a pelvic examination. Factors that increase the risk of cervical cancer include HIV or HPV infection, history of STBBI, becoming sexually active at a young age, having multiple sex partners, smoking, multiparity, use of oral contraceptives, and daughters whose mothers took diethylstilbestrol (DES) (Canadian Cancer Society, 2019a). As routine pelvic examinations and Pap smears are no longer recommended for adolescents, routine cervical cancer screening begins for sexually active females at the age of 21 and is repeated every 1 to 3 years, depending on risk factors and previous test results (Canadian Cancer Society, 2019a).

HPV is known to cause genital warts, cervical cancer, penile cancer, anal cancer, and oropharyngeal cancer. A safe and effective vaccine against nine HPV types is available and, since 2006, has been routinely administered to all males and females between the ages of 9 and 13 years of age. Ideally, youth should receive the vaccine before they become sexually active. All youth who have not previously received the vaccine in a routine program should receive the vaccine in a "catch-up" program (CPS, 2018e).

Testicular cancer is the number one cancer in adolescent and young adult males and the annual incidence is steadily increasing (Canadian Cancer Society, 2019b). Known risk factors include an undescended testicle, personal or family history of testicular cancer, calcium deposits in the testicle, and tall adult height. Testicular cancer occurs more often in White males and less often in males of African or Asian ancestry. It is also linked to a higher socioeconomic status. Adolescent males should learn to perform a testicular self-examination and should continue this practice monthly (see Quality and Safety Scenario box, earlier). Nurses introduce and teach methods of self-examination to adolescents, who naturally are interested in their developing bodies.

## ◆ Chemical Agents

### Substance Use and Abuse

Adolescents are influenced by a complicated interaction between biological and psychosocial development, environmental messages, and societal attitudes regarding the use of substances such as alcohol, tobacco, or cannabis. Society as a whole is increasingly oriented toward using chemicals such as drugs, alcohol, and tobacco to feel better, look better, act more sociable, stay awake, sleep, be sexy or erect, or lose weight. Some of the most famous music, movie, and sports stars openly model substance use and abuse. It is no surprise that adolescents are making the choice to experiment with and use substances at younger and younger ages.

Alcohol is the substance most commonly abused by teenagers. Although it is illegal to sell alcohol to anyone under the age of 19 in the majority of Canadian jurisdictions, 70% of Canadian youth aged 12 to 17 reported consuming an alcoholic beverage in the previous 12 months (Drug Free Kids Canada, 2019). For adolescent problem drinkers, Alcoholics Anonymous has pamphlets and other resources, including meetings, for young people who are ready to begin recovery.

After alcohol, cannabis is the most widely used psychoactive substance among Canadian youth aged 15–19. Cannabis, more commonly called marijuana, is a green or brown material consisting of the dried flowers, tops, and leaves of the cannabis plant. Hashish is the dark brown or black resinous secretion of the flowering tops and can be further processed to produce hashish oil or wax. Cannabis is usually smoked as a cigarette ("joint") and may be laced with other substances, such as cocaine. Cannabis can also be smoked as a resin in a pipe or bong, referred to as "dabbing," or inhaled through a vaporizer.

Cannabis can also be baked into foods and orally ingested, known as "edibles."

Up to one third of Canadian students in Grades 7 to 12 reported using cannabis, although overall use has steadily decreased over the past decade (Canadian Centre on Substance Use and Addiction, 2019). Males are more likely to use cannabis and are more likely to report driving after use. Regular use of cannabis before the age of 16 has been linked to greater risk of mental illness, including schizophrenia, bipolar disorders, and anxiety, as well as greater likelihood of impairment of cognitive development among youth (Canadian Centre of Substance Use and Addiction, 2019). Because Canada has recently legalized the nonmedical use of cannabis, further research is required to provide a clearer understanding of the use and harms of cannabis use among Canadian youth.

Inhalant abuse, also known as volatile substance abuse, solvent abuse, sniffing, or bagging, is the deliberate inhalation of a volatile substance to achieve an altered mental state (CPS, 2018f). Given that inhalants are legal, inexpensive, and easy to obtain, there is a high abuse potential among youth. Usually starting as children, 1.3% of Canadian youth 15 years of age and older reported lifetime use of inhalants. Inhalant abuse is more common in rural and isolated communities with high rates of unemployment, poverty, and violence, among those who have been physically or sexually abused, or neglected, the incarcerated or homeless, as well as in Indigenous communities.

In a national survey, 1.6% of Canadians in Grades 7 to 9 and 3.5% of students in Grades 10 to 12 reported the use of opioids to get high, and not for medicinal purposes (Health Canada, 2016). Among Indigenous youth aged 12 to 17, 1.3% used illicit or prescription opioids to get high.

Overdose occurs when someone takes one or more drugs in a quantity or combination that exceeds what their body can handle. Overdoses may occur with many types of drugs, including those used recreationally, bought over-the-counter, legally prescribed, or obtained illicitly (CMHA, 2019b). Some drugs, such as opioids, are central nervous system depressants, meaning that they slow normal functions like breathing and heart rate to the point that they stop altogether. Other drugs such as amphetamines, cocaine, and MDMA (ecstasy) have an opposite effect: they speed up the central nervous system and may lead to heart attack, stroke, or seizure. Overdoses can have serious consequences, including permanent brain injury or even death. Youth aged 15 to 24 is one of the groups with the fastest-growing rates of hospitalization for overdoses, as young people may experiment with different substances and engage in riskier substance-use behaviours. They are also more likely to binge-drink, which poses a higher risk of toxicity. In 2016, Health Canada made naloxone (Narcan) available without a prescription to temporarily reduce the effects of an opioid overdose. This is one part of an overdose prevention strategy that also includes The Good Samaritan Overdose Act, opiod public awareness initiatives, financial support for substance use and addictions programs, provincial and territorial emergency treatment funds, and supervised consumption sites.

Substance use is a precursor to abuse, which emphasizes the need for health care providers to be alert for and screen individuals for its presence. Identifying adolescent substance users or abusers requires a careful nursing assessment that is conducted in an accepting manner (Boxes 15.5 and 15.6) and referral for appropriate management. The CPS (2016a) recommends individuals be screened for substance use at every well visit during adolescence using the CRAFFT mnemonic.

## Tobacco Use

In 2017, smoking prevalence among students in Grades 7 to 9 was 1.0% overall, while among adolescents aged 15 to 19, 7.9% were current smokers. However, there was substantial growth by age, as 11.2% of 18- and 19-year-olds were current smokers. Between 2014 and 2016, there was no significant change in smoking prevalence among youth (Statistics Canada, 2018a). Indigenous and LGBTQ2 youth have higher-than-average smoking rates. They were also more likely to be exposed to second-hand smoke at home and in vehicles (37% and 51%, respectively) than their mainstream peers (20% and 30%) (Harvey, et al., 2016). Adolescents begin using tobacco for a variety of reasons, including wanting to look older or wanting to imitate their friends, adult role models, or media images. Advertising by the tobacco industry directed at adolescents has also been shown to encourage adolescent smoking.

Another form of tobacco use is smokeless tobacco (SLT), also known as snuff or chew. Two common forms are sold in Canada: chewing tobacco comes in leaves and is chewed, and snuff is loosely ground tobacco that is placed between the gingival and buccal mucosa. The user sucks on the tobacco and then spits out the juices. SLT is heavily sweetened with sugar and flavouring salts and, because it is held next to the teeth, promotes tooth decay and periodontal disease. Furthermore, the gritty material scratches soft tissues, allowing nicotine and other chemicals to directly enter the bloodstream. Given that holding one pinch of SLT in your mouth for 30 minutes delivers as much nicotine as four cigarettes, SLT carries significant health risks and is not a safe substitute for smoking. In addition, use of any form of tobacco increases the risk of oral cancer (Canadian Cancer Society, 2019c).

Recently, adolescents have begun using electronic cigarettes (e-cigarettes, vaping). Electronic cigarettes, which are battery operated, vaporize liquid for inhalation through an appliance that resembles a cigarette; there is no smoke involved (Health Canada, 2019b). Flavoured liquid in cartridges, either with or without nicotine, is attractive and legally available to adolescents over the age of 18 years. In 2017, 23% of Canadian youth in Grades 7 to 12 reported vaping at least once (Statistics Canada, 2018a). Vaping devices are frequently disguised to look like everyday objects (e.g., a USB key) to prevent awareness among parents and teachers. Furthermore, dual use of tobacco and e-cigarettes is common among Canadian youth. Because of the newness of this trend, there is little evidence to determine whether e-cigarette use will contribute to tobacco use or may be used as a safe substitute for smoking.

Smoking with a hookah or waterpipe, also called a nargile or shisha, is becoming more common among adolescents in Canada. Specially made tobacco is heated and the smoke passes through water and is then drawn through a rubber hose to a mouthpiece (MyHealth Alberta, 2019). Traditionally used by older men in India and Persia, hookah smoking can be found in

restaurants and hookah bars across Canada. Contrary to public opinion, using a hookah is not a safe alternative to smoking because it carries the same health risks as smoking cigarettes.

Through their work in public health, the nurse's primary prevention focus is on keeping nonsmokers from starting smoking and helping smokers to stop. Some of the most effective measures to reduce smoking rates in teens are already in place across Canada, such as high taxes, labelling deterrents, bans on point-of-sale displays and advertising to minors, and smoke-free spaces (including vehicles transporting minors). And while most jurisdictions have banned smoking in enclosed public spaces and in vehicles when children or youth are present, there is still much work to be done. Given that more adolescents have tried

---

**BOX 15.5  Major Signs of Substance Abuse**

Depending on the substance used, the signs can include the following:
- Agitation
- Altered sleep
- Appetite loss
- Blackouts
- Depression
- Diarrhea
- Distorted perception
- Drowsiness/lethargy
- Dry mucous membranes
- Euphoria
- Hallucinations
- Inability to concentrate or solve problems
- Inability to perform regular work or social activities
- Memory loss
- Nausea
- Poor coordination
- Respiratory depression
- Unintentional injuries
- Weight loss
- Withdrawal

Source: HealthLink BC. (n.d.). *Signs of substance use*. Retrieved from https://www.healthlinkbc.ca/health-topics/aa52544.

---

**BOX 15.6  CRAFFT: Adolescent Substance Abuse Screening Test**

A brief screening test for adolescent substance abuse developed by the Center for Adolescent Substance Abuse Research at the Boston Children's Hospital uses the acronym CRAFFT to guide health care providers when they are interviewing adolescents about substance abuse:

C—Have you ever ridden in a CAR driven by someone, including yourself, who was "high" or had been using alcohol or drugs?

R—Do you ever use alcohol or drugs to RELAX, feel better about yourself, or fit in?

A—Do you ever use alcohol or drugs when you are by yourself, ALONE?

F—Do you ever FORGET things you did while using alcohol or drugs?

F—Does your family or do your FRIENDS ever tell you that you should cut down on your drinking or drug use?

T—Have you gotten into TROUBLE while you were using alcohol or drugs?

Two or more affirmative answers suggest a significant problem and warrant referral and follow-up.

Reprinted with permission from the Center for Adolescent Substance Abuse Research, Boston Children's Hospital © 2009.

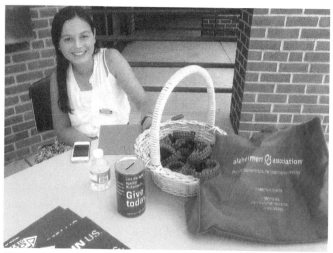

Fig. 15.6 Adolescents participate in school-sponsored community service.

e-cigarettes than traditional cigarettes, governments are being urged to treat e-cigarettes the same way as traditional tobacco products and to expand all current smoking restrictions in public spaces and workplaces to include them (Harvey, et al., 2016).

## ❖ DETERMINANTS OF HEALTH

### ◆ Social Factors and Environment

#### School

Middle school or junior high and high school bring new social experiences, introducing the adolescent to changing classes, multiple teachers and teaching styles, variable class schedules, homework load, and a variety of peer influences. School populations may be significantly larger than the child has experienced previously, and making and solidifying new friendships may be more difficult. Yet, despite these challenges, these school settings also provide meaningful in-school and after-school learning, peer contact, intellectual stimulation, and social or volunteer community service activities (Fig. 15.6).

Schools and peers, as opposed to home and parents, become the primary setting through which expectations are shared and standards communicated. During health-promotion visits, nurses ask adolescents about school and their friends and how they are doing with both. The nurse can also monitor adolescents as they prepare for and make the transition to their next social arena and role, whether it is university or college, apprenticeship training, the military, or another career choice.

#### Culture and Ethnicity

Cultural and ethnic influences operate throughout childhood and continue into adolescence. The primary difference in adolescence is that teens question, modify, or reject these influences, exchanging them for those of their peers or of the dominant cultural group. First-generation adolescents of immigrant parents have to negotiate two cultures: languages and sets of expectations. These adolescents often live a double life that might result in increased stress. Adolescents from minority groups, such as Indigenous people, Asians, Muslims,

or Africans might experience discrimination and rejection if they try to fit in to the dominant adolescent culture, which is often middle class, White, and Protestant. Advertising is directed to middle-class or affluent teens, not the economically depressed, and media images might not include attractive ethnic-looking models. Adolescents from different cultures might experience additional stress when their attempts to fit in to the dominant culture are contrary to the values and beliefs of their own culture.

The growing ethnic diversity in the adolescent population influences how adolescent health will be approached. For example, Statistics Canada (2018b) reports that the number of immigrant and visible minority Canadians will grow by 2031. With fast growth in the numbers of Asian, Arab, and Indigenous Canadian youth, cultural awareness of health care needs and the highlighted attention to health inequalities and academic outcomes, especially among adolescents from racial minorities and ethnic groups, are required (Diversity Awareness). Nurses need to recognize the additional stresses experienced by adolescents and assess them for those stresses as they wrestle not only with their own identities but also with their cultural identities.

### 🌐 DIVERSITY AWARENESS

#### *Integration of Indigenous Ways of Knowing During a Concussion Awareness Educational Workshop for Indigenous Communities*

Sports activities are the leading causes of health injury in Canadian youth, with higher rates of head injuries occurring among Indigenous individuals. Since participation in hockey is common among Indigenous youth, there is an expected incidence of 5–20 concussions per 100 players per season, and more than 15% of all injuries in youth hockey are due to this injury. However, concussions are considered to be a hidden epidemic due to the lack of recognition of them among players, coaches, and parents. Moreover, there is no word in Indigenous languages for concussion, further limiting the reporting, treatment, and recovery from this injury. An unidentified and untreated concussion may negatively impact physical, cognitive, and emotional health that may disrupt school, family, and community life. It has been suggested that there is an imperative need to deliver Indigenous-sensitive programs for concussion awareness and early identification.

The purpose of this article was to describe collaboration of nurses from both an urban setting and from a remote, Indigenous setting to develop and implement a culturally sensitive educational workshop of concussion awareness for a local Indigenous community. The team enacted the principle of "two-eyed seeing," in which strengths of both Indigenous and Western ways of knowing were brought together. The participants reported high levels of concussion knowledge both before and after the workshop, suggesting that concussion-related information may also have come from hockey organizations and recent media reports. Participants who were hockey players indicated that the three reasons for not reporting a concussion were fear of not being able to play, lack of knowledge about concussion, and feeling that the team was counting on them to win.

Providing similar educational programs over time may enhance behavioural change that can reduce concussion injuries, as well as examine the relationship between concussion education and incidence of concussion.

Source: Hunt, C., Michalak, A., Lefkimmiatis, C., et al. (2018). Exploring concussion awareness in hockey with a First Nations community in Canada. *Public Health Nursing, 35*, 202–201. https://doi.org/10.1111/phn.12407

## ◆ Levels of Policymaking and Health

Many laws and regulations are aimed at adolescents and deal with the minimum age at which they can assume adult responsibilities and decision making. The rationale for these restrictions is that adolescents, although capable, lack the experience, perspective, and judgement to recognize and avoid choices that might be detrimental to them, so they require protection. A question raised frequently when minimum age is considered is whether strict age criteria are appropriate for any adolescent, particularly because development is variable and experiences are diverse.

Certain provincial laws may allow a 16- or 17-year-old youth to decide to live independently and assume adult responsibilities. Except for the province of Quebec, there are no laws in Canada that specifically provide for emancipation of a minor, where the individual is economically and emotionally separate from the family or guardian (Justice for Youth and Children, 2013).

Most often, confidentiality is the more important issue for adolescents. The nurse can assure them that information shared will be kept confidential unless the teens pose a risk to themselves or others, or state or public health reporting mandates that the information be shared. For example, abuse must be reported, STBBIs need to be reported, and some provinces require adolescent sexual activity to be reported if an age difference of 3 years or more exists between the sexual partners.

Nurses need to familiarize themselves with the legal rights of adolescents in their jurisdiction and the resources available in their community.

### Economics

Identification with peers, the essence of self-image during adolescence, includes dressing alike, having similar possessions, and doing similar activities, all of which require economic resources. This can cause a major conflict between parents and adolescents. Parents may think that they should have the power to decide how their adolescent spends money. Adolescents may believe, just as strongly, that they know the best ways to allocate resources and determine the amount of money they need.

Ideally, parents and adolescents should negotiate economic questions, with the parents becoming less controlling as the teen gains more experience and expertise in these matters. However, the family with limited economic resources has fewer choices, and adolescents from these families may feel trapped by their circumstances. Poverty is particularly hard on children, and as they become adolescents, they often develop a fatalistic view of life.

Some adolescents seek employment to earn their own money and have control over it. Others work because their families need the income. It is important for the nurse to assess the economic resources of each adolescent's family and work within them when partnering with the adolescent in health care planning.

## ◆ Health Services/Delivery System

Many health care resources are available to the adolescent. Teens can continue to see their child health care providers in a pediatric centre as they did as younger children, but this setting is usually rejected because of the young-child atmosphere.

Adolescents can also make use of services such as family planning clinics. These settings may designate certain days and hours for teens, whereas other facilities integrate them into the adult-oriented protocols. The pregnant adolescent typically finds prenatal care in an adult-focused setting, although more adolescent-specific programs are being developed. The physical needs of pregnant adolescents may be the same as those of the pregnant adult, but the psychosocial needs are different and should be approached by a professional who has comprehensive knowledge of their development and responses to stress.

The adolescent is a rapidly changing individual. The public health nurse should have a thorough understanding of adolescent physical and psychosocial growth and development and recognize each teen as a person.

Adolescents not only tend to be fearful about procedures or possible diagnoses but also need to stay in control of the situation. These conflicting feelings can be difficult to manage simultaneously. By establishing the adolescent as a partner with the health care providers in promoting good health and screening the adolescent for health risks, the nurse facilitates the adolescent's sense of control (Box 15.7).

The adolescent's questions should be answered thoroughly and honestly. In many instances the adolescent is hesitant to voice concerns, so information is offered even when questions are not asked. An effective indirect approach to learning about adolescent concerns, especially about potentially embarrassing or stressful topics, is to say "Many teenagers ask me about [a topic]. Have you ever thought about this?" or "A lot of young people want to know about [a topic]."

Direct questions are also important, even about sensitive topics: "Have you ever thought about suicide?" "Are you depressed?" "Are you sexually active?" "Do you use birth control and/or protection?" However, asking first about friends and the adolescent's feelings about them may be a good

---

### BOX 15.7 HEADSSS Assessment

The HEADSSS assessment provides a mnemonic that guides health care providers through an adolescent's psychosocial assessment. Responses should be interpreted as those that are indicators of strengths or protection from risk and those that are indicators of risky behaviour or situations.

Home
Education, employment, eating
Activities
Drugs
Sexuality
Suicide or depression
Safety

Source: Klein, D., Goldenring, J., & Adelman, W. (2014). *HEADSSS 3.0: The psychosocial interview for adolescents updated for a new century fueled by media*. Retrieved from https://www.contemporarypediatrics.com/modern-medicine-feature-articles/heeadsss-30-psychosocial-interview-adolescents-updated-new-century-fueled-media.

lead-in approach: "Are any of your friends doing drugs?" "How do you feel about it?" Vague or circuitous questions may be interpreted as a sign of discomfort or lack of understanding and may cause the adolescent to be equally vague when responding.

Correct anatomical terms and descriptions of laboratory tests, disease processes, and possible outcomes are essential components in treating adolescents as individuals who are capable of being responsible for their own bodies.

## ❖ NURSING APPLICATION

Adolescence is a period of rapid growth and development, with changes occurring physically and psychosocially. Nurses play a pivotal role in influencing health-promotion, preventive-screening, and disease-prevention activities. The primary responsibility for the nurse dealing with the important period known as the transition from childhood to adulthood is to provide education about some of the expected changes and how to deal with them.

Primary prevention methods are effective when the nurse is able to partner with the adolescent in recognizing his or her health needs. Treating the teen in a respectful manner enables the teen to assume more responsibility. Nurses must remain sensitive to the changes the adolescent is encountering and understand the need for guided independence.

Some important health-education topics for the adolescent population include proper nutrition, exercise, teen pregnancy and protection against STBBIs, and no-cost access to contraception (CPS, 2016a, 2018d, 2019). Teens are taught about the significance of their lifestyle choices with regard to future health. Drug and alcohol use, injury prevention, violence, and tobacco use are all behaviours that are known to contribute to illness and death among teens. Nurses use educational tools that appeal to the age group by conducting Internet searches for resources. Teens are able to relate to Internet resources, celebrities, and social media sites. Peers have the greatest influence on teenagers.

Nurses need to educate teens, in partnership with their parents, about the fact that unintentional injuries are the leading cause of death in the adolescent population. Nurses should reinforce research regarding distracted driving, seat-belt use, and texting, adjusting the radio, and listening to loud music while driving.

Adolescent girls are educated about breast self-examinations, cervical cancer, and human papillomavirus. Adolescent males are educated about testicular self-examination. Both sexes are encouraged to undergo physical examinations and follow the recommended vaccination schedule.

Various screenings are used by the nurse as a secondary prevention measure for the adolescent. Nurses also screen adolescents for hypertension, eating disorders, type 2 diabetes, pregnancy, and STBBIs.

Adolescents respond better when they feel that they are regarded as young adults and a partner in their health-promotion efforts. The nurse needs to become skilled at discussing difficult or embarrassing topics with teenagers. It is essential that adolescents feel that they are treated with respect and regarded as an individual.

## CASE STUDY

### Drug-Facilitated Sexual Assault: Jessica

Sexual assault includes any type of sexual activity to which an individual does not agree. Because of the effects of some drugs, commonly called "date rape drugs," victims may be physically helpless, unable to refuse, or even unable to remember what happened.

During a preparticipation evaluation for a summer sports camp, Jessica, a 16-year-old high school student, expresses concern to the nurse that she knows someone who might have had sex "without knowing it." How can the nurse answer these common questions?

#### Reflective Questions

- What are date rape drugs and how can a person be unaware that such a drug has been ingested?
- What can you do to protect yourself?
- What do you do if you think you have been sexually assaulted?
- What can you do when someone you care about has been sexually assaulted?

## CARE PLAN

### Drug-Facilitated Sexual Assault: Jessica

**Nursing Issue**
Potential for powerlessness related to suspected rape/rape trauma syndrome

**Definition**
At risk of perceived lack of control over a situation and/or one's ability to significantly affect an outcome

**Risk Factors**
- Suspected date rape/rape trauma syndrome
- Acute injury (rape)
- Insufficient knowledge
- Disturbed body image
- Situational low self-esteem

**Expected Outcomes**
- Acknowledges personal strength
- Perceived control
- Perceived resources
- Participation in health care decisions
- Increase healthy lifestyle choices

*Goal:* increase individual's sense of power over potential/actual situation for self/others.

**Interventions**
- Active listening
- Risk identification
- Health care information exchange
- Support system enhancement
- Rape trauma treatment and referral
- Decision-making support
- Health education

## SUMMARY

Adolescence is a period of rapid change, when the integration of family, peer, educational, social, cultural, and community experiences begins to take form in the teen's sense of self. Many view adolescence as a construction site in its early stages. Onlookers assume that eventually a recognizable structure will emerge but have no idea what that structure will be. Although many parents, teachers, and health care providers feel that hard hats and steel-reinforced shoes are needed, each is better equipped with an understanding of and respect for the adolescent's developmental struggles with physical and cognitive changes, autonomy, body image, peer relations, and identity. The goal, after all, is for the teen to emerge in young adulthood with a healthy body, mind, and spirit.

### Evolve Chapter Features

http://evolve.elsevier.com/Canada/Edelman/healthpromotion/
• Review Questions

## REFERENCES

American Academy of Dermatology (AAD). (2016). *Caring for tattooed skin: Tips from dermatologists.* Retrieved from http://www.aad.org.

Association of Professional Piercers. (2019). *Suggested aftercare for body piercing.* Retrieved from https://www.safepiercing.org/aftercare.php.

Austin, K., & Lane, M. (2018). The prevention of firearm injuries in Canadian youth. *Paediatrics and Child Health*, 23(1), 35–42. https://doi.org/10.1093/pch/pxx164.

Banerji, A., Canadian Paediatric Society (CPS), & First Nations, Inuit, and Métis Health Committee (2012). Preventing unintentional injuries in Indigenous children and youth in Canada. *Pediatrics and Child Health*, 17(7), 393. https://doi.org/10.1093/pch/17.7.393.

Bottorff, J., Struik, L., Bissell, L., et al. (2014). A social media approach to inform youth about breast cancer and smoking: An exploratory descriptive study. *Collegian*, 21(2), 159–168.

Canadian AIDS Treatment Information Exchange (CATIE). (2016). *HIV: A primer for service providers.* Retrieved from https://www.catie.ca/en/hiv-canada/2/2-3/2-3-4.

Canadian Cancer Society. (2019a). *Risk factors for cervical cancer.* Retrieved from http://www.cancer.ca/en/cancer-information/cancer-type/cervical/risks/?region=ab#Sexual_activity.

Canadian Cancer Society. (2019b). *Risk factors for testicular cancer.* Retrieved from http://www.cancer.ca/en/cancer-information/cancer-type/testicular/risks/?region=ab.

Canadian Cancer Society. (2019c). *Six other ways tobacco increases your risk of getting cancer.* Retrieved from http://www.cancer.ca/en/prevention-and-screening/reduce-cancer-risk/make-healthy-choices/live-smoke-free/6-other-ways-that-tobacco-increases-your-risk-of-cancer/?region=ab.

Canadian Centre for Cybersecurity. (2018). *Get cyber safe.* Retrieved from https://www.getcybersafe.gc.ca/index-en.aspx.

Canadian Centre on Substance Use and Addiction. (2019). *Regular cannabis use linked to increased risk of mental illness.* Retrieved from https://www.ccsa.ca/regular-cannabis-use-linked-increased-risk-mental-illness.

Canadian Children's Rights Council. (2019). *Reflections on youth suicide.* Retrieved from http://www.canadiancrc.com/Youth_Suicide_in_Canada.aspx.

Canadian Dermatology Association. (2019). *Acne.* Retrieved from https://dermatology.ca/public-patients/skin/acne/.

Canadian Mental Health Association (CMHA). (2019a). *Children, youth, and depression.* Retrieved from https://cmha.ca/resources/children-youth-and-depression.

Canadian Mental Health Association (CMHA). (2019b). *Overdose prevention.* Retrieved from https://cmha.ca/documents/overdose-prevention.

Canadian Paediatric Society (CPS). (2012a). *Healthy active living: Physical activity guidelines for children and adolescents.* Retrieved from https://www.cps.ca/en/documents/position/physical-activity-guidelines.

Canadian Paediatric Society (CPS). (2012b). *Child and youth injury prevention: A public health approach.* Retrieved from https://www.cps.ca/en/documents/position/child-and-youth-injury-prevention.

Canadian Paediatric Society. (2014). *Sports-related concussion: Evaluation and management.* Retrieved from https://www.cps.ca/en/documents/position/sport-related-concussion-evaluation-management.

Canadian Paediatric Society (CPS). (2016a). *An update to the Greig Health Record: Preventive health care visits for children and adolescents aged 6 to 17 years.* Retrieved from https://www.cps.ca/en/documents/position/greig-health-record-technical-report#ref71.

Canadian Paediatric Society (CPS). (2016b). *Meeting the needs of adolescent parents and their children.* Retrieved from https://www.cps.ca/en/documents/position/adolescent-parents.

Canadian Paediatric Society (CPS). (2017a). *Guidelines for genetic testing in healthy children.* Retrieved from https://www.cps.ca/en/documents/position/guidelines-for-genetic-testing-of-healthy-children.

Canadian Paediatric Society (CPS). (2017b). *Screen time and young children: Promoting growth and development in a digital world.* Retrieved from https://www.cps.ca/en/documents/position/screen-time-and-young-children.

Canadian Paediatric Society (CPS). (2018a). *Harm reduction: An approach to reducing risky health behaviours in adolescents.* Retrieved from https://www.cps.ca/en/documents/position/harm-reduction-risky-health-behaviours.

Canadian Paediatric Society (CPS). (2018b). *Vegetarian diets in children and adolescents.* Retrieved from https://www.cps.ca/en/documents/position/vegetarian-diets.

Canadian Paediatric Society (CPS). (2018c). *Update on meningococcal vaccination for Canadian children and youth.* Retrieved from https://www.cps.ca/en/documents/position/invasive-meningococcal-vaccination.

Canadian Paediatric Society (CPS). (2018d). *Sexually transmitted infections in adolescents: Maximizing opportunities for optimal care.* Retrieved from https://www.cps.ca/en/documents/position/sexually-transmitted-infections.

Canadian Paediatric Society (CPS). (2018e). *Human papillomavirus vaccine for children and adolescents.* Retrieved from https://www.cps.ca/en/documents/position/HPV.

Canadian Paediatric Society (CPS). (2018f). Inhalant abuse. Retrieved from https://www.cps.ca/en/documents/position/inhalant-abuse.

Canadian Paediatric Society (CPS). (2019). *Universal no-cost access to contraception for youth in Canada.* Retrieved from https://www.cps.ca/en/documents/position/universal-access-to-no-cost-contraception-for-youth-in-canada.

Canadian Safety Council. (2019). *Sports and active living safety.* Retrieved from https://canadasafetycouncil.org/category/sports-active-living.

Canadian Society for Exercise Physiology (CSEP). (2019). *Canadian 24-hour movement guidelines for children and youth (ages 5–17).* Retrieved from https://csepguidelines.ca/children-and-youth-5-17.

Copstead, L., & Banasik, J. (2013). *Pathophysiology* (5th ed.). St. Louis: Saunders.

Department of Justice. (2017). *Age of consent to sexual activity.* Retrieved from https://www.justice.gc.ca/eng/rp-pr/other-autre/clp/faq.html.

Diabetes Canada. (2018). *Type 2 diabetes and Indigenous peoples.* Retrieved from https://guidelines.diabetes.ca/cpg/chapter38.

Drug Free Kids Canada. (2019). *Alcohol and youth.* Retrieved from https://www.drugfreekidscanada.org/prevention/drug-info/alcohol/.

Duval Smith, F. (2016). Caring for surgical patients with piercings. *Association of Perioperative Nurses Journal, 103*(6), 584–593. https://doi.org/10.1016/j.aorn.2016.04.005.

Egale Canada Human Rights Trust. (2019). Egale youth services. Retrieved from https://egale.ca/youthservices/.

Erikson, E. (1968). *Identity: Youth and crisis.* New York: Norton. [Seminal Reference].

Goodwill, A., & Ishiyama, F. I. (2015). Finding the door: Critical incidents facilitating gang exit among Indigenous men. *Journal of Cultural Diversity and Ethnic Minority Psychology, 21*(4), 1–8.

Government of Canada. (2013). *Clinical guidelines for nurses in primary care: Pediatric and adolescent health.* Retrieved from https://www.canada.ca/en/indigenous-services-canada/services/first-nations-inuit-health/health-care-services/nursing/clinical-practice-guidelines-nurses-primary-care/pediatric-adolescent-care/chapter-19-adolescent-health.html#a33.

Grekul, J., & LaBoucane-Benson, P. (2008). Aboriginal gangs and their (dis)placement: Contextualizing recruitment, membership, and status. *Canadian Journal of Criminology and Criminal Justice, 50*(1), 59–82. https://doi.org/10.3138/cjccj.50.1.59.

Guyton, A. C., & Hall, J. E. (2011). *Textbook of medical physiology* (12th ed.). Philadelphia: W. B. Saunders.

Harvey, J., Chadi, N., & Canadian Paediatric Society (2016). *The Canadian Pediatric Society (CPS) preventing smoking in children and adolescents: Recommendations for practice and policy.* Retrieved from https://www.cps.ca/en/documents/position/preventing-smoking.

Health Canada. (2016). *Summary of results: Canadian student tobacco, alcohol and drug use survey.* Retrieved from https://www.canada.ca/en/health-canada/services/canadian-student-tobacco-alcohol-drugs-survey/2014-2015-summary.html.

Health Canada. (2018). *Concussion: Sports and recreation.* Retrieved from https://www.canada.ca/en/public-health/services/diseases/concussion-sign-symptoms/sport-recreation.html.

Health Canada. (2019a). *Canada food guide.* Retrieved from https://food-guide.canada.ca/en/.

Health Canada. (2019b). *About vaping.* Retrieved from https://www.canada.ca/en/health-canada/services/smoking-tobacco/vaping.html.

Hobin, E., So, J., Rosella, L., et al. (2014). Trajectories of objectively measured physical activity among secondary students in the context of a province-wide physical education policy: A longitudinal analysis. *Journal of Obesity, 2014,* 958645. https://doi.org/10.1155/2014/958645.

Justice for Youth and Children. (2013). *Leaving home rights.* Retrieved from https://jfcy.org/en/rights/leaving-home-rights/.

Kohlberg, L. (1981). *The philosophy of moral development.* San Francisco, CA: Harper & Row.

Kreipe, R. (2016). Eating disorders. In R. M. Kliegman, B. M. D. Stanton, J. S. Geme, et al. (Eds.), *Nelson textbook of pediatrics* (20th ed., Chapter 28.). St. Louis: Elsevier.

Landstedt, E., Hammarström, A., & Winefield, H. (2015). How well do parental and peer relationships in adolescence predict health in adulthood? *Scandinavian Journal of Public Health,* 1–9. https://doi.org/10.1177/1403494815576360.

Mental Health Commission of Canada. (2018). *Annual report: Building for the future.* Retrieved from https://www.mentalhealthcommission.ca/English/who-we-are/annual-report.

Mental Health Commission of Canada. (2019). *First Nations, Inuit, and Metis.* Retrieved from https://www.mentalhealthcommission.ca/English/what-we-do/first-nations-inuit-and-metis.

Merck Manual. (2019). *Delayed puberty.* Retrieved from https://www.merckmanuals.com/en-ca/professional/pediatrics/endocrine-disorders-in-children/delayed-puberty.

Moilanen, K., & Manuel, M. (2019). Helicopter parenting and adjustment outcomes in young adulthood: A consideration of the mediating roles of mastery and self-regulation. *Journal of Child and Family Studies,* 1–14. https://doi.org/10.1007/s10826-019-01433-5.

MyHealth Alberta. (2019). *Hookah and waterpipe smoking.* Retrieved from https://myhealth.alberta.ca/Alberta/Pages/Hookah-and-waterpipe-smoking.aspx.

National Eating Disorder Information Centre (NEDIC). (2014). *Eating disorders: Know the facts.* Retrieved from http://nedic.ca/know-facts/overview.

National Initiative for Eating Disorders (NIED). (2018). *About eating disorders in Canada.* Retrieved from https://nied.ca/about-eating-disorders-in-canada.

O'Connor, D. L., Blake, J., Bell, R., Bowen, J., Callum, K., Fenton, S., et al. (2018). Canadian consensus on female nutrition: Adolescence, reproduction, menopause, and beyond. *Journal of Obstetrics and Gynaecology Canada, 48*(6), 508–554. https://doi.org/10.1016/j.jogc.2016.01.001.

Piaget, J. (1969). *The theory of stages in cognitive development.* New York: McGraw-Hill. [Seminal Reference].

Public Health Agency of Canada (PHAC). (2010). *Stages of childhood: Adolescence.* Retrieved from https://www.canada.ca/en/public-health/services/health-promotion/childhood-adolescence/stages-childhood.html.

Public Health Agency of Canada (PHAC). (2016). *Health behaviour in school-aged children.* Retrieved from https://www.canada.ca/en/public-health/services/health-promotion/childhood-adolescence/programs-initiatives/school-health/health-behaviour-school-aged-children.html.

Public Health Agency of Canada (PHAC). (2018). *A framework for action on STBBIs.* Retrieved from https://www.canada.ca/en/public-health/services/reports-publications/canada-communicable-disease-report-ccdr/monthly-issue/2018-44/issue-7-8-july-5-2018/article-5-framework-action-sexually-transmitted-blood-borne-infections.html.

Public Health Agency of Canada (PHAC). (2019a). *Building a youth policy for Canada.* Retrieved from https://www.canada.ca/en/youth/programs/policy.html.

Public Health Agency of Canada (PHAC). (2019b). *Canadian guidelines on sexually transmitted infections.* Retrieved from https://www.canada.ca/en/public-health/services/infectious-diseases/sexual-health-sexually-transmitted-infections/canadian-guidelines/sexually-transmitted-infections.html.

Public Safety Canada. (2014). *Youth gangs in Canada: A review of current topics and issues.* Retrieved from https://www.publicsafety.gc.ca/cnt/rsrcs/pblctns/2017-r001/index-en.aspx.

Public Safety Canada. (2018). *Bullying prevention: Nature and extent of bullying in Canada.* Retrieved from https://www.publicsafety.gc.ca/cnt/rsrcs/pblctns/bllng-prvntn/index-en.aspx#a05.

Registered Nurses Association of Ontario (RNAO). (2007). *Position statement: Respecting sexual orientation and gender identify.* Retrieved from https://rnao.ca/policy/position-statements/sexual-orientation-gender-identity.

Roggenkamp, H., Nicholls, A., & Pierre, J. M. (2017). Tattoos as a window to the psyche: How talking about skin art can inform psychiatric practice. *World Journal of Psychiatry, 7*(3), 148–158. https://doi.org/10.5498/wjp.v7.i3.148.

Royal Canadian Mounted Police (RCMP). (2018). *Just the facts: Gangs.* Retrieved from http://www.rcmp-grc.gc.ca/en/gazette/gangs.

Royal Canadian Mounted Police (RCMP). (2019). *Bullying and cyberbullying.* Retrieved from http://www.rcmp-grc.gc.ca/cycp-cpcj/bull-inti/index-eng.htm.

Scoliosis Research Society. (2019). *What is scoliosis?* Retrieved from https://www.srs.org/patients-and-families/conditions-and-treatments/adolescents.

Statistics Canada. (2014). *Self-reported sexual assault in Canada.* Retrieved from https://www150.statcan.gc.ca/n1/pub/85-002-x/2017001/article/14842-eng.htm.

Statistics Canada. (2016a). *The health of girls and women in Canada.* Retrieved from https://www150.statcan.gc.ca/n1/pub/89-503-x/2015001/article/14324-eng.htm.

Statistics Canada. (2016b). *Victimization of Aboriginal people in Canada, 2014.* Retrieved from https://www150.statcan.gc.ca/n1/pub/85-002-x/2016001/article/14631-eng.htm.

Statistics Canada. (2018a). *Smoking: 2017.* Retrieved from https://www150.statcan.gc.ca/n1/pub/82-625-x/2018001/article/54974-eng.htm.

Statistics Canada. (2018b). *Ethnic diversity and immigration.* Retrieved from https://www150.statcan.gc.ca/n1/pub/11-402-x/2011000/chap/imm/imm-eng.htm.

Statistics Canada. (2019a). *Death and mortality rates by age group.* Retrieved from https://www150.statcan.gc.ca/t1/tbl1/en/tv.action?pid=1310071001.

Statistics Canada. (2019b). *Live births, by age of mother.* Retrieved from https://www150.statcan.gc.ca/t1/tbl1/en/tv.action?pid=1310041601.

Tremblay, M. S., Carson, V., Chaput, J. P., et al. (2016). Canadian 24-hour movement guidelines for children and youth: An integration of physical activity, sedentary behaviour, and sleep. *Applied Physiology Nutrition and Metabolism, 41*(6, Suppl. 3), S311–S327. https://doi.org/10.1139/apnm-2016-0151.

Tylka, T., & Wood-Barcalow, N. (2015). What is and what is not positive body image? Conceptual foundations and construct definition. *Body Image, 14*, 118–129. https://doi.org/10.1016/j.bodyim.2015.04.001.

University of Toronto. (2019). *Researching for LGBTQ2S+ health!* Toronto: Dalla Lana School of Public Health. Retrieved from http://lgbtqhealth.ca/.

# 16

# Young Adult

*Barbara Wilson-Keates, RN, MS, PhD*

Originating US chapter by *Elizabeth Connelly Kudzma, CNL, MPH, WHNP-BC, DNSc*

## INTENDED LEARNING OUTCOMES

*After completing this chapter, the reader will be able to:*

- Analyze specific health recommendations for the young adult.
- Identify attitudes, behaviours, and habits that compose the lifestyles of young adults.
- Define tasks that are consistent with adult development.
- Describe the nurse's role in reducing the rate of unintentional pregnancies in young adult women.
- Determine occupational hazards that interfere with the young adult's welfare.

- Evaluate strategies that the nurse can use to reduce the risks associated with young adult behaviours.
- Analyze occupational, cultural, and ethnic risk factors that may affect young adults.
- Delineate nursing roles in preventive intervention for healthy young adults in home and community environments.
- Discuss proposed suggestions for preconceptional care.

## KEY TERMS

Achievement-oriented stress
Aerobic exercise
Basal metabolic rate
Binge drinking
Cardiovascular disease
Congenital defects
Fetal neural tube defects (NTDs)
Hepatitis B

Hepatitis C
Human immunodeficiency virus (HIV)
Human papillomavirus (HPV)
Hypertension
Infertility
Intimacy versus isolation
Metabolic syndrome
Orchitis

Papanicolaou (Pap) smear
Postconventional level of moral reasoning
Sexual consent
sudden arrhythmia death syndromes (SADS)
Stress
Sun protection factor (SPF)
Testicular self-examination (TSE)

---

### ⁇ THINK ABOUT IT

#### Using Private Information in Shared Living Arrangements

Young adults in communal living arrangements (university or college dormitories, co-operative housing) are often placed with other individuals who have different cultural, language, or other values. The use of cell phones and computers with video and audio recording capabilities has opened the possibility that private behaviour may be recorded without consent and then may be shared through a form of social networking (Facebook, Twitter, instant messaging, apps, and other shared computer sites). There are even instances where recording has occurred in classrooms without the permission of the instructor or others in the class.

These situations are expected to become more prevalent.

- What are the implications of this for violation of privacy for individuals and even groups (e.g., students, fraternities, sororities)?
- What are the legal implications? (Provinces have laws against most cases of unauthorized recording.)
- How might unauthorized recording alter classroom, dormitory, and communal living dynamics?

The young adult period encompasses the ages from 18 to 34 years, a time that spans the end of adolescence to the beginning of middle adulthood (Statistics Canada, 2018a). Completion of formal education, commencing full-time employment, getting married, and parenthood are all major milestones that may occur in this phase of development (Zacarés, Serra, & Torres, 2015). The major task accomplished in this period is preparing for and assuming full adult responsibilities, rights, and privileges. This is a potentially difficult period as young adults are not totally independent and are learning to separate from the home and their parents (Zacarés et al., 2015).

## BIOLOGY

The young adult period is a time of many physical and emotional changes and is an opportunity for learning by experience and experimentation (Quality and Safety Scenario). Young adulthood is characterized by greater complexity of thinking, further organization of emotional and cognitive development, and decision making based on the impact on others and future consequences. All phases of young adult development garner considerable interest. Judging by the increase in the number of books on self-development, more young adults are exploring topics in holistic healing and spiritual health and development. Health behaviours, safety practices, diet, exercise, weight control, sexuality, and addictions are widely discussed topics. Preventive health concerns for young adults can be separated into two categories: developing behaviours that promote a healthy lifestyle and decreasing the incidence of accidents, injuries, and acts of violence. Among Canadians aged 25 to 34, more than half the deaths are attributed to accidents (36%), suicide (18%), and cancer (11%) (Statistics Canada, 2015a). Deaths from medication overdoses doubled in the 25 to 39 age group across Canada (Statistics Canada, 2017a).

## ⚡ QUALITY AND SAFETY SCENARIO

### Examining Problematic Drinking Behaviours in Young Adults

A study of 507 post-secondary students indicated that 67% of males and 71% of females engaged in binge drinking (five or more drinks in one session for males; four or more drinks in one session for females) at least once in the previous 30 days (Edkins, Edgerton, & Roberts, 2017).

You are the nurse at a community college student health centre. Arya, a 19-year-old first-year student, has generally been a good student, easily making the adjustment to living away from home during her first 2 months in the residence. She comes to you to talk about an episode that occurred the previous weekend and that frightened her. On Saturday night, she was at a party at a private residence in a rural, wooded setting away from the campus. She remembers consuming five or six alcoholic drinks; however, any memory after midnight is missing. She woke up in a fellow female student's residence room without any memory of leaving the party or returning to the residence. She was able to piece together information from her friends, who told her that she had consumed at least nine alcoholic drinks that night and that she had left the party with others who were returning to the residence, but they were not the friends with whom she had been seen all evening. She is concerned that she may have been drugged or that she may be having memory lapses. Assessment of her previous alcohol use reveals that she can recount at least four occasions during which she drank more than seven drinks at a party or family gathering. She describes her family as "social drinkers." On days that she anticipates drinking, she restricts her caloric intake. Last June, she was involved in a minor car accident that might have been related to her consumption of at least three drinks that afternoon. To further analyze Arya's situation, you formulate the following questions:

- Do you think that Arya has a problem with drinking? Would you classify her as a binge drinker? How do you clarify what she values?
- Is Arya engaging in risky behaviour, especially if she drives while drinking?
- What kind of physical assessment might assist you to make a determination that Arya has a drinking problem?
- What kinds of preventive educational programs could you advise?
- What kinds of monitoring and follow-up mechanisms might assist Arya in keeping her safe and in a treatment plan?

Source: Edkins, T., Edgerton, J. D., & Roberts, L. W. (2017). Correlates of binge drinking in a sample of Canadian university students. *International Journal of Child, Youth & Family Studies, 8*(1). https://doi.org/10.18357/ijcyfs81201716944.

In 2016, approximately 25% of the Canadian population were composed of adults aged 15 to 34 (Statistics Canada, 2018a). Among Canadian young adults, 14% do not live in a town or a large urban centre, 27% belong to a visible minority group, and 75% report having a friend from another ethnic group. The number of Indigenous people aged 15 to 24 increased 40% over the previous 10 years, compared with a 6.5% increase among non-Indigenous young adults over the same time period. Almost 100% of young adults use the Internet on a daily basis. Young adults in Canada will continue to be a large and important group within the Canadian population. They are very different from younger generations before them and from their parents and grandparents today as they are more diverse, educated, and socially connected than past young adults. However, not all young adults are sharing these benefits. Many are unemployed or employed in temporary jobs and may be struggling with mental health challenges, addictions, and homelessness. Health-promotion efforts are particularly important for young adults because health teaching for this age group has the significant potential to directly influence overall health outcomes for this current and subsequent generations

Young adulthood is generally the healthiest time of life. Physical growth is mostly complete by the age of 20 years; most concerns related to physiological development are focused on ensuring optimal functioning of body systems. The young adult's physical abilities are in peak condition, and compensatory mechanisms operate optimally during illness to provide minimal disruption in health patterns. Nursing goals for individuals of this age group are oriented toward prolonging this period of optimal physical energy; developing the mental, emotional, spiritual, and social potential; encouraging proper health habits; anticipating and screening individuals for the onset of chronic disease and therefore being able to treat it at an early stage; and treating disease when appropriate.

Full adult stature in men is reached at approximately age 21 years; in women, full growth occurs earlier, typically by age 17 years. Optimal muscle strength occurs from age 25 years to age 30 years, and then gradually declines by approximately 10% from age 30 years to age 60 years. Manual dexterity peaks in young adulthood and begins to decline in the mid-30s.

Women have greater longevity than men. In 2018, the life expectancy for the total Canadian population was 79.8 years for men and 83.9 years for women (Statistics Canada, 2018b). Among Indigenous people, the Inuit have the lowest projected life expectancy of 64 years for men and 73 years for women. The Métis and First Nations populations have similar life expectancies, at 73–74 years for men and 78–80 years for women (Statistics Canada, 2017b). Reasons for a lower life expectancy among Indigenous people include lack of access to health care services, higher rates of chronic diseases such as heart disease and diabetes, poorer living conditions, and higher rates of suicide and medication overdoses (Truth and Reconciliation Commission [TRC], 2015).

# ❖ GORDON'S FUNCTIONAL HEALTH PATTERNS

## ◆ Health Perception–Health Management Pattern

Because excellent physical health is frequently taken for granted, concern about health and well-being is relatively low among individuals in their 20s, but begins to increase in individuals in their 30s. Monitoring of specific health parameters is both necessary and appropriate to determine health needs and incipient problems. After the mid-30s, an increased sense of the finiteness of life develops. with limitations imposed by work choices, well-being, monetary resources, and the deterioration of physical abilities. Specific health care management in the young adult age span is generally split into health care management for various age groups according to the preventive services that are required.

In 2017, the Canadian Task Force on Preventive Health Care recommended that annual checkups be replaced with focused age-appropriate health prevention activities and screening that emphasized the early identification and possible treatment of health conditions. The decision was based on evidence that patients who have annual checkups do not achieve better health outcomes than those who do not. The Task Force also expressed concern that annual nonspecific examinations may lead to overdiagnosis and conditions of uncertain clinical importance, which can lead to anxiety and unnecessary medical intervention (Canadian Task Force on Preventive Health Care, 2017).

### Behavioural Health History

A health history inclusive of behaviour is particularly important for young adults. This type of history focuses on risk factors for unintentional injuries, such as accidents, seat-belt use, and alcohol and drug consumption, which are major causes of death and disability in this age group. Adults aged 20 to 39 years were the most likely to die from overdoses because they had the highest medication overdose mortality rate among all age groups (Statistics Canada, 2017a). Because more men than women consume illicit drugs, a higher percentage of men than women die from overdose deaths. Suicide and self-inflicted injuries are the leading cause of death for Indigenous people up to 44 years of age. The safety focus of nursing health promotion for the younger adult takes different forms, from the simple—monitoring helmet and seat-belt use—to more complex concerns—threats such as climate change, protecting the environment, and increasing globalization. Fig. 16.1 lists questions and content that may be appropriately included in a health history for young adults, focusing on probable age-specific behaviours.

Young adults are comfortable with the use of technology to answer their health questions and tend to not believe in the infallibility of health care providers and the current health care system. Up to 93% do not schedule preventive health care provider visits, and about half of these individuals visit a primary care health care provider less than once a year. They are much more likely to use social media to pose questions about their health and receive answers from a large audience in real time. They are more apt to join social support groups for 24-hour support from others who are experiencing the same health issues and are more likely to search for information about alternative medicine, supplements, and organic food (Arnold, 2018).

### Preventive Care

The basic goals of preventive care are to maximize the period of optimal health status and detect incipient health problems. The Preventive Care Checklist (Table 16.1) is an evidence-informed tool to screen average-risk adults at the periodic health examination. The periodic health examination consists of a summary of history taking, physical examination, counselling, immunizations, and appropriate investigations relevant to preventive health care. However, it is important to remember that increased screening does not translate to improved health outcomes. Clinical judgement is required along with the preventive care form to manage symptomatic patients or patients with established diseases or health conditions. Subsequent counselling sessions focus on rechecking and updating information gathered in earlier meetings. (Ridley, Ischayek, Dubey, et al., 2016).

A physical examination includes measurements of height, weight, body mass index (BMI), and blood pressure (BP), with an emphasis on the need to avoid inactivity and obesity, which are risk factors for many health problems. The Canadian Task Force on Preventive Health Care (2018) currently recommends against teaching breast self-examination, and concludes that the current evidence is insufficient to assess the additional benefits and harm of clinical breast examination beyond screening mammography for women aged 50 to 74 years. Screening for cervical cancer is strongly recommended in women who have been sexually active (Papanicolaou [Pap] smear). The Canadian Cancer Society (2019) recommends that by age 15 all men should know how their testicles normally look and feel and that men should talk to their primary care provider if they notice any changes in their testicles. Testicular self-examination (TSE) may detect testicular cancer at an early stage and it may be taught to adult men. However, there is scant evidence to evaluate the accuracy, benefits, or effectiveness of this activity because early testicular cancers often present as benign inflammations (epididymitis or testicular trauma).

The typical young adult health examination also looks for signs of chronic disease. One in 25 Canadian adults aged 20 and older reported having a mood and anxiety disorder and at least one of the four major chronic diseases: cardiovascular disease (CVD), hypertension, diabetes, chronic obstructive pulmonary disease (COPD), and cancer (Health Canada, 2017a). Among Canadian adults, mental illness is the leading case of workplace disability. Approximately 4 in 5 Canadian adults have at least one modifiable risk factor for chronic disease such as self-reported tobacco smoking, physical inactivity, unhealthy eating, and harmful use of alcohol. Overall, Canada ranks among the worst of OECD (Organization of Economic Co-operation and Development) countries for adult obesity rates. Indigenous people experience

**Well Young Adult Behavioural Health History Content**

**Sociodemographic content and questions:**

What organizations (community, religious, lodge, social, professional, etc.) are you involved in? _____

How would you describe your community?_____

Hobbies, skills, interests, and recreational activities? _____

Military service? No_____ Yes_____ From ____ to_____

Overseas assignment? No_____ Yes_____

Close friends or immediate family members who have died within the past two years? _____

Names and addresses of relatives or close friends in the area. _____

Marital status:  S  M  D  W    Length of time _____

**Environmental content and questions:**

Do you live alone? No_____ Yes_____

When did you last move? _____

Describe your living situation. _____

Number of years of education completed: _____

Elementary?_____ High school?_____ Post-secondary?_____

Occupation?_____ Employer?_____

How long have you worked for this employer? _____

Are you satisfied with your work situation? No_____ Yes_____

Do you consider your work risky or dangerous? No_____ Yes_____

Is your work stressful? No_____ Yes_____

Over the past two weeks, have you felt depressed or hopeless? No_____ Yes_____

**Biophysical content questions:**

Have you smoked cigarettes? No_____ Yes_____

How much? Less than ½ pack per day? About one pack per day? More than 1 ½ packs per day?

Are you smoking now? No_____ Yes_____ Length of time smoking?_____

Have you ever smoked cigars or a pipe? No_____ Yes_____

If yes, how long?_____ Do you smoke cigars or a pipe now? No_____ Yes_____

Do you drink alcohol (wine, beer, or whiskey)? No_____ Yes_____

If you do, how much each day on the average?_____ Each week?_____

Do you consume large amounts occasionally (binge drinking)? No_____ Yes_____

Have you been drunk on work days? No_____ Yes_____

Have you had alcoholic drinks in the morning sometime in the past year? No_____ Yes_____

How much coffee, tea, or cola do you drink? _____

Do you use seat or lap belts? No_____ Yes_____

What type of exercise do you do each week? Describe type and amount. _____

Are you satisfied with your weight? No_____ Yes_____ Body image? No_____ Yes_____

Do you use a bicycle or motorcycle helmet? No_____ Yes_____ Helmet and pads while rollerblading? No_____ Yes_____

How much sleep do you usually get each night? _____

Meals: Do you generally eat: three regular meals per day? two meals per day? irregular meals?

Are you sexually active? No_____ Yes_____

If so, are you aware of the risks of sexually transmitted infections? No_____ Yes_____

**Fig. 16.1** Common well young adult behavioural health history content. (From Somers, A. R., & Breslow, L. [1979]. Lifetime health monitoring program. *Nurse Practitioner, 4*[40], 50–54; US Preventive Services Task Force. [2015]. *Published recommendations.* Rockville, MD: Agency for Healthcare Research and Quality.)

## TABLE 16.1    Preventive Care Checklist for Adults

| | AGE 18 TO 34 YEARS | |
| Health Issue | Intervention | Frequency |
| --- | --- | --- |
| **Lifestyle and Habits** | | |
| Family planning | Counsel about age-related infertility, and that assisted reproductive technology cannot assist with age-related decline | Each visit |
| Poverty | No validated screening question but recognize that poverty is a social determinant of health | |
| **Functional Inquiry** | | |
| Depression | Do not routinely screen for depression if no past history or asymptomatic | Each visit |
| **Education/Counselling** | | |
| Obesity/nutrition/body mass index (BMI) | 1. Record height, weight, and BMI<br>2. BMI ≥25 kg/m$^2$ but <40 kg/m$^2$: offer structured behavioural interventions aimed at weight loss<br>3. BMI of 30 to 39 kg/m$^2$ or high risk of diabetes: offer structured behavioural interventions aimed at weight loss | Each visit |
| **Physical Examination** | | |
| Blood pressure (BP) | 1. Measure BP at all appropriate visits<br>2. Target BP 140/90 mm Hg; 130/80 mm Hg in those with diabetes | Each visit |
| Cervical cancer in women | Screen with Papanicolaou (Pap) tests if ever sexually active | Every 3 years |
| Breast cancer in women | 1. Do not routinely screen<br>2. Do not screen with breast mammography or magnetic resonance imaging (MRI)<br>3. Do not perform clinical breast examination or self-examination on a regular basis | |
| **Laboratory Tests and Investigations** | | |
| Type 2 diabetes | 1. Screen every 1 to 5 years, depending on risk determined using a calculator or other risk factors<br>2. HbA$_{1c}$ level is the preferred screening test (FPG level or OGTT are acceptable alternatives)<br>3. HbA$_{1c}$ level of ≥6.5%, FPG level ≥7 mmol/L, or 2-hour plasma glucose level in an OGTT of ≥11.1 mmol/L are diagnostic | Individually determined |
| Dyslipidemia | 1. Screening fasting lipid profile if at increased risk<br>2. Screen with Framingham risk score every 3–5 years if 10-year risk is <5%, or every year if 10-year risk is ≥5%<br>3. Framingham risk score should be doubled if positive family history for premature cardiovascular disease<br>4. Discuss "cardiovascular age" | Individually determined |
| Sexually transmitted infections (STIs) | Screen for STIs if risk factors are present<br>Screen for HIV if risk factors are present, patient was ever sexually active, or patient wants test | Individually determined |
| **Immunizations** | | |
| Human papillomavirus (HVD) vaccination | 1. Women up to and including 26 years—bivalent (HPV2) or quadrivalent (HPV4) or nonvalent (HPV9) vaccine<br>2. Men up to and including 26 years of age— HPV4 or HPV9 vaccine<br>3. Recommended for men who have sex with men | Individually determined |
| Diphtheria, Tetanus | Primary series for previously unimmunized adults<br>Booster dose every 10 years | |
| Influenza | Annually | |
| Meningococcal conjugate | Adults up to and including 24 years of age not immunized in adolescence—one dose | |

## TABLE 16.1   Preventive Care Checklist for Adults—cont'd

### AGE 18 TO 34 YEARS

| Health Issue | Intervention | Frequency |
|---|---|---|
| Pertussis | 1. One dose of acellular pertussis-containing vaccine in adulthood<br>2. Adults who will be in close contact with young infants should be immunized as early as possible<br>3. One dose of Tdap vaccine should be administered in every pregnancy, ideally between 27 and 32 weeks of gestation. | |
| Measles, Mumps | Susceptible adults born in or after 1970—one dose | |
| Polio | Primary series for previously unimmunized adults when a primary series of tetanus toxoid- and diphtheria toxoid-containing vaccine is being given or with routine tetanus toxoid- and diphtheria toxoid-containing vaccine booster doses | |
| Rubella | 1. Susceptible adults—one dose<br>2. If vaccine is indicated, pregnant women should be immunized after delivery | |
| Varicella (chickenpox) | Susceptible adults up to and including 49 years of age—two doses; if only one dose was previously received, a second dose should be provided | |

*BMI,* Body mass index; *BP,* blood pressure; *FPG,* fasting plasma glucose; *HbA$_{1c}$,* glycated hemoglobin; *HIV,* human immunodeficiency virus; *OGTT,* oral glucose tolerance test; *Tdap,* tetanus, diphtheria, acellular pertussis.
Modified from, Ridley J., Ischayek, A., Dubey, V., et al. (2016). Adult health checkup: Update on the Preventive Care Checklist Form®. *Canadian Family Physician 62*(4), 307–313; Health Canada. (2018). *Canadian immunization guide: Immunization of adults.* Retrieved from https://www.canada.ca/en/public-health/services/publications/healthy-living/canadian-immunization-guide-part-3-vaccination-specific-populations/page-2-immunization-of-adults.html#p3c1t1.

higher rates of chronic diseases when compared with the non-Indigenous population, largely due to the range of social, geographical, and physical factors embodied in the social determinants of health. Chronic diseases are currently the major cause of morbidity, mortality, and disability among Indigenous people (Government of Canada, 2017). In addition, recent non-European and low-income immigrants and refugees also reported higher rates of chronic diseases, particularly hypertension and diabetes (Creatore, Moineddin, Booth, et al., 2010). For all ethnic groups, cardiovascular risk-factor profiles (i.e., the percentage of people with two or more major cardiovascular risk factors, such as smoking, obesity, diabetes, and hypertension) were worse among those with longer duration of residency in Canada, particularly among Chinese and Black immigrants (Chiu, Austin, Manuel, et al., 2012). The prevalence of cardiovascular disease did not differ significantly between recent immigrants and long-term residents, irrespective of ethnic group.

The outcome was least favourable for younger women and men aged 20 to 39 with ischemic heart disease (IHD), who were about 18 and 11 times more likely to die of any cause, respectively, than individuals of the same age without IHD (Health Canada, 2018a).

The Canadian Cardiovascular Society (Anderson, Grégoire, Pearson, et al., 2016) recommends that screening for CVD and identification and management of risk factors should begin for men and women after the age of 40. However, there are age exceptions to this overall standard. Providers may consider screening earlier in ethnic groups that have an increased risk, such as South Asian or Indigenous people. Among individuals aged 30 to 39 without diabetes, the presence of a positive parental history of premature CVD (onset younger than 55 years of age in first-degree male relatives and younger than 65 years of age in female relatives) increases an individual's Framingham risk score twofold.

Adoption of and engagement in low-risk lifestyle behaviours remain the cornerstone of prevention of CVD and are recommended for all age groups. As well as the management of traditional risk factors (hypertension, dyslipidemia, diabetes, and smoking), abdominal obesity, physical inactivity, and alcohol consumption are all modifiable risk factors in preventing CVD. Promotion of health behaviours, including smoking cessation, regular physical activity, a healthy diet, achieving a healthy weight, moderate alcohol consumption, and moderate sleep duration, are promoted to attain maximal CVD risk reduction. Smoking cessation is considered the most important health behaviour for CVD prevention. Achievement of smoking cessation along with pharmacotherapy is associated with long-term abstinence.

The primary goal of nutrition therapy is an emphasis on the reduction of cholesterol, replacement of saturated fats with polyunsaturated fats, and avoidance of trans fats. Adherence to a specific food plan, such as the Mediterranean diet, the Dietary Approaches to Stop Hypertension (DASH) diet, or a low glycemic index diet, have all been shown to help reduce the risk of CVD. The Mediterranean diet is high in monounsaturated fats, mainly from olive oil, high in complex carbohydrates from legumes and grains, high in fibre, and high in fish. This diet limits foods with refined carbohydrates, processed or fast food, red meat, and animal fat. Individuals are encouraged to select a dietary pattern that best fits with their values and preferences. Addition of omega-3 polyunsaturated fatty acid supplement is not recommended because it does not reduce the risk of CVD events.

Along with adoption of a healthy dietary intake, individuals are encouraged to consume a moderate caloric intake in order to achieve and maintain a healthy body weight. Individuals are further encouraged to accumulate 150 minutes of moderate-to-vigorous aerobic physical activity per week, in bouts of 10 minutes or more.

Young adults are at risk of sudden arrhythmia death syndromes (SADS) that refer to a variety of cardiac arrhythmia disorders which are often genetic and can cause sudden death in young, apparently healthy people. In Canada, 1 in 2500 babies are born with long QT syndrome and at least 600 Canadians under the age of 35 years die annually from SADS (Canadian Sudden Arrhythmia Death Syndrome Foundation [CSADSF], 2019). Up to 50% of affected individuals report warning signs, which include fainting (syncope) or seizure during physical activity, fainting (syncope) or seizure resulting from emotional excitement, emotional distress, and a family history of unexpected sudden death during physical activity or during a seizure, or any other unexplained sudden death of an otherwise healthy young person. Ready access to an automated external defibrillator (AED) in sports arenas, gymnasiums, and other community gathering places can prevent sudden death.

Nurses can assist in gathering a comprehensive health history, including pertinent information about hypertension, cardiovascular disease, and SADS in parents and relatives. Cardiovascular assessment of the young adult includes determination of the presence of hyperlipidemia, hypertension, obesity, diabetes, chest pain, heart disease, or unexpected syncope. Nurses can also promote healthy lifestyle behaviours to further reduce the risk of CVD and advocate for the presence of accessible AED in public places with responsible personnel who are trained in cardiopulmonary respiration (CPR).

In women, a history of pregnancy-induced hypertension or pre-eclampsia is important and a risk factor for CVD (Research for Evidence-Informed Practice).

Hypertension results from increases in cardiac output or increases in peripheral resistance, or a combination of both, and is one of the most common chronic diseases affecting almost 160,000 Canadians aged 18 to 34 (Statistics Canada, 2019a). It has broad health implications through its association with obesity, chronic kidney disease, CVD, and death. In Canada, hypertension is 80% attributed to dietary factors and 20% related to physical inactivity. Tobacco use, genetics, and stress may also play a role. According to *2018 Hypertension Canada Guidelines*, the emphasis of BP assessment is screening for hypertension to reduce cardiovascular risk, to monitor antihypertensive treatment, and to engage the patient in risk-reduction strategies. Ambulatory or home measurement is preferred over BP measurement in-office to reduce the influence of "white coat" or masked hypertension. Regardless of the setting, measurement using an electronic (oscillometric) device is preferred over auscultatory methods. Validated wrist devices with arm and wrist support at heart level may be used to measure BP in young adults with obesity or large arm circumferences.

In adults without diabetes, hypertension is considered with BP ≥135/85 mm Hg for an automated measurement in

## RESEARCH FOR EVIDENCE-INFORMED PRACTICE

### Effectiveness-Informed Guidelines for the Prevention of Cardiovascular Disease in Women—Update

During the last decade, the Canadian Heart and Stroke Foundation (CHSF) has developed and promoted a public campaign, *Time to See Red*, in an to attempt to differentiate how cardiovascular disease (CVD) preventive strategies should be altered for women (CHSF, 2019). The myth that CVD is a "man's" disease has been abolished. Heart attack and stroke is the number one cause of premature death in Canadian women and 53% of Canadian women have cardiac symptoms that go unrecognized. Frequently, women do not experience the classic "chest pressure or pain" symptoms and may experience a heart attack without chest pressure. Women may report shortness of breath, pressure or pain in the lower chest or upper abdomen, dizziness, lightheadedness or fainting, upper back pressure, or extreme fatigue. Moreover, two-thirds of all clinical research funding for CVD disease focuses on men. This is also a global problem. Heart disease is the leading cause of death in women worldwide.

An important newer recommendation of these guidelines is that pregnancy history provides the health care provider, with a criterion to predict future CVD risk. Women with a history of hypertensive disorders of pregnancy (HDP), such as pregnancy-induced hypertension or pre-eclampsia, have a significantly higher risk of CVD. The panel reviewed a large meta-analysis of women with a history of HDP and discovered that the women have approximately twice the risk of developing heart disease, stroke, and thrombolytic events in the decades after pregnancy. Pregnancy may induce a temporary state that is similar to early metabolic syndrome and, as such, could be considered a failed stress test for the development of CVD in the future. Therefore it is highly recommended that the delivering health care personnel refer pre-eclamptic women after delivery to the primary health care provider or cardiologist so that risk factors for CVD can be observed and adjusted to be more in accord with the "ideal cardiovascular health" pattern. Health care providers who are seeing females during a first visit should carefully review previous pregnancy complications, including pre-eclampsia and gestational diabetes, preterm birth, and birth of an infant small for its gestational age. Therefore women diagnosed with HDP should be approached with screening of a lipid panel, with a discussion of possible medication therapy. In addition, other health disorders, such as depression and autoimmune diseases (systemic lupus erythematosus and rheumatoid arthritis), may also elevate the risk of CVD.

Sources: Guidelines from Nerenberg, K., Daskalopoulou, S. S., & Dasguta, K. (2014). Gestational diabetes and hypertensive disorders of pregnancy as vascular risk signals: An overview and grading of the evidence. *Canadian Journal of Cardiology, 30*(7), 765–773. Anderson, T. J., Grégoire, J., Pearson, G. J., et al. (2016). 2016 Canadian Cardiovascular Society Guidelines for the management of dyslipidemia for the prevention of cardiovascular disease in the adult. *Canadian Journal of Cardiology, 32*(11), 1263–1282. Retrieved from https://www.onlinecjc.ca/article/S0828-282X(16)30732-2/pdf.

an ambulatory, home or office setting or ≥140/90 mm Hg in a non-automated office setting. In adults with diabetes, hypertension is diagnosed when BP is ≥130/80 mm Hg with either non-automated or automated measurement in any setting. Treatment consists of modifying health behaviour (e.g., smoking cessation, weight loss, becoming more physically active) and/or pharmacological treatment with a target BP of ≤135/85 mm Hg for adults without diabetes and ≤130/80 mm Hg for young adults with diabetes. Young adults with hypertension are encouraged to reduce dietary sodium intake to 2000 mg per day (5 g of salt or 87 mmol of sodium). Furthermore, when stress may be contributing to hypertension, cognitive behavioural interventions are more likely to be effective if relaxation techniques are used as well (Hypertension Canada, 2018).

There are also noticeable disparities in the development of hypertension in various population subgroups. Hypertension rates are lower in Indigenous populations compared with the non-Indigenous population, possibly due to the Indigenous population being younger overall. The First Nations Information Governance Centre (FNIGC, 2019) is a federally mandated entity that uses First Nations principles to create Indigenous models of research. Future community projects are planned based on research and survey data.

Canadians who self-report as Black, South Asian, socioeconomically disadvantaged, and those who live in Atlantic Canada have a higher prevalence of hypertension. These results indicate a higher incidence of hypertensive risk factors (e.g., unhealthy diets, obesity, sedentary lifestyles). Other disadvantaged groups, such as homeless individuals, are less aware of the hypertensive status and have worse BP control. South Asian Canadians and Chinese Canadian populations have been found to have poorer antihypertensive medication adherence than the general Canadian population (Liu, Quan, Chen, et al., 2014). Initiatives led by federal and provincial health authorities and charitable organizations address hypertension and reduction of cardiovascular risk factors for disadvantaged populations with some success, particularly South Asian populations. However, best evidence-informed practices must be shared, programs need to have assurances of long-term funding, and adequate surveillance data are required to truly assess and reduce hypertension for disadvantaged Canadians.

Metabolic syndrome (MetS) is a health disorder that, left untreated, greatly increases the risk of many chronic illnesses, including diabetes and CVD (Metabolic Syndrome Canada, 2019). This syndrome includes the lethal risks of high lipid levels, insulin resistance, hypertension, and abdominal obesity. MetS is diagnosed when a patient has three of the following conditions:

- High BP (≥130/85 mm Hg, or receiving medication)
- High blood glucose levels (≥5.6 mmol/L, or receiving medication)
- High triglycerides (≥ 1.7mmol/L, or receiving medication)
- Low high-density lipoprotein (HDL)-cholesterol (<1.0 mmol/L in men, or <1.3 mmol/L in women)
- Large waist circumference (≥102 cm in men, 88 cm in women)

Currently, 17% of Canadian adults aged 18 to 39 have this combination of metabolic risk factors and the prevalence increases with age. Support is growing for the CHANGE Program, a unique evidence-informed lifestyle intervention that uses a team approach of family doctors, nurses, dietitians, and kinesiologists. Participants are encouraged to adhere to the Mediterranean diet, engage in physical activity, and other lifestyle interventions over a 1-year period. From the pilot project, most participants reduced their 10-year risk from CVD and 25% of participants demonstrated reversal of MetS at 12 months.

In 2018, 2.3 million (7.3%) Canadians over the age of 12 have been diagnosed with diabetes and 75,000 Canadians aged 18 to 39 self-reported as having type 1 or type 2 diabetes. Approximately one in four Canadians are living with type 2 diabetes, either diagnosed or undiagnosed, or its precursor, referred to as prediabetes. This number is expected to rise to one in three by 2020 (Rosella, Lebenbaum, Fitzpatrick, et al., 2015). The excess costs due to diabetes are large, resulting in a substantial burden on the health care system as a result of serious microvascular and macrovascular complications (e.g., blindness, cardiovascular disease, myocardial infarction, renal disease, depression, oral disease, nerve damage, and stroke). The financial burden of diabetes is expected to continue, to reach $3.8 billion by 2020.

Diabetes is usually not the primary cause of death, but many of its complications are associated with premature death (Public Health Agency of Canada [PHAC], 2014). It is estimated that 12% of all deaths in Canada are attributable to diabetes and that people with diabetes are more likely to die prematurely than people without diabetes in every age group. In younger Canadians (aged 20 to 39), all-cause mortality rates were 4.2 to 5.8 times higher among individuals with diabetes. Diabetes lowers life expectancy by 5 to 11 years for adults.

Indigenous peoples living in Canada are among the highest-risk populations for diabetes and related complications. Screening for diabetes should be carried out earlier and at more frequent intervals (Canadian Diabetes Association [CDA], 2018). Particular attention is needed for Indigenous women and girls of child-bearing age as the high incidence of hyperglycemia in pregnancy, both gestational and type 2 diabetes, and maternal obesity increase the risk of childhood obesity and diabetes in the next generation. Prenatal screening for gestational diabetes as well as postpartum screening for women with a history of gestational diabetes are recommended along with appropriate follow-up. Effective preventive strategies that are grounded in Indigenous-specific social, culture, and health services contexts of each community are necessary. It is vital that health care providers acknowledge the legacy of colonization and its ongoing adverse influences on Indigenous health, including maintenance of socioeconomic disadvantages that limit healthy choices (healthy diets, physical activity opportunities), stir experience of shame and stigma with a diagnosis of diabetes, and recall residential school-like conditions with expectations that Indigenous peoples with diabetes will acquire diabetes knowledge and produce "test" results.

### Decision Making and Risk Taking

The decision making of a young adult directly affects health and well-being. Peak physical skills stimulate young adults to be venturesome, daring, enterprising, and aggressive. Young adults have less experience with the death of significant people in their lives, and they may take inordinate risks. The leading causes of death in individuals aged 18 to 34 are unintentional injuries, such as accidents, seat-belt use, alcohol and drug consumption, and possibly overdose (Statistics Canada, 2017a). Suicide and self-inflicted injuries are the leading cause of death for Indigenous people up to 44 years of age. The prevalence of adverse behaviours associated with sudden death illustrates a developmental lack of fear in young adults. Underuse of seat belts and helmets by motorcyclists and bicyclists is a cause of many accidental injuries and deaths. In 2017, 25.3% of Canadian cyclists aged 18 to 24 reported they always used a helmet, while this number increased to 44% for Canadians aged 25 to 49 (Statistics Canada, 2017c). Cyclists who "always" wore a helmet were more likely than other cyclists to always use a seat belt when driving or as a passenger (90% vs. 76%) and to have had a flu shot in the past year (33% vs. 20%), as well as being less likely than non-users to smoke (10% vs. 21%) or to engage in heavy episodic drinking (17% vs. 27%). Helmet users were also more likely to adopt other safety practices, such as having a household smoke detector and a fire escape plan, and to receive the seasonal influenza vaccine.

## Communicable Diseases and Adult Immunization

Although the increased availability of better medication treatments and/or vaccines, improved hygiene and food handling, and provision of cleaner water supplies have promoted prevention and control of infectious disease, new disease threats are continually emerging. Much of this increase is due to improvements in travel and changes in social, sexual, and other behaviours that expose broader populations of individuals to emerging pathogens.

Consequently, adults require immunization to restore waning immunity against some vaccine-preventable diseases and to establish immunity against other diseases that are more common in adults (Health Canada, 2018b). In addition, immunization of adults prevents infection and, therefore, subsequent exposure of young children and others at increased risk of contracting vaccine-preventable diseases. Vaccines may also be required due to individual risk resulting from occupation, travel, underlying illness, or lifestyle. Despite the need, adult vaccination rates remain low, resulting in adults being vulnerable to vaccine-preventable diseases. Common reasons for incomplete immunization in adulthood include lack of recognition of the importance of adult immunization, missed opportunities for vaccination, and lack of coordinated immunization programs for adults. Opportunities to review and improve vaccination uptake for adults involve new patient encounters, periodic health examinations, pregnancy and the immediate postpartum period, assessment of new immigrants, and parents attending their child's vaccination visits.

Although Canada has one of the lowest rates of active tuberculosis (TB), Indigenous people and foreign-born Canadians account for more than 75% of new cases (PHAC, 2018a). In 2017, the rate of active TB has remained steady, at 4.9 per 100,000 population, while the rate among Indigenous people is much higher, at 21.5 per 100,000 population, due to overcrowding, inadequate sanitation, lack of access to fresh water, and malnutrition. Other risk factors for TB include human immunodeficiency virus (HIV) infection, smoking, alcohol use, having diabetes, and being immunocompromised. Given that Canada is committed to meeting the World Health Organization (WHO) goal of less than one TB case per 100,000 by 2035, preventive activities must emphasize the reduction of health inequities, awareness and education, medical advancements, community-led TB initiatives, and global TB elimination efforts. In addition, the focus of tuberculosis surveillance needs to maintain tracking of full completion of medication protocols and treatment of medication-resistant types.

Cases of acute hepatitis B have declined in young adults because of vaccination programs aimed at children, adolescents, and adults in high-risk groups, and use of personal protective equipment in health care settings (PHAC, 2011). However, rates of acute hepatitis B infection remain high among Indigenous people and immigrants from countries where hepatitis B infection is endemic. In addition, hepatitis B infection rates among female Indigenous people were four times higher than among non-Indigenous females, while infection rates for Indigenous males were almost twice the rate of non-Indigenous males. Sexual transmission is the most common mode of transmission, followed by injection and insufflation drug use. Hepatitis B vaccination is recommended for high-risk populations such as health care workers, individuals with chronic liver or kidney disease, travellers to hepatitis B-endemic areas, or immunocompromised individuals. Approximately 250,000 Canadians are infected with the hepatitis C virus and individuals aged 25 to 39 are the second highest age group infected (PHAC, 2018b). The individuals most at risk are those who have injected illicit drugs, are undergoing hemodialysis, and who are seropositive for viral hepatitis B or HIV. Disproportionately affected populations include gay, bisexual, and other men who have sex with men, Indigenous people, and individuals from countries with high hepatitis C prevalence. Recent curative advances in antiviral medication treatment for hepatitis C results in undetectable viral load in the blood. Clinicians should consult with their provincial/territorial hepatitis C programs for more information on coverage of treatment through provincial/territorial formularies (Health Canada, 2019a).

The human papillomavirus (HPV), affects 75% of sexually active men and women in their lifetime and the prevalence of infection is highest among 20- to 24-year-olds (Health Canada, 2017b). HPV is spread through sexual contact, is responsible for almost all cervical cancers, and is linked to cancer of the throat, oral cavity, penis, anus, vagina, or vulva. Three vaccines are effective against the virus and its subtypes and are recommended for girls and women aged 9 to less than 27 years, including those who have had previous Pap test abnormalities, cervical cancer, or genital warts. Vaccination is also recommended for boys and men aged 9 to less than 27 years. In addition, the vaccine may also be given to women and men 27 years of age and older who are at ongoing risk of exposure to HPV. Vaccination prior to onset of sexual activity and exposure to HPV is recommended to maximize the benefit of the vaccine.

Pertussis (whooping cough) vaccination is part of the original vaccine series offered to infants. As it is now known that the antibody titre protection for pertussis diminishes with age, pertussis vaccination is recommended with the 10-year tetanus booster injection. This newly formulated vaccine recommended for adults is known as Tdap (tetanus, diphtheria, acellular pertussis). Adults younger than 65 years who have never received

Tdap should substitute it for their next 10-year interval booster dose (Health Canada, 2018b).

## ◆ Nutritional-Metabolic Pattern

Young adults value slimness, defined muscle tone, and athletic ability. Emphasis on body "thinness" can lead to improper eating. Regular physical activity increases muscle and bone strength, decreases body fat, aids in weight control, enhances well-being, and reduces depression. Physical activity levels are positively influenced by structural environmental improvements, such as sidewalks, bike lanes, and parks, and by legislative policies that improve access to physical activity facilities (Canadian Society for Exercise Physiology [CSEP], 2019). An optimally functioning basal metabolic rate in the young adult allows adequate oxygen intake during normal activity and rest periods. An average woman needs to eat about 1800 calories per day, while an average man needs 2250 calories daily.

During the young adult years, caloric intake increases substantially, particularly in men. Increased caloric intake without a corresponding increase in energy expenditure can lead to obesity, a progressive chronic disease that is characterized by abnormal or excessive fat accumulation that impairs health (Statistics Canada, 2018c). As a leading cause of type 2 diabetes, hypertension, and CVD, it is estimated that 1 in 10 premature deaths among Canadian adults aged 20 to 64 years is directly attributed to obesity. Obesity stigma often leads to significant inequities in access to health care, employment, and education, often due to negative stereotypes that people with obesity are lazy, unmotivated, or lacking in self-discipline. Among non-Indigenous Canadians, the prevalence of overweight was higher than among Indigenous people (34% vs. 30%), but lower for the prevalence of obesity (27% vs. 37%). Adult Indigenous males had higher overweight prevalence than females (34.6% vs. 26.6%), but lower obesity prevalence (31.6% vs. 40.6%) (Kolahdooz, Sadeghirad, Corriveau, et al., 2017). Immigrants tend to have lower rates of being overweight or obese. Whereas diet, medications, and bariatric surgery may be advised for cases of severe obesity, these treatments must be evaluated for risks and benefits (Obesity Canada, 2019).

For many Canadians, food sources are abundant, portion sizes have increased, and lifestyles are becoming increasingly sedentary. More specifically, young adult diets should contain a variety of nutrient-dense foods, especially whole grains, fruits, vegetables, low-fat or fat-free milk, lean meats, and protein sources. Caloric intake and the intake of saturated and trans fats, cholesterol, added sugars, sodium, and alcohol should be limited. Food-label information (now includes trans fats) should be read on all processed and packaged foods. Another challenge is the increasing consumption of food prepared and eaten away from home, which is generally higher in fats, cholesterol, and sodium and lower in fibre and calcium than that prepared in the home (Health Canada, 2019b). This suggests that the composition of food prepared outside the home promotes weight gain. Some provinces have legislation that requires restaurants and fast food outlets to list food composition on menus.

"Food deserts" have emerged over the past 20 years as spaces of concern for communities, public health authorities, and researchers because of their potential negative impact on dietary quality and subsequent health outcomes (Slater, Epp-Koop, Jakilazek, et al., 2017). *Food deserts* are residential geographic spaces, typically in urban settings, where low-income residents have limited or no access to retail food establishments with a sufficient variety of healthy foods at affordable cost. The situation may be further worsened because residents may lack the financial resources to own a car and have limited or no access to public transit. Residents of northern Indigenous communities may also experience many problems in accessing healthy, accessible, and nutritious foods. Northern residents may pay exorbitant prices for healthy, nutritious foods but regular, "southern" prices for junk food and pop.

Nurses and other health providers can investigate weight problems by measuring waist circumference, BP, cholesterol levels, and activity levels rather than using weight alone. Assessments of weight and height are used to calculate BMI. Whereas the BMI may be a good indicator for population screening, it may not be the best measurement for predicting health risks, as in each individual fitness level, lifestyle habits, and presence or absence of other health-risk conditions must be considered (Health Canada, 2016). Individuals with a BMI of $25 \text{ kg/m}^2$ or less (male waist size of less than 102 cm, female waist size of less than 88 cm) have the least risk of developing health problems and should have weight-maintenance teaching. Individuals with a BMI of $30 \text{ kg/m}^2$ or greater who have tried diets and exercise may be considered for weight-reducing medications (Health Canada, 2016). A BMI of 35 to $40 \text{ kg/m}^2$ or above may meet the criteria for bariatric surgery (Ontario Bariatric Network, 2015). However, the focus of nursing advice is conservative at first, recommending lifestyle management, careful diet appraisal, and increase in exercise patterns (Health Canada, 2016). Use of activity monitors such as Fitbit, heart-rate monitors (Apple Watch), and fat/muscle calculators may provide incentives for healthy eating and exercise patterns. Long-term weight management is a frustrating process. However, a winning solution for long-term benefits and weight loss is to adopt a healthy, enjoyable lifestyle with increased physical activity rather than trying to lose large amounts of weight too quickly through a restrictive diet (Obesity Canada, 2019). The nurse should use people-first and nonjudgemental language that refers to the person before the condition (a person with obesity) rather than identifying the person on the basis of the disability (an obese person).

Proper nutrition is particularly necessary for the young adult female during the child-bearing years. The factors contributing to iron deficiency in this age group are regular loss of blood (during menses) and pregnancy. Young women in a lower income bracket, who do not eat a healthy diet and have heavy periods or use nonsteroidal anti-inflammatory medications, are specifically at risk of iron-deficiency anemia. Iron supplementation is recommended during pregnancy for optimal growth of the fetus and supporting structures (Perry, Hockenberry, Lowdermilk, et al., 2014). Health Canada (2018c) recommends that all women of child-bearing age take a supplement of 0.4 mg folic acid every day, a B vitamin found in dark green leafy vegetables, fruits, nuts, beans, dairy products, meat, grains, and eggs, to reduce the risk of fetal neural tube defects (NTDs), including spina bifida. The supplementation period should begin ideally before conception, or at least 3 months before pregnancy, and continue for the duration of breastfeeding. Although the rate of children born with an NTD has significantly decreased since promotion of folic acid supplementation, at least 25% of North American women of child-bearing age do not have sufficient folate intake to optimally protect their offspring from NTDs. Women of lower socioeconomic status are less well protected by folate and, as a result, bear the greatest burden of this serious congenital anomaly (Noam, Bernstein, Boucher, et al., 2016).

Most adolescents and adult women fail to meet their calcium requirements, placing them at risk of osteoporosis and bone fractures in later life. Low calcium intake is a direct result of low milk consumption related to soft drink ingestion. An increase in intake of calcium-containing foods is therefore recommended, particularly for teens and young women (see Chapter 21).

## ◆ Elimination Pattern

Patterns of elimination are generally well established by young adulthood. Although eating disorders (anorexia and bulimia) typically begin at an earlier stage of development, they can persist during young adulthood. The fashion industry is widely criticized for using underweight women as young female models, thereby emphasizing excessive thinness as the ideal female standard.

Assessment of young adults is also directed toward teaching about the common complaints of constipation, hemorrhoids, and occasional diarrhea. Although the risk of colon cancer is low in this age group, young adults should be aware that changes in elimination patterns or blood in the stool should be reported to their primary care provider. Nurses can counsel young adults on the benefits of drinking adequate amounts of fluid and eating fruits and vegetables, which are sources of fibre, to promote normal bowel activity.

## ◆ Activity-Exercise Pattern

Inactivity is a factor predisposing to CVD and obesity; increasing access to and promoting locations for physical activity are increasingly emphasized. The CSEP (2019) recommends that Canadians aged 18 to 64 accumulate at least 150 minutes of moderate-to-vigorous-intensity physical aerobic activity per week, in bouts of 10 minutes or more, as well as muscle- and bone-strengthening activities at least 2 days a week. Recently, 64% of Canadians aged 18 to 34 self-reported 150 minutes of physical activity per week (Health Canada, 2019b). However, in a 2017 survey, only 16% of monitored Canadian adults met the recommended physical activity guidelines (Statistics Canada, 2019b). Major barriers for young adults are lack of time, lack of access to exercise facilities, and lack of financial resources to participate in physical activities.

### Radiation and Excessive Sun Exposure

Nurses need to educate young adults about the risks of sun exposure and tanning, the preventive use of sun-blocking agents, and the awareness of skin symptoms that might indicate cancer. Sun-blocking agents reduce sunburn or other skin damage, with the goal of lowering the risk of skin cancer. A number of the agents are rated on the basis of skin type and sensitivity to burning. Many lotions and creams are available, with differing radiation protection levels. Sun protection factor (SPF) index is a measure of the effectiveness of various preparations and is measured by Health Canada. For example, a rating of SPF 30 means the sunscreen blocks 97% of ultraviolet B (UVB) rays, while a rating of SPF 50 blocks 98% of UVB rays. The best protection is achieved by application of broad-spectrum, water-resistant agents 15 to 30 minutes before exposure and then reapplying every 15 to 30 minutes during exposure to the sun. Further application may be necessary if activities involve swimming, sweating, or rubbing of skin. Sunscreens that block both ultraviolet A (UVA) rays and UVB rays are more effective in preventing cancer than those that block only UVB rays. Women's makeup preparations and moisturizers may include sun-blocking agents. Wearing sunglasses that block both UVA and UVB rays and wearing sun-protective clothing are also recommended. Young adults should avoid sunbathing during the 2-hour period before and after noon, because two-thirds of the day's UV light comes through the Earth's atmosphere during this time. The nurse considers that the most effective skin cancer prevention activities for young adults include primary care counselling, sun protection, and avoiding the use of tanning beds (Health Canada, 2017c).

### Sports

Bicycling and motorcycling are encouraged by environmentalists to decrease automobile pollution; this trend is also promoted to relieve traffic congestion, avoid the high costs of fuel and car maintenance, and increase interest in healthy exercise. Cyclists are at risk of being involved in accidents with automobiles. Head injury is responsible for many bicycle-related fatalities. Currently, many provinces have mandatory helmet laws for riders younger than 18 years. Motorcycles have less occupant protection than do automobiles but are appealing to young adults, primarily because they have high-performance and speed capabilities. Helmets for cycling and motorcycling are the single most effective preventive measure to decrease the incidence of brain and head injury.

Each year, hundreds of preventable head injuries are reported on Canadian ski, snowboard, and toboggan hills. Injuries such as fractures and sprains are also common. Most of these injuries can be prevented by wearing appropriate gear or obtaining proper training and knowledge. A helmet cannot prevent all head injuries, but it can significantly reduce the risk of a head injury.

There are 10 million boaters in Canada. Most fatal boating incidents (78%) occur during recreational activities, with half of Canadian boating deaths occurring on lakes (53%); 91% of boating victims are male. In addition, one-third of boating deaths are alcohol related (Canada Safety Council, 2018). The second highest number of drowning deaths is consistently found among Canadians aged 20 to 34, with 1.6 deaths per 100,000. Mountain climbing, hiking in poor weather conditions, use of an all-terrain vehicle (ATV) or a snowmobile are other hazardous activities. Many so-called accidents are not random, uncontrollable events, but are predictable and preventable if precautions and risks are analyzed (Canada Safety Council, 2018).

Amateur and professional sports activities generally pose few hazards when rules and safety precautions are observed. Relatively few fatalities are associated with the professionally organized contact sports, such as hockey, football, or lacrosse, but chronic injuries and concussions can cause degenerative brain diseases. In addition, sports-related health injuries and, specifically, concussions have been linked to an increase the incidence of dementia, memory-related diseases, and chronic traumatic encephalopathy. This has resulted in significant changes in professional sports policies and sports concussion protocols, which have been for amateur and community sports leagues as well (Parachute Canada, 2019).

A comprehensive history of recreational activities alerts the nurse to specific needs about safety education. Young adults are encouraged to learn and abide by the rules of the sport in which they are engaged. Rules in many sports have evolved from health and safety concerns, enabling the individual to learn the sport well with appropriate instruction.

## ◆ Sleep-Rest Pattern

Young adults are subject to fatigue induced by work, stress, or inactivity. Changes in activity or stressors can help reduce fatigue. Attempting new and challenging tasks can help reduce mental stress. New physical activities, such as learning a new sport or form of exercise, can also provide stimulation. A number of digital devices now record sleep as well as activity patterns.

## ◆ Cognitive-Perceptual Pattern

### Physical and Mental Patterns

Visual acuity is highest at approximately age 20 years and begins to decline at approximately age 40 years, when farsightedness frequently develops. Hearing is also best at age 20 years; the ability to distinguish high-pitched tones decreases with age. The other senses—taste, smell, touch, and awareness of temperature and pain—remain stable until age 45 to 50 years.

Further maturation requires young adults to learn skills and behaviours that increase the performance abilities gained as adolescents. The factors that an individual young adult may perceive as essential to learn will depend on specific goals, values, attitudes, and practices as influenced by intrinsic (constitutional) and extrinsic (environmental or community) factors. Executive decision making becomes better developed: calculation of risks versus rewards, prioritizing, self-evaluation, self-correction, and long-term planning become more sophisticated. The development of intellectual maturity influences the selection of behaviours and attitudes that affect health and well-being practices.

### Piaget's Theory

Several stage theorists have described the growth of young adult thought and moral development. It is important to note that these stages are fluid, and individual differences occur. Within Piaget's cognitive-developmental theory, formal operational thought evolves from concrete operational thought in adolescence and extends through the reasoning process of young adults (Piaget, 1972). Although more recent developmental theorists dispute Piaget's findings, this scheme of cognitive development assists the nurse in learning about and understanding young adult reasoning. Achievement of formal operational thinking allows young adults to analyze all combinations of possibilities and construct hypotheses. Young adult thought becomes more perceptive and insightful; issues can therefore be evaluated realistically and objectively. Young adults are energetic and can therefore contribute substantially to social and occupational decision making. Although they tend to take greater risks, young adults typically demonstrate the use of appropriate reasoning, anticipation, and analytical approaches.

### Intellectual Growth

Organization of information influences memory. Evidence shows that recall performance diminishes with age: at its peak in the 20s, memory starts to diminish during the 30s. Improved strategies for organization of information, however, can enhance recall, and limitation of memory with increasing age is likely a result of retrieval rather than storage mechanisms. Recent evidence from brain development research indicates that during the early years of young adulthood important frontal lobe brain development is still occurring; this is important for control of emotions and later full adult rational decision making (Neinstein, 2013).

### Erikson's Theory

Erikson (1993), another widely cited psychological theorist, reported that the most important goal for young adults is the development of an increased sense of competency and self-esteem. In developing self-esteem, the young person learns to be truly open and capable of trust through the formation of intimate relationships that are characteristic of this period. This stage is described as a phase of psychosocial development termed intimacy versus isolation and loneliness.

Erikson's concept of genuine intimacy extends beyond sexual relations to a broader view of mutual psychosocial intimacy with a spouse or lover, parents, children, and friends. Characterized by the reciprocal expression of affection, intimacy requires mutual trust. These interchanges are spontaneous for the young adult; relationships should be free and allow self-disclosure. Young adults who are unsure of their identity may avoid intimate contact or engage in promiscuous behaviour lacking in true intimacy, which can result in isolation and consequent self-absorption. Healthy adults search for continuity, regularity, or unity of meaningful relationships, while avoiding situations of little commitment.

### Moral Development

Young adults who have successfully mastered the previous cognitive, social, and moral stages are usually able to recognize or use principled reasoning. Kohlberg identifies this ability as the postconventional level of moral reasoning (Kohlberg & Lickons, 1986). During this phase the individual is able to differentiate the self from the rules and expectations of others and to define principles regarding rights in terms of self-chosen principles. The interests of individuals can be weighed against the needs of society and the state, and violations of law can be justified when individual interests are in accord with principles.

Although development of principled moral reasoning is possible during young adulthood, it may never occur if the cognitive and social factors that stimulate higher reasoning are not present. Acts of personal violence representative of lower moral reasoning should not be present; however, such acts do occur during this period, illustrating the need for moral developmental concerns to be addressed at earlier stages of education and socialization.

## ◆ Self-Perception–Self-Concept Pattern

In non-Western cultures the entrance to adulthood is generally defined and marked by social events such as marriage. In Western societies, maturation is defined through the individual's achievement of financial and residential independence, and is a more drawn-out, gradual process. There is evidence that young adults have recently been attaining traditional life milestones later; this includes completing school and leaving home, attaining financial independence, marrying, and having the first child (Neinstein, 2013).

Two emotional themes regarding the value of work and financial independence become evident during young adulthood. During their 20s, young adults yearn to explore and experiment, keeping structures temporary and reversible. These individuals may move from job to job and relationship to relationship, remaining in a transient state. At the opposite extreme is the urge to prepare for the future by making firm commitments. During this period, both men and women question their value to society, the merit of their accomplishments, their success as sexual beings, and the probability of attaining their unfulfilled goals.

In 2017, more than 65% of women aged 25 to 34 were employed full time, an increase from 23% in 1950 (Statistics Canada, 2018d). The increase in labour force participation for women has been driven by higher attainment of postsecondary education, decrease in propensity of employed women to withdraw from the workforce due to marriage or motherhood, and maternal leave job protection, as well as legislation addressing unfair labour practices. Yet gender pay inequity remains a problem, with women earning $0.87 for every dollar earned by men. The federal and provincial governments have enacted various forms of legislation and statutory mechanisms in the area of labour standards or human rights to address the problem of gender wage discrimination (Pay Equity Commission, 2019). However, access to benefits may not be available, especially to high-risk groups such as immigrants or employees receiving the minimum wage. In addition, some types of employment expose individuals to occupational risks and hazards. The Government of Canada has begun to modernize the *Canada Labour Code*, for example, by introducing stronger adherence and enforcement provisions, a right to request flexible work arrangements, new unpaid leaves for family responsibilities, to participate in traditional Indigenous practices, and for victims of family violence, as well as to limit unpaid internships (Employment and Social Development Canada, 2019). Many young adults are high achievers and seek opportunities to be challenged. Employment

problems are stressful and traumatic to an individual's self-esteem and self-worth, particularly in the current economic environment. The failure to obtain promotions or pay rises can accelerate the degree of stress. Employment is more than a source of income; it provides self-esteem and social interaction. Because the adjustment to the job market influences many other aspects of daily living, young adults frequently require assistance in developing coping mechanisms to manage stress. Properly managing the initial stress prevents further complications that can arise if the young adult uses unhealthy stress relievers such as alcohol or drugs.

Young women have many of the same concerns about employment and success as do young men. Many young women postpone child-bearing until they have established their careers; many are absent from the job for only a standard maternity leave. Women who return to work when their children are very young frequently risk the emotional strain caused by guilt feelings and role strain. In addition to helping parents cope with the stress of being absent from their children, nurses can help them identify ways to provide high-quality supervision in their absence, through private babysitters, day care programs, or through neighbours, friends, and relatives. The implementation of more affordable public day care has contributed to an increased employment participation rate for women by almost 30% since 2000. However, the participation rate of young adult women remains below the labour market participation rate for men by 9% (Employment and Social Development Canada, 2017). The labour market participation rate for Indigenous people is currently 8% below the rate for other Canadians. Immigrants to Canada who have a university degree attained outside of Canada tend to be underemployed. Almost 30% of immigrant men are working in a job that requires only high-school education, and 44% of immigrant women are employed in a job that requires only a high-school education (Statistics Canada, 2018a).

The Canadian workforce is changing dramatically as companies merge, restructure, downsize (right size), and shift employees around to meet changing market conditions, company mergers, and buyouts. The fundamental nature of work is changing with ever-increasing global competition, rapid technological changes, and increased use of contracted and temporary workers (Employment and Social Development Canada, 2018). There is increasing concern about "globalization," outsourcing, and moving jobs overseas, especially in manufacturing, the pharmaceutical industry, and the computer industry. Unemployment or underemployment for young adults is a particular concern after recovery from the prolonged recession beginning in 2008 (Employment and Social Development Canada, 2018). There is concern that even with better job prospects, this young adult population will be behind in wages for years, and this may impact overall lifetime earnings. Younger hires may start at lower salaries and begin their employed years with firms that pay less or have less potential for advancement. Among young adults, 12% are low-income earners, compared with 25% of Indigenous young adults and 29% of young adults with a disability (Statistics Canada, 2018a). Nursing activity in occupational and industrial settings can be directed toward improving both working conditions and employer–employee relationships. When nurses advocate healthy work sites, this increases the chance that young adults will have access to comprehensive health-promotion programs.

## ◆ Roles-Relationships Pattern

Young adult friendships are more enduring than are earlier relationships. The focus of the relationship is the sharing of feelings or confidences as well as common interests. True friendship is characteristic of a person who wants to give rather than receive. Friendships are necessary in a constantly changing society; they provide a source of emotional support and a basis of stability for developing the self-concept. Social networking sites such as Facebook, Instagram, Twitter, and social apps allow young adults to interact quickly with one another to organize events/dates and share photos, experiences, thoughts, and perceptions. Young adults use Internet dating services to widen access to potential dating candidates (Statistics Canada, 2018a).

Establishing interpersonal relationships involves agreeable and purposeful interactions with other people. Interpersonal relationships can be created with people of the same or the opposite sex. Age is typically a less important factor than it was during adolescence. The formation of intimate relationships develops within or outside a family context, the school setting, or work environment. High-speed cell phone and wireless Internet access facilitate maintenance of relationships from high-school and university settings with mostly text messaging.

For some the significant other is a person of the same sex. About 4 to 10% of Canadian young adults consider themselves to be either same-sex or bisexual (Statistics Canada, 2015b). Same-sex couples represent 0.9% of all Canadian couples and one-third of these were legally married. In 2005, Canada became the first non-European country to enact the Civil Marriage Act, which gives married same-sex partners the same legal recognition as other married couples. In addition, the *Civil Marriage Act* gave same-sex parents the same rights as heterosexual parents and some provinces have also made it legal for same-sex parents to adopt children in Canada (Library of Parliament, 2005).

Transgender issues and rights have been headlines in the news recently. Transgender issues arise when one's gender identity or expression does not match the individual's assigned sex. Transgender expression is independent of sexual orientation, as individuals may be heterosexual, same sex, or bisexual. This category includes individuals who have reassigned their sexual identity different from that assigned at birth.

In addition to achieving intimacy, the young adult must accomplish other developmental tasks to achieve true psychosocial maturation (Fig. 16.2). Decision making about life and career directions is the developmental milestone that heralds the transition from adolescence to adulthood. Decisions usually entail establishing independence from the family of origin. This transition may involve an actual physical move from the parents' home (going away to community college or university, travelling abroad, or getting an apartment); however, movement away is not the sole indicator of independence. In 2017, 35% of young adults were living with their parents, up from 31% in

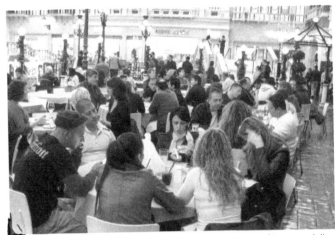

**Fig. 16.2** Young adults enjoy gathering in a local café to socialize together.

2001. The increase was largest for youth aged 25 to 29 (Statistics Canada, 2018a). Young adults frequently remain in their parents' home for economic reasons, particularly when life choices involve continued schooling, unemployment, or remaining unmarried. In some cultures, unmarried adults live with their parents until they are married, and newly married young adults share the home of their parents until they begin having their own children.

In 2016, 9% of men and 5% of women aged 25 to 34 had not completed high school, compared with 22% and 19%, respectively, in 1990. In 2011, 31% of Indigenous men and 25% of Indigenous women had not completed high school. Furthermore, a large gap in postsecondary enrollment remains between youth from lower and higher income families. Nonfinancial factors, such as academic performance and parental education, play a significant role (Statistics Canada, 2018a).

A greater proportion of young adults are enrolled in higher education than ever before (Statistics Canada, 2018a). In 2017, almost 30% of male young adults had a college certificate or a Bachelor's degree or higher, while 42% of female young adults had a college certificate or a Bachelor's degree of higher (Statistics Canada, 2018a). Postsecondary fields of study tend to differ between men and women, with more men entering business administration and engineering and more women entering social sciences and humanities. The growing technology industry provides employment in a wide variety of occupations and start-up companies. Work styles within these companies tend to be different from those in the traditional workplace, including an expectation of longer and more fluid workdays.

As tuition fees for full-time undergraduate students have increased faster than the rate of inflation over the past decade, 50% of graduates will have an average student debt of $26,300 (Statistics Canada, 2018a). Because student loan repayment typically begins 6 months after graduation, new graduates have to face the harsh realities of trying to find employment and ways to begin loan repayment, and this may involve moving home for a short time. Others will start or attend graduate school to obtain better work skills.

Individuals in the later years of this age group typically choose life partners and begin families; they make decisions about child-bearing and the number and education of children. Additional consideration must be given to decisions related to child-bearing, such as finances, safety, family support, where to live, the relationship with extended family members, and the roles and responsibilities within the family unit. Young adults who are establishing a family must have open communication about self-development, which includes issues of dual careers, child-rearing practices, and domestic duties.

Family harmony and development are major goals for many young adults. Although family size and structure have undergone dramatic changes in recent decades, concern about each member's health and safety continues to be a primary focus. Family life is influenced by the qualities of individual family members. Typically, economic security, status, place in the community, and healthy patterns of living, such as good nutrition, personal hygiene, and physical fitness, are associated with healthy family adjustment.

### Separation and Divorce

Approximately 38% of marriages in Canada end in divorce (Statistics Canada, 2019c), and many young adults do not marry but have children. Although dissatisfaction and unhappiness are frequent precursors to separation and divorce, the decision to dissolve a marriage is not easy. Considerable emotional strain exists for both partners, their children, their families, and their close friends. Divorce requires that young adults re-evaluate their basic values, individual personality, spiritual beliefs, and ego strength, job potential, and socioeconomic factors to ensure future security for themselves and their children.

Of Canada's 9.4 million families, 16% lived in lone-parent families in 2011, with 8 in 10 being led by women (Statistics Canada, 2015c). Lone-parent families often face financial challenges that two-parent households don't. However, the term "lone" may be misleading because support can come from other family members, including grandparents. Lone mothers may be in committed relationships with a partner who contributes to their family life, but choose to live in "living apart together" (LAT) couples. According to Statistics Canada (2019c), 8% of women aged 20 and over (1.9 million) are in LAT couples. In addition, multigenerational living is increasing and is relatively common among immigrant and Indigenous families. As 75% of grandparents in lone-parent homes report some responsibilities for household costs, living together makes it easier to share costs and provide care (Vanier Institute, 2019).

Nurses can assist young adults to identify sources of assistance and support (Innovative Practice). Nursing care and assessment can help to identify the feelings of guilt, grief, and loss that young adults experience during a separation or divorce. Suggesting that young adults read articles or books on issues related to divorce is helpful, because they provide a reference point for their experiences. The nurse recommends marital counselling by a qualified professional; this may be the most beneficial source of support.

### Male and Female Risk of Violence

Intimate partner violence has serious health consequences for women and men; however, because of social and legal factors,

## INNOVATIVE PRACTICE

### Social Media and Use of Internet and Cell Phone Delivery Systems for Preventive Health Information

Today's use of technology is changing practice patterns and the way that health communications may be transmitted. Wearables and mobile apps today support fitness, health education, symptom tracking, and collaborative disease management and care coordination.

Some biomedical innovations for Pap test understanding and prevention of sexually transmitted infections (STIs) and human immunodeficiency virus (HIV) infection have been adopted (such as use of electronic health records and cell phones/Internet to trace contacts), but full adherence by the person seeking care is often hindered by behavioural factors. Technological interventions allow behavioural supports and educational programs to be delivered with less cost and more convenience. These include STI/HIV testing and partner interventions, behavioural interventions, self-management strategies, and provider care information. Text messaging is also possible. As smartphones are connecting individuals domestically and globally, a new category of "personalized preventive health coaches" or digital health advisors will develop and grow to allow the dissemination of more active engaging health diagnosis, treatment, and counselling.

Source: Christensen, S. & Morelli, R. (2012). MyPapp: A mobile app to enhance understanding of Pap testing. *Computers, Informatics and Nursing, 30*(12), 627–631; Dimitrov, D. V. (2016). Medical Internet of things and big data in healthcare. *Healthcare Informatics Research, 22*(3), 156–163.

it is probably the most under-reported form of abuse (Diversity Awareness). Of all reported violent crime in Canada, more than 25% resulted from family violence, with two-thirds of victims being women. Family violence and abuse crosses all socioeconomic, racial, ethnic, religious, gender, and age boundaries. Women were also four times more likely than men to be victims of intimate partner violence (IPV) (PHAC, 2018c). However, rates of IPV are believed to be under-reported, since victims are often less willing to report violence because of the stigma associated with it. Compared with men, women who experience spousal violence are more likely to report being sexually assaulted, beaten, choked, or threatened with a gun or a knife, to have higher rates of injury caused by abuse, and to experience long-term post-traumatic stress disorder (PTSD). Indigenous women are more likely to experience IPV and nearly 60% of Indigenous women are more likely to report being physically injured as a result of it as compared with 41% of non-Indigenous women. In addition, women who self-identify as lesbian or bisexual and women with disabilities were more likely to be victims of IPV than heterosexual women. One in four college or university students have been a victim of sexual assault (Quinlan, Quinlan, Fogel, et al., 2017). Identification of, education about, and strategies to prevent bullying, dating violence, and sexual violence among young adults require active attention and participation from federal, provincial, community, and academic stakeholders. Nurses and other primary health care providers assist in detecting or treating violence or abuse in an optimal manner. However, more efforts must be made to recognize the scope of the problem and to provide appropriate counselling (see Diversity Awareness box).

**DIVERSITY AWARENESS**

## Partner and Family Violence: Gender and Culture Differences

### Assessing the Problem

Epidemiological researchers have attempted to determine the risks for intimate partner and family violence. Intimate partner violence includes four behaviours: physical violence, sexual violence, threats of physical or sexual violence, and/or emotional abuse. Understanding the roots of partner violence has been more difficult than ascertaining determinants of physical disease. The victims of family violence are usually children, the female spouse, intimate partners, and older persons (Canadian Women's Foundation, 2019). Factors associated with intimate partner violence include young age, low income, pregnancy, mental health disorders, separation or divorce, and a history of abuse. The unequal position of women in a relationship and the manner in which conflict is managed, as well as differences in culture, education, and prestige associated with the partners' occupations, are related to the risk of violence. Domestic violence is a problem in all age, ethnic, and religious groups; in some cultures, attitudes toward women even legitimize the practice. Women who have gained positions of respect and power outside the home through activities in their neighbourhood or community are less likely to be abused. In men and women, viewing abuse as a child increases the likelihood that abusive behaviours are used by these same individuals as adults (PHAC, 2018c).

### Are Nurses Willing to Take Action?

Some studies indicate that nurses have been reluctant to take action regarding violence against women or men. Some of the traditional reasons for not taking action are based on paternalistic attitudes, in which the victim is blamed for his or her part in the social situation that becomes violent. Nursing's strong advocacy stance and emphasis on the communication of nonjudgemental, genuine concern should provide a strong foundation to avoid blaming the victim and to focus on pathological factors that have been identified by much of the health profession's research in this area.

### How Can Nurses Recognize Abuse?

Research demonstrates that nurses should be more aware of indicators of partner violence. These include the presence, as revealed by a health history, of separation or divorce, alcoholism, frequent verbal disagreements, and high levels of conflict. Other warning signs include repeated visits to emergency departments, complaints of headaches or backaches, psychiatric illness, and incidents of bruises, sprains, and lacerations. Abusers are more likely to have hostile personality styles with aggressive tendencies. As children, they may have had unattainable goals, and their achievements may have been met with harsh criticism and toxic and depersonalizing behaviour. Abusers may also use passive aggressive tactics, turning passive withdrawal and blaming behaviours against the helping individual in an effort to portray the abuser as a victim.

### Reflective Questions

- Are nurses less than helpful in their detection and management of domestic violence? Why do you think this occurs?
- Are nurses, because of their education and sensitization to people with mental health disorders, more or less likely than others to experience violence in their own domestic settings? Explain why.

Sources: Centre for Public Legal Education in Alberta. (2018). *Learning about abuse*. Retrieved from https://www.willownet.ca/just-the-facts/learning-about/; Landenburger, K. M., & Campbell, J. C. (2012). Violence and human abuse. In M. Stanhope, & J. Lancaster (Eds.). *Public health nursing: Population-centered health care in the community* (pp. 828–853). St. Louis: Elsevier; Public Health Agency of Canada. (2018). *Family violence: How big is the problem in Canada?* Retrieved from https://www.canada.ca/en/public-health/services/health-promotion/stop-family-violence/problem-canada.html.

## ◆ Sexuality-Reproductive Pattern

By young adulthood the menstrual cycle is generally well established in the woman. Cyclical hormonal function is responsible for regularity of the cycle and normal functioning of the ovaries and uterus. The normal duration of menses is 4 to 5 days (range of 2 to 7 days, with a blood loss of 40 mL). Blood loss greater than 80 mL per cycle is abnormal and may lead to anemia. Irregularities such as painful menstruation, premenstrual syndrome, and prolonged or heavy bleeding need further assessment. Although these problems are not always abnormal, the symptoms and the individual's reaction to them can signal functional disorders and the need for further investigation and treatment.

### Reproductive Problems

Infertility is defined as the lack of conception in the presence of unprotected sexual intercourse for at least 12 months. Approximately 16% of couples of reproductive age in Canada are believed to be infertile (PHAC, 2019a). Infertility has become more of a public issue since the advance of assisted reproductive technologies, such as in vitro fertilization and gamete intrafallopian transfer, which can enable couples with known reproductive problems to conceive children. These technologies frequently create great stress for the couple and often result in marital conflicts and distress. Infertility is not an issue for those in the 18- to 25-year age range, as peak fertility is from age 20 years to age 35 years; however, after the age of 30 years, infertility is more common and a more specific diagnostic workup or referral for some type of assisted reproductive strategy may be indicated.

Common problems of the male reproductive system include orchitis, epididymitis, and varicoceles and hydroceles. Mumps in the postpubertal male can cause swelling of the testes, orchitis, and subfertility. Even with appropriate vaccination, mumps cases are becoming more prevalent as the mumps vaccine is not fully effective (Health Canada, 2018b). External conditions such as fungal infections, contact dermatitis, and eczema; parasites such as mites (scabies) and lice; and nonvenereal diseases such as erysipelas, abscesses, and fistulas can occur in the scrotum.

### Unintended Pregnancy

Researchers believe that up to 40% of pregnancies in Canada are unintended, with women aged 20 to 24 having the highest rate of unintended pregnancy (Society of Obstetricians and Gynaecologists of Canada [SOGC], 2019). Unintended pregnancy is an important public health issue and relates to increased risks of delayed prenatal care, depression, and other personal and relationship problems. Family planning is one of

**TABLE 16.2 Summary of Risks and Noncontraceptive Benefits of Selected Contraceptive Methods**

| Contraceptive Method | Risks of Use | Noncontraceptive Health Benefits |
|---|---|---|
| Oral contraceptives (various formulations: extended, combined, monophasic, biphasic, triphasic, multiphasic, and progestin only) | Thromboembolic disorders, CVA, coronary artery disease especially with smoking, hypertension, diabetes, breast cancer | Reduced risk of functional pelvic inflammation, endometriosis, uterine fibroids, endometrial cancer, ovarian cancer, iron-deficiency anemia, ectopic pregnancy, irregular cycles |
| Transdermal (contraceptive patch: Ortho Evra) | Similar to oral contraceptives | Easy verification of presence, weekly application |
| Injectable progestin (Depo-Provera) | Prolonged amenorrhea, venous thrombosis, thromboembolism | Bone loss especially in adolescents, unsure of lifetime risk of osteoporosis |
| Vaginal ring (NuvaRing) | Similar to oral contraceptives, increased risks of cardiovascular events | Vaginal ring hormonal option |
| Intrauterine contraceptive device (IUD: Mirena) | Bleeding, anemia, difficult removal, PID, ectopic pregnancy, cramping | Reduced risk of anemia, low cost for long term |
| Emergency contraception (Plan B) | Nausea, abdominal pain, delay of menses | Not for routine use |
| Diaphragm (non-latex silicone only) | Toxic shock syndrome, allergy to spermicide, urinary tract infection | Reduced risk of vaginitis, cervicitis |
| Condom | Allergy to rubber, latex, or spermicide | Reduced risk of STI and HIV transmission |
| Spermicides[a] | Sensitivity to agent | Antiviral activity against HPV, decreased activity of other STIs, decreased risk of PID |
| Sponge | Toxic shock syndrome | Decreased activity of STI organisms |
| Female sterilization (tubal ligation) | Anesthesia, infection, hemorrhage | One-time procedure |
| Male sterilization (vasectomy) | Complication rates low, reversal may be difficult | One-time procedure |

[a]Often used in combination with other methods.

*CVA,* Cerebrovascular accident; *HPV,* human papillomavirus; *IUD,* intrauterine device; *PID,* pelvic inflammatory disease; *STI,* sexually transmitted infection.

Source: Black, A., Guilbert, E., Costescu, D., et al. (2015). Canadian contraception consensus (Part 1 of 4). *Journal of Obstetrics and Gynaecology Canada, 37*(10), 936–942.

the biggest public health achievements of the twentieth century. Although many Canadian adults get the cost of contraception covered through supplemental insurance from their employer, 25% of Canadians do not have access to employer group plans and some plans limit or exclude contraceptive coverage completely (Motluk, 2016).

Women enrolled in community colleges and universities have high rates of reported sexual violence, of sexually transmitted infections (STIs), and unintended pregnancy that result most often from the influence of alcohol on risky behaviour, lack of negotiation for sexual consent, and haphazard contraceptive use (Quinlan et al., 2017). First-year students are particularly vulnerable. To address these problems, colleges and universities have adopted stricter institutional policies and educational programs aimed at making students fully aware of what an authentic sexual consent entails to protect victims. The recent reporting on the inadequacies of college/university policies on sexual consent has forced higher education institutions to be more proactive and forthcoming, with early incoming student counselling and elaborate policies governing appropriate student campus behaviour.

Approximately half of unintended pregnancies are the result of contraceptive failure. Both married and unmarried young adults need information about contraceptives (Table 16.2) to decrease the number of unwanted pregnancies and the need for abortions. The nurse's role in contraceptive counselling involves helping individuals to choose the method most appropriate to their needs. Laws and policies in some settings restrict nurses and other health care providers from engaging in certain types of counselling, including providing abortion information.

Emergency contraception (EC) helps to prevent pregnancy after unprotected sex or failed birth control. It does not terminate an existing pregnancy or protect against an STI. Two types of emergency contraception are available: emergency contraceptive pills (ECPs) or an intrauterine device (IUD). ECPs are most effective when taken within 72 hours after having sex, but may be taken up to 5 days after having sex. They contain hormones that prevent ovulation or fertilization of the egg. A copper IUD is a small, T-shaped plastic device wrapped in copper and it is inserted into the uterus by a health care provider. When inserted within 7 days of unprotected sex, it causes a chemical change that damages sperm before they can meet the ovum. A benefit of the IUD is that it can remain in the uterus for up to 5 years as an ongoing form of birth control. Like any birth control method, neither type of emergency contraception is 100% effective (Black, Guilbert, Costescu, et al., 2015). The choice to use emergency contraception is frequently made with the partner and may involve complex decision making, centring on responsibility, relationship power, and a woman's right to choose and have autonomy over her body (Black et al., 2015).

### Prenatal Care

Among Canadian women, Indigenous women struggle more to achieve optimal maternal and infant outcomes (PHAC, 2017). Poverty is one of the strongest determinants of health and is associated with food insecurity, poor nutrition, obesity, and increased rates of smoking and recreational drug use, crowded living conditions, and increased exposure to environmental hazards and violence. Women who live in poverty and experience these associated conditions are less likely to initiate prenatal care and are at higher risk of poorer pregnancy outcomes, including preterm birth and intrauterine growth restriction. Optimal outcomes may be further hindered when women live in remote or northern communities and have less access to prenatal health care services. Immigrant women are another key population to consider, because this population may be less aware of the health care system, may have limited social networks, or limited access to or eligibility for services.

Nurses can play a vital role in identifying those with inadequate income and assist them to access the resources to which they qualify. They can also connect women and their families with community networks that provide social and financial support, as well as identifying and overcoming institutional and organizational barriers.

### Sexually Transmitted Infections

STIs describe diseases that are transmitted sexually and include chlamydia, syphilis, gonorrhea, genital warts, and HPV (Table 16.3). STIs continue to be a significant public health concern in Canada. Rates of reported cases of chlamydia, gonorrhea, and infectious syphilis have risen significantly since 2005 (Health Canada, 2017d). Males and females aged 20 to 24 had the highest rates of chlamydia, while rates of gonorrhea were highest among males aged 20 to 29. Since 2005, infectious syphilis rates have increased 115% among males. Males aged 25 to 29 had the highest rates of infectious syphilis; in females, rates were highest among those aged 20 to 24. Rates for STIs, particularly gonorrhea, were higher among Indigenous people (Gatrix, Plitt, Turnbull, et al., 2017).

The causes of increasing STI rates are complex and include changing sexual attitudes regarding risky sexual behaviour, the use of recreational drugs that decrease inhibitions and impair sexual decision making, and the practice of seeking sexual partners through the Internet. The increase in syphilis rates partially results from increasing rates of men who have sex with men (MSM). Syphilis infection in women of child-bearing age is of concern because of the potential of congenital syphilis in infants exposed to *Treponema pallidum* prenatally or during child-birth. Screening for syphilis as part of comprehensive prenatal care for all pregnant women is key to preventing congenital syphilis.

### Human Immunodeficiency Virus

More than 60,000 Canadians are estimated to have HIV infection and approximately 14% of those with HIV are unaware that they have the disease (PHAC, 2019b). Indigenous populations have incidence rates 2.7 times higher than non-Indigenous Canadians. In addition, immigrants from HIV-endemic countries have incidence rates 6.4 times higher than Canadians of other ethnicities. Increased incidence rates are also seen in men who have sex with other men and people who inject drugs. Improved longevity of infected persons and better treatment have made HIV infection more like a chronic disease. HIV is transmitted by sexual intercourse (oral, vaginal, anal), shared needles, and infected blood. Another less common source of transmission is from the mother to the baby across the placental barrier or through breast milk. The higher level of worry about contracting HIV and other STIs in young adults is correlated with the implementation of risk-reduction behaviours. The incidence of STIs is greatly reduced with proper use of condoms.

The WHO has developed a global health strategy to eliminate this disease by 2030. To endorse this strategy, Canada developed a specific set of 90-90-90 targets with the goal that by 2020, 90% of all people living with HIV know their status, 90% of those diagnosed receive antiretroviral treatment, and 90% of those on treatment achieve viral suppression. Prevention education is aimed at all sexually active individuals to counsel them about the hazards of unprotected sexual activity and on the effective use and limitations of condoms, stressing that they must be used properly and can fail. Condom failures occur at an estimated rate of 10% to 15%; therefore, counselling should stress that condom use is not foolproof. Another success is the decline in perinatal transmission. The rates of HIV perinatal transmission are greatly reduced by medication therapy during pregnancy, changes in obstetric practice, and prohibition of breastfeeding in infected mothers. In 2018, the SOGC highly recommended voluntary testing for HIV and counselling as a part of basic prenatal care (Loutfy, Kennedy, Poliquin, et al., 2018).

The nurse's role in intervening with regard to STIs includes providing treatment, early diagnosis, and education. When an individual is suspected of having an STI, the nurse obtains a complete history, including sexual history, sexual contacts, previous treatment and test results, any signs or symptoms of a current infection, recent use of antibiotics, and allergic reactions to antibiotics. When treatment is required, the nurse ensures that the person understands the goals of treatment in an attempt to gain cooperation, including follow-up care with partners and adherence to the care plan. Appropriate health education for the individual with an STI also includes the mode of transmission, incubation periods, signs and symptoms, methods of treatment, complications resulting from lack of treatment, and signs of recurrent infections.

## ◆ Coping–Stress Tolerance Pattern

### Assessment of Stress Levels

Stress, the result of forces operating on the individual that disrupt physiological or psychological equilibrium, is an integral part of young adulthood; therefore, a comprehensive health assessment should include questions to determine stress levels. Anxiety, nervousness, depression, or somatic complaints are indicators of stress, as are events such as divorce, loss of employment, failure to be promoted, or financial difficulties. The role of the nurse is to listen, offer support, and demonstrate concern. The nurse also suggests referrals to appropriate health providers and support groups.

### Achievement-Oriented Stress

Achievement-oriented stress differs from the stress of situational crises in that the stress of an overachiever is derived from internal pressures to succeed as measured by self-defined goals.

## TABLE 16.3    Summary of Selected Sexually Transmitted Infections (STIs)

| Infections | Causative Agent | Diagnostic Methods | Treatment | Risks or Complications | Nursing Teaching |
|---|---|---|---|---|---|
| Viral diseases | Treatment does not eradicate underlying infection | | | | |
| AIDS | HIV | Enzyme immune assay, Western blot, viral tests | Current recommendations | Opportunistic infections, perinatal transmission | Monitor CD4 T-lymphocyte analysis and HIV plasma viral load, monitor men who have sex with men, early pregnancy testing strongly recommended |
| Hepatitis B | Hepatitis B virus | Hepatitis B antibody test | No specific therapy available | Perinatal transmission | Routine vaccination or vaccine before pregnancy |
| Genital herpes | Herpes simplex virus | Herpes simplex virus antibody test, culture, viral test | Acyclovir at first diagnosis or episode | Urethral stricture, lymph node enlargement | Examine partners, abstain from sex while symptomatic |
| Genital warts | Human papilloma virus | Clinical inspection, colposcopy, biopsy | Podophyllin, trichloroacetic acid, cryotherapy/laser, valacyclovir, famciclovir | Cervical dysplasia, cervical cancer | Offer Gardasil or Cervarix vaccine and counselling, return for treatment as necessary, treat partner |
| **Bacterial/Other STIs** | | | | | |
| Gonorrhea | *Neisseria gonorrhoeae* | Culture | Ceftriaxone, cefixime, some strains becoming resistant | PID, infertility, ectopic pregnancy | Monitor antibiotic treatment, examine partner, repeat culture, check for chlamydia |
| Syphilis | *Treponema pallidum* | Fluorescent antibody tests of lesion or exudates, VDRL, RPR | Benzathine penicillin G | Secondary/late syphilis | Monitor treatment, test and monitor partner |
| Chlamydia | *Chlamydia trachomatis* | Culture, chlamydia monoclonal antibody test | Azithromycin, doxycycline | Infertility, ectopic pregnancy, urethral scarring, PID, endocervicitis, neonatal infection | Refer partners for evaluation, condoms to prevent future infection |
| Bacterial vaginosis | *Gardnerella vaginalis* | Clinical criteria, wet mount (clue cells) | Metronidazole (Flagyl) | Asymptomatic infection | Sexual transmission not proven |
| Trichomoniasis | *Trichomonas vaginalis* | Trichomonas rapid test, culture (protozoa) | Metronidazole (Flagyl) | Recurrence, excoriation of genital area | Use condoms to prevent new infection |
| Vulvovaginal candidiasis | *Candida albicans*, non–*C. albicans* | Wet mount/potassium hydroxide test (hyphae and spores) | Antifungal medication: butoconazole, miconazole, clotrimazole | Recurrence of disease | Reduce moisture/heat in genital area, recheck in 14 days |

*PID*, Pelvic inflammatory disease; *RPR*, rapid plasma reagin (test); *VDRL*, Venereal Disease Research Laboratory (test).
Sources: Based on information from Health Canada. (2019). *Canadian guidelines on sexually transmitted infections*. Retrieved from https://www.canada.ca/en/public-health/services/infectious-diseases/sexual-health-sexually-transmitted-infections/canadian-guidelines/sexually-transmitted-infections.html; Perry, S., Hockenberry, M., Lowdermilk, D., et al. (2014). *Maternal-child nursing care* (5th ed.). St. Louis: Elsevier.

Among many other stressors, young adults are often engaged in higher education programs at the undergraduate or graduate level. Achievement-oriented stress frequently causes workaholic habits, including loss of sleep and omission of meals. When this behaviour becomes extreme, there can be serious physical and emotional consequences, such as nutrition problems or burnout, which, in turn, leads to severe emotional and physical exhaustion. Workaholic behaviours may not be perceived by the individual and may not be apparent until changes in body functions or behaviour occur. Young adults are generally health conscious and willing to alter personal lifestyles and behaviour patterns to reduce stress and become healthier.

### Suicide and Depression

Suicide is a leading cause of death among young adults. Young adults may be thought of as "young invincibles"; however, they are in an age group exposed to new stressors (Canadian Association for Suicide Prevention [CASP], 2018). Suicide occurs because many young adults are unable to cope with the pressures of adulthood. For some people, pressure arises when they are dealing with interpersonal conflicts such as marital problems, family discord, or the loss of a close relationship; for others, the precipitating event is a lack of personal resources, unemployment, or dissatisfaction with work or school. Many young adults try to solve their problems before the fatal incident but see no positive solutions; in many cases, a prior suicide attempt was a signal for help.

Suicide rates are higher for men than for women; males account for 75% of suicides in Canada (Statistics Canada, 2017d). However, more women are known to have depressive disorders and to unsuccessfully attempt suicide. Young adults are more likely as a group to attempt suicide than are older individuals, and professionals are more likely to attempt suicide than are nonprofessionals. Suicide is more common among single, widowed, and divorced individuals. Chronically ill young adult males may also be more at risk of depression than young adult females because social support systems are more robust within female relationship networks. Indigenous people have significantly higher rates of suicide and suicide ideation than non-Indigenous Canadians.

Nursing interventions are directed toward identifying behaviours in individuals who may be contemplating suicide. Presuicidal individuals also tend to exhibit impaired reality testing; feelings of hopelessness, helplessness, and rejection; impaired judgement and decision making; anxiety; weight loss; insomnia; or a radically changed affect. In addition to identifying presuicidal behaviours, the nurse also investigates relationship patterns to determine behaviours that are complicated by feelings of worthlessness and defeat. When the nurse identifies a young adult at risk of a suicide attempt, referrals to other professionals are indicated.

## ◆ Values-Beliefs Pattern

Young adults enter their 20s with habits, values, and beliefs acquired during childhood and adolescence. Many acquired habits foster continuance of practices that are hazardous to health and well-being in later life. Prevention is directed toward altering value and belief patterns that encourage poor health practices, and reorienting them toward those that support optimal health behaviours. Nursing care is more effective when the nurse can describe, discriminate, identify, and align value and belief patterns consistent with practices known to maximize health.

### Values Involved in Parenting

Parenthood is envisioned as an important developmental stage by most young adults; therefore, health-promotion and health-protection activities to ensure healthy offspring are crucial (see the Case Study and Care Plan at the end of this chapter). Genetic impairments or congenital defects caused by abnormal chromosomes are responsible for 4 to 6% of perinatal deaths (Perry et al., 2014). Tests are available for approximately 200 genetic diseases (Perry et al., 2014). Most of the genetic testing offered is for single-gene impairment to mothers and fathers who have a family history of genetic disease. Young adults with a genetic disease must make many important decisions; predicting the transmission of the disease to potential offspring is essential to future planning.

### Values Regarding Prenatal Diagnosis and Genetic Impairment

Extensive prenatal diagnostic procedures have been available since the mid-1960s. This capability has enabled the identification of high-risk pregnancies and requires the cooperation and education of child-bearing women and their partners, both of whom must provide accurate family health and obstetrical histories and comply with suggested screening and follow-up measures. Decisions about the advisability of reproduction are based on current information on genetics and known deleterious genetic factors.

The finding of a malformed or genetically impaired fetus may result in a parental decision to terminate the pregnancy. Genetic counselling is an important nursing intervention for young adults. A genetic specialist gives technical explanations of genetic disorders; however, nurses have a strong supportive role in helping young adults decide whether to have children or to carry through a pregnancy that is at risk.

## ❖ ENVIRONMENTAL PROCESSES

### ◆ Physical Agents

#### Ethnicity, Race, and Culture

The young adult whose ethnic background is different from that of the dominant culture may encounter prejudice and discrimination, which can occur because of differences in race, creed, language, attitudes, values, preferences, or behaviours. The young adult is susceptible to these prejudices at work, at school, in health care delivery systems, and in the community.

Race and ethnicity are closely connected to educational and work-related decisions, which subsequently affect the choice of residence. Many minority families live in substandard housing or crowded living spaces. A lifestyle on the margins, when combined with insufficient economic resources, frequently affects health. Poverty is more common among Indigenous families, which may often lead to unmet basic needs of food, clothing, and housing and, in turn, leads to decreased regard for health needs.

#### Accidents

Injuries are the leading cause of death in young adults and individuals younger than 34 years (Statistics Canada, 2019d). Motor vehicle accidents cause more fatalities than all other causes of death combined. Reducing speed limits contributes to lower fatality rates. All Canadian provinces and territories have seatbelt laws and require appropriate child safety seats for passengers under the age of 16 (Insurance Corporation of British Columbia [ICBC], 2019). Distracted driving, texting while driving, and cell phone use are the cause of many motor vehicle crashes. All provinces and territories have enacted legislation that limits the use of hand-held cell phones while driving. The continued high incidence of vehicle accidents in the young adult age group is related to accessibility of cars to young adults and peer pressure on driving behaviour; reckless driving and driving under the influence of alcohol and drugs are now viewed as closely connected to violent and abusive behaviour.

Accident-prevention education is an important part of young adult driving instruction. Most young licensed drivers have participated in driver education courses, and provinces have adopted a graduated driver licensing program. This is a staged program designed to help new drivers, regardless of age, acquire the knowledge and skill needed to safely operate a motor vehicle under a variety of driving conditions (Manitoba Public Insurance, 2019).

## ◆ Biological Agents

### Noise Pollution

Young adults are exposed to high levels of noise in occupational and recreational settings (concerts and nightclubs). Long-term exposure to loud noise is directly related to impaired hearing and can increase irritability and stress. Young adults can be exposed to noises in the work setting from industrial machinery and equipment. Although industrial exposure can be difficult to mitigate, many young adults worsen the situation through recreational exposure, by listening to music or music videos at excessively high decibel levels. Ear protection is necessary to prevent hearing disability. Recognition of hazards and corresponding appropriate preventive education are early nursing strategies for decreasing excessive noise exposure.

### Air Pollution

Motor vehicles are the largest source of air pollution; vehicles release tons of particles and noxious gases each year, most of which is either carbon monoxide or hydrocarbons. Carbon monoxide in high concentrations is deadly; in lower concentrations, it causes headaches, dizziness, and heart palpitations. In sunlight and low-lying areas, automobile exhaust becomes photochemical smog that contains ozone, which irritates the eyes and the respiratory tract. Although air pollution is not a problem only for young adults, they frequently work in dirty, entry-level jobs in industrial settings and may be among the age group that is most affected.

### Occupational Hazards and Stressors

Occupational hazards pose a threat of illness, injury, or death in all age groups, and occupational safety standards have contributed greatly to the reduction of work-related accidents. The 1986 Canadian *Occupational Health and Safety Act* (Department of Justice, 2019) has resulted in the improvement of work conditions, along with the provision of health care facilities, in many companies.

Young adults should not be allowed to work in certain industrial settings without vocational training to reduce hazards. Young adults frequently want a challenge and high wages; therefore, they work in hazardous jobs—for example, on offshore drilling rigs, on construction sites, or on high bridges. Because of their age, physical stamina, and agility, young adults are suitable candidates for positions that require extreme physical abilities. Occupational training should include education about personal exposure risks, identification of work-related hazards, and identification of situations in which the severity of accidents is connected to personal behaviors or habits. For example, drivers of heavy construction machinery should be particularly observant, avoid reckless behaviours, and avoid fast driving. Working women who are pregnant can expose their fetuses to industrial chemicals. Proper evaluation and temporary reassignment may be necessary.

Occupational preventive intervention requires that known work hazards and risks be identified early. Health histories should include questions about the place of work, type of work, and young adults' understanding of the risks associated with their occupations. Occupational risk and health are closely related; stress associated with work, the use of alcohol or drugs, and a negative attitude toward work are predictive of occupational injuries. Job counselling aimed at changing the nature of employment can be an appropriate referral for some people with health conditions. Nurses in occupational settings can provide periodic health assessments, updates of the health history, and counselling.

## ◆ Chemical Agents

### Drug Use

Canada continues to experience a serious opioid crisis, with devastating effects on families and communities. Misuse of opioids, such as morphine, fentanyl, oxycodone, and codeine, has emerged following a rise in opioid-related harms, including increased hospitalizations and deaths linked to overdose (Canadian Community Health Survey [CCHS], 2018). More female than male young adults had taken opioids (12% vs. 8%, respectively), while Indigenous people report a higher rate of use. However, opioids have an increased potential to be used in a nontherapeutic manner because of the associated psychoactive properties. Problematic use of opioids is defined as taking the medication in greater amounts than prescribed or more often than directed, intentionally taking the medication to get high to help cope with stress or other problems, or tampering with a product before taking it, such as crushing the tablet to swallow, snort, or inject. Of Canadians who regularly take opioids, 10% engaged in some problematic use of these substances. Problematic use is linked to injury, disability, criminal behaviour, suicide, addiction and death.

Mental health disorders frequently co-occur with problematic use of opioids (CCHS, 2018). In 2017, 17 adults were hospitalized daily for opioid poisoning, an increase of 27% since 2013. Between 2016 and 2018, an estimated 10,300 Canadians died from opioid overdose, with the majority occurring in the 20–39 age group. Fentanyl was the opioid responsible for most deaths, and 75% of deaths were accidental or non-intentional. Injecting opioid is also linked to HIV or hepatitis infection. The highest rate of increase for opioid poisonings occurred in community hospitals rather than large, urban centres (Canadian Institute for Health Information [CIHI], 2018).

Concerned with the rise in overdose death, Health Canada (2019c) has recommended a comprehensive, multipronged strategy to address the opioid crisis, including addressing drug safety, monitoring and optimal prescribing, access to pain management and addiction services, as well as public and professional education. The opioid crisis has also lead to consideration of radical community interventions, such as safe consumption sites and take-home naloxone to reverse the effects of opioids (CIHI, 2018). Nursing activities include preventive strategies to curb the problem of drug misuse. Distribution of current drug literature, early treatment of complications, public access to non-prescription naloxone, and information regarding drug treatment centres are only part of the answer.

## Alcohol Use

In 2017, Canadian Centre on Substance Use and Addiction (CCSA) reported that 83% of young adults consumed alcohol at least once during the past year. The highest rate of drinking for males was among those aged 25 to 34 (91%) and for females aged 18 to 24 (92%). Binge alcohol consumption (i.e., having five or more drinks in one sitting) is becoming more common in the young adult population. Male and female young adults (aged 18 to 24) are more likely to report heavy drinking than adults over the age of 25 (80% versus 63% for males, and 77% versus 49% for females) (CCSA, 2017). Alcohol use and misuse play a contributing role to the development of diabetes, cancers of the oral cavity, colon, and esophagus, ischemic heart disease, and liver cirrhosis. In 2016, 57,000 hospitalizations were due to a condition entirely caused by alcohol. Alcohol-related accidents among individuals aged 18 to 24 years continue to be a leading cause of preventable morbidity, disability, and death (CCSA, 2017). All provinces and territories have set a maximum blood alcohol concentration of 0.08% for driving. Modifying alcohol consumption in young adults can decrease the frequency of chronic and disabling conditions in later life.

## Tobacco Use

Smoking is a leading cause of preventable death in Canada; therefore, smoking cessation is the single most important counselling topic for all people because of its potential to lower the risk of contracting many preventable diseases. Cigarette smoking rates have declined to 16% for Canadians aged 20 to 24, and 18% for individuals aged 25 to 34 (Reid, Hammond, Tariq, et al., 2019). More than one half of smokers aged 20 to 24 intend to quit in the next 6 months, while 48% of smokers aged 25 to 34 intend to quit during this time period. In 2017, 16% of young adults had successfully quit smoking in the previous year. Regarding e-cigarette use, 29% of adults aged 20 to 24 and 26% of those aged 25 to 34 reported trying an e-cigarette. However, less than 1% of Canadian adults were daily users. Most adults used them in an attempt to quit smoking with limited success. Less than 2% of adults have used alternative tobacco products, such as cigarillos, cigars, waterpipes, or snuff.

Individuals employed in high-risk occupations (e.g., mining, construction) are informed of the synergistic relationship between smoking and other environmental exposures, including exposure to asbestos, coal dust, and radiation. Fear tactics, nagging, preaching, and threats are generally ineffective in convincing people to stop smoking. A major barrier to smoking cessation is the presence of other smokers, particularly in situations where alcohol is also being consumed. Tobacco control measures are strongly correlated with smoking cessation rates of young adults (Health Canada, 2018a). Nurses are familiar with the antismoking resources in their communities, enabling them to make the appropriate referrals.

## Cannabis Use

As of October 17, 2018, Canada became the second country in the world to legalize the nonmedical use of cannabis for adults (Statistics Canada, 2019e). Impacts of legalization on the use of cannabis in Canada remain uncertain because the Cannabis Act has been in place only for a short period of time and because the framework for legalization makes comparisons to other jurisdictions difficult due to varying regional access, different provincial/territorial retail sales models, and restrictions on product type of potency. During 2019, 27% of Canadians aged 15 to 24 while approximately 30% for individuals aged 25 to 44 used cannibus (Statistics Canada, 2019e). Not much is currently known about the specific type of cannabis products being consumed. Consequently, emergent literature suggests that quantity may be a better predictor of cannabis-related harms than frequency. This, in turn, could have public health policy implications for health, health care service use, revenues, and crime.

## ❖ DETERMINANTS OF HEALTH

### ◆ Social Factors and Environment
#### Neighbourhood Resources

The environment of the community strongly influences the well-being of the young adult and sets the standard for the health of people and families living within a neighbourhood. Neighbours can be an excellent source of support, which can be especially important to a young mother who does not have immediate family nearby. Nurses working in community settings facilitate the contact of individuals with common interests through community activities and support groups. Community resources for exercise and recreation can make important contributions to the young adult's physical and emotional health. When these resources are available, the young adult can have the opportunity to exercise and release stress in a positive fashion.

### ◆ Levels of Policymaking and Health

Young adults comprise a major political constituency in Canada, as seen in their involvement in recent federal elections; 69% of 15 to 24 years olds are members of a group, organization or association, while 42% of adults aged 20 to 34 volunteer, and 81% say they financially support a charitable or nonprofit organization (Statistics Canada, 2018a). Some public policy issues are unemployment, sustainability, pollution, the environment, and war. Through these efforts, young adults can influence and improve living conditions for future generations.

One of the young adult's age-related tasks is to choose and develop a lifelong career. This choice is directly related to economic factors; young adults want satisfying occupations that also yield adequate economic returns. To manage financially and maintain a lifestyle in which personal needs can be met, young adults may elect to have fewer children. Caring for aging parents can also cause physical, psychosocial, spiritual, and economic stress.

Although goals differ greatly among young adult couples, they are generally concerned with acquiring material comforts; the desire for housing, transportation, clothing, or recreation generally necessitates that both partners are employed to meet financial obligations. This desire necessitates the changing of roles and the sharing of responsibilities, and open communication becomes a crucial component.

Because of the high cost of housing, many young adults have multiple roommates, creating additional demands and health risks.

For many young adult couples, problems of unemployment for one or both, different careers, friends, and differing maturity levels place additional strains on their relationship. These circumstances can provide a basis for domestic difficulty. Domestic arguments can precede family disruption, leading to marital separation or divorce. In addition to the emotional strain placed on family members, domestic arguments can result in aggressive acts of abuse and personal injury. Young adults can also be faced with decisions about day care facilities; the couple or mother may need support to resolve guilt feelings related to the separation from the child. Some young adults may also bear responsibilities for caring for aging parents or relatives.

Lifestyles may also include living arrangements with individuals of the same sex or the opposite sex. Although these lifestyles are becoming more acceptable in today's society, attitudes toward varied lifestyles contribute pressures that lead to further stress and uncertainty.

### ◆ Health Services/Delivery System

For Indigenous people, recent immigrants, disabled, or LGBTQ2 Canadians, health services may be lacking or, when available, are not culturally sensitive or adapted to the customs and beliefs of the people who are served. Access to public transportation can be a critical problem, affecting the ability of the young adult to keep appointments.

Health delivery methods in Canada are based primarily on Western belief systems, which tend to be rigid in their applications. For example, women seeking birth control information and prescriptions are expected to use health clinics and adhere to a set schedule of return visits. Nurses need to be able to identify health practices and health system gaps that are barriers to care and harmful to people.

However, nurses may not be able to deliver care optimally within changing health care settings because of barriers to practice and ineffective workforce planning, data, and information infrastructure. The Canadian Nurses Association (CNA, 2019) strongly promotes active involvement of nursing expertise when decision makers are considering changes or reforms to health policy. The nursing profession cannot contribute optimally unless nurses fully participate in team planning and health care redesign with government, health care organizations, and other health care providers. (see the Case Study and Care Plan at the end of this chapter).

### ❖ NURSING APPLICATION

Young adulthood is generally considered to be the most healthful period of life. In terms of physical changes, growth is complete by this stage. The physical abilities of the young adult are in peak condition, so the goals of the nurse are aimed at maintaining optimal physical condition, encouraging healthy habits, screening individuals for disease, and treating illnesses. Health examinations at recommended intervals are a crucial component of screening individuals for potential health concerns and providing education about measures to avoid disease and disability.

It is necessary to screen individuals for cardiovascular conditions after the age of 25 years as well as to provide education about risk factor modification. Intervention efforts should reflect diversity of age, sex, ethnicity, and socioeconomic status. As the nurse obtains an assessment of the individual and family history, the necessity of further screening, education, or monitoring is determined. Elements of education include smoking cessation and dietary modifications.

Young adults are encouraged to engage in physical activity and muscle-strengthening exercise. Lack of time or lack of access may be barriers to increased physical activity. The nurse working with the young adult population should consider implementing work-site wellness programs. Group fitness or weight-loss programs can be an effective means of promoting wellness at work while increasing employee satisfaction and productivity. Some companies encourage the formation of facility-sponsored sports teams for charities or sports such as bowling leagues, hockey teams, or a running club. This encourages camaraderie among colleagues and increases participation for people who respond well to group motivation. Nonworking young adults looking for a group fitness or sports program should be directed to resources within the community via Internet research.

The nurse working with young adults provides education about skin cancer risk, the need for adequate sunscreen, and signs and symptoms of skin cancer. Safety education is provided about recreational and sports-related injuries and how to prevent them. Additional education is required for both young males and females for contraception and prevention of STIs and HIV infection. It is imperative that women receive preconceptional and early prenatal care to maintain optimal health for themselves and the unborn child.

The nurse working with the young adult population often becomes a counsellor. It is important to assess stressors, as prolonged stress, anxiety, or depression can negatively affect the health of the individual. Stressors may be related to relationships, divorce, employment, layoffs, or financial concerns. The nurse listens, offers support and concern, and provides the individual or family with resources or support groups specific to the stressor.

In order to make safe and effective judgements using the nursing diagnoses, it is essential that nurses understand defining characteristics of the nursing diagnoses to focus on goals, interventions, and effective outcomes.

## CASE STUDY

### Preparing for Child-bearing: Kirsten

Kirsten is a healthy 24-year-old woman whose favourite sport is running. Most of the time she runs outside, but she also uses gym treadmills. Since this spring, Kirsten has believed that her breathing capacity is diminishing and her levels of energy are decreasing. During her period these symptoms appear to worsen. Last week, while running up a rather steep course, Kirsten became much weaker, dizzier, and more fatigued than usual, and her best friend and running partner recommended that she make a health care provider's appointment for a physical examination. Kirsten's running partner also noted that she has appeared pale lately.

In the health care provider's office, Kirsten is noted to have a normal temperature, elevated heart and respiratory rates, and a BP of 90/60 mm Hg. Kirsten's description of her period is that it tends to be heavy and has been this way for 5 years. For muscle aches and pains caused by running, she usually takes two aspirin tablets every 3 to 4 hours for as long as 7 days. When her running increases during the summer, she takes aspirin or ibuprofen continually for 2 to 3 months. Diagnostic testing indicates that her hemoglobin level is 70 g/L, and her red blood cells are pale and small. Kirsten has been in a long-term relationship for several years, her wedding is in several months, and there has been discussion of preconceptional health planning and future children.

#### Reflective Questions
- What common health alteration in young adult women is most likely for Kirsten?
- What contributing factors place Kirsten at risk?
- What lifestyle modifications can Kirsten implement to decrease her risk?

## CARE PLAN

### Preparing for Child-bearing: Kirsten

#### Nursing Issue
Health-seeking needs resulting from preconceptional assessment and preparation for child-bearing

#### Defining Characteristics
- Expressed desire to improve overall health to prepare for child-bearing
- Expressed thoughts about planning for pregnancy soon
- Desire to improve nutritional status before child-bearing
- Desire to improve nutritional intake of essential vitamins and minerals (iron and calcium)
- Plan to take a multivitamin each day
- Plan to limit consumption of foods high in sodium and fat
- Plan to limit alcohol consumption
- Plan for exercise program to increase stamina and flexibility
- Seeks physical examination to rule out problems that might negatively affect pregnancy
- Seeks information on pregnancy risk factors (biophysical, psychosocial, sociodemographic, and environmental)

#### Related Factors
- Expressed desire to improve the quality of relationship with husband or partner
- Desire to attend education classes to improve knowledge of child-bearing and positive health practices
- Plan for room or housing for a young couple that might accommodate children in the future
- Plan for employment arrangements that accommodate child care

#### Expected Outcomes
- Increase in indices of well-being in person
- Healthy pregnancy and future child
- Increase in self-confidence and awareness preparation for child-bearing
- Management of pregnancy risk factors before becoming pregnant
- Making the person aware of resources available for pregnancy and child care

#### Interventions
- Assess current level of wellness regarding preparation for child-bearing.
- Identify community resources that provide information regarding preconceptional planning and preparation.
- Identify primary health provider, midwife, or obstetrician, and hospitals with delivery services.
- Assess biophysical risk factors (genetic–genomic disorders, nutrition problems, and current medical problems).
- Assess for history of pregnancy loss.
- Test for blood type and rhesus (Rh) factor.
- Screen for STI, tuberculosis, rubella titre, sickle cell trait.
- Review immunization status.
- Assess need to augment diet, particularly to increase intake of calcium and iron.
- Take a multivitamin daily.
- Assess for psychosocial risk factors (mental health disorders; use of drugs, alcohol, and caffeine; and smoking).
- Counsel to avoid alcohol consumption.
- Assess for possible sociodemographic risk factors (poverty, first pregnancy risks of dystocia or pregnancy-induced hypertension, residence [rural or urban], and ethnicity).
- Assess for environmental risks (exposures to chemicals, medications, pesticides, pollution, smoke, stress, and radiation).
- Assess current employment situation.
- Identify child care arrangements.

From Gordon, M. (2016). *Manual of nursing diagnosis* (13th ed.). Burlington, MA: Jones & Bartlett Learning.

## SUMMARY

Nurses promote health care measures and behaviours at all places where young adults come into contact with the health care delivery system. In community college and university settings, efforts can be directed toward health-education curricula, with an emphasis on implementation of positive health behaviours, use of appropriate social networking skills, establishment of peer counselling groups, and better utilization of sports and exercise facilities. Workshops on alcoholism, substance abuse, sports or exercise, mental health and self-expression, relationships, and various aspects of sexual care are effective in postsecondary school populations. At the work site, the occupational nurse is involved with employee counselling, BP monitoring and treatment, exercise recommendations, smoking reduction, lifestyle modifications, and stress-reduction techniques. Preventive care, mental health, dental health, and maternity and infertility benefits are being analyzed when necessary. Young adults are generally healthy, which challenges the nurse to be even more creative, sensitive, and insightful in implementing care for individuals within this age group.

**Evolve Chapter Features**

hhttp://evolve.elsevier.com/Canada/Edelman/healthpromotion/

- Review Questions

## REFERENCES

Anderson, T. J., Grégoire, J., Pearson, G. J., et al. (2016). Canadian Cardiovascular Society guidelines for the management for the prevention of cardiovascular disease in the adult. *Canadian Journal of Cardiology, 32*(11), 1263–1282. https://doi.org/10.1016/j.cjca.2016.07.510.

Arnold, A. (2018). *Millennials and healthy living: It's about online content, not doctor's visits.* Retrieved from https://www.forbes.com/sites/andrewarnold/2018/02/25/millennials-and-healthy-living-its-about-online-content-not-doctors-visits/#2ea96d9432f2.

Black, A., Guilbert, E., Costescu, D., et al. (2015). Canadian contraception consensus. *Journal of Obstetrics and Gynaecology Canada, 37*(10), 936–938. https://doi.org/10.1016/S1701-2163(16)30033-0.

Canadian Association for Suicide Prevention (CASP). (2019). *About suicide and life promotion.* Retrieved from https://suicideprevention.ca/page-18154.

Canadian Cancer Society. (2019). *Finding testicular cancer early.* Retrieved from https://www.cancer.ca/en/cancer-information/cancer-type/testicular/finding-cancer-early/?region=on.

Canadian Centre on Substance Use and Addiction (CCSA). (2017). *Alcohol (Canadian drug summary).* Retrieved from https://www.ccsa.ca/alcohol-canadian-drug-summary.

Canadian Community Health Survey (CCHS). (2018). *Pain medication containing opioids.* Retrieved from https://www150.statcan.gc.ca/n1/pub/82-625-x/2019001/article/00008-eng.htm.

Canadian Diabetes Association (CDA). (2018). *Guidelines for type II diabetes and Indigenous care.* Retrieved from https://guidelines.diabetes.ca/cpg/chapter38.

Canadian Heart and Stroke Foundation (CHSF). (2019). *#TimetoSeeRed.* Retrieved from https://www.heartandstroke.ca/women.

Canadian Institute for Health Information (CIHI). (2018). *Smaller communities feeling impact of opioid crisis in Canada.* Retrieved from https://www.cihi.ca/en/opioids-in-canada/2018/opioid-related-harms-in-canada/smaller-communities-feeling-impact-of-opioid-crisis-in-canada.

Canadian Nurses Association (CNA). (2019). *Policy support resources.* Retrieved from https://www.cna-aiic.ca/en/policy-advocacy/policy-support-resources.

Canada Safety Council. (2018). *Sports safety.* Retrieved from https://canadasafetycouncil.org/?s=sportshttps://canadasafetycouncil.org/?s=sports.

Canadian Society for Exercise Physiology (CSEP). (2019). *About CSEP.* Retrieved from https://www.csep.ca/home.

Canadian Sudden Arrhythmia Death Syndrome Foundation (CSADSF). (2019). *Who we are.* Retrieved from https://www.canadianwomen.org/the-facts/gender-based-violence/.

Canadian Task Force on Preventive Health Care. (2017). *Annual check-ups not recommended.* Retrieved from https://canadiantaskforce.ca/annual-checkups-do-not-result-in-better-health-outcomes-national-task-force-reaffirms/.

Canadian Task Force on Preventive Health Care. (2018). *Breast cancer update.* Retrieved from https://canadiantaskforce.ca/guidelines/published-guidelines/breast-cancer-update/.

Canadian Women's Foundation. (2019). *The facts about gender-based violence.* Retrieved from https://www.canadianwomen.org/the-facts/gender-based-violence/.

Chiu, M., Austin, P. C., Manuel, D. G., et al. (2012). Cardiovascular risk factor profiles of recent immigrants vs. long-term residents of Ontario: A multi-ethnic study. *Canadian Journal of Cardiology, 28*(1), 20–26. https://doi.org/10.1016/j.cjca.2011.06.002.

Creatore, M. I., Moineddin, R., Booth, G., et al. (2010). Age- and sex-related prevalence of diabetes mellitus among immigrants to Ontario, Canada. *Canadian Medical Association Journal, 182*(8), 781–789. https://doi.org/10.1503/cmaj.091551.

Department of Justice. (2019). *Canadian Occupational Health and Safety Regulations.* Retrieved from https://laws-lois.justice.gc.ca/eng/regulations/sor-86-304/index.html.

Edkins, T., Edgerton, J. D., & Roberts, L. W. (2017). Correlates of binge drinking in a sample of Canadian university students. *International Journal of Child, Youth, & Family Studies, 8*(1), 112–144. https://doi.org/10.18357/ijcyfs81201716944.

Employment and Social Development Canada. (2017). *Employment insurance monitoring and assessment 2016–2017.* Retrieved from https://www.canada.ca/en/employment-social-development/programs/ei/ei-list/reports/monitoring2017/chapter1.html.

Employment and Social Development Canada. (2018). *The way Canadians work has changed.* Retrieved from https://www.canada.ca/en/employment-social-development/news/2018/08/what-we-heard-the-way-canadians-work-has-changed.html.

Employment and Social Development Canada. (2019). *Work standards.* Retrieved from https://www.canada.ca/en/services/jobs/workplace.html.

Erikson, E. H. (1993). *Childhood and society.* New York: W. W. Norton. [Seminal Reference].

First Nations Information Governance Centre (FNIGC). (2019). *FNIGC data online.* Retrieved from http://fnigc.ca/dataonline/.

Gatrix, J., Plitt, S., Turnbull, L., et al. (2017). Prevalence and antibiotic resistance of Mycoplasma genitalium among STI clinic attendees in Western Canada: A cross-sectional analysis. *BMJ Open, 7,* e016300. https://doi.org/10.1136/bmjopen-2017-016300.

Government of Canada. (2017). *Preventing and managing chronic disease in First Nations communities: A guidance framework.* Retrieved from http://publications.gc.ca/site/eng/9.840825/publication.html.

Health Canada. (2016). *Canadian guidelines for body weight classification in adults.* Retrieved from https://www.canada.ca/en/health-canada/services/food-nutrition/healthy-eating/healthy-weights/canadian-guidelines-body-weight-classification-adults/quick-reference-tool-professionals.html.

Health Canada. (2017a). *How healthy are Canadians?* Retrieved from https://www.canada.ca/en/public-health/services/publications/healthy-living/how-healthy-canadians.html.

Health Canada. (2017b). *Human papilloma virus.* Retrieved from https://www.canada.ca/en/public-health/services/diseases/human-papillomavirus-hpv.html.

Health Canada. (2017c). *Stay sun safe.* Retrieved from https://www.canada.ca/en/health-canada/services/publications/healthy-living/sun-safety-infographic.html.

Health Canada. (2017d). *Report on sexually transmitted infections in Canada: 2013–2014.* Retrieved from https://www.canada.ca/en/public-health/services/publications/diseases-conditions/report-sexually-transmitted-infections-canada-2013-14.html#s3.

Health Canada. (2018a). *Report from the Canadian Chronic Disease Surveillance System: Health disease in Canada, 2018.* Retrieved from https://www.canada.ca/en/public-health/services/publications/diseases-conditions/report-heart-disease-Canada-2018.html#s2-3.

Health Canada. (2018b). *Canadian immunization guide part 3: Vaccination of specific populations.* Retrieved from https://www.canada.ca/en/public-health/services/publications/healthy-living/canadian-immunization-guide-part-3-vaccination-specific-populations/page-2-immunization-of-adults.html.

Health Canada. (2018c). *Folic acid and neural tube defects.* Retrieved from https://www.canada.ca/en/public-health/services/pregnancy/folic-acid.html.

Health Canada. (2019a). *Hepatitis C.* Retrieved from https://www.canada.ca/en/public-health/services/diseases/hepatitis-c/health-professionals-hepatitis-c.html.

Health Canada. (2019b). *Nutrition and healthy eating.* Retrieved from https://www.canada.ca/en/health-canada/services/food-nutrition/healthy-eating.html.

Health Canada. (2019c). *Responding to Canada's opioid crisis.* Retrieved from https://www.canada.ca/en/health-canada/services/substance-use/problematic-prescription-drug-use/opioids/responding-canada-opioid-crisis.html.

Hypertension Canada. (2018). *Hypertension guidelines for adults and children, 2018.* Retrieved from https://guidelines.hypertension.ca/chep-resources/.

Insurance Corporation of British Columbia (ICBC). (2019). *Road safety.* Retrieved from https://www.icbc.com/road-safety/safer-drivers/Pages/Seatbelts.aspx.

Kohlberg, L., & Lickons, T. (1986). *The stages of ethical development: From childhood through old age.* San Francisco: Harper. [Seminal Reference].

Kolahdooz, F., Sadeghirad, B., Corriveau, A., et al. (2017). Prevalence of overweight and obesity among Indigenous populations in Canada: A systematic review and meta-analysis. *Critical Reviews in Food Science and Nutrition, 57*(7), 1316–1327. https://doi.org/10.1080/10408398.2014.913003.

Library of Parliament. (2005). *Bill C-38: Civil Marriage Act.* Retrieved from https://lop.parl.ca/sites/PublicWebsite/default/en_CA/ResearchPublications/LegislativeSummaries/381LS502E. [Seminal Reference].

Liu, Q., Quan, H., Chen, G., et al. (2014). Antihypertensive medication adherence and mortality according to ethnicity: A cohort study. *Canadian Journal of Cardiology, 30*(8), 925–931. https://doi.org/10.1016/j.cjca.2014.04.017.

Loutfy, M., Kennedy, V. L., Poliquin, V., et al. (2018). No. 354—Canadian HIV pregnancy planning guidelines. *Journal of Obstetrics and Gynaecology Canada, 40*(1), 94–114. https://doi.org/10.1016/j.jogc.2017.06.033.

Manitoba Public Insurance. (2019). *Graduated driver licensing.* Retrieved from https://www.mpi.mb.ca/Pages/graduated-driver-licensing.aspx.

Metabolic Syndrome Canada. (2019). *About metabolic syndrome.* Retrieved from https://www.metabolicsyndromecanada.ca/about-metabolic-syndrome.

Motluk, A. (2016). Birth control often not covered by Canadian insurers. *Canadian Medical Association Journal, 188*(14), 1001–1002. https://doi.org/10.1503/cmaj.109-5313.

Neinstein, L. (2013). *The new adolescents: An analysis of health conditions, behaviors, risks, and access to services among emerging young adults.* Retrieved from https://eshc.usc.edu/thenewadolescents/doc/TheNewAdolescents_Final_Locked.pdf.

Noam, A., Bernstein, M., Boucher, F., et al. (2016). Folate and neural tube defects: The role of supplements and food fortification. *Paediatrics & Child Health, 21*(3), 145–149. https://doi.org/10.1093/pch/21.3.145.

Obesity Canada. (2019). *About Obesity Canada.* Retrieved from https://obesitycanada.ca/.

Ontario Bariatric Network. (2015). *Bariatric surgery program.* Retrieved from http://www.ontariobariatricnetwork.ca/our-programs/surgical-program.

Parachute Canada. (2019). *After a concussion: Guidelines for return to play.* Retrieved from http://www.parachutecanada.org/downloads/resources/return-to-play-guidelines.pdf.

Pay Equity Commission. (2019). *An overview of pay equity in various Canadian jurisdictions 2018.* Retrieved from http://www.payequity.gov.on.ca/en/GWG/Pages/overview_pe.aspx.

Perry, S., Hockenberry, M., Lowdermilk, D., et al. (2014). *Maternal-child nursing care* (5th ed.). St. Louis: Elsevier.

Piaget, J. (1972). Intellectual evolution from adolescence to adulthood. *Human Development, 15*, 1–12. [Seminal Reference].

Public Health Agency of Canada (PHAC). (2011). *Hepatitis B: An overview.* Retrieved from https://www.canada.ca/en/public-health/services/infectious-diseases/hepatitis-b-infection-canada.html.

Public Health Agency of Canada (PHAC). (2014). *Diabetes in Canada: Facts and figures from a public health perspective—A health impact.* Retrieved from https://www.canada.ca/en/public-health/services/chronic-diseases/reports-publications/diabetes/diabetes-canada-facts-figures-a-public-health-perspective/chapter-2.html.

Public Health Agency of Canada (PHAC). (2017). *Preconception care.* Retrieved from https://www.canada.ca/en/public-health/services/publications/healthy-living/maternity-newborn-care-guidelines-chapter-2.html#a2.

Public Health Agency of Canada (PHAC). (2018a). *The time is now to eliminate TB in Canada.* Retrieved from https://www.canada.ca/en/public-health/corporate/publications/chief-public-health-officer-reports-state-public-health-canada/eliminating-tuberculosis.html.

Public Health Agency of Canada (PHAC). (2018b). *Hepatitis C: An overview.* Retrieved from https://www.canada.ca/en/public-health/services/reports-publications/canada-communicable-disease-report-ccdr/monthly-issue/2018-44/issue-7-8-july-5-2018/article-7-hepatitis-c-canada-2018-infographic.html.

Public Health Agency of Canada (PHAC). (2018c). *Family violence: How big is the problem in Canada?* Retrieved from https://www.canada.ca/en/public-health/services/health-promotion/stop-family-violence/problem-canada.html.

Public Health Agency of Canada (PHAC). (2019a). *Fertility.* Retrieved from https://www.canada.ca/en/public-health/services/fertility/fertility.html.

Public Health Agency of Canada (PHAC). (2019b). *Summary: Estimates of HIV incidence, prevalence, and Canada's progress on meeting the 90-90-90 HIV targets, 2016.* Retrieved from https://www.canada.ca/en/public-health/services/publications/diseases-conditions/summary-estimates-hiv-incidence-prevalence-canadas-progress-90-90-90.html.

Quinlan, E., Quinlan, A., Fogel, C., et al. (2017). *Sexual violence at Canadian universities: Activism, institutional responses, and strategies for change.* Waterloo: Wilfrid Laurier University Press.

Reid, J. L., Hammond, D., Tariq, U., et al. (2019). *Tobacco use in Canada: Patterns and trends* (2019 Ed.). Waterloo, ON: Propel Centre for Population Health Impact, University of Waterloo. Retrieved from https://uwaterloo.ca/tobacco-use-canada/tobacco-use-canada-patterns-and-trends.

Ridley, J., Ischayek, A., Dubey, V., et al. (2016). Adult health checkup: Update on the Preventive Care Checklist Form®. *Canadian Family Physician, 62*(2), 307–313.

Rosella, L. C., Lebenbaum, M., Fitzpatrick, T., et al. (2015). Prevalence of prediabetes and undiagnosed diabetes in Canada (2007–2011) according to the fasting plasma glucose and $HBA_{1C}$ screening criteria. *Diabetes Care, 38*(7), 1299–1305. https://doi.org/10.2337/dc14-2474.

Slater, J., Epp-Koop, S., Jakilazek, M., et al. (2017). Food deserts in Winnipeg, Canada: A novel method for measuring a complex and contested construct. *Health Promotion and Chronic Disease Prevention in Canada, 37*(10), 350–356. https://doi.org/10.24095/hpcdp.37.10.05.

Society of Obstetricians and Gynaecologists of Canada (SOGC). (2019). *Your pregnancy: Special considerations.* Retrieved from https://www.pregnancyinfo.ca/your-pregnancy/special-consideration/unintended-pregnancy/.

Statistics Canada. (2015a). *Leading causes of death in Canada 2015.* Retrieved from https://www150.statcan.gc.ca/n1/pub/84-215-x/2012001/table-tableau/tbl003-eng.htm.

Statistics Canada. (2015b). *Same-sex couples and sexual orientation by the numbers.* Retrieved from https://www.statcan.gc.ca/eng/dai/smr08/2015/smr08_203_2015#a3.

Statistics Canada. (2015c). *Lone-parent families.* Retrieved from https://www150.statcan.gc.ca/n1/pub/75-006-x/2015001/article/14202/parent-eng.htm.

Statistics Canada. (2017a). *Causes of death in Canada 2017.* Retrieved from https://www150.statcan.gc.ca/n1/daily-quotidien/190530/dq190530c-eng.htm.

Statistics Canada. (2017b). *Projected life expectancy at birth by Aboriginal identity.* Retrieved from https://www150.statcan.gc.ca/n1/pub/89-645-x/2010001/life-expectancy-esperance-vie-eng.htm.

Statistics Canada. (2017c). *Health reports: Cycling in Canada.* Retrieved from https://www150.statcan.gc.ca/n1/pub/82-003-x/2017004/article/14788-eng.htm.

Statistics Canada. (2017d). *Suicide: An overview.* Retrieved from https://www150.statcan.gc.ca/n1/pub/82-624-x/2012001/article/11696-eng.htm.

Statistics Canada. (2018a). *A portrait of Canadian youth.* Retrieved from https://www150.statcan.gc.ca/n1/pub/11-631-x/11-631-x2018001-eng.htm.

Statistics Canada. (2018b). *Health-related life-expectancy in Canada.* Retrieved from https://www150.statcan.gc.ca/n1/pub/82-003-x/2018004/article/54950-eng.htm.

Statistics Canada. (2018c). *Obesity in Canada.* Retrieved from Canadian Community Health Survey https://www150.statcan.gc.ca/n1/pub/11-627-m/11-627-m2018033-eng.htm.

Statistics Canada. (2018d). *The gender wage gap and equal pay day 2018.* Retrieved from https://www150.statcan.gc.ca/n1/pub/89-28-0001/2018001/article/00010-eng.htm.

Statistics Canada. (2019a). *High blood pressure.* Retrieved from https://www150.statcan.gc.ca/t1/tbl1/en/tv.action?pid=1310009609.

Statistics Canada. (2019b). *Tracking physical activity levels of Canadians.* Retrieved from https://www150.statcan.gc.ca/n1/daily-quotidien/190417/dq190417g-eng.htm.

Statistics Canada. (2019c). *Divorce rates by year of marriage.* Retrieved from https://www150.statcan.gc.ca/t1/tbl1/en/tv.action?pid=3910002801.

Statistics Canada. (2019d). *Death and age-specific mortality rates.* Retrieved from https://www150.statcan.gc.ca/t1/tbl1/en/tv.action?pid=1310039201&pickMembers%5B0%5D=2.9&pickMembers%5B1%5D=3.1.

Statistics Canada. (2019e). *Analysis of trends in the prevalence of cannabis use and related metrics in Canada.* Retrieved from https://www150.statcan.gc.ca/n1/pub/82-003-x/2019006/article/00001-eng.htm.

Truth and Reconciliation Commission. (2015). *Honouring the truth: Reconciling for the future.* Retrieved from http://nctr.ca/reports.php.

Vanier Institute. (2019). *Lone mothers and their families in Canada.* Retrieved from https://vanierinstitute.ca/lone-mothers-families-canada-diverse-resilient-strong/.

Zacarés, J. J., Serra, E., & Torres, F. (2015). Becoming an adult: A proposed typology of adult status based on a study of Spanish youth. *Scandinavian Journal of Psychology, 56*(3). https://doi.org/10.1111/sjop.12205.

# 17

# Middle-Aged Adult

*Marti Harder, RN, MSN*

Originating US chapter by *Maureen Murphy, CNM, RN, MEd, MSN, PhD*

## INTENDED LEARNING OUTCOMES

*After completing this chapter, the reader will be able to:*

- Name three psychosocial and spiritual changes that frequently occur during middle age.
- Explain the normal biological changes that occur as a result of the aging process.
- Identify the major causes of death in the middle-aged adult.
- Describe frequently occurring health patterns of middle-aged adults.

- Discuss the unique health problems related to the occupations of the adult between age 35 years and age 65 years.
- Analyze the influence of psychosocial stressors on the middle-aged adult and the ways the individual's culture and occupation can affect these stressors.

## KEY TERMS

Advance directive
Body mass index (BMI)
Calcium
Cardiac output
Cataract
Constipation
Degenerative joint disease
Durable power of attorney
Empty nest syndrome
Functional aerobic capacity
Generativity versus stagnation

Gingivitis
Glaucoma
Health care agent
High blood pressure
Kyphosis
Living will
Macular degeneration
Menopause
Midlife crisis
Obesity
Osteoarthritis

Osteopenia
Osteoporosis
Overweight
Perimenopause
Periodontitis
Presbycusis
Presbyopia
Sleep disorders
Vitamin D

## ❓ THINK ABOUT IT

### The "Sandwich Generation"

Charlie Shelton is 48 years old and has been in excellent health. He operates heavy machinery for a construction team that clears environmentally polluted sites in an inner city. These sites are known to be contaminated (lead, mercury, other chemicals), so he visits the occupational health nurse, who supervises intermittent blood testing and physical examinations. He has never smoked and tries to follow the best health advice. He has two children (aged 15 and 18 years). His wife Sarah was working as a licensed practical nurse in a skilled nursing facility until she injured her back and is now receiving disability insurance payments. The elder child plans to enter university next fall, but the Sheltons wonder how they will afford and manage this. Sarah is also the sole caretaker of her mother, who is 80 years old and is in need of increasing assistance. Although Charlie and Sarah worked hard and saved money all their lives, they are worried about university costs, funding an eventual retirement, and the cost of care for Sarah's mother. In addition, Sarah's injury has made them far more conscious about workplace hazards and exposures. The occupational health nurse sees Charlie to assess his physical health; she is also a source for additional referral and support.

- What types of health care providers and referrals are needed by the Sheltons?
- What can health care providers do to guide and support the Sheltons during this stressful time?
- What other health-promotion and wellness strategies might be suggested and implemented to help them?
- Viewed through the lens of social determinants of health and health inequities, what community organizations might the health care provider recommend to meet the needs of this family?
- What responsibilities do health care providers and policymakers have to provide health promotion to middle-aged adults?

An excellent resource for these questions that includes national demonstrations of small work-site health programs may be found at Canadian Centre for Occupational Health and Safety (CCOHS, 2019): https://www.ccohs.ca/topics/wellness/promotion/.

During their midlife years, many adults experience expanded responsibilities and increased productivity. In most cases, there is a concomitant increased sense of accomplishment. Middle adulthood spans a 30-year interval between 35 and 65 years of age. Within this age interval, significant biological, physiological, social, psychological, and spiritual changes occur. Vital statistics reports published by Statistics Canada (2017a, 2017b) divide the middle-aged adult into six categories for ease of describing mortality and morbidity data. These are 35 to 39 years, 40 to 44 years, 45 to 49 years, 50 to 54 years, 55 to 59 years, and 60 to 64 years. This age group (30-year span) comprises 40% of the population of Canada (Statistics Canada, 2017c).

Many changes related to aging and health that occur during this time frame will be discussed in this chapter. Health promotion addresses social determinants of health, which affect choices in behaviour and practices that optimize health and well-being for the adult in midlife. This concept is the central focus of the presentation of materials and related figures and study aids. The role of nurses will be interwoven throughout the text. Nurses are integral to the health of Canadian people, and hence to fostering health promotion and health maintenance.

## BIOLOGY AND GENETICS

Although their onset differs, biological changes come to the forefront during the middle years, affecting most body systems. The hair of the adult begins to thin and turn grey. The skin's moisture and turgor decrease, and with the loss of subcutaneous fat, wrinkling occurs. Excessive sun exposure through the years makes some changes more pronounced, especially increased coarseness of facial features.

Fat deposition increases during these years, often with concomitant increases in weight. Body height decreases as a result of decreased bone density and mass. This combination of changes results in increased body mass index (BMI). The body contour changes as love handles and saddlebags appear. Sedentary lifestyles and unchanged dietary habits contribute considerably to these changes.

The inactive lifestyle is further compromised by a decrease in energy; "I'm not as young as I used to be" is a common remark. This proclamation is legitimate because the capacity for physical work actually decreases. As functional aerobic capacity decreases, there is a resulting decrease in cardiac output. For individuals who maintain regular exercise programs that provide stretching and strengthening of skeletal muscle, cardiac output remains essentially undiminished for many years.

In the musculoskeletal system, bone density and mass progressively decrease. When 55-year-old adults say that they were 2.5 cm taller when they were 18 years of age, the observation is likely to be true. A 2.5- to 10-cm loss in height occurs as a person ages; thinning of the intervertebral discs accounts for approximately 2.5 cm. However, dramatic losses in height (more than 10 cm) can occur with thoracic kyphosis, an angulation of the posterior spine (commonly known as *hunchback*). The wear and tear on joints predisposes the adult to degenerative joint disease, deterioration of the joint(s), with more frequent painful backaches. The general decrease in muscle tone reduces physical agility.

Degenerative joint disease, specifically osteoarthritis, has its peak onset in middle age and can greatly influence activity and endurance, which impacts employment. Most frequently, the knees and hands, followed by the hips, spine, shoulders, and ankles, are involved. Osteopenia is a condition of subnormally mineralized bone, usually as a result of a rate of bone lysis that exceeds the rate of bone matrix synthesis. Osteoporosis is a disorder characterized by abnormal loss of bone density and deterioration of bone tissue, with an increased fracture risk. It occurs most frequently in postmenopausal women who have fair complexions and are small, in sedentary individuals, and in people using corticosteroids on a long-term basis. Furthermore, osteoporosis increases with age.

The functional capacity of all organ systems generally decreases. For example, in the gastrointestinal tract, the following chain of events occurs: decreased metabolism leads to less enzyme production, resulting in lower hydrochloric acid levels, which decreases tone in the large intestine. As a result, the middle-aged adult may experience acid indigestion with increased belching.

When the adult leads a sedentary lifestyle, the effects of the diminished motility through the gastrointestinal tract can be more pronounced. It is well known that North Americans eat more refined foods (foods that are low in bulk) than residents of developing nations. A low-bulk diet can contribute to the problem of constipation, a change in bowel habits characterized by decreased frequency or passage of hard, drier stools and difficult defecation, and is believed to be a primary contributor to the increased incidence of colon cancer in Canada. Between age 25 years and age 85 years, a 35% loss of nephron units occurs. The remaining nephrons increase in size and undergo degenerative changes. The entire weight of the kidneys decreases. Because blood supply is also diminished, the glomerular filtration rate is decreased by nearly half.

Significant changes occur in the cardiovascular system as the blood vessels lose elasticity and become thicker. This process predisposes middle-aged adults to coronary artery disease, hypertension, myocardial infarctions, and strokes. Heart disease is the second leading cause of death in middle-aged adults (Statistics Canada, 2017a).

Menopause is the cessation of menses. It is an expected physiological change related to aging, and it marks the end of a woman's reproductive function. Menopause is determined retrospectively after cessation of menses for 12 consecutive months. In North America the median age for menopause is 50.5 to 51.4 years (Palacious, Henderson, Siseles, et al., 2010). Women now expect to live one-third of their lives after menopause. A great deal more must be learned about what causes many of the symptoms that occur in menopause. Sheehy (1993) conducted interviews of 100 women from their mid-40s to their 60s and also interviewed 75 physicians and other experts. Her analysis showed that many of these people felt there was a renewed sexual vitality and surge of mental energy for menopausal women. She characterized menopause as a gateway to a second adulthood. Northrup (2012) and King and colleagues (2013) propose that many women make menopause a time of personal inventiveness while gradually adapting to the many expected biological, psychological, social, and spiritual changes of menopause. During menopause,

## BOX 17.1  Leading Causes of Death in Middle-Aged Adults

**Age 35 to 44 Years**
- Unintentional injuries (1391 deaths)
- Malignant neoplasms (1114 deaths)
- Intentional self-harm (640 deaths)

**Age 45 to 54 Years**
- Malignant neoplasms (4271 deaths)
- Heart disease (1729 deaths)
- Unintentional injuries (1553 deaths)

**Age 55 to 64 Years**
- Malignant neoplasms (13180 deaths)
- Heart disease (4992 deaths)
- Unintentional injuries (1490 deaths)

Canada's estimated population in 2017 was 36,708,083.

Sources: Data from Statistics Canada. (2017). *Leading causes of death, total population, by age group*. Retrieved from https://www150.statcan.gc.ca/t1/tbl1/en/tv.action?pid=1310039401&pick; Statistics Canada. (2018). *Population*. Retrieved from https://www150.statcan.gc.ca/n1/pub/12-581-x/2018000/pop-eng.htm.

## BOX 17.2  Examples of Health-Promotion and Disease-Prevention Objectives for the Middle-Aged Adult

**Overall Goals**
- Improve access to high-quality health services.
- Improve health and well-being for all age groups.
- Reduce inequities across all racial and ethnic groups of Canadians.

**Objectives**
- Increase the proportion of adults who have a consistent source for their primary care needs.
- Reduce the proportion of adults aged 18 years or older who experience a limitation in activity due to chronic health conditions.
- Reduce the annual number of new cases of diagnosed diabetes. Reduce the proportion of persons with diabetes with a hemoglobin $A_{1c}$ value greater than 9%.
- Reduce deaths from work-related injuries in all industries.
- Reduce the overall cancer death rate.
- Reduce the proportion of adults with hypertension.
- Reduce coronary heart disease deaths.
- Reduce the proportion of adults who are obese. Increase the proportion of adults who engage in aerobic physical activity of moderate intensity on a regular, preferably daily, basis.
- Increase smoking cessation success for adult smokers.

production of ovarian estrogen and progesterone ceases; the remaining estrogen is produced by the adrenal glands. As a result of the diminished estrogen level, a woman's secondary sex characteristics regress, evident as, for example, loss of pubic hair and decrease in breast size. The female reproductive organs shrink, and vaginal secretions decrease, requiring additional lubrication.

As men approach the end of the middle years, they experience changes in their sexual response cycle as testosterone levels plateau and then decrease. The testes undergo degenerative changes, the number of viable spermatozoa diminishes, and the volume and viscosity of semen decrease. In men, sexual energy gradually declines; achieving an erection takes longer, but it is sustained longer. Stress, however, can significantly diminish function (Pines, 2011).

### Life Expectancy and Mortality Rates

In the previous decade (2001–2010), life expectancy increased for all groups of Canadians in the middle adult years. Across the 30-year age span, there was a decrease in mortality for all racial and ethnic groups, with the most significant decreases noted between age 35 years and age 44 years. Life expectancies for Canadian men and women are now at record highs: 83 years for women and 79 years for men (Statistics Canada, 2017d).

The leading causes of death during middle adulthood are heart disease, cancer, and accidents (Statistics Canada, 2017b). Box 17.1 shows a breakdown for each decile or 10-year interval for the middle-aged adult. Reducing disabilities and deaths from these chronic conditions are national health-promotion and disease-prevention objectives.

The Public Health Agency of Canada (PHAC) uses a multifaceted approach to mitigate the chronic disease burden: epidemiology and surveillance to monitor trends, environmental strategies to promote healthy behaviours, health system interventions to advance clinical and preventive services, and community

resources to improve clinical management of chronic conditions (PHAC, 2019). In Box 17.2, leading health indicators are outlined to give the reader some perspective of the many health-related goals, tasks, and opportunities that lie ahead for Canadians.

The PHAC (2017) identifies that most of the leading indicators identified above are preventable, or at least modifiable. Having a working knowledge of social determinants of health and research–based health-improvement strategies enables health professionals to modify their practice and health-promotion education efforts to best help Canadians achieve their target goals. Doing so also supports the goals of the PHAC to support Canada's public health priorities (PHAC, 2017). Health education, coupled with an understanding of social determinants of health, often conducted by professional nurses, has been effective with adults who want to or must change their lifestyle behaviours. Nursing professionals have contributed extensively in helping the nation to meet the target goals for heart disease, stroke, and many types of cancer.

Whereas the Statistics Canada (2017b) morbidity-related data showed some reduction of illnesses in recent years, there were a number of areas where there is backsliding. Most notably, greater proportions of Canadians are obese and have symptoms of high blood pressure compared with previous years. Hypertension and obesity are conditions that significantly affect the middle-aged adult. They often lead to heart disease, stroke, and the development of diabetes. The most recent national data from 2017 on obesity prevalence indicate obesity was higher among middle-aged adults (31.9%) than among younger (19.7%) or older (28%) adults (Statistics Canada, 2017e).

Areas of improvement in some illnesses were encouraging. For instance, decreases were noted in the number of cancer deaths for individuals aged 55 to 64 years (Statistics Canada, 2017b).

Furthermore, laws that discourage or forbid smoking continue to have significant health-promotion impact across populations.

Projecting ahead, efforts must be directed toward the following: increasing awareness to improve the overall health of Canadians; expanding knowledge of the initiative in schools, Indigenous communities, and local health agencies through the use of public service announcements carried on radio, television, and Internet-based programs; and linking goals to preventive health provisions associated with work sites (occupational health programs) and health insurance policies. In addition to addressing social determinants of health and heath inequities, health counselling, and behaviour-modification strategies provided by nurses, advanced practice nurses, and mental health nursing specialists, physicians may assist in making progress in the health of Canadian people.

## Sex and Marital Status

In the midlife years, the death rate for men is higher. Men are more likely than women to die of heart disease for all age groups (35–44, 45–54, and 55–65 years) and all racial and ethnic groups (Statistics Canada, 2017b). Although cardiovascular disease death rates are declining for both sexes, heart disease remains one of the primary causes of death. The risk factors for heart disease include obesity, lack of physical activity, smoking, high total cholesterol level, hypertension, and genetics. Obesity is common, serious, and costly. Just under one-third of Canadian adults were reported to be obese in 2016 and 2017 (Statistics Canada, 2017e). Among Canadian adults, the prevalence of obesity among middle-aged men was higher (30%) than among women (27%) (Statistics Canada, 2017e). (See Chapter 21 for a discussion of overweight, obesity, and the PHAC's target goals.)

Nearly 40% of adults in Canada are married. Findings from the 2011 census (Statistics Canada, 2011) show that the number of interracial and interethnic married couples has increased from the preceding decade. Married adults report better health than divorced, widowed, or never-married adults. In 2005, same-sex marriages became legal in Canada and they tripled in number between 2006 and 2011. Same-sex common-law relationships increased by 15% (Statistics Canada, 2015d). Furthermore, according to international studies, just over 4% of the general population may be transgender, or were assigned one gender at birth but now identify as another (Canadian Professional Association for Transgender Health [CPATH], 2015).

## Race and Ethnicity

In 2016, Indigenous people represented 4.9% of the total Canadian population (Statistics Canada, 2016a). The Indigenous population has increased by 42.5% since 2006, more than four times the rate of the non-Indigenous Canadian population. The largest numbers of Indigenous people reside in Ontario and the western Canadian provinces, and make up the bulk of the population in Nunavut and the Northwest Territories.

According to the Aboriginal Peoples Survey (Statistics Canada, 2011), more than 40% of Indigenous people considered their health to be excellent or very good. Cancer and circulatory system diseases are the two leading causes of death for Indigenous people, with the latter being elevated for both men

and women compared with the non-Indigenous Canadian population. Diabetes is one of the fastest growing diseases among Indigenous populations in Canada (Government of Canada, 2018). In Canada, the Indigenous population's average annual income of $47,102 (Statistics Canada, 2016b) is lower than that of the non-Indigenous population ($58,900) (Statistics Canada, 2016c).

According to the 2016 census, 21.9% of the Canadian population were immigrants, 76.6% were Canadian-born, and 1.5% were non-permanent residents. The largest percentage of recent immigrants (2011 to 2016) reside in the large metropolitan areas (Toronto, 29.4%; Montreal, 14.8%; and Vancouver, 11.8%) (Statistics Canada, 2016d). The census further identifies 22.3% of the Canadian population as belonging to the visible minority population, with the two largest of those groups being South Asian and Chinese. As compared with the majority population, the South Asian group has an increased risk of diabetes and hypertension. The prevalence of smoking is almost three times lower in the visible minority population, and obesity is five times more prevalent in the majority population. Cardiovascular illness was almost twice as prevalent in South Asians as it was in the Chinese population.

## Access to Health Care

Individuals who are low income may have greater vulnerabilities in relation to their psychological and physical health status. When people are unemployed, they may lose medical benefits. In some Canadian provinces, employers pay the fees for medical services plans, whereas in other provinces these fees are covered by the provincial governments.

Individuals who reside in remote or northern regions of Canada often struggle to access health care resources. Doctors may not visit some regions, and communities may rely on nurse practitioners to meet their needs. Sometimes those nurse practitioners will rotate through a series of remote communities, and visit each community once per week, or less often. When people need the attention of specialist care, transportation to the closest major city is required, and this often is a hardship for many people.

## Genetics

The middle-aged adult is at greater risk than the young adult of diseases known to be associated with genetics (i.e., familial characteristics). These conditions include diabetes, hypertension, Huntington's chorea, arteriosclerosis, gout, obesity, heart disease, and alcoholism. There are some malignancies that are related to genetics: for example, women with a personal or family history of breast cancer are at a higher risk of developing this type of malignancy. In addition, individuals with a family history of colorectal cancer, rectal or colon polyps, or ulcerative colitis have an increased risk of developing this type of cancer (Genomics).

# ❖ GORDON'S FUNCTIONAL HEALTH PATTERNS

## ◆ Health Perception–Health Management Pattern

To promote health in the middle-aged adult, the nurse performs a health assessment that includes the person's values and beliefs,

## GENOMICS

### Genotype-Targeted Therapies for Lung Cancer

Lung cancer remains the leading cause of cancer-related deaths worldwide and the most common cancer (excluding non-melanoma skin cancers) among both men and women in Canada. In 2017, 28,600 people in Canada (14,400 men and 14,200 women) were diagnosed with lung cancer and 21,100 people (11,100 men and 10,000 women) died of lung cancer. The incidence rates of lung cancer levelled off in the mid-1980s and has been on the decline since then. Men continue to have a higher rate of lung cancer death than women, likely due to the differences in tobacco use (Canadian Cancer Society, 2017). Several types of cancer treatment are available—surgery, radiation therapy, chemotherapy, immunotherapy, hormone therapy, and stem cell transplant—yet the 5-year survival rate has not increased in several decades. Molecular and genomic profiling of lung tumours has revolutionized the treatment of metastatic non–small cell lung cancer (NSCLC). The Adjuvant Lung Cancer Enrichment Marker Identification and Sequencing Trials (ALCHEMIST) involve genetic screening of resected NSCLC specimens (Cardarella & Johnson, 2013). Patients whose tumours test positive for either epidermal growth factor receptor gene (EGFR) or anaplastic lymphoma kinase gene (ALK) mutations will be referred to the ALCHEMIST for genotype-directed targeted therapies (Govindan, Mandrekar, Gerber, et al., 2015). Adjuvant targeted therapy, based on tumour mutation genotyping, will likely improve outcomes for all NSCLC patients.

Sources: Cardarella, S., & Johnson, B. E. (2013). The impact of genomic changes on treatment of lung cancer. American Journal of Respiratory and Critical Care Medicine, 188(7), 770–775; Canadian Cancer Society. (2017). Lung cancer statistics. Retrieved from http://www.cancer.ca/en/cancer-information/cancer-type/lung/statistics/?region=pe; Govindan, R., Mandrekar, S. J., Gerber, D. E., et al. (2015). ALCHEMIST trials: A golden opportunity to transform outcomes in early-stage non-small cell lung cancer. Clinical Cancer Research, 24, 5439–5444.

lifestyle patterns, general perceptions of health, and health practices (Pender, Murdaugh, & Parsons, 2015).

### Risk Factors

The major risk factors for adults in the middle years are environmental and behavioural; they can be changed by bolstering social determinants of health, addressing health inequities, and through teaching, counselling, and use of other nursing interventions. Helping adults to take care of themselves and to change, when indicated, can be accomplished on an individual or a group basis.

Some of the health-promotion needs of the middle-aged adult include acceptance of aging, the need to exercise, and weight control. Decreasing or stopping cigarette smoking and alcohol consumption can also be identified needs. Preventive health screening is vital. The adult needs input into and control of as many of these behaviours as possible.

The health risks of middle-aged adults overall are categorized as group risks (age, sex, race) and personal risks. Precritical secondary prevention includes periodic selective screening for the detection of disease before it becomes clinically apparent, such as a breast self-examination. A suggested screening examination appears in Box 17.3.

Chronic conditions are defined as those that last for more than 3 months. The leading chronic diseases found in the middle-aged adult include cardiovascular disease, cancer, diabetes, obesity, arthritis, hepatitis, weak or failing kidney function, and chronic respiratory disease, all of which are among the most common, costly, and preventable of all health problems (Lubkin & Larsen, 2013). As of 2014, three out of five Canadian adults have at least one chronic condition, and four out of five people are at risk for one. Four major chronic conditions (cancer, diabetes, cardiovascular disease, and chronic respiratory disease) are the cause of 67% of all deaths each year. More middle-aged adults are living with chronic diseases that affect their health and well-being. The cost of treating people with chronic diseases is substantial, with an economic burden exceeding $100 billion in both direct health care costs and indirect lost productivity costs (Government of Canada, 2013a).

### ◆ Nutritional-Metabolic Pattern

Dietary factors and unhealthy weights are correlated with five of the 10 leading causes of death in Canada: coronary heart disease, some cancers, stroke, non–insulin-dependent diabetes mellitus, and atherosclerosis.

Physical activities and nutritional patterns are frequently correlated. The middle-aged adult typically leads a more sedentary lifestyle than does the young adult, primarily because of increased responsibilities at work and home and the many convenience devices that are found in homes and workplaces. Linked with less activity is the lack of attention to modification of food intake and calorie consumption, resulting in obesity, which globally is one of the major health problems of the middle years.

### Obesity

One in four adult Canadians (approximately 6.3 million people) are obese (Obesity Canada, 2017), with the highest levels found in men and in the middle-aged population. Obesity-related conditions (heart disease, stroke, type 2 diabetes, and certain types of cancer) contribute to the leading causes of preventable death. Body mass index (BMI) is used as a screening tool for overweight or obesity. BMI is a person's weight in kilograms divided by the square of height in metres. Overweight is defined as having a BMI of 25 to <30. A BMI of ≥30.0 falls within the obese range. Obesity is frequently subdivided into categories: obesity (BMI of 30 to <40) and severe obesity (BMI of ≥40) (Obesity Canada, 2017). Statistics show that there was a 17.5% increase in the incidence of obesity in Canada compared with a decade ago (Statistics Canada, 2015a).

Overweight and obesity are major risks factors for preventable, noncommunicable conditions that contribute to increased health costs, morbidity, and death. An increased BMI substantially raises the risk of coronary heart disease, high blood pressure, high cholesterol, stroke, type 2 (non–insulin dependent) diabetes, gallbladder disease, osteoarthritis, sleep apnea, obesity hypoventilation syndrome, and endometrial, breast, prostate, and colon cancers (Government of Canada, 2013a; World Health Organization, 2016). Individuals who are obese often suffer from social stigmatization, discrimination, and lowered self-esteem (Hunger & Major, 2015). Obesity Canada (2017) recommends that all adults be screened for obesity. For patients with a BMI of 30 kg/m², it is recommended that people

## BOX 17.3   Screening Examination: Age 35 to 65 Years

**Database**
- Health history
- Health hazard appraisal
- Psychological inventories as needed

**Physical Examination Emphasizing**
- Weight and height
- Blood pressure, pulse rate
- Breasts
- Pelvis
- Prostate
- Testicles
- Eyes
- Mouth
- Skin

**Laboratory Procedures**
- Papanicolaou smear and human papillomavirus test: every 5 years
- Hemoccult test: three stools for the Hemoccult test with physical examination after age 50 years
- Colonoscopy or sigmoidoscopy every 5 to 10 years after age 50 years as indicated
- Mammography: initial screening at age 40 years, annually at age 45 to 54 years, then every 2 years at age 55 years or older
- Urinalysis: examined at the time of physical examination
- Lipid profile: all men aged 35 years or older; women aged 20 years or older who have heart disease or risk factors for heart disease

- Chest radiograph with physical examination if heavy smoker
- Tetanus and diphtheria booster every 10 years
- Influenza vaccine: follow current recommendations
- Counselling and testing for human immunodeficiency virus (HIV) as indicated
- Rubella serological test (women of child-bearing age)

**Self-Care Education and Counselling**
- With physical examination; individualized according to individual's risk factors
- Injury prevention: seat belts, helmets, firearms, smoke detectors
- Stress reduction
- Exercise
- Diet: cholesterol, fat, sodium, fibre, multivitamins with folic acid (women of child-bearing age)
- Calcium
- Breast self-examination
- Testicular self-examination
- Dental care
- Mouth care
- Sexually transmitted infections
- Contraception
- Skin protection from ultraviolet light
- Alcohol and other substance abuse
- Smoking cessation
- Possible hormone prophylaxis (perimenopausal and postmenopausal women)

Source: Canadian Cancer Society. (2017). *Find cancer early*. Retrieved from http://www.cancer.ca/en/prevention-and-screening/reduce-cancer-risk/find-cancer-early/?region=pe.

be moved toward more intensive, multicomponent behavioural interventions.

Social determinants of health and health inequities have a profound impact on one's health. For example, women with less education and low incomes are at an increased risk of being overweight. In addition to sex, race, and socioeconomic status, genetics may be a contributing factor. The most significant variables, however, are health behaviours, particularly food intake and exercise and activity patterns. Although an abundance of health information is available, these challenges persist.

Losing weight and maintaining weight loss may require an individual to change eating and activity behaviours, but the social, food preparation, and consumption behaviours of the family must change as well. Prevention of obesity is the goal of weight management during the middle years. When the adult is obese, a clear-cut history of the onset is imperative. A lifelong history of obesity is significantly more arduous to alter than that of adult-onset obesity. A decrease in calories should be accompanied by at least 30 minutes of exercise five times a week. When calories are reduced and exercise is increased, weight loss is achieved and maintained.

The weight-management resources available to the adult are plentiful. Weight-management programs using behaviour modification can be found in various settings, such as universities and work sites, Weight Watchers, Overeaters Anonymous, and Take Off Pounds Sensibly. If the nurse identifies a need for weight management and no program is available, a self-help

group can be started. A suggested list of topics generated by the group is assembled. A discussion of basic nutrition with appropriate handouts is a good place to start. Having adults record their individual goals and keep a 1-week diet log is nonthreatening and helpful for future planning; it also gives the participants some responsibility in the program. Food intake journals assist the individuals in maintaining weight-loss outcomes.

### High Saturated Fat Diet

Cholesterol levels and ratios have a significant influence on cardiovascular and cerebrovascular morbidity and mortality rates. Health Canada (2018) considers the following to be ideal guidelines for healthy cholesterol levels: total cholesterol of less than 5.2 mmol/L, high-density lipoprotein (HDL) levels more than 0.9 mmol/L, and low-density lipoprotein (LDL) levels of less than 3.5 mmol/L. In the middle-aged population, 40% of Canadians live with dyslipidemia (Statistics Canada, 2015b), and this percentage has remained steady in the past decade.

The fact that the numbers haven't risen is attributed to the use of statin medications that lower the level of LDLs in the blood. Some studies demonstrate the beneficial effects of estrogen administration on heart health (Mikkola, Tuomikoski, Lyytinen, et al., 2015). The Coronary Primary Prevention Trial demonstrates that men at high risk of coronary heart disease are able to reduce the risk by approximately 2% for every 1% lower blood cholesterol level. Before using medication to reduce cholesterol level, individuals with high cholesterol levels are advised

## TABLE 17.1   Dietary Reference Intake for Calcium and Vitamin D

### DIETARY REFERENCE INTAKES FOR CALCIUM AND VITAMIN D

| List Stage Group | CALCIUM | | | VITAMIN D | | |
|---|---|---|---|---|---|---|
| | Estimated Average Requirement (mg/day) | Recommended Dietary Allowance (mg/day) | Upper Level Intake (mg/day) | Estimated Average Requirement (IU/day) | Recommended Dietary Allowance (IU/day) | Upper Level Intake (IU/day) |
| Infants 0 to 6 months | * | * | 1000 | ** | ** | 1000 |
| Infants 6 to 12 months | * | * | 1500 | ** | ** | 1500 |
| 1–3 years old | 500 | 700 | 2500 | 400 | 600 | 2500 |
| 4–8 years old | 800 | 1000 | 2500 | 400 | 600 | 3000 |
| 9–13 years old | 1100 | 1300 | 3000 | 400 | 600 | 4000 |
| 14–18 years old | 1100 | 1300 | 3000 | 400 | 600 | 4000 |
| 19–30 years old | 800 | 1000 | 2500 | 400 | 600 | 4000 |
| 31–50 years old | 800 | 1000 | 2500 | 400 | 600 | 4000 |
| 51–70 years old (males) | 800 | 1000 | 2000 | 400 | 600 | 4000 |
| 51–70 years old (females) | 1000 | 1200 | 2000 | 400 | 600 | 4000 |
| >70 years old | 1000 | 1200 | 2000 | 400 | 800 | 4000 |
| 14–18 years old, pregnant/lactating | 1100 | 1300 | 3000 | 400 | 600 | 4000 |
| 19–50 years old, pregnant/lactating | 800 | 1000 | 2500 | 400 | 600 | 4000 |

*For infants. Adequate intake is 200 mg/day for 0 to 6 months of age and 260 mg/day for 6 to 12 months of age.
**For infants. Adequate intake is 400 IU/day for 0 to 6 months of age and 400 IU/day for 6 to 12 months of age.
Sources: Government of Canada. (2010). *Vitamin D and calcium: Updated dietary reference intakes.* Retrieved from http://www.hc-sc.gc.ca/fn-an/ nutrition/vitamin/vita-d-eng.php; The National Academies of Sciences, Engineering, and Medicine, Health and Medicine Division. (2010). *Dietary reference intakes for calcium and vitamin D as recommended by the Institute of Medicine.* Retrieved from http://www.nationalacademies.org/hmd/ Reports/2010/Dietary-Reference-Intakes-for-Calcium-and-Vitamin-D.aspx.

to reduce their intakes of saturated fat, total fat, and dietary cholesterol; normalize their weight; and increase their level of physical activity. If lifestyle changes are not successful, medication is often advised.

## Calcium and Vitamin D

Adequate calcium intake is essential for developing and maintaining bone mass. Additionally, calcium is needed for other physiological processes, including muscle contraction and blood pressure regulation. Men and women need a minimal daily intake of 1000 mg of calcium. Pregnant and nursing women need 1200 mg, and postmenopausal women need either 1000 mg (when taking estrogen) or 1500 mg (when not taking estrogen). When daily intake of calcium is less than adequate, the serum calcium level will be maintained by leaching calcium from bone, resulting in osteoporosis. Weight-bearing exercise contributes to bone mass by increasing mechanical stress on the bones, whereas vitamin D promotes calcium absorption and regulates serum calcium and phosphate concentrations to maintain bone health (Heaney, 2013). Together with calcium, vitamin D helps to protect older adults from osteoporosis.

Vitamin D also plays an important role in overall health and the prevention of chronic diseases. Emerging studies suggest an association between inadequate levels of vitamin D and an increased risk of chronic diseases, such as in osteoporosis, diabetes, heart disease, hypertension, cancers, obesity, depression, cognitive decline, fractures and falls, and autoimmunity (LaFevre, 2015; Nair & Maseeh, 2012). Worldwide, across all ethnic, sex, and age groups, an estimated 1 billion people have inadequate levels of vitamin D (Holick, 2012; Palacios &

Gonzalez, 2014). Possible causes of vitamin D deficiency include an insufficient consumption of vitamin D–fortified foods, lack of dietary supplements, and limited exposure to sunlight. It is very difficult to achieve sufficient vitamin D intake through dietary sources alone as few foods naturally contain vitamin D. The food sources that provide vitamin D include fatty fish, dairy products, liver, and fortified cereals and beverages. The best way to ensure adequate vitamin D serum levels is through supplementation (Health Canada, 2012).

Vitamin D is unique because it can be synthesized endogenously when the skin is exposed to ultraviolet B (UVB) radiation. Many factors can interfere with UVB exposure and the body's ability to synthesize vitamin D from sunlight: seasons, time of day, length of day, location, cloud cover, smog, the skin's melanin content, and use of sunscreen (Nair & Maseeh, 2012). Aging may also impede cutaneous synthesis of vitamin D. As people age, the skin cannot synthesize vitamin D as efficiently as when they are younger. Older adults are also more likely to spend more time indoors (homebound or occupations that limit sun exposure). Prolonged sun exposure to prevent vitamin D deficiency is not generally recommended because exposure to UV radiation increases the risk of skin cancer. The exact definition of a low vitamin D level is not well established. Daily vitamin D intake of 600 IU in adults aged 18 to 70 years and 800 IU in adults older than 70 years will meet the needs of most adults (Institute of Medicine, 2011) (Table 17.1).

## Caffeine

Caffeine is a popular stimulant found in coffee, tea, and some soft drinks, such as colas. Caffeine prolongs the amount of time that physical work can be performed and appears to decrease boredom and increase attention span. On the negative side, coffee has recently been the subject of significant scrutiny from the media, with reports of a link between cancer of the pancreas and coffee consumption. There is controversy regarding whether daily moderate intake of caffeine has any detrimental effects.

Like alcohol and nicotine, caffeine is readily available and has become an accepted part of daily living. Because caffeine is a strong stimulant with effects that are typically taken for granted, its importance as an addictive substance must be emphasized. Ingestion of 0.5 g of caffeine (three to four cups of coffee) can increase the basal metabolic rate by an average of 10%, and possibly as much as 25% for some people.

Long-term stimulation of the central nervous system results in restlessness, sleep disturbances, cardiac stimulation, and withdrawal effects. Nurses' assessment should screen individuals for stimulating and addictive substances that may be producing these symptoms.

### High-Sodium Diet

High-sodium diets play a significant role in hypertension, especially when consumed over many years. The result may be an increase in the amount of total body fluids, which increases peripheral vascular resistance. Salt contains approximately 40% sodium and is a contributing factor for hypertension in the 10% to 20% of Canadians who are at risk. On average, 92% of middle-aged men and 70% of women consume more than the tolerable upper intake level of sodium. A major contributor to dietary sodium is the salt found in processed foods.

In the past three decades, many clinical studies have demonstrated the effectiveness of lowering blood pressure by reducing dietary sodium intake. Other studies have described the relationships between urinary and sodium excretion and the change of blood pressure with age (Pöss, Ewen, Schmeider, et al., 2015).

### Alcohol Abuse

Substance abuse can be a devastating habit. Many adults abuse prescription and illicit drugs and, especially, alcohol. Alcohol is frequently treated as a nondrug, but alcohol addiction is second only to nicotine addiction. Alcohol is readily available, reasonably inexpensive, and considered a part of social exchange; its long-range physiological and psychological effects are well documented. It is estimated that 5.8 million adults in Canada struggle with alcohol use. This affects men (23.8%) more than women (14.2%) (Statistics Canada, 2017f).

*Canada's Low-Risk Alcohol Drinking Guidelines,* issued by the Canadian Centre on Substance Use and Addiction (2018), define moderate drinking as no more than two drinks a day for women and no more than three drinks a day for men. Women are more vulnerable than men to the effects of alcohol because, kilogram for kilogram, women have less water in their bodies, and they tend to weigh less than men. This means that identical doses of alcohol per kilogram of body weight will result in significantly higher blood alcohol levels in women. A woman's brain and other organs are exposed to more alcohol and to the toxic by-products of alcohol as it is metabolized. Excessive

drinking can be affected by risk factors such as family histories of alcoholism, gender (men exhibit higher rates than women), ethnicities (due to genetic differences in the way that alcohol is metabolized; Indigenous people show higher rates of alcoholism), and mental health issues (Searidge Foundation, 2016).

Alcohol use disorders are associated with motor vehicle accidents, violence, homicides, suicides, drownings, heart disease, strokes, liver disease, pancreatitis, and fetal alcohol syndrome. Fetal alcohol syndrome is the most common known preventable cause of mental impairment. The brain damage that occurs with fetal alcohol syndrome can result in lifelong problems with learning, memory, attention, and problem solving (Health Canada, 2017).

Initially, alcohol appears to be a stimulant, but it is actually a central nervous system depressant and anaesthetic. Long-term alcohol use produces tolerance, thereby necessitating a gradual increase in dose to achieve the same effect. Alcohol contributes to problems with safety because of decreased reaction time and depression of the central nervous system. Individuals experiencing alcohol use disorders may report symptoms such as heartburn and gas, stomach distension, poor eating habits, nausea and vomiting, gastric pain, right upper quadrant pain, and irritation of the mouth, throat, and esophagus. Two additional subtle findings are spider angiomas and palmar erythema.

Primary prevention for substance and alcohol abuse is complex, especially because adults consume these agents for many reasons, including peer pressure, loneliness, alienation, frustration, anxiety, and low self-esteem. Heavy drinkers may also be following the example established by influential people in their lives. Merely telling people about the potential physical, emotional, and legal hazards appears to have little effect as a preventive measure. Promotion of more realistic portrayals of substance abuse through the media is difficult to implement. Although techniques such as assertiveness training and teaching adults to resist persuasion are helpful, more useful approaches might include helping them learn to manage anxiety and increase their self-esteem. Less anxious and more confident people have greater skills in resisting peer influences to participate in substance abuse; they also are more likely to have fewer episodes of isolation and loneliness.

Early detection and intervention can decrease ongoing and future physical and psychosocial problems resulting from alcohol abuse. Nurses use a variety of screening strategies to identify individuals' perceptions and consequences of drinking. The CAGE questionnaire is one of the most popular screening tools used in primary care. The Michigan Alcohol Screening Test (http://counselingresource.com/quizzes/alcohol/-mast/index.html) and the Alcohol Use Disorders Identification Test (https://www.drugabuse.gov/sites/default/files/files/AUDIT.pdf) are examples of other screening instruments.

Abnormal laboratory test results, including elevations in aspartate aminotransferase level, erythrocyte mean corpuscular volume, and serum glutamyltransferase level, are not adequately sensitive and specific enough to detect alcohol use disorders as these may be a result of other causes, including trauma, disease, and medications.

A variety of treatments are known to be effective, but no single "best" intervention has been identified. Effective treatments may be to address other problems with use of interventions such as pharmacological agents, stress management, acupuncture, individual and family therapy, and supportive environments.

## Oral Health

*Gingivitis.* Gingivitis is found commonly among adults who fail to brush their teeth and use dental floss regularly. Redness and swelling develop around the teeth. Bleeding of the gums, while the teeth are being brushed, is an early sign of gingivitis. The gums may or may not be tender. When inflammation is not adequately treated and controlled, periodontitis, involving bone destruction, can develop in addition to tooth loss.

*Dental hygiene and decay.* Dental health is essential to overall health. Brushing the teeth and flossing after eating, receiving routine dental checkups, and consuming fewer carbohydrates (especially simple sugars) are important interventions to prevent dental caries. Adults in the middle years have responsibility not only for their own regular dental care but also for the care of their children and parents. Fluoridation of water (versus bottled or tap water) and use of applied sealants are additional health choices that support prevention of dental caries and, possibly, tooth loss.

There is increasing evidence to show that periodontal, or gum disease, is closely linked to diabetes, heart disease, and stroke. For the middle-aged woman, poor oral health can cause premature births and low-birth-weight infants (Bensley, Van Eehwyk, & Ossiander, 2011).

There are many conditions that begin with changes in the oropharyngeal mucosa, such as cancer of the mouth and esophageal cancer. Consequently, annual dental checkups are important because dental professionals (dentists or dental hygienists) may be the first to detect a symptom or irregularity that points to a potentially dangerous condition.

Findings of the Canadian Dental Association (2017) regarding the state of oral health indicate that approximately 64.6% of Canadians with average income receive annual health care by a dentist. For those individuals in the lower income brackets, 46.5% receive dental care, and 78.5% of those with higher income receive annual care. People who are in vulnerable populations (individuals whose annual income is below the poverty line, others who are chronically ill or disabled, or still others whose medical or psychiatric treatment plans are very complicated) may not receive adequate or proper oral health care. While there is evidence of progress being made to increase access to oral health services for a greater proportion of the population, those who are vulnerable because of illnesses still find difficulty in obtaining proper and adequate oral health care (Benjamin, 2012; Canadian Dental Association, 2017). The factors that frequently deter oral health care in this population include lack of dental insurance, lack of transportation, limitations of disability, increasing costs of treatment, and inability to afford the cost of oral health care. National data indicate that the cost of dental care is a deterrent to sustained oral health. Findings from the Canadian Dental Association indicate that one out of six Canadians reported an unmet dental need because of cost in the previous 12 months. Among adults aged 18 to 64 years, the main reason to forego a dental visit for an oral health problem in the previous year was cost. Overall, Canadians from lower-income families had two times worse dental outcomes compared with higher-income families.

Tobacco use in any form (cigarettes, pipes, and smokeless [spit] tobacco) increases the risk of gum disease. Findings from Bloom, Simile, Adams, and colleagues (2012) indicate that dental health is often poor among smokers (currently smoking) compared with former smokers and with those who have never smoked. Smokers who were interviewed said that they had three or more dental problems. In addition, current smokers reported infrequent visits to their dentist (in some cases, more than 5 years) or never seeing a dentist. Research findings indicate the prevalence of gum disease is two times greater in individuals who smoke cigarettes compared with individuals who have never smoked (Canadian Dental Association, 2017).

In summary, oral disease is preventable. Regularly scheduled dental care with a dentist and dental hygienist is highly recommended for good dental hygiene and early treatment of dental decay and periodontal diseases, such as gingivitis. In addition, dentists can provide screening for oropharyngeal cancer. Oral health is essential in the overall digestive and elimination processes.

## ◆ Elimination Pattern

Aging brings a gradual decrease of tone in the large intestine. This change, accompanied by a sedentary lifestyle, lack of fibre in the diet, and inadequate fluid intake, can predispose the adult to constipation. Advertising on television and other forms of media present strong arguments that encourage individuals to rely on external controls rather than on exercise and dietary means to solve this problem. Consequently, many adults are dependent on taking fibre products, as well as laxatives, for regular bowel movements.

In the kidneys, degenerative changes in the nephron units gradually increase during the middle years. In most cases, adults do not have any appreciable alteration in kidney function unless the person has experienced repeated infections, trauma, or the long-term effects of diabetes mellitus or hypertension.

Alteration in bladder control (incontinence) can occur in both women and men because of weakening of the muscles of the pelvic floor or damage to pelvic nerves. Urinary incontinence is problematic in women who have experienced multiple births. In men, urinary incontinence frequently occurs as a complication of surgery for prostate cancer. Incontinence can be socially embarrassing, but the condition can be relieved with Kegel exercises (Santacreu & Fernández-Ballesteros, 2011; Siegel, 2014).

## ◆ Activity-Exercise Pattern

Regular physical activity increases life expectancy and the quality of life. Exercise helps to prevent coronary heart disease, hypertension, diabetes, osteoporosis, and depression. Research findings show there is a strong correlation between physical exercise and lower rates of osteoporosis (Osteoporosis Canada, 2018), back injury, stroke, and colon cancer. Weight-loss programs that incorporate physical activities also make significant contributions to health promotion, as evidenced by increased life expectancy and quality of life.

One of the objectives of the PHAC (2017) is to continue to decrease deaths related to heart disease. Evidence suggests that a significant percentage of Canadians in the middle-aged adult bracket do not engage in regular moderate physical activity for at least 30 minutes on 5 or more days a week. Only a fraction of adults perform the recommended level. Sedentary behaviour increases with aging. This finding may be due to the onset of conditions that affect mobility and strength.

Continuous, rhythmic exercise maintained for a period sufficient to stress the cardiac system (increase heart rate and blood pressure) is desirable. Some suggested activities include brisk walking, jogging, swimming, bicycling, and skipping rope, as well as walking or biking to work. Activities that focus on skill and coordination should be attempted by the adult older than 40 years rather than activities necessitating speed and strength. Moderation is key for all groups of individuals. Caution is recommended for adults nearing age 65 years to prevent muscle strains and/or falls. Overexertion, as evidenced by dizziness, chest pressure or chest pain, and unresolved shortness of breath, should be avoided. Additionally, in hot weather, strenuous exercise should be balanced with rest periods and increased intake of fluids to prevent heat stroke.

Nurses play significant roles in assessing, teaching, and evaluating individuals relative to activity-exercise programs. Advanced practice nurses are often instrumental in creating and guiding weight-loss programs; nurses working in the community may see local citizens at health fairs or health-promotion events; and other nurses or therapists visit individuals at home for care following hospitalization for surgery or acute illness as home health professionals. Activity programs are initiated to restore health (following heart attack) or to improve cardiac function (such as cardiac and pulmonary rehabilitation), and in some cases to control blood glucose levels. A thorough assessment, including a cardiac stress test, is necessary when an individual has not exercised regularly in the past. Parameters for heart rate, blood pressure, and length and frequency of exercise sessions are set in advance by a cardiologist. Nurses support and guide individuals by helping them determine program goals, by monitoring their progress, and by teaching individuals how to modify lifestyle behaviours to obtain particular objectives.

To achieve maximal effectiveness, physical exercise should involve as many muscles as possible and be performed on a regular basis. Adults should spend 30 minutes or more in brisk physical activity every day for a total of 3 to 4 hours per week. The optimal performance level differs for each individual and should be based on parameters set by the individual's physician in advance of the individual starting a fitness program. The following formula to calculate the target heart rate is shown on the Canadian Heart and Stroke Foundation website. Begin by subtracting one's age from 220 and then multiply this number by 0.75 to determine a heart rate that is within safe limits. For example, for an individual who is 50 years old, $(220 - 50) = 170$; $170 \times 0.75 = 127.5$ (or 128 beats per minute) for the optimal heart rate. Comparatively, the cardiac muscle capacity of a person younger than 50 years would be greater than 128 beats per minute; as the functional aerobic capacity is increased, the target heart rate required to tone the cardiac muscle will increase.

To summarize, routine exercise is essential to the health of the heart and overall muscle strength. The type of activity and style is an individual choice. Program goals are achieved more readily when exercise is incorporated into leisure activities or is a part of a group activity.

## ◆ Sleep-Rest Pattern

Viewed through the lens of the social determinants of health, middle-aged Canadians may not get as much sleep as young adults because of increased demands in their lives. Caring for immediate family, children, and sometimes parents, as well as employment responsibilities, consume most of a 24-hour period.

Insomnia is a common finding in this age category. It may be the result of overstimulation, resulting from drinking too many caffeinated beverages, strenuous exercise within 2 hours of bedtime, or failure to have a regular sleep–wake schedule in a 24-hour period (Canadian Sleep Society, 2018). Frequently occurring insomnia can lead to distractibility, irritability, and fatigue during the daytime hours.

Sleep apnea is a common disorder during which normal breathing is disrupted by breathing pauses or shallow breaths. Breathing pauses may occur 30 times or more each hour and may last from a few seconds to minutes. Because of collapsed or blocked airways, a loud snorting or snoring sound is produced when normal breathing resumes. This pattern of pauses and shallow breathing is typical for the most common type of sleep apnea: obstructive sleep apnea. Although obstructive sleep apnea may be experienced by all, this type of sleep apnea commonly affects obese adults. Central sleep apnea is the less common type of sleep apnea. It occurs because of a disruption of central nerve signals to the diaphragm, resulting in brief periods of not breathing while asleep.

Sleep apnea is a chronic condition and may increase the risk of myocardial infarction, stroke, arrhythmias, and heart failure. Treatments include lifestyle changes such as weight loss, continuous positive airway pressure therapy, the use of mouthpieces, or surgical intervention (Government of Canada, 2013b).

Rest is essential to allow restorative functions of the body to occur. The effects of insomnia can be counteracted by regularly scheduled, high-quality sleep, and occasional napping when fatigued. If insomnia becomes a chronic problem, cognitive behavioural therapy has also been demonstrated to be an effective treatment option (Kaldo, Jernelöv, Blom, et al., 2015). The Canadian Sleep Society (2018) offers detailed information about treating insomnia and other sleep disorders with medications if that modality is indicated.

## ◆ Cognitive-Perceptual Pattern

Learning is a phenomenon that occurs across the life span. The need to increase knowledge or information and the need to acquire new skills are constants, as adults develop through a variety of experiences. Employment demands or

## BOX 17.4  Developmental Tasks of Middle Age

- Helping children become responsible, happy adults
- Rediscovering or developing new satisfaction in the relationship with one's spouse (for the single adult, this can occur in a relationship with a sibling or significant other)
- Developing an affectionate, but independent, relationship with aging parents
- Reaching the peak in one's career
- Achieving mature social and civic responsibility
- Accepting and adapting to biological changes
- Maintaining or developing friendships
- Developing leisure-time activities

new roles in life, such as becoming a parent or suddenly needing to care for an older family member, thrust the middle-aged adult into numerous different learning situations. The ability to learn a range of skills or to acquire knowledge through observing, performing, or participating in play activities begins in childhood, as described by Gardner (1983, 1993), and extends into the middle years and beyond. The capacity to perform intellectually (i.e., reason through critical thinking, use/increase vocabulary, and apply spatial perception skills) stays constant through the 35- to 65-year-old age range. However, some decreases in reaction time and cognitive flexibility become more apparent as age increases.

### Intellectual Ability

The ability to acquire new knowledge or skills, or "learning intelligence," accumulates through formal education and life experiences and continues to increase throughout life. The evidence of this phenomenon is demonstrated by the many scholars and artists who become more productive in their middle years than when they were young adults. Some individuals discover "new talents" later in life because they have more leisure time or motivation to explore new areas or interests.

The theories of Piaget (1970), Bloom (1984), and Havighurst and Orr (1956) are relevant to the middle-aged adult. These theorists conclude that the prime time to be in the learner role is when the developmental task for that role is to be accomplished. The adult in the middle years as the learner-performer is a case in point. For example, to balance the responsibilities of caring for children and parents and being employed outside the home, the adult may explore new career options or creative endeavours.

Havighurst and Orr (1956) define developmental tasks as the basic tasks of living that must be achieved for the adult to live successfully. These tasks are dictated by the expectations of society, the physiological changes of the body throughout life, and the individual's own value system and goals. Although initially described in 1956, Havighurst and Orr's developmental tasks of middle age remain timely (Box 17.4).

If career goals have been previously identified, then attaining them can be highly rewarding, both psychologically and financially. In addition to career activities, the mature adult has an increased social awareness and often assumes more civic responsibility.

In Piaget's theory of cognitive development, formal operations are the highest or most complex level. This stage begins at approximately age 12 years and continues throughout life. Piaget describes the thoughts of adults as being both flexible and effective. The adult can deal efficiently with complex problems of reasoning, including hypothesis testing (Piaget, 1970).

Bloom (1984) developed a hierarchy of cognitive levels in the adult learner. Knowledge is the simplest or most basic cognitive level. Knowledge is the acquisition of information. The adult learner defines "high blood pressure" in lay terms.

Comprehension is the second level, as indicated by the learner grasping the meaning of the communicated message and relating the term(s) to other material. For example, the individual can state one way that obesity influences high blood pressure.

The third level is application of knowledge. At this level the learner demonstrates an understanding of ideas and concepts by extending them to describe or relate them to real-life situations. For example, the individual with hypertension becomes involved in an exercise program.

The fourth level is analysis. At this level, all aspects of learning are united in thought, and the individual is cognizant of the relationships and interactions of all the parts. For example, the individual considers his or her values and life goals when making decisions about taking action in regard to understanding health care needs.

The highest order of learning involves synthesis and evaluation. The person is able to combine various elements to form a plan and then is able to judge the extent to which the actions and results satisfy the original objectives. For example, people may develop plans to improve their health status and increase their disease self-management responsibilities. The next step is to validate the results of ongoing health care programs in relation to their projected expectations. Genetic and personality factors, in combination with environmental conditions and lifestyle practices, account for the large difference in the ways in which individuals maintain mental abilities. Schaie and Willis (2005) have identified seven factors that maintain cognitive function in later life:

- Absence of chronic diseases
- Living with favourable socioeconomic factors, including maximal occupational complexity, a low degree of routine, and an intact family
- Involvement in complex social activities
- Flexible personality style
- Marriage to a spouse with high cognitive function
- Maintaining high levels of performance speed
- Personal satisfaction with accomplishments in midlife and early old age (see Box 17.4)

### Perceptual Changes

Presbyopia (farsightedness) is common in middle-aged adults, even in individuals who have had no previous problems with their vision. This condition occurs because of the loss of elasticity in the lens of the eye so that the adult cannot focus on objects that are in close range, such as reading without using prescription lenses.

Presbyopia is corrected with prescription lenses, which may be needed only for reading or for close work. LASIK surgery, a surgical intervention to correct refraction, is currently widely used and is favoured by individuals who do not want to use standard eyeglasses.

Other visual conditions that may not be as easily corrected include decreased peripheral vision and decreased visual sensitivity in the dark. Both conditions are slow and insidious in their development and occur as the cornea becomes less transparent. Because all these conditions are not readily detected by the individual, middle-aged adults should undergo a routine professional eye examination every year.

Glaucoma occurs as a result of increased intraocular pressure, which can damage the optic nerve, resulting in vision loss and blindness (Canadian Association of Optometrists, 2018). Loss of peripheral vision, or tunnel vision, is a common condition associated with glaucoma. Damage to the optic nerve is irreversible, but visual loss can be prevented if damage is identified early and treatment is initiated. Information available at the Canadian National Institute of the Blind (CNIB) website shows that glaucoma is the third highest leading cause of blindness in Canada (after cataracts and age-related macular degeneration) (CNIB, 2017). In a study of newly diagnosed glaucoma in Canadians, nearly half of the patients had moderate or advanced disease at the initial diagnosis; a late diagnosis was associated with socioeconomic deprivation (Buys, Gaspo, & Kwok, 2012). The importance of regular eye examinations by an ophthalmologist cannot be underestimated.

A cataract, opacity of the lens, can develop and cloud the vision in the later years of middle age. Often cataracts develop in people who have diabetes. Another disorder, diabetic retinopathy, gradually causes rupture of vessels in the retina, which leak into the eye, causing lack of colour differentiation and central vision changes.

Macular degeneration is often referred to as age-related macular degeneration (AMD). This age-related disorder is a progressive deterioration of the maculae of the retina and choroid structures of the eye and results in damaged sharp and central vision. Approximately 1 million Canadians aged 50 years or older are affected by AMD, and the number of people with AMD is estimated to reach 2 million by 2020 (CNIB, 2017). This condition is very serious because it represents the effects of several disorders. Once a diagnosis of macular degeneration has been made, retinal ophthalmologists should be involved in the care of the individual.

Another common perceptual change in middle age is presbycusis (impaired auditory acuity). The first sounds to be lost are higher frequencies, such as a woman's voice. This is important in the work environment and situations that require social interaction. Because this process is subtle, middle age is a time for auditory evaluations as a part of routine examinations.

Beginning in the middle years, the sense of taste diminishes in a progressive and predictable manner. The taste buds located more anteriorly on the tongue are the first to be affected, causing an inability to detect sweet and salt. When the effectiveness of the posterior taste buds declines, detection of bitter and sour flavours is lost. Consequently, this change can alter a person's food preferences and present problems for people who insist on adding salt to compensate for the deficit. Nurses involved in the care of the middle-aged adult, perhaps in the community or in home health, can show the individual how the use of various herbs and spices can enhance flavour.

## ◆ Self-Perception–Self-Concept Pattern

### Levinson's Theory

In Levinson's research on men (Levinson, 1986a, 1986b) and women (Levinson, 1996), a theory on "individual life structures" is posed. Levinson describes age-associated seasons or eras. The midlife transition, beginning at age 38 to 40 years, appears to include reappraising one's life, integrating the polarities, and modifying one's life structure toward being who one wants to be. Middle-aged adults struggle with meaning, value, and direction of their lives.

### Erikson's Theory

In Erikson's eight stages of the life cycle (Erikson & Erikson, 1998), the last three stages are related to adulthood. Stage 7, generativity versus stagnation or self-absorption, is most frequently associated with the middle years.

Erikson identifies generativity as the primary task to achieve during adulthood. Generativity includes a sense of productivity and creativity as evidenced by reaching previously established goals versus stagnation, the failure to achieve lifelong goals (Hornstein, 1986; Reifman, Biernat, & Lang, 1991; Thomas, 1995). Generativity also encompasses a desire to care for others versus self-absorption, the tendency to direct most of one's interest and attention to oneself, thereby excluding others.

Middle age is a time of critical self-review. For some, this review may prompt sadness, disappointment, self-doubt, and regret if the desired and expected life goals have not been met. Both women and men question their value to society, the merit of their accomplishments, their success as sexual beings, and the probability of attaining yet unfilled life goals. Women generally make this life assessment between 35 and 50 years or age, whereas men do not usually begin until approximately age 40 years. Women typically begin earlier to look for changes they may want to make in their lives (Apter, 1995), whereas men remain content with the status quo. Because the male life assessment tends to begin later, there is potential for couples of approximately the same age to experience conflict within the relationship. This type of self-review and lack of effective communication of personal needs with a spouse or life partner is a threat to marital stability (Erikson & Erikson, 1998; Vaillant & Vaillant, 1990).

### Physiological Changes

The effect of physiological changes on mental health is nearly as critical during the middle years as it is during adolescence. Some of the most obvious changes that influence self-esteem are greying hair, an increase in the number of wrinkles, decreased visual and auditory acuity, and changes in body shape. The extent to which these changes are tolerated depends largely on the person's level of self-satisfaction and acceptance. Some people try to "hold on" to youth by dressing as more youthful counterparts dress, whereas others adapt their attire to their age and position in life.

Before 2002, hormone replacement therapy (estrogen alone, or estrogen and progesterone) was given to millions of postmenopausal women. Millions of women took hormone therapy not only to relieve hot flashes but also in the hope that it might prevent heart disease, the number one cause of death in postmenopausal women. All of that changed in 2002, however, when data from the Women's Health Initiative (WHI) showed that postmenopausal women who took estrogen and progesterone actually had higher rates of heart attacks and other health problems, including stroke, blood clots, and breast cancer.

Follow-up analysis of the WHI data showed that the effects of hormone therapy depend on a woman's age and the length of time since menopause. In younger postmenopausal women, between 50 and 59 years of age, hormone use did not increase the risk of cardiac events, as it did in older women. There is new evidence that hormone therapy may actually be beneficial for younger postmenopausal women, but, for now, hormone therapy is not recommended for the prevention of heart disease (Whayne & Mukherjee, 2015).

Health benefits of hormone therapy include decreased risk of osteoporosis and decreased rates of colorectal cancer (Whayne & Mukherjee, 2015). Research is ongoing regarding the risks and benefits of hormone therapy. Currently, the only approved indication for postmenopausal hormone therapy is for the relief of moderate to severe vasomotor symptoms (hot flashes). Only short-term use is advised (1–3 years) (Lowdermilk & Perry, 2012). Increasing numbers of women are now using non-hormonal ways to treat hot flashes and other symptoms associated with menopause. Caution needs to be exercised as natural health products are not as closely regulated as prescription medications.

Because there are few scientific data, many midlife women find it difficult to make decisions about using alternative products. Black cohosh, soy, and vitamin E are just a few of the products marketed to women. Even if these products are effective, women must be cautious about medication interactions that may occur. The use of prescription medication increases with age. The benefits of using alternative therapy may outweigh the risks, but more research is needed on the safety profile of natural remedies.

It is difficult to separate menopause from the physical and psychological changes that women experience as they age. The stressors common to women in their 40s and 50s include raising a family, helping parents as they age, coping with divorce or death of a spouse, retirement, and financial insecurity. Menopause happens in the midst of this. All the events in a woman's life influence her experience of menopause and the perimenopause, a period that precedes menopause and lasts approximately 4 years. Symptoms such as mood swings, nervousness, agitation, fatigue, and depression are often ascribed to the decline in estrogen levels that occurs during this time. The physiological changes are important, but a woman's experience in menopause is profoundly affected by all the events in her life (Lowdermilk & Perry, 2012).

## RESEARCH FOR EVIDENCE-INFORMED PRACTICE

### "Regrets are the natural property of grey hairs,"—Charles Dickens

Disappointment and regret are common emotions experienced across all ages. Life-span theorists suggest that regret-producing consequences are associated with low levels of life satisfaction, low levels of subjective well-being, and high levels of biological age–related changes among midlife and older adults more often than among younger adults (Wrosch, Bauer, & Scheier, 2005). Time lived was understood to intensify the degree of angst associated with perceived regrettable situations, because middle-aged and older adults have less time to take corrective action or make amends.

The latest research suggests that middle-aged and older adults are less likely to engage in remorseful rumination than are younger adults (Brassen, Gamer, & Peters, 2012; Charles, 2010; Mather, 2012). Despite normative age-related physical decline, middle-aged and older adults typically report greater life satisfaction and remarkably higher levels of emotional well-being than young adults, including a decline in their experience of negative emotions (Chowdhury, Sharot, Wolfe, et al., 2014). Even in the presence of physical comorbidities, decreased cognitive agility, a diminishing social circle, and perhaps the death of a spouse, family member, or close friends, middle-aged and older adults have harnessed strategies that preserve emotional well-being, even as they continue to age (Mather, 2012). According to Mather (2012), age-related emotional processing has a biological basis that helps explains why patterns of coping with regret differ between young adults and those in the middle years and beyond.

Sources: Brassen, S., Gamer, M., Peters, J., et al. (2012). Don't look back in anger! Responsiveness to missed changes in successful and nonsuccessful aging. *Science, 336*(6081), 612–614; Charles, S. T. (2010). Strength and vulnerability integration: A model of emotional well-being across adulthood. *Psychological Bulletin, 136*(6), 1068–1091; Chowdhury, R., Sharot, T., Wolfe, T., et al. (2014). Optimistic update bias increases in older age. *Psychological Medicine, 44*(9), 2003–2012; Mather, M. (2012). The emotion paradox in the aging brain. *Annals of the New York Academy of Sciences, 1251*(1), 33–49; Wrosch, C., Bauer, I., & Scheier, M. F. (2005). Regret and quality of life across the adult life span: The influence of disengagement and available future goals. *Psychology and Aging, 20*(4), 657–670.

Men also experience physical and psychological reactions to middle age. The hormonal changes in men are gradual, typically beginning between 40 and 55 years of age. The symptoms are similar to those experienced by women with the emotional effects related to other life events, past coping patterns, and general feelings of self-esteem.

### ◆ Roles-Relationships Pattern

Middle age is frequently a time of reassessment, turmoil, and change, a time that has been called "midlife crisis." The turning point occurs for several reasons. Over time, middle-aged adults become aware of subtle and compromising changes in physical, cognitive, and emotional agility. Furthermore, the inevitability of one's own death is recognized, perhaps for the first time. Middle-aged adults must accept that lifestyle choices have been made, unintended consequences may have lasting repercussions, and the opportunity to amend prior decisions may no longer be possible. Alternatively, middle-aged adults may be quite satisfied with prior life choices and the resultant personal satisfaction and contentment (Research for Evidence-Informed Practice).

## Family

Duvall and Miller (1985) delineate eight stages of the family life cycle, with stages 5, 6, and 7 in the middle years :

- Stage 5: families with children, with the oldest child aged 13 to 20 years; lasts approximately 7 years
- Stage 6: families launching young adults, from the first leaving until the last; lasts approximately 8 years
- Stage 7: families from empty nest to retirement; lasts approximately 15 years

The developmental tasks identified for the families in stages 6 and 7 are similar to those described by Havighurst and Orr (1956); they focus on changes from a nuclear family to a marital couple with other responsibilities. For example, in stage 6, the parents who are helping their children become independent may also be caring for their aging parents. Additionally, middle-aged adults fulfill multiple complex responsibilities within a variety of career, social, and civic positions.

These transitions can be even more challenging for the family headed by a single parent. In 2016, 19.2% of Canadian children (approximately 1.3 million) were part of lone-parent families (Statistics Canada, 2019a), with the lone parent most typically being the mother. The proportion of children in single-parent families was higher in the territories, Nova Scotia, and New Brunswick. The single most significant health risk in families headed by a single mother is low income. Of those children living in low-income households, 42% resided with a lone mother (approximately 1.1 million children), and 25.5% with a lone father (approximately 260,000 children). Comparatively, 85% of children who lived with couple parents (i.e., married) were in households that were at least 200% above the poverty level (Statistics Canada, 2019b). Inadequate resources make it extremely difficult for middle-aged mothers to fulfill their responsibilities.

Families with young adolescents or young adult children have been described in research studies as both *postparental* and *launching families*. In contrast, criticism of this emphasis on the separation of children (regardless of age) from their families is increasing. Gilligan (1982) criticizes the work of many human development theorists who identify human development in terms of separation from the family. Apter (1990) also challenges the conventional view that adolescent girls must reject their mothers as part of a healthy development. Middle-aged parents are encouraged to continue to care for and nurture their adolescent and adult children while recognizing the increasing interdependence of their relationships.

By supporting their children's efforts, parents can increase the self-esteem of their children while being effective role models. The parent assumes less of a parent–child relationship while interacting more on an adult-to-adult level. As the children are "launched," the parents may have uninterrupted time alone and time to share activities. Family life may also be threatened by older children living at home, opposition to a child's partner, or the inability to establish satisfactory relationships with potential or actual partners or sons-in-law and daughters-in-law. For many parents, the idea of their children leaving home is anticipated with relief that the heavy care responsibilities of parenting are over or with dread over having to fill the void of time and inactivity. The empty nest syndrome may be exacerbated if the couple has never learned to communicate effectively and to enjoy each other's company without the children.

At the other end of the family spectrum, aging parents can place demands on the adult child primarily because older adults are frequently beset with health problems. A caring relationship is in order, in which the aging parent's need for independence is recognized.

Because of society's emphasis on youth, the middle-aged adult must associate feelings of self-worth with personal integrity rather than with body appearance or physical prowess. Friends can provide invaluable support systems. With the newly found free time after children have left home, the middle-aged adult can share favourite activities and learn new ones. Middle-aged adults should remind themselves how much and how well they are doing, especially considering the complexity of the demands placed on them. Never before in history have families pursued such varied and individual-oriented goals as they do today.

Although for many Canadians the concept of family remains of major importance, the perceptions are different from those held by previous generations. Parents and children in most families are involved in numerous activities, as evidenced by a "let's-hurry-or-we'll-be-late" orientation. Even younger children frequently have schedules that must be met if they are to get to their dance, drama, play, or enrichment classes. None of these activities necessarily have a negative effect, but the cumulative influence places heavy demands on all family members. Additionally, many activities in which both children and adults are involved have a certain degree of competitiveness. For example, parents frequently become emotionally involved in the athletic activities of their children to the extent that the failure of a 6-year-old child to play a winning hockey game causes a great deal of parental anguish. One only has to listen to the cheering of parents at a Timbits hockey game to note whose self-esteem is at stake. Shouts of "Kill her," "Grab the forward," and so on do not tend to engender feelings of team spirit or a notion of playing for the sake of having a good time (Erikson & Erikson, 1998).

## Work

Perhaps the most common role that middle-aged adults share is that of a worker. Much of their pride and sense of satisfaction is derived from their work. Work is equated with being "grown up." One can easily recall the "What do you want to be when you grow up?" questioning of youth. Success and achievement are evaluated in terms of careers and family life. The work ethic still persists, especially for individuals born during the Great Depression, and for many of their offspring as well. Much of their conversation evolves from what they do, such as "My name is Leslie Smith. I am a real estate agent." To be mature is to be a responsible, hard-working individual (Erikson & Erikson, 1998). Research has shown that middle-aged adults are more satisfied with their jobs than are younger adults.

Middle-aged adults constitute most of the Canadian workforce. For many, vocations play a major role in defining personal levels of wellness. There were approximately 240,000 nonfatal workplace injuries and illnesses in 2016, an increase from 232,000 in 2015, and from 239,000 in 2014 (Association of Workers' Compensation Boards of Canada, 2016). The highest rates of nonfatal injuries occur in construction, manufacturing, and health services. Thirty percent of nonfatal injuries and

## ⚡ QUALITY AND SAFETY SCENARIO

### *Examples of Prevention Strategies to Address Cardiovascular Disease in Women*

Social determinants of health and health inequities can have a profound impact on one's daily health choices. While the list of recommendations noted below provides helpful prevention strategies to reduce cardiovascular disease, it is also important to acknowledge how these social determinants of health can impact and even inform one's daily choices.

- *Eat a healthy diet* with fruits, vegetables, whole grains, and fat-free or low-fat milk and milk products. Choose foods low in saturated fats, cholesterol, salt (sodium), and added sugars.
- *Exercise regularly.* Adults need 2 hours and 30 minutes (or 150 minutes total) of exercise each week. You can spread your activity out during the week, and can break it up into smaller chunks of time during the day.
- *Be smoke-free.* If you are ready to quit smoking, call Health Canada at 1-866-366-3667 for free resources, including free quit coaching, a free quit plan, free educational materials, and referrals to other resources where you live.
- *Limit alcohol use,* which can lead to long-term health problems, including heart disease and cancer. If you do choose to drink alcohol, do so in moderation, which is no more than one drink a day for women. Do not drink at all if you are pregnant.
- *Know your family history.* There may be factors that could increase your risk for heart disease and stroke.
- *Manage any medical condition* you might have. Learn the ABCs of heart health. Keep them in mind every day and especially when you talk to your health care provider:
  - Appropriate aspirin therapy for those who need it
  - Blood pressure control
  - Cholesterol management
  - Smoking cessation.

Source: Heart & Stroke Foundation Canada. (2018). *Women's unique risk factors.* Retrieved from https://www.heartandstroke.ca/heart/risk-and-prevention/womens-unique-risk-factors.

illnesses requiring days away from work continue to be due to overexertion and repetitive motion (Nicholson, 2011).

A total of 904 workers died from a work-related injury in Canada during 2016, compared with 852 in 2015 and 919 in 2014. Approximately one-third of the 2016 fatally injured workers died as a result of traumatic injuries and disorders, while almost half of the deaths were related to neoplasms, tumours, and cancers (Association of Workers' Compensation Boards of Canada, 2016). In decreasing order, workers in mining, agriculture, forestry, fishing, construction, and transportation are at an increased risk of dying from a work-related injury (Nicholson, 2011). Poor housekeeping and poor design predispose workers to falls and other accidents; exposure to noise and toxic chemicals also make employees susceptible to injury and illness. Many injuries that contribute significantly to the morbidity and mortality of adults can be prevented. Fixing faulty steps, repairing faulty electrical wires, and securing carpets are only a few of the many preventive measures. Other work-related problems include exposure to harmful substances, resulting in lung diseases, cancers, and workplace violence (Quality and Safety Scenario).

The effect of life events on mental health depends on the personal strength of the individual, the availability of supports, and the nature and number of events and their significance for the person. Three common examples of life events with potential disruptive effects are marital separation or divorce, having two or more jobs, and caring for aging parents. Their negative effects may be alleviated if assistance is provided early in the process of a change. In some organizations, resources for managing problems of addiction, life transitions, emotional issues, financial problems, stress reduction, and grief counselling are available off-site to all employees. These resources are offered without cost to the individual and, in some cases, to their family members or support persons.

### The Two-or-More-Job Family: Family and Work Responsibilities

More and more women are in the workforce for their own financial well-being or that of their family, especially with the increased cost of living, insurance, and postsecondary education expenses and the decreased availability of employer-sponsored pension. Other women, who are postmenopausal and have launched their last child, have a new-found freedom and begin to rediscover themselves, sometimes through a new career. The husband may be a support person in this venture or he may feel threatened by his wife's new pursuits. These role changes and life transitions can be stressors to the family.

The balance between marital status, with or without children at home, caring for older parents, and employment obligations can significantly affect the psychological well-being of the woman in her middle years. In recent years, changes in family patterns with adult children moving back into their parents' home, sometimes with their offspring, bring new challenges to relationships, resources, and responsibilities within the home.

Historically, women worked with their husbands within the family farm or business. Only in the few decades immediately after World War II did many middle-class women stay at home while their husbands went to work. Currently, women make up a significant portion of the workforce. Additionally, many women have become highly educated and motivated to pursue careers. Both men and women are increasingly taking jobs that do not end at 5:00 p.m. The problems and challenges of the workplace are experienced at home as adults bring projects and problems home with them.

Job-related travel has also increased during the last few years for both men and women. Travel by either partner means additional responsibilities for the one who remains at home. Additionally, if one spouse travels far more than the other travels, feelings of resentment may develop, or the common ground for discussion of work events may be altered. The one who stays at home may feel "put upon" when the spouse is perceived as having fun. In contrast, travel is tiring and is not usually as exciting as it appears to observers. The travelling spouse can come home tired and irritable and desire peace and quiet, which may conflict with the expectations of other family members.

Men may feel threatened by highly successful and visible women. For some families, the post–World War II prototype was for the husband to support the family financially and gain status through achievements of work outside the home. As women gain recognition and acclaim for their career accomplishments, even the most "enlightened" man may experience twinges of envy and discomfort. Men have few role models from whom to learn how best to be a participant in a successful two-career family. Men may need as much, if not more, support than women in adapting to contemporary family styles. Opportunities to discuss what it means to be a man in today's society can be helpful, such as in support groups with volunteers or professionals who provide services to various agencies and community resources.

In addition to the changes in women and the effect on families of each adult working at one or more jobs, the nature of the parental work environment is critical to family coping ability. Work that is emotionally draining, particularly when it is filled with conflict, poses special threats to family stability. When parents come home tired, angry, or frustrated from their experiences at work, they probably have limited emotional support to share with other family members. When people gain self-esteem from their jobs and generally enjoy going to work, they tend to experience less frustration and dissatisfaction with themselves and their positions, enabling them to give more of themselves to other members of the family.

Middle age is important when one is looking at the career clock. Issues that need to be considered include mid-career changes and preretirement planning. Retirement is a major turning point; to many people, it is the transition from middle age to old age and the period of work to the period of leisure or different work.

Adults are working up to and beyond the age of retirement. Many are entering new careers later in life because they are living longer and are in need of more financial resources to successfully enter the older adult years. As adults progress through the middle years, they become increasingly aware of the time remaining until retirement: "Can I readjust my goals?" "Is there disparity between where I am in my career and where I would like to be?" An example might be the 60-year-old veteran nightclub singer whose goal to record a solo album remains to be achieved. The heightened awareness of age and the decreased likelihood of finding another suitable job can precipitate increased anxiety or depression in this singer.

### Caring for Aging Parents

The needs of aging parents and of the middle-aged adult's own children can create additional demands during the middle years (Fig. 17.1). The middle-aged adult can feel caught between the children and the parents. Both children and older parents can present unrealistic, excessive demands and be difficult to please.

Middle-aged adults may be faced with having frail and ill parents live within their own family unit or placing them in a nursing home. These dilemmas are complicated by the reality that their parents are growing older and may not have long to live. The recognition of the parents' impending death heightens middle-aged adults' awareness of their own aging and mortality.

Difficulties in caring for older parents can be somewhat lessened when potential situations are discussed before a crisis arises. This is particularly true when all members of the middle-aged adult family are working, space in their home is limited, and

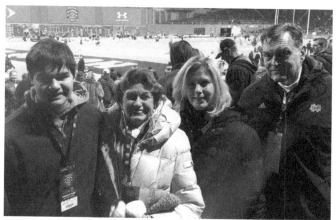

**Fig. 17.1** Middle-aged adults, young adults, and older adults can enjoy meaningful relationships with one another.

the community has few resources for the well or ill older adults. Although institutionalization is undesirable to many families, the care of ill, older parents may eventually require it. By anticipating these needs and preparing for them, middle-aged adults and their parents can develop further meaningful relationships with one another.

### Divorce

Divorce is a major disruption to the marriage and family and to each individual's short-term and long-term health. As the divorce rate has risen in recent years, individuals and families have been challenged to find solutions to new and multiple problems. When a divorce occurs, each family member must confront the necessity to examine and, in many cases, modify an accustomed style of living and adapting.

In the early 1970s, Wallerstein, Lewis, and Blakeslee (2000) began a longitudinal study of 131 children of divorced parents through extensive interviews with the children and their parents. The children are now adults with families of their own. The most significant findings of this ongoing study are the long-lasting, cumulative, and demonstrative effects of divorce that continue for decades. Although Wallerstein et al. (2000) found healing in adults is more or less complete 3 years after divorce, this is not so for the children, who experience the divorce differently from their parents.

Some of the limitations of this research are anecdotal methods versus double-blind interviews; the children are primarily White, educated, and upper middle class; and the findings are not differentiated from those of high-conflict families, nor are distinctions made between the influences of conflict that caused the divorce and the actual divorce itself. Continuing research is being done to illuminate these initial findings on the long-term effects of divorce. Sumnera (2013) suggests that parental midlife divorce also impacts children who are adults at the time of parental separation. Therapeutic interventions that assist adult children of divorced parents to reconcile the divorce experience of their parents should be offered and available.

### Death

Similarly to divorce, death of a spouse can result in grieving for the loss of companionship and the loss of an anticipated future free from the responsibilities of work and children. The surviving spouse may be unprepared to be single again, to be the only parent, or to live alone. The loneliness may be exacerbated by ill or dying peers or parents. Middle-aged adults become increasingly aware of the finite nature of life, thinking not only of the number of years since birth but also of the number of years left to live. The midlife review is a common outcome of this recognition.

◆ **Sexuality-Reproductive Pattern**

Research suggests that a high proportion of men and women remain sexually active well into later life (Lochlainn & Kenny, 2013). Men and women can continue to have a satisfactory pattern of sexual functioning throughout the middle and older adult years. As they would in any other developmental phase, middle-aged adults may need counselling to make health-promoting decisions about their sexual and reproductive behaviours and health.

Unintended pregnancies are high across all ages of Canadian women, but are highest in middle-aged women. Fertility begins to decline for women between 35 and 40 years of age; however, perimenopausal women are still at risk of an unintended pregnancy (Nelson, 2011). Nearly 30% of pregnancies in women older than 35 years are unintended (Godfrey, Chin, Fielding, et al., 2011). In their 2016 study, the Sex Information and Education Council of Canada (SIECCAN) found that more than 60% of single Canadian adults between the ages of 40 and 59 failed to use a contraceptive during sexual intercourse (SIECCAN, 2016). In contrast, women planning to have children during the fourth and fifth decades of life should know that fertility rates decrease and infant mortality rates increase, especially when mothers are aged 45 years or older. The average age of women at first birth is rising, and stillbirths occur more frequently in middle-age women (Johnson & Tough 2012).

The pregnancy-related mortality rate for all women in Canada has fluctuated over the years. In 2011, it was 4.8 deaths per 100,000 live births, as compared with 9.0 deaths per 100,000 live births in 2008, 2.5 per 100,000 in 1990, and 7.6 per 100,000 in 1980 (Verstraeten, Mijovik-Kondejewski, Takeda, et al., 2015). Further research needs to be done on maternal mortality rates among Indigenous people of Canada to assess the comparisons with the rest of the Canadian maternal population. Achieving the goal of reducing maternal deaths will require that national, provincial, and local policies address women's needs before and during pregnancy, and that gaps in research and prevention programs be identified through improved monitoring.

Changes in the reproductive systems of men and women result in changes in sexual function throughout adulthood. During middle adulthood, sexual arousal is slower, orgasms are less intense, and a return to pre-arousal levels is more rapid, with men having longer refractory periods between erection and ejaculation. When a person continues to be sexually active, these functional changes occur over decades and are minimally noticeable until later in adulthood, unless external factors are present, such as the negative effects of some antihypertensive and antidepressant agents.

After menopause, many women enjoy sex more, especially because the risk of pregnancy no longer exists. Conversely, menopause can bring many challenges to a woman. Canadian culture values women largely for their youth, beauty, and child-bearing ability. Middle-aged women may confront their own aging for the first time and may be perplexed as to the symptomatic factors and possibly changing roles. Women can experience vaginal dryness, difficulty finding a partner, less interest in initiating sex, and longer times to reach orgasm. However, perceived emotional closeness during sex was found to be associated with more frequent arousal, lubrication, and orgasm (Trompeter, Bettencourt, & Barrett-Connor, 2012).

Although men and women frequently enjoy satisfactory sexual relationships throughout the middle adult years, men in their middle age are more vulnerable to sexual dysfunction than are women. Erectile dysfunction, the inability to attain or maintain an erection sufficient enough for sexual activity, is a common disorder among older men. The gradual decline of age-related physiological function combined with chronic comorbidities may impair erectile function (Hockenberry & Masson, 2015). Common disorders related to erectile dysfunction include cardiovascular disease, diabetes, lower urinary tract symptoms, and depression—all of which should be considered by health care providers when assessing middle-aged men experiencing erectile dysfunction. Several readily available, nonsurgical treatments for erectile dysfunction exist: medications, supplements, hormonal therapy, penile injection, and external vacuum devices. The successful treatment of erectile dysfunction has the potential to increase sexual performance satisfaction, intimacy between partners, and overall quality and satisfaction with life. Although the risk of pregnancy is no longer a concern for middle-aged consenting adults, improved sexual function may increase the frequency of sexual activity and perhaps with more than one partner. Health care providers should not hesitate to initiate a sexual wellness assessment with middle-aged adults. Discussions should include specific sexual wellness strategies designed to prevent sexually transmitted infections (STIs).

Abnormal genital bleeding and secondary amenorrhea are common gynecological conditions that indicate serious physical problems. Abnormal genital bleeding is the most common reason for gynecological office visits by adult women. Although pregnancy and menopause are the most common causes of secondary amenorrhea, other conditions related to abnormal pregnancy, functional disorders, physiological changes, and pathological factors must be considered (Eliopoulos, 2010).

As for adolescents and young adults, STIs continue to be a major public health problem for middle-aged adults. Women and children bear an inordinate share of the burden: sterility, ectopic pregnancy, fetal and infant deaths, birth defects, and mental development delay. Virtually all cases of cervical cancer involve women who also are infected by human papillomavirus (HPV), but HPV does not always cause the cancer by itself. Other risk factors, such as age (most cases occur in women younger than 50 years of age), ethnicity (it affects women of African ancestry more than White women), and lower income and education (which may result in less cervical screening) may also increase the chance for the cancer to develop (Canadian Cancer Society, 2019a). As with many other health behaviours and diseases, the full effect on the life of an individual and the family may not be realized until middle age.

Adults in middle age have many of the same HIV/AIDS (human immunodeficiency virus/ acquired immunodeficiency syndrome) risk factors as younger people, but they may be less aware of their risk. In 2013, people aged 50 years or older accounted for 19% of the positive HIV diagnoses in Canada for that year. More than 50% of new HIV infections occur as a result of people who have HIV but do not know it (PHAC, 2013). The actual numbers may be higher, because HIV/AIDS is often misdiagnosed, underreported, and undertested in this population. Middle-aged Canadians are more likely to receive a diagnosis of HIV infection later in the course of their disease, which can lead to a poorer prognosis and shorter survival after an HIV infection diagnosis (PHAC, 2013).

More than three-fourths of all people currently with HIV/AIDS in Canada are men. Although anyone can be affected by HIV, it continues to be concentrated in specific populations in Canada, with gay men continuing to be the most affected population (PHAC, 2013). Transgender women who have sex with men are among the groups at highest risk of HIV infection, followed by injection drug users, who remain at significant risk of getting HIV. The PHAC now recommends HIV screening for adolescents and adults between 15 and 64 years, those who engage in risky behaviours, and all pregnant women, including those who present in labour whose HIV status is unknown (PHAC, 2013).

## ◆ Coping–Stress Tolerance Pattern

Kobasa (1979) was the first to investigate the concept of stress hardiness. She identified hardiness as an aspect of personality that included control, commitment, and challenge. Her theory is clinically relevant because it suggests hardiness acts as a mediator between perceived stress and self-efficacy across many dimensions: physical, psychological, mental, and emotional. According to Kobasa, individuals who demonstrate hardiness, across the health continuum, appear to be more resistant to the effects of stress.

Stress is an unavoidable human life experience that triggers a reactive physiological response often derived from perceived psychological stressors. The many negative effects of perceived stress on physical health are well documented. Physiologically, stress causes the hormones cortisol, epinephrine, and norepinephrine to activate or exacerbate a number of conditions, including chronic physical, mental, and comorbid health conditions (Manchanda & Madan, 2014; Vranceanu, Gonzalez, Niles, et al., 2014). Stress tolerance is a learned behaviour. More than 35 years ago, Benson first described the "relaxation response" as a reproducible state of deep rest (Benson & Klipper, 1975). The immediate and long-lasting effects of stress can be mitigated with effective coping skills,

 **INNOVATIVE PRACTICE**

### The Benson–Henry Institute for Mind Body Medicine at Massachusetts General Hospital, Harvard Medical School Mind/Body Medical Symptom Reduction Programs

Research demonstrates that 60% to 90% of health care visits are for symptoms such as headaches, insomnia, weakness or fatigue, and gastrointestinal symptoms, all of which are frequently stress related. The Mind/Body Medical Symptom Reduction Programs are designed to help individuals who have chronic illnesses (including life-threatening illnesses) or stress-related symptoms to better manage their health problems and optimize their quality of life. The interventions combine conventional medical care with knowledge of the effects of behaviours and attitudes on health. The following interventions are included in the biopsychosocial-spiritual approach of the assessment and treatment plans:

- Eliciting the relaxation response, a state of deep rest that changes responses to stress (decreases vital signs and muscle tenseness, increases mindfulness)
- Enhancing coping skills through cognitive-behavioural strategies
- Encouraging exercise or physical activity
- Providing nutritional counselling
- Monitoring and adjusting medication, when necessary, in consultation with the physician

Research demonstrates the following results may occur after these interventions:

- Persons with pain reduced their number of physician visits by 36%.
- Visits to a health maintenance organization were reduced by approximately 50% after a relaxation response–based intervention, resulting in significant cost savings.
- Blood pressure was lowered and use of medications decreased in 80% of hypertensive persons; 16% were able to discontinue all of their medications.
- Sleep patterns were improved for 100% of persons with insomnia; 90% reduced or eliminated the use of sleep medication.
- Infertile women reported decreased levels of depression, anxiety, and anger, along with a 35% conception rate.
- Women with severe premenstrual syndrome experienced a 57% reduction in physical and psychological symptoms.
- Health-promoting behaviours, such as nutrition, social supports, self-esteem, health responsibility, and exercise, increased after the program and were maintained by the 6-month follow-up visit.
- Six months after the program, 80% of persons continued to experience reduction of their physical symptoms.
- Anxiety and depression normalized for most participants and were maintained for 6 months following the program.
- Women with menopause reported fewer hot flashes, lower blood pressure, improved sleep, and decreased depression, anxiety, and anger.

including holistic mind–body interventions such as meditation, yoga, tai chi, and deep breathing (Manchanda & Madan, 2014; Wang, Lee, Wu, et al., 2014). Evidence-informed research demonstrates how the mind–body connection helps individuals to cope with a wide range of illnesses and stressful life events (Innovative Practice).

In a 45-year longitudinal study of 173 men, Vaillant (2003) and Vaillant and Vaillant (1990) found that the extent of tranquilizer use before age 50 years was the most powerful negative predictor of both mental and physical health outcomes at age 65 years. Another important predictor for health outcomes was the maturity of defences against stress such as sublimation, anticipation, altruism, and humour.

## Stress and Heart Disease

As reiterated throughout this chapter, heart disease is the second leading cause of death in the middle-aged adult. In landmark studies, Haynes, Levine, Scotch, and colleagues (1978) and Haynes, Feinleib, and Kannel (1980) described the relationship of psychosocial factors to coronary heart disease using the Framingham study. In the study, 24 measures of psychosocial stress were used. In men, aging worries correlated significantly with systolic and diastolic blood pressure. Marital disagreement and personal worries correlated significantly with diastolic blood pressure. Both diastolic and systolic pressure correlated significantly with work changes and anxiety in employed women between 45 and 64 years of age. Anger suppressed, anger discussed, tension, and anger symptoms correlated significantly with diastolic blood pressure in this age group.

Among white-collar men in this age group, the Framingham type A and ambitiousness scales also correlated significantly with elevated diastolic blood pressure. The correlation of anger symptoms and anger discussed with diastolic pressures was significant for white-collar women aged between 45 and 65 years. The initial findings of Haynes and her colleagues have been supported by many other studies, including those of Spielberger, Jacobs, Russell, et al. (1983), Kawachi, Sparrow, Spirolli, et al. (1996), Williams, Patton, Siegler, et al. (2000), and Sanchez-Gonzalez, May, Koutnik, et al., (2015).

The death of a parent enhances awareness of one's vulnerability to illness and death. The more opportunities and time people have to prepare for these stressful events, the more likely they will be to feel in control and the less likely they will be to feel anxious and helpless. When individuals assume more responsibility for their life, decisions lead to concrete behaviours, such as drafting a will, developing an advance directive (which includes living will, health care agent, and granting a durable power of attorney), and making funeral prearrangements. An advance directive is a legal document prepared when an individual is alive, competent, and able to make decisions to provide guidelines for health care providers in the future, when the individual is not able to make decisions because of physical disability (being unconscious) or mental incompetence. By granting a power of attorney, the individual designates another person (spouse, son, daughter, or friend) to make health care decisions (especially about how aggressive treatment should be in forestalling death) when an individual becomes unable to make such decisions. The nurse helps middle-aged adults anticipate stressors so that they are better prepared to cope with and to prevent additional physical, psychosocial, and spiritual stressors, thereby optimizing their health.

## ◆ Values-Beliefs Pattern

When adults make decisions affecting their lives, this is usually the result of a personal, complex pattern of values and beliefs. Much of what people value or believe to be true is formed early in life and can be the most difficult to alter. Usually, people do not spend a great deal of conscious thought on abstract explanations of the meaning of life and why certain things are valued. However, during times of illness or crisis, most people will take time to review their value systems and seek meaning about what is important.

A crisis at any age can be a turning point during which both increased vulnerability and increased potential are present. When the crisis is managed successfully, a virtue or strength will evolve. Erikson and Erikson (1998) identified *caring* as a middle-aged adult virtue that is often developed during times of crisis.

Committed responsibilities for the care and welfare of others promote moral development. When middle age is lived with generativity, many opportunities are afforded to live life by one's higher principles. The middle-aged adult can differentiate among personal wants and needs, duties demanded by society, and principles by which to live. Kohlberg's work on moral development delineated these phases as conventional and postconventional. His studies of men described stage 3 as an interpersonal definition of morality, whereas stage 4 is a societal definition based on law and order. Kohlberg concludes that most Canadian adults are in these phases of moral development. In contrast, stage 5 is the concern and willingness to sacrifice oneself for the well-being of others (Kohlberg & Lickona, 1986). Subsequent studies by Gilligan (1982) on moral development in women and men demonstrate sex differences when describing high morality. Women discussed issues of selfishness versus responsibility, of exercising care with decision making, and avoiding hurting others. Men described terms of *justice, fairness,* and *rights of individuals.* Gilligan (1982, 1990) concluded that women possess a process of moral development different from that of men.

Valuing others, having relationships, and being responsible to others enable middle-aged adults to make the transitions of moral development. This process is accomplished through raising children, developing more junior employees, and serving the community. As people fulfill these commitments, they increasingly treat others as equals and gradually develop a sensitivity and desire to change barriers to human worth and equality such as racial prejudice, homelessness, and inadequate access to health care.

## ❖ ENVIRONMENTAL PROCESSES

Environmental factors are significant variables in health promotion. Cleanliness in home, work, and school environments helps control the spread of infectious diseases such as influenza. The effect of handwashing in controlling illness cannot be overstated. In a larger context, continued efforts at improving sanitation and controlling pollution (air, water, noise) will result in a reduction of health problems such as lung disease, transmission of bacterial and viral infections, and hearing loss.

Because there are approximately 18 million workers in Canada (Statistics Canada, 2019c), occupational hazards are a serious threat to national health. Exposures to toxic chemicals, asbestos, mining dust, ionizing radiation, physical hazards, excessive noise, and stress can precipitate numerous health problems (Canadian Centre for Occupational Health and Safety [CCOHS], 2018a). For the middle-aged worker, these problems include cancers, lung and heart diseases, decreased hearing, physical injuries, and mental health disorders (CCOHS, 2018b).

## ◆ Physical Agents

Ionizing radiation is a physical agent that can cause cancer. One example of this is cancer caused by medical procedures that include the use of diagnostic radiography and therapeutic radiation.

Water pollution has become another major concern. Many industrial and agricultural wastes, such as benzene and chlordane, have been recovered in rivers and lakes from which drinking water is obtained. These substances can potentially lead to carcinomas and other health problems.

Air pollution from automobile emissions, burning fuels, and industrial incineration has warranted smog alerts and air pollution indices. This issue is especially important to the individual with chronic diseases such as bronchitis, emphysema, and asthma (CCOHS, 2017).

Noise pollution in industry is a potential problem for the middle-aged adult worker. Hearing loss is the most common occupational disease, but it can be prevented if federal guidelines are followed with regard to noise exposure levels and hearing conservation programs, especially prevention activities aimed at miners and construction workers, for whom hearing loss is a major problem. Exposure to excessive noise, radon, radiation, sunlight, and vibration can produce problems such as chronic obstructive lung disease, cancer, and degenerative diseases (Nissenbaum, Aramini, & Hanning, 2012).

## ◆ Biological Agents

As noted throughout this text, health and disease are influenced by the interactions among the agent, host, and environment. Agent factors can be biological, physical, chemical, or psychological. The biological causes of diseases include bacteria, viruses, rickettsiae, fungi, parasites, and food poisoning. Because these causes are often limited to identifiable occupations, they can be readily diagnosed, treated, and prevented. Many of these agents are transmitted through the air or by contact with certain media, such as water, food, blood, or feces.

Hepatitis A is caused by viral infection, with transmission occurring primarily through the fecal–oral route. This host–agent interaction typically occurs in the middle-aged adult living in an environment with poor sanitation and having close contact with an infected person. The person may also be exposed through contaminated food and water. The hepatitis B viral agent is transmitted primarily in the blood or plasma of the infected individuals, which is particularly significant for the adult who is employed in a health care setting. Among medical and dental personnel (with surgeons, oral surgeons, and pathologists at the highest risk), the risk of contracting hepatitis B is six times higher than that of the general population.

There are two other infections that are of particular concern for middle-aged adults: pneumonia and varicella/herpes zoster ("shingles"). Both can be prevented through vaccinations, which adults aged 60 and 50 years or older, respectively, are advised to receive (PHAC, 2018).

## ◆ Chemical Agents

Chemical agents include a wide variety of substances that increase the risk of morbidity and death in the middle-aged adult. When a home is located near an industry, there is the risk of exposure to toxic chemicals that pollute the air. Contaminants can also be carried home on the clothing from the workplace.

Workers at increased risk include coal miners, wood handlers, and those who work with asbestos. Pneumoconiosis is found in approximately 15% of coal miners, with "black lung disease," and continues to contribute to mortality rates from various respiratory diseases. Wood handlers have increased the risk of certain cancers. The asbestos worker has an increased risk of mesothelioma and asbestosis. Many workers each year are exposed to benzene and vinyl chloride, which may be carcinogens. Canadian industrial workers may also be inadequately protected from exposure to at least 10 of the 163 most common hazardous chemicals. More than 2000 of the 50,000 chemicals found in the workplace are suspected human carcinogens. Following Canadian regulations, all workplace chemicals must be specifically labelled in order to protect workers from accidental injury or exposure (Workplace Hazardous Material Information System [WHMIS], 2018).

### Tobacco

Cigarette smoking is the leading cause of preventable death, disease, and disability in Canada. In 2017, an estimated 5 million people over the age of 12 smoked cigarettes in Canada. In the middle-aged population, approximately 25% of men and 15% of women in Canada smoke. The proportion of smokers varies by income levels. Among those with the lowest income, one in five Canadians are smokers, and in households with the highest income, one in 10 are smokers (Statistics Canada, 2018a). Among Canadians, cigarette smoking, and exposure to second-hand smoke, is responsible for more than 45,000 premature deaths annually, which is nearly 1 in 5 of all deaths in the country (Canadian Cancer Society, 2019b). Smoke recipients are at increased risks of heart disease as well as colds, chronic bronchitis, emphysema, and cancers of the mouth, lungs, esophagus, pancreas, and bladder. Many 50-year-old adults have a 30-plus-year history of cigarette smoking. The life expectancy for smokers is at least 10 years less than that of nonsmokers; however, quitting smoking, and not having smoked for 20 years, reduces the risk of dying of smoking-related disease dramatically. Five years after quitting smoking an individual reduces their risk of lung cancer by 30 to 60% (Lung Cancer Canada, 2018).

Few smokers realize that cigarettes contain 2000 known chemicals, including tar, nicotine, hydrogen cyanide, formaldehyde, and ammonia. Cigarette smoking is, for most smokers, an addiction to nicotine, which is absorbed into the bloodstream. Nicotine acts on the two divisions of the nervous system: central (brain and the spinal cord) and peripheral (autonomic nervous system and motor and sensory fibres to the arms and legs). The effects of nicotine stimulation can be observed both in electroencephalographic changes and in hand tremors. Nicotine also stimulates the heart, leading to an increased pulse rate and elevated blood pressure. Although smokers frequently believe that cigarettes have a calming effect, this notion is misleading. Nicotine stimulates the body, whereas carbon monoxide causes lethargy. Smokers may feel calm, although they are actually having their sensations dulled by carbon monoxide. Additive effects such as those from chlorine, cotton dust, and γ-radiation can lower mid-expiratory flow values. Profound effects can also be observed with asbestos interaction.

## ❖ DETERMINANTS OF HEALTH

### ◆ Social Factors and Environment

Culture is a set of beliefs, practices, norms, customs, rituals, and assumptions about life that are first learned from one's parents and extended family during the early years of socialization (Spector, 2012). Spector further relates the ways in which one's cultural background is a component of one's ethnic background.

Nurses understand the potential influences their own ethnic cultures have on those of others. The middle-aged adult may not interpret dizziness as a possible symptom of hypertension: for example, it may be described simply as a spell. People from different ethnic backgrounds may have completely different definitions of health. The obese adult who has received positive reinforcement throughout life for being pleasingly plump is less motivated to lose weight than is the adult who defines health as being svelte.

The health problems of middle-aged adults, even within major ethnic groups, are varied. Recent immigrants to Canada have a much lower death rate than non-immigrants, even among those who lived in neighbourhoods classified as having low socioeconomic conditions (Khan, Urquia, Kornas, et al., 2017). This "healthy immigrant effect" tends to decline over time and successive generations. Immigrant men have a slight advantage in mortality over female immigrants, which might be caused by barriers for the women in accessing health care services in some provinces.

Poverty rates are important indicators of community well-being and the health status of community members. According to the 2016 Canadian census, 4.8 million visible minority people, or 14.2% of the Canadian population, were in the low-income bracket. By ethnicity, the highest national low-income rates were for Arabs (36.2%), West Asians (34.7%), and Koreans (32.6%) (Statistics Canada, 2018b).

Economic adversity, disproportionate access to health services, and cultural differences may contribute to lower life expectancy and the disproportionate disease burden for Indigenous Canadian people. The Indigenous person in Canada's life expectancy (64 years for males and 73 years for females) is considerably lower than that for the Canadian general population (82.3 years). Mortality rates are significantly higher in many areas for Indigenous Canadian people compared with the Canadian general population, including those from tuberculosis, pneumonia, diabetes mellitus, unintentional injuries, intentional self-harm, breast cancer, and alcohol and drug abuse (Statistics Canada, 2015c).

*Culture also determines acceptable gender-specific and age-specific attitudes and behaviours.* Accepted gender-specific attitudes and behaviours associated with life-defining rituals (birth, marriage, illness, and death) are particularly important for stabilizing and preserving one's culture. Aging confers vast decline and compromise for both sexes. Middle-aged adults who

---

### 🌐 DIVERSITY AWARENESS

#### *Health Care for Middle-Aged Indigenous People*

Culturally safe and effective health care is imperative for all, especially people with several comorbid conditions who do not have a consistent primary care provider or clinic. Middle-aged Indigenous people are in need of consistent health care. The Indigenous are a large and sometimes vulnerable population in Canada. Many Indigenous people live in remote or rural Canadian locations, and are considered "underserved" in their health care. Barriers to adequate care delivery include socioeconomic status, geography, lack of infrastructure and staff, and language or cultural barriers. While some barriers can be similar between different groups of Indigenous people, others may vary significantly based on location of residence and status. Health care providers need to understand their beliefs so that the episodic interactions will be most productive. Furthermore, it is important for health care providers to consider use of language, community, family, and cultural traditions as part of the health care process. It may also be important to assess the preference for family involvement when it comes to decisions about health. A family member should be allowed to participate in interactions with health providers. Involvement of the family may increase the person's ability to engage in health-promotion and health care activities.

#### Reflective Questions
- Given the context from which you live and work, how is diversity viewed or acknowledged in health care settings?
- What are a few questions that you might want to ask to determine care preferences from a culturally safe lens?

Source: National Collaborating Centre for Aboriginal Health. (2011). *Access to health services as a social determinant of First Nations, Inuit and Métis health*. Retrieved from https://www.ccnsa-nccah.ca/docs/determinants/FS-AccessHealthServicesSDOH-EN.pdf.

---

conform to stereotypical patterns of expected role behaviours often receive continued communal support and reverence even as their health status and abilities decline. Conversely, those who choose not to conform to expected changes in behaviours and roles risk exclusion, isolation, loneliness, and compromised health. Nurses who promote cultural safety can ensure that appropriate health promotion is provided, especially for vulnerable populations and those individuals, families, and communities who have special health care needs (**Diversity Awareness**).

### ◆ Levels of Policymaking and Health

Adults in the middle years are frequently at the peak of their careers. Although their net income may be greater than it was during early adulthood, they frequently have significant additional financial obligations. For many individuals in their late 50s or early 60s, retirement is a life stage they have dreamt about and anticipated for years (Fig. 17.2). Leaving full-time employment for a less strenuous daily routine may not be possible for many middle-aged adults. A number of reasons are offered to account for this relatively new trend:

- The high quality of health care in Canada provides technological advances that extend the limits for life expectancy. Individuals are living longer than previous generations, and therefore they cannot "afford" to retire in their mid-50s to early 60s because they have a financial need to "fund" another 25 to 30 years of life.

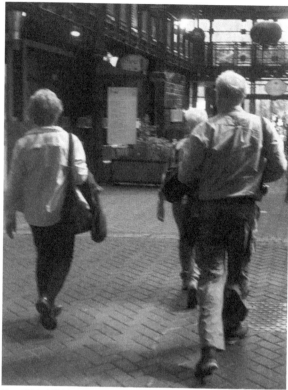

**Fig. 17.2** Middle-aged adults may enjoy travel after retirement.

- Changes in the Canadian economy in the past 10 years have necessitated significant changes in family patterns. Increasingly, more than one generation lives together in the same home so as to afford the rising costs of commodities that have been taken for granted. For example, the costs of a university education funded by middle-aged adults are not necessarily balanced by a full-time position at the end of the 4 or 5 years needed to obtain a university degree. Young adults may not be leaving home in their early 20s, as previous generations have done. Consequently, their parents, if still employed, may be required to continue to work to support adult children and also to pay the debt of the university educational experience.

- Individuals may have increasing health care expenses as this is becoming more costly. As people develop health conditions that are related to accumulated stress and the aging process, they require more use of their benefits from their extended health insurance companies. Since many Canadians do not have extended health benefit plans (through their workplaces), for them, health expenses from prescriptions, therapies, and other services not covered by their province's government-funded medical service plan can add up. Because of the cost, some Canadians may not be able to receive the best possible treatment since they cannot afford it. In addition, some Canadians may be supporting older parents, whose health conditions result in increased costs for their parents' medications, private care, and/or long-term care expenses. When the adult or family members have ongoing health problems, the economic status of the family can be compromised further (see **Diversity Awareness** box).

- While the national unemployment statistics have been fairly steady since 2016, with even some slight improvements in recent years, provincial levels show variations, with Newfoundland and Labrador having the highest unemployment, and the southwest region of British Columbia having the lowest levels (Statistics Canada, 2018c). When people lose their jobs, they are often without extended health benefits, and when they develop illnesses or conditions that are associated with the middle years, it can cause additional expenses and mental strain and possibly lead to mental health problems. The individual's economic status plays a role in the incidence of mental illness, with higher rates of anxiety, depression, and phobias evident in adults at the lower socioeconomic level.

- Technological changes have opened opportunities for individuals to work at home and/or remote sites. These extensions of the workplace often necessitate individuals to change their routines, and to take educational courses to keep current with job requirements, or to be competent to take on more responsibilities. Training to increase skills or knowledge can be expensive and often must be funded by the individual.

## ◆ Health Services/Delivery System

Numerous agencies are geared to providing information and other resources for the middle-aged adult. Councils of community services frequently publish a directory, outlining the various available services. The main structure of the Canadian health care system includes services that are provincially funded, such as hospitals and family physicians. Voluntary agencies include the Heart and Stroke Foundation, the Canadian Cancer Society, the Lung Association, and Alcoholics Anonymous. Many educational and self-help programs are sponsored by these organizations. The Lung Association sponsors a smoking cessation program, which can be conducted individually, or on a group basis in a work or community setting. Service agencies include professional organizations, such as provincial/territorial nursing regulatory bodies and associations, the Canadian Medical Association, bar associations, Young Men's Christian Association (YMCA), and hospice programs.

Canada's medicare system provides access to health care for all Canadians. The implications of this statute are most significant for middle-aged adults, who often have pre-existing health conditions. Preventive screening will allow individuals to receive testing for the detection of cancer and other conditions that can influence initiation of treatment at an earlier stage of illness. The financial expense of such treatments is generally covered by citizens' respective provincial medical services plans. However, long wait times often exist for such treatments, which may result in anxiety and a deterioration of patients' health conditions. Those Canadians who have the financial means may choose to pursue more prompt treatment at private care agencies where costs are fully borne by the consumer and/or only partially covered by the provincial Medical Services Plan. Usually, seeking treatment at private agencies allows people to avoid the long waiting time for treatment in the public system. Private care agencies exist in various formats in each Canadian province.

## ❖ NURSING APPLICATION

Interventions focused on health promotion span the gamut for nurses working in the community or on location at work sites. Consequently, there are many ways nurses interact with middle-aged adults.

Individuals in this middle-age range will probably need the services of a professional nurse *several times* before they reach their 60s. They may meet a nurse when seeking care for themselves in a physician's office or primary care centre. As a parent, they are likely to accompany their school-age child or their own older parent to the emergency department to obtain care for a sports-related injury or trauma following a fall. In the employment realm, some individuals will have their initial experience with a nurse through a pre-employment evaluation visit. As a company employee, the same person may receive first aid for a minor injury or have his or her blood pressure monitored periodically by a nurse working in the occupational health department.

If individuals need surgery or hospitalization, they may meet a home health nurse after discharge. Nurses are also available in rehabilitation settings to instruct and coach people regarding lifestyle changes following a heart attack or other acute events. Community health nurses provide health-promotion activities such as senior health fairs that include "flu clinics," where adults are vaccinated against influenza. Life events such as the death of a partner, sudden unemployment, or disability may cause anxiety, depression, or other stress-related symptoms. Nurses who specialize in mental health can provide counselling and other forms of treatment for grief support or mental health disorders resulting from trauma or sudden losses.

In a variety of settings, nurses are health educators. For example, the nurse who works in the community or in occupational health initiates events that raise awareness to identify health risks among middle-aged adults. In that role, the nurse teaches strategies for controlling symptoms and accepting responsibility for changing potentially dangerous health habits. These interventions can be provided on a one-to-one or group basis or as a lecture presented in a health seminar.

The target groups identified by occupational health nurses frequently have common needs for information, interventions, and periodic monitoring. Common concerns in the workplace are exposure to chemical or toxic substances, tobacco and substance abuse and addiction, and ongoing problems with fatigue attributable to frequent changes in scheduled shifts.

Occupational health nurses have a wide range of responsibilities. For example, they may evaluate patterns of absenteeism to identify a source for infection that is affecting a group of employees. The nurse participates in policy development focused on preventing or reducing the incidence of work-site injuries or incidents. In another instance, the nurse provides clarification of the CCOHS regulations when new machinery is incorporated into operation. The nurse is wise to invite a broad spectrum of employee participants to join a company safety committee. Their primary purpose is focused on keeping the work site safe for employees. Strategies to achieve that objective include determining health hazards that exist in each department of the company and developing or refining procedures that promote safety, such as creating policies that address infection control or procedures for fire drills. If nurses have the appropriate certification, they can also offer classes in cardiopulmonary resuscitation and the use of the automated external defibrillator.

The scope of practice for community health nurses (CHNs) differs from province to province. They may be employed by a city or town, or derive their authority through a health jurisdiction. The role of the CHN focuses on health promotion and disease prevention for a population living in a specific area. The CHN interfaces with nurses working in the municipality and surrounding areas such as in health clinics, provincial/territorial health agencies and ministries, hospitals, urgent care clinics, schools, emergency services, and local businesses. Frequently, lectures or demonstrations are involved with service organizations in communities such as the Lions or Kiwanis Clubs. The CHN may combine efforts with nurses who volunteer as parish nurses. Together they may present health fairs to serve a broad scope of health-information needs of the local community. The features of the fair could include any of the following: demonstrations in the use of car seats and seat belts; short presentations on fall prevention; screening measures to identify risk factors for heart disease, cancer, and diabetes; community planning guides for emergency preparedness; massage therapy for stress reduction; and informational guides for the regional poison control centre. Such events allow the CHN and service organizations to generate interest and enthusiasm among people who are interested in improving the health and well-being of residents living in their local community.

Health-promotion strategies will become more widely recognized as the objectives of the PHAC are incorporated into health plans supported by health policies, employers, wellness programs, and health care providers. Nurses are in leadership roles to organize and implement early detection and screening programs. They survey communities and identify needs of the specific populations, and evaluate the effectiveness of public health measures already in place. They are called on to develop educational programs and create online information sites that disseminate current medical research findings to the public, showing how changes in lifestyle behaviours can positively influence health outcomes. Progress toward the national objectives of the PHAC are incorporated in websites so that Canadian people can see, and learn first hand, how important changes in their own lifestyle will affect the overall health of Canada.

In summary, better health and enhanced well-being of Canadian people are expected outcomes of health promotion. The PHAC objectives provide the framework and direction for improving health awareness and practices among Canadian residents.

In this chapter, health needs and potential diseases and conditions relevant to middle-aged adults have been addressed along with strategies to mitigate symptoms, prevent complications, and foster well-being. Normal changes expected with the aging process were also presented. Selected objectives of the PHAC were compared with findings published for health outcomes of Canadians. In addition, the impact of social processes, such as relationships, family, work, values and belief systems, disability and death, and finances, completed the discussion.

Nurses provide important strategies for fostering health promotion. They are employed in most settings where middle-aged adults live, work, play, and raise their families. Because of this integral position in society, nurses are highly influential in identifying health concerns, organizing interventions, and evaluating the effectiveness of program outcomes. The PHAC health objectives are presented as one approach for health professionals to use in their mission to improve the health and well-being of the Canadian people.

The CCOHS mandates that employees have a healthy and safe work environment; therefore a complete health history is essential, and may be mandatory in some workplaces. Is there a history of hypertension, arthritis, cancer, or hernia? Is there significant family history? Is the person a smoker? How many packs per day are smoked? Does the person take medications? Medical limitations must be addressed: for example, decreased visual acuity may mean no driving, and dermatitis means no skin exposure to oils, chemicals, or solvents. Removing a worker from a particular job (or moving them to another work area) may be indicated if the worker might endanger coworkers, if the worker has a disease condition that might be aggravated by the job, or if the worker is taking prescribed medications with potentially harmful side effects.

The nurse in the community and in industry should reiterate key safety directives to the middle-aged adult. For example, wear seat belts and observe speed limits, use only hands-free phone communication, and avoid texting while driving. The middle-aged adult's reaction time is also decreasing, which reinforces the need for periodic driving testing as required by several provincial driver licensing agencies.

With an increase in leisure time, the middle-aged adult is at greater risk of recreational accidents. As noted, moderation should be stressed. Alcohol is a depressant and should be avoided in activities that require attentiveness.

Protection from burns is essential; 56% of fatal residential fires are directly related to cigarette smoking while in bed. Falls can occur at any age; safety measures should be considered for the entire family, including specific preparatory planning for the very young and aging parents. A few suggestions to the middle-aged adult might be to avoid highly waxed floors, correct poor environmental lighting, avoid high beds, and avoid bathtubs lacking nonslip bottoms.

The CCOHS was designed to ensure that workers are employed under safe and healthy working conditions. Their policies are applicable to every employer who is engaged in a business that affects commerce. The employer must ascertain that the workplace is free from recognized hazards and must comply with the national policies. The CCOHS has offices in most major cities and can provide recommended standards for occupational agents.

Nurses can participate actively in the safety committee of the industry in which they are employed. When no such committee exists, many protection measures will fall on the nurse. The following are some suggestions:

- Tour the facilities on a regular basis. Be familiar with resource books, laws, and codes.
- Develop a toxicology chart with symptoms of overexposure and recommended treatment. Update this chart frequently.
- Be a role model in safety issues; wear safety glasses, protective footwear, and gloves; and do not smoke.
- Discuss the pre-employment physical examination with the employee, with an emphasis on risk factors. Monitor health problems and exposure levels in the work setting.

The worker must be aware of the protective clothing that should be worn, sanitation measures for the work environment, general hygiene measures, and proper immunization. The food handler, for instance, should have an annual tuberculosis skin test, wear clean clothing and appropriate hair protection, and use good handwashing techniques. The nurse should not assume that workers know how to protect themselves and others.

A major challenge for the nurse is to encourage workers to assume responsibility for protecting their own health. Increasingly, organizations are interested in promoting the health of their employees for many reasons, including enhancing their recruiting efforts and minimizing lateness, absenteeism, turnover, physical and emotional inability to work, disability costs, and health and life insurance costs. Health-promotion programs are increasingly recognized for their vital contributions to the financial viability of organizations.

Health-promotion programs within an organizational setting can be categorized in one of three levels: awareness, lifestyle change, and supportive environment. The goal of a health program, at the level of awareness, is to increase the individual's knowledge or interest in a particular health issue, such as smoking cessation. Examples of awareness programs include special events, flyers, lunch seminars, meetings, and newsletters. Changing health behaviours or status is not the goal of awareness programs, but is the goal of lifestyle change programs.

Lifestyle change programs last at least 8 to 12 weeks and include assessment, education, and evaluation components to help individuals implement long-term modifications in health behaviour and experience the results of their instituted changes. To maintain these long-term changes and to develop a healthy lifestyle, a supportive organizational environment is needed. This type of environment may include health-promoting physical settings, corporate policies and culture, ongoing programs, and employee ownership of programs.

## CASE STUDY

### Caregiver Role Strain: Ms. Sandra A.

Sandra, a 47-year-old divorced woman, received a diagnosis of stage III ovarian cancer 4 years ago, for which she had a total hysterectomy, bilateral salpingo-oophorectomy, omentectomy, lymphadenectomy, and tumour debulking followed by chemotherapy, consisting of cisplatin (Platinol), paclitaxel (Taxol), and doxorubicin (Adriamycin). She did well for 2 years and then moved back to her hometown near her family and underwent three more rounds of second-line chemotherapy. She accepted a less stressful job, bought a house, renewed old friendships, and became more involved with her two sisters and their families.

Sandra developed several complications, including metastasis to the lungs. Then she could no longer work, drive, or care for herself. She had been told by her oncologist that there was nothing else that could be done and that she should consider entering a hospice. She met her attorney and prepared an advance directive and completed her will. She decided to have hospice care at home and, with the help of her family, set up her first floor as a living and sleeping area. She was cared for by family members around the clock for approximately 3 days.

Sandra observed that she was tiring everyone out so much that they could not really enjoy each other's company. At this time, she contacted the local home care agency to seek assistance. Her plan was to try to enjoy her family and friend's visits. After assessment, the home care nurse prioritized her problems to include fatigue and caregiver role strain. Other potential problem areas that may need to be incorporated into the care plan include anticipatory grieving and impaired comfort.

#### Reflective Questions

* Viewed through the lens of social determinants of health and health inequities, what are some of the stresses on Sandra's middle-aged sisters and their families?
* What resources are available to manage these stresses and support the sisters while caring for their dying sister Sandra?
* Describe Sandra's feelings about dependency and loss of autonomy because she is unable to do her own activities of daily living any longer.

## CARE PLAN

### Caregiver Role Strain: Ms. Sandra A.

#### Nursing Issue
Potential for caregiver role strain related to sister's terminal cancer

#### Defining Characteristics
* Sandra's sisters are weary from doing all of the daily care for Sandra.
* Sandra and her family are at a point where they are accepting her terminal status.
* Sandra and her family want to prepare for a death at home.

#### Related Factors
* The sisters are missing work and neglecting their own families.
* The sisters need assistance to care for Sandra as she continues to become compromised.

#### Intended Outcomes
* Sandra and her sisters will contact the home care nurse to assist in planning daily hospice care at home.

* The home care nurse and the family will plan realistic care.
* Sandra will have quality time with her sisters and friends as her condition allows.
* The sisters will be able to voice their grief and anger about Sandra's upcoming death.

#### Interventions
* Home health aides are scheduled for 24 hours a day.
* A psychiatric nurse practitioner will meet Sandra and her family to schedule therapy time for anticipatory grieving.
* The sisters will attend a support group for families involved in hospice care at home.
* A schedule will be made to allow each sister time at home, one-on-one time with Sandra, and time for rest.

## SUMMARY

Nurses help middle-aged adults improve their quality of life, both for the present and for the future, by acknowledging how social determinants of health and health inequities impact health status and risk factors, through health promotion, and other nursing interventions. Nurses work in a variety of health care settings available to middle-aged adults: outpatient clinics, occupational health clinics, and private practice.

Health promotion and disease prevention are aimed at the personal habits and lifestyles of adults to improve their biological, spiritual, and psychosocial development. The strategies to help an adult achieve a higher level of health include individual and group counselling based on identified risk factors, providing self-help information that is most relevant to the middle-aged adult, and describing available resources. Using these strategies, the nurse can motivate middle-aged adults to prioritize their own health and quality of life, including it as a prerequisite for their own present and future health and particularly preceding the responsibilities in promoting the health and quality of life of younger and older generations. After years of poor health practices, adults can make changes that reduce their risk of disability from chronic disease and promote functioning and quality of life.

### Evolve Chapter Features
http://evolve.elsevier.com/Canada/Edelman/healthpromotion//
* Review Questions

# REFERENCES

Apter, T. (1990). *Altered loves: Mothers and daughters during adolescence.* New York: Ballantine Books.

Apter, T. (1995). *Secret paths: Women in the new midlife.* New York: Norton.

Association of Workers' Compensation Boards of Canada. (2016). *2016 lost time claims in Canada.* Retrieved from http://awcbc.org/?page_id=14.

Benjamin, R. M. (2012). Oral health care for persons living with HIV/AIDS. *Public Health Reports, 127*(Suppl. 2), 1–2.

Bensley, L., Van Eehwyk, J., & Ossiander, E. M. (2011). Association of self-reported periodontal disease with metabolic syndrome and a number of self-reported chronic conditions. *Prevention of Chronic Disease, 8*(30), A50.

Benson, H., & Klipper, M. Z. (1975). *The relaxation response.* New York: Hapertorch.

Bloom, B. S. (1984). *Taxonomy of educational objectives: Handbook 1, Cognitive domain.* New York: Longman.

Bloom, B., Simile, C. M., Adams, P. F., et al. (2012). Oral health status and access to oral health care for U.S. adults aged 18-64: National health interview survey, 2008, National Center for Health Statistics. *Vital Health Statistics, 10*(253), 1–22.

Brassen, S., Gamer, M., Peters, J., et al. (2012). Don't look back in anger! Responsiveness to missed changes in successful and nonsuccessful aging. *Science, 336*(6081), 612–614. https://doi.org/10.1126/science.1217516.

Buys, Y., Gaspo, R., & Kwok, K. (2012). Referral source, symptoms, and severity at diagnosis of ocular hypertension or open-angle glaucoma in various practices. *Canadian Journal of Ophthalmology, 47*(3), 217–222.

Canadian Association of Optometrists. (2018). *Glaucoma.* Retrieved from https://opto.ca/health-library/about-glaucoma.

Canadian Cancer Society. (2017). *Lung cancer statistics.* Retrieved from https://www.cancer.ca/en/cancer-information/cancer-type/lung/statistics/?region=mb.

Canadian Cancer Society. (2019a). *Risk factors for cervical cancer.* Retrieved from http://www.cancer.ca/en/cancer-information/cancer-type/cervical/risks/?region=on.

Canadian Cancer Society. (2019b). *Smoking causes 1 in 5 of all deaths, costs $6.5 billion in healthcare in Canada each year: Study.* Retrieved from http://www.cancer.ca/en/about-us/for-media/media-releases/national/2017/cost-of-tobacco/?region=on.

Canadian Centre for Occupational Health and Safety (CCOHS). (2017). *Air quality.* Retrieved from https://www.ccohs.ca/newsletters/hsreport/issues/2009/06/ezine.html.

Canadian Centre for Occupational Health and Safety (CCOHS). (2018a). *Hazards.* Retrieved from https://www.ccohs.ca/topics/hazards/.

Canadian Centre for Occupational Health and Safety (CCOHS). (2018b). *Effects on the body.* Retrieved from https://www.ccohs.ca/topics/hazards/chemical/effects/.

Canadian Centre for Occupational Health and Safety (CCOHS). (2019). *Promotion.* Retrieved from https://www.ccohs.ca/topics/wellness/promotion/.

Canadian Centre on Substance Use and Addiction. (2018). *Drinking guidelines.* Retrieved from http://www.ccdus.ca/Eng/topics/alcohol/drinking-guidelines/Pages/default.aspx.

Canadian Dental Association. (2017). *The state of oral health in Canada.* Retrieved from https://www.cda-adc.ca/stateoforalhealth/_files/thestateoforalhealthincanada.pdf.

Canadian National Institute of the Blind (CNIB). (2017). *Blindness in Canada.* Retrieved from https://cnib.ca/en/sight-loss-info/blindness/blindness-canada?region=bc.

Canadian Professional Association for Transgender Health (CPATH). (2015). *Literature review to support health service planning for transgender people.* Retrieved from http://www.cpath.ca/resources/documents/.

Canadian Sleep Society. (2018). *Healthy sleep for healthy Canadians.* Retrieved from https://css-scs.ca/.

Cardarella, S., & Johnson, B. E. (2013). The impact of genomic changes on treatment of lung cancer. *American Journal of Respiratory and Critical Care Medicine, 188*(7), 770–775. https://doi.org/10.1164/rccm.201305-0843PP.

Charles, S. T. (2010). Strength and vulnerability integration: A model of emotional well-being across adulthood. *Psychological Bulletin, 136*(6), 1068–1091.

Chowdhury, R., Sharot, T., Wolfe, T., et al. (2014). Optimistic update bias increases in older age. *Psychological Medicine, 44*(9), 2003–2012. https://doi.org/10.1017/S0033291713002602.

Duvall, E. M., & Miller, B. (1985). *Marriage and family development* (6th ed.). New York: Harper Collins.

Eliopoulos, C. (2010). *Gerontological nursing: Common aging changes.* Philadelphia: Wolters Kluwer.

Erikson, E. H., & Erikson, G. M. (1998). *Life cycle completed.* New York: W. W. Norton.

Gardner, H. (1983). *Frames of mind: The theory of multiple intelligences.* New York: Basic Books.

Gardner, H. (1993). *Multiple intelligences: The theory in practice.* New York: Basic Books.

Gilligan, C. (1982). *A different voice: Psychological theory and women's development.* Cambridge, MA: Harvard University Press.

Gilligan, C. (1990). *Mapping the moral domain.* Cambridge: Harvard University Press.

Godfrey, E. M., Chin, N. P., Fielding, S. L., et al. (2011). Contraceptive methods and use by women aged 35 and over: A qualitative study of perspectives. *BMC Women's Health, 11*, 5.

Government of Canada. (2013a). *Preventing chronic disease strategic plan, 2013–2016.* Retrieved from http://publications.gc.ca/collections/collection_2014/aspc-phac/HP35-39-2013-eng.pdf.

Government of Canada. (2013b). *Sleep apnea.* Retrieved from https://www.canada.ca/en/public-health/services/chronic-diseases/sleep-apnea.html.

Government of Canada. (2018). *Type 2 diabetes.* Retrieved from https://www.canada.ca/en/public-health/services/diseases/type-2-diabetes.html.

Govindan, R., Mandrekar, S. J., Gerber, D. E., et al. (2015). ALCHEMIST trials: A golden opportunity to transform outcomes in early-stage non-small cell lung cancer. *Clinical Cancer Research, 24*, 5439–5444. https://doi.org/10.1158/1078-0432.CCR-15-0354.

Havighurst, R. I., & Orr, B. (1956). *Adult education and adult needs.* Chicago: Center for Study of Liberal Education for Adults.

Haynes, S. G., Feinleib, M., & Kannel, W. B. (1980). The relationship of psychosocial factors to coronary heart disease in the Framingham Study. III. Eight-year incidence of coronary heart disease. *American Journal of Epidemiology, 111*(1), 37–58.

Haynes, S. G., Levine, S., Scotch, N., et al. (1978). The relationship of psychosocial factors to coronary heart disease in the Framingham Study. I. Methods and risk factors. *American Journal of Epidemiology, 107*(5), 362–383.

Health Canada. (2012). *Vitamin D and calcium: Updated dietary reference intakes.* Retrieved from https://www.canada.ca/en/health-canada/services/food-nutrition/healthy-eating/vitamins-minerals/vitamin-calcium-updated-dietary-reference-intakes-nutrition.html.

Health Canada. (2017). *Fetal alcohol spectrum disorder.* Retrieved from https://www.canada.ca/en/health-canada/services/healthy-living/your-health/diseases/fetal-alcohol-spectrum-disorder.html.

Health Canada. (2018). *Cholesterol guidelines*. Retrieved from https://www.canada.ca/en/health-canada/services/nutrients/cholesterol.html.

Heaney, R. B. (2013). Vitamin D and calcium absorption: Toward a new model. In P. Burckhardt, B. Dawson-Hughes, & C. M. Weaver (Eds.), *Nutritional influences on bone health* (pp. 261–272). London: Springer.

Hockenberry, M. S., & Masson, P. (2015). Erectile dysfunction in the elderly. *Geriatric Urology, 4*(1), 33–43. https://doi.org/10.1007/s13670-014-0107-4.

Holick, M. F. (2012). Vitamin D: Extraskeletal health. *Rheumatic Diseases Clinics of North America, 38*(1), 141–160.

Hornstein, G. (1986). The structuring of identity among midlife women as a function of their degree of involvement in employment. *Journal of Personality, 54*, 551–575.

Hunger, J. M., & Major, B. (2015). Weight stigma mediates the association between BMI and self-reported health. *Health Psychology, 34*(2), 172–175.

Institute of Medicine (US) Committee to Review Dietary Reference Intakes for Vitamin D and Calcium. (2011). In A. C. Ross, et al. (Eds.), *Dietary reference intakes for calcium and vitamin D*. Washington, DC: National Academies Press (US). doi:10.17226/13050. Retrieved from https://www.ncbi.nlm.nih.gov/books/NBK56070/.

Kaldo, V., Jernelöv, S., Blom, K., et al. (2015). Guided internet cognitive behavioral therapy for insomnia compared to a control treatment—a randomized trial. *Behaviour Research and Therapy, 71*, 90–100. https://doi.org/10.1016/j.brat.2015.06.001.

Kawachi, I., Sparrow, D., Spirolli, A., et al. (1996). A prospective study of anger and coronary heart disease: The Normative Aging Study. *Circulation, 94*, 2090–2095. https://doi.org/10.1161/01.CIR.94.9.2090.

Khan, A., Urquia, M., Kornas, K., et al. (2017). Socioeconomic gradients in all-cause, premature and avoidable mortality among immigrants and long-term residents using linked death records in Ontario, Canada. *Journal of Epidemiology & Community Health, 71*(7), 625–632. https://doi.org/10.1136/jech-2016-208525.

King, D. E., Hunter, M., Harris, J., et al. (2013). *Dealing with the psychological and spiritual aspects of menopause: Finding hope in the midlife*. New York: Routledge.

Kobasa, S. (1979). Stressful life events, personality and health: An inquiry into hardiness. *Journal of Personality and Social Psychology, 37*, 1–11.

Kohlberg, L., & Lickona, T. (1986). *The stages of ethical development: From childhood through old age*. New York: Harper Collins.

Lafevre, M. L. (2015). Screening for vitamin D deficiency in adults: US Preventive Services Task Force recommendation statement. *Annals of Internal Medicine, 162*(2), 133–140.

Levinson, D. (1986a). A conception of adult development. *American Psychologist, 41*, 3–13.

Levinson, D. (1986b). *The seasons of a man's life*. New York: Ballantine.

Levinson, D. (1996). *The seasons of a woman's life*. New York: Knopf.

Lochlainn, M. N., & Kenny, R. A. (2013). Sexual activity and aging. *Journal of the American Medical Directors Association, 14*(8), 565–572.

Lowdermilk, D., & Perry, S. (2012). *Reproductive system concerns. Maternity and women's health care* (10th ed.). St. Louis: Mosby.

Lubkin, I. M., & Larsen, P. D. (2013). *Chronic illness: Impact and intervention* (8th ed.). Burlington, MA: Jones & Bartlett.

Lung Cancer Canada. (2018). *Lung cancer*. Retrieved from http://www.lungcancercanada.ca/Lung-Cancer.aspx.

Manchanda, S. C., & Madan, K. (2014). Yoga and meditation in cardiovascular disease. *Clinical Research in Cardiology, 103*(9), 675–680. Retrieved from https://www.cdc.gov/nchs/data/nvsr/nvsr64/nvsr64_08.pdf.

Mather, M. (2012). The emotion paradox in the aging brain. *Annals of the New York Academy of Sciences, 1251*(1), 33–49.

Mikkola, T. S., Tuomikoski, P., Lyytinen, H., et al. (2015). Estradiol-based postmenopausal hormone therapy and risk of cardiovascular and all-cause mortality. *Menopause (New York), 22*(9), 976–983. https://doi.org/10.1097/GME.0000000000000450.

Nair, R., & Maseeh, A. (2012). Vitamin D: The "sunshine" vitamin. *Journal of Pharmacology and Pharmacotherapeutics, 3*(2), 118–126.

Nelson, A. L. (2011). Perimenopause, menopause, and postmenopause: Health promotion strategies. In R. A. Hatcher, et al. (Ed.), *Contraceptive technology* (20th ed.) (pp. 737–777). New York: Ardent Media.

Nicholson, J. (2011). *Five leading causes of workplace injury*. Retrieved from http://www.ehow.com/info_7933497.

Nissenbaum, M. A., Aramini, J. J., & Hanning, C. D. (2012). Effects of industrial wind turbine noise on sleep and health. *Noise and Health, 60*, 237–243.

Northrup, C. (2012). *The wisdom of menopause: Creating physical and emotional health during the change*. New York: Random House.

Obesity Canada. (2017). *Obesity in Canada*. Retrieved from https://obesitycanada.ca/obesity-in-canada/.

Osteoporosis Canada. (2018). *What is osteoporosis?* Retrieved from https://osteoporosis.ca/.

Palacios, C., & Gonzalez, L. (2014). Is vitamin D deficiency a major global public health problem? *The Journal of Steroid Biochemistry and Molecular Biology, 144*(Pt A), 138–145. https://doi.org/10.1016/j.jsbmb.2013.11.003.

Palacious, S., Henderson, V. W., Siseles, N., et al. (2010). Age of menopause and impact of climacteric symptoms by geographical region. *Climacteric: The Journal of the International Menopause Society, 13*(5), 419–428. https://doi.org/10.3109/13697137.2010.507886.

Pender, N., Murdaugh, C. L., & Parsons, M. A. (2015). *Health promotion in nursing practice* (7th ed.). Upper Saddle River, NJ: Pearson.

Piaget, J. (1970). *Structuralism*. New York: Basic Books.

Pines, A. (2011). Male menopause: Is it a real clinical syndrome? *Climacteric: The Journal of the International Menopause Society, 14*(1), 15–17.

Pöss, J., Ewen, S., Schmeider, R. E., et al. (2015). Effects of renal sympathetic denervation on urinary sodium excretion in patients with resistant hypertension. *Clinical Research in Cardiology, 104*(8), 672–678. https://doi.org/10.1007/s00392-015-0832-5.

Public Health Agency of Canada (PHAC). (2013). *Population-specific HIV/AIDS status report: People living with HIV/AIDS*. Retrieved from https://www.catie.ca/sites/default/files/SR-People-Living-with-HIV.pdf.

Public Health Agency of Canada (PHAC). (2017). *Departmental results report 2016–2017*. Retrieved from https://www.canada.ca/en/public-health/corporate/transparency/corporate-management-reporting/departmental-performance-reports.html.

Public Health Agency of Canada (PHAC). (2018). *Canadian immunization guide*. Retrieved from https://www.canada.ca/en/public-health/services/canadian-immunization-guide.html.

Public Health Agency of Canada (PHAC). (2019). *Public health notices*. Retrieved from https://www.canada.ca/en/public-health/services/public-health-notices.html.

Reifman, A., Biernat, M., & Lang, E. (1991). Stress, social support, and health in married professional women with small children. *Psychology of Women Quarterly, 15*, 431–445.

Sanchez-Gonzalez, M. A., May, R. W., Koutnik, A. P., et al. (2015). Impact of negative affectivity and trait forgiveness on aortic blood pressure and coronary circulation. *Psychophysiology, 52*(2), 296–303. https://doi.org/10.1111/psyp.12325.

Santacreu, M., & Fernández-Ballesteros, R. (2011). Evaluation of a behavioral treatment for female urinary incontinence. *Journal of Clinical Interventions in Aging, 6*, 133–139.

Schaie, K. W., & Willis, S. L. (2005). *Intellectual functioning in adulthood: Growth, maintenance, decline, and modifiability*. Philadelphia: American Society on Aging.

Searidge Foundation. (2016). *Alcoholism: Contributing factors*. Retrieved from https://www.searidgealcoholrehab.com/alcoholism-factors.php.

Sex Information & Education Council of Canada (SIECCAN). (2016). *Preliminary report: Sexually transmitted infection (STI) risk among single adults in the Trojan/SIECCAN sexual health at midlife study*. Retrieved from http://sieccan.org/wp/wp-content/uploads/2016/05/Trojan-SIECCAN-STI-report.pdf.

Sheehy, G. (1993). *Menopause: The silent passage*. New York: Random House.

Siegel, A. L. (2014). Pelvic floor muscle training in males: Practical applications. *Urology, 84*(1), 1–7.

Spector, R. E. (2012). *Cultural diversity in health and illness* (8th ed.). Upper Saddle River, NJ: Prentice Hall.

Spielberger, C. D., Jacobs, G., Russell, S., et al. (1983). Assessment of anger: The state-trait anger scale. In J. N. Butcher, & C. D. Spielberger (Eds.), *Advances in personality assessment* (Vol. 2) (pp. 159–187). Hillsdale, NJ: Lawrence Erlbaum Associates.

Statistics Canada. (2011). *Aboriginal peoples in Canada: First nations people, Métis and Inuit*. Retrieved from https://www12.statcan.gc.ca/nhs-enm/2011/as-sa/99-011-x/99-011-x2011001-eng.cfm.

Statistics Canada. (2015a). *Health at a glance*. Retrieved from https://www150.statcan.gc.ca/n1/pub/82-624-x/2014001/article/11922-eng.htm.

Statistics Canada. (2015b). *Cholesterol levels of adults, 2012 to 2013*. Retrieved from https://www150.statcan.gc.ca/n1/pub/82-625-x/2014001/article/14122-eng.htm.

Statistics Canada. (2015c). *Avoidable mortality among first nations adults in Canada: A cohort analysis*. Retrieved from https://www150.statcan.gc.ca/n1/pub/82-003-x/2015008/article/14216-eng.htm.

Statistics Canada. (2015d). *Same-sex couples across Canada*. Retrieved from https://www.statcan.gc.ca/eng/dai/smr08/2015/smr08_203_2015.

Statistics Canada. (2016a). *Aboriginal peoples in Canada: Key results from the 2016 census*. Retrieved from https://www150.statcan.gc.ca/n1/daily-quotidien/171025/dq171025a-eng.htm.

Statistics Canada. (2016b). *Data tables, 2016 census: Employment income statistics*. Retrieved from https://www12.statcan.gc.ca/census-recensement/2016/dp-pd/dt-td/Rp-eng.cfm?TABID=2&Lang=E&APATH=3&DETAIL=0&DIM=0&FL=A&FREE=0&GC=0&GID=1334853&GK=0&GRP=1&PID=110682&PRID=10&PTYPE=109445&S=0&SHOWALL=0&SUB=0&Temporal=2017&THEME=123&VID=0&VNAMEE=&VNAMEF=&D1=0&D2=0&D3=0&D4=0&D5=0&D6=0.

Statistics Canada. (2016c). *Income of individuals by age group, sex and income source; Canada, provinces and selected census metropolitan areas*. Retrieved from https://www150.statcan.gc.ca/t1/tbl1/en/tv.action?pid=1110023901&pickMembers%5B0%5D=1.1&pickMembers%5B1%5D=2.6&pickMembers%5B2%5D=3.1&pickMembers%5B3%5D=4.1.

Statistics Canada. (2016d). *Focus on geography series, 2016 census*. Retrieved from https://www12.statcan.gc.ca/census-recensement/2016/as-sa/fogs-spg/Facts-can-eng.cfm?Lang=Eng&GK=CAN&GC=01&TOPIC=7.

Statistics Canada. (2017a). *Deaths and mortality rates by age group*. Retrieved from https://www150.statcan.gc.ca/t1/tbl1/en/tv.action?pid=1310071001.

Statistics Canada. (2017b). *Leading causes of death, total population by age group*. Retrieved from https://www150.statcan.gc.ca/t1/tbl1/en/tv.action?pid=1310039401.

Statistics Canada. (2017c). *Population estimates on July 1st, by age and sex* Retrieved from. https://www150.statcan.gc.ca/t1/tbl1/en/tv.action?pid=1710000501.

Statistics Canada. (2017d). *Life expectancy*. Retrieved from https://www150.statcan.gc.ca/n1/pub/89-645-x/2010001/life-expectancy-esperance-vie-eng.htm.

Statistics Canada. (2017e). *Body mass index, overweight or obese, self-reported, adult, age groups* (18 years and older). Retrieved from https://www150.statcan.gc.ca/t1/tbl1/en/tv.action?pid=1310009620.

Statistics Canada. (2017f). *Heavy drinking, 2016*. Retrieved from https://www150.statcan.gc.ca/n1/pub/82-625-x/2017001/article/54861-eng.htm.

Statistics Canada. (2018a). *Smoking, 2017*. Retrieved from https://www150.statcan.gc.ca/n1/pub/82-625-x/2018001/article/54974-eng.htm.

Statistics Canada. (2018b). *Visible minority, individual low-income status, low-income indicators, generation status, age and sex for the population in private households in Canada, provinces and territories, census metropolitan areas and census agglomerations, 2016 census—25% sample data*. Retrieved from https://www12.statcan.gc.ca/census-recensement/2016/dp-pd/dt-td/Rp-eng.cfm?LANG=E&APATH=3&DETAIL=0&DIM=0&FL=A&FREE=0&GC=0&GID=0&GK=0&GRP=1&PID=110563&PRID=10&PTYPE=109445&S=0&SHOWALL=0&SUB=0&Temporal=2017&THEME=120&VID=0&VNAMEE=&VNAMEF=.

Statistics Canada. (2018c). *Recent trends in Canada's labour market: A rising tide or a passing wave?* Retrieved from https://www150.statcan.gc.ca/n1/pub/71-222-x/71-222-x2018001-eng.htm.

Statistics Canada. (2019a). *Portrait of children' family life in Canada in 2016*. Retrieved from https://www12.statcan.gc.ca/census-recensement/2016/as-sa/98-200-x/2016006/98-200-x2016006-eng.cfm.

Statistics Canada. (2019b). *Distribution of total income by census family type and age of older partner, parent or individual*. Retrieved from https://www150.statcan.gc.ca/t1/tbl1/en/tv.action?pid=1110001201.

Statistics Canada. (2019c). *Employment and unemployment*. Retrieved from https://www150.statcan.gc.ca/n1/en/subjects/labour/employment_and_unemployment.

Sumnera, C. C. (2013). Adult children of divorce: Awareness and intervention. *Journal of Divorce & Remarriage, 54*(4), 271–281.

Thomas, S. P. (1995). Psychosocial correlates of women's health in middle adulthood. *Issues in Mental Health Nursing, 16*, 285–314.

Trompeter, S. E., Bettencourt, R., & Barrett-Connor, E. (2012). Sexual activity and satisfaction in healthy community-dwelling older women. *The American Journal of Medicine, 125*(1), 37–43.

Johnson, J. & Tough, S. (2012). Delayed child-bearing. *Journal of Obstetrics and Gynaecology Canada, 271*(January), 80–93.

Vaillant, G. (2003). *Aging well: Surprising guideposts to a happier life from the landmark Harvard study of adult development*. New York: Little, Brown.

Vaillant, G., & Vaillant, C. (1990). Natural history of male psychological health, XII: A 45-year study of predictors of successful aging at age 65. *American Journal of Psychiatry, 147*(1), 31–37.

Verstraeten, B., Mijovic-Kondejewski, J., Takeda, J., et al. (2015). Canada's pregnancy-related mortality rates: Doing well but room for improvement. *Clinical & Investigative Medicine, 38*(1), 15–36.

Vranceanu, A. M., Gonzalez, A., Niles, H., et al. (2014). Exploring the effectiveness of a modified comprehensive mind-body intervention for medical and psychologic symptom relief. *Psychosomatics, 55*(4), 386–391. https://doi.org/10.1016/j.psym.2014.01.005.

Wallerstein, J. S., Lewis, J., & Blakeslee, S. (2000). *The unexpected legacy of divorce: A 25 year landmark study*. New York: Hyperion.

Wang, F., Lee, E. K., Wu, T., et al. (2014). The effects of tai chi on depression, anxiety, and psychological well-being: A systematic review and meta-analysis. *International Journal of Behavioral Medicine, 21*(4), 605–617. https://doi.org/10.1007/s12529-013-9351-9.

Whayne, T. F., & Mukherjee, D. (2015). Women, the menopause, hormone replacement therapy and coronary heart disease. *Current Opinion in Cardiology, 30*(4), 432–438. https://doi.org/10.1097/HCO.0000000000000157.

Williams, J. E., Patton, C. C., Siegler, I. C., et al. (2000). Anger proneness predicts coronary heart disease risk: Prospective analysis from the Atherosclerosis Risk in Communities (ARIC) study. *Circulation, 101*(17), 2034–2039.

Workplace Hazardous Material Information System (WHMIS). (2018). *Canada's national WHMIS portal*. Retrieved from http://whmis.org/.

World Health Organization (WHO). (2016). *Obesity and overweight*. Retrieved from http://www.who.int/mediacentre/factsheets/fs311/en/.

Wrosch, C., Bauer, I., & Scheier, M. F. (2005). Regret and quality of life across the adult life span: The influence of disengagement and available future goals. *Psychology and Aging, 20*(4), 657–670.

# 18

# Older Persons

*Dianne Groll, RN, MSc, PhD*

Originating US chapter by *Jeanne Merkle Sorrell, FAAN, RN, PhD*

## INTENDED LEARNING OUTCOMES

*After completing this chapter, the reader will be able to:*

- Discuss how the population of older persons has changed in recent years.
- Describe health-promotion activities specifically targeted to older persons.
- Discuss various theories of aging.
- Describe how normal aging changes in the older person relate to health-promotion strategies.
- Discuss nutritional factors that promote healthy living for the older person.
- Discuss preventive strategies related to risk factors that could lead to health problems in older persons.
- Describe health-promotion strategies for the five most prevalent health conditions and the five leading causes of death among older persons.
- Discuss how health-promotion activities can impact problems related to environmental, physical, biological, and chemical agents that contribute to disability, morbidity, and death in later adulthood.
- Analyze social and political issues that influence the well-being of older persons.
- Identify major resources for healthy living that are available for older persons.

## KEY TERMS

Activities of daily living
Alzheimer's disease
Atrophy
Cognition
Delirium
Dementia
Depression
Euthanasia
Glaucoma
Health literacy
Erectile dysfunction
Influenza

Instrumental activities of daily living
Life review
Medical assistance in dying (MAID)
Mild cognitive impairment
Mini-Mental State Examination (MMSE)
Nutritional screening
Osteoporosis
Polypharmacy
Postoperative cognitive dysfunction (POCD)
Presbycusis

Presbyopia
Pressure injury
Reminiscence
Sclerosis
Social portfolio
Stress incontinence
Theories of aging
Urge incontinence
Willis–Ekbom disease (formerly restless legs syndrome)

## ? THINK ABOUT IT

### Older Smokers

You are the director of an older persons' centre in which 10 of your 40 members smoke. Several of the smoking individuals currently experience health problems. One older woman has chronic obstructive pulmonary disease and avoids using her oxygen because she is not supposed to smoke while the oxygen tank is in the room. One older man has high blood pressure; lung cancer has been diagnosed in another one of the smokers. As director of the centre, you would like to help these older persons to stop smoking. You have referred them to their health care provider to obtain assistance with smoking cessation. All involved are on limited incomes and cannot afford to pay the charge for either a behaviour-management class or nicotine-replacement therapy.

- What additional information do you need to determine if a smoking cessation program in your centre has been successful?
- What types of resources are available to help you obtain the necessary assistance for these smokers?
- What provisions are available under provincial or territorial health care plans to assist a person with smoking cessation?
- What policy changes might be instituted within the older persons' centre to prevent second-hand smoke from harming the residents in the facility's care?

There is a popular poster featuring an older man with an impressive muscular physique that is obviously the result of hours and hours of working out. The poster's title carries a strong message: "Aging is not for sissies." Because older persons are living longer and healthier as a result of health-promotion and technological advances, health care providers often enjoy the gift of caring for older persons who are active and still making important contributions to society. To be caring for a group of human beings that was virtually non-existent 100 years ago is truly extraordinary. It is important to help ensure, however, that these individuals are not only living longer but also that their lives are fulfilling and lived in dignity with as much independence as possible.

Who is the older person today? Older people are living longer and working longer. In 2015, approximately one in five Canadians aged 65 or older reported working during the year. This is the largest increase of employed older persons in Canada since 1995. Within this group, about 30% reported working full time, primarily in agriculture, retail, administration, property management, and transportation (Statistics Canada, 2017a).

The population of older persons in Canada is also becoming more culturally diverse. By 2036, it is projected that immigrants will represent approximately 27.3% of the Canadian population, compared with 20% in 2011. Of these immigrants, it is estimated that the larges waves of immigration will be from Asian countries (56.8%) and European countries (16.6%). In the next 15 years, it is projected that nearly one in two Canadians will be immigrants or of second generation (Statistics Canada, 2017b). These shifts in population characteristics mean that the aging population in Canada will become more diverse. This has important implications for person-centred care, as nurses need to develop an awareness of the cultural diversity of this population and identify the cultural beliefs that influence their health care decisions.

There are many positive changes for older persons today. In general, Canadians are much better educated and more proficient in using technology than in the past—a trend which will become increasingly visible as our population ages. In 1951, 7.8% of individuals aged 18–24 were enrolled in an undergraduate university program, compared with 27% in 2013 (Statistics Canada, 2013; Vanderkamp, 1984). The poverty rate for older persons in Canada is also decreasing, as 4.9% were living in poverty in 2016, which reduced to 3.9% in 2017. These figures are even more impressive for older persons who live alone, as rates declined from 11% in 2016 to 8.4% in 2017 (Statistics Canada, 2019a). More older persons are "aging in place" in the community, with new living options that include retirement communities and independent living facilities or assisted living facilities, as well as skilled care institutions.

On the other hand, there are new challenges for health promotion in older persons. Widening health inequality between Indigenous and non-Indigenous people is a relevant, pressing example. In Canada, Indigenous people have the poorest overall health compared with any other ethnic group; a disparity which has *grown* in past decades. The proportion of Indigenous peoples with self-reported poor/fair health status rose from 18% in 2001 to 22% in 2014 (Hajizadeh, Hu, Bombay, et al., 2018). Other challenges exist for health promotion planning and interventions, such as changing patterns of family structure and cohabitation of older persons. Specifically, there has been an increase in divorce rates, and more women are living alone: 25% of women aged 65 are living alone; the proportion jumps to 55% for those who are 85 years of age or older (Statistics Canada, 2016a). All these changes have implications, as they highlight how health promotion and intervention initiatives should be delivered.

On July 1, 2018, approximately 6 million Canadians (17.2% of the population) were 65 years or older (Statistics Canada, 2019c). By 2063 the number of older persons aged 65 years or older is expected to be 13 million, with 4.95 million aged 80 years or older (Statistics Canada, 2015a). The 65 years or older population is expected to increase from 17% today to 25.6% by 2063 (Statistics Canada, 2015b). Persons aged 80 years or older are the fastest-growing group within the population of older persons, which means that nurses in the community, acute care settings, and long-term facilities will increasingly be caring for these individuals. Many factors have come together to help older persons live longer and healthier. These include continued vaccination development, health-promotion activities, injury prevention, decreases in smoking, and less air pollution. Women comprise the vast majority of centenarians, with approximately 7100 women aged 100 and over in 2015, compared with 900 men, although this disparity is expected to decrease steadily in the next 45 years (Statistics Canada, 2016b).

Aside from these direct factors influencing physical health, there are a number of indirect factors which should also be considered. For instance, increasing the health literacy of older persons in Canada is essential for effective health promotion. This involves the ability to understand, analyze, and communicate information that is necessary to make informed decisions about one's health (Rootman & Gordon-El-Bihbety, 2008). This can involve properly following prescription dosage instructions, understanding nutrition facts and labels, and being able to understand which behaviours will maintain and improve health over time. Despite its importance, only one in eight persons (12%) over the age of 65 is adequately health literate (Sinha, Griffin, Ringer, et al., 2016). In addition, misconceptions surrounding health promotion for older persons can impede the ability of nurses and other health providers to offer care that will enhance healthy aging. These misconceptions need to be overcome so that older persons receive health-promotion interventions that help to keep them active and healthy, while taking into account each individual's level of health literacy.

Health promotion is as important in later adulthood as it is in childhood. Older persons derive the same benefits from health-promotion activities as do their younger counterparts; they are not "too old" to stop smoking, start exercising, change their diet, or relinquish other bad health habits. Specific health-promotion strategies may differ for the young old (55–75 years), the middle old (75–85 years), and the very old, or oldest old (85 years or older). For example, strength training may be very appropriate for the young and middle old groups but may not be feasible for the oldest old. Balance exercises need to be addressed especially for those in the older two age groups. The potential for improvement with all groups is great, and nurses have a key role in changing common societal misconceptions and in creating new understandings regarding health promotion for older persons.

The diversity of cultural backgrounds in Canada influences the many biological, psychological, social, and economic changes as well as the spiritual and life transitions associated with aging that will be discussed in this chapter. Older persons who have immigrated to Canada have brought with them different languages, spiritual and cultural beliefs, eating preferences, and views about health and illness that may seem strange to younger Canadians. Furthermore, people of different cultures may value older persons differently on the basis of their cultural perspective. Many cultures view older persons as a source of family and cultural history and wisdom. Throughout this chapter, cultural norms and behaviours will be discussed within each functional health pattern.

As the population of older persons continues to increase, the cultural diversity within this population will also increase. Cultural background and race have an effect on the prevalence of disease in Canada, although much more research is needed. Aside from data on the health of Indigenous peoples, there is a serious lack of research on the health of other visible minority groups in Canada: particularly, the health of older persons within these groups. Of equal concern is that fact that existing research examines health outcomes related to immigration status, which conflates the status of immigrant health to visible minority health—not all immigrants are members of a visible minority (Khan, Kobayashi, Lee, et al., 2015). Some preliminary findings from the existing, reliable research are that South Asians are at higher risk of heart disease and diabetes, and older Chinese persons are at much higher risk of depression, both compared with Whites (Khan et al., 2015). Racial and ethnic discrimination and access to health care are the most pressing determinants of minority health to be addressed in Canada (Khan et al., 2015).

## BIOLOGY AND GENETICS

Although there is a serious need to promote the health of the older population, there are numerous challenges in meeting this need. One of the great challenges to health promotion for older persons lies in the misconceptions about the benefits of disease prevention and health promotion. Another challenge relates to the difficulty in separating normal changes of aging from pathological processes and illness. Age-related changes are frequently regarded as inevitable and irreversible. However, there is a large amount of variability in age-related changes within each individual. Environmental, economic, physiological, genetic, psychological, social, and cultural factors combine to influence the aging process. Many older persons have an interest in learning about their genetic makeup and how this may influence their aging process and

## GENOMICS

### Personal Genetic Testing

Older persons are increasingly interested in learning about their own DNA to find clues about their heritage and about factors that may affect their future health. With technological developments in recent years, it is now possible to purchase low-cost genetic kits for as little as $100. Do the results of these tests prompt older persons to change their habits to more healthy lifestyles?

Health-related genetic tests include predictive tests for alterations in genes known to be strongly associated with disease onset (e.g., Alzheimer's disease and several cancer syndromes), along with susceptibility tests that give feedback of much lower increased risk of developing common health conditions (e.g., type 2 diabetes).

An important advantage of direct-to-consumer (DTC) testing is the potential that the results could motivate consumers to make lifestyle changes to reduce their disease risk. Consumers state that genetic susceptibility tests for conditions such as obesity would motivate them to adopt a healthier lifestyle and could also provide information that could help their primary care provider monitor their health.

Very few studies have evaluated whether individuals change their lifestyle after receiving genetic risk results. Early evidence suggests, however, that, thus far, genetic test results have not had a demoralizing effect on consumers' efforts or desire to change health habits. There is mixed evidence on how susceptibility testing may influence use of health services. The bottom line is that when consumers receive the results of their testing, they often find that their personalized risk results are matched with the same health recommendations they already know. Most experts believe that potential breakthroughs that could enable genomic risk information to be used routinely to prevent disease and foster healthy aging are still in the future.

Source: McBride, C. (2015). Personal genomic tests for healthy aging: Neither feast nor foul. *Generations. Journal of the American Society on Aging.* Retrieved from http://www.asaging.org/blog/personal-genomic-tests-healthy-aging-neither-feast-nor-foul.

development of disease. The Genomics box provides information about personal genomic testing.

Most researchers agree that biological changes show that growth and development peak during early adulthood, with subsequent linear decline until death. These normal changes must be distinguished from pathological changes to focus health-promotion interventions on behaviours that can be changed. For example, it is normal for older persons to experience a decline in their respiratory vital capacity. Therefore, when nurses are recommending exercise programs, older people must start gradually, allowing them to experience the exercise free from respiratory distress. Selected changes are discussed specifically in the Gordon's Functional Health Patterns section later.

Another challenge in promoting the health of older persons relates to the prevalence of chronic illness and multiple health problems. Although chronic illness is not a normal part of aging, years of environmental assault, poor health behaviours, and stress have placed older persons at a high risk of developing these illnesses. Table 18.1 lists the percentage of older persons with chronic conditions. Illness influences the older person's capacity and motivation to learn new behaviours, so health-promotion activities need to be individualized to fit functional abilities. According to Public Health Agency of Canada (PHAC, 2019), 44% of adults aged

**TABLE 18.1   Average Percentage of People Aged 65 Years or Older Who Have Chronic Health Conditions**

| Chronic Condition | % Age ≥65 years |
| --- | --- |
| Arthritis | 46.9 |
| Hypertension | 43.7 |
| Cancer | 22.6 |
| Diabetes | 17.9 |
| Chronic obstructive pulmonary disease | 8.3 |
| Asthma | 7.5 |
| Dementia | 7.0 |

Source: Statistics Canada. (2019). *Diseases and physical health conditions.* (Data from the 2017 Canadian Community Health Survey.) Retrieved from https://www150.statcan.gc.ca/n1/en/subjects/health/diseases_and_physical_health_conditions.

20 or older have at least one chronic condition. Some of the most common conditions for persons aged 65 and above are listed in Table 18.1. The prevalence of preventable illness and the concomitant physical limitations associated with chronic disease clearly indicate that there is a great need for health-promotion and disease/injury-prevention activities in this population. It is important to note that health-promotion practices among older persons may vary because of the individual's self-perception of health status and the individual's economic and cultural background (Diversity Awareness).

### Theories of Aging

The study of how and why people age has continued over many years and has been the source of a great deal of debate. For many years, the cause of death on many older persons' death certificates was listed simply as "old age." At the 55th Annual Meeting of the Gerontological Society of America, Butler and Olshansky (2002) explored this mindset in a presentation entitled "Has Anyone Ever Died of Old Age?" As the specialization of gerontology has progressed, researchers have clarified the physiological, social, and psychological reasons related to why people die.

There is no formula to predict how a person will age or how long that individual will live. Many theories of aging continue to be examined today, including those regarding metabolism, free radicals, stress, the role of the immune system, genetics, epigenetics (the blending of nature/genetics and nurture/environment), and diet. It is postulated that genetic markers may predict the development of disease and play a large role in determining how a person will age and how long the person will live. In addition, researchers report that calorie-restricted diets have resulted in an increase in longevity in animals; however, there is debate regarding whether calorie restriction alone or calorie restriction in the presence of genetic markers increases longevity. The role of antioxidants in binding free radicals is also being researched as an important influence on increasing longevity. Although no consensus has yet been reached that describes the entire aging process, exciting theories continue to be forthcoming (National Institute on Aging,

*Perceived Health Status of Indigenous People*

The Public Health Agency of Canada's 2016 *Health Status of Canadians* report provides interesting information about the ways that perceived health differs based on ethnicity. Data from 2010 revealed that First Nations living off reserves, Inuit, and Métis were less likely than non-Indigenous people to report being in good or excellent health.

More specifically, 63% of non-Indigenous Canadians reported that they felt they had good or excellent health. However, only 50% of First Nations living off reserve, 54% of Métis, and 55% of Inuit people perceived their health in the desirable range of good to excellent. In all groups, health perceptions rose dramatically as income status rose, with about 40% of Canadians in the lowest income bracket reporting good to excellent health, compared with 80% in the highest bracket. With the goal of person-centred care in mind, it is essential to listen to these needs, and help communicate them to other health care providers on your team to ensure each patient is receiving care with dignity and respect. Trust will be greatly improved when time is taken to consider the unique needs of each patient. Older persons play a particularly important role as cultural mentors in Indigenous communities; therefore, their unique point of view is essential for the relevant promotion of healthy aging practices. Once one feels that one's needs are being appropriately considered, self-efficacy (belief in one's ability to meet goals) increases, potentially leading to improved perceptions of one's health, and hopefully, increases in healthy behaviours.

Source: Public Health Agency of Canada. (2016). *Health Status of Canadians 2016.* Ottawa: Author. Retrieved from http://healthycanadians.gc.ca/publications/department-ministere/state-public-health-status-2016-etat-sante-publique-statut/alt/pdf-eng.pdf.

2011). Some of the theories used to explain aging are briefly described in Box 18.1.

## ❖ GORDON'S FUNCTIONAL HEALTH PATTERNS

### ◆ Health Perception–Health Management Pattern

Motivation is an important factor in maintaining health. Nurses who care for older persons know that the best nursing in the world cannot make individuals do something they believe to be unnecessary. A primary factor in the older person's motivation to promote personal health is the perception of health and its subsequent management. For older persons who have always been healthy and then receive a diagnosis of a serious disease, it is important that they find ways to promote health while living with the disease. For example, new research shows that many of the debilitating aspects of Parkinson's disease can be minimized through active exercise, including bicycling (Paddock, 2012). Older persons with a diagnosis of spinal stenosis or back pain that prevents them from walking long distances may think they can no longer travel. New mobile devices such as scooters, which allow the person to ride through the airport and then check the scooter at the gate, help to make travel to visit friends or family or dreamed-of adventures possible. These devices also provide independence for older persons to go out in their neighbourhood to socialize (Fig. 18.1).

Nurses can be very helpful in talking with older persons to learn their goals for health and what motivates them. If they dislike group activity, it may not be effective to encourage

## BOX 18.1 Theories of Aging

### Biological Theories of Aging

- Programmed theories of aging: Aging is the result of predictable cellular death.
  - Immunity theory: Aging is a programmed accumulation of damage and decline in the function of the immune system, resulting from oxidative stress.
  - Neuroendocrine control/pacemaker theory: Aging is a programmed decline in the functioning of the nervous, endocrine, and immune systems. The cells lose their ability to reproduce.
  - Gene theory: Longevity may be associated with a genetic trait or a "longevity gene": "juvenescent" genes mediate youthful vigor and mature adult well-being, and "senescent" genes promote functional decline and structural deterioration.
- Error theories of aging: Aging is the result of an accumulation of random errors in the synthesis of cellular DNA and RNA.
  - Oxidative stress theory (free radical theory): Errors are a result of random damage from free radicals.
  - Cross-linkage theory: Aging is a product of accumulated damage from errors associated with cross-linked proteins where cross-linked proteins become stiff and thick.
  - Wear-and-tear theory: Cellular errors are the result of deterioration over time because of continued use.
- Calorie restriction theory: In animal models, calorie restriction increased the life span and the health of the animals.

### Sociological Theories of Aging

- Activity theory: Continued activity is an indicator of successful aging.
- Disengagement theory: In the course of aging, the individual slowly withdraws from former roles and activities.
- Role theory: The ability of an individual to adapt to changing roles throughout life is predictive of adjustment to the changing roles associated with aging.
- Continuity theory: In normal aging, personality remains consistent. Personality influences role activity and life satisfaction.
- Age stratification theory: The relationship between age as an element of social structure and aging people as a cohort.
- Subculture theory: Older people have their own norms, habits, and beliefs and interact better among age peers than with other age groups.

### Developmental Theories of Aging

- Erikson's developmental theory: There is a predetermined order of development, and specific tasks are associated with specific periods in a person's life. For older persons, the developmental stage is integrity versus despair.
- Peck's developmental theory: This theory expanded on Erikson's theory with identification of discrete tasks of late life that when accomplished together result in ego integrity.
- Havighurst's developmental theory: There are specific tasks associated with aging, including adjusting to the losses of aging (e.g., health, income, death of spouse and peers), adapting to change and new roles, and accepting life's experiences.
- Tornstam's theory of gerotranscendence: Aging is viewed as the movement from birth to death and maturation toward wisdom. Gerotranscendence involves achieving wisdom through personal transformation.

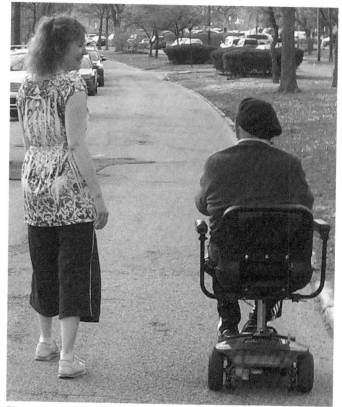

**Fig. 18.1** Mobile devices such as scooters provide independence for older persons with limited mobility.

chronic illnesses do not need to prevent health-promotion activities. Older persons should be encouraged to continue with self-care activities rather than to relinquish them to caregivers. Because some memory impairment may be present in cognitively healthy older persons, memory aids and familiar environments should be encouraged so that they keep their minds active, continue learning, and maintain their self-confidence.

A variety of activities promote health and prevent frailty. These include maintaining healthy weight and diet; staying active; practicing fall prevention; maintaining relationships; and keeping regular medical appointments. Age-appropriate preventive measures for Canadian primary care providers (Shimizu, Bouchard, & Mavriplis, 2016) recommend clinical preventive services for older persons that include immunizations (influenza and pneumococcal) and screenings for early detection of breast cancer, colorectal cancer, diabetes, lipid disorders, and osteoporosis; and smoking-cessation counselling for those who smoke. Canada's health care system covers these necessary preventive services, which can be accessed by request when visiting primary health care providers. Provincial and territorial health care plans provide exercise and fall-prevention programs free of charge to assist older persons to stay active and mobile (e.g., Government of Ontario, 2019). There are also many different online and mobile applications that aid in monitoring exercise and may be fun for older persons to use. Helping an older person to understand the importance of learning or maintaining healthy behaviours is an essential nursing role.

them to take exercise or nutrition classes. Suggesting an exercise DVD that can be used at home or reading about nutrition may be more helpful. It is important not to underestimate older persons' abilities; many older persons continue to actively participate in competitive sports. Even

Health-maintenance behaviours include exercise, good nutrition, sexual safety, and appropriate sleep-rest patterns. Health-maintenance practices also include regular health care checkups, which will provide early detection and management of disease. Although these behaviours are important for all older persons, the perception of these activities and the ability to practice good health behaviours differ by cultural group. It is essential that nurses are culturally sensitive and understand that cultural values guide behaviour. In so doing, the nurse will be most effective in helping the older person form a positive health perception and practice good health behaviours (Innovative Practice).

## Nutritional-Metabolic Pattern

Proper nutrition helps prevent cancer, obesity, and gastro-intestinal disorders and provides older persons with the energy required to function in all activities of daily living. One can measure good nutrition by determining whether the individual is meeting the recommended daily allowance (RDA) for caloric intake. Energy intake needs differ, depending on age, with adults aged 65 or older typically requiring fewer calories than younger adults. Although fewer calories are needed, older persons require more nutrition from these calories to promote and protect health. This means paying closer attention to important micro- and macronutrients to ensure that older persons are getting the most out of their food (PHAC, 2006). The most recent version of Canada's Food Guide (*Canada's Dietary Guidelines*, released in 2019) provides specific dietary recommendations for older persons. It emphasizes eating with others to diversify diet and provide important social contact, creating an emergency food supply in case of situations which may make it hard to leave the house, and taking advantage of community resources such as grocery delivery, cooking classes, and lunch clubs or meal programs to encourage a healthy relationship with food (Health Canada, 2019a).

Poor nutrition in older persons not only affects their overall health but also contributes to higher health care costs. Specific nutritional risk factors for older persons include solitary living, being of a particular race/ethnicity, low income, social isolation, and low social support (Tyler, Corvin, McNab, et al., 2014). According to a report released in the *Canadian Medical Association Journal*, one-third (34%) of Canadians aged 65 or older are on the cusp of malnutrition (Lange-Chenier, 2013). This data underscores the problems of maintaining good nutrition. For independent older persons, the barriers that may interfere with the ability to obtain adequate and nutritional food include diminished attitude, medications, limited mobility, social isolation, and poverty.

## INNOVATIVE PRACTICE

### Geriatric Assessment

The health care system, with its emphasis on acute care, busy office schedules, and fragmented delivery systems, often frustrates older people and their families. The very old or frail person's health problems are often overlooked, ignored, or only partially treated. Many communities have a health care service that uses a team approach to meet the special needs of older persons. This service is known as geriatric assessment.

#### Goals of Geriatric Assessment
- Maintain health and health-maintenance practices:
  - Promote disease prevention through routine immunizations and health screenings.
  - Implement fall-prevention strategies to decrease the incidence of falls and fall-related injuries.
- Minimize hospitalizations.
- Establish complete diagnoses that are often missed or overlooked, including hearing impairment, vision deficits, early dementia, depression, and poor nutrition.
- Decrease overprescription and misuse of medications, including prescription medications, over-the-counter medications, vitamins/minerals/supplements, and herbal remedies.

Geriatric assessment uses an interdisciplinary team consisting of a geriatric nurse practitioner, a physiotherapist, and a social worker. Each member of the team evaluates the person from a health care, functional, cognitive, or psychosocial perspective. Additional members of the team might include a geriatric psychiatrist, geriatrician, nutritionist, pharmacist, dentist, or podiatrist. The program team evaluates the home environment, risk of falls, incontinence, vision and hearing impairments, memory loss, depression and anxiety, functional decline, physical deconditioning, caregiver stress, economic resources, advance directives, and quality-of-life issues. The team is coordinated by the geriatric nurse practitioner.

Geriatric assessment is not meant for all older people. The people who benefit are those who are frail. An older person who might benefit from geriatric assessment is one who:
- Is older than 80 years
- Has a history of frequent falls
- Is losing weight
- Is depressed
- Has mild memory loss
- Has been hospitalized three times in 2 months
- Takes more than five medications regularly and frequently gets them confused
- Has no close family or other support persons in the community
- Is in need of health teaching

Geriatric assessment usually identifies the strengths and weaknesses of the older person and evaluates that person's situation, including family and other social support. Following the assessment, the geriatric nurse practitioner begins developing a care plan to incorporate usable strengths and assist with weaknesses.

The primary care physician, family physician, internist, geriatrician, or geriatric nurse practitioner is a key link between the geriatric assessment team and the individual, primarily because this provider carries out the team's recommendation and monitors the person's progress. In most cases the nurse practitioner coordinates between the team and the person's primary physician and family.

Geriatric assessment clinics are available in many larger cities, and access is typically gained through primary care referral. As the Canadian health care system moves toward favouring prevention over intervention, geriatric assessment will play a key role in identifying individual strengths, correcting problems, and maintaining the health and quality of life of older citizens.

Problems with access to food are compounded by the effect of normal changes of aging. Declines in gastro-intestinal organ function can lead to changes in digestive metabolism and the absorption and elimination of nutrients. A deterioration of the smell, vision, and taste senses and the high frequency of dental and swallowing problems make maintaining adequate daily nutrition even more difficult. Additionally, adverse effects of required medications may affect appetite. Cultural food preferences and lifelong eating habits, such as diets high in fat and cholesterol, are other obstacles to maintaining optimal nutrition.

Because of physiological and metabolic changes associated with aging, nutritional problems are more difficult to quantify and evaluate in older persons (Mueller, 2015). A nutritional assessment for an older person entails a comprehensive approach that includes a health history, physical examination, laboratory data, dietary data, and measurement of functional status. Initial nutritional screening, however, is more straightforward. Nutritional screening evaluates the risk of malnutrition and may identify the need for a more formal nutrition assessment. There are a variety of tools, such as the Mini Nutritional Assessment (MNA), that can be used for nutritional screening in older persons. The MNA contains an initial set of questions that if scored below 11 indicates risk of malnutrition and requires the completion of additional questions to confirm the likelihood of malnutrition (Mueller, 2015). The MNA and other screening tools can identify the risk of malnutrition, but a formal nutritional assessment is needed to establish a diagnosis of malnutrition and appropriate interventions.

The living environment further affects nutritional status. Community-dwelling older persons are at high risk of nutritional disorders because access to food may be limited. Older persons in long-term care facilities do not have a problem with availability of food, but the meals may contain excessive fat, cholesterol, or salt, and may lack sufficient fibre. Additionally, fresh fruit and vegetables are less available. Institutional food may be unappealing, and institutions may not be able to adapt their meals to the cultural and religious preferences of their residents. Encouraging family members to bring in special foods that the resident enjoys is helpful. Nurses who work in institutional settings make an important difference for older persons by assessing the person's food preferences and any difficulties in eating, followed by careful planning of an appropriate menu, to encourage healthy eating.

A pleasant setting with social interaction enhances the desire to eat. In one study an expert panel of nutrition practitioners concluded that the two most important enablers of healthy eating among older persons are accessibility and social support (Tyler et al., 2014). Many older persons want to age in their own home without having to relocate to a long-term care facility. Research suggests that nutritional supports play a critical role in the older persons' ability to remain in their homes (Tyler et al., 2014). Food assistance from friends and family in the form of cooking or food sharing is an important facilitator of nutritional health and being able to age in place. One study focused on how social lives and community environmental supports and barriers affected older persons' nutritional health (Tyler et al., 2014). The researchers conducted 29 focus group discussions with 144 residents of one of the largest retirement communities in the United States. The findings revealed that the high social connectedness of residents was associated with both positive and negative influences. The high degree of social support in the retirement community positively influenced the nutritional health of the participants. Social gatherings, however, also appeared to encourage residents to eat more than they would by themselves and to eat less nutritious foods. The findings also suggested that friends and neighbours provide an excellent point of entry for nutritional interventions such as information about food-assistance strategies and other types of educational programs for health promotion.

Lack of appetite may also accompany disease. Medications, poor dentition, difficulty swallowing, or a lack of dentures can also cause older people to eat less than is optimal. Those in acute care hospitals or long-term care facilities may experience a lack of appetite as a result of illness. The hospital stay is a time during which good nutrition is most important to heal wounds and to restore energy; however, a lack of interest in or energy for eating during hospitalization places the older person at a high risk of developing nutritional disorders.

Obesity is also a problem for older persons. According to data from the Canadian Health Measures Survey (Statistics Canada, 2018a), 31% of those aged 40 to 59 years and 33% of those aged 65 years or older are considered obese. Obesity is associated with several chronic health conditions, including hypertension, diabetes, and heart disease. It is important to recognize, however, that scientists have described a phenomenon called "the obesity paradox," in which obesity in older persons, unlike in younger individuals, does not appear to be clearly associated with a shorter life span. Some studies have suggested that the "ideal" protective weight might be higher in the older population (Pietrzykowska, 2016). It is interesting to consider this theory in the context of the above statistics, demonstrating a slight increase in rates with age. There is still much debate about this, however, and because obesity is clearly linked to a lesser quality of life, it is important to discuss options for weight reduction. During weight loss, muscle is lost as well as fat. This is an important consideration when one is planning a weight-loss program for older persons because, as a result of normal aging and often deconditioning, they are likely to have less muscle mass and more fat than when they were younger. Studies have found, however, that a moderate weight loss of 5% to 10% results in significant health benefits and that even a weight loss of 3% in older persons significantly reduces inflammation, blood pressure, cholesterol levels, and blood glucose levels (Pietrzykowska, 2016). For nurses working with older persons who are trying to lose weight, it is important to recognize that these individuals may have struggled with trying to lose weight for years and may be very frustrated with their unsuccessful efforts to achieve an ideal weight. Factors such as living alone and not wanting to cook for one person, the expense and short shelf life of fresh fruits and vegetables, medications, fast food, lack of motivation, and difficulty exercising make losing weight difficult. Nurses can help empower older persons by identifying realistic strategies for them to attain and maintain a healthy weight.

Nurses assist older persons in maintaining the highest possible nutritional level by teaching them about the food needed to maintain optimal nutritional status and by providing information about resources to help purchase food. There are currently no federal nutrition assistance programs offered to Canadians; however, older people may be eligible for a number of other general financial benefits. Examples include the Old Age Security (OAS) pension and the Guaranteed Income Supplement (older persons are automatically enrolled if their income meets requirements, and they are receiving the OAS pension). Data from 2018 on the use of the government programs show that 6.1 million Canadians (96% of older persons) are using OAS, and 1.3 million (19% of older persons) are using the Guaranteed Income Supplement. These numbers are promising, suggesting that the majority of those who are eligible are taking advantage of these resources.

In addition to financial benefits, there are other federally supported nutrition assistance programs available to older persons, including Meals on Wheels, or other local meal delivery services run by community organizations. Additionally, certain provincial and territorial programs, such as EatRight Ontario or Dial-a-Dietitian in Manitoba, connect older persons with registered dietitians via telephone. Detailed information about these programs, as well as other important nutritional information related to older persons, is given in Chapter 21.

## ◆ Elimination Pattern

Bowel and bladder functions in the older person are altered by normal changes of aging. The bladder retains its tonus, but its capacity decreases. Gastro-intestinal motility decreases as people age. In addition to some of the normal changes of aging, diet plays a significant role in problems with intestinal motility and constipation. Decreased intake of fluids and fibre contribute in large part to constipation. Many medications taken by older persons also cause elimination concerns. Lack of physical activity and changes in the environment that decrease privacy also contribute to elimination problems. Many older persons may believe elimination problems are an unavoidable part of aging and may be embarrassed to mention their concerns to health care providers. It is important to reassure them that through diet and exercise they can gain control of most elimination problems.

Constipation is often a major problem for older persons and has far-reaching effects on their quality of life. There are several bowel elimination problems that are described by people as constipation: hard stools, infrequent stools, the need for excessive straining, and a feeling of incomplete bowel evacuation often associated with abdominal cramping or feeling bloated. Although inadequate diet and inactivity are common causes of constipation, it is important to consider whether constipation is related to metabolic disease such as hypothyroidism, neurological disease such as Parkinson's disease, psychological illness such as depression, or medications. Nurses can assess the cause of constipation and develop an appropriate plan of care. Encouraging older persons to exercise and increase their fluid intake helps reduce the incidence of constipation. Integrating more fibre into the diet and eating prunes each day can also be very effective for preventing constipation.

According to Yoo and Spencer (2018), 58% of people over age 65 in Canada report having had at least one instance of urinary incontinence, though this figure is expected to rise as the population ages in coming years. Further, the College of Family Physicians of Canada's Frailty 5 Checklist (Freedman & McDougall, 2019) cites that up to 70% of older women experience some form of regular urinary incontinence. Incontinence is classified as either acute (transient) or chronic (established) (Touhy & Jett, 2012). Acute incontinence has a sudden onset, has been present for less than 6 months, and is usually secondary to a treatable condition. Chronic incontinence has either a sudden or a gradual onset and is categorized into four major types: stress incontinence is the most common and occurs during exercise, laughing, coughing, or sneezing; urge incontinence, or the inability to delay voiding after the bladder is full; urge, mixed, or stress urinary incontinence with high postvoid residual incontinence occurs when the bladder does not empty completely and becomes overdistended, which may be caused by an obstruction in the urinary elimination tract, such as that caused by an enlarged prostate gland; and functional incontinence, which is associated with environmental barriers, physical limitations, or cognitive impairment where the person is unable to reach the toilet.

Incontinence results in threats to both psychological and physical health, including depression, urinary tract infections, skin breakdown, and falls. Nurses can help older persons to understand incontinence as a manageable problem. Implementing appropriate management is important for the older person's continued good health and self-esteem. Pelvic floor or Kegel exercises can be taught to strengthen the musculature of the urinary system (Mayo Clinic, 2015a, 2015b). Pilates exercises have also been demonstrated to be effective in treating incontinence (Crawford, 2013). Management programs may include scheduling regular times to void, improving access to toileting facilities, management of diet and fluids, and the use of disposable absorbent undergarments. Voiding schedules are most effective when the person selects specific times during the day for urination. Eliminating dietary caffeine helps people with urge incontinence and increasing fibre in the diet helps those whose incontinence is related to constipation.

## ◆ Activity-Exercise Pattern

According to data obtained via self-report questionnaires, 40.6% of Canadians aged 65 or older regularly meet the recommended 150 minutes of physical activity per week, with a higher proportion of men reporting regular participation in exercise than women (Statistics Canada, 2017c). However, data collected from the Canadian Health Measures survey (Statistics Canada, 2017d) tells a very different story, estimating that only 16.9% of adults in the 60+ age group are meeting the recommended weekly activity guidelines. The discrepancy between these statistics highlights how some self-report data can produce less-than-accurate results. This makes it particularly important for nurses to ask patients specific, practical questions about a patient's activity levels (e.g., "What do you normally do to get active? Do you like to participate with friends?" etc.) to get a good idea of how physically active a patient likely is on

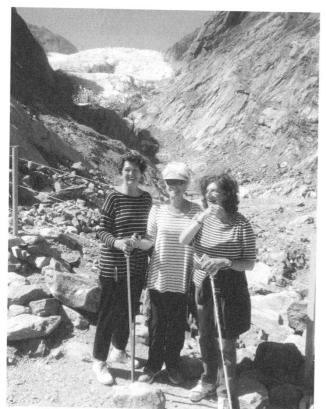

Fig. 18.2 Normal changes of aging and environmental deterrents do not prevent older persons from exercising.

a day-to-day basis. The benefits of regular exercise in promoting health and preventing disease are widely accepted. Regular physical activity helps, and may even prevent, many chronic health problems associated with aging, including hypertension, obesity, diabetes, and depression. Regular physical activity can increase both the years of life and the quality of those years. Strength training can improve balance and reduce the risk of falls, strengthen bones, and reduce blood glucose levels. Normal changes of aging, pathological conditions, and environmental deterrents do not need to prevent the older person from exercising (Fig. 18.2).

The Canadian Society for Exercise Physiology (CSEP, 2011) recommends that older persons aged 65 and older should perform a combination of aerobic exercise and muscle-strengthening activities every week. They recommend at least 150 minutes of aerobic exercise, ranging from moderate intensity to vigorous intensity, depending on the older person's level of fitness, and muscle-strengthening activities can include exercises that work all the major muscle groups. Teaching the many benefits of exercise is the first lesson in motivating older persons to engage. With respect to the role that culture plays on the value of exercise, individual counselling is needed to identify exercises that can be enjoyed and continued (Fig. 18.3). The nurse or physiotherapist assists in designing an appropriate exercise program that will help to maintain strength, flexibility, and balance. Walking, which can be done in both community settings and health care facilities, is a popular form of exercise among older persons.

Other popular activities for older persons include swimming, weight-bearing exercises, and aquatic exercises. Weight-bearing and muscle-building exercises help to maintain functional mobility, promote independence, and prevent falls. Weight-bearing exercises are shown to be highly effective in reducing bone wasting associated with osteoporosis. Regular exercise promotes maintenance of bone mineral density in older persons. People with conditions such as spinal stenosis and arthritis often find that they can exercise in a swimming pool without pain, so this is an important way for them to maintain an exercise plan and increase their functional ability. Box 18.2 lists many benefits that can be derived from participation in an exercise program.

Before beginning any exercise program, an older person who has not been exercising should consult a health care provider. After the program begins, activity levels can be increased gradually. Adherence to an exercise program is a major problem for all populations. The best strategies to encourage continued exercise among older persons are to communicate the importance of exercise in maintaining quality of life and to help them choose an exercise that they enjoy and is easily accessible. Exercising with a family member or friend is also helpful in motivating older persons to exercise.

## ◆ Sleep-Rest Pattern

Inability to sleep is a frequent concern of older persons. Chaput, Wong, and Michaud (2017) report that 53.3% of men and 70.0% of women aged 65–79 fall short of the recommended 7–9 hours of sleep either sometimes, most of the time, or all the time. Sleep difficulties may include sleep apnea, the inability to fall asleep, the inability to stay asleep, the inability to fall back to sleep when awakening in the night, or the feeling of not being refreshed when awakening in the morning. Sleep-disordered breathing, or sleep apnea, may affect up to 13% of persons aged 70 to 79, with significantly more men reporting the disorder than women. It is a concern not only due to deficits in sleep but also because it is associated with various cardiovascular diseases, diabetes, and depression (Statistics Canada, 2018b). Willis–Ekbom disease (formerly restless legs syndrome), characterized by unpleasant throbbing, pulling, or creeping sensations in the legs and an almost uncontrollable urge to move the legs, is a neurological disorder that affects many older persons (National Institute of Neurological Disorders and Stroke, 2015). As the sensations are worse when the person is lying down and trying to sleep, the disorder can seriously limit sleep quality. Older persons are more likely to report excessive daytime sleepiness, which means that they find it difficult to remain awake or alert at appropriate times during the day (Chervin, 2015). The high prevalence of sleep disorders in older persons indicates that it is an important area for health care providers to address.

The benefits of a good night's sleep are numerous. Quality sleep results in overall increases in energy, motivation to continue a high quality of life, and improved immune function. Nurses assist older persons in achieving a good night's sleep through assessment that might reveal

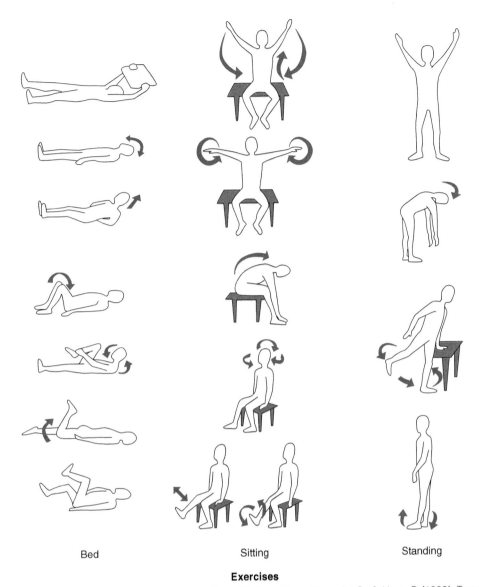

Bed                    Sitting                    Standing

**Exercises**

**Fig. 18.3** Bed-lying, sitting, and standing exercises. (Redrawn from Ebersole, P., & Hess, P. [1998]. Toward healthy aging: Human need and nursing response [3rd ed.]. St. Louis: Mosby.)

| BOX 18.2   Benefits of Exercise for Older Persons | |
| --- | --- |
| • Better sleep | • Better digestion |
| • Reduced constipation | • Weight loss |
| • Lower cholesterol level | • Socializing opportunities |
| • Lower blood pressure | • Greater sense of well-being |

possible causes of sleep disturbances. The Pittsburgh Sleep Quality Index is a subjective tool that is helpful in assessing the quality and patterns of sleep in older persons (Smyth, 2012). The tool measures seven areas: subjective sleep quality, sleep latency, sleep duration, habitual sleep efficiency, sleep disturbances, use of sleeping medication, and daytime dysfunction. Teaching older persons about normal changes reassures them that their sleep patterns have changed but are not necessarily harmful. Having this information may decrease anxiety. Identifying normal bedtime rituals, such

as drinking a glass of milk, taking a relaxing bath, reading, or meditating, and ensuring that the person is able to continue these practices may help to establish normal sleep routines. Increasing physical activity during the day also helps them fall asleep more readily at night. Taking pain medication or using alternative pain-relief methods before going to bed can help those who suffer from painful conditions obtain better rest at night.

Residents of long-term care facilities or people in acute-care facilities may have difficulty adjusting to the environment at night. Adjustments in noise and lighting help these individuals sleep better. Emotional disorders frequently interfering with sleep can be identified, and therapy and medication can be administered during the day to help people experiencing these problems sleep peacefully at night. Although a nap may be beneficial, it is important to ensure that daytime napping is not interfering with night-time sleep (Innovative Practice).

## INNOVATIVE PRACTICE

### Measures to Promote Sleep

Sleep problems can be caused by many things, including stress; medications; medical conditions such as angina, asthma, anxiety, or depression; poor sleeping habits; and sleep disorders. The following are some suggestions to improve sleep in older persons.

**Do**

- Plan a regular bedtime and wake-up schedule.
- Participate in exercise, hobbies, and other activities during the day.
- Develop specific bedtime rituals, such as reading, meditating, drinking a glass of milk, or taking a warm bath. These tell the body it is almost time for sleep.
- Ensure a comfortable and quiet sleep environment, which is dark except for night safety lights.
- Sleep on a comfortably firm mattress with comfortable pillows and bedclothes.
- Use the bed only for sleep and sexual activities.
- Check with a health care provider about prescription and over-the-counter medications that may interfere with sleep.

**Avoid**

- Long daytime naps that may interfere with night-time sleep
- Exercise or vigorous activity immediately before bedtime
- Caffeine after mid-morning
- Drinking alcohol before going to bed
- Sleep medications
- Tobacco products
- Driving when tired or sleepy

**When Sleep Problems Persist**

- Keep a sleep log, recording times and duration of sleep throughout the 24-hour period for at least 1 week.
- Ask sleep companion about sleep habits, such as snoring or restlessness.
- See health care provider.

Sleep medications may be helpful for short-term use; however, numerous studies assert that they are not a recommended long-term solution (American Geriatrics Society, Beers Criteria Update Expert Panel, Fick, et al., 2015; Praharaj, Gupta, & Gaur, 2018; Voight, Gottschall, Köberlein-Neu, et al., 2016). In particular, long-term use of benzodiazepines, barbiturates, and chloral hydrate for treatment of insomnia in older persons because of older persons' increased sensitivity to these medications and increased risk of dependency, and the decreased metabolism of long-term medications, resulting in an increased risk of cognitive impairment, falls, and overdose. Similarly, over-the-counter medications such as antihistamines, or herbal supplements such as melatonin, which are often used to assist with sleep, are to be used with caution in older persons (Schroeck, Ford, Conway, et al., 2016). Instead, sleep hygiene education, stimulus control (i.e., teaching the patient to limit bedroom activities to sleep and sexual activities to maintain the association of the bedroom with sleep), and relaxation training are a few recommendations for appropriate long-term sleep solutions for older persons (Praharaj et al., 2018).

## ◆ Cognitive-Perceptual Pattern
### Cognition

Thinking processes (cognition) in old age have been the subject of intensive study in the past few decades. Brain weight decreases with aging, and a shift occurs in the proportion of grey matter to white matter. The ways in which these changes are manifested in individuals differ because of culture, heredity, lifestyle, environmental exposures, and many other factors. These changes can manifest as differences in processing of information, memory, comprehension, problem solving, and decision making. It is important to think about how even subtle changes in cognition may affect older persons in their day-to-day activities. For example, older persons are often targeted by scams that ask them to send money or personally identifiable information to callers who appeal to their sense of fear or the promise of a reward.

There is a common belief that most older persons will eventually develop dementia; however, cognitive problems are not a normal change of aging, and many individuals live well into old age without ever experiencing dementia. It is important to be cautious in assessing older people who present with confusion, because confusion is not always indicative of dementia, but can be the result of many treatable health problems, including electrolyte imbalances, diabetic ketoacidosis, and hypoxia. Mild cognitive impairment is a pathological collection of symptoms that results in memory loss, language difficulties, and impairments in judgement and reasoning. A review of instrumental activities of daily living will help identify changes in tasks requiring higher executive functions, such as paying bills, taking medications as ordered, using the phone, and driving safely.

A condition that is receiving increased attention in older persons is postoperative cognitive dysfunction (POCD). POCD is a temporary deterioration in cognition that is associated with surgery and anaesthesia (Sorrell, 2014). As the population of older persons has increased dramatically in recent years, surgery is more common at advanced ages. Individuals with POCD experience postoperative cognitive changes that may include anxiety, blurred vision, inability to sleep, hallucinations, and depression. POCD is not the same as delirium, which is a short-term change in cognition that may develop in the immediate postoperative period. Cognitive changes in POCD are more subtle and extend over a longer period—sometimes for months after discharge from the hospital. These changes can be very distressing to the older person and the older person's family. POCD is thought to be related to the type or amount of anaesthesia administered during surgery, but more research needs to be done to establish the cause of POCD and how to prevent it. It is important for nurses in all health care contexts to be aware of the possibility of POCD in older persons and to identify ways in which they can intervene. Because there is no specific treatment for POCD, nurses need to anticipate the needs of older persons and also their families. Educating the older persons, their families, and those who care for them about POCD and emphasizing that it is usually temporary helps to decrease anxiety.

Dementia is not accepted as being a normal change of aging. Dementia is an umbrella term for a group of cognitive disorders that affect memory and lead to difficulty in areas of language, motor activity, object recognition, and ability to plan

---

**Mini Mental Status Examination Sample Items**

**Orientation to Time**

"What is the date?"

**Naming**

"What is this?"

[Point to a pencil or pen.]

**Reading**

"Please read this and do what it says."

[Show examinee the words on the stimulus form.]

CLOSE YOUR EYES

---

**Fig. 18.4** Mini-Mental State Examination sample items. (Reproduced by special permission of the Publisher, Psychological Assessment Resources, Inc., 16204 North Florida Avenue, Lutz, Florida 33549, from the Mini Mental State Examination, by Marshal Folstein and Susan Folstein, Copyright 1975, 1998, 2001 by Mini Mental LLC, Inc. Published 2001 by Psychological Assessment Resources, Inc. Further reproduction is prohibited without permission of PAR, Inc. The MMSE can be purchased from PAR, Inc. by calling (813) 968-3003.)

and organize. Dementias include Alzheimer's disease, the most common dementia, as well as Parkinson's-related dementia, Huntington's disease, Creutzfeldt–Jakob disease, Pick's disease, and Lewy body dementia. The Alzheimer's Society of Canada (2016) estimates that approximately 560,000 people in Canada are living with some form of dementia, 68.8% of whom are over the age of 65.

The symptoms of dementia include forgetfulness, inattentiveness, disorganized thinking, altered levels of consciousness, perceptual disturbances, sleep-wake disorders, psychomotor disturbances, and disorientation. Assessment for dementia can be made part of the routine assessment of older persons, especially if any of these symptoms arise. One tool that has been used successfully to screen older persons for cognitive impairments is the Mini-Mental State Examination (MMSE) (Folstein, Folstein, & McHugh, 1975; Yellowlees, 2015) (Fig. 18.4).

The MMSE was developed to assess the baseline mental status of older persons and to evaluate change or decline in mental functioning. The instrument is based on a 30-point scale that measures the level of awareness and orientation, appearance and behaviour, speech and communication, mood and affect, disturbances in thinking, problems with perception, and abstract thinking and judgement. The higher the older person scores on the examination, the more intact the mental status is presumed to be. When the result of the examination is 23 or lower, the individual is determined to have a problem with cognition. It is important to note that this instrument has been criticized for its cultural insensitivity, and it is difficult to use among individuals who speak languages other than English and among those with visual impairment and low literacy.

The MMSE is relatively easy to perform after a little practice and has been used for initial and subsequent evaluation of older persons in a variety of settings. The most effective way to perform the assessment is to make the person comfortable and establish a rapport. Eliminating extraneous noise and promoting attention and concentration will allow individuals to answer questions to the best of their ability. After the examination the score can be computed and used as a basis for care planning and further evaluation.

While there is currently no cure for Alzheimer's disease (Alzheimer's Society of Canada, 2016), treatment of Alzheimer's disease includes the use of medications for memory loss, including cholinesterase inhibitors and memantine, treatments for behavioural changes associated with Alzheimer's disease, and treatment for sleep changes. Medications to treat Alzheimer's disease are known as cholinesterase inhibitors. These medications are most effective during the early stages of the disease and act by increasing the levels of acetylcholine in the brain to prevent further loss of cognition and improve cognitive status.

Nonpharmacological techniques for managing the problems associated with dementia include developing and keeping routines; working in a calm, gentle, and unhurried manner; encouraging self-care activity; and reducing sensory overload. Interventions to keep the older person safe include curtailing wandering behaviour and preventing falls and other injury.

### Sensory Factors

Older persons experience age-related changes in vision, hearing, taste, smell, and touch sensation. Because of the normal changes and potential pathological changes associated with the senses, older persons of all cultural backgrounds and in all settings benefit from routine assessment and appropriate nursing interventions. Safety, particularly while driving, is a concern for older persons and society. Sensory changes affect a person's ability to drive safely. Nurses can encourage older persons to take senior driving classes to learn how to become safer drivers as these changes occur.

A variety of structural changes cause visual acuity to decrease, colour discrimination to become less acute, pupil size and constriction ability to decrease, and peripheral vision to diminish. Presbyopia is a loss of accommodation that occurs as people age and results in the inability to maintain focus on objects close to the eye. The lens of the eye thickens and becomes yellow and predisposes the older person to cataracts. The older person is also at increased risk of glaucoma, a group of eye disorders characterized by increased intraocular pressure. Because of the normal changes in the aging eye and the high risk of disease, a baseline eye assessment should be done to identify age-related changes and any disease processes. Follow-up eye appointments should be scheduled annually.

The nurse routinely assesses the older person for the accumulation of cerumen (earwax) to ensure optimal hearing (see the Case Study and Care Plan at the end of this chapter). Hearing deficits are common in old age, resulting from inner ear atrophy or sclerosis of the tympanic membrane. The inner ear also undergoes a number of changes, including those that are cell degenerative and nerve related. Presbycusis is a progressive sensorineural hearing loss associated with aging, and results in difficulty filtering background noise and understanding higher-pitched voices. Sound threshold changes, with an associated difficulty in understanding what others are saying. Similar to the changes of the eye, changes in hearing and the increased risk of pathological conditions indicate that older persons should have ear and hearing screening. Approximately 80% of those aged 60 to 79 years old experience some degree of hearing loss, defined as a loss of 15 decibels in at least 1 year (Statistics Canada, 2016c). Loss of hearing can result in decreased quality of life, as it may lead to miscommunication, loss of self-esteem, depression, falls, safety risks, and cognitive decline. Hearing aids assist those with hearing loss to communicate more effectively.

Taste changes with aging because of a loss of taste buds. The flavours of sweet, sour, salty, and bitter become blurred with this loss. The sensations brought about by touch may also diminish with the decrease in sensory nerve endings, especially in the presence of debilitating diseases such as diabetes, stroke, or Parkinson's disease. The ability to smell and the acuity of the olfactory nerve also decrease with age. Because of the loss of smell and taste sensations, older persons have the tendency to increase the amounts of salt and sugar in their food, possibly negatively affecting chronic health conditions. Teaching older persons about safe cooking and the use of alternative seasonings in food may help them adjust to these sensory changes. Additionally, the sense of smell is impaired, which may result in the inability to sense common warning signals such as smoke or rotten food. It is helpful to teach older persons to check the dates on their food packages frequently and to be attentive when cooking and preparing meals so as to ensure safety.

The decline in taste and smell sensations, combined with problems of obtaining adequate nutrition, makes dental care of vital importance to this population. Lack of fluoridated water and preventive dentistry during the developmental years may have led to tooth and periodontal problems in the older population. Periodontitis, or gum disease leading to tooth loss, is a common contributor to decreased taste sensation and poor nutrition. The inability to chew and swallow food in a comfortable manner works synergistically with decreased smell and taste sensations and other problems that inhibit proper nutrition. The Canadian Dental Association (2019) recommends that adults be seen for oral hygiene checks and counselling at least twice a year. During the initial evaluation, follow-up visits are scheduled to ensure that teeth and gums remain in good condition and that appropriate dental care devices are being used.

The skin of the older person changes, becoming thinner, less elastic, wrinkled, and more fragile. Although sweating decreases and injuries take longer to heal, the skin remains capable of sensing and performing its protective role. Chronic disease, however, can place an individual at risk of decreased sensation throughout the body. Cerebrovascular accidents (strokes) and neuropathies resulting from diabetes are two examples of diseases that disrupt the ability to feel pain and pressure through the skin. This lack of sensation can threaten safety. Older persons benefit from information about safety when cooking on a hot stove and the appropriate temperature for bathing and showering to prevent burns.

Nurses should perform frequent skin assessments to detect alterations in skin integrity at an early stage and implement appropriate interventions. The potential for skin impairment is common for those who have sensory impairment from physical disease or dementia. A pressure injury is a localized area of tissue necrosis that develops when soft tissue is compressed between two bony prominences or between a bony prominence and an external surface for a prolonged period. In addition to prolonged pressure on the skin, friction, moisture, shearing, and inadequate nutrition place the older person at risk of developing a pressure injury, which is difficult to treat. Preventing the injury is the best method for maintaining intact skin. People at risk of pressure injury should change their position at least every 2 hours to redistribute pressure appropriately throughout all areas of the skin. Elevating the lower extremities and maintaining proper body alignment are imperative to prevent pressure injury. Specialty beds are readily available in most care settings to decrease pressure and assist in positioning individuals who are at risk. Positioning pillows and other orthopedic devices provide ways to help maintain the proper support of body parts and body alignment. Proper nutrition, including adequate amounts of zinc and vitamins C and E, will help prevent this skin problem.

## ◆ Self-Perception–Self-Concept Pattern

The variability of self-concept in the older person is similar to the variability that is seen in the general population. As in all aspects of health, culture, environment, family, lifestyle factors, and heredity combine to form self-concept. Self-concept includes an individual's attitudes, perception of abilities (cognitive, affective, or physical), body image, identity, general sense of worth, and general emotional pattern. Personality traits tend to remain constant throughout life.

## Developmental Theories of Aging

Many people believe that adults no longer grow emotionally or physically in their later years. In truth, although the rate of physical decline exceeds the rate of physical growth, no evidence has been found that emotional growth declines in any way. One need only view the classic film *Driving Miss Daisy* to understand that older persons go through many developmental changes in the 30 to 40 years that often make up older adulthood. Erikson's (1982) theory of development asserts that older persons must pass through developmental stages as do infants, children, and younger adults. As in all stages of psychosocial development, unsuccessful passage through a stage can result in psychological illness, and successful passage through the stage promotes health (Erikson, 1982).

Ego integrity versus despair is the developmental stage of older persons (Erikson, 1982). The quality associated with successful passage of this stage is to achieve a balance between integrity and despair. "The process of bringing into balance feelings of integrity and despair involves a review of and a coming to terms with the life one has lived thus far" (Erikson, Erikson, & Kivnick, 1986). On the basis of the increasing life span, this stage of development was expanded into three additional stages: ego differentiation versus work role preoccupation, which involves achieving identity apart from work; body transcendence versus body preoccupation, which focuses on adjusting to normal aging changes; and ego transcendence versus ego preoccupation, which involves accepting death (Erikson, 1997).

Other developmental theorists have built upon Erikson's work. Some of these theories of aging are included in Box 18.1. Levinson moved away from Erikson's focus on the role of tensions that emerge during successive stages and, instead, emphasized that major life transitions are influenced by evolving physiological, psychological, and role-oriented life changes (Agronin, 2013). Vaillant also moved from an emphasis on "stages" to focus on developmental tasks of life. Vaillant theorized that generativity grows out of one's career. His studies suggested that successful generativity tripled the chances for a person to experience more joy than despair in their 70s (Agronin, 2013). Gilligan criticized Erikson, Levinson, and Vaillant for proposing theories that addressed only male development and focused her work primarily on the unique role of interpersonal connections in female development (Agronin, 2013).

Cohen is considered a founding father of geriatric psychiatry, bringing forth a modern conception of old age. He focused on the continued potential for growth that occurs not in spite of old age but because of it. His work demonstrated how the brain continually re-sculpts itself in response to experience and learning. Cohen also emphasized the role of creativity, which he believed persisted and even increased in old age. He proposed that older persons can develop a social portfolio to enhance moving through various phases. The social portfolio comprises individualized lists of vital activities that a person can engage in through an active review of lifelong personal assets. The social portfolio should include vital activities than a person can engage in even when faced with serious disability or loss (Agronin, 2013).

Nurses working in all settings are charged with helping older persons accomplish the task of balancing ego integrity and despair. Two successful methods of support for older persons at all cognitive levels are reminiscence and life review. An increasing number of researchers have found that there are substantial psychosocial health benefits for older persons who participate in reminiscence programs, with beneficial outcomes of enhanced mood, increased socialization, improved cognitive functioning, and enhanced well-being (Chippendale & Bear-Lehman, 2012; Smiraglia, 2015). There are many different types of reminiscence programs that are designed to engage participants in discussing their memories, sometimes with reflection prompts such as food or objects from the person's past. Life review is a more formal therapy technique taking the person through his or her life in a structured and chronological order. Both of these therapeutic approaches can be done individually or in groups, orally or through writing.

## ◆ Roles-Relationships Pattern

Although the general framework of self-perception remains constant throughout the life span, the source of an individual's self-perception often changes with older adulthood. The formation of the self that has focused on a person's role in the family changes when one's children become independent or a spouse dies. Roles such as daughter, son, sister, brother, wife, or husband may be lost because of death or illness. The loss of these roles can result in grieving, sadness, and, potentially, depression in the older person. In contrast with the loss of these roles, however, new roles, such as grandparenting, evolve (Fig. 18.5).

The most recent Canada-wide data on the diversity of grandparents living with grandchildren states that around 600,000 grandparents (8%) live in the same home as their grandchildren (Milan, Laflamme, & Wong, 2015). This study also provided interesting data on the influence of culture on familial living arrangements. Most of the grandparents living with grandchildren were of South and East Asian descent (Punjabi, Philippines, Chinese), followed by those of European descent (Spanish, Portuguese, Italian, German), and North African/Middle Eastern descent. The role of grandparent frequently brings great joy and happiness at a time when the older person feels loss; however, grandparents who rear grandchildren encounter both emotional and physical stress. Their new role as grandparent–caregiver may lead to role confusion and increased health-related problems (Bundy-Fazioli, Fruhauf, & Miller, 2013). Researchers have also found, however, that these grandparents may show positive levels of physical activity and self-care, especially if they do not perceive the caretaking responsibility as highly stressful (Bundy-Fazioli et al., 2013). Thus, it is important for nurses to explore with these individuals what activities may help to reduce stress. Coping strategies such as accepting responsibility, self-control, positive reappraisal, planned problem solving, and distancing may be helpful. Support groups, counselling, and education to help them manage stress more effectively are other resources that should be explored. Encouraging and supporting older persons in their caregiving role is important to help them ease the stress and strain of changes that come with the caregiving experience.

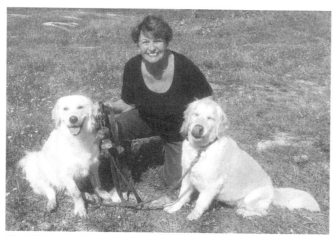

**Fig. 18.5** Loss of some roles can provide an opportunity for new roles. As family members grow up and move away, the older person may decide to devote time to training dogs to be pet therapy dogs.

With the average life span increasing, older persons can spend many more years in retirement than previous generations. Hooyman and Kiyak (2011) noted a variety of factors that were predictors of satisfaction with retirement. Those factors included good health and functional ability, adequate income, a suitable living environment, a strong social support system, and a positive outlook. An important factor was the autonomy of the retiree in choosing retirement and the preparation for the retirement while still working. For married retirees, having a good marital relationship and sharing similar interests with the spouse supported satisfaction with retirement. Having retirement activities that provide an opportunity to feel useful, to learn and grow, and to enjoy oneself are important. Many retirees enjoy sports and hobbies developed during their working years, whereas others become actively involved in volunteerism and other community and civic activities.

Volunteering can be an effective method for older persons to continue to feel engaged in the community as a productive, contributing member of society. Older persons who volunteer have an external incentive for getting dressed and going out of the house in the morning; they take a great amount of pride in their work. Filling a volunteer position provides a feeling of self-worth and helps to change negative feelings about retirement and other role changes. It also makes important contributions to society.

Downsizing from the family home to a smaller residence, widowhood, retirement, and relocation can elicit profound feelings of loss. Older persons who remain engaged in a variety of activities and relationships are happier and healthier. Personality, and its expression over time, is considered a major determinant of how engaged or active a person will be late in life. Other variables such as culture, health, bereavement, and habit affect activity as well.

Health-promotion activities centre on an understanding of the individual's usual behaviour and any unexpected or unexplained deviation from that behaviour. Nurses can help older persons identify the meaning of their lost roles and the results of those losses, and work through reactions to the losses. In more traumatic cases, support groups, such as bereavement groups,

can be helpful. The nurse supports people going through role changes by eliciting reactions and facilitating communication about these reactions. Significant others, such as children, neighbours, and friends, can provide important support. The nurse is integral in helping older persons develop and explore their new roles in their older years.

### ◆ Sexuality-Reproductive Pattern

The World Health Organization (WHO) defines sexual health as "a state of physical, emotional, mental and social well-being in relation to sexuality" (WHO, 2006). In older persons, as in all adults, sexual health is characterized by an approach to sexual relationships that is positive and respectful. In order for nurses and other health care providers to provide the most effective and comprehensive care for older persons, it is critical to abandon preconceptions and biases regarding sexuality in this population.

Older persons who are not cisgender (meaning that their gender corresponds with their birth sex, e.g., female sex, identifies as a woman) or heterosexual may experience health inequalities as a result of their gender identities or sexual and affectional orientations. Demographic estimates for the Canadian LGBTQ2S+ (lesbian, gay, bisexual, transgender, queer or questioning, and two-spirit) population are inconsistent and require further study. Existing data on the health care experiences of these individuals show that this population continues to face health inequities inked to social stigma, discrimination, and denial of their civil and human rights (Charles, Haaland, Kulkarni, et al., 2015; Colpitts & Gahagan, 2016). The Canadian Federation of Medical Students (Charles et al., 2015) specifically state that Canadian medical schools "have the responsibility to provide comprehensive and prejudice-free curricula in the care of LGBTQ2S+ individuals" (p. 2). This sentiment must extend to the education patient-care practices of nurses in order to ensure that all members of this community feel safe and cared for when seeking medical treatment. The population of older LGBTQ2S+ persons is more likely to delay seeking treatment for health problems and has a higher incidence of psychosocial problems. Nurses who use a nonjudgemental approach and open-ended questions related to marital status and sexual orientation can be very supportive in encouraging LGBTQ2S+ individuals to openly express their concerns about their health and well-being.

The most accurate predictor of sexual interest in older adulthood is the enjoyment and frequency of sex at a younger age. More than 50% of adults aged over 75 continue to engage in sexual activity three or more times a month. Surely, there are physiological changes associated with aging which can change some aspects of one's sexual life, but this does not mean that older people cannot adapt their sexual scripts accordingly. Older persons also need to fulfill the human need for intimacy and love, and to touch and be touched. Sexual activity may become more focused on quality than quantity, with more focus on intimate touching, caressing, and kissing. What was once considered foreplay may become mainplay for older persons, bringing changes which can still be satisfying and fulfilling. Although the need to express sexuality continues, older persons are susceptible to many chronic medical conditions, such as cardiac problems, arthritis, and normal aging changes that can make sexual intercourse difficult. In both sexes, reduced availability of sex hormones results in less rapid and less extreme vascular responses to sexual arousal. The lack of circulating hormones in both men and women results in changes in four areas of the sexual system: arousal, orgasm, postorgasm, and extragenital changes. Men experience less intense and slower erections, increased difficulty regaining an erection, decreased force of ejaculation, and an extended refractory time. Medications and other measures to manage medical conditions can also hinder sexual response. Erectile dysfunction may also occur, though this is not limited to older persons and can be experienced much earlier in life. For women, many changes begin at the perimenopausal age (the period before menopause begins), as the production of estrogen decreases. With age, the vagina becomes narrower, shorter, and thinner, and there is less natural lubrication. Future research must investigate potential psychosocial changes in sexuality over the life span, as most research has focused on physical changes exclusively.

Nurses are in an ideal position to help older persons find ways to improve their sexual health by assessing whether individuals are experiencing any challenges, or have any questions. It is important to remember that people may not bring these topics up on their own: so, asking questions in a sensitive, professional manner can be invaluable. Knowledge is essential to the successful fulfillment of sexuality needs. After making a sexual assessment, nurses can intervene to prevent or correct problems, but they frequently choose not to consider sexuality when planning care. One of the reasons for this is that nurses may believe the societal myths about older persons' sexuality, causing them to view it as less important. With proper education and experience, nurses can become sufficiently confident to venture into this delicate area.

One way in which nurses can gain knowledge of the sexual needs of older persons is through a staff development program using role play to discuss and process feelings associated with an older person's limitations in fulfilling intimate and sexual relationships. The expression of intimacy and sexuality among older persons results in a higher quality of life achieved through fulfilling a natural desire. In long-term care facilities, the need to address sexual needs of residents is great because of difficulties related to their chronic illnesses and because of a lack of resident privacy to engage in intimate and sexual relationships. Long-term care facilities can develop policies to assist residents in effectively fulfilling the need for intimacy and sexuality.

Many nurses believe that acquired immunodeficiency syndrome (AIDS) and other sexually transmitted infections (STIs) are not problems for older persons. However, the number of cases of human immunodeficiency virus (HIV) infection and AIDS in older persons continues to increase because greater numbers of older persons are becoming newly infected with HIV and an increasing proportion of those who have HIV are reaching their older years (Haddad, Li, Totten, et al., 2018). Two areas that are so important for successful aging—cognition and social engagement—are of particular concern for those

aging with HIV, as declines in both of these areas have been observed in this population (Vance, 2013). Approximately 50% of individuals with HIV experience cognitive problems, and as people age they may be at increased risk of developing cognitive changes. Social support and engagement often decline for many older persons and may be exacerbated by stigma and depression in older persons with HIV (Vance, 2013). It is important for nurses to suggest ways to promote social engagement, as this may help to improve both mood and cognitive functioning.

Older persons are just as susceptible to STI as younger adults. Yet one survey showed that only 5.1% of men older than 61 years had used a condom in recent sex (Esposito, 2016). There seems to be a lack-of-awareness population of older persons about the risks of STIs in their sexual relationships. Esposito (2016) noted that if you go into an STI clinic and look at the brochures about AIDS or STIs, you do not see people with wrinkles and grey hair on the front of those brochures. There are several reasons for which sexual safety practices are not followed by older persons. For example, some find themselves single after years of monogamy, and are not up to date with STI prevention practices and where to go for resources. Older persons may also fall behind in terms of general sex education, depending on when they were last educated in the area. Furthermore, older individuals at high risk of HIV (e.g., men who have sex with men, transgender women who have sex with men, etc.) may not be aware or be up to date on resources such as pre-exposure prophylaxis (PrEP). It is important that older persons become more aware of risks in their sexual relationships and follow the safer sex guidelines recommended by the Public Health Agency of Canada (PHAC, 2015). With all of this information in mind, it is critical that nurses ask respectful, open-ended questions about all aspects of health, including sexual health. Nurses are accessible points of contact who are capable of providing information on physiological changes affecting sexuality associated with age, resources for safer sex, and further referral for where to turn if issues require specific attention.

## ◆ Coping–Stress Tolerance Pattern

An individual's ability to cope with the common stresses of older adulthood is a key factor in maintaining self-concept. As people age, they tend to encounter many losses, such as the loss of a home, spouses, friends, siblings, and even children. They also experience declines in income and in health and physical functioning. The nurse who cares for the older person can provide support during the coping process related to these losses. Trying to find the positive and developmental benefits of losses is preferable to continually thinking about a loss or bad event. Negative associations have been found between depressive symptoms and rumination, catastrophizing, and self-blame. After assessing the most appropriate way in which the individual desires to cope with a situation, the nurse may help create a suitable environment for coping.

The spirituality of older persons is also an important consideration in helping them cope with stressful situations. Spirituality is very individual and may be exercised privately or through a religious framework. However, the impact of spirituality on quality of life has been well documented among older persons and often has a strong relationship with older persons' ability to cope with the changes and losses of aging.

## Depression

Among older persons, depression may mainly affect those with chronic illnesses and cognitive impairment and result in suffering, family disruption, and disability. Depression can worsen the outcomes of many illnesses and increase mortality. Aging-related and disease-related processes, including arteriosclerosis and endocrine and immune system changes, compromise the integrity of frontostriatal pathways, the amygdala, and the hippocampus, and increase vulnerability to depression. Heredity factors may also play a part. Psychosocial adversity—economic impoverishment, disability, isolation, relocation, caregiving, and bereavement—contributes to physiological changes, further increasing susceptibility to depression or triggering depression in already vulnerable older individuals.

It is important to know that most older persons are *not* depressed. Estimates of major depression in community-dwelling older persons fall around 3 to 5%, although 15% experience elevated depressive symptoms (Canadian Psychological Association, 2015). The National Institute of Mental Health (n.d.) noted that the risk of depression increases in older persons as they experience chronic illnesses and when their ability to function becomes impaired. The numerous losses experienced by older people may be partly to blame. Depression is also caused by physiological changes in the aging body. Although depression appears to affect older persons in much the same way that it affects younger individuals, certain patterns of symptoms and older persons' overall susceptibility are different from those of younger counterparts.

Nurses are integral in helping to diagnose and manage depression in older persons. Depression can be found in all care environments. Some common behaviours include sullen affect, lack of appetite and weight loss, sleep disturbances, fatigue, decreased ability to think or concentrate, psychomotor agitation, decreased participation in daily living and social activities, social withdrawal, and suicidal ideation. Many instruments are available to assist nurses in assessing older persons for this commonly occurring disorder. The Geriatric Depression Scale (Yesavage, Brink, Rose, et al., 1983) is available in several formats, with 30, 15, 5, or 1 question, and is easily administered. Positive results on the screening examinations require referral to social services for a diagnostic workup. After depression has been diagnosed, successful management may include psychotherapy, behavioural therapy, and, if necessary, antidepressant medication.

## Suicide

Suicide is the ninth leading cause of death in Canada, and twelfth leading cause for persons aged 65 and over. Males account for 80% of deaths by suicide in this age group, and females account for 52% of hospitalizations for self-inflicted injury (PHAC, 2016). Hanging, firearms, and poisoning are the most common methods of suicide used by older persons (Navaneelan, 2015).

The reason for the high number of suicides in the population of older persons continues to be explored. The elevated rate of depression helps the medical community understand the motive of many older persons. Many older persons have serious medical illnesses that provide an explanation for wanting to die. Risk factors for suicide include social isolation, alcohol and substance abuse, psychosis, bereavement, and serious medical illness. Many individuals who committed suicide were found to have alcohol and/or pain-killing medications in their bodies on autopsy.

The importance of different aspects of life also differs by culture. Some older persons may visit a health care provider with a somatic problem before the suicide attempt as, perhaps, a final call for help. Nurses working with older persons must be aware of the high rate of suicide in this age group and be alert for the risk factors. Older persons exhibiting signs of depression must be asked about possible suicidal thoughts. Suicide threats must be taken seriously, and appropriate interventions must be implemented to keep the older person safe.

The incidence of chronic illness that frequently accompanies old age raises a concern for ethical care. Many members of society believe that with the increased life span, individuals may be subjected to more suffering. A solution to ending the suffering of those with chronic illness has been voluntary euthanasia, or medical assistance in dying (MAID). In 2016, federal legislation was passed in Canada to legalize MAID. Physicians, and in some provinces and territories, nurse practitioners (e.g., Ontario) are able to provide assistance during this process, which can occur in two ways: (1) direct administration of a substance known to cause death, clinician-administered, or (2) ingestion of a prescribed medication that the eligible person takes themselves, in order to bring about their own death. In order to be eligible for medically assisted death, a person must be eligible for Canadian health insurance (i.e., not a visitor to Canada), be at least 18 years old and mentally competent, have an irremediable medical condition, make a voluntary request, and be able to give informed consent in the process of MAID (Health Canada, 2019b). Nurses help society to understand the many benefits of older adulthood and celebrate the extended life span. Nurses caring for chronically ill older persons have the added responsibility of determining who is at a higher likelihood of requesting medically assisted death, and helping them to be as comfortable as possible and free of pain through the use of pharmacological and nonpharmacological interventions. Nurses are instrumental in ensuring that the older person experiences a pain-free death by advocating an appropriate pain-management program and working with other health care providers toward this goal.

## ◆ Values-Beliefs Pattern

Every person who nurses care for will have a different sense of spirituality, which will have an influence on the way the person chooses to live, and the decisions made by the person about health care. Hodge, Bonifa, and Chou (2010) found that most older persons describe themselves as both spiritual and religious. The life of the spirit may help older persons to overcome the pain and suffering of chronic health and psychosocial problems encountered in their later years.

Nurses may find themselves in the providential but difficult position of attempting to promote the spiritual health of individuals. One reason for this perceived difficulty may be the nurse's discomfort with the person's belief system. Spirituality plays a significant role in meaning-making in relation to attitudes and beliefs about the world, self, and others.

There may be as many different spiritual values and beliefs as there are individuals. Differing spiritual values make helping older persons actualize their spirituality, and thus acquire a high quality of life, difficult for nurses. Because of the highly personal quality of spirituality, an unobtrusive and sensitive presence by the nurse is needed to allow the person in any setting to achieve spiritual health. Spiritual assessment tools are available to guide nurses with questions to better understand the person's spirituality. Open-ended questions such as "What is your perception of a higher being and spirituality?" encourage discussions about the person's innermost spirituality. The nurse can provide an environment that is supportive to the practice of the person's spirituality. Assisting older persons to actualize their spirituality can provide great comfort to the person and lead nurses to a deeper understanding of their own spirituality.

## ❖ ENVIRONMENTAL PROCESSES

### ◆ Physical Agents

#### Accidents

One important focus for injury prevention in older persons is falls. The most recent statistics show that falls are the leading cause of injury-related hospitalization for older persons in Canada, with 20 to 30% of this population experiencing a fall each year (PHAC, 2014). Over one-third of reported falls resulted in broken or fractured hips, injuries which put increasing demands on health care providers in Canada. It is essential that nurses are knowledgeable about interventions for prevention (Quality and Safety Scenario).

Some of the causes of falls in older persons are neuromuscular dysfunction, osteoporosis, stroke, and sensory impairment. Falls can result in decreased mobility, decreased ability to live independently, and increased risk of an early death. Although a fall in a younger individual may not be problematic, a fall in an older person can have devastating consequences. Falls account for 40% of admissions to long-term care facilities each year. Even if older persons are not injured in a fall, they may develop a fear of falling, and therefore limit their activities and increase their risk of future falls.

Because of the higher risk of osteoporosis in the older population, a fall can result in a fracture. Osteoporosis is a disease of bone loss common to women aged 70 years or older and men aged 80 years or older. The disease develops six times more frequently in women than it does in men. The rapid decline in estrogen secretion at the onset of menopause signals the calcium in the bones to move into the bloodstream, which causes the bones to become weak and brittle. Because of this weakness, falls in older persons with osteoporosis frequently result in fractures, which place these individuals in a spiral of iatrogenic risk, beginning

### ⚡ QUALITY AND SAFETY SCENARIO

**Fall Prevention for Older Persons in the Community: Ontario's Example**

Falls in community-dwelling older persons are a critical problem for nurses to address, as falls are the leading cause of injury in older persons. The Registered Nurses' Association of Ontario (RNAO) has created a guide for preventing falls and reducing injury from falls, which is periodically updated via newly released editions (RNAO, 2017). The guide's recommendations are based on research of evidence-informed practices, and each recommendation is ranked, based on the existing level (or quality) of research to support its effectiveness. These recommendations are intended to provide helpful information for clinicians, though clinical decisions involve more considerations than evidence alone and clinicians need to individualize decision making for a specific patient.

The RNAO notes that various approaches to identify people at increased risk are helpful. There is no single evidence-informed instrument that accurately identifies older persons at increased risk of falling. Clinicians need to assess risk on the basis of a variety of factors, such as a history of falls and impaired mobility and balance. Early intervention is important for people assessed to be at risk, as these interventions can prevent serious injury. The RNAO states that more research is needed for clinical validation of tools to identify older persons at risk of falling.

**Summary of Recommendations**
- All adults should be screened for risk of falls at least annually, or upon admission for injury.
- Screening should involve inquiry about potential history of falls, identification of gait, balance, or mobility difficulties, and clinical judgement.
- For those patients at risk of falls, conduct an in-depth assessment of risk factors using validated measures appropriate for the patient.
- Those patients with multiple risk factors or a long history of falls should be referred to appropriate medical or community resources, such as exercise and balance physiotherapy.
- In order to uphold the patient's self-efficacy, use positive messaging and an open conversational style.
- Self-support options should be discussed, and the family should be engaged where appropriate to augment person-centred care. Individualized plans can be made using this information.

Source: Registered Nurses' Association of Ontario. (2017). *Preventing falls and reducing injury from falls* (Fourth Edition). Toronto: Author. Retrieved from https://rnao.ca/sites/rnao-ca/files/bpg/FALL_PREVENTION_WEB_1207-17.pdf.

with weeks of decreased mobility and possibly resulting in pressure injuries, psychological trauma, pneumonia, and even death.

The risk factors for osteoporosis include a small, thin frame; White or Asian ancestry; family history of osteoporosis; excessive thyroid medication or high doses of cortisone-like medications for treatment of asthma, arthritis, or cancer; a diet low in dairy products and other sources of calcium; physical inactivity; smoking cigarettes; and drinking alcohol. Osteoporosis is typically diagnosed after an older person sustains a fracture. However, bone density testing is readily available to determine individuals at risk before a fracture occurs. Sufficient calcium intake remains vitally important and will continue to reduce the normal bone loss of aging. Health care providers frequently monitor calcium and vitamin D levels as a part of wellness care in older persons. Most women need 1000 mg daily before menopause and 1500 mg daily after menopause. Consuming this amount of calcium from today's average diet is difficult; therefore, a calcium supplement is essential. Vitamin D is also essential for bone health. Although one can obtain adequate vitamin D by daily exposure to the sun, because of concerns about the amount of sun exposure necessary, 400 to 800 IU of vitamin D supplements is usually recommended in conjunction with calcium. For the prevention of osteoporosis and the optimal maintenance of both psychological and physical well-being in the older person, regular physical activity is necessary.

Less than half of older persons tell their health care provider about a fall, so it is important for nurses to inquire about falls. Because many factors contribute to falls, risk assessment is essential. If a fall has been sustained, the older person is at increased risk of falling again and fall-prevention strategies must be implemented. Several fall risk assessment tools have been developed, but more research is needed to validate their use in different settings. By identifying the risks of falls and assessing an older person's vision, hearing, medication use, blood pressure, mobility, and other factors, nurses can predict and prevent many falls.

Table 18.2 lists frequent causes of accidents that occur in the home and nursing interventions to prevent them. Nurses who provide care in the community are in an ideal position to prevent injuries. During the initial and subsequent assessments, the nurse can evaluate individuals' homes for common factors leading to fires, poisoning, and falls, such as frayed wires on electrical appliances that can produce sparks and start fires, improperly labelled cleaning products that can be accidentally ingested, loose rugs on the floor, absence of handrails on stairs or in bathrooms, and poor lighting that can cause falls. Appropriate health teaching incorporates the concept of accident prevention for all older persons living not only in the community but also in acute care facilities and long-term care facilities.

### Preventing Injury

Falls and fires are leading causes of unintentional injury and death in people 65 years or older. Other unintentional injuries and deaths in older persons are caused by motor vehicle accidents, suffocation, and poisoning. Because of normal age-related changes and the increased incidence of chronic illness, older persons can experience decreased muscle strength and delayed reaction time

| TABLE 18.2   Safety Risk Areas and Related Interventions | |
|---|---|
| **Area of Attention** | **Intervention** |
| Stairways | Secure handrails<br>Illuminate stairways with light switches at both top and bottom<br>Eliminate clutter on all steps and stair landings<br>Use nonskid treads on steps |
| Bedroom | Use nightlights<br>Tack down carpet<br>Discourage use of throw rugs<br>Arrange furniture so that it will not obstruct clear pathways<br>Secure extension cords and telephone wires and remove them from walking areas<br>For smokers, never smoke in bed |
| Bathroom | Use handrails near tub and toilet<br>Use nonskid mats in tub area and on floor<br>Use a bath thermometer to measure hot water in tub<br>Use nightlights |
| Kitchen | Wear nonflammable, lightweight clothing when cooking<br>Place dishes and cooking utensils at reasonable heights<br>Use stepstools with a handrail according to specifications and only when not alone<br>Keep off wet floor and refrain from using slippery wax<br>Never climb on chairs<br>Keep emergency numbers near the telephone<br>Ensure locks can be easily opened in times of emergency<br>Cook at front of the stove rather than at the back<br>Do not use electrical appliances with frayed cords |
| Living room | Use furniture that is easy to get in and out of Eliminate clutter on all floor areas<br>Install fire detectors at appropriate places |
| Outdoors | Make sure stairs are free of breaks and cracks, and clear of snow and ice<br>Use safe handrails<br>Provide good lighting for stairs and walkways |

The older person's ability to feel changes in heat and cold may be impaired as a result of normal and pathological changes of aging. This process can cause older persons to die of the effects of excessive heat or cold. During periods of high temperature and humidity, older people should increase fluid and salt intake, stay in a cool and shaded environment, remain calm, have more rest periods, and refrain from going outdoors when the temperature is higher than 32.2°C (90°F). Sweating, which is reduced in older persons, can be accommodated by the wearing of light-coloured, lightweight cotton clothing. If sweating ceases or is inadequate, the older person is at risk of heat stroke. Heat stroke can contribute to sepsis, myocardial infarction, and cerebrovascular accidents, particularly in people with diabetes. Reduced body heat can also present problems in the older person. Symptoms of and interventions for hypothermia are listed in Box 18.3.

---

**BOX 18.3 Nursing Interventions for Hypothermia**

**Symptoms**
- Cold to touch
- Slow respiration
- Bradycardia
- Low blood pressure
- Slurred speech
- Drowsiness
- Temperature 32.2°C rectally

**Interventions**
- Warm hands and feet
- Cover with blanket
- Set room temperature to 21°C
- Wear cap to bed at night
- Wear socks to bed at night
- Wear several layers of clothing
- Increase activity
- Decrease alcohol intake
- Use extreme caution with space heaters, heating pads, or electric blankets

---

and, subsequently, become more vulnerable to environmental hazards. Decreased sensory acuity and impaired balance further diminish their ability to interpret the environment.

As the percentage of older persons living in Canada increases, the number of older drivers also increases. Transport Canada releases annual statistics on driving demographics and patterns. Their latest published numbers state that there were 4.7 million licensed drivers aged 65 years and over in 2017. In the same year, this group accounted for 18% of all fatalities and 14.2% of serious injuries for drivers; fatality rates falling just behind the most at-risk group of drivers (those aged 25–34 years), who made up 18.9% of fatalities and 21% of serious injuries (Transport Canada, 2019). Additionally, older persons are less likely to survive major trauma compared with middle aged or younger adults, making it more dangerous if serious injuries do occur. Age-related changes in vision, joint mobility, and cognitive changes may affect the older person's ability to drive. Because of these changes, older persons often avoid driving at night, in bad weather, in heavy traffic, on long trips, or on highways or high-speed roads.

Older individuals are at increased risk of severe injury resulting in hospitalization, disability, or death from motor vehicle injuries because of the many changes in their neuromuscular and sensory abilities, which slow response time in emergency situations. The majority of collisions in Canada occur in urban areas, with drivers being the most at risk of death or serious injury compared with passengers, pedestrians, and cyclists (Transport Canada, 2019). Most traffic fatalities involving older persons occur during the daytime and involve other vehicles. In two-vehicle fatal crashes involving both older and younger drivers, the older driver's vehicle was more than twice as likely to be struck than the younger person's, indicating a decline in defensive driving as opposed to an increase in aggressive driving among older persons.

Older persons are encouraged to take a seniors' driving safety course to learn how aging changes can affect their driving and strategies for safer driving. Nurses working in the community may encourage older drivers to contact the Canadian Automobile Association (CAA) for driving classes designed to meet their needs. In addition, attending these classes often provides savings on vehicle insurance. CAA also provides information about aging and driving, and the effect of certain medications on one's ability to drive. These are good resources to share with older persons or those involved in their care as reference points (CAA, 2019a). At some point, it may be better for older persons to stop driving. Box 18.4 offers warning signs that suggest when an older person should limit or stop driving. Older persons are often highly resistant to requests to stop driving, as being able to drive is an important sign of independence. Many families find out only after a car accident that the older person has not heeded their warning and has been driving without their knowledge. In the case of an older person with dementia, health care providers may need to talk with family members to find a way to prevent the person from driving. If an older person has been found to be an unsafe driver and refuses to stop driving, a family member may take away the car keys or mechanically disable the car so that it cannot be driven. It is important, however, to find ways for the older person to continue to participate in pleasurable activities and not to become isolated. For example, a loss of spiritual connections may occur when older persons can no longer drive to their place of worship. In rural areas, there are many older persons managing farms and dependent on being able to drive to obtain needed supplies and services. Family members or friends may be able to set up a schedule to alternate driving the person to the grocery store, church, and other places. This can also help to provide important social interactions. Additionally, the CAA lists resources available in each province to support older persons. Examples include Manitoba's Driving Angels program, where volunteers offer to drive older persons to appointments, events, and to run errands. Ontario offers a Mature Drivers Workshop to refresh safe, defensive driving techniques (CAA, 2019b).

### Elder Mistreatment

Elder abuse (elder mistreatment) refers to intentional or neglectful acts by a caregiver or "trusted" person that results in, or may lead to, harm of a vulnerable elder. The Government of Canada lists the following forms of elder abuse and mistreatment: physical abuse, sexual abuse, psychological abuse, financial abuse, and neglect (Government of Canada, 2016). The most recent Canada-wide statistics on elder abuse were released in 2015, reporting that one-third of perpetrators of elder abuse are family members. Grown children of the older person are the most common perpetrators, followed by spouses, siblings, and extended family. Instances of abuse were most common in rural areas, with the territories, Saskatchewan, New Brunswick, and Alberta reporting the highest incidence of family violence in Canada (Statistics Canada, 2015c). According to the Canadian Association of Retired Persons (CARP, 2018), the most common

## BOX 18.4 Signs That Driving Habits Should Change

Poor driving skills that are warning signs of unsafe driving include:

- *Has the driver been issued two or more traffic tickets or warnings in the past two years?* Tickets can predict a greater risk for collision.
- *Has the driver been involved in two or more collisions or "near-misses" in the past two years?* Rear-end crashes, parking lot fender-benders, and side collisions while turning across traffic rank as the most common mishaps for drivers with diminishing skills, depth perception, or reaction time.
- *Does the driver have difficulty working the brake and gas pedals?* Drivers who lift their legs to move from the accelerator to the brake, rather than keeping a heel on the floor and pressing with the toes, may have waning leg strength.
- *Does the driver sometimes miss stop signs and other traffic signals?* Perhaps the driver is inattentive or cannot spot the signs in a crowded, constantly moving visual field.
- *Does the driver weave between or straddle lanes?* Signalling incorrectly or not at all when changing lanes can be particularly dangerous, especially if the driver fails to check mirrors or blind spots.
- *Do other drivers honk or pass frequently, even when the traffic stream is moving relatively slowly?* This may indicate difficulty keeping pace with fast-changing conditions.
- *Does the driver get lost or disoriented easily, even in familiar places?* This could indicate problems with working memory or early cognitive decline.

Source: Canadian Automobile Association (CAA). (2019). *Signs that driving skills are declining.* Retrieved from https://www.caa.ca/seniors/signs-that-driving-habits-should-change/, as summarized from Canadian Medical Association. (2019). *Determining medical fitness to operate motor vehicles* (CMA Driver's Guide, 9th ed.). Ottawa: Joule. Retrieved from https://optometrists.sk.ca/wp-content/uploads/2018/09/CMA_Driveru2019s_Guide_9th_edition.pdf.

forms of abuse among its members are emotional (64%), financial abuse (34%), institutional abuse (including neglect in long-term care facilities, 29%), physical abuse (18%), and neglect (18%).

Victims of elder abuse are more likely to be single women older than 75 years who are dependent on the caregiver for food and shelter. They are more likely to be frail, to be incontinent, or to have a mental health disorder. The abuser is usually the adult son or daughter of the victim, who has poor impulse control and low self-esteem (Nies & McEwan, 2011). Nurses have a responsibility to identify abuse, provide appropriate care for injuries, and report suspected abuse to appropriate state agencies or law enforcement personnel. The nurse may consult social services to find a more suitable living arrangement for the victim. The most important consideration is to provide a safe environment for the older person who is in immediate danger.

## ◆ Biological Agents

Because of decreased immune system response, older persons are susceptible to bacterial and viral disease. In many cases, older persons have not received primary immunization against diphtheria and tetanus. A large emphasis is placed on immunizing young children against communicable disease; however, older persons can also be protected by commonly available vaccines that have been shown to lower both morbidity and

mortality. Influenza and pneumonia are two disease processes that are associated with higher mortality and morbidity.

### Influenza

Influenza is among the top 10 most common causes of death in older persons (Statistics Canada, 2019b). Health Canada (2018) reports that, per year, 12,000 hospitalizations and 3000 deaths occur due to influenza alone. They state that people over the age of 65, and residents of long-term care facilities are at particularly high risk of experiencing complications or hospitalizations. Additionally, many chronic diseases (for which prevalence increases with age), such as cardiac or pulmonary disorders and diabetes mellitus, also put individuals at higher risk of flu-related health complications. The group with the highest rates of influenza vaccination in Canada are those aged 50 to 64 (34.1%), and those aged 65 and above (61.1%). This may be due to the increased availability of vaccination clinics and programs for older persons, as they are recognized, and therefore prioritized, as an at-risk group (Health Canada, 2019c). However, this should not downplay the importance of increasing vaccination rates in younger age groups to strengthen the effect of herd immunity (critically important for the protection of anyone who cannot be vaccinated). The vaccine, composed of inactivated whole virus or viral subunits grown in chick embryo cells, is given annually to older persons, especially those with chronic conditions such as pulmonary or cardiac problems and those in long-term care facilities. Vaccination is contraindicated in people who have experienced a reaction to the vaccine, and caution must be exercised in administering the vaccine to people who have allergies to eggs.

### Pneumococcal Infections

Deaths from pneumococcal infections has declined in previous years, indicating the value of public health initiatives to make information widespread about the importance of immunization against pneumonia and influenza. Implementation of immunization programs in public places such as supermarkets and drugstores, in addition to health care providers' offices and clinics, has enhanced access to this preventive measure. Nevertheless, many older persons remain unvaccinated. The Public Health Agency of Canada (PHAC, 2019) recommends that older persons aged 65 years or older receive the pneumococcal vaccination. It is important that nurses inform the public about the importance of immunizations and counteract the myth that receiving the vaccination will result in the disease, which often prevents older persons from receiving immunization.

### Cancer

Cancer is the leading cause of death in Canada and was expected to claim an estimated 82,100 Canadians in 2019 (Canadian Cancer Society, 2019). It is estimated that approximately one in two Canadians (49% of men and 45% of women) will be diagnosed with cancer at some point in their lifetime, with 220,400 new diagnoses in 2019 alone (Canadian Cancer Society, 2019). About 90% of cases occur in persons aged 50 years or over, and prevalence increases with age (Canadian Cancer Society, 2019). The reason for

## TABLE 18.3   Top Five Cancers in Canada, by Sex

| | Rank | Percent of all Cancers |
|---|---|---|
| **All cancers combined, both sexes:** | ... | 100 |
| Lung and bronchus | 1 | 13.5 |
| Breast | 2 | 13.0 |
| Colorectal | 3 | 12.2 |
| Prostate | 4 | 10.9 |
| Urinary bladder (including in situ) | 5 | 5.3 |
| **All cancers combined, males:** | ... | 100 |
| Prostate | 1 | 21.4 |
| Lung and bronchus | 2 | 13.8 |
| Colorectal | 3 | 13.2 |
| Urinary bladder (including in situ) | 4 | 7.9 |
| Non-Hodgkin's lymphoma | 5 | 4.7 |
| **All cancers combined, females:** | ... | 100 |
| Breast | 1 | 26.2 |
| Lung and bronchus | 2 | 13.2 |
| Colorectal | 3 | 11.2 |
| Corpus uteri | 4 | 6.2 |
| Thyroid | 5 | 5.1 |

Source: Statistics Canada. (2016). *Cancer incidence in Canada, 2013*. Ottawa: Author. Retrieved from https://www150.statcan.gc.ca/n1/en/daily-quotidien/160315/dq160315a-eng.pdf?st=I70An10Q.

the increased prevalence of cancer in this population is unknown; however, theories include longer exposure to carcinogens, increased susceptibility to cancer in the older body, decreased cellular healing ability, loss of tumour-suppressing genes, and decreased immune function. Although the exact cause cannot be determined, cancer is a significant issue for older persons in Canada.

The most common types of cancer are listed by sex in Table 18.3. Prostate cancer is the leading cancer among men of all races and ages and is clearly the most common male cancer, constituting 21% of all diagnoses. Early detection of prostate cancer allows treatment while it is still localized in the prostate gland and highly curable. Evidence suggests that by use of a combination of screening techniques more cases of prostate cancer can be detected earlier. There are three key components of an appropriate prostate screen: symptomatology, prostate-specific antigen level measurement, and a digital rectal examination. The four major treatment options for prostate cancer are surgery, radiation therapy, watchful waiting, and hormone therapy.

Breast cancer is the most common cancer in females of all ages and ethnicities in Canada, accounting for 26.2% of all cancer diagnoses. Three-quarters of all breast cancers occur in women older than 50 years. The risk is increased in women whose close female relatives (mothers or sisters) have had the disease. Women who have never had children or who had their first child after age 30 years appear to have an increased risk. The causes of breast cancer remain unclear. The best protection is early detection and prompt treatment. The Canadian Task Force on Preventive Health Care (2018) recommends screening (via mammogram) once every 2 to 3 years for women aged 50 to 74 years old. These guidelines do not apply to women at high risk due to personal or familial risk, and screening should be conducted before age 50 years based on the instruction of a health care provider.

Nurses help older persons change the habits that place them at high risk of developing cancer. Following nutritional guidelines (as suggested earlier in this chapter), reducing stress, adopting a program of regular exercise, and stopping smoking and other use of tobacco products are a few of the approaches that nurses can advise to promote individual wellness. Periodic monitoring and screening in the form of regular visits to a primary health care provider or community screening can alert older persons to early signs and symptoms of cancers that occur during the later years.

## ◆ Chemical Agents

Chemical agents can be both therapeutic and harmful, depending on their use. The increased use of prescription and over-the-counter medications can result in increased adverse effects. The use of alcohol and tobacco products can be especially harmful for older persons.

### Medication Use

Normal changes of aging have a significant effect on the pharmacodynamics of medications in older persons. The ways in which medications are absorbed, distributed, metabolized, and excreted from the body are affected by normal physiological changes and by illness. Even when medications are taken as prescribed, age-related changes and disease increase the risk of undesirable adverse effects. Older persons are more likely to take multiple medications, resulting in increased risk of serious medication interactions. In addition to potential adverse effects caused by prescription medications, older persons take many types of nonprescription substances, including over-the-counter medications; vitamins, minerals, and supplements; herbal remedies; and foods and other traditional remedies used to resolve common ailments. Polypharmacy, or the use of multiple medications for the same or for different health problems, is a major concern for older persons. Around 82.6% of persons aged 65 to 79 years old regularly take prescription medication, with 29.9% prescribed five or more (Rotermann, Sanmartin, Hennessy, et al., 2014). The higher rate of polypharmacy in older persons as compared with younger groups is related to increased health problems in older persons and new medications that effectively treat these conditions.

Many older persons who reside at home take their medications independently. Although self-medication with prescription and nonprescription substances is an effective method of disease management, little is known about the process of taking medications after the person leaves the health care practice or facility. Although it is generally assumed that medications are taken as prescribed, sensory disturbances, lack of knowledge, and alternative medication, alcohol, and nutrition practices may present challenges to medication self-administration that interfere with medical management of health problems. Nurses should take a thorough medication history to assess the individual for past reactions to medications and identify all currently prescribed and nonprescription substances taken. New medications should be started at their lowest effective dose, and the dose should be increased slowly as necessary.

One of the major barriers to medication adherence in the older person is affordability. As discussed in the Nutrition-Metabolic Pattern section, programs such as OAS pension can help to supplement the income of older persons. Unfortunately, this is not always adequate for covering life's many expenses; in particular, the cost of prescription medication. Canada is the only country with a universal health care program that does not cover the cost of prescription medications (Morgan, Law, Daw, et al., 2015). In fact, Morgan and Lee's (2017) review of cost-related medication non-adherence in developed countries found that one in 12 older Canadians are not taking all (or any) of their prescriptions because they cannot afford them. They state that among countries included in their study, those with lower medication adherence (United States and Canada) had lower availability of coverage options and higher direct patient charges for prescriptions. All countries that provided coverage for outpatient prescriptions had comparable, very low (~3%) levels of cost-related non-adherence. Of particular importance is the fact that Canadians aged 55 to 64 years old are most affected by lack of prescription coverage, as they do not qualify for public plans aimed specifically at older persons (minimum age of 65 years old). These programs vary by province and territory, so it is important for nurses to ask patients about their ability to access coverage and point them to necessary resources if they are experiencing challenges.

### Alcohol and Drug Abuse

According to Sacco, Kuerbis, Goge, and colleagues (2013), the prevalence of alcohol use disorder will increase in older persons as the baby boomer generation ages. In the next 20 years, psychoactive drugs (e.g., benzodiazepines) will accompany alcohol as the most abused substances among older persons (Wang & Andrade, 2013). Older persons may be classified as moderate drinkers but frequently consume large amounts of alcohol at a time. Alcohol and drug abuse in older persons is often unreported and unnoticed because the symptoms can be similar to those of other common problems of aging, and health care providers often do not ask people about alcohol or nonprescription drug use. The longer the problem remains undetected, the greater it becomes and the more the potential harm related to other chronic health problems.

Older persons are more vulnerable to the effects of alcohol and illicit medications because their detoxification and excretion systems are not as efficient as those of younger people. Alcoholism and drug abuse predispose older persons to accidents and injury, cognitive decline, physical debility, nutritional deficiencies, disease, and decreased function. Additionally, alcohol use while taking medications can interfere with the desired effect of the medication. Loneliness, cognitive decline (e.g., memory problems), and a high incidence of mood disorders put older persons at increased risk of substance abuse; thus, screening for substance-use patterns must be prioritized in this group.

### Tobacco Use

Tobacco use includes cigarette smoking, cigar smoking, pipe smoking, and chewing tobacco. Use of tobacco products is associated with cardiovascular disease, several types of cancer, and chronic lung disease (Alam, Lam, Drucker, et al., 2019). Some older men and women today may be the first generation to have smoked throughout their lives, starting in their teens or 20s when smoking seemed fashionable. The results of smoking occur slowly over time, and problems are usually not experienced until signs and symptoms of smoking-related health problems occur. Because smoking can initiate and promote disease processes, it is one of the most important negative predictors of longevity. Smoking is a particular problem for older persons because of the large number of medications they take and the potential for medication interactions. Nicotine–drug interactions can potentiate or interfere with a desired medication effect.

Older persons can experience the benefits of smoking cessation even after the age of 65 years. These people may be more motivated to quit smoking than when they were younger, because they are likely to see some of the damage that smoking has caused and anticipate that smoking cessation will restore or improve their health. Nurses can assist older persons in making the commitment to quit smoking through education and referral to smoking cessation programs.

## ❖ DETERMINANTS OF HEALTH

### ◆ Social Factors and Environment

The incidence of chronic and acute illnesses, the subsequent decline in functional status, changes in economic status, and changes in family structure frequently place older persons in situations for which they are admitted to acute care facilities or must make a temporary or permanent move into a residential facility or a long-term care facility. When providing health-promotion services to older persons, nurses must take into account the type of setting in which the person lives. The Research for Evidence-Informed Practice box provides helpful information about transitional care for older persons with chronic illness, as well as their caregivers.

When older persons leave their homes, they may enter a continuum of care extending from an independent living centre and assisted living facilities to skilled care facilities, with possible short-term stays in acute care settings. Nurses who work in each of the settings on the continuum can promote health to this population in many ways. From the acute care setting through each stage of the continuum, opportunities are available for nurses to introduce older persons and their families to community resources (Table 18.4). The acute care nurse has the opportunity to present health-promotion strategies at a time during which individuals may perceive the greatest need to change their lifestyle behaviours so that they can return to an improved health state. In most cases an acute care admission is an opportunity to introduce health-promotion teaching. However, the acute care nurse may feel frustrated by the inability to see the results of this teaching and may therefore give it a low priority in the care plan.

## RESEARCH FOR EVIDENCE-INFORMED PRACTICE

### Evidence-Informed Transitional Care for Chronically Ill Older Persons and Their Caregivers

Unplanned readmissions within 30 days of discharge are estimated to be at 90%. A multidisciplinary research team developed a transitional care model (TCM) to focus on the needs of very high-risk chronically ill older persons who are transitioning from the hospital to the home following an acute illness. The TCM is led by an advanced practice nurse (APN) using a holistic person-centred and family-care–centred approach. The APN acts as the "point person" throughout the episode of care, facilitating timely exchange of information across all settings. The criteria identified to determine high-risk persons include those who are 80 years or older, those who have moderate-to-severe functional deficits, and those who are unable to complete self-care or manage daily tasks.

The tools used to assess potentially affected persons include the Hospital Admission Risk Profile, the Katz Index of Independence in Activities of Daily Living or the Lawton Instrumental Activities of Daily Living Scale, and the Mental Status Assessment of Older Adults (Mini-Cog). Potentially affected persons are also screened with use of the Geriatric Depression Scale (Short Form) to assess symptoms of depression. The following risks associated with readmission have been identified: having four or more active coexisting health problems, being treated with six or more prescribed standing medications, having two or more hospitalizations within the previous 6 months, being hospitalized within the previous 30 days, having been hospitalized with baseline dementia, being treated for delirium, lacking formal or informal family caregiver support, and having low health literacy.

With APN services under the TCM, mutual goals are developed, there is improved communication and collaboration among health care providers, there is improved medication and dietary adherence, there are decreased numbers of rehospitalizations during the 52 weeks of follow-up, and there is high person, caregiver, and health care provider satisfaction. The barriers to widespread adoption of the TCM identified include the organization of current systems of care, barriers of regulation, lack of quality and financial incentives, and culture of care issues.

Source: Bixby, M. B. (2011). Evidence-informed transitional care for chronically ill older persons and their caregivers. *Journal of Geriatric Care Management, 21*(2), 20–24.

Some older persons will rapidly grasp material that they believe will prevent future hospital admissions and restore their health. Home health nursing appointments, transportation services, housekeeping services, adult day care, and assistance with grocery shopping or home-delivered meals will help older persons return to the home environment better prepared to recover from the illness. Helping older persons and their families locate adult day care programs, smoking-cessation programs, stress-management workshops, or weight-loss and exercise programs before leaving the hospital will encourage older persons to enter these programs immediately after discharge, while they are motivated.

Long-term care nurses are able to locate and plan community resources during the resident's stay. Some community services will enable an older person to return home to an environment in which active health promotion continues. Community resources that may help older persons who are discharged from long-term care facilities include adult day care programs, support groups and medical resources, telephone and Internet information, and referral services. In addition to their role in individual care planning, long-term care nurses can be more involved in institutional policy changes. Recommendations about smoking policies, healthy diets, and exercise programs may prompt interdisciplinary changes that will result in improved health for the entire institution.

The geriatric care manager who visits older persons in their home or in other residential facilities may be charged with individual health-promotion planning. Nurses who provide care in the community deliver health care information and services to individuals and their families. The resources available to community health nurses are frequently rich and enable the nurses to draw on a variety of sources to assist in promoting the health of community-dwelling older persons. Transportation options, home-delivered meals, assistance with housekeeping, socialization activities, exercise programs, and self-help groups are only a few of the health-promotion resources available within the community. Nurses in all settings can consult a social worker or contact the community services office for older persons for information on available resources.

As discussed in the introduction of this chapter, it is important for the nurse to consider the health literacy level of older persons and their families when providing information and health teaching. It is important to keep in mind that those at risk of low health literacy are older persons, minorities, people of low socioeconomic level, and the medically underserved. Older persons with low health literacy may have difficulty finding appropriate health care providers, seeking preventive health care, filling out health forms, managing chronic illness, following directions, understanding the relationship between risk behaviours and health problems, and following medication and treatment plans. It is important for nurses to identify older persons who have low health literacy and develop instructional materials that use simple language and short sentences, avoiding or defining technical terms. Nurses can provide assistance for older persons who have difficulty completing forms. For older persons who have limited English language skills, written and oral instruction can be provided in their native language.

In recent years there has been a substantial increase in the use of palliative and hospice care by older persons. Palliative care is provided for people with a serious illness who will continue to receive curative treatment and symptom relief. Whereas palliative care is available to anyone with a serious illness, hospice care requires a terminal prognosis with an expected death within 6 months. Once the person is placed in hospice care, treatment to relieve pain and other symptoms is continued but the person and health care provider have decided to end all curative treatment. According to the Canadian Hospice Palliative Care Association (CHPCA, 2014), chronic diseases account for 70% of deaths in Canada. They state that as chronic illnesses become more common with age, demand and support for hospices also increase over the life span. Although there is both a need and a desire for this service, only 16 to 30% of Canadian individuals who have died were using hospice care while critically ill, while the other 70% died in a hospital. The CHPCA (2014) notes that only six out of the 13 provinces and territories

## TABLE 18.4  Long-Term Care Housing and Assessment Continuum

| | Independent Living | Retirement Community | Assisted Living | Long-Term Care Facility |
|---|---|---|---|---|
| Description | Covers a broad range of housing options (residential houses, apartments, condominiums, townhouses, subsidized older persons housing) for older persons who are functionally and socially independent | Provides a living arrangement that integrates shelter and services for older persons who do not need 24-hr protective oversight | Provides a living arrangement that integrates shelter and services for frail older persons who are functionally and/or socially impaired and require 24-hr protective oversight | Provides a living arrangement that integrates shelter with medical, nursing, psychosocial, and rehabilitation services for older persons who require 24-hr nursing supervision |
| Primary services | **A** Environmental security. Possibly, coordination of resident services (transportation, activities, housekeeping) *OR* no services are available | **B** A plus: Meals (one to three per day). Transportation. Activities. Housekeeping assistance. Assistance with coordination of community-based services | **C** A and B plus: Assistance with activities of daily living. Medication monitoring, 24-hr protective oversight | **D** A, B, and C plus: Medication administration, 24-hr nursing supervision |
| Mobility | Capable of moving about independently *OR* ambulatory with cane or walker Independent with wheelchair, but needs help in an emergency | Capable of moving about independently Able to seek and follow directions Able to evacuate independently in emergency *OR* ambulatory with cane or walker Independent with wheelchair, but needs help in an emergency | Mobile, but may require escort or assistance resulting from confusion, poor vision, weakness, or poor motivation *OR* requires occasional assistance to move about, but is usually independent | May require assistance with transfers from bed, chair, and toilet *OR* requires transfer and transport assistance Requires turning and positioning in bed and wheelchair |
| Nutrition | Able to prepare own meals; eats without assistance | Able to prepare own meals; eats without assistance. Generally, a minimum of one meal a day is available | All meals and snacks are provided. May require assistance getting to dining room or requires minimal assistance (opening cartons or other packages, cutting food, or preparing trays) | May be unable or unwilling to go to dining room. May be dependent on staff for eating or feeding needs *OR* may be fully dependent on staff for nourishment (includes reminders to eat) |
| Hygiene | Independent in all care, including bathing | Independent in all care, including bathing and personal laundry | May require assistance with bathing or hygiene *OR* may require assistance, initiation, structure, or reminders. Resident may be able to complete tasks | May be dependent on staff for all personal hygiene |
| Housekeeping | Independent in performing housekeeping functions (includes making bed, vacuuming, cleaning, and laundry) | Independent in performing housekeeping functions (includes making bed, vacuuming, cleaning, and laundry) *OR* may need assistance with heavy housekeeping, vacuuming, laundry, and linens | Housekeeping and laundry services provided | Housekeeping and laundry services provided |
| Dressing | Independent and dresses appropriately | Independent and dresses appropriately | May require occasional assistance with shoelaces, zippers, or medical appliances or garments *OR* may require reminders, initiation, or motivation | May be dependent on staff for dressing |
| Toileting | Independent and continent | Independent and completely continent *OR* may have incontinence, colostomy, or catheter, but independent in caring for self through proper use of supplies | Same as for retirement community *OR* may have occasional problem with incontinence, colostomy, or catheter and may require assistance in caring for self through proper use of supplies | May have problem with incontinence, colostomy, or catheter and requires assistance *OR* may be dependent and unable to communicate needs |

## TABLE 18.4  Long-Term Care Housing and Assessment Continuum—cont'd

| | Independent Living | Retirement Community | Assisted Living | Long-Term Care Facility |
|---|---|---|---|---|
| Medications | Responsible for self-administration of all medications | Responsible for self-administration of all medications OR may arrange for family or home health employer to establish a medication administration system | Able to self-administer medications OR facility staff may remind the person about or monitor the actual process OR facility staffed by registered nurses or licensed practical nurses who administer medications | Medications administered by staff personnel or self if assessed as capable |
| Mental status | Oriented to person, place, and time. Memory intact, but has occasional forgetfulness AND able to reason and plan and organize daily events. Mentally capable of identifying needs and meeting them | Oriented to person, place, and time AND memory is intact, but has occasional forgetfulness without consistent pattern of memory loss AND is able to reason and plan and organize daily events. Mentally capable of identifying environmental needs and meeting them | May require occasional direction or guidance in getting from place to place OR may have difficulty with occasional confusion that may result in anxiety, social withdrawal, or depression OR orientation to time or place or person may be impaired | Judgement can be poor and may attempt tasks that are not within capabilities OR may require strong orientation and reminder program. May need guidance in getting from place to place OR disoriented to time, place, and person OR memory is severely impaired |
| Behavioural status | Deals appropriately with emotions and uses available resources to cope with inner stress | Deals appropriately with emotions and uses available resources to cope with inner stress AND deals appropriately with other residents and staff OR may require periodic intervention from staff to resolve conflicts with others to cope with situational stress | May require periodic intervention from staff to facilitate expression of feelings to cope with inner stress OR may require periodic intervention from staff to resolve conflicts with others to cope with situational stress | May require regular intervention from staff to facilitate expression of feelings and to deal with periodic outbursts of anxiety or agitation OR maximal staff intervention is required to manage behaviour |

have policies to help with access to care 24 hours a day, 7 days a week, and that families and loved ones routinely end up carrying 25% of the cost of end-of-life care. Despite this, out of 2976 Canadian adults surveyed, 96% were in support of access to hospice and palliative care, highlighting this care as a priority for the individuals and families of those facing death.

Individuals in a hospice are empowered to live with dignity, alert, and free of pain. The goal of hospice care is to facilitate a "good death" for individuals. Families and loved ones are consistently engaged in caregiving for the dying and helping them maintain the highest possible quality of life. The hospice environment promotes quality of life within the context of differing cultural and spiritual values and beliefs. Nurses in all settings may identify and refer individuals for palliative or hospice care and facilitate use of these services to promote wellness during serious or terminal illness.

Older persons can be overwhelmed with the amount of advertising that is directed at them about such "necessities" as nutritional supplements, medications, hearing aids, alarms to use if they fall, phones, Internet sites, and digital devices. Nurses can help them sort out the confusion related to this advertising and direct them to reliable sources of information. CARP (formerly the Canadian Association of Retired Persons) is an advocacy group that provides many services to people older than 50 years, including excellent educational materials and community resources. Individuals can become members; it provides benefits such as access to discounts on health and lifestyle expenses, such as vision care or pharmacy

discounts. For the public, CARP offers tips and resources covering health, happiness, and safety for the older Canadian; for example, they share tips for financial and cyber security, retirement income security, and pension protection. CARP also participates in political advocacy to amplify the voice of the older population in Canada, with campaigns on issues such as the unaffordability of hydro bills for those living alone, increasing financial benefits for caregivers, and pension protection. All information is accessible on the CARP website, and topics are written in lay terms (easily understood language) and are printed in large print to accommodate vision changes. This self-help method is especially important for those who feel uncomfortable addressing questions on finances or sensitive health topics to nurses and other health care providers, as information is available directly to the older person.

Two additional environments of care emerged in the second half of the twentieth century: continuing care retirement communities (CCRCs) and assisted living facilities (ALFs). CCRCs are full-service communities offering long-term contracts that provide older persons with a continuum of care, extending from retirement services through assisted living to skilled nursing, all in one location. The mission behind CCRCs is "aging in place." CCRCs are expensive and require an entrance fee and a monthly payment. Residence in a CCRC requires commitment to a long-term contract that specifies the housing, services, and nursing care provided. ALFs are defined as homelike settings that promote resident autonomy, privacy, independence, dignity, and respect while providing necessary support. The lower cost of ALFs in comparison with skilled long-term care facilities and the greater emphasis on functional autonomy make these facilities appealing to older consumers and their families. Although residents of ALFs have many long-term health care needs, it is important to understand that the role and availability of nurses in these facilities differ greatly in each facility.

One additional social factor should be considered—that of age discrimination. Even today when many older persons are active contributors to society, they experience discrimination in seeking employment and in many other areas. Older persons have described situations where they seek medical care and, instead of health care providers speaking directly to them, they direct their inquiries to a family member who is present. Many of these older persons are highly educated, cognitively aware, and perfectly capable of implementing advice from health care providers to maintain their health. Getting old should not carry a stigma. Older persons are in a position to enrich the lives of others through the wealth of knowledge and experience that they have accumulated through the years.

### Diversity Awareness

Ethnocultural diversity will increase dramatically in Canada in the next decade alone, meaning our aging population will become more and more diverse. These changes in diversity bring unprecedented challenges to the health care delivery system. Challenges will continue to present themselves in the way that each culture perceives the status of the older person within society, the way health is maintained or improved, the causes and meanings of disease throughout life, and the ways in which disease and injury are managed from the cultural perspective versus how they are managed according to the health care system.

Nurses must be aware of the cultural diversity of older persons for whom they care and the cultural beliefs that influence health care decisions of older persons. Cultural humility efers to the ability of nurses to accept the cultural backgrounds of individuals and provide care that best meets the persons' needs, not the nurses' needs. To develop cultural humility the first step is to examine personal beliefs and the effect of these beliefs on professional behaviour. Nurses may best accomplish this by conducting personal cultural assessments. After identifying personal cultural biases that influence care, nurses must bracket these beliefs to make sure they do not affect delivery of care. It is important to remember that although an older person may be part of a cultural group, the individual may have become acculturated while living in Canada. A cultural history is therefore an essential first step in determining the person's health care beliefs and practices. When conducting cultural assessments, the nurse must remember that some of the standardized assessment tools, such as the Geriatric Depression Scale and the MMSE, are available in languages other than English. Caution must be taken in interpreting a tool that has not been formally translated, because the meanings of many words and phrases may not have an appropriate translation. The nurse must also be cautious when using assessment tools that have not been tested and validated with people of different cultures and nationalities. It is also essential to note that not all assessment materials are effective cross-culturally, which should be considered when choosing materials based on varying cultural belief systems.

Different cultures perceive health and wellness differently, making cultural awareness an essential part of patient-centred care.

The final stage in attaining cultural humility is to develop skills for working with culturally diverse populations. This entails the development of knowledge in working with culturally diverse populations and consistently using those skills with older persons. Conducting cultural assessments, using translation services, and providing culturally humble care are integral components to developing culturally safe and improving care.

### ◆ Levels of Policymaking and Health

This chapter has attempted to emphasize the need for health-promotion services for older persons. The PHAC has a Best Practices Portal to keep up to date on recent, empirically supported evidence-informed health-promotion practices. Nurses who do not work specifically in public health can benefit greatly from this information, as it can help anyone in need of credible resources and information to disseminate to patients.

Older persons continue to be able to choose their own health care provider. Preventive immunizations include those for influenza, pneumonia, and hepatitis B. Preventive screening examinations include those for diabetes, cholesterol and cardiovascular diseases, colorectal cancer, breast cancer, cervical cancer, and prostate cancer. Counselling services for smoking cessation and for medical nutrition therapy for those with diabetes or kidney disease are also available.

It is estimated that Canada spends approximately 11.5% of its gross domestic product (GDP) on health care, amounting to $6604 per Canadian resident (Canadian Institute for Health Information [CIHI], n.d.). Although this is in line with spending from other economically powerful countries (who also have medicare programs), there are many areas requiring improvement for better health care outcomes and affordability. Older persons in Canada require an average of $12,000 in health care spending annually, compared with $2700 for the rest of the population (Canadian Medical Association [CMA], 2018). As one ages, rising health expenditures can put older persons at risk of financial distress. On a more general note, in a study of 11 developed countries (United Kingdom, Australia, the Netherlands, New Zealand, Norway, Switzerland, Sweden, Germany, Canada, France, and the United States), Canada's health care system placed second to last based on average performance in care process, access, administrative efficiency, equity, and health care outcomes (Commonwealth Fund, 2016). The same study highlighted the following areas in need of improvement: one in five Canadians waited 7+ days for their last primary care appointment; one in three waited 3+ hours at their last visit to the emergency department; and one in two Canadians waited more than 4 weeks for their last appointment with a specialist. Aside from cost-related barriers to health care (primarily to medications, vision, dental, and forms of therapy such as physiotherapy or psychotherapy), these wait times are essential to recognize and understand as a health care provider. With these obstacles in mind, nurses continue to play a key role in promoting health not only to prevent illness and injury but also to prevent older persons from losing all their savings and becoming impoverished.

Nongovernmental organizations also influence policy decisions affecting older persons and health. Professional health care provider organizations, such as the Canadian Nurses Association, the Canadian Gerontological Nurses Association, and the CMA, conduct research to determine best practices in older persons care and to provide information to policymakers. CARP and the National Incentive for Care of the Elderly (NICE) are examples of two consumer organizations that gather information, fund research related to issues of older persons, and act as advocates for older persons in policymaking organizations.

### ◆ Health Services/Delivery Systems

Unfortunately, many people are not financially prepared for older adulthood. Although some individuals receive supplemental income from pensions or individual retirement accounts, many do not, and the amount of income from these sources is often very limited. Most older persons live on limited incomes. This can be especially troubling, as health care costs tend to increase with age. Programs such as the OAS pension and the Guaranteed Income Supplement (both previously discussed in this chapter) are available to supplement income, although these are not always sufficient to cover all necessary prescriptions and specialty services such as care in the community.

In Canada, basic medical and hospital care is provided through a universal health care system paid for through taxes. Each province and territory has its own health insurance plan. Individuals may get extra coverage through their workplace to pay for health care services that government plans don't fully cover such as prescription medications, dental care, and physiotherapy. Many older Canadians lose their extended health insurance benefits when they retire and may not be able to afford additional private insurance, and thus may struggle to meet routine and unexpected medical expenses. Completing advance directives, including naming a conservator in advance of illness, assists caregivers, health care providers, clergy, and the family in making difficult decisions at the end of life, when the affected person is no longer able to make them. The better prepared the older person is, the easier it is to receive appropriate care and treatment during times of illness. Reverse annuity mortgages are one option for increased income during the later years. A reverse annuity mortgage is obtained when a bank or private business purchases the home of an older person. The bank pays the person a set amount of money each month until the house is paid for in its entirety. The older person continues to live in the home. This approach provides the person with necessary funds and negates the need to move and sell the house if an illness arises. When the older person (mortgagee) dies, the bank or mortgager then owns the property.

Long-term care insurance is an option for those planning for the possibility of long-term care. As with other insurance programs, younger adults can purchase a policy, now widely available from insurance agents. A premium is paid each month that entitles the beneficiary to receive long-term care benefits at home, in an assisted living facility, in a day care facility, or in a long-term care facility. Older individuals are cautioned to explore the many options available for this type of insurance. The benefits and coverage differ, and exclusions are frequently written into the contract to prevent care in certain situations. An important feature of these policies is the option to hire a personal caregiver if the need arises.

The nurse who specializes in the care of older persons helps a great deal to promote their health and well-being through education, research, and practice. Educational curricula must be evaluated continually to ensure that content is appropriate and accurate with respect to aging. The quality of care depends on the clinician's knowledge base. Education for the older person is equally important and begins with an assessment of the individual's level of understanding of health-promotion activities.

Health-promotion and illness/injury-prevention research for this population is only beginning. Much more remains to be done in exploring the concepts of health promotion, relating these concepts, and developing and testing hypotheses. Research is needed to debunk commonly held beliefs, myths, and stereotypes about aging. Defining some of the concepts of health promotion, such as quality of life and functional ability, will yield immeasurable amounts of information that can be tested. Eventually, with the commitment of qualified nurses, health promotion will be respected for the integral role it plays in the quality of life of older persons.

## ❖ NURSING APPLICATION

Nurses in a position of providing care to older persons focus on promoting quality of life, promoting the health of the population, maintaining self-care, and preventing disease and its complications. Nursing activities with the older person often focus on the management of chronic conditions. While concentrating on healing, the nurse delivers care in a holistic manner that addresses the functional and psychosocial needs of the older person.

Nurses assist older persons by engaging them in health-promotion activities. Some of the major areas of focus are healthy weight and diet, activity, fall prevention and home safety, and medical appointments for screening. Pneumococcal and seasonal influenza immunizations are extremely important for the older person. Additionally, the older person is educated about cancer screenings and other screenings aimed at detecting diabetes, late-onset heart disease, osteoporosis, and hypertension. An effective method of ensuring that older persons participate in screenings is to coordinate health fairs in older persons' centres. The nurse is able to provide a common location where the older person can obtain vaccinations, necessary education, blood pressure checks, and fingerstick glucose monitoring. The nurse offers counselling, as needed, and refers the older person to a primary care provider for follow-up.

## ▌ SUMMARY

Life expectancy is now beyond 75 years for both men and women, with the fastest-growing age group being those older than 85 years. This phenomenon is indeed wonderful. However, as noted at the beginning of this chapter, aging is not for sissies.

The aging process causes physiological changes in many body functions, and older persons have a higher frequency of illness than the younger population. The many physical, emotional, and role changes of aging are complicated by the increased diversity in cultural and spiritual backgrounds. Older persons who have immigrated to Canada have brought with them different languages, values and beliefs, spiritual patterns, eating habits, and of course, views toward Western medicine. Culturally safe health-promotion services are therefore integral to helping older persons lead high-quality lives throughout their extended life spans.

Some of the dysfunctional aspects of aging have extrinsic causes, such as environmental pollution. Older persons are as susceptible as any age group to society's problems, such as homelessness, mistreatment, and drug and alcohol abuse. In conjunction with physiological and pathological changes, multiple acute and chronic diseases can result. Internal and public policy changes will continue to help older persons live in a world in which old age can be the most rewarding stage of life.

Many problems of old age are related to lifestyle. Changes in nutritional needs, sleep patterns, and activity level are required to adapt to normal and pathological processes. Psychological health depends on reassessing spirituality, self-concept, and role functions. Change and adaptation are possible. Aging healthfully is hard work, but with the assistance of nurses and other health care providers, older persons can be empowered to live their final years with a sense of peace in their life review of happy memories and accomplishments.

**Evolve Chapter Features**

http://evolve.elsevier.com/Canada/Edelman/healthpromotion/
- Review Questions

## CASE STUDY

### *Unsafe Driving: Perminder Dhaliwal*

Perminder Dhaliwal, a healthy 75-year-old man, lives in his own apartment and is completely independent in activities of daily living and instrumental activities of daily living. Last Friday morning, Perminder left his apartment complex at 8:00 a.m. to go to the store. While backing out of his driveway, he failed to see a school bus passing on the intersecting street, and his car struck the bus. Although no one was injured, this incident indicated the need for a sensory and neurological assessment. The assessment revealed both hearing and visual deficits.

**Reflective Questions**
- What would the nurse do to help with the results of the assessment?
- Should this person undergo further neuropsychological tests?
- How best can the nurse support this person during this difficult time in his life?
- In what ways might the family be helpful in this situation?

## CARE PLAN

### *Unsafe Driving: Perminder Dhaliwal*

**Nursing Issue**
Possible risk of injury related to unsafe driving

**Defining Characteristics**
- Altered response time
- Change in vision or hearing

**Related Factors**
- Past accident
- Stressful life events
- Receipt of traffic tickets
- Witnessed poor driving

**Expected Outcomes**
- Person will have realistic expectations of ability to drive.

- Person and nurse will set appropriate limitations on driving.
- Person will take a driver refresher course.
- Family will help to monitor driving competencies.
- Person will have no further accidents.

**Interventions**
- Assist Perminder in registering for a renewal driving program.
- Meet Perminder and a family member to discuss ways to ensure consistent safe driving.
- Assist Perminder in finding alternative modes of transportation until visual and hearing alterations are corrected and instead of driving in the evening.
- Schedule hearing and vision appointments for Perminder and assist in transportation to appointments.

# REFERENCES

Agronin, M. E. (2013). From Cicero to Cohen: Developmental theories of aging, from antiquity to the present. *The Gerontologist*, *54*(1), 30–39.

Alam, S., Lang, J. J., Drucker, A. M., et al. (2019). Assessment of the burden of diseases and injuries attributable to risk factors in Canada from 1990 to 2016: An analysis of the Global Burden of Disease Study. *Canadian Medical Association Journal Open*, *7*(1), E140.

Alzheimer's Society of Canada. (2016). *Dementia numbers in Canada*. Retrieved from https://alzheimer.ca/en/Home/About-dementia/What-is-dementia/Dementia-numbers#main-content.

American Geriatrics Society, Beers Criteria Update Expert Panel, Fick, D. M., et al. (2015). American Geriatrics Society 2015 updated beers criteria for potentially inappropriate medication use in older adults. *Journal of the American Geriatrics Society*, *63*(11), 2227–2246.

Bundy-Fazioli, K., Fruhauf, C. A., & Miller, J. L. (2013). Grandparents caregivers' perceptions of emotional stress and well-being. *Journal of Family Social Work*, *16*, 447–462.

Butler, R., & Olshansky, S. J. (2002). Has anybody ever died of old age? *The Gerontologist*, *42*(Special 1), 285–286. [Seminal Reference].

Canadian Association of Retired Persons (CARP). (2018). *Elder abuse*. Retrieved from http://www.carp.ca/2018/05/30/89-per-cent-say-government-must-address-elder-abuse-yet-hardly-registered-election/.

Canadian Automobile Association (CAA). (2019a). *Signs that driving skills are declining*. Retrieved from https://www.caa.ca/seniors/signs-that-driving-habits-should-change/.

Canadian Automobile Association (CAA). (2019b). *Refresher courses*. Retrieved from https://www.caa.ca/seniors/refresher-courses/.

Canadian Cancer Society. (2019). *Canadian cancer statistics: 2019*. Retrieved from https://www.cancer.ca/en/cancer-information/cancer-101/canadian-cancer-statistics-publication/?region=on.

Canadian Dental Association. (2019). *Dental care FAQs*. Retrieved from https://www.cda-adc.ca/en/oral_health/faqs/dental_care_faqs.asp.

Canadian Hospice Palliative Care Association (CHPCA). (2014). *Fact sheet: Hospice palliative care in Canada*. Retrieved from http://www.chpca.net/media/330558/Fact_Sheet_HPC_in_Canada%20Spring%202014%20Final.pdf.

Canadian Institute for Health Information (CIHI). (n.d.). *How much does Canada spend on health care?* Retrieved from https://www.cihi.ca/en/how-much-does-canada-spend-on-health-care-2017.

Canadian Medical Association (CMA). (2018). *Seniors' care*. Retrieved from https://www.cma.ca/seniors-care.

Canadian Psychological Association. (2015). *"Psychology works" fact sheet: Depression among seniors*. Retrieved from https://cpa.ca/docs/File/Publications/FactSheets/PsychologyWorksFactSheet_DepressionAmongSeniors.pdf.

Canadian Society for Exercise Physiology (CSEP). (2011). *Canadian physical activity guidelines*. Retrieved from https://www.csep.ca/CMFiles/Guidelines/CSEP_PAGuidelines_older-adults_en.pdf.

Canadian Task Force on Preventive Health Care. (2018). *Breast cancer update, 2018*. Retrieved from https://canadiantaskforce.ca/guidelines/published-guidelines/breast-cancer-update/.

Chaput, J. P., Wong, S. L., & Michaud, I. (2017). Duration and quality of sleep among Canadians aged 18 to 79. *Statistics Canada Health Reports*, *28*(9), 28–33.

Charles, C., Haaland, M., Kulkarni, A., et al. (2015). *Improving healthcare for LGBTQ populations*. Ottawa: Canadian Federation of Medical Students. Retrieved from https://www.cfms.org/files/position-papers/2015%20Improving%20Healthcare%20for%20LGBTQ%20Populations.pdf.

Chervin, R. D. (2015). *Approach to the patient with excessive daytime sleepiness*. Retrieved from http://www.uptodate.com/contents/approach-to-the-patient-with-excessive-daytime-sleepiness.

Chippendale, T., & Bear-Lehman, J. (2012). Effect of life review writing on depressive symptoms in older adults: A randomized controlled trial. *American Journal of Occupational Therapy*, *66*, 438–446.

Colpitts, E., & Gahagan, J. (2016). "I feel like I am surviving the health care system": Understanding LGBTQ health in Nova Scotia, Canada. *BMC Public Health*, *16*(1), 1005.

Commonwealth Fund. (2016). *2016 Commonwealth Fund International Health Policy survey of adults*. Retrieved from https://www.commonwealthfund.org/publications/surveys/2016/nov/2016-commonwealth-fund-international-health-policy-survey-adults.

Crawford, B. (2013). Pilates and the pelvic floor. *Advance Healthcare Network*, *24*(16), 25.

Erikson, E. H. (1982). *Life cycle completed: A review*. New York: W. W. Norton. [Seminal Reference].

Erikson, E. H. (1997). *The life cycle completed*. New York: W.W. Norton. [Seminal Reference].

Erikson, E. H., Erikson, J. H., & Kivnick, H. Q. (1986). *Vital involvement in old age: The experience of old age in our time*. New York: W.W. Norton. [Seminal Reference].

Esposito, L. (2016). Seniors and sexual health: What older adults should know. *U.S. News and World Report*. Health. Retrieved from http://health.usnews.com/health-news/patient-advice/articles/2016-03-16/seniors-and-sexual-health-what-older-adults-should-know.

Folstein, M. E., Folstein, S. E., & McHugh, P. (1975). "Mini-mental state." A practical method for grading the cognitive state of patients for the clinician. *Journal of Psychiatric Research*, *12*, 189–198. [Seminal Reference].

Freedman, A., & McDougall, L. (2019). Frailty 5 Checklist: Teaching primary care of frail older adults. *Canadian Family Physician*, *65*(1), 74.

Government of Canada. (2016). Elder abuse: It's time to face the reality. Retrieved from https://www.canada.ca/en/employment-social-development/campaigns/elder-abuse/reality.html#a.

Government of Ontario. (2019). *Exercise and falls prevention programs: How seniors can join free classes to help maintain balance and strength or prevent falls*. Retrieved from https://www.ontario.ca/page/exercise-and-falls-prevention-programs#section-3.

Haddad, N., Li, J. S., Totten, S., et al. (2018). HIV in Canada–surveillance report, 2017. *Canadian Communicable Disease Report*, *44*(12), 324–332. https://doi.org/10.14745/ccdr.v44i12a03.

Hajizadeh, M., Hu, M., Bombay, A., et al. (2018). Socioeconomic inequalities in health among Indigenous Peoples living off-reserve in Canada: Trends and determinants. *Health Policy*, *122*(8), 854–865. https://doi.org/10.1016/j.healthpol.2018.06.011.

Health Canada. (2018). *Flu: Influenza for health professionals*. Retrieved from https://www.canada.ca/en/public-health/services/diseases/flu-influenza/health-professionals.html#a5.

Health Canada. (2019a). *Healthy eating for seniors*. Retrieved from https://food-guide.canada.ca/en/tips-for-healthy-eating/seniors/.

Health Canada. (2019b). *Medical assistance in dying*. Retrieved from https://www.canada.ca/en/health-canada/services/medical-assistance-dying.html.

Health Canada. (2019c). *Influenza immunization in the past 12 months, by age group*. Retrieved from https://www150.statcan.gc.ca/t1/tbl1/en/tv.action?pid=1310009625.

Hodge, D., Bonifas, R., & Chou, R. (2010). Spirituality and older persons: Ethical guidelines to enhance service provision. *Advances in Social Work*, *11*, 1.

Hooyman, N., & Kiyak, H. (2011). *Social gerontology: A multidisciplinary perspective* (9th ed.). Boston, MA: Allyn & Bacon.

Khan, M., Kobayashi, K., Lee, S. M., et al. (2015). (In)Visible minorities in Canadian health data and research. *Population Change and Lifecourse Strategic Knowledge Cluster Discussion Paper Series, 3*(1), 5. Retrieved from https://ir.lib.uwo.ca/cgi/viewcontent.cgi?article=1013&context=pclc.

Lange-Chenier, H. (2013). Older Canadians at risk of undernourishment. *Canadian Medical Association Journal, 185*(10), E473. https://doi.org/10.1503/cmaj.109-4482.

Mayo Clinic. (2015a). *Kegel exercises: A how-to guide for women*. Retrieved from http://www.mayoclinic.org/healthy-lifestyle/womens-health/in-depth/kegel-exercises/art-20045283?pg=1.

Mayo Clinic. (2015b). *Kegel exercises for men: Understand the benefits*. Retrieved from http://www.mayoclinic.org/healthy-lifestyle/mens-health/in-depth/kegel-exercises-for-men/art-20045074.

Milan, A., Laflamme, N., & Wong, I. (2015). *Diversity of grandparents living with their grandchildren* (Catalogue no 75-006-X, no. 2015001). Ottawa: Statistics Canada.

Morgan, S. G., & Lee, A. (2017). Cost-related non-adherence to prescribed medicines among older adults: A cross-sectional analysis of a survey in 11 developed countries. *BMJ Open, 7*(1), e014287. https://doi.org/10.1136/bmjopen-2016-014287.

Morgan, S. G., Law, M., Daw, J. R., et al. (2015). Estimated cost of universal public coverage of prescription drugs in Canada. *Canadian Medical Association Journal, 187*(7), 491–497. https://doi.org/10.1503/cmaj.141564.

Mueller, C. M. (2015). Nutrition assessment in older adults. *Topics in Clinical Nutrition, 30*(1), 94–102. https://doi.org/10.1097/TIN.0000000000000022.

National Institute of Mental Health. (n.d.). *Older adults and depression*. Retrieved from https://www.nimh.nih.gov/health/publications/older-adults-and-depression/index.shtml.

National Institute of Neurological Disorders and Stroke. (2015). *Restless legs syndrome fact sheet*. Retrieved from http://www.ninds.nih.gov/disorders/restless_legs/detail_restless_legs.htm.

National Institute on Aging. (2011). *Biology of aging: Research today for a healthier tomorrow*. Retrieved from http://www.nia.nih.gov/sites/default/files/biology_of_aging.pdf.

Navaneelan, T. (2015). *Suicide rates: An overview* (Catalogue no. 82-624-X). Ottawa: Statistics Canada.

Nies, M. A., & McEwan, M. (2011). *Community/public health nursing: Promoting the health of populations* (6th ed.). Philadelphia: Saunders.

Paddock, C. (2012). *Fast cycling benefits Parkinson's patients. Medical News Today*. Retrieved from http://www.medicalnewstoday.com/articles/253197.php.

Pietrzykowska, N. B. (2016). Obesity in the elderly. *Obesity Action Coalition*. Retrieved from http://www.obesityaction.org/educational-resources/resource-articles-2/general-articles/obesity-in-the-elderly.

Praharaj, S. K., Gupta, R., & Gaur, N. (2018). Clinical practice guideline on management of sleep disorders in the elderly. *Indian Journal of Psychiatry, 60*(3), S383.

Public Health Agency of Canada (PHAC). (2006). *Healthy aging in Canada: A new vision, a vital investment*. Retrieved from http://www.phac-aspc.gc.ca/seniors-aines/alt-formats/pdf/publications/public/healthy-sante/vision/vision-eng.pdf.

Public Health Agency of Canada (PHAC). (2014). Seniors' falls in Canada: Second report. Retrieved from https://www.canada.ca/en/public-health/services/health-promotion/aging-seniors/publications/publications-general-public/seniors-falls-canada-second-report.html.

Public Health Agency of Canada (PHAC). (2015). *Questions & answers: Prevention of sexually transmitted and blood borne infections among older adults*. Retrieved from https://www.canada.ca/en/public-health/services/infectious-diseases/sexual-health-sexually-transmitted-infections/reports-publications/questions-answers-adults.html.

Public Health Agency of Canada (PHAC). (2016). *Suicide in Canada: Current context*. Retrieved from https://www.canada.ca/content/dam/canada/health-canada/migration/healthy-canadians/publications/healthy-living-vie-saine/suicide-canada-infographic/alt/infographic-infographique-eng.pdf.

Public Health Agency of Canada (PHAC). (2019). *Update on the use of pneumococcal vaccines in adults 65 years of age and older—A public health perspective*. Retrieved from https://www.canada.ca/en/public-health/services/publications/healthy-living/update-on-the-use-of-pneumococcal-vaccines-in-adult.html.

Registered Nurses' Association of Ontario (RNAO). (2017). *Preventing falls and reducing injury from falls* (4th ed.). Toronto: Author. Retrieved from. https://rnao.ca/sites/rnao-ca/files/bpg/FALL_PREVENTION_WEB_1207-17.pdf.

Rootman, I., & Gordon-El-Bihbety, D. (2008). *A vision for a health literate Canada: Report of the expert panel on health literacy*. Ottawa: Canadian Public Health Association. [Seminal Reference].

Rotermann, M., Sanmartin, C., Hennessy, D., et al. (2014). *Prescription medication use by Canadians aged 6 to 79* (Catalogue no 82-003-X). Ottawa: Statistics Canada.

Sacco, P., Kuerbis, A., Goge, N., et al. (2013). Help seeking for drug and alcohol problems among adults age 50 and older: A comparison of the NLAES and NESARC surveys. *Drug and Alcohol Dependence, 131*(1–2), 157–161. https://doi.org/10.1016/j.drugalcdep.2012.10.008.

Schroeck, J. L., Ford, J., Conway, E. L., et al. (2016). Review of safety and efficacy of sleep medicines in older adults. *Clinical Therapeutics, 38*(11), 2340–2372. https://doi.org/10.1016/j.clinthera.2016.09.010.

Shimizu, T., Bouchard, M., & Mavriplis, C. (2016). Update on age-appropriate preventive measures and screening for Canadian primary care providers. *Canadian Family Physician, 62*(2), 131–138.

Sinha, S. K., Griffin, B., Ringer, T., et al. (2016). *An evidence-informed national seniors' strategy for Canada* (2nd ed.). Toronto: Alliance for a National Seniors Strategy.

Smiraglia, C. (2015). Qualities of the participant experience in an object-based museum outreach program to retirement communities. *Educational Gerontology, 41*(3), 238–248.

Smyth, C. A. (2012). *The Pittsburgh Sleep Quality Index (PSQI)*. Retrieved from http://consultgerirn.org/uploads/File/trythis/try_this_6_1.pdf.

Sorrell, J. M. (2014). Postoperative cognitive dysfunction in older adults. A call for nursing involvement. *Journal of Psychosocial Nursing and Mental Health Services, 52*(11), 17–20. https://doi.org/10.3928/02793695-20141021-03.

Statistics Canada. (2013). *Participation rate in education, population aged 15 to 29, by age and type of institution attended, Canada, 1995/1996, 2000/2001, 2005/2006, and 2011/2012 to 2012/2013*. Ottawa: Author. Retrieved from https://www150.statcan.gc.ca/n1/pub/81-582-x/2014001/tbl/tble1.1-eng.htm.

Statistics Canada. (2015a). Number of persons aged 80 and over, observed (1921 to 2013) and projected (2014 to 2063), according to the low-growth (L), medium-growth (M1) and high-growth (H) scenarios, Canada. *Population projections for Canada, provinces, and territories* (Cat. no. 91-520-X). Retrieved from https://

www150.statcan.gc.ca/n1/pub/91-520-x/2014001/c-g/desc/desc2.11-eng.htm.

Statistics Canada. (2015b). Table 2.4: Selected age structure indicators, observed (1923 to 2013) and projected (2023 to 2063) according to the low-growth (L), medium-growth (M1) and high-growth (H) scenarios, Canada. *Population projections for Canada, provinces, and territories* (Cat. no. 91-520-X). Retrieved from https://www150.statcan.gc.ca/n1/pub/91-520-x/2014001/tbl/tbl2.4-eng.htm.

Statistics Canada. (2015c). *Family violence in Canada: A statistical profile, 2013* (Cat. No. 85-002-X). Ottawa: Canadian Centre for Justice Statistics.

Statistics Canada. (2016a). *Insights on Canadian Society: Living alone in Canada*. Ottawa: Author. Retrieved from https://www150.statcan.gc.ca/n1/pub/75-006-x/2019001/article/00003-eng.htm.

Statistics Canada. (2016b). *Number of centenarians, by sex, Canada, 2001 to 2061*. Ottawa: Author. Retrieved from https://www150.statcan.gc.ca/n1/pub/89-503-x/2015001/article/14316/c-g/c-g03-eng.htm.

Statistics Canada. (2016c). *Health fact sheets: Hearing loss of Canadians, 2012 to 2015*. Ottawa: Author. Retrieved from https://www150.statcan.gc.ca/n1/pub/82-625-x/2016001/article/14658-eng.htm.

Statistics Canada. (2017a). *Census in brief: Working seniors in Canada* (Cat. no. 98-200-X2016027). Ottawa: Author. Retrieved from https://www12.statcan.gc.ca/census-recensement/2016/as-sa/98-200-x/2016027/98-200-x2016027-eng.pdf.

Statistics Canada. (2017b). *Immigration and diversity: Population projections for Canada and its regions, 2011 to 2036* (Cat. no 91-551-X). Ottawa: Author. Retrieved from https://www150.statcan.gc.ca/n1/en/pub/91-551-x/91-551-x2017001-eng.pdf?st=iHuUXAny.

Statistics Canada. (2017c). *Physical activity, self-reported, adult, by age group*. Ottawa: Author. Retrieved from https://www150.statcan.gc.ca/t1/tbl1/en/tv.action?pid=1310009613&pickMembers%5B0%5D=1.1&pickMembers%5B1%5D=3.3.

Statistics Canada. (2017d). *Household population meeting/not meeting the Canadian physical activity guidelines*. Ottawa: Author. Retrieved from https://www150.statcan.gc.ca/t1/tbl1/en/tv.action?pid=1310038801.

Statistics Canada. (2018a). *Obesity in Canadian adults, 2016 and 2017*. (Data from Canadian Health Measures Survey). Ottawa: Author. Retrieved from https://www150.statcan.gc.ca/n1/pub/11-627-m/11-627-m2018033-eng.htm.

Statistics Canada. (2018b). *Health fact sheets: Sleep apnea in Canada, 2016 and 2017*. Ottawa: Author. Retrieved from https://www150.statcan.gc.ca/n1/pub/82-625-x/2018001/article/54979-eng.htm.

Statistics Canada. (2019a). *Canadian income survey, 2017*. Ottawa: Author. Retrieved from https://www150.statcan.gc.ca/n1/daily-quotidien/190226/dq190226b-eng.htm.

Statistics Canada. (2019b). *Leading causes of death, total population, by age group*. Ottawa: Author. Retrieved from https://www150.statcan.gc.ca/t1/tbl1/en/tv.action?pid=1310039401.

Statistics Canada. (2019c). *Canada's population estimates: Age and sex. The Daily*, January 25. Retrieved from https://www150.statcan.gc.ca/n1/daily-quotidien/190125/dq190125a-eng.htm.

Touhy, T., & Jett, K. (2012). *Toward healthy aging: Human needs & nursing response* (8th ed.). St. Louis: Mosby.

Transport Canada. (2019). *Canadian motor vehicle traffic collision statistics: 2017*. Ottawa: Author. Retrieved from http://www.tc.gc.ca/eng/motorvehiclesafety/canadian-motor-vehicle-traffic-collision-statistics-2017.html.

Tyler, S., Corvin, J., McNab, P., et al. (2014). "You can't get a side of willpower": Nutritional supports and barriers in The Villages, Florida. *Journal of Nutrition in Gerontology and Geriatrics, 33*, 108–125.

Vance, D. (2013). The cognitive consequences of stigma, social withdrawal, and depression in adults aging with HIV. *Journal of Psychosocial Nursing and Mental Health Services, 51*(5), 18–20. https://doi.org/10.3928/02793695-20130315-01.

Vanderkamp, J. (1984). University enrollment in Canada 1951-83 and beyond. *Canadian Journal of Higher Education, 14*(2), 49–62. [Seminal Reference].

Voight, K., Gottschall, M., Köberlein-Neu, J., et al. (2016). Why do family doctors prescribe potentially inappropriate medication to elderly patients? *BMC Family Practice, 17*(1), 93. https://doi.org/10.1186/s12875-016-0482-3.

Wang, Y. P., & Andrade, L. H. (2013). Epidemiology of alcohol and drug use in the elderly. *Current Opinion in Psychiatry, 26*(4), 343–348. https://doi.org/10.1097/YCO.0b013e328360eafd.

World Health Organization (WHO). (2006). *Defining sexual health: Report of a technical consultation on sexual health, 28–31 January 2002*. Geneva. Retrieved from https://www.who.int/reproductivehealth/publications/sexual_health/defining_sh/en/.

Yesavage, J., Brink, T. L., Rose, T. L., et al. (1983). Development and validation of a geriatric depression screening scale: A preliminary report. *Journal of Psychiatric Research, 17*, 37–49. [Seminal Reference].

Yellowlees, P. M. (2015). *The value of the Mini-Mental State Exam*. Retrieved from http://www.medscape.com/viewarticle/844603.

Yoo, R., & Spencer, M. (2018). Continence promotion and successful aging: The role of the multidisciplinary continence clinic. *Geriatrics, 3*(4), 91. https://doi.org/10.3390/geriatrics3040091.

# 19

# Screening

*Shannon Dames, MPH, EdD, and Alexa Garrey, RN*

Originating US chapter by *Elizabeth Connelly Kudzma, CNL, MPH, WHNP-BC, DNSc*

## INTENDED LEARNING OUTCOMES

*After completing this chapter, the reader will be able to:*
- Discuss screening and its role in secondary prevention and health promotion.
- Analyze criteria to determine if a disease has evidence-informed guidelines for screening.
- Identify health care, economic, and ethical implications related to the screening process.

- Discuss how collaborative community and national partnerships and policies assist in the development and implementation of a screening program.
- Describe elements of the nursing role in the screening process.

## KEY TERMS

Asymptomatic pathogenesis
Community assessment
Community resources
Cost–benefit ratio analysis
Cost-effectiveness analysis
Cost-efficiency analysis
Disability-adjusted life year (DALY)
Efficacy
Efficiency
Epidemiology
False negative test results
False positive test results
Group or mass screening
Iatrogenic
Incidence
Individual screening
Interobserver reliability
Interprofessional education
Intraobserver reliability
Key community individuals

Lead agency
Morbidity
Mortality
Multiple test screening
One-test disease-specific screening
Point-of-care testing (POCT)
Prevalence
Quality-adjusted life year (QALY)
Quality of life
Quantity of life
Racial and Ethnic Approaches to Community Health
Reliability
Secondary prevention
Sensitivity
Significance
Specificity
Stakeholders
Target community
Validity

## ? THINK ABOUT IT

### Screening Then and Today

In the 1920s, educators started to investigate the concepts of intelligence quotient, lower intelligence, and mental handicaps. Intelligence categories were separated numerically, and "cretin" became a medical term used to describe a lower level of intelligence. Neonatal hypothyroidism (cretinism) was more common in mountainous inland areas away from sea salt sources of iodine. It is very rare in the modern world because of the required screening of all infants at birth (blood tests measure levels of thyroid-stimulating hormone and thyroxine). Screening testing of mothers during pregnancy and of infants shortly after birth with dried blood spot (DBS) technology allows treatment and lifetime monitoring before the serious signs of thyroxine deficiency occur. This disorder and others (e.g., phenylketonuria [PKU]) are health screenings' modern success stories. Neonatal hypothyroidism has virtually disappeared in the developed world as a result of the screening of babies (target population) followed by appropriate treatment for affected individuals. However, the storage and research use of DBS technology raises significant controversy over lack of parental knowledge and consent for research activities. Regulations vary greatly from province to province. For example, in British Colombia, parents are presented with the opportunity to request the sample be destroyed, whereas Ontario has no official policy and procedure (Canadian Agency for Drugs and Technologies in Health [CADTH], 2011).

Very recently, biotechnology companies have developed tests that aim to screen an individual's DNA for genes associated with diseases or population subgroups (Nickolich, Farahi, Jones, et al., 2016). DNA testing examines a person's genetic code to provide information about genealogy or ancestry that may be helpful in assessing a person's risk of disease. Personalized DNA testing kits are available to help consumers discover their risks of developing disorders (such as Alzheimer's disease, diabetes, and breast cancer). An over-the-counter home test for human immunodeficiency virus (HIV) was approved by the US Food and Drug Administration and was marketed to consumers in 2012. Although this product is not approved for sale in Canada, it may be purchased online. The availability of screening options that may be novel, but unproven, raises new questions about media information provided to the public, the politics involved (Lin & Gostin, 2016), and the reliability and validity of screening methods and associated necessary counselling.

- Why has the newborn period been identified as an important time to require screening tests?
- Each government regulates a list of mandated screening for newborns. Do you know what your government/province/ministry of health requires?
- The availability and feasibility of screening tests is constantly changing. How are new screening tests evaluated and added to the mandated requirements?
- What characteristics of screening tests have to be considered for neonates? What characteristics of screening tests have to be considered for individuals of any age?
- How is the margin of error further defined for screening tests/instruments?
- What aspects of screening program development should nurses participate in: assessment, data analysis, implementation, evaluation of health outcomes?

Evidence-informed preventive services *are effective in reducing death and disability, and are cost-effective or even cost-saving. Preventive services consist of screening tests, counselling, immunizations, or medications used to prevent disease, detect health problems early, or provide people with the information they need to make good decisions about their health. While preventive services are traditionally delivered in clinical settings, some can be delivered within communities, work sites, schools, residential treatment centres, or homes (National Prevention Council, 2011, p. 18).*

Clinical and community preventive services are vital to health promotion and disease prevention. Most adults are not up to date on the core set of clinical preventive services recommended at various ages, and the proportion of older people who are current with their screening or are unwilling to be screened diminishes as more screening strategies are added (Bynum, Davis, Green, et al., 2012; Davis, Bynum, Katz, et al., 2012). Screening is an important component of clinical preventive services because it is a valuable tool for health care providers to identify chronic conditions and risk factors before the condition becomes costly both in financial terms and for quality of life. This is particularly important as the health care paradigm shifts from medical and volume-based to a health-promotion and value-based model of care. Although health education about screening is categorized as part of the rubric of primary prevention, the actual process of screening is part of secondary prevention.

The primary goal of screening is to detect risk factors and a condition early, to prevent or treat it, and to deter its progression. An important assumption underlying the use of screening is that detection early in the asymptomatic period allows treatment at a time when the eventual course of the disease can

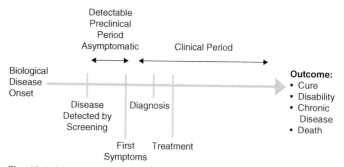

**Fig. 19.1** Screening Periods

be altered significantly. (see Box 19.1) Similarly, identifying risk factors assists in identifying the populations needing screening and focuses attention on needed behaviour change before disease develops. Screening strategies are based on the principle that the selected disease is preceded by a period of asymptomatic pathogenesis or latency (disease development before symptoms first appear) when risk factors predisposing a person to the disease are building toward full manifestation of the disease (Fig. 19.1). Screening takes advantage of the prepathogenic state and the early pathogenic state—identifying risks relating to disease in the earliest and most treatable stages.

Screening strategies are essential to the core of the health-promotion metaphor—the upstream/downstream narrative. When health care providers are so preoccupied with managing the acute care (ill/dying) of the drowning downstream, they have little time to focus on why individuals become ill and fall into the river upstream. Screening tests focus attention on going upstream to the source to better identify valid determinants of health status. Identification of valid health status measures involves accurate screening tests.

At the time this textbook was written, a global pandemic emerged from a novel coronavirus (COVID-19). While Canada's screening strategies will continue to evolve, in the first few months there was a twofold approach to screening for COVID-19: (1) the self-screener, and (2) a nasopharyngeal swab. The self-screener is an online tool that asks a series of symptom-related questions. Depending on how the questions are answered, the user is then provided with recommendations on how best to proceed. Those who fit the criteria for clinical screening are then provided with instructions to contact local screening service providers.

As the global pandemic unfolds, the complexity and importance of screening has become increasingly apparent. Widescale screening efforts are providing invaluable insights into the virus and its spread. Countries with the most proactive screening methods are proving to have better control of the spread. This demonstrates how screening and data collection are imperative to tracking and controlling novel and highly contagious diseases.

Widescale screening may be the most prudent approach to monitor and prevent the spread of disease. However, many countries are limited in their screening capacity due to supply and personnel shortages. This is a common issue with many screening initiatives, which is why many end up on wait lists for a variety of common screening procedures such as colonoscopies and mammograms. COVID-19 reminds us that despite the challenges of screening, it is imperative to track and prevent the development and spread of disease.

Administration of screening tests, some of which might be fairly simple and relatively inexpensive when compared with the burden of disease, provides value in improved quality of care and decreased health care costs. Screening is not generally a diagnostic measure, nor is it curative. It is a preliminary step to identify (upstream) individuals who need more diagnostic workup to prevent further development of the condition or disease and to ameliorate adverse disease outcomes. More importantly, it is a step toward empowering individuals to make more informed choices about their health and health behaviours. A second, but equally important, objective of screening is to reduce the costs of managing the disease by avoiding more intensive interventions required in later disease stages. A cost-conscious approach to health care mandates that health care providers, at all levels, acquire a basic understanding of the screening process and its application. Unfortunately, upstream screening and the application of screening processes involves complicated decision making, and is entangled with social policy, communication and media information, and personal choice.

## ADVANTAGES AND DISADVANTAGES OF SCREENING

### Advantages

Some screenings are very simple and performed at home (blood pressure, heart rate, weight, and oxygen saturation), and nurses are involved in promoting their use and educating people about their use. This chapter, however, will focus more on the efficacy and efficiency of clinical, procedural, and laboratory-based tests. Screening tests offer several advantages. Although some screening procedures are simple and relatively inexpensive, others are expensive and may not be cost-effective. The simplicity

of some screening procedures decreases the time and cost of the health care personnel involved, especially when compared with the cost of treating the disease after symptoms appear, and enables less skilled technicians to administer the test.

A second advantage is the ability to apply the screening process to both individuals and larger populations. In an individual screening program, one person is tested by a health care provider who has selected the individual as high risk (such as prior hypertension). The practitioner can make this decision independently; the health care agency can define a specific policy; or legislative bodies can require the screening by law, as in the case of HIV screening for refugee and immigration applicants (Bisaillon, 2011).

HIV is a contagious virus that can be spread through contact with infected blood, pre-ejaculate, semen, and vaginal fluid. The virus attacks the body's CD4 cells, leaving the infected person with a weakened immune system. If left untreated, the person's immune system depletes and acquired immunodeficiency syndrome (AIDS) may develop. At this stage of the disease process, the affected person is highly susceptible to opportunistic infections. When HIV and AIDS first emerged in the 1980s, there was no known cure or treatment and it was considered a "death sentence." With the advent of antiretroviral therapy this is no longer the case. HIV-positive people who follow strict adherence to their medical treatment are able to live full lives to nearly full life expectancy (CATIE, 2018).

The Canadian *Immigration and Refugee Protection Act* does not explicitly deny entry to applicants who are HIV positive; however, in "Section 33: Inadmissibility," the government maintains the right to refuse entry to those who "might reasonably be expected to cause excessive demand on health or social services" (Government of Canada, 2001).

Group or mass screening occurs when a target population is selected on the basis of an increased incidence of a condition or a recognized element of high risk within an identified group. For example, the target population may be invited to a central location on a designated day to be tested for the selected disorders (elevated levels of lipids and cholesterol, hypertension, osteoporosis, elevated blood glucose level).

A third advantage is the ability to provide one-test disease-specific screening or multiple test screenings. A one-test disease-specific screening is the administration of a single test that searches for a characteristic that indicates a high risk of developing a disorder. An example of this would be blood pressure screening to evaluate hypertension (Yoon, Fryar, & Carroll, 2015). Multiple test screening is the administration of two or more tests to detect more than one disease. In some cases, one sample can be used to evaluate an individual for several conditions, saving time and money and making the process efficient and economical. For example, a blood sample can be assessed for a number of components, including glucose and cholesterol levels. The combination of the relatively low-cost screening test and flexibility makes screenings adaptable to all levels within the health care delivery system. Other multiple test screenings of importance are for substance abuse, mental health disorders and depression, and sexually transmitted infections (STIs).

A final advantage of screening is that it creates an opportunity for providing health education to a group of individuals who may not otherwise receive it. In some situations, it is possible to establish a clinical relationship during the screening process that leads to preventive visits and includes educating people about healthy lifestyles, risk reduction, developmental needs, activities of daily living, and preventive self-care. Individual behaviours are one of the contributors to today's chronic illnesses. This makes awareness one of the first steps in prevention. If better awareness is combined with health-education and health-promotion tools, individuals have a better opportunity to manage their own risks. Taking advantage of a potential health-promotion teachable moment should never be overlooked.

The commonly recommended 6-month dental screening is an example. Although the individual is at the dentist's office to be screened for cavities and to have teeth cleaned to avoid gum disease, the hygienist provides education and reminders on the correct way and the necessity to brush and floss teeth correctly, and a check is provided for oral cancer. Another example is in the recommended counselling for tobacco cessation—ask, advise, assist, arrange (Registered Nurses Association of Ontario [RNAO], 2017). It is not enough to simply screen an individual with the question, "Do you use tobacco?" Readiness to quit should also be determined and combined with cessation treatment assistance (Government of Canada, 2009). Nurses who are familiar with community resources can then refer individuals to smoking cessation programs that fit with the person's preferences and values.

## Disadvantages

The primary disadvantages of screening stem largely from uncertainties in scientific evidence, which sets normal testing ranges and therefore also ranges of error for screening tests. When effectiveness depends on the screening program's ability to distinguish those who probably have the disease from those who do not, any margin of error can result in serious consequences. Some individuals who do not have the condition will be referred for further tests, and some who do have the disease will not get needed referrals. Those incorrectly referred (false positive) suffer needless anxiety and unnecessary medical interventions, some of which can be harmful, while awaiting more definitive diagnosis (e.g., high levels of prostate-specific antigen [PSA]). False positive osteoporosis screening results can lead to unnecessary bone building medication treatment that may have side effects. Some noninvasive prenatal strategies test for very rare disorders, so the predictive value may be questioned (Nickolich et al., 2016; Vora & O'Brien, 2014). Mammography screening for breast microcalcifications identifies a significant number of women (who may be false positives) who later undergo medically invasive breast biopsies. Women with false positive results bear the burden of the follow-up visits, time off work, and long-term psychological consequences (Brodersen & Siersma, 2013) to determine whether the disease is actually present.

The effects on those whose diseases have been overlooked (false negative) are even more important. For example, Canada's current two-tier method of testing for Lyme disease is vulnerable to false negatives (Lloyd & Hawkins, 2018). These individuals have a false assurance of health that is shattered when the illness becomes obvious. They lose the opportunity to receive earlier treatment that could prevent irreversible damage. The difficulty of balancing the benefits to some against the burdens to others may be an ethical issue underlying many screening programs. The significance of this disadvantage can vary; therefore, it should be assessed for each screening program, disease, and population.

## SELECTION OF A SCREENED DISEASE

The selection of a screened disease goes beyond examination of any disease alone. The selection process must also encompass less-tangible factors, such as the emotional impact (HIV infection) (Nayak, Roberts, & Greenspan, 2011) of the disease's detection on the screened population. Even after data have been gathered and the critical issues have been reviewed, the final decision of whether to screen individuals must often be reached with incomplete evidence or with answers that raise ethical issues, on an epidemiological and a personal level.

The potential uncertainties confounding the decision to screen individuals emphasize the need to conduct an analysis of available material to obtain a decision that is as objective and scientific as possible. Answers to the following questions may provide a basis for determining whether a disease is screenable:

- Does the significance of the disorder warrant its consideration as a community problem?
- Can the disease be detected by screening?
- Should screening for the disease be done?
- What are the health benefits? For example, can it be treated?

As simplistic as these questions may appear, the answers or lack of answers, in addition to individual preferences, may expose complex issues that determine whether a well-informed decision can be made on screening.

### Significance of the Disease for Screening

According to the Centers for Disease Control and Prevention (CDC), epidemiology is the method used to find the causes of health outcomes and diseases in populations. In epidemiology, the patient is the community and individuals are viewed collectively. By definition, epidemiology is the study (scientific, systematic, and data driven) of the distribution (frequency, pattern) and determinants (causes, risk factors) of health-related states and events (not just diseases) in specified populations (neighbourhood, school, city, province, country, global) (CDC, 2015)

Health information on both morbidity and mortality may be used to identify the most important diseases affecting populations. The term morbidity refers to a diseased state or disability from any cause; however, the view of morbidity can be broader, including a range or degree of the illness that affects the person. Mortality statistics (deaths) in a given population can be easier to use as end-outcome indices, as long as statistical collection measures are accurate.

The significance of a disease refers to the level of priority assigned to the disease as a public health concern. Although the opinions of political and public interest groups may influence this evaluation, significance is generally determined by incidence and prevalence, and by the quantity (severity) and quality of life affected by the disorder (CDC, 2012). The media may also have a role in defining a public health problem that should be screened for, or addressed, as the media provides a place for compelling storytelling about the impact of disease and potential screening (Dorfman & Krasnow, 2014). In a time where rates of adherence to vaccinations have dropped off, the resurgence of measles is a prime example of how the media is able to alert the general population and provide mass information on how to keep Canadians and their families safe.

Key factors in assessing the need for screening criteria are quantifying measures of disease frequency. The two measures most used in epidemiology are incidence and prevalence (CDC, 2012; Lundy & Janes, 2014). Incidence indicates the rate of a new population problem and estimates the risk of an individual developing a disease or condition during a specific period or over a lifetime. Prevalence is the proportion of a given population with the disease or condition at any one point in time. It provides the best estimate of whether a person is likely to become ill during a specific period. In short, incidence is new cases, and prevalence is all cases within a set period of time. Chronic conditions are usually measured by their prevalence (generally existing), whereas acute conditions are assessed by their incidence (rate of new occurrences). Both are used in assessing the need for community services and screenings, and help develop the criteria for evidence-informed practice screening guidelines that include the age at which screening should be performed, the frequency and manner of screening, and the person who should perform the screening. The greater the physical and psychological harm experienced by the population, the greater is the urgency to designate the condition/disease as a priority health problem. A first step in assessing screening feasibility is evaluation of disease significance to decide if the disorder warrants the time, effort, and financial resources that must be allocated. For example, there has been a significant decline in the incidence of late-stage colorectal cancer in Canada since 2000, and this is attributed to increased rates of screening (Canadian Cancer Society, Statistics Canada, & Public Health Agency of Canada [PHAC], 2017).

Estimating the quality of life affected by a disease presents problems but is also a necessary step. The perception of quality of life is subjective, and individual evaluations may differ. For example, not all people equally perceive the disability resulting from a disease; some may make adjustments and cope, whereas others do not. Those who do not may be more likely to say that the quality of their lives is significantly lower than that of other people.

Two epidemiological measures are used to estimate quality of life. A quality-adjusted life year (QALY) is a measurement of quality of life. It is defined as perfect health minus the disability-adjusted life year (DALY). The QALY assumes that 1 year of excellent health is 1 QALY (1 year of life × 1 utility value = 1 QALY). It also assumes that 1 year spent in a less perfect state of health or with disease (or comorbidities) is worth less. A determination of the QALY value involves multiplication of the utility value associated with a state of health by the number of years lived in that state of health. Following this thinking, half a year lived in excellent health is 0.5 QALY (0.5 year of life × 1 utility

value), which is the same as 1 full year of life lived in a disease state (1 year × 0.5 utility value). A disease state that halves utility value includes those diseases that cause significant challenges to the point where they limit mobility or result in persistent pain, extreme fatigue, etc.

A second measure, the disability-adjusted life year (DALY), refers to 1 year spent in less than healthy life. It is a measure of the burden of disease, and measures the gap between the current health status and excellent health status. It also accounts for life lost and life quality diminished through disability. The QALY and DALY measures may both be used, depending on whether the outcome of the screening measure is intended to maximize health or minimize disability (Airoldi & Morton, 2009; Costello, 2014).

There is currently greater focus on quantifying measurements of health outcomes so as to weigh the costs of screening, treatment, and effects on populations. The QALY incorporates morbidity and mortality in a single arithmetic measure. It allows computation, estimation, and comparisons of screening decisions. However, the estimation of formulas association with utility and disability is difficult. QALYs assist in analyzing the gap between strict treatment decisions and their economic costs, informing public health decision making (Costello, 2014).

By contrast, measures of the quantity of life affected by the disease are more readily obtainable. In addition to prevalence and incidence rates, disease-specific mortality rates present different aspects of the disease for analysis. Disease-specific mortality may be linked to the severity of an incident occurring or the long-time health burden cost associated with management of the disease. There is some evidence that mandatory screening of athletes reduces the incidence of sudden cardiac death in athletes who are supposedly young and fit; the cost of comprehensive cardiac screening is high and controversial (Anderson, Grenier, Edwards, et al., 2014; Shephard, 2011); a death in a young athletically fit person is a very untoward, severe event. With other diseases, the prevalence of the disorder may not be high, but the problem requires disproportionate amounts spent on maintenance or management after the condition is fully expressed. For PKU, a case undetected at birth means a lifetime of suboptimal development and neurological disease management.

## Detection

With the relative significance of the disease established, the next step is to determine if health professionals can screen individuals for the disease. Are there well-documented diagnostic criteria for the disorder? Is there a valid and reliable screening instrument? Are sufficient community resources and treatment modalities available to support a screening program?

### Diagnostic Criteria

Detection of a disease requires knowledge of the characteristics that indicate its presence or, as in screening, its early pathogenic, asymptomatic state, and is often based on risk factors such as heredity, age, sex, and family history. For example, screening tests may be recommended for men or women (Canadian Task Force on Preventive Health Care [CTFPHC], 2017). Selected

**BOX 19.2 Point-of-Care Testing and Hepatitis C**

Point-of-care testing (POCT) is a diagnostic test performed outside of a clinical setting; in Canada, this type of testing is most commonly performed by nurses. This is a type of low-barrier health care. The results of POCT are often instant and, thus, create the opportunity for treatment to begin sooner. However, this resource also comes with its challenges. At the moment there is no national standard with regard to POCT and laboratory accreditation, training is not widely regulated, and reporting mechanisms need to be improved. Through the work of stakeholders, however, these issues can be addressed (CADTH, 2017).

In 2017, Health Canada approved the use of OraQuick HCV POCT for hepatitis C. This test does not provide definitive proof of disease, but detects whether the person has been exposed to the virus in the past. To confirm a diagnosis, a laboratory blood test must then be done. Studies done have shown that many people who are at risk for hepatitis C report not being tested due to lack of time or access to the test, lack of knowledge of disease and risk factors, and lack of culturally safe care. POCT removes some of these barriers and creates the opportunity for health care providers to open up a conversation and increase awareness (Fish, 2017).

disease diagnostic criteria should be well documented and defined and not merely accepted as commonly used indicators. The impact of uncertainty in detecting disease is amplified when the application of the screening design is considered. Some diseases, such as sickle cell anemia or PKU, are defined by the presence or absence of a single, isolated gene or enzyme. Other conditions, such as high blood glucose levels (diabetes), are measured according to numerical values for which a normal range has been set. Although there may be some disagreements over normal parameters, diabetes is a serious disease, and early treatment has been shown to decrease the incidence of morbidity and death attributable to vascular diseases and stroke.

## Screening Measures

The next step is to determine if methods exist to detect the disease during an early stage. If screening measures are available, an analysis should determine if any of them fulfill the requirements for the screening process: available, easy to administer, safe with minimal discomfort, cost-effective, and accurate. Ultimately the decision to use a screening test will depend on how well the measure can distinguish those individuals who probably do not have and will not develop the condition from those who are likely to develop the condition. The variables that aid in a screening instrument's evaluation include reliability, validity, and reproducibility, which are a measure of the accuracy of the instrument.

Reliability is an assessment of the reproducibility of the test's results when different individuals with the same level of skill perform the test during different periods and under different conditions. The instrument or measure should yield consistent or stable results over time. If the same result emerges when two individuals perform the test, interobserver reliability is shown. If the same individual is able to reproduce the results several times, intraobserver reliability is demonstrated.

From this information, health professionals can determine the amount of training required for health care providers, technicians, or personnel who administer the test. For example, if

interobserver reliability is low, additional training might be required to work toward a more consistent method of screening test delivery. This is frequently necessary in blood pressure cuff hypertension screening (Ringrose, Millay, Babwick, et al., 2015) or in weight measurements, where the scale may not function properly. If intraobserver reliability is low, the health professional might surmise that the instrument, and not the individual, is at fault. Some screening measures are of necessity more qualitative, and intraobserver reliability may be very important in the case of substance abuse or mental health/depression screening. Finally, for a screening test to be valid, which is the next requirement, it must first be reliable, but reliability is only a necessary condition and is not entirely sufficient for validity.

Validity reflects the accuracy or truthfulness of the test or instrument itself. In a controlled setting, one evaluates validity by testing the instrument on a group of individuals who have positive or negative results. A valid test correctly distinguishes individuals who have preclinical disease from those without preclinical disease. The ideal result is to have the instrument identify 100% of the diseased individuals (positive reactions) and 100% of the nondiseased individuals (negative reactions).

There are also ranges of measurement for disease reliability and validity. Perfectly accurate categorization of validity rarely occurs in practice. Therefore, the measure of validity has been divided into two components that quantify the margin of error in screening instruments. Sensitivity measures the first component. This refers to the proportion of people with a condition who correctly test positive when screened. If a test has good sensitivity, the number of individuals with the disease who are missed through inaccurate categorization as false negatives will decrease. Conversely, a test with poor sensitivity will overlook individuals with the condition, and there will be a large number of false negative test results: individuals who actually have the condition but were told they are disease-free or tested negative for the disease.

Specificity is the second component. Specificity measures the test's ability to recognize negative reactions or individuals in whom disease is absent. A test with excellent specificity will rarely produce a positive result if the disease is not present. A test with poor specificity could result in false positive test results. Individuals with false positive test results are told that they have a disease or condition when in actuality they do not. Specific epidemiological formulas are used to measure both sensitivity and specificity.

Ideally, tests should be highly sensitive and highly specific; however, this is usually not the case, and some balance is reached between the two concepts. For some tests, there may also be an indeterminate zone in which the individual does not test strictly negative or positive. In these tests, the numerical cut-off may be subject to interpretation or a more arbitrary decision. A cut-off decision may be made so that the screening instrument is less likely to miss actual cases of disease at the cost of erroneously identifying cases of disease (false positives) that will need more diagnostic work, which may be expensive and invasive.

Consider the issues that a public health nurse faces when using a newly developed screening test with low specificity and moderate sensitivity. Low specificity means few true negative test results and more false positive test results. This is the current situation with mammography screening. The nurse and other health professionals (also health advocacy groups, such as those involved in breast cancer awareness) must then consider the cost, inconvenience, and psychological stress experienced by the people with false positive results during the period after their incorrect screening test, the unnecessary additional referrals, and the ability of the existing follow-up services to meet these needs. With only moderate sensitivity, a number of false negative results could occur, which may ignore individuals who could benefit from treatment. Medical, economic, political, and ethical issues are involved; that is, should a screening program be implemented when it is known that the tests may involve avoidable harms such as additional biopsies and excessive treatment.

A broader issue concerns large health fair screening programs and point-of-care testing (POCT; Box 19.2); for example, where a targeted population such as older persons is sought for a mass screening. The efficiency and efficacy of such programs must be analyzed. The following are examples of questions that address efficiency and efficacy: Is the targeted population prepared in an appropriate way before engaging in the screening tests? Are the health care practitioners who are administering the test educated (and certified) according to the standard protocols of test administration? Are follow-up measures and appropriate referral access instituted in the program? There are times when an older person lacks the cognitive ability or physical independence to follow-up on positive screening results. Patients and health care providers may overestimate the benefits and underestimate the harm of screening and associated treatment (Hoffmann & Del Mar, 2015). Answers to these questions challenge health care providers in the development, implementation, and follow-up processes identified so that screening efficiency and efficacy is enhanced.

Very recently, a number of for-profit genomic and biotechnology companies have marketed genetic tests to identify genes and ancestry associated with risk factors and diseases. A number are available on the Internet. One of the leading companies providing this service reports that its DNA analysis can provide information on about 100 health disorders and traits, including carrier risk, medication response, and disease risk (e.g., Parkinson's disease, cholesterol levels, presence of diabetes). Noninvasive prenatal tests are currently marketed to identify neonatal chromosomal abnormalities, including Down syndrome, very early in gestation with a simple blood test (Nickolich et al., 2016); these tests are less invasive than amniocentesis, but positive test results require confirmation by amniocentesis. These tests are becoming common and dramatically less expensive. The advent of these at-home tests offers the opportunity for people to become more involved and take control of their health, but may also come at a cost to their privacy (Office of the Privacy Commissioner of Canada, 2017).

Consumer-available tests can involve issues of standardization, cost, and privacy, and failure to make reports fully explainable or understandable. Comprehensive research on screening tests significantly influences the efficacy of the entire process. Data on the reliability and validity of individual tests and screening programs in general provides valuable information to evaluate, anticipate, and ideally control these influences, enabling the program to work effectively toward its established goal and positive health care outcomes.

## Primary Care and Community Screening Resources

Screening is often done in an outpatient primary care setting. Implementing a screening program depends on availability of appropriate community resources, such as funds, health care workers, and follow-up services, including access, referrals, treatment sources, and administrative personnel. Nurses can provide structure and design for screening programs as seamless organization of a program is essential to success. Knowledge of a disease's characteristics and an effective screening instrument are useless without financial and organized human support to use them. Many screening programs are of necessity complex, requiring intense efforts in the area of partner development.

A lead agency or group may be identified to oversee the development of the community health program. The origins of the lead agency range from a community service organization to local public health departments responding to regulations or a mandate at the provincial or federal level. Regardless of its origin, the agency must perform a self-evaluation to compare its level of expertise with what is required to supervise the process of the screening effort. Early identification of the lead agency, along with potential partnerships, allows the effective use of talents and the division of labour.

For the lead agency to develop and oversee the development of any community health program, such as the delivery of a screening program, partnerships and coalitions are essential. The agency must contact and organize necessary stakeholders. Stakeholders are individuals or groups who have a legitimate interest in the topic. Examples of stakeholders include key community individuals; hospitals; health and social service agencies, such as primary health care centres; and community organizations, including houses of worship, community centres, schools, transportation agencies, and volunteer organizations. Key community individuals are those people who are considered leaders within the community. The primary rule is to never assume that what is appropriate and effective for one community will be appropriate and effective for another.

Stakeholders and partners, along with nurses, perform the community assessment together. A community assessment is a systematic method of data collection that provides a detailed account, first identifying need and subsequently determining the type, quantity, and quality of resources. Review of demographic, vital statistics, and morbidity and mortality data may identify the assessed need. Resources might come from an eclectic variety of support sources, including government entities such as public health departments, social services, and even safety and transportation in the case of car seat safety screenings. Schools, private businesses, churches, and places of social gatherings might provide resource support, either in screening support or in the actual administration of the screening.

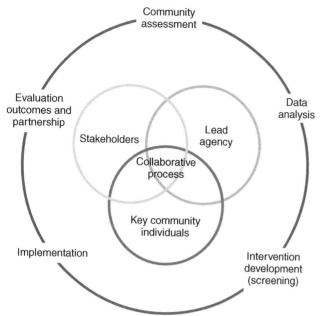

Community
assessment

Evaluation
outcomes and
partnership

Data
analysis

Stakeholders

Lead
agency

Collaborative
process

Key community
individuals

Implementation

Intervention
development
(screening)

**Fig. 19.2** Collaborative Partnership: Community Health Program Development

After the assessment has been completed, the data analysis will reveal the target community or high-risk population, the available health care resources, and the health needs of the high-risk population. The identified partners collaborate, review, and analyze the data, leading to the development of health-improvement strategies (in this case a screening program), with methods of implementation to move the target population smoothly through the screening process. Finally, monitoring and evaluating outcomes is essential to determine the effectiveness of the program and the achievement of stated goals. Evaluation includes monitoring of the entire process, including the successful workings of the partnership. Fig. 19.2 presents a model of collaborative partnership: community health program development. Population health nursing is an important component of the partnership.

The constraints affecting the operation of a screening program include financial concerns, political issues, cultural constraints, follow-up and referral services, and accessible treatment facilities. All partners are aware that responses from the target community are affected partly by their experience with other screening programs, such as the means used to inform them, the accessibility of the location, the availability of transportation, the convenience of the program's hours, and the cultural safety of the delivery and design of the program. A public health nursing approach identifies the necessary community resources and defines how these resources interact and may be mobilized to achieve maximal benefits and positive outcomes. Financial support of a screening program is a constraint that can influence all points in the system. Although some programs are delivered entirely on a voluntary basis, organizers of others must submit grant proposals to local, provincial/territorial, or federal departments when consideration of medical and economic ethics is involved.

Planners must look beyond the screening day and investigate financial resources for follow-up care and treatment.

In addition to financial accessibility, follow-up services need to be accessible in terms of convenient locations and open hours. For example, an evening clinic may reach those who are reluctant or financially unable to miss work. Nurse practitioner clinics facilitate access to preventive health services at convenient times for various population groups. An efficient referral system links the follow-up resources to the screening program, providing continuity of care. A method must be devised to encourage the participant to take positive action on the referral. Public health nurses will facilitate this process with a variety of communication techniques, such as emails, telephone or in-person counselling, mailings, and home visits.

Another example is that a college of health sciences organizes a health fair which includes screening. This also creates opportunities for interprofessional education and practice (Uden-Holman, Curry, & Benz, 2015). Nursing students and medical students manage physical assessments and laboratory screenings. Pharmacists screen individuals for medical use of inappropriate or contraindicated medications. Social workers may assess individuals for mental health issues. There is a plan for continuation of care if disease issues and risks are identified: for example, individuals needing immediate referrals for hypertension control. In this instance the college may agree to assist in referrals to providers who will donate time to assist in this effort.

## Should Screening for the Disease Be Done?

After it has been determined that the disease is significant and can be screened for, establishing whether health professionals should do so is the final step. Screening for a particular disorder and ultimately treating those with the early-identified disorder improve the chances of a favourable outcome in comparison with those whose disorder is not found until signs and symptoms become evident. Therefore, several questions must be considered. If a test accurately identifies a condition in the early stages, is there any benefit to the individual? Are there effective treatment modalities for the condition? The Canadian Task Force on Preventive Health Care may recommend against routine screening (CTFPHC, 2014). In 2014, the CTFPHC recommended against PSA screening for prostate cancer because the balance of harms from early treatment (urinary incontinence, bowel control, erectile dysfunction) outweighed the benefits of early diagnosis. As noted before, recommendations for mammography screening have changed several times within the last decade because of high rates of false positive test results, overdiagnosis, too many normal/benign biopsy specimens, and overtreatment (Kidd & Colbert, 2015; Lin & Gostin, 2016; Thompson, Eklund, & Esserman, 2015). A woman with microcalcifications found on mammography may have to undergo an open or core biopsy to determine if cancer cells are truly present; this may involve several days' absence from work or having to find child care.

It is necessary for the health care provider to remain aware of changes in screening guidelines. Screening is based on the disease's asymptomatic period. Therefore, adequate information must exist concerning the optimal time for screening, specific intervention during this time, and knowledge regarding the effect of early detection and treatment on the prognosis. Without this knowledge, health care providers are unable to explain how the outcomes of those with early detected disease differ from those with undetected disease, and they cannot support the health benefits derived from the screening program.

Follow-up is critical to determine if the intervention strategies prescribed are in fact happening. Should screening be done if there is no follow-up in terms of medical or social services? A prescribed follow-up regimen may be very broad and include a wide variety of intervention strategies, such as diet, exercise, and medication therapy. Follow-up services may include an evaluation and review of the literature that discusses evidence-informed practice pertaining to a particular medication, as well as the identification of intervention characteristics that impair follow-up, such as cost, inconvenience, or side effects. Consideration must also be given to those factors that enhance follow-up. For example, nurses can provide ongoing counselling and education about a medication and assist individuals in lifestyle transformations that include health-promoting behaviours.

The safety of a potential intervention is a concern when the widespread application of further medical interventions or invasive diagnostic tests after a screening program is considered. Risks or harmful side effects can be costly in terms of human health and the increased medical care required to correct iatrogenic or interventional effects (e.g., additional surgical procedures or emotional distress). As an example, Georgia, who is aged 54 years and has a low risk of breast cancer, attends a community clinic and wants more information about the optimal interval between breast cancer screenings. She found some discrepancies between recommendations from the Canadian Cancer Society, the CTFPHC, and other trusted health resources. The nurse, using an evidence-informed practice model, helps Georgia to find or review the most recent and best sources of information that would answer her question (Mandelblatt, Stout, Schechter, et al., 2016). In addition to the scientific literature, the nurse locates consumer information for Georgia. In this case the nurse would assist women to make informed health choices about screening tests.

The bottom line is that to be effective, a high-quality, cost-effective, research/evidence-informed screening tool or technique is needed that identifies a real or potential "problem." Screening must provide real and workable "solutions," in which the tangible and intangible costs of the screening are less than the risk of the disease and result in measurable health benefits.

## ETHICAL CONSIDERATIONS

Improving health is considered a just and moral act integral to values endorsed throughout the health care system. Screening activities are separate from interventions offered for established disease (e.g., myocardial infarction). Rather than treating those who have established disease, a screening program invites seemingly well individuals to be tested to determine their disease risk and the need for follow-up. This request for voluntary participation implies an expectation of a health benefit, although at this stage nothing is said about what it will be, the cost, or what the participant must do to obtain it. Screening programs need to clarify expectations and inform participants as contingent issues occur. Screening participants need to know whether the ultimate benefit is preventive, ameliorative, or curative, and what responsibility they assume to secure this outcome.

### Borderline Cases and Cut-off Points

A screening program measurement is often based on a numerical value, so a question often arises about the use of cut-off points for the screening instrument and borderline cases. The goal of a screening program, identifying an individual as having high risk or not having high risk, depends on this numerical value. When the clinical parameters are not clear, a cut-off point is used. Above this point, the person is considered to be disease positive; below this point, the individual is disease negative. Consequently, readjusting the cut-off point can become a highly controversial issue, as the cut-off point controls the percentage of positive and negative results. If the disease were potentially life-threatening, even though there is a high risk of false positive results with a lower cut-off point/threshold, keeping it low is still preferred to missing individuals who may have the disease. In addition, if a disease is relatively benign in terms of potential stigmatization, anxiety, and problems with treatment, lowering the cut-off point could again be safe and ethical.

Examples of problems related to identifying cut-off points and borderline cases are common in community nursing practice. Hypertension is a common disease in which a variance of 5 to 10 mm Hg can make the difference in identifying a person as having high risk of hypertension. Lipid and cholesterol level cut-offs and ratios are always subject to further examination. Recommendations change as new evidence emerges. Sophisticated approaches may discriminate between borderline cases that should be referred and ones that should not. Nurses can assist in identifying other risk factors associated with hypertension or lipid-level evaluation, such as family history, diet, and smoking, as criteria for deciding whether to refer an individual. An updated literature review is imperative before these issues are reviewed in relation to a particular screenable disease.

### Economic Costs and Ethics

In the past, the tendency was to disregard the cost of promoting a healthy, disease-free, or disease-controlled status; this results in a philosophical stand that all care should be given to all individuals at all costs. There is now a fuller recognition of the enormous costs that could be involved with many screening programs. Allocating community funds to a large screening event may result in a lack of funds for other projects.

Populations benefiting from a screening test will be balanced by those suffering in terms of decreases in service for other medical or social needs.

The initial operational costs must be considered, including buying or renting screening equipment, floor space, and engaging professionals or technicians to administer the tests and interpret the results. These costs are encountered a second time when individuals are referred for further evaluation. Patient costs include time and income that are lost. Given the combined operational and patient costs, questions are raised:

- Do the costs result in improved health outcomes?
- Are the benefits worth the expenditures required?

The answers are influenced partly by the values (other than monetary ones) attributed to the benefit. Saving lives in a young population may be judged more valuable than screening older populations with more chronic illnesses. A strictly economic approach, however, may eliminate the intangible variables and require the use of more objective data for decision making.

When program designs are reviewed, three main approaches may be used to evaluate the economic resources affected: cost–benefit ratio, cost-effectiveness, and cost-efficiency analyses. The current relevance and use of such concepts require a basic understanding of their role in the selection of a condition for screening. They tend to be separate methods and most frequently are used independently of one another.

### Cost–Benefit Ratio

Cost–benefit ratio analysis is performed first, because it allows the comparison of various outcomes in monetary terms. This comparison is necessary in health planning when the initial consideration is dependent on whether the expected health outcome (such as reduction in the incidences of cardiovascular disease, decrease in infant mortality, or reduction of the detection of a visual problem) will be most beneficial to the community at the most reasonable cost. The cost of the screening versus the cost of long-term care management may be weighed. For example, what is the cost–benefit ratio of blood pressure screenings, compared with the medical and financial cost of a stroke caused by undiagnosed hypertension, to the individual, the community, and the health care system? The cost of screening is weighed against other factors, such as the cost and feasibility of vaccination programs, as in the case of screening individuals for human papilloma virus for cervical cancer (Maine, Hurlburt, & Greeson, 2011).

### Cost Effectiveness

If the reduction of cardiovascular disease is chosen as the desired outcome, the next step is a cost-effectiveness analysis, which determines the optimal use of resources to reach a predetermined, constant end-point or the desired health outcome. The screening benefit remains the same; the best method of getting to the target outcome is the focus of the investigation. For example, for reduction of cardiovascular disease, various methods might be used. These methods include screening

**RESEARCH FOR EVIDENCE-INFORMED PRACTICE**

**The Registered Nurses Association of Ontario's Nursing Best Practice Guidelines Program**

In 1999, the Registered Nurses Association of Ontario (RNAO) received funding from the Ontario government to create the *Nursing Best Practice Guidelines* Program. The program proved to be a success and continues to grow. Today there are 50 research-backed guidelines that cover five areas of practice: Gerontology, Primary Health Care, Home Health Care, Mental Health Care, and Emergency Care (Canadian Nurses Association, 2019). Every 3 years, each guideline is reassessed by a team of experts who make changes or confirm that the guideline is still up to date and in line with the most current research and recommendations. The RNAO offers a toolkit to aid nurses in implementing these guidelines into their practice.

An example of one of RNAO's guidelines is the *Engaging Clients Who Use Substances* guideline. The 118-page document offers health care providers with up-to-date, research-informed information to help them better care for their patients who have substance use issues. The guideline introduces the topic at a novice level and builds up in complexity from there. It weaves in the social determinants of health, stages of change, harm reduction, and trauma-informed care.

The *Nursing Best Practice Guidelines* are a comprehensive tool that provide nurses and other health care providers with the opportunity to carry out evidence-informed practice.

Source: Registered Nurses Association of Ontario (RNAO). (n.d.). *Nursing Best Practice Guidelines*. Retrieved from https://rnao.ca/bpg.

individuals for hypertension and cholesterol, performing electrocardiograms on all individuals aged 25 years or older who are admitted to the hospital, screening young athletes for cardiovascular disease, sponsoring an antismoking campaign, or providing nutrition counselling. Implementation of all these options would be ideal, but with limited resources some choices are made.

### Cost Efficiency

The last approach to help bring the economic resources into perspective is cost-efficiency analysis. The purpose is to be efficient and budget a limited amount of money toward achieving as much of the desired outcome as possible. The funds are the focus, not the health benefit.

## SELECTION OF SCREENABLE POPULATIONS

The selection of a screenable population is as important as the selection of a screenable disease and is often based on incidence and prevalence data. The objective is to identify a high-risk group that, when tested, will yield a significant number of diseased individuals. With a well-planned selection approach, the efforts and cost of screening the population are minimized and the health benefit is maximized. The main criterion used to define an appropriate population is the definitive presence of risk factors related to the disorder. Within community settings, nurses can ensure a thorough examination of possible risk factors, including both person-dependent and environment-dependent factors (Research for Evidence-Informed Practice).

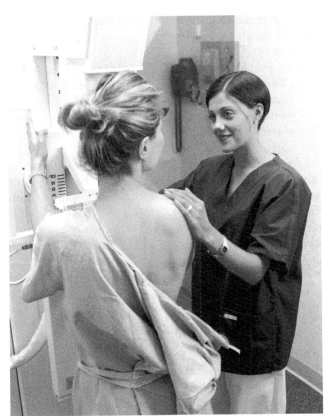

Fig. 19.3 Mammography Screening (Courtesy John Foxx; from Stockbyte/Thinkstock.)

## Person-Dependent Factors

The person's age is important because of age-dependent changes in the levels of risk factors throughout the population. For example, the risk of many cancers increases as a person grows older (Weir, Thompson, Soman, et al., 2015). A high priority is placed on screening vulnerable populations, especially women, infants, and children, as the outcomes obtained affect long-range growth and development patterns. As the average life span increases, however, the effects of risk factors in young adults and middle-aged adults are becoming more apparent, making certain prevalent and costly chronic conditions equally important to control. The middle-aged adult population may be screened for hypertension, diabetes, breast cancer, glaucoma, and heart disease; this population is requiring earlier screening, as some of these disease conditions are becoming apparent in early adulthood and even teenage years. Older people may be screened for cognitive decline, although screening for the asymptomatic older person is controversial because of lack of effective dementia treatment. Routine genetic screening for various biomarkers, such as β-amyloid peptide, β$_2$-microglobulin and tau proteins, amyloid plaques, and *APOE-e4* is under investigation (Alzheimer Society of Canada, 2018; Sutphen, Jasielec, Shah, et al., 2015).

Gender has obvious implications for screening programs. For example, women are tested frequently for two reproductive-related conditions: breast cancer and cervical cancer (Fig. 19.3). Screening a population from a particular ethnic or racial group is appropriate, as some disorders occur more frequently in certain racial or ethnic groups. On a national and provincial level, Statistics Canada, the Canadian Cancer Agency, and provincial cancer health authorities all do not account for ethnicity in their statistics. It is possible to find some Canadian-specific research on certain cancer rates relating to ethnicity. For example, a health report completed in 2018 suggests that female immigrants of East or Southeast Asian descent are at a higher risk of developing thyroid cancer (Bushnik & Evans, 2018). Using existing statistics of breast cancer rates in Ontario and applying a surname algorithm, one study posits that women from South Asian descent are diagnosed at a later stage and women of Chinese descent at an earlier stage than the general population (Ginsburg, Fischer, Shah, et al., 2015). However, the fact that health authorities and organizations generally do not account for ethnicity in their statistics makes it difficult for nurses to lobby and advocate for specific groups to have more targeted screenings, particularly in communities that have large numbers of ethnic or racial minority women (Diversity Awareness).

Health inequalities disproportionality affect Canadians who live below the poverty line (Mikkonen & Raphael, 2010). The World Health Organization has outlined a list of economic and social factors which greatly influence health and health inequalities. They are known as the social determinants of health (SDH) and are as follows (Canadian Public Health Association [CPHA], n.d.):

- Income and income distribution
- Food insecurity
- Disability
- Indigenous status
- Housing
- Early childhood development
- Education
- Unemployment and job security
- Employment and working conditions
- Social exclusion
- Social safety network
- Health services
- Gender
- Race

Many of the SDH are affected by an individual's socioeconomic status, either directly or indirectly, and affect the individual's behaviour (CPHA, n.d.).

Personal behavioural characteristics related to lifestyle may suggest the need to screen a particular individual or group. When health care practitioners review lifestyle, they are looking at daily habits that affect health and wellness, such as nutrition, fitness level, tobacco use, alcohol and drug use, sexual practices (HIV), stress management, adequate rest, immunizations, periodic examinations, use of seat belts, and other safety factors. Engaging in some of these behaviours while avoiding others is essential for living a healthy life. Therefore, screening for personal behavioural characteristics that are considered risky assesses the likelihood of a longer, disease-free life. Once screening recommends elimination of risky behaviours, the development of healthy behaviours via programming and transformation of lifestyles is crucial. Health care providers have a responsibility to educate and empower individuals about

## 🌐 DIVERSITY AWARENESS

### *Eliminating Health Inequities Among Ethnically Diverse Groups*

Diversity is acknowledged as a strength of Canada, but it is apparent that inequities exist among the various racial and ethnic groups in the attainment and maintenance of health. The minority populations of Canada include, but are not limited to, First Nations, Chinese, East Indian, Inuit, Black Canadians, Japanese, and South Asians. These categories oversimplify the reality of the multicultural nature of assessing health status, screening, and making plans to improve health. These particular racial groupings are not absolute, because there are subgroups within each.

Inequities and factors such as access to care need to be taken into consideration when screening programs are being planned. To plan, implement, and evaluate a screening program that targets a specific population, the provider must have an awareness of the target population that includes components such as lifestyle, socioeconomic characteristics, education, heredity, environmental factors, values, religious and cultural beliefs, communication style, and language. Partnering with key individuals and organizations in the community through the entire process is important for any screening program to be successful, as the following scenario illustrates.

Hospital administrators in a town located outside a city in the Pacific Northwest are concerned about the health status of a new immigrant population. Recent census data indicate that the number of immigrants from Syria has grown. The census data also reveal that this population is primarily young adults and children under 14 years of age. The officials of the town and the hospital are aware that many of the refugees will not have immunization records and, due to exposure to trauma, may require psychosocial supports.

On the basis of this data, the hospital officials decide to plan a health and screening day for this population. The hospital distributes flyers in the community in the primary native language of the target population. The day of the screening arrives, and the number of participants is very low. The hospital officials are very concerned. They had good intentions. They do not know what to do next.

#### Reflective Questions

- What critical actions did the hospital officials perform that might be considered positive in the planning of the health and screening day?
- What critical actions did the hospital officials not perform that might have contributed to the poor turnout at the health and screening function?
- What might the hospital officials consider in their planning for the next health and screening day?
- How might they engage the community and the target population in planning the health and screening day?
- What local community agencies and groups might be invited to participate as partners when the health and screening day is being planned and implemented?
- Can you identify any creative ways to bring the health and screening day to the targeted population, making the program more accessible?

the next step in the evaluation of their potential condition once screening has been completed. Those being screened have a responsibility to seek treatment and follow-up services, and ultimately engage in behavioural change toward a healthy lifestyle if the screening is to serve a purpose.

Regional inequities exist and include many of the previously mentioned inequities. These are of great concern, but identifying the causes is complex. Research is being done on interrelationships between the determinants of health, to include biology and genetics, individual behaviours, the social environment, the physical environment, and health services (access and quality).

Many people who engage in high-risk behaviours—which can lead to a variety of health issues—have experienced trauma. By implementing upstream programs into our health care system, we have the opportunity to mitigate exposure to potentially preventable trauma. One such program has been created with help from the Public Health Agency of Canada (PHAC). The Women's Resource Centre and Sexual Assault Services Association in Antigonish, Nova Scotia, has been given funding to carry out their Healthy Relationship for Youth Initiative. This program provides the opportunity for teenagers who live in rural, Mi'Kmaq, and African Nova Scotian communities to learn about dating violence and the complicated factors that play a part in it. This local initiative is a part of Canada's larger strategy to prevent and address gender-based violence and the mental and physical health consequences that are borne from the issue (PHAC, 2019).

## Environment-Dependent Factors

The area of environmental health and protection has expanded over the years and is becoming more complex. Environmental health and protection has been defined as the science that is concerned with elements of the environment that influence people's health and well-being. These factors include conditions of the workplace, home, and communities, including chemical, physical, and psychological forces (Allender, Rector, & Warner, 2014). Environment-related risk factors relevant to screening designs are associated with an individual's surroundings. Areas that may be considered include overpopulation; indoor and outdoor air pollution; water pollution; safe drinking water; noise pollution; radiation exposure; biological pollutants; hazardous waste management and disposal of garbage; vector and pesticide control; deforestation, wetlands destruction and desertification; energy depletion; inadequate housing; contaminated food and foods with toxic additives; safety in the home, at the work site, and in the community; and psychological hazards (Allender et al., 2014; Roelofs, Shoemaker, Skogstrom, et al., 2010).

In occupational health, a legitimate population for screening includes those in high-risk work areas, where harmful chemicals, airborne particles, or high-decibel machinery puts the workers at risk of cancer, respiratory conditions, or auditory problems. At the other extreme is the sedentary executive work life, where the lack of exercise is prevalent, placing the worker at risk of obesity and obesity-related conditions such as diabetes. The use of an occupational health nurse to provide individual and mass screening for such problems, in addition to routinely recommended screening, is recognized as integral in promoting better business practices.

## National Guidance and Health Care Reform

### Screening for Type 2 Diabetes in the Canadian Indigenous Population

The prevalence of type 2 diabetes (DM2) in Canada is growing. The Canadian Indigenous population sees rates of this disease

## BOX 19.3 Important Considerations in Screening for Type 2 Diabetes in the Canadian Indigenous Population

- Recognizing the continuing effects of colonization, which include but are not limited to: distrust of the medical system, intergenerational trauma, socioeconomic inequities, and limited access to health resources
- Creating culturally appropriate initiatives by working with community leaders and stakeholders
- Building local capacity to create and implement future programs to empower communities and individuals, which can also ensure better adherence through better understanding of the disease and the importance of screening
- Screening adults with a family history of the disease over the age of 18, regardless of the presence of symptoms
- Providing proper point-of-care training for local health care providers to increase the availability of screening in rural and/or remote communities
- Creating high-quality education programs which focus on the content of the material and the medium or mediums of dissemination; considering print materials, visual aids, and storytelling as possible options
- Increasing the proportion of elementary, middle, and senior high schools that provide school health education to promote personal health and wellness in the following areas: nutrition; signs and symptoms; historical and genetic factors; and the importance of health screenings and checkups
- Increasing the proportion of children with a diagnosed condition identified through screening between 6 weeks and 6 months who have an annual assessment of services needed and received
- Increasing depression screening by primary care providers, as depression has been linked to the disease
- Providing sustainable funding to ensure that efforts are not lost and can continue

Sources: Halseth, R. (2019). *The prevalence of Type 2 diabetes among First Nations and considerations for prevention.* Prince George, BC: National Collaborating Centre for Aboriginal Health; Diabetes Canada Clinical Practice Guidelines Expert Committee. (2018). Diabetes Canada 2018 Clinical Practice Guidelines for the Prevention and Management of Diabetes in Canada. *Canadian Journal of Diabetes, 42*(Suppl 1), S1–S325.

## BOX 19.4 Preventive Services for Older Persons (Examples)

- Abdominal Aortic Aneurysm (2017)
- Breast Cancer (2011)
- Breast Cancer Update (2018)
- Cervical Cancer (2013)
- Cognitive Impairment (2015)
- Colorectal Cancer (2016)
- Diabetes, Type 2 (2012)
- Hepatitis C (2017)
- Hypertension (2012)
- Impaired Vision (2018)

## BOX 19.5 Guidelines for Children (Examples)

- Developmental Delay
- Obesity
- Tobacco Use
- Vision Impairments
- Hearing Impairments
- Newborn Screening Tests (tests vary by province):
  - Galactosemia test
  - Hearing tests
  - Phenylketonuria (PKU) screen
  - Sickle cell disease test
  - Thyroid hormone tests (for congenital hypothyroidism)

### INNOVATIVE PRACTICE

#### Informatics, Technology, and Newborn Screening

Health information technology will allow health care to better assess and manage quality health care with the streamlining of efficient and effective information. Access to digital medical records allows the sharing of results and follow-up findings between clinicians, testing laboratories, and health delivery providers.

- How does access to newborn electronic screening results benefit the clinician? How does it benefit the person seeking care? How does it benefit public health?
- Where else do you think health care could benefit from similar abilities?
- What do you think is necessary for this to happen (think about differences in data collection requirements)?

continued to implement screening programs which work to level out this disparity, with varying levels of success. Box 19.3 examines what has been done and how these programs can better work to serve our Indigenous communities.

### The Canadian Task Force on Preventive Health Care

The Public Health Agency of Canada (PHAC) developed the Canadian Task Force on Preventive Health Care (CTFPHC) to support primary care providers in delivering preventive health care. Their screening recommendations evolve as new scientific evidence becomes available, so this chapter will not provide specific details on the recommended screenings. Boxes 19.4 and 19.5 list examples of screening services for older persons and children (CTFPHC, 2019; HealthlinkBC, 2019). For a brief look at how evolving technology may enhance health care delivery, see the Innovative Practice box. See Quality and Safety Scenario for an example of a health-promotion model.

In 2010, the PHAC started the CTFPHC to ensure primary care providers are able to carry out research-informed preventive care. The Task Force has created guidelines for many health topics, including but not limited to, breast cancer, cognitive impairment, hypertension, and obesity. Knowledge translation is an important part of the Task Force's role. Each guideline is accompanied by educational tools intended for both clinicians and patients. These tools include videos,

that are disproportionately higher. DM2 is, in fact, on the rise globally among Indigenous children (Dean & Sellers, 2015). The reasons for this health inequality are complex and are related to the population's history of colonization (Diabetes Canada Clinical Practice Guidelines Expert Committee, 2018; Halseth, 2019). Over the last 20 years, the government of Canada has algorithms, and FAQ sheets. By creating tools that are accessible and comprehensible to patients, the CTFPHC empowers individuals to make informed choices about their health and well-being (CTFPHC, 2019). Fig. 19.4 is an example of one of the CTFPHC's patient algorithm tools.

## THE NURSE'S ROLE

As one of the important stakeholders (Institute of Medicine, 2011), nurses play a role in every aspect of the screening program development process, including assessment, data analysis, planning, implementation, evaluation of the health outcomes, and evaluation of the process (including the workings of the partnership; see Fig. 19.2). One aspect of this health process is the development and implementation of screening programs for targeted groups. As nurses use higher decision-making skills based on advancing education and expertise (Institute of Medicine, 2011), they will face questions such as "Should this condition be screened for or not?" In the role of decision maker and planner, the nurse is responsible for reviewing all issues concerned with screening individuals for an appropriate disease, including the criteria specific to the disease, the medical and economic ethics, and the community resources that are affected. If the choice is to screen individuals, the participation of nurses and other partnering groups is essential in the development of a care plan. The last step integral to the nursing role is the planning and development of an efficient referral system to enhance continuity of care and to ensure follow-up.

Because some preventive care services are provided through extended health care coverage, the nurse collaborates with other health providers to ensure that preventive services, along with the required education and counselling, are available through primary care or community services such as a primary care clinic, a person-centred medical home, or a community health centre or even at the work site. These services may include:

- Blood pressure, diabetes, and cholesterol tests
- Cancer screenings, including mammograms and colonoscopies
- Counselling on topics such as quitting smoking, losing weight, eating healthily, treating depression, and reducing alcohol use
- Routine vaccinations against diseases
- Flu and pneumonia immunizations
- Counselling, screening, and vaccines to ensure healthy pregnancies
- Regular well-baby and well-child visits, from birth to age 21 years

Nurses have long been responsible for screening individuals and educating people about healthy lifestyles and decreased risks as part of the ordinary primary care assessment process. Questions concerning nutrition, coping, and self-care are all assessment or screening questions, leading to moments of opportunity or "teachable moments" for health promotion. These evaluation activities are invaluable for gauging risk and potential areas for screening. Teaching individuals the meaning and limitation of screening test results is an important element of this role, as is informing them of their part in obtaining implied benefits.

Nursing staff, at all levels, are important in applying preventive services to include screening and education. The concept of the person-centred medical home encourages the use of each member of the primary health care team to the highest level of their professional and licensing abilities. The combined nursing roles of health educator and screener mean that the nurse continues to educate individuals about risk factors and teach them ways to alter and reduce risks generally through lifestyle changes, such as proper diet, exercise, and stress management, and by limiting the use of alcohol, illicit drugs, and tobacco. The role as educator is essential in the screening process because nurses provide individuals with the information necessary for choices they will make regarding healthy behavioural change. The nurse is actually

## ⚡ QUALITY AND SAFETY SCENARIO

### *Pender's Health-Promotion Model*

A health care provider's responsibility is to assess, plan, implement, and evaluate a screening program. Part of this responsibility includes teaching individuals, families, and populations about the importance of participating in these programs and ultimately engaging in safe behaviours that promote health. The health-promotion model is a useful guide for practice (Pender, Murdaugh, & Parsons, 2015). The model presents the interrelationship among behaviour-specific cognitions and affective factors and individual characteristics and experiences that motivate individuals to engage in behaviours that promote health and decrease unsafe habits and practices. The health care provider may find that the application of this model in practice influences the relationship between the provider and the individual in a positive way. The model is a framework that assists the provider in assessing factors believed to influence health behaviour changes. Once the provider has an accurate assessment, obtained via questions, decisions may be made concerning factors that inhibit health-promoting behaviours and, ultimately, potential interventions to assist individuals in achieving positive health outcomes. This information will assist the provider to develop appropriate teaching methods.

**Health-Promotion Assessment Questions**
- How do you define health?
- What does health mean to you?
- How would you describe your health now?
- Do the choices you make and the actions you take affect your health?
- Can you give examples when choices and actions created a positive change in health for you?
- Can you give examples when choices and actions created a negative or unsafe change in health for you?
- What factors facilitated choices and actions that created a positive change in health?
- What factors created barriers to choices and actions that led to a negative or unsafe change in health?
- Are there any supportive personal influences in your life that would assist you in choices and actions that would create a positive change in your health (e.g., family, friends, and health care providers)?
- Are there any supportive situational influences, such as more than one plan of action, pertaining to the health change available to you?

Source: Modified from Pender, N., Murdaugh, C., & Parsons, M. A. (2015). *Health promotion in nursing practice* (7th ed.). Upper Saddle River, NJ: Pearson.

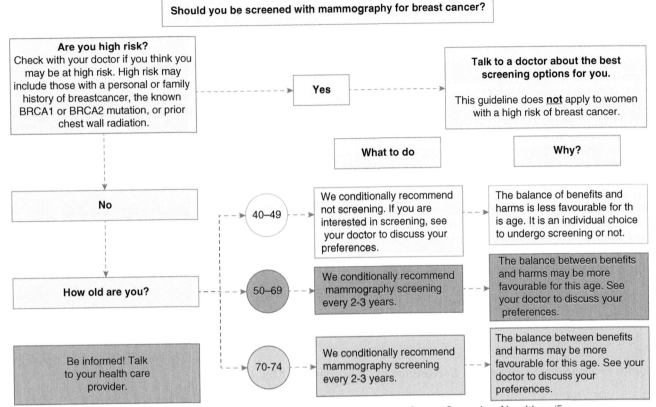

Fig. 19.4 Canadian Task Force on Preventive Health Care: Breast Cancer Screening Algorithm. (From Canadian Task Force on Preventive Health Care. *Breast cancer screening 2020.* Retrieved from https://canadiantaskforce.ca/.)

---

**BOX 19.6    Equitable Approaches to Community Health**

***Trust: Build a Culture of Collaboration With Communities That Is Based on Trust***

- *Empowerment.* Give individuals and communities the knowledge and tools needed to create change by seeking and demanding better health and building on local resources.
- *Culture and history.* Design health initiatives that are grounded in the unique historical and cultural context of racial and ethnic minority communities in Canada.
- *Focus on causes.* Assess and focus on the underlying causes of poor community health and implement solutions that will stay embedded in the community infrastructure.
- *Community investment and expertise.* Recognize and invest in local community expertise and motivate communities to mobilize and organize existing resources.

- *Trusted organizations.* Enlist organizations within the community that are valued by community members, including groups with a primary mission unrelated to health.
- *Community leaders.* Help community leaders and key organizations forge unique partnerships and act as catalysts for change in the community.
- *Ownership.* Develop a collective outlook to promote shared interest in a healthy future through widespread community engagement and leadership.
- *Sustainability.* Make changes to organizations, community environments, and policies to help ensure that health improvements are long-lasting and community activities and programs are self-sustaining.
- *Hope.* Foster optimism, pride, and a promising vision for a healthier future.

Source: From Centers for Disease Control and Prevention. (2016). *Racial and ethnic approaches to community health.* Retrieved from http://www.cdc.gov/reach.

---

practicing primary prevention interventions, but this is done in coordination with a secondary preventive role.

## EQUITABLE APPROACHES TO COMMUNITY HEALTH

The Centers for Disease Control (CDC), a US-based health organization, is currently utilizing a program called REACH (Racial and Ethnic Approaches to Community Health). This program supports effective community-level programs

to reduce health inequities in minority communities across the United States. Data from the REACH (Centers for Disease Control and Prevention, 2020) Risk Factor Survey (2009), focusing on breast and cervical cancer prevention, cardiovascular health, and diabetes management, have shown that changing health behaviours in minority communities has improved health and reduced community inequities. Here in Canada we tend to approach population health through the lens of inequity, regardless of a person's ethnic background. How do you think these approaches differ? (Box 19.6.)

## CASE STUDY

### Screening

Mrs. C. is an 82-year-old White widow. Six years ago, she moved from her house into a one-bedroom apartment. She maintains her apartment and does all her errands without assistance, all of which she is very proud. She reports that occasionally she has fallen, probably because of some degree of decreasing vision, especially when moving from direct sunlight into shadows and when walking at night. The only medications she takes are an analgesic for pain management of osteoarthritis, an antihypertensive medication, and a daily vitamin and cranberry supplement. Her antihypertensive medication has recently been changed.

Today, she is going to her annual "checkup" with nurse practitioner (NP) Kelly, who is part of a new practice of "integrative medicine." The collaborative practice of registered nurses, NPs, and physicians emphasizes the role of prevention, including screenings. While Kelly is assessing Mrs. C.'s health status, she is also reflecting on how to better care for the practice's ever-enlarging older person population. Kelly has access to a large referral group, including medical specialists.

### Reflective Questions

- What data will nurse practitioner Kelly collect to assess Mrs. C.'s health? Why?
- What risk factors will Kelly most likely evaluate? Why?
- What screening tests will Kelly suggest? Why?
- Propose several possible nursing diagnoses for Mrs. C. What possible etiological factors from Mrs. C., her family, and her community might be involved?
- What questions will Kelly ask to evaluate Mrs. C.'s health status?
- Compare and contrast these different (individual, family, and community) approaches to health promotion, emphasizing screening and cost effectiveness.
- Discuss the advantages and disadvantages of screening older people.

## CARE PLAN

### Health Promotion, Emphasizing Screenings of Older People: Mrs. C.

Caring for older people is challenging and rewarding. New ways of caring need to be developed, especially considering the increasing number of the older "baby boomer generation" in Canada.

### Nursing Issue
Adequate community therapeutic regimen management

### Definition
The pattern in which an individual, family, and/or community experiences (or is at risk of experiencing) difficulty integrating screening programs for the promotion of health and reduction of risk factors

### Defining Characteristics
#### Major
- The individual, family, and/or community verbalizes the desire to manage health promotion with the assistance of the family and community, including a nurse practitioner.
- The individual and family verbalize inadequate knowledge of health-promotion strategies, especially risk factors identified through screening methods.

#### Minor
- What are Mrs. C.'s screening and health-promotion needs?
- What is Mrs. C's understanding of aging and of accelerated risk factors for illness?

### Related Factors
- Complexity, including discomfort, of some screenings (e.g., mammograms, osteoporosis testing)

- New ways of thinking about and delivering health promotion, including periodic screening recommended for older people
- Shifts of resources and costs from individual providers to the community and family (e.g., self-screenings, transportation)

### Interventions
- Promote attitudes of openness to new health information.
- For elevated blood pressure readings, repeat blood pressure screening on three different visits.
- Develop a more detailed activity/experience log with special attention to physical safety (falls) and vision problems.
- Explore nutritional and activity strategies that are more appealing to each individual.
- Begin the program slowly.
- Follow up on additional risk factors.
- Offer resources to support goals and interventions.

### Expected Outcomes
- The person may experience anxiety.
- The person may experience despair.
Mrs. C., her family, and her community will:
- Verbalize a full understanding of health promotion, especially screenings.
Mrs. C. will:
- Identify and discuss her own risk factors and other data obtained from screenings.
- Establish appropriate goals to decrease the unhealthy findings of her screenings.
- Design and implement a modification program to fulfill these goals.
- Evaluate the efficacy of this care plan with nurse practitioner Kelly.

## SUMMARY

Screening is the administration of measures or tests to distinguish individuals who may have a condition from those who probably do not have it. It is an effective, efficient tool in preventive health care if used for conditions applicable to the screening model and specifically directed toward an at-risk population.

Implementing screening programs requires coordination and planning and provides numerous places for nursing intervention, especially within the currently evolving health care environment, which is emphasizing prevention activities. Nurses can provide individuals, communities, and populations with valuable preventive, health-promotion, and health-education support in the care of healthy individuals and populations. Through education and resource sharing, nurses have the opportunity to support their patients to make empowered and informed choices and take control of their health.

**Evolve Chapter Features**

http://evolve.elsevier.com/Canada/Edelman/healthpromotion/
- Review Questions

## REFERENCES

Airoldi, M., & Morton, A. (2009). Adjusting life for quality or disability: Stylistic difference or substantial dispute? *Health Economics, 18*(11), 1237–1247.

Allender, J., Rector, C., & Warner, K. (2014). *Community health nursing: Promoting and protecting the public's health* (8th ed.). Philadelphia: Lippincott, Williams & Wilkins.

Alzheimer Society of Canada. (2018). *Amyloid imaging.* Retrieved from https://alzheimer.ca/en/Home/News-and-Events/feature-stories/amyloid-imaging.

Anderson, J. B., Grenier, M., Edwards, N. M., et al. (2014). Usefulness of combined history, physical examination, electrocardiogram, and limited echocardiogram in screening adolescent athletes for risk for sudden cardiac death. *The American Journal of Cardiology, 114*(11), 1763–1767.

Bisaillon, L. (2011). Mandatory HIV screening policy & everyday life: A look inside the Canadian immigration medical examination. *Aporia: Nursing Journal, 3*(4), 5–14.

Brodersen, J., & Siersma, V. D. (2013). Long-term psychosocial consequences of false-positive screening mammography. *The Annals of Family Medicine, 11*(2), 106–115.

Bushnik, T., & Evans, W. K. (2018). Sociodemographic characteristics associated with thyroid cancer risk in Canada. *Health Reports, 29*(10). Retrieved from https://www150.statcan.gc.ca/n1/pub/82-003-x/2018010/article/00001-eng.htm.

Bynum, S. A., Davis, J. L., Green, B. L., et al. (2012). Unwillingness to participate in colorectal cancer screenings: Examining fears, attitudes, and medical mistrust in an ethnically diverse sample of adults 50 years and older. *American Journal of Health Promotion, 26*(5), 295–300.

Canadian Agency for Drugs and Technologies in Health (CADTH). (2011). *Newborn screenings for abnormalities in Canada.* Retrieved from https://cadth.ca/sites/default/files/pdf/Newborn_Screening_es-26_e.pdf.

Canadian Agency for Drugs and Technologies in Health (CADTH). (2017). Point-of-care testing. *Environmental Scan, 10.* Retrieved from https://www.cadth.ca/sites/default/files/pdf/es0308_point_of_care_testing.pdf.

Canadian Cancer Society, Statistics Canada, & Public Health Agency of Canada. (2017). *Canadian cancer statistics 2017.* Retrieved from http://www.cancer.ca/~/media/cancer.ca/CW/cancer%20information/cancer%20101/Canadian%20cancer%20statistics/Canadian-Cancer-Statistics-2017-EN.pdf.

Canadian Nurses Association (CNA). (2019). *Evidence-based practice.* Retrieved from https://www.cna-aiic.ca/en/nursing-practice/evidence-based-practice.

Canadian Public Health Association (CPHA). (n.d.). *What are the social determinants of health?* Retrieved from https://www.cpha.ca/what-are-social-determinants-health.

Canadian Task Force on Preventive Health Care (CTFPHC). (2014). *Prostate cancer.* Retrieved from https://canadiantaskforce.ca/guidelines/published-guidelines/prostate-cancer/.

Canadian Task Force on Preventive Health Care (CTFPHC). (2017). *CTFPHC releases AAA screening guideline.* Retrieved from https://canadiantaskforce.ca/ctfphcs-releases-aaa-screening-guideline/.

Canadian Task Force on Preventive Health Care (CTFPHC). (2019). *Published guidelines.* Retrieved from https://canadiantaskforce.ca/guidelines/published-guidelines/.

CATIE. (2018). *HIV in Canada: A primer for health service providers.* Retrieved from https://www.catie.ca/en/hiv-canada.

Centers for Disease Control and Prevention (CDC). (2012). *Introduction to epidemiology.* Retrieved from http://www.cdc.gov/ophss/csels/dsepd/ss1978/lesson1/section/.html/.

Centers for Disease Control and Prevention (CDC). (2015). *What is epidemiology?* Retrieved from http://www.cdc.gov/excite/epidemiology.

Centers for Disease Control and Prevention. (2020, February 20). *Racial and Ethnic Approaches to Community Health.* Retrieved from http://www.cdc.gov/nccdphp/dnpao/state-local-programs/reach/index.htm.

Costello, J. (2014). *Measuring benefits.* Retrieved from https://www.givingwhatwecan.org/blog/2014-03-04/measuring-benefits.

Davis, J. L., Bynum, S. A., Katz, R. V., et al. (2012). Sociodemographic differences in fears and mistrust contributing to unwillingness to participate in cancer screenings. *Journal of Health Care for the Poor and Underserved, 23*(4 Suppl. l), 67–76.

Dean, H. J., & Sellers, E. A. (2015). Children have type 2 diabetes too: An historical perspective. *Biochemistry and Cell Biology, 93*(5), 425–429. https://doi.org/10.1139/bcb-2014-0152.

Diabetes Canada Clinical Practice Guidelines Expert Committee. (2018). Diabetes Canada 2018 clinical practice guidelines for the prevention and management of diabetes in Canada. *Canadian Journal of Diabetes, 42*(Suppl. 1), S1–S325. https://doi.org/10.1016/j.jcjd.2017.10.

Dorfman, L., & Krasnow, I. D. (2014). Public health and media advocacy. *Annual Review of Public Health, 35,* 293–306.

Fish, S. (2017). *Hepatitis C point of care testing: What is its impact on testing and linkage to care?* Retrieved from https://www.catie.ca/en/pif/spring-2017/hepatitis-c-point-care-testing-what-its-impact-testing-and-linkage-care.

Ginsburg, O. M., Fischer, H. D., Shah, B. R., et al. (2015). A population-based study of ethnicity and breast cancer stage at diagnosis in Ontario. *Current Oncology, 22*(2), 97. https://doi.org/10.3747/co.22.2359.

Government of Canada. (2001). *Immigration and refugee protection act, Part 1: Immigration to Canada*. Ottawa: Author. Retrieved from https://laws.justice.gc.ca/eng/acts/i-2.5/page-8.html#docCont.

Government of Canada. (2009). *5 stages to quitting*. Retrieved from https://www.canada.ca/en/health-canada/services/health-concerns/tobacco/quit-smoking/faqs-facts/five-stages-quitting.html.

Halseth, R. (2019). *The prevalence of Type 2 diabetes among First Nations and considerations for prevention*. Prince George, BC: National Collaborating Centre for Aboriginal Health.

HealthlinkBC. (2019). *Health screening*. Retrieved from https://www.healthlinkbc.ca/health-topics/tc4037#tc4040.

Hoffmann, T. C., & Del Mar, C. (2015). Patients' expectations of the benefits and harms of treatments, screening, and tests: A systematic review. *Journal of the American Medical Association Internal Medicine, 175*(2), 274–286. https://doi.org/10.1001/jamainternmed.2014.6016.

Institute of Medicine. (2011). *The future of nursing: Leading change, advancing health*. Retrieved from http://www.iom.edu/Reports/2010/The-Future-of-Nursing-Leading-Change-Advancing-Health.aspx/.

Kidd, A. D., & Colbert, A. M. (2015). Mammography: Review of the controversy, health disparities, and impact on young African American women. *Clinical Journal of Oncology Nursing, 19*(3), E52–E58. https://doi.org/10.1188/15.CJON.E52-E58.

Lin, K. W., & Gostin, L. O. (2016). A public health framework for screening mammography: Evidence-based vs politically mandated care. *Journal of the American Medical Association, 315*(10), 977–978. https://doi.org/10.1001/jama.2016.0322.

Lloyd, V. K., & Hawkins, R. G. (2018). Under-detection of Lyme disease in Canada. *Healthcare (Basel, Switzerland), 6*(4), 125. https://doi.org/10.3390/healthcare6040125.

Lundy, K., & Janes, S. (2014). *Community health nursing: Caring for the public's health* (3rd ed.). Boston, MA: Jones & Bartlett.

Maine, D., Hurlburt, S., & Greeson, D. (2011). Cervical cancer prevention in the 21st century: Cost is not the only issue. *American Journal of Public Health, 101*(9), 1549–1555.

Mandelblatt, J., Stout, N. K., Schechter, C. B., et al. (2016). Collaborative modeling of the benefits and harms associated with different US breast cancer screening strategies. *Annals of Internal Medicine, 164*(4), 215–225. https://doi.org/10.7326/M15-1536.

Mikkonen, J., & Raphael, D. (2010). *Social determinants of health: The Canadian facts*. Toronto: York University School of Health Policy and Management.

National Prevention Council. (2011). *National prevention strategy*. Washington, DC: US Department of Health and Human Services, Office of the Surgeon General. Retrieved from https://www.surgeongeneral.gov/priorities/prevention/strategy/report.pdf.

Nayak, S., Roberts, M., & Greenspan, S. (2011). Cost-effectiveness of different screening strategies for osteoporosis in postmenopausal women. *Annals of Internal Medicine, 155*, 751–761.

Nickolich, S., Farahi, N., Jones, K., et al. (2016). PURLs: Aneuploidy screening: Newer noninvasive test gains traction. *Clinician Reviews, 26*(2), 29–30 26.

Office of the Privacy Commissioner of Canada. (2017). *Direct-to-consumer genetic testing and privacy*. Retrieved from https://www.priv.gc.ca/en/privacy-topics/health-genetic-and-other-body-information/02_05_d_69_gen/.

Pender, N., Murdaugh, C., & Parsons, M. A. (2015). *Health promotion in nursing practice* (7th ed.). Upper Saddle River, NJ: Pearson.

Public Health Agency of Canada (PHAC). (2019). *Government of Canada announces funding for the Antigonish Women's resource centre and sexual Assault services association*. Retrieved from https://www.canada.ca/en/public-health/news/2019/03/government-of-canada-announces-funding-for-the-antigonish-womens-resource-centre-and-sexual-assault-services-association.html.

Registered Nurses Association of Ontario (RNAO). (2017). *Best practice guideline implementation to reduce smoking*. Retrieved from https://rnao.ca/sites/rnao-ca/files/Evidence_Booster-Autumn_2017_smoking_FINAL_0.pdf.

Ringrose, J., Millay, J., Babwick, S. A., et al. (2015). Effect of overcuffing on the accuracy of oscillometric blood pressure measurements. *Journal of the American Society of Hypertension, 9*(7), 563–568. https://doi.org/10.1016/j.jash.2015.04.007.

Roelofs, C., Shoemaker, P., Skogstrom, T., et al. (2010). The Boston Safe Shops model: An integrated approach to community environmental and occupational health. *American Journal of Public Health, 100*(Suppl. 1), S52–S55. https://doi.org/10.2105/AJPH.2009.176511.

Shephard, R. (2011). Mandatory ECG screening of athletes: Is this question now resolved? *Sports Medicine, 41*(12), 989–1002.

Sutphen, C. L., Jasielec, M. S., Shah, A. R., et al. (2015). Longitudinal cerebrospinal fluid biomarker changes in preclinical Alzheimer's disease during middle age. *Journal of the American Medical Association Neurology, 72*(9), 1029–1042. https://doi.org/10.1001/jamaneurol.2015.1285.

Thompson, C. K., Eklund, M., & Esserman, L. J. (2015). Putting the "great mammography debate" to rest. *American Journal of Hematology/Oncology, 11*(9), 21–22.

Uden-Holman, T. M., Curry, S. J., & Benz, L. (2015). Public health as a catalyst for interprofessional education on a health sciences campus. *American Journal of Public Health, 105*(S1), S104–S105. https://doi.org/10.2105/AJPH.2014.302501.

Vora, N. L., & O'Brien, B. M. (2014). Noninvasive prenatal testing for microdeletion syndromes and expanded trisomies: Proceed with caution. *Obstetrics & Gynecology, 123*(5), 1097–1099.

Weir, H. K., Thompson, T. D., Soman, A., et al. (2015). The past, present, and future of cancer incidence in the US: 1975–2020. *Cancer, 121*(11), 1827–1837. https://doi.org/10.1002/cncr.29258.

Yoon, S. S., Fryar, C. D., & Carroll, M. S. (2015). *Hypertension prevalence and control among adults: US, 2011–2014*. NCHS data brief, no 220. Hyattsville, MD: National Center for Health Statistics.

# 20

# Health Education

*Collette Tattman-Melo, MN-ANP, CCRN, CCN, NP(f)*

Originating US chapter by *Susan A. Heady, RN, PhD*

## INTENDED LEARNING OUTCOMES

*After completing this chapter, the reader will be able to:*
- Analyze the goals of health education.
- Discuss learning principles that affect health education.
- Apply teaching and learning concepts to teaching.
- Describe selected theoretical models and strategies used in health education to influence the behaviour change process.
- Explain the steps in preparing a health teaching plan.
- Propose learning strategies appropriate to each learning domain using a variety of resources.
- Discuss the importance of evaluating the educational process.

## KEY TERMS

Ambivalence
Autonomy
Behaviour change
Ecological model
Empowerment
Health belief model
Health education
Health inequities

Health literacy
Health promotion
Health-promoting behaviours
Motivational interviewing
Pedagogy
Protection motivation theory (PMT)
Quality and safety
Self-efficacy

Shared decision making
Social cognitive theory
Social justice
Social marketing
Transtheoretical model (Stages of change)
Victim blaming

## ❓ THINK ABOUT IT

### The Challenges of Health Education

With personal health behaviour patterns linked closely to the current causes of morbidity and death, health education is fundamental to promoting lifestyle change. People may lack the knowledge needed for making lifestyle changes, such as awareness of risks. In addition, they may not be aware of, or be able to access, effective health-promotion strategies and resources in the community. In each encounter, the nurse has the opportunity to (1) assess the learner's needs for education related to primary, secondary, and/or tertiary prevention, and (2) assess the underlying structural and social determinants of health that impact the learner's ability to learn or make change. Whether the target audience is an individual or a community, the nurse considers these questions in addressing the health-education needs:
- What can people do to improve their health in the context of lifestyles?
- How can individuals, families, and communities make healthier choices?
- How is the nurse able to promote healthy behavioural change?
- What is the nurse's role in facilitating health through education and program planning?

Reflect on the following scenario. Tonya is a 14-year-old girl who lives with her mother and older brothers. Her after-school activities focus on texting her friends and watching television. Tonya is obese for her age and height. According to the school nurse, many of her peers are also overweight or obese. Consider the following:
- What does Tonya know about healthy nutrition and exercise?
- What factors may promote or interfere with Tonya's learning or adopting a change in lifestyle?
- How can the nurse best address Tonya's health-education needs?
- What resources to support learning are—or should be—made available to Tonya, her family, and/or the community?
- What are the health-education needs of other students in the school?
- What information is relevant to teaching Tonya or planning programs for the middle school students in this neighbourhood?
- Which theories can be used in planning health-education programs?
- How might families or the community be involved in supporting obesity prevention and reduction for these teens?
- What are the needs of other residents of the community?

Health education is a vital component in promoting individual and community health. However, information alone does not change behaviour. One cannot assume that poor health is related only to a lack of information or education and that by providing this, recipients will experience improved outcomes. Individual behaviours such as diet, physical activity level, and substance misuse play a significant, but not the only, role in health outcomes. Addressing social determinants of health that affect these individual behaviours, and supporting patients in self-management of positive lifestyle changes, can be effective, not only in preventing chronic diseases but also in reversing their progression and significantly reducing health care costs (Liddy, Johnston, Nash, et al., 2016).

Health education must be designed to reduce barriers to the adoption of lifestyle behaviour changes. Nurse educators must also focus on examining ways to prompt positive individual *and* community behaviour change through policy and program development that address the social determinants of health, thereby reducing health inequities. As our population ages, chronic health concerns become more prevalent. There is a greater need to shift the focus from acute, individualized interventions, to community-based interventions that include programming improvement, advocacy, and education in health promotion, illness prevention, and chronic disease management (Canadian Foundation for Healthcare Improvement, 2019, bullet 2). The 1984 *Canada Health Act* set out the main priorities of health care, which remain to this day: "to protect, promote and restore the physical and mental well-being of residents of Canada and to facilitate reasonable access to health services without financial or other barriers" (Government of Canada, 2017a, p. 5). These priorities involve promoting positive health behaviours, increasing health literacy and collaboration, and reducing health inequities. Achievement of these objectives provides challenges and opportunities for health promotion.

Although many health goals are affected by individual lifestyle practices, health is influenced significantly by social, environmental, economic, physical, and political factors, all of which can be significantly impacted by education, particularly if education includes advocacy. The Public Health Agency of Canada's (PHAC) vision for health education includes a commitment to providing early health literacy and prevention education, beginning with preschool, then continuing throughout the K–12 education continuum and beyond. This involves an approach to developing healthy citizens not only by delivering basic health-promotion and disease-prevention concepts and encouraging risk-reduction behaviours but also by advocating for community resources that support young people and their families, thereby decreasing health inequities—systematic, potentially avoidable differences in health status or health resources between population groups. The Ottawa Charter for Health Promotion states that health promotion must occur "within the settings of their everyday life; where they learn, work, play and love" (World Health Organization [WHO], 1986, p. 3). Box 20.1 outlines the four main approaches to building healthy school communities.

Nursing, with its unique contributions to health care, is a professional resource that can help facilitate these changes through health-education and advocacy strategies. Nurses, in partnership with other health care providers, can be the link between the goals of the PHAC and the people who need to hear its messages and act on those messages.

# NURSING AND HEALTH EDUCATION

Educating people is an integral part of the nurse's role in every practice setting—schools, communities, work sites, health care delivery sites, and homes. Health education involves not only providing relevant information but also facilitating health-related behaviour change. The nurse, using Miller and Rollnick's (1991) motivational interviewing strategies, can assist people in achieving their health goals in a way that is consistent with their personal lifestyles, values, and beliefs.

Nurses also work to remove barriers to the successful achievement of these goals: barriers such as, but not limited to, perceived or actual racism and discrimination, poor living conditions, lack of support, time or knowledge. Removing barriers and calling attention to health inequities prevents "victim blaming" (Groleau, Benady-Chorney, Panaitoiu, et al., 2019), where the cause of ill health is largely focused on the individual rather than on social or economic causes, thus negatively emphasizing the individual being responsible for the "wrong" health choices.

The roles of Registered Nurses in Canada are regulated at a jurisdictional level (i.e., by the provinces and territories in which nurses work); however, the principles of nursing practice in the document *The Framework for the Practice of Registered Nurses in Canada* (Canadian Nurses Association [CNA], 2015, p. 3) reflects a pan-Canadian approach describing health teaching and health promotion as primary nursing responsibilities. This includes educating people about healthy lifestyles, risk reduction, developmental needs, activities of daily living, and preventive self-care. This responsibility to teach individuals is balanced by their right, their desire, their ability, and their readiness to receive information about their health status, risks, and ways to reduce their risks—all basic tenants of motivational interviewing that is foundational to health-education principles.

Nurses often function as health care coordinators for individuals in their care. Depending on the interests and needs of a person, nurses establish a partnership to guide the individual in the selection and use of relevant, credible health resources and services. Health-education principles provide the nurse with strategies and tools for assessing an individual's readiness for health teaching, offering support for practicing healthy behaviours, and evaluating technological information and resources. These strategies also help the nurse facilitate behaviour change while satisfying the person's right to relevant health information and the freedom for people to make decisions about their own health. Health education encourages self-care, self-empowerment, and, ultimately, less dependence on the health care system.

Nurses have long been involved in public health education, taking on the role of coordinating the educational services provided by a health agency or institution. As a health educator, the nurse may use marketing strategies to enhance the effectiveness of health-education programs that are focused on certain target populations. The health-education specialist helps other nurses and health professionals improve their skills in developing and delivering teaching plans.

## Definition

*Health education* is "any combination of learning experiences designed to help individuals and communities improve their

## BOX 20.1  Comprehensive School Health

### Selected Health-Promotion and Disease-Prevention Objectives Related to Educational and Community-Based Programs

**Goal**

To support the wellness of all community members and improve health and education outcomes through engaging students, applying evidence-informed practices and supporting sustainability and development of healthy social and physical environments.

**Social and Physical Environment**

The social environment is:

- The quality of relationships among and between staff and students in the school
- The emotional well-being of students
- Influenced by relationships with families and the wider community
- Supportive of the school community in making healthy choices by building competence, autonomy, and connectedness
  The physical environment is:
- The buildings, grounds, play space, and equipment in and surrounding the school
- Basic amenities such as sanitation, air cleanliness, and healthy foods
- Spaces designed to promote student safety and connectedness and minimize injury
- Safe, accessible, and supportive of healthy resources for all members of the school community

**Teaching and Learning**

- Formal and informal provincial/territorial curriculum, resources, and associated activities
- Knowledge, understanding, and skills for students to improve their health and well-being and enhance their learning outcomes
- Professional development opportunities for staff related to health and well-being

**Healthy School Policy**

- Policies, guidelines, and practices that promote and support student well-being and achievement and shape a respectful, welcoming, and caring school environment for all members of the school community

**Partnerships and Services**

Partnerships are:

- The connections between the school and student's families
- Supportive working relationships among schools, and among schools and other community organizations and representative groups
- Health, education, and other sectors working together to advance school health  Services are:
- Community and school-based services that support and promote student and staff health and well-being, such as school lunch programs and food-banks to promote nutrition and food security

Source: Joint Consortium for School Health (2016). *What is comprehensive school health?* Retrieved from http://www.jcsh-cces.ca/images/What_is_Comprehensive_School_Health_-_2-pager_-_July_2016.pdf.

health, by increasing their knowledge or influencing their attitudes" (WHO, 2019, para 1). This process involves several key components. First, health education involves the use of teaching–learning strategies. Second, learners maintain voluntary control over the decision to make changes in their actions. Third, health education focuses on behaviour changes that have been found to improve health and well-being. Health education facilitates the development of health knowledge, skills, and attitudes through the application of theories or models. Commonly used theories of individual and community behaviour change, and strategies to promote them will be discussed later in this chapter. Generally, health-education strategies help ensure that individuals, as consumers of health services, are satisfied and have received the health information that is most relevant to them, as determined by them. From a public health perspective, health-education programs are intended not only to enhance individuals' abilities to make positive lifestyle changes but also to support social and political actions that promote health and quality of life in communities.

The following scenario is an example of a therapeutic situation in which a health-education approach may be used to meet an individual's health needs.

Sada Thompson, a 21-year-old university senior, visits university health services because she wants to change her method of birth control. She has experienced side effects from the birth control pill that she has been taking for the past year and knows little about other options. She has recently started dating John after breaking up with Steven 3 months ago. Having decided to be sexually active with John, Sada is feeling uncertain about what she needs to do to take care of herself and how to discuss this uncertainty with John. She is aware of all the talk about sexually transmitted infections (STIs) on campus, and she knows that John is popular and has dated several other women in school, which concerns her.

Sada is seeking new information, she may need to acquire new skills, and she is best served by clarifying any feelings or attitudes that affect her decision to use a new birth control method while meeting her continued safety. After recording her health assessment history, assessing her need for a gynecological examination and arranging for laboratory tests, the nurse develops a teaching plan. Selecting one or more strategies for helping Sada review all her contraceptive options, the nurse establishes an environment in which Sada can choose to try a new method or request a change in her prescription for oral contraceptives. Together, they identify actions Sada can take to use the method properly. They also anticipate and identify ways that Sada can solve problems of adjusting to the new method.

The nurse answers Sada's immediate questions about safe sex, gives her several pamphlets and evidence-informed websites developed for post-secondary students about this topic, and suggests that she participate in the peer counselling night on STIs that will be held on campus in 2 weeks. The peer counselling hotline number and drop-in hours are given to Sada. The nurse explains that the students who provide the peer counselling are trained to help other students talk about and deal with this important issue. The nurse invites Sada to call or come back to the office for additional help, information, and problem-solving discussion.

This example illustrates that educational interventions, in addition to direct health resources and services, are necessary to meet the individual's goal. Although health care providers prefer that people choose to take actions that will promote health and not detract from it, the individual determines the level of application of health recommendations based upon personal values and goals.

## Goals

The goal of health education is to help individuals, families, and communities achieve, through their own actions and initiative, optimal states of health. Health education facilitates voluntary actions to promote health. Another important goal of health education is improving health literacy.

*Functional literacy* was defined in 1995 by the Organization for Economic Co-operation and Development and Statistics Canada (OECD & Statistics Canada, 1995), who maintain that literacy is a practice-based skill, as more than a basic reading ability to include the understanding and use of printed information that is fundamental to daily life at work, at home, and in the community. Therefore building upon functional literacy, health literacy is the ability to apply these skills to health situations for the purpose of achieving healthier outcomes.

Despite achieving the highest international rates of adult post-secondary education (Statistics Canada, 2018a, para 1), approximately 48.5% of Canadian adults have lower literacy than is needed to understand everyday reading, or be competent in most jobs (Statistics Canada, 2018b). This can translate into experiencing difficulty with common health tasks, such as following directions on a prescription drug label or adhering to a childhood immunization schedule using a standard chart. With the rise of chronic illness, health literacy is crucial for health maintenance and disease prevention. For example, an individual who is diagnosed with diabetes must have the ability to read, understand, and apply information about diet and nutrition, medication administration, and blood glucose monitoring.

Nurses contribute to improving health literacy by assisting care recipients to obtain and decipher educational materials such as forms and instructions and electronic medical records (EMR), and help navigate clients through the mass of information found on the Internet. Further discussion regarding the selection and evaluation of materials will be presented later on in this chapter.

Social justice, the solution to health inequities, refers to fair treatment, equal access to resources, and the right to autonomy and cultural expression for all people. Groups affected by inequities are those with lower socioeconomic status and include "Indigenous peoples, sexual and racial/ethnic minorities, immigrants and people living with functional limitations" (PHAC, 2018, p. 8). The *Canadian Poverty Reduction Strategy* reports that over 3 million Canadians live in poverty and "an estimated 35,000 people are homeless on any given night" (Government of Canada, 2017b, p. 8). Strategies, such as those to reduce poverty, are best supported by partnering with provincial, territorial and municipal stakeholders, Indigenous people, and community groups. Perhaps, most importantly, initiatives that embrace public input, particularly from those who live with health inequities, create upstream approaches to obtaining social justice. Nurses work as advocates to reduce inequities by taking part in strategies and initiatives which are key components of "nursing's professional responsibility to address unjust systems and structures" (Thurman & Pfitzinger-Lippe, 2017, p. 187).

Community initiatives that work toward reducing health inequities include those that exercise leadership in monitoring health status. Nurses play a role in this, for example, by advocating for and participating in the development of immunization clinics, needle exchange programs, and home health monitoring. The nursing role consists of reporting progress and identifying what is successful and what is not within the programs they work.

Collaborative, people-centred care is an essential component of quality and safety whether health promotion is directed toward an individual, family, or community. In the planning and implementation of health education, nurses must ensure that health care recipient's dignity, values, and needs are at the forefront of the management of their health. Programs, and the professionals that represent them, must show respect for cultural, ethnic, and social diversity by honouring choices and decisions, and incorporating cultural norms into care delivery, all while promoting a climate of self-management, improved information and understanding, and collaborative participation (British Columbia Ministry of Health, 2015, p. 1). Use of health-education strategies that are person-centred can have a significant impact on the outcomes of health care recipients, and fit with the standards of the Canadian Patient Safety Institute (2018, p. 4), of providing person-centred care, care that supports teamwork, and communication. The Quality and Safety Scenario provides an example of person-centred health-promotion strategies.

Health education and motivational interviewing encourage positive, evidence-informed changes in lifestyle behaviours that prevent acute and chronic disease, decrease disability, and enhance wellness. Another goal of these two activities that

---

### ⚡ QUALITY AND SAFETY SCENARIO

#### *A Community-Based Person-Centred Health Promotion*

The HANS KAI intervention was designed to address chronic disease prevention and management in socioeconomically challenged communities. HANS KAI is based upon the Japanese concepts of *han*, meaning "group," and *kai*, meaning "meeting." A study of a Manitoba-based health care co-operative sought to analyze the effects of peer support groups on the health of participants. Peer groups consisting of 10 members, who were matched based upon commonalities of community area and age, were encouraged to meet regularly and participate in required components such as physical activity, healthy snack preparation, and goal setting for healthy living.

A survey was conducted to measure the effects of the group on health-related topics such as knowledge of common chronic conditions, physical activity and nutrition, smoking, social isolation, and mental health status. The most common responses regarding the benefits of the HANS group was the interconnectedness between participants and the positive outcomes this had on mental health through the effects of motivation, inspiration, and accountability; 66% of participants were able to describe positive behavioural changes, such as stress-reduction techniques, healthier cooking strategies, and increase in physical activity, the benefits of which flowed over into other members of participants' households.

Although the group was participant led, facilitators of the HANS group were available to provide information regarding various support services within participant communities, resulting in increased accessibility, usability, and collaboration of services.

Source: Henteleff, A. & Wall, H. (2018). The HANS KAI project: A community-based approach to improving health and well-being through peer support. *Health Promotion and Chronic Disease Prevention in Canada*, 38(3). https://doi.org/10.24095/hpcdp.38.3.04. Retrieved from https://www.canada.ca/en/public-health/services/reports-publications/health-promotion-chronic-disease-prevention-canada-research-policy-practice/vol-38-no-3-2018/hans-kai-project-community-based-approach-improving-health.html.

fosters successful changes in health behaviour is empowerment, through the use of positive affirmations and reflective listening, both strategies of motivational interviewing. People who believe they have autonomy—the ability to take control over their own lives in order to improve their health—and who are involved in decision making are more likely to experience an improvement in mental and physical health outcomes (Legate, Ryan, & Rogge, 2017, p. 862).

Two main objectives of health education and motivational interviewing are to change health behaviours and to improve health status. *Health education*, the act of providing information (teacher-driven), and *motivational interviewing*, the act of discussing information (participant-driven), are mutually supportive activities (Logren, Ruusuvuori, & Laitinen, 2017, p. 1840).

Health educators use one-to-one and group counselling techniques as strategies for active health learning and may refer people to health-education resources or assist them in acquiring information pertinent to solving health concerns. The following example helps illustrate the goals of health education. The general principles of learning that are found in Box 20.2 are fundamental to the planning of successful health-education programs.

Kate Hanson, aged 22 years, visits the local family health centre for fatigue and symptoms similar to influenza. During the assessment with the nurse, Kate discloses that she has missed her last two periods.

The physical examination findings, the laboratory test findings, and the health assessment pattern confirm Kate's suspicions of pregnancy. Psychosocial evaluation reveals that Kate works part-time as an administrative assistant and lives in an apartment with her recently unemployed partner, Jim. Further interviewing reveals that Kate has minimal knowledge of prenatal care; she has a diet of take-out food that is high in fat, sodium, and sugar, with infrequent consumption of fresh fruits or vegetables, and she has three or four beers on the weekends. Kate has never taken vitamin supplements, she leads a sedentary lifestyle, and she is obviously overwhelmed by the news that she is pregnant.

The nurse first takes steps to create a safe and trusting atmosphere in which Kate can feel free to share her concerns and apprehensions; the nurse does this by asking open-ended questions, affirming her abilities, and using reflective statements (OAR). When Kate expresses concerns about telling her partner about the pregnancy, the nurse uses reflective listening to evoke revelations in Kate regarding ways she can problem solve this herself. The nurse is sure to offer a nonjudgemental, patient value–driven approach to Kate's choice regarding whether or not to maintain the pregnancy. Kate is advised of her options, then, based upon her decisions to proceed with the pregnancy, she is taught the importance of taking a multiple vitamin with an iron supplement daily, discontinuing the consumption of alcohol, checking with her primary care provider (PCP) before taking medications, and making time for more rest during the day. Sensing that this is all that can be accomplished at this time, the nurse offers Kate three resources that accommodate a variety of learning styles and level of education: a web link to evidence-informed prenatal care and fetal development; an app for tracking stages of fetal growth; and a pamphlet on prenatal care. An appointment is made for her to return in 1 week with her partner, with goals to discuss the pregnancy with both Kate and her partner at that time. Kate acknowledges that she understands the instructions, and the nurse documents the teaching and recommendations in Kate's medical record.

During the next visit, the nurse meets Kate and her partner, Jim. Together, they explore the meaning of the pregnancy in their lives, and the nurse helps them identify actions they will need to take. The recommendations that were made during Kate's first visit are reviewed and reinforced. The nurse then uses motivational interviewing techniques to help the couple establish ways to improve their diet and exercise. The nurse reinforces Kate's need for proper rest and regular prenatal PCP checkups, and uses OAR strategies to help the couple come up with potential solutions to problems while they adjust to these new responsibilities. Most importantly, the nurse gives them information on the clinic's weekly prenatal classes, which are free of charge and covered by their provincial health insurance. The classes include information about physical changes, psychosocial changes, and nutritional needs during the pregnancy, the labour and delivery period, and the newborn and postpartum periods. A nurse practitioner conducts the classes at the clinic, which are given in a group format to facilitate social support and problem solving among expectant parents.

At Kate's request, the nurse gives Kate and Jim further written and web-based educational information to review at home regarding how to make healthy food choices on a limited income. The couple is encouraged to meet the social worker to explore their financial needs and options because Jim was recently laid off. Another clinic appointment is made for Kate in a couple of weeks, Jim is supported in his value-based decision to look for work while Kate attends the next appointment, and the couple is encouraged to call if questions or concerns arise in the interim. A schedule of the prenatal classes is reviewed, and a date for the next session is made. Kate and Jim acknowledge that

---

**BOX 20.2  How to Facilitate Learning**

- Use methods that stimulate a variety of senses to accommodate all learning styles.
- Involve the person actively in the learning process, enabling the participant to be engaged in at least 50% of the conversation (avoid lecturing).
- Establish a comfortable, appropriate learning environment.
- Assess the readiness of the learner, which may be affected by physical, social, emotional, and financial factors.
- Connect with the existing needs, values, and interests of the learner; remove your own agenda.
- Use repetition. Review and reinforce concepts several times in a variety of ways.
- Structure the learning encounter to achieve progress recognizable by the individual and provide frequent, positive, and specific affirmations and feedback.
- Start with what is known and proceed to what is unknown, moving from simple to complex.
- Apply the concepts to several settings to facilitate generalization.
- Pace the learning appropriately for the individual.

they understand what they need to do, and the nurse documents what was taught and discussed in Kate's health care record.

This example illustrates the goal of health education: to help individuals achieve optimal health and well-being through their own value-driven actions and initiative. Through health education, individuals can learn to make informed decisions about personal and family health practices and to use health services in the community. The couple in this example receive educational assistance from the nurse that will promote better health and well-being for Kate, her partner, and their baby.

## Learning Assumptions

Chapters 10 to 18 in this book address the factors one should consider when teaching different age groups and the learners' respective characteristics to consider when one is developing a teaching plan.

The nurse considers the developmental stage, cognitive level, and interests of the individual. The level of information to be conveyed and the skills and abilities of the individual will guide the methods and resources used.

## Family/Caregiver Health Teaching

The terms *family* and *caregiver* are used here interchangeably; they play an important role in health and illness. Because the caregiving unit is one within which health values, abilities, habits, and health-risk perceptions are developed, an individual's health, understanding, and interaction with the family is essential to promote health and reduce health risks in individuals and communities (Wright & Leahey, 2013). Skills in caregiver interviewing and assessment are valuable tools for nurses.

Family health assessment and health teaching are closely related. The assessment model in Chapter 6 provides a comprehensive approach to identifying problems, strengths, and health-education needs. The goal is to empower members to achieve optimal states of health while guiding them through problem solving and decision making.

In clarifying the health-teaching needs of a family, the nurse might ask:

How does the learner define family, and who is in it?
What health-related tasks are they performing?
How are they functioning and how are they meeting each other's needs?
How well are they communicating?
What do these caregivers need to know?
What do they need to know now?
What do they think they need to know?
How can they learn what they need to know?

The nurse works with caregivers to set broad health-promotion goals, then directs the health teaching toward a more specific area. It is essential that caregivers agree with the goals and teaching needs. As families participate in the assessment interview, perhaps members can identify their own health-teaching needs. Health teaching includes all family members, with learning activities appropriate for each individual. The general teaching goal will be the same for all members, but the approaches and specific goals for each member or subsystem will be different. Children, adolescents, and older person members require a

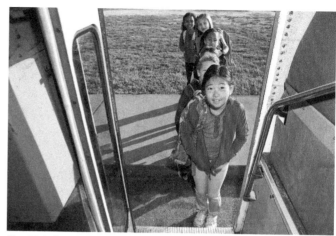

Fig. 20.1 School-age children will engage in safe travel. (iStockphoto/ Kali9.)

flexible and varied approach to teaching, due to their differences in life stages, experiences, and abilities, more so than when teaching young or middle-aged adults (Fig. 20.1).

## Health Behaviour Change

The process of health education directs people toward voluntary changes of their health behaviours. Viewing health behaviour through an ecological model, the nurse recognizes the complex interaction of individuals with their environment and the multiple influences of the individual, the interpersonal group, and the community on health behaviour. This section examines the use of commonly used models of individual health behaviour change. Community and group models in health-education planning are addressed later in this chapter.

Individual models of health behaviour help explain factors influencing and interfering with positive health behaviours. In addition, they contribute to understanding how educational intervention supports behaviour change.

Beliefs, social relationships, values, and information contribute to motivation and behaviour and are underlying factors in the making of any decision to change behaviour (Kebbe, Perez, Buchholz, et al., 2018). Health-promoting behaviours are any activities that an individual undertakes to enhance health, healthy environments, prevent disease, and detect and control the symptoms of a disease. Identifying and teaching people about lifestyle behaviours that need to be changed is only the first step in the process of assisting individuals in moving from knowledge to action. Nurses apply concepts from the protection motivation theory, social learning theory, and the transtheoretical model in subsequent steps to formulate an action plan that meets the needs and capabilities of each person in making healthy behaviour changes.

### Protection Motivation Theory

Behaviour can be influenced by intra- and interpersonal beliefs, social norms, and networks (including online influences), as well as by policies. The protection motivation theory (PMT) was developed by Ronald W. Rogers' (1975). He extended the health belief model in 1983, with several adaptations in 1984

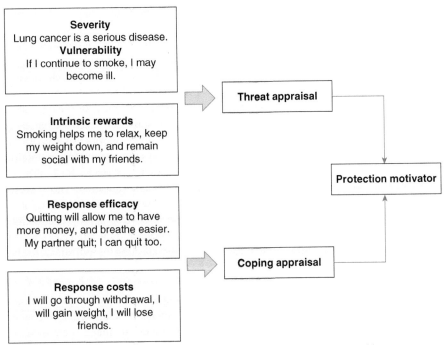

Fig. 20.2 Protection motivation theory process for quitting smoking.

and 1985, which surmises that engagement in health-promoting behaviour is based upon three factors: one's beliefs about the severity of the illness; perceived benefits of change; and barriers and confidence levels (self-efficacy) in creating change. PMT theory builds upon this and focuses on how fear influences change. The perceived severity and vulnerability of the threat is the first appraisal, and the perceived coping of the threat is the second appraisal the individual processes before attempting change. Social marketing is an example of how the use of fear utilizes the PMT, such as with stop-smoking campaigns, where the threat to health is a stimulus to protection motivation. Fig. 20.2 provides an example of the analytical processes one goes through using the PMT.

## Social Cognitive Theory

Bandura's (1997) social cognitive theory, or social learning theory, describes three interacting, reciprocal factors—behaviour (role modelling), cognition (what we think and feel), and environment (social influences)—which people learn from. The interplay between these factors is tridirectional, where people are both observers and producers of behaviour that occurs as a result of the environment; however, behaviour also influences cognition and social environment.

This theory emphasizes the influence of self-efficacy, or efficacy beliefs, on health behaviour. Self-efficacy refers to the confidence in one's ability to successfully perform and maintain change behaviours (see the Case Study and the Care Plan at the end of this chapter). When social support and resources are limited or unfavourable, confidence levels decrease (Bandura, 1982). The nurse educator facilitates behaviour change by role modelling and providing social support and resources so that all three domains of the theory are supported.

## Transtheoretical Model of Change

The transtheoretical model (TTM), or "stages of change model," is useful for determining where a person is in relation to making a behaviour change (Prochaska & DiClemente, 1984). According to the TTM, health-related behaviour change progresses through the following five stages, regardless of whether an individual is quitting or adopting a behaviour:

- *Precontemplation.* The person is not thinking about or considering quitting or adopting a behaviour change within the next 6 months (not intending to make changes).
- *Contemplation.* The person is seriously considering making a specific behaviour change within the next 6 months (considering a change).
- *Planning or preparation.* The person who has made a behaviour change is seriously thinking about making a change within the next month (making small or sporadic changes).
- *Action.* The person has made a behaviour change, and it has persisted for 6 months (actively engaged in behaviour change).
- *Maintenance.* The period beginning 6 months after the action has started and continuing indefinitely (sustaining the change over time) (Prochaska, Redding, & Everset, 2015).

The TTM is useful in determining the person's readiness for learning in relation to changing a behaviour, so that health education or behaviour-change interventions can be matched to the stage. Self-efficacy is a key construct in this model. This model also acknowledges the importance of continuing reflection and intervention to maintaining behaviour change long term. The TTM has been used by health professionals in planning interventions with a wide variety of people at risk.

Regardless of the quality of nurses' assessment methods and educational strategies, people do not always make the choices recommended to them by health professionals or adhere to the healthy changes. Naturally, health professionals want people to choose the recommended course of action, but each individual must be supported in their right to choose not to follow advice. Nurse educators must resist what motivational interviewing theorists Rollnick, Miller, and Butler (2008) refer to as the "righting reflex": the desire to correct the individual through providing unsolicited advice. The nurse, in an effort to project what is best or right for the learner, can come across as pressuring, which results in pushback (Canadian Centre on Substance Use and Addiction, 2017, p.1).

Enlisting the individual's partnership or cooperation achieves better results. This can be done by exploring the learner's ambivalence: the simultaneous conflict that occurs when considering change. The nurse acknowledges the difficulties and drawbacks of the change process, and even discusses the learner's reasons *not* to change. By discussing the downside to change, such as moving away from familiarity and comfort, the nurse is able to establish a rapport of understanding, and assist the individual to appreciate the discrepancy between the life that is being lived and the life that is desired, thus creating intrinsic motivation to move toward change. Effective health education requires an understanding of the influential factors affecting the individual's decision making, including the comforts that the current behaviour holds.

Another key factor in the ability to comply with health education is the barriers that occur as a result of the social determinants of health. The individual may not have the resources to pay for a proper diet or may not feel safe exercising at a public facility due to their ethnicity, gender, or sexual orientation. It is important to assess the impact that the social determinants of health may have on the individual's ability and confidence for change, and seek ways for the learner to navigate barriers with the nurse's assistance, thus increasing confidence levels and reducing victim blaming.

Many health professionals tend to view a person's cooperation with the health care regimen as a single choice, when this cooperation often involves many choices every day. For example, following a low-processed food diet involves constant, and often inconvenient, costlier choices that must be considered each day. The expectation is that people will do this every day for the rest of their lives, even when the nurse cannot guarantee health as a result.

Nurses can increase an individual's motivation and capabilities to change by involving the individual in planning and goal setting, providing information that is understandable and acceptable, and assisting the person in developing new skills. The use of Doran's (1981) SMART goals provides the framework for goal setting:

- Specific
- Measurable
- Attainable
- Relevant/realistic
- Time-based

After establishing that the individual has voiced a desire to change, the nurse can use the following key action points for developing interventions for behaviour change:

- Assess the behaviour for the role it plays in the person's life.
- Assess readiness to receive information.
- Assess the confidence level the person has in the ability to change.
- Assess driving factors or values that influence priorities and perceived need for change.
- Motivate and enhance self-efficacy by using personalized messages and affirmations.
- Support autonomy for the type and degree of change.
- Offer resources to decrease barriers to change.
- Assist the person with using SMART goals to modify behaviour.
- Plan ways to monitor and maintain the behaviour change.

Theories and strategies for health behaviour change are at the heart of health education. Those presented in this section help nurses to assess an individual's stage in the behaviour-change process and to develop appropriate teaching plans. The goals of the teaching plans and the strategies selected will differ, depending on the factors affecting the individual's readiness to learn and to change.

## Ethics

Applying principles of respect, autonomy, justice, and beneficence, nurses have an active role as advocates in empowering care recipients to make their own informed decisions about their health and care. The nurse works collaboratively with the individual and family to make optimal health care decisions that align with the needs, goals, and values of the individual and family, a process called shared decision making (SDM) (National Quality Forum, 2018, p. 1).

Research is proving that the use of SDM increases clinician awareness and skills in addressing issues that may not be uncovered in an information-giving style of education. This is particularly true for groups such as lesbian, gay, bisexual, transgender, queer/questioning, and two-spirit (LGBTQ2) persons who may not feel comfortable disclosing their sexual identity or who avoid care altogether for fear they will be misunderstood or discriminated against (Chin, Lopez, Nathan, et al., 2016, p. 591), for example, a transgender man who resists undergoing a Pap test, a test that is associated with being female. Understanding the complex inter- and intrapersonal dynamics fosters open communication and shared decision making, leading to the nurse providing informative, unbiased, and relevant care that respects the individual's goals and concerns.

Although the focus of health education may be on the behaviour-change process, the nurse must exercise caution when trying to persuade the individual to consider healthy alternatives. The potential for inadvertent manipulation and coercion exists, particularly when addressing different cultural or minority groups who may not feel empowered, may not have proficient use of the English language, or who have conflicting traditional practices, to voice their wants or opinions. All competent people have the right to autonomous choice. Nurses must respect decisions made by the individual and their caregivers, even when the choice is considered "unhealthy" or not what the nurse might suggest or do. This can become particularly difficult in tripartite interactions—those that involve the nurse, the individual and another caregiver—such as with parents and children. Box 20.3 provides a case example of how easy it is to inadvertently coerce individuals into conforming to the expert's ideals, and how using SDM can avoid this.

## BOX 20.3   Case Example: Shared Decision Making, Immunization, and Ethics

A father brought his 13-year-old son to the nurse to seek advice about immunizations. All immunizations had previously been refused by the mother and the father was unsure of the benefits of immunization because he only had the information from his ex-partner about the negative aspects of immunization. All contact had been lost between the father and his ex-partner since he had been granted full custody and decision-making rights of the child. The child expressed apprehension regarding the vaccines because of the physical pain associated with the injections, and the decision to go against his mother's wishes. The nurse, concerned that the child was immunization-naive, discussed the need for immediate vaccination as well as the risks associated with exposure to vaccine-preventable diseases. The father agreed to immunize the child that day, following the catch-up immunization schedule which calls for multiple immunizations in one visit.

In this instance, the nurse's well-intentioned prompt advice and action resulted in a lack of information regarding the risks and benefits of the vaccines as well as a disregard for the child's concerns. Had shared decision-making (SDM) occurred, the nurse would have assisted this family in working through the conflict regarding the mother's wishes and discussed how this might impact the child's relationship with his mother; risks, benefits, side effects, and concerns would have been discussed in greater detail, as well. At that time, the decision of whether or not to immunize would have been supported by all parties. By not using an SDM approach and instead focusing on the nurse's own agenda, crucial information was missed, resulting in the potential for nurse liability had a negative outcome ensued.

## BOX 20.4   Advocating, Educating, and Assessing: Jordan's Principle

Indigenous people often face health challenges, such as limited access to care, poverty, and increased rates of obesity. Indigenous children are more often than non-Indigenous children left waiting for services they need, or are denied services that are available to other children, because of funding conflicts between provincial and federal governments. Jordan's Principle is a child-first principle named in memory of Jordan River Anderson, a First Nations child from Norway House Cree Nation in Manitoba, who died at the age of 5 in hospital from a rare disorder, never having gone home from hospital since birth.

Jordan's Principle ensures that no Indigenous children experience delays, denials, or disruptions in services while government agencies work through administrative and jurisdictional disputes (First Nations Child and Family Caring Society of Canada, 2018). In 2016 the Canadian Indigenous Nurses Association (then ANAC) and the Canadian Nurses Association (CNA) signed a partnership to further develop their collaborative Indigenous health and nursing work. As a result, the two associations together endorse Jordan's Principle and support innovation in this area (CNA, 2019). The nurses' role is to advocate for Indigenous children and youth who have a suspected or confirmed developmental disability or complex medical needs and report a case of Jordan's Principle so that prompt care can be implemented (First Nations Health Authority [FNHA], 2019). Education and assessment of the child and caregivers affected by this principle are also a part of the nursing role.

Sources: First Nations Child and Family Caring Society of Canada. (2018). *Jordan's Principle: Ensuring First Nations children receive the public services they need when they need them*. Retrieved from https://fncaringsociety.com/sites/default/files/jordans_principle_information_sheet_november_2018.pdf; Canadian Nurses Association (CNA). (2019). *Indigenous health*. Retrieved from https://www.cna-aiic.ca/en/policy-advocacy/indigenous-health; First Nations Health Authority (FNHA). (2019). *Jordan's Principle*. Retrieved from http://www.fnha.ca/what-we-do/maternal-child-and-family-health/jordans-principle.

## Genomics and Health Education

Advances in genetics and genomics present new opportunities and responsibilities for nurses in health education. Over-the-counter or mail-in use of genetic and genomic technologies requires nurses to incorporate information and implications of the technologies into educational programs for vulnerable individuals, families, and populations. The Canadian Nurses Association (CNA) supports the role of nurses providing unbiased genetic counselling to clients, which includes deciphering technical medical jargon to those who struggle to make decisions about reproductive and genetic technologies. As such, nurses who have in-depth preparation and experience in this field have a crucial role to play in not only advocating for the client but also "in shaping policies about assisted human reproduction; genetic testing; genetic therapy; genetic enhancements; the human genome project and privacy concerns; and human cloning" (CNA, 2002, p. 1). Although an increasingly wide range of situations include the need for the nurse to be prepared to discuss genetics and genomics, the primary focus for nursing is health promotion, symptom management, and disease prevention.

## Diversity and Health Teaching

Diversity extends beyond race and ethnicity and includes economic status, language, gender, religion, and sexual orientation, all coinciding with the social determinants of health, and contributing to the potential for health inequity. This diversity can influence beliefs about health, perceptions of disease and illness, health-seeking behaviours, and attitudes toward health providers, and plays a role in the use of traditional and complementary healing practices. Nurses must recognize how the key determinants of health, including experiences of discrimination or historical trauma, influence the health and well-being of specific population groups (Government of Canada, 2018, para. 2). Advocacy to address these influences, as well as to support each group's unique and diverse experiences, must occur, while noting the impact of language, literacy level, sexual orientation, age, educational background, and culture on the abilities of the individual to apply health education strategies (Box 20.4).

Nurses also need to provide a safe, nonjudgmental environment for the LGBTQ2 community. This involves using inclusive language (such as "partner" rather than "spouse" and "relationship status" instead of "marital status"), identifying oneself by their pronoun, and asking which pronouns clients associate with so as to generate appropriate and sensitive communication. Finally, nurses assist those to remove obstacles to living a life of enjoyment. Researchers who have studied the experiences of LGBTQ2 people have found that as a result of living with intolerance, they suffer from threats of, or actual experience of, violence from strangers, peers, and family, and experience barriers to education and employment, resulting in increased homelessness, substance misuse, and the development of mental health concerns (OK2BME, 2019).

### Cultural Aspects of Health Teaching

**When There Is a Language Barrier**
- Use courtesy and a formal approach.
- Address the person by his or her last name; then clarify how the person wishes to be addressed, including clarification of the use of pronouns.
- Introduce yourself, pointing to yourself as you give your name.
- Avoid overgeneralizing, stereotyping, or other culturally biased assumptions.
- Attempt to use words in the person's language, indicating respect for the individual's culture.
- Use simple, everyday words rather than complex words, medical jargon, or colloquialisms.
- Use hand gestures to help the person understand, but be aware that differences in both verbal and nonverbal communication can influence care.
- Instruct the person in small increments.
- Have the person demonstrate understanding of the message.
- Provide written instructions for the person to take home, preferably in their own language.
- When available, provide written material in other languages.
- Use qualified health care interpreters.

**Areas to Consider in Cultural Assessment**
- How does the individual identify with a particular cultural group?
- What are their habits, customs, values, and beliefs?
- Are there any cultural sanctions or restrictions?
- Do they have any spiritual or religious beliefs and practices?
- Are they a part of any specific social networks that support their culture?
- Are there any nutritional beliefs, food preferences, and restrictions?

**Reflective Questions**
- What are my own cultural assumptions, beliefs, and biases that need to be challenged? How do these affect my provision of care?
- How can I obtain and use materials (such as magazines, brochures, artwork) in my work that reflect the social and cultural diversity of the people I serve?

Sources: Adapted from Canadian Pediatric Society. (2019). *Caring for kids new to Canada: A guide for health professionals working with immigrant and refugee children and youth*. Retrieved from https://www.kidsnewtocanada.ca/culture/competence#key-points; Andrews, M. M., & Boyle, J. S. (2016). *Transcultural concepts in nursing care* (7th ed.). Philadelphia: Wolters Kluwer/Lippincott.

The CNA's position statement on cultural humility requires nurses to reflect on their own privilege and determine how their values and experiences impact the way they provide care (CNA, 2018, p. 3). When teaching people of different cultural, racial, sexual, and ethnic groups, the nurse endeavours to provide culturally safe education. Nurses recognize that the person's or group's background, beliefs, and knowledge may differ significantly from their own and seek to respect different world views, openness to traditional healing practices, and maintain flexibility in integrating cultural practices in the plan of care (Debs-Ivall, 2018, para. 4) (Diversity Awareness).

## COMMUNITY AND GROUP HEALTH EDUCATION

When nurses begin to teach groups of people, they automatically enter a program planning and administrative process. When an organization wants to offer an ongoing health-education program for a target population, social marketing provides a strategy for reaching members of the group and implementing a service that will satisfy these members as consumers. Community-based social marketing is defined as marketing principles and techniques—such as prompts, messaging, and images—that those who develop and deliver programs use to promote sustainability and benefit the individual and society. It involves "identifying barriers to a behaviour, developing and piloting a program to overcome these barriers, implementing the program across a community and evaluating the effectiveness of a program" (Government of Canada, 2013, bullets 4–7). An example of social marketing in Canada is Worksafe Saskatchewan's Mission Zero sticker campaign, which promotes the goals of achieving zero workplace injuries, fatalities, and suffering by families. The campaign was initiated in 2008 in response to Saskatchewan having the second worst workplace injury rates in Canada (Safe Saskatchewan, 2018, p. 3). Principles of social marketing and health-education strategies are combined, along with concepts from community group health behaviour-change models and health-education strategies, to promote population-based changes in behaviour to improve health. Social marketing provides a strategy for reaching members of the group and implementing a service that will satisfy these members as consumers.

Social marketing communication reaches beyond the individual level to influence social conditions, policy, legislation, and normative group behaviour. Key attributes of a social marketing approach are the offering of benefits and the reduction of barriers to influence the target group's behaviour. Social marketing strategies could be used in designing programs for health promotion (tobacco use, obesity), injury prevention (seat-belt wearing, helmet use), and environmental protection (reducing engine idling, water conservation). Any results of the social marketing campaign that impacts the target population will improve the nurse's ability to develop effective educational interventions.

Another model commonly used in community health-education planning is the diffusion of innovations model (Rogers, 2003), which explains how an idea or product is adopted and spreads through a social system. In public health, diffusion of innovations is used to address the factors that support or inhibit the adoption of effective, evidence-informed interventions to improve community health. Practical application of the model involves addressing factors such as ease of use, trialability, and advantageous benefit, understanding the target population and recognizing the importance of achieving a good fit among the characteristics of the innovation, the community adopting it, and the context or environment for change (Brownson, Tabak, Stamatakis, et al., 2015).

## TEACHING PLAN

Preparation for teaching a group program, such as a seminar or course, begins after the marketing and administrative plans are well under way. These activities ensure that there are enough participants for the program, and they provide the structure for developing the teaching plan—the program objectives, available time, human and material resources, and so on. When the marketing and administrative functions have been provided by others, and when educational strategies are developed for one person at a time, the nurse can concentrate efforts on developing the teaching plan.

A health-teaching plan may emphasize a phase of the behaviour-change process that is related to the individual's or group's health-promotion needs or problems. The written teaching plan represents a package of educational services provided to a consumer or student. The plan is written from the learner's point of view.

The process of generating a teaching plan helps the nurse recognize and use methods of learning that involve the individual as an active participant. The plan includes a list of specific actions or abilities that the person may perform at intervals during and at the end of the educational intervention. Teaching plans help nurses clarify intended outcomes. Preparing a teaching plan involves the steps of the teaching–learning process outlined in Box 20.5.

## Assessment

Assessment, the first step in the process, involves determining the characteristics of the learner and identifying learning needs. The following characteristics of the learner are important for the nurse to identify and consider in planning:

- Age, developmental stage in the life cycle, and level of education
- Health beliefs
- Motivation and readiness to learn
- Health risks and problems
- Current knowledge and skills
  Barriers and facilitators to learning:
- The reader is encouraged to refer to the chapters (see Unit 3) about individual development

Assessment of the learner can be accomplished by answering the following five questions:

- What are the characteristics and learning capabilities of the individual?
- What are the learner's needs for health promotion, risk reduction, or health problems?
- What does the person already know and what skills can the person already perform that are relevant to the health needs?
- Is the learner motivated to change any unhealthy behaviours?

---

### BOX 20.5   Steps in the Teaching–Learning Process

Assessment:
- Learner characteristics
- Learning needs

Development of intended learning outcomes

Development of a teaching plan:
- Content
- Teaching strategies, learning activities
- Use of technology

Implementation of the teaching plan

Evaluation of expected outcomes:
- Achievement of learning outcomes

Evaluation of the teaching process

---

- What are the barriers to and facilitators of health behaviour change?

When preparing a teaching plan for one person in a primary care setting, the nurse may learn background information about the individual from that person's record and agency reports that include descriptions of the person's population group. Nurses often agree to teach health classes that others have organized. In this case the nurse asks for project reports that provide marketing and needs-assessment information about the students who are expected to attend the classes (see the Care Plan at the end of the chapter).

## Program Goals

The program goals of a health-education project reflect the desire to facilitate improvement in a larger-scale health problem or social living conditions. Program goals are broad statements on long-range expected accomplishments that provide direction; they establish criteria and standards for which performance is measured, evaluated, and improved.

## Learning Goals

Learning goals are best established when the student and the nurse work together. These goals reflect the health behaviour or health status change that the person will have achieved by the end of an educational intervention. Learning goals relate to the program goals and are learner or community needs driven.

## Determining Intended Learning Outcomes

To determine the intended learning outcomes of a health-education intervention, the nurse answers the following questions:

- What broad public health and social goals guide the proposed educational program?
- What are the participant's learning goals?
- What does the learner need to know, do, and believe to progress through the behaviour-change process?

Intended learning outcomes indicate the steps to be taken by the individual toward meeting the learning goal, and may involve the development of knowledge, skill, or change in attitude. Learning outcomes are often used interchangeably with learning objectives. However, learning objectives signify what the teacher intends to teach (teacher-driven), whereas learning outcomes project the expectations of the student's learning as far as what the learner will achieve, understand, or perform after being educated.

Regardless of terminology, objectives or outcomes are most useful when stated in behavioural terms and when they contain the following components: a precise action verb indicating what the learner will be able to do; the conditions under which the task is performed; and the level of performance expected. Learning outcomes guide the selection of content and methods and help narrow the focus of a teaching plan to more achievable steps; they also aid in setting standards of performance and suggesting evaluation strategies (Centre for Teaching Support & Innovation, University of Toronto, 2019, para. 2).

## TABLE 20.1   Examples of Nonmeasurable and Measurable Outcomes

| Domain | Outcomes |
|---|---|
| Cognitive | **Not measurable:** Dan will understand the correct food choices for following a low-salt diet<br>**Measurable:** Dan will correctly *select* low-salt foods from the options provided |
| Affective | **Not measurable:** Dan will demonstrate the importance of low salt intake<br>**Measurable:** Dan will *verbalize* the importance of low salt intake by *discussing* the impact this will have on his health |
| Psychomotor | **Not measurable:** Dan will know how to determine a serving<br>**Measurable:** Dan will *demonstrate* correct measurement of a one-serving portion |

## TABLE 20.2   Domains of Learning, Teaching Strategies, and Examples of Desired Outcomes Related to a Behaviour Change

| Domains of Learning | Teaching Strategies | Examples of Desired Outcomes Related to a Behaviour Change |
|---|---|---|
| Cognitive (thinking) | Lecture<br>One-to-one instruction<br>Discussion<br>Audiovisual or print<br>Computer-assisted/ simulation | Describes and/or explains information relevant to the behaviour change |
| Affective (feeling) | Role modelling<br>Discussion<br>Role playing<br>Simulation gaming/ virtual reality | Expresses positive feeling, attitudes, values toward changing the behaviour |
| Psychomotor (acting) | Demonstration<br>Practice<br>Mental imaging | Demonstrates performance of skills related to the behaviour change |

## Examples of Learning Outcomes

In writing learning outcomes, the nurse selects action verbs from taxonomies that indicate observable learning. In Table 20.1, examples are given for outcomes in each domain of learning. The first objective listed for each domain is incorrect because the verb does not indicate observable learning. The second example for each domain is measurable because the verb used (indicated in boldface, italic type) allows the learning to be observed.

When preparing a teaching plan, the nurse differentiates information the individual *needs to know* from information considered *helpful to know* in order to develop appropriate learning objectives. This process provides cues to the nurse for planning effective strategies for the necessary level of learning. As the level of learning to be achieved becomes complex, the educational strategies and methods selected involve the individuals in more active application and analysis of the content.

## Three Domains of Learning

A key component of a health-education program is content. When selecting content, the nurse considers what information, skills, and attitudes need to be taught and the level of learning to be achieved.

Content is commonly divided into three domains: cognitive; psychomotor; and affective. Cognitive learning refers to the development of new facts or concepts, and building on or applying knowledge to new situations. Psychomotor learning involves developing physical skills from simple to complex actions. Affective learning alludes to the recognition of values, religious and spiritual beliefs, family interaction patterns and relationships, and personal attitudes that affect decisions and problem-solving progress.

To learn or change a health behaviour, a person may need to acquire new information, practice some physical techniques, and clarify the ways in which the new behaviour may affect relationships with others. The nurse's role is to select a combination of content from the three domains that is appropriate to meet the behavioural objective. To find samples of content for a teaching plan, the nurse researches resource materials, such as books, teaching guides, journal articles, pamphlets, and flyers created by nonprofit agencies and professional organizations. The nurse is careful about giving students materials with technical vocabulary that is too complex for the audience.

## Designing Learning Strategies

Designing the learning strategies for an educational intervention involves selecting the methods and tools and structuring the sequence of activities. The teaching plan to this point provides the foundation on which to base the activity selection and sequence. The following questions guide the design of learning strategies:

- What are some basic considerations for selecting teaching methods for health-education programs?
- How does the nurse, as instructor, establish and maintain a learning climate?
- What actions can the nurse perform to increase the effectiveness of the learning methods?
- How can the use of technology (virtual reality, simulation, apps) support the learning experience?
- What methods tend to promote behaviour change?

## Teaching Strategies

Numerous strategies for teaching are available (Table 20.2). A few of those most commonly used are listed and described here. Lecture is a well-known method in which the teacher verbally presents information and instructions to the person or audience and where the term 'learning objectives' might be most appropriate. Lecture provides a way to present a large amount of information to a number of people in a nonthreatening way. This can be an effective method if active learning strategies such as learner participation through questioning are integrated. Discussion involves interaction between the nurse educator and the individuals. The nurse may prepare questions in advance to guide the discussion. This method allows an opportunity for the nurse to gain a better perception of the individuals' understanding of the topic and to clarify the information and learning goals; the term "learning outcomes" is most appropriate for this style of teaching.

Demonstration and practice are used in learning psychomotor skills such as performing exercises. The nurse demonstrates the expected behaviour while the person observes. Then the nurse watches and provides feedback and encouragement while the person performs the behaviour. Using the actual equipment that individuals will use in their home facilitates successful performance. For complex tasks, teaching a few steps at a time, in sequence, and that build upon one another, aids skill development.

Simulation gaming may involve computer "apps" or role play. An example might be providing an app that compares *Canada's Dietary Guidelines* recommendations to home grocery lists. Role play involves acting out a potential scenario, allowing individuals to practice appropriate responses to challenging situations. For example, a person restricted to a low-sugar diet can act out a response to being offered dessert by an insistent family member or friend played by the nurse.

### Considerations for Selecting Methods

The nurse's first consideration is to use methods that promote self-directed learning. An active participant usually learns more.

Factoring in the characteristics of the population (developmental stage, age, and knowledge of the topic and learning styles), the nurse selects teaching methods that best support the goals of the educational program, and varies the teaching methods in a given session. The nurse is sensitive to the energy level and anxiety of the audience when presenting content that requires strong concentration or causes anxiety.

### Learning Climate

For group presentations the nurse addresses several activities when seeking to establish an environment that is conducive to health behaviour change. The first activity is creating a sense of preparedness and organization by providing physical facilities with adequate furnishings and suitable audiovisual materials and handouts. Even the instructor's appearance will lend credibility or distraction to the presentation; first impressions count!

The second activity involves anticipating the needs of the group and communicating information about the schedule and the facilities. This action alleviates the group's apprehension and makes the group members more comfortable.

The third activity focuses on the nurse's assessment of the individual and group learning needs, possibly through questions and dialogue. Members of the group need to believe that the program will be beneficial and relevant to their situations. The instructor watches for and reinforces signs of motivation to participate in the experience.

Fourth, having established a positive learning climate, the nurse seeks to maintain a high level of motivation, a sense of individualized attention, and a progression. As a check, the nurse might ask for periodic feedback from the group about the effectiveness of the program and its relevance to group needs.

Finally, the nurse works with the group to maintain the learning climate. This process involves observing group interactions, helping individuals to participate, intervening to help the group deal with controlling its members, and remaining cognizant of dynamics in the group process that will facilitate or inhibit learning.

### Teaching for Each Learning Domain

As mentioned, teaching is directed toward one or more of three learning domains: cognitive, psychomotor, and affective. Examples of appropriate teaching strategies for each domain and the expected outcomes in relation to behaviour change are summarized in Table 20.2.

### Evaluating the Teaching–Learning Process

The teacher can evaluate the learning, or measure achievement of learning outcomes in all domains through the use of written or oral testing, demonstrations, observation, self-reports, and self-monitoring.

The nurse can incorporate techniques for obtaining feedback about teaching performance into the teaching plan. Confidential, end-of-program questionnaires are the usual method for obtaining written feedback. The nurse may ask for verbal feedback at various times from the group, from individual students, and from observers of the class. Nonverbal communication cues from participants may indicate their satisfaction, fatigue, or frustration with the educational intervention. Word-of-mouth referrals to future programs and support from other community agencies and professionals may also indicate approval of the program format.

The overall process of the teaching–learning experience needs to be evaluated. The procedures used to organize and promote an educational program can affect its ultimate success. The nurse (or a program administration committee) records activities such as advertising, registration, fee collection, and availability and repair of equipment and materials. This evaluative information can then be used to improve subsequent programs.

Occasionally, the nurse is asked to justify a health-education program in terms of its effect on the community's public health goals or social problems. Health promotion involves a combination of health-protection activities, preventive health services, and health-education programs; therefore, drawing a direct correlation between one particular educational intervention and the statistical improvement of the health problem can be difficult. Statistics, such as the number of people served each year, the percentage of the target population reached, the number of service providers used, and the number and cost of programs, are important and need to be preserved. As these statistics change over time, the data will provide cues to program successes and problems. Nurses can also describe the pedagogy, the theory and practice of education and its effects on health and social problems and behaviours.

### Evaluating Resources

The end of a teaching plan includes resources for people to use for continuing education, counselling, peer support, and health services; providing additional resources reinforces and sustains the initial teaching. The Internet as a health-education tool may either positively or negatively influence a person's health practices, but can prove to be beneficial because it reduces barriers to accessing health information. With a wealth of information widely and readily available to many, the nurse educator must establish the validity and reliability of resources that are used by the nurse, or presented by the learner to the nurse, for review.

Peer-reviewed, evidence-informed resources are the most reliable sources of information, whereas general Internet sites can project bias and lack evidence. Regardless of the type of resource used, tools such as Blakeslee's (2004, p. 6) CRAAP method for evaluation: currency, relevance/reputability, appropriateness (cultural), accuracy and purpose.

Reliable, scholarly Internet resources are most easily determined by looking at the site domain, the ending of the URL address. Generally speaking, .edu, .gov, or .org reflect reliable educational, governmental, and organizational institutions, whereas, .com and .net reflect commercial businesses or organizations related to the Internet, and do not necessarily offer unbiased information.

Use of particular types of search tools can also set the stage for the validity of information retrieved, such as general Internet search engines versus scholarly library databases or using "Health on the Net" toolbars that facilitate access to reliable health information (HON, 2018).

Electronic peer-reviewed journals, pdf client teaching information sheets from reputable sources, and providing websites hosted by accredited organizations, (e.g., Toronto Hospital for Sick Children's *AboutKidsHealth.ca* website) are some of ways informatics is used in nursing to provide reliable information (Fig. 20.3).

## TEACHING AND ORGANIZING SKILLS

To develop teaching and organizing skills in health education, the nurse often needs to learn new behaviours. Nurses can systematically perform steps to assist in obtaining these skills:

- Seek self-assessment opportunities.
- Identify, list, and prioritize learning needs.
- Begin to identify the resources that are available for reading, instructor training, and practice teaching.
- Select the target population and the general topic.
- Draft an initial set of learning goals.
- Work through the steps of the teaching–learning process, including the development of a teaching plan.
- Identify other people or a project team to help.

After implementing the educational intervention, the nurse sets time aside to discuss the outcomes, review what worked and what didn't work, and revise the teaching for the next session.

In addition, health-education research evaluates teaching interventions. This contributes to the evidence base from which nurses can implement new teaching strategies or question the effectiveness of traditional approaches. An example of a study of interdisciplinary pedagogy in the field of sustainable

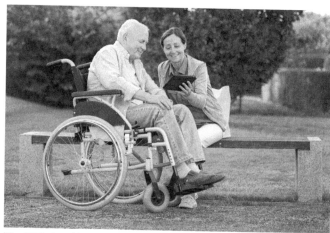

**Fig. 20.3** An older person using computer-based information for education. (iStockphoto/FredFroese.)

food systems is provided in Research for Evidence-Informed Practice.

As additional programs on either an individual or a group basis are provided, the nurse will be able to clarify specific instructor teaching and organizing skills that come naturally.

These skills tend to improve a program's effectiveness and enable the logistics to run smoothly. The teacher is first a learner; this is true in health education and any other form of education.

## RESEARCH FOR EVIDENCE-INFORMED PRACTICE

### *Emergent Themes From Sustainable Food Systems Education Resulting in Signature Pedagogy*

There is a growing concern about the ways in which our current food system matches population need at the risk of negatively impacting the environment. Concepts of food security and environmental sustainability have often been taught separately from one another, despite growing evidence that this disconnect serves as a barrier to food systems transformation. To address this concern, educators at University of British Columbia developed new interdisciplinary educational programs, termed sustainable food system education (SFSE), that link these two concepts together to address the complexities of the modern food system.

Educators who participated in the SFSE programs evaluated the programs and identified common pedagogical themes that emerged. These themes, consisting of systems thinking, multi-, inter-, and transdisciplinary experimental learning approaches and participatory learning were then used to develop a signature teaching model for use in future SFSE programs. Presenting this model to scholars and practitioners for review allows the dialogue on SFSE theory and practice to advance, and addresses challenges encountered during the process of educating varying disciplines.

Source: Valley, W., Wittman, H., Jordan, N., et al. (2018). An emerging signature pedagogy for sustainable food systems education. *Renewable Agriculture and Food Systems, 33*(5), 467–480. https://doi.org/10.1017/S1742170517000199

## CASE STUDY

### Albert

Albert Mitchell is a 36-year-old man who will be travelling to Dubai to give a business presentation in 3 months. Although he has travelled widely in Canada as a consultant, this is his first trip to the Middle East. He requests information regarding immunizations needed before his trip. Albert states that as he will only be in Dubai for few days, he is unlikely to contract a disease in such a short time and therefore believes that it is illogical to obtain immunizations. Albert states that he has heard the side effects of the immunizations might be worse than the diseases they prevent. He is also concerned about leaving his wife at home alone because she is 6 months pregnant.

**Reflective Questions**

- How would you address Albert's beliefs?
- What learning, for you and for Albert, would be needed in each domain?
- What learning theories would you consider?
- How might his family concerns be addressed?

## CARE PLAN

### Preparing a Teaching Plan

**Nursing Issue**
Deficient knowledge (specify area)

**Defining Characteristics**
- Verbalization of inadequate information or an inadequate recall of information
- Verbalization of misunderstanding or misconception
- Request for information
- Instructions followed inaccurately
- Inadequate performance on a test
- Inadequate demonstration of a skill

**Related Factors**
- Pathophysiological states
- Sensory deficits
- Memory loss
- Intellectual limitations
- Interfering coping strategies (denial or anxiety)
- Lack of exposure to accurate information
- Lack of motivation to learn
- Inattention
- Cultural or language barriers

**Intended Outcomes**
The learner will:
- Express an interest in learning.
- Correctly state the information on the specific topic.
- Correctly demonstrate skills needed to practice health-related behaviour.
- Modify health behaviour on the basis of the acquisition of new knowledge.
- List resources for more information or support.
- The individual and the family will explain how to incorporate new information into their lifestyle.

**Interventions**
- Provide accurate and culturally relevant information related to the specific topic.
- Select teaching techniques appropriate to the individual's learning needs.
- Explore the individual's interpretation of the information and its meaning in the context of the person's life.
- Demonstrate and then have the individual practise new skills.
- Assist the person in identifying and implementing alternative strategies when initial choices are not successful.
- Include significant others as appropriate.
- Provide names, telephone numbers, Internet sources of resource people, or organizations.

## SUMMARY

Of all health care providers, nurses spend the most time in direct contact with individuals; they have many opportunities to recognize a need for knowledge and a readiness to learn new information and behaviours. The more accurate the assessment of the learner's needs and barriers, and the more flexible and diverse components of a health-promotion program are, the more effective an educational intervention will be in influencing health behaviours.

Planning to teach one person is different from planning to teach a group. One-to-one interventions tend to follow a counselling or problem-solving approach. Group interventions can range from guided discussions on concerns that evolve from the group to a more structured learning experience involving presentations, skill practice, and attitude-awareness exercises. The range of health-education strategies provides nurses with techniques and methods applicable to health service settings, schools, work sites, and other community facilities.

**Evolve Chapter Features**
http://evolve.elsevier.com/Canada/Edelman/healthpromotion/
- Review Questions

# REFERENCES

Bandura, A. (1982). The psychology of chance encounters and life paths. *American Psychologist, 37,* 747–755. [Seminal Reference].

Bandura, A. (1997). *Self-efficacy: The exercise of control.* New York: W. H. Freeman. [Seminal Reference].

Blakeslee, S. (2004). The CRAAP test. *LOEX Quarterly, 31*(3). Retrieved from https://commons.emich.edu/loexquarterly/vol31/iss3/4/.

British Columbia Ministry of Health. (2015). *The British Columbia Patient-Centred Care Framework.* Retrieved from http://www.health.gov.bc.ca/library/publications/year/2015_a/pt-centred-care-framework.pdf.

Brownson, R. C., Tabak, R. G., Stamatakis, K. A., et al. (2015). Implementation, diffusion, & dissemination of public health interventions. In K. Glanz, B. K. Rimer, & K. Viswanath (Eds.), *Health behaviour and health education: Theory, research, and practice* (5th ed.). (pp. 301–326). San Francisco: Jossey-Bass.

Canadian Centre on Substance Use and Addiction. (2017). *Motivational interviewing.* Retrieved from http://ccsa.ca/Resource%20Library/CCSA-Motivational-Interviewing-Summary-2017-en.pdf.

Canadian Foundation for Healthcare Improvement. (2019). *Better how? Our commitment to a culture of engagement.* Retrieved from https://www.cfhi-fcass.ca/OurImpact/better-how.

Canadian Nurses Association (CNA). (2002). *The role of the nurse in reproductive and genetic technologies.* [pdf file]. Retrieved from https://www.cna-aiic.ca/~/media/cna/page-content/pdf-fr/ps58_role_nurse_reproductive_genetic_technologies_march_2002_e.pdf?la=en.

Canadian Nurses Association (CNA). (2015). *Framework for the practice of registered nurses in Canada.* Retrieved from https://www.cna-aiic.ca/-/media/cna/page-content/pdf-en/position_statement_promoting_cultural_competence_in_nursing.pdf?la=en&hash=4B-394DAE5C2138E7F6134D59E505DCB059754BA9.

Canadian Nurses Association (CNA). (2018). *Promoting cultural competence in nursing.* [pdf file]. Retrieved from https://www.cna-aiic.ca/-/media/cna/page-content/pdfen/position_statement_promoting_cultural_competence_in_nursing.pdf?la=en&hash=4B394DAE-5C2138E7F6134D59E505DCB059754BA9.

Canadian Nurses Association (CNA). (2019). *Indigenous health.* Retrieved from https://www.cna-aiic.ca/en/policy-advocacy/indigenous-health.

Canadian Patient Safety Institute (CPSI). (2018). *Engaging patients in patient safety: A Canadian guide* [pdf file]. Retrieved from https://www.patientsafetyinstitute.ca/en/toolsResources/Patient-Engagement-in-Patient-Safety-Guide/Documents/Engaging%20Patients%20in%20Patient%20Safety.pdf.

Centre for Teaching Support & Innovation, University of Toronto. (2019). *What are learning outcomes?* Retrieved from https://teaching.utoronto.ca/teaching-support/course-design/developing-learning-outcomes/what-are-learning-outcomes/.

Chin, M., Lopez, F., Nathan, A., et al. (2016). Improving shared decision making with LGBT racial and ethnic minority patients. *Journal of General Internal Medicine, 31*(6), 591–593. https://doi.org/10.1007/s11606-016-3607-4.

Debs-Ivall, S. (2018). Do you value difference and embrace diversity a strength? *Canadian Nurse* (May 4). Retrieved from https://canadian-nurse.com/en/articles/issues/2018/may-june-2018/do-you-value-difference-and-embrace-diversity-as-a-strength.

Doran, G. T. (1981). There's a S.M.A.R.T. way to write management's goals and objectives. *Management Review, 70*(35). [Seminal Reference].

First Nations Child and Family Caring Society of Canada. (2018). *Jordan's Principle: Ensuring First Nations children receive the public services they need when they need them.* Retrieved from https://fncaringsociety.com/sites/default/files/jordans_principle_information_sheet_november_2018.pdf.

First Nations Health Authority (FNHA). (2019). *Jordan's Principle.* Retrieved from http://www.fnha.ca/what-we-do/maternal-child-and-family-health/jordans-principle.

Government of Canada. (2013). *An overview of community-based social marketing.* Retrieved from https://www.nrcan.gc.ca/energy/efficiency/communities-infrastructure/transportation/municipal-communities/4401.

Government of Canada. (2017a). *Canada Health Act* [PDF file]. Ottawa: Minister of Justice. Retrieved from https://laws-lois.justice.gc.ca/PDF/C-6.pdf.

Government of Canada. (2017b). *Towards a poverty reduction strategy—Discussion paper* [pdf file]. Retrieved from http://publications.gc.ca/collections/collection_2016/edsc-esdc/Em20-53-2016-eng.pdf.

Government of Canada. (2018). *Social determinants of health and health inequalities.* Retrieved from https://www.canada.ca/en/public-health/services/health-promotion/population-health/what-determines-health.html.

Groleau, D., Benady-Chorney, J., Panaitoiu, A., et al. (2019). Hyperemesis gravidarum in the context of migration: When the absence of cultural meaning gives rise to "blaming the victim. *BMC Pregnancy and Childbirth, 19*(1), 197. https://doi.org/10.1186/s12884-019-2344-1.

HON. (2018). *Medical professional.* Retrieved from https://www.hon.ch/med.html.

Kebbe, M., Perez, A., Buchholz, A., et al. (2018). Barriers and enablers for adopting lifestyle behavior changes in adolescents with obesity: A multicentre, qualitative study. *PLoS ONE, 13*(12), e0209219. https://doi.org/10.1371/journal.pone.0209219.

Legate, N., Ryan, R., & Rogge, R. (2017). Daily autonomy support and sexual identity disclosure predicts daily mental and physical health outcomes. *Personality and Social Psychology Bulletin, 43*(6), 860–873. https://doi.org/10.1177/0146167217700399.

Liddy, C., Johnston, S., Nash, K., et al. (2016). Implementation and evolution of a regional chronic disease self-management program. *Canadian Journal of Public Health, 107*(2), e194–e201. https://doi.org/10.17269/cjph.107.5126.

Logren, A., Ruusuvuori, J., & Laitinen, J. (2017). Group members' questions shape participation in health counselling and health education. *Patient Education and Counseling, 100*(10), 1828–1841. https://doi.org/10.1016/j.pec.2017.05.003.

Miller, W. R., & Rollnick, S. (1991). *Motivational interviewing: Preparing people to change addictive behavior.* New York: Guilford Press. https://doi.org/10.1002/casp.2450020410. [Seminal Reference].

National Quality Forum. (2018). *Shared decision making: A standard of care for all patients.* Retrieved from https://www.policymed.com/2018/04/nqp-playbook-released-on-shared-decision-making-in-health-care-settings.html.

OK2BME. (2019). *Potential obstacles for the LGBTQ+ community.* Retrieved from https://ok2bme.ca/resources/parents-educators/potential-obstacles/#title.

Organization for Economic Co-operation and Development, & Statistics Canada. (1995). *Literacy, economy and society: Results of the first international adult literacy survey* [Abstract]. Retrieved from https://www.voced.edu.au/content/ngv%3A40154.

Public Health Agency of Canada. (2018). *Key health inequalities in Canada: A national portrait.* Retrieved from https://www.canada

.ca/content/dam/phac-aspc/documents/services/publications /science-research/hir-full-report-eng_Original_version.pdf.

Prochaska, J. O., & DiClemente, C. C. (1984). *The transtheoretical approach: Crossing traditional boundaries of change*. Homewood, NJ: Dow Jones-Irwin. [Seminal Reference].

Prochaska, J. O., Redding, C. A., & Evers, K. E. (2015). The transtheoretical model and stages of change. In K. Glanz, B. K. Rimer, & K. Viswanath (Eds.), *Health behaviour and health education: Theory, research, and practice* (5th ed.). San Francisco: Jossey-Bass. [Seminal Reference].

Rogers, E. M. (2003). *Diffusion of innovations* (5th ed.). New York: Free Press. [Seminal Reference].

Rogers, R. W. (1975). A protection motivation theory of fear appeals and attitude change. *Journal of Psychology, 91*, 93–114. https://doi. org/10.1080/00223980.1975.9915803. [Seminal Reference].

Rollnick, S., Miller, W. R., & Butler, C. C. (2008). *Motivational interviewing in health care: Helping patients change behavior*. New York, NY: Guilford Press. [Seminal Reference].

Rosenstock, I. M., Strecher, K. J., & Becker, M. H. (1988). The social learning theory and health belief model. *Health Education Quarterly, 15*, 175–183 [Seminal Reference].

Saskatchewan, Safe. (2018). *Strategic framework: Communication safety education strategy*. Retrieved from https://safesask.com/wp-content /uploads/2018/12/Community-Safety-Education-Strategy -Revised-December-2018-1.pdf.

Statistics Canada. (2018a). *Education indicators in Canada: An international perspective*. Retrieved from https://www150.statcan.gc.ca/ n1/pub/81-604-x/2018001/hl-fs-eng.htm.

Statistics Canada. (2018b). *Table 37-10-0047-01. Literacy, numeracy— Average scores and distribution of proficiency levels, by sex and age group*. Retrieved from https://www150.statcan.gc.ca/t1/tbl1/en/ tv.action?pid=3710004701.

Thurman, W., & Pfitzinger-Lippe, M. (2017). Returning to the profession's roots. *Advances in Nursing Science, 40*(2), 184–193. https:// doi.org/10.1097/ANS.0000000000000140.

World Health Organization (WHO). (1986). *The Ottawa Charter for Health Promotion*. Retrieved from https://www.canada.ca /content/dam/phac-aspc/documents/services/health-promotion /population-health/ottawa-charter-health-promotion -international-conference-on-health-promotion/charter.pdf. [Seminal Reference].

World Health Organization (WHO). (2019). *Health education*. Retrieved from http://www.who.int/topics/health_education/en/.

Wright, L., & Leahey, M. (2013). *Nurses and families: A guide to family assessment and intervention* (6th ed.). Philadelphia: F.A. Davis Company.

# 21

# Nutrition and Health Promotion

*Emily MacLeod, RN, MN, Jane Tyerman, RN, PhD, CCSNE*

Originating US chapter by *Myrtle McCulloch, RDN, MS, EdD, Staci McIntosh, RD, MS*

## INTENDED LEARNING OUTCOMES

*After completing this chapter, the reader will be able to:*

- Evaluate the objectives outlined in Health Canada's healthy eating strategy.
- Analyze the leading diet-related causes of illness and death in Canada and the corresponding nutrients specific to each.
- Summarize and evaluate the rationale behind the recommendations contained in *Canada's Dietary Guidelines*.
- Compare proportions of food and food choices recommended in Health Canada's *Eat Well Plate*, with food proportions featured currently in the marketplace.
- Analyze food aid programs for marginalized groups, those living in poverty, Indigenous people, and older persons in Canada.
- Evaluate personal diet intakes over a 24- to 48-hour period, using the *Eat Well Plate* to learn how to guide and create healthy meals and snacks for any stage in the life cycle.

## KEY TERMS

Body mass index (BMI)
Botanicals
Canada's Dietary Guidelines
Canada's Food Guide Eat Well Plate
Cancer
Cardiovascular diseases (CVDs)
Cholesterol
Cirrhosis
Coronary heart disease (CHD)
Diabetes mellitus (DM)
Dietary Approaches to Stop Hypertension (DASH)
Dietary reference intakes (DRIs)
Dyslipidemia
Fibre
Food insecurity
Food secure
Heart disease
Hemolytic uremic syndrome
Hemorrhagic colitis
Herbals
High-density lipoprotein cholesterol
Human immunodeficiency virus
Hyperglycemia
Hyperlipidemia
Hypertension

Incidence
Lacto-ovo vegetarian
Low-density lipoprotein cholesterol
Metabolic syndrome
Micronutrients
Microbiome
Nutrition screening
Nutrigenomics
Nutritional genomics
Obese
Osteoporosis
Overweight
Prediabetes
Prehypertension
Prevalence
Salmonellosis
Serving sizes
Stroke
Sugar
Teratogenic
Trans fat
Triglyceride
Type 2 diabetes
Underweight
Vegan

### Evaluating Nutrition Intake

The following format may be used to evaluate your own nutrition intake as well to obtain a diet history from a care recipient.

Use Health Canada's Eat Well Plate (https://food-guide.canada.ca/en/tips-for-healthy-eating/make-healthy-meals-with-the-eat-well-plate/).

1. Ask the individual which food from each of the following food groups he or she has consumed in one 24-hour period. Use a household plate to make accurate estimations of proportions and food choices, where possible. Start with this question: In the past 24 hours how many foods did you eat from each of the following groups?

**Vegetable and Fruits** (make half your plate vegetables and fruits)
Try a variety of vegetables and fruits, such as: carrots, mushrooms, sliced peppers, cabbage, leafy greens, pears, apples, berries, bananas.

**Whole Grain Foods** (make one quarter of your plate whole grain foods)
Choose whole grain foods, such as: whole grain pasta, whole grain bread, whole oats or oatmeal, whole grain brown or wild rice, quinoa, whole grain cereal, whole grain crackers.

**Protein Foods** (make one quarter of your plate protein foods)
Choose protein foods, such as: eggs, lean meats and poultry, nuts and seeds, fish and shellfish, lower fat dairy products, beans, peas, and lentils, soy beverages, tofu, soybeans, and other soy products.

2. Use a plate to estimate proportions from each group and insert them in the corresponding boxes. Recommendations for each food group are listed.
3. Use this information to identify what elements of a balanced diet are missing and explain how to improve the diet or make any other changes that may be of benefit.
4. Teach yourself and your patients how to compare the nutrition facts table on foods to choose products that are lower in sodium, sugars or saturated fat.

## NUTRITION IN CANADA: LOOKING FORWARD FROM THE PAST

### Classic Vitamin-Deficiency Diseases

Food and nutrition have always been important to health. Until as recently as the mid-twentieth century, many nutrient-deficiency diseases, such as rickets, pellagra, scurvy, beriberi, xerophthalmia (eye fails to produce tears), and goitre were still prevalent globally (Mozaffarian, Rosenberg, & Uauy, 2018). Although these conditions continue to persist in some low- and middle-income countries (LMIC), they have virtually disappeared from high-income areas of the world. The availability of an abundant food supply, the fortification of some foods with critical nutrients, and the implementation of better methods of determining and increasing the nutrient contents of foods have contributed to the decline of nutrient-deficiency diseases.

The mandatory iodization of salt for table or household use in 1949, for example, contributed greatly to elimination of goitre as a public health problem in Canada (Canadian Public Health Association [CPHA], n.d.). Similarly, beriberi and pellagra disappeared after the discovery that inadequate thiamine and niacin levels respectively contribute to these diseases. Today, nutrient deficiencies are mostly seen as iron and calcium deficits, with osteoporosis and anemia, respectively, being the most common, as well as malnutrition related to obesity and its related comorbidities. The

few cases of protein-energy malnutrition that are listed annually as causes of death generally occur as secondary results of severe illness or injury, premature birth, child neglect, problems of the homebound aged, alcoholism, or some combination of these factors. Although undernutrition still occurs in some groups of people in Canada, including those who are isolated or poor, these once-prevalent diseases of nutritional deficiency have been replaced by diseases of dietary excess and imbalance (Table 21.1).

### Dietary Inadequacy

Calorie inadequacies can have devastating effects in children in developing countries leading to wasting and stunting syndromes. Although not to the same degree, many households and communities in Canada experience food insecurity and show some degree of these imbalances. Food insecurities are especially high in northern and Indigenous communities in Canada, due to economic access to adequate food, the high cost of food in isolated communities and concerns about the safety and sustainability of the food supply (Dachner & Tarasuk, 2018).

Although there are differences as to their causes, eating disorders are also classified as calorie imbalances. These can be seen in any sex and age group, with some starting in elementary school children. For diagnostic purposes, there are four conditions: anorexia nervosa, bulimia nervosa, binge eating disorder, and disordered eating not otherwise specified. The latter may include binge eating, compulsive overeating, or overexercising with respect to the calories consumed.

Depending on the length of time and the age of the individual, the physiological consequences, especially for anorexia nervosa, are life threatening. Long-term complications may include alterations in the heart rate and blood pressure, depletion of lean mass, anemia, bone loss, amenorrhea, hypoglycemia, and psychological symptoms. Early diagnosis and treatment are critical to the success of recovery.

### Dietary Excesses

Problems resulting from dietary imbalances (i.e., overconsumption of some food groups and inadequate consumption of other food groups) now rank among the leading causes of illness and death in Canada. As stated in 2016 by Health Canada in their *Healthy Eating Strategy* (Health Canada, 2016), "We have seen obesity rates and diet-related chronic diseases increase over the past few decades, even as our awareness and knowledge about healthy eating have increased."

In Canada, chronic diseases directly associated with diet—namely ischemic heart disease, stroke, colorectal cancer, diabetes mellitus (DM) and breast cancer—are among the leading causes of premature death (Institute for Health Metrics and Evaluation, 2018). Four other major causes of death—accidents, cirrhosis, suicide, and homicide—are often associated with excessive alcohol intake.

Current statistics show that more than one in four adults in Canada has obesity (Canadian Obesity Network, 2017). Although adult levels of overweight/obesity on their own are alarming, excess weight among youth has been linked to health problems that until now were seen only in adults: high blood pressure, type 2 diabetes, high cholesterol levels, depression, and sleep apnea (Rao, Kropac, Do, et al., 2016). There remains

## TABLE 21.1   Health Problems Related to Poor Nutrition

| Health Problem[a] | Contributing Lifestyle and Nutrition Practices[b] |
|---|---|
| Anemia | Diet with inadequate iron, folate, or vitamin $B_{12}$ intake (depending on type of anemia); excessive alcohol intake |
| Cancer (breast, cervical, and colon) | Excessive calorie intake, belly fat; low fibre intake; excessive alcohol intake (linked to colon, and possibly breast cancer) |
| Cirrhosis | Excessive alcohol intake |
| Constipation | Inadequate fibre or fluid intake; high fat intake; sedentary lifestyle |
| Dental caries | Excessive, frequent consumption of concentrated sweets or sugar-sweetened beverages; lack of fluoride; poor dental hygiene |
| Type 2 diabetes | Excessive calorie intake; excessive fat intake (in particular saturated fat, trans fat); sedentary lifestyle |
| Cardiovascular/ heart disease | Excessive calorie intake; excessive fat intake (in particular saturated fat, trans fat); excessive carbohydrate intake; excessive sodium intake, inadequate fibre intake; sedentary lifestyle |
| Hypertension | Excessive sodium and insufficient potassium intake; excessive calorie intake; possible excess alcohol intake; sedentary lifestyle |
| Obesity | Excessive calorie intake; excessive fat and carbohydrate intake; sedentary lifestyle |
| Osteoporosis | Low calcium intake; low vitamin D intake; excessive intake of protein, sodium, and caffeine; sedentary lifestyle; excessive alcohol intake |
| Underweight and growth failure | Inadequate calorie intake; poor diet |

[a]A number of health problems are caused or exacerbated by poor nutrition. Health care providers strive to prevent or delay these health problems.
[b]Not all may apply in every case.

a persistently high rate of obesity among Canadian youth, with approximately one in five youths aged 12 to 17 being classified according to reported height and weight as overweight or obese (Statistics Canada, 2015a).

Reducing the incidence of obesity in any age group is vital to overall health. Although excess weight or obesity is commonly viewed as an imbalance between energy intake and energy expenditure, other factors need to be considered, such as the environment, race, and socioeconomic status. For example, genes are involved in the process of energy balance and a connection has been made between microbial gut alterations and obesity (Romieu, Dossus, Barquera, et al., 2017). Recent evidence is also showing obesity as a cause of gene mutations which are responsible for controlling appetite and metabolism (Singh, Kumar, & Mahalingam, 2017). Although a genetic link to obesity has been noted, the evidence continues to be unclear and there is a risk that over-reliance on the attribution of obesity to genetics may decrease focus on policies and interventions that address the complex social aspects to the obesity epidemic.

*Canada's Dietary Guidelines* (Health Canada, 2019) state: "Decisions about healthy eating are influenced by many aspects of our social and physical environments, from household income and food skills to government food policies. All sectors—including agriculture, environment, education, housing, transportation, the food industry, trade, as well as child, family and social services—have a role to play for *Canada's Dietary Guidelines* to have far-reaching and longstanding effects on the nutritional health of Canadians." The guidelines acknowledge the importance of a coordinated, system-wide approach that engages all sectors of influence. Fig. 21.1 demonstrates the complex layers of influence that shape a person's food and physical activity choices. Creating and supporting a healthy eating pattern means that such influential factors have been taken into consideration and that healthy food options should be made available and should be accessible to all individuals. In support of this guideline, the Centers for Disease Control and Prevention (CDC) has proposed strategies for both providing healthy food and preventing obesity in the United States (see Innovative Practice for examples).

### INNOVATIVE PRACTICE

#### Health Canada's Healthy Eating Strategy

Health Canada's Healthy Eating Strategy aims to improve the food environment in Canada to make it easier for Canadian's to make the healthier choices by:

**Improving Healthy Eating Information**
Canada's new dietary guidelines, released in January 2019, are a mobile-friendly web application that provides Canadians with easier access to dietary guidance.

**Improving Nutrition Quality of Foods**
Canadians as a whole continue to eat too much trans fats. Eating foods high in trans fats increases the risk of heart disease, one of the leading causes of death in Canada. On September 17, 2018, Health Canada banned the use of partially hydrogenated oils in foods, the main source of industrially produced trans fat. It is now illegal for manufacturers to add partially hydrogenated oils to foods sold in Canada.

**Protecting Vulnerable Populations**
Children's eating habits and taste preferences are highly influenced by advertising. In order to protect children, Health Canada is working to restrict advertising to children under 13 years of age of foods that meet criteria for:
- Sugars
- Sodium
- Saturated fat

**Supporting Increased Access to and Vulnerability of Nutritious Foods**
The Nutrition North Canada program is one way in which Canada works to support increased access and availability to nutritious foods by providing retail subsidy in partnership with Crown-Indigenous Relations and Northern Affairs Canada. Effective October 1, 2016, the Nutrition North Canada program was expanded to an additional 37 isolated northern communities.

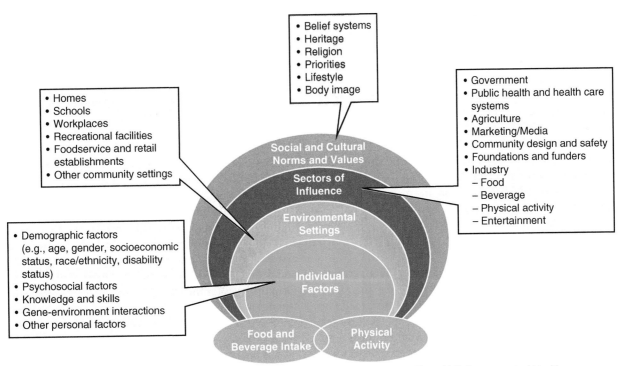

**Fig. 21.1** Social-ecological framework for food and physical activity decisions. (From U.S. Department of Health and Human Services & U.S. Department of Agriculture. [2015]. *Dietary guidelines for Americans 2015–2020* [8th ed.]. Retrieved from https://health.gov/dietaryguidelines/2015/guidelines/chapter-3/social-ecological-model/.)

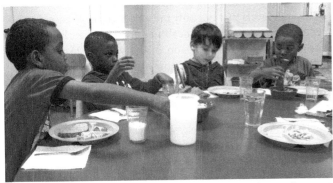

**Fig. 21.2** Children who eat with each other in an appropriate environment often eat more nutritiously and try a wider variety of foods than when eating alone or at home. (From Mahan, L. K., & Raymond, J. L. [2017]. *Krause's food & the nutrition care process* [14th ed.]. St Louis: Elsevier.)

Encouraging healthy choices in diet, exercise, and weight control are the major focus of The Integrated Pan-Canadian Healthy Living Strategy (Government of Canada, 2005) (Fig. 21.2). In 2010, the Pan-Canadian Healthy Living Strategy framework was strengthened, with additional emphasis on risk factors and conditions, as well as focus on new areas of opportunity, including overweight and obesity prevention, mental health promotion, and injury prevention.

## Nutrition-Related Health Status

A variety of diet-related factors exact a heavy toll on the Canadian population as the following key points illustrate. The following statements give a broad-based view of the health status of Canadians:

- Almost 50% of deaths from cardiovascular disease were attributed to dietary risks in 2017 (Institute for Health Metrics and Evaluation, 2018). Dietary risks include low intake of nutritious foods, such as vegetables and fruit. In Canada, vegetable and fruit intakes remain consistently low (Colapinto, Graham, & St-Pierre, 2018).
- In the Canadian population, 58% of all Canadians and 72% of children between the ages of 4 and 13 years of age consumed sodium above the recommended limits (Health Canada, 2017a).
- One in two Canadians consume saturated fat above the recommended limit (Health Canada, 2015).
- In 2015, sugary drinks were the main sources of total sugars in the diet of Canadians, with children and adolescents (ages 9–18 years) having the highest average daily intake (Langlois, Garriguet, Gonzalez, Sinclair, et al., 2019).
- Canadians get most of their daily energy intake from carbohydrates including children and youth. In 2015, Canadian children received 53.4% of their daily energy from carbohydrates and only 15.6% from protein (Statistics Canada, 2017a).
- Canadian households spend approximately 30% of their food budget on meals and snacks purchased from full-service restaurants, fast-food retailers, as well as refreshment stands, snack bars, vending machines, canteens, caterers, and food trucks (Health Canada, 2019).

- Household food insecurity is prevalent throughout Canada where 12.6% of households experience "inadequate or insecure access to food because of financial constraints" (Dietitians of Canada, 2016).
- Rates of food insecurity are high among Indigenous households compared to non-Indigenous households. Rates of moderate to severe food insecurity range from 22 to 63% of Indigenous households depending on which population has been surveyed (Health Canada, 2019).
- Only 26% of mothers report exclusive breastfeeding for the first 6 months, as recommended by the World Health Organization (WHO) and Health Canada, the majority of whom are 30 years of age or older and have a postsecondary education (Gionet, 2015).

## Nutrition Objectives for Canada

As can be seen already, a considerable gap exists between public health recommendations and consumer practices. The overarching goal for nutrition in the second decade of the millennium is that food intake patterns change in order to improve overall health. Although Canada has lacked an integrated national food policy that supports an intersectoral approach to food and health, the government's *A Food Policy for Canada* has recently been developed around four pillars: (1) food security, (2) health, (3) environment, and (4) sustainable growth of the agriculture and food sector (Government of Canada, 2017). As Food Secure Canada (2017) states: "In order to create a better food system, we need to start thinking more comprehensively about how we govern our food, from farm to fork" (p. 3).

## FOOD AND NUTRITION RECOMMENDATIONS

Food and nutrition guidelines are introduced in this chapter with the intent of motivating the reader to achieve three principal goals. The first goal is to encourage individual interest in the health-promoting power of good nutrition and to promote self-evaluation and comparison of one's own food habits and choices with respect to the dietary recommendations presented here. The second goal is to understand the many systemic factors that have contributed to the current nutrition-related health issues. These problems are so pervasive that many health authorities believe a multisectoral approach, beyond traditional education about healthy food choices, is required. The following reports provide the foundation for national nutrition recommendations that have been translated into law, policy, programs, and many consumer messages. In addition, *Canada's Food Guide 2019* snapshot has also been translated into over 30 languages including several Indigenous languages such as Ojibwe, Michif, and Inuinnaqtun. Health Canada and Indigenous Services Canada are committed to working with Indigenous peoples to support the development of healthy eating tools for First Nations, Inuit, and Métis:

- *Intakes: The Essential Guide to Nutrient Requirements* (National Research Council, 2006) and *Dietary Reference Intakes for Calcium and Vitamin D* (National Research Council, 2010)
- *Canada's Food Guide* 2019 (Health Canada, 2019) (Fig. 21.3)
- Eating Well with Canada's Food Guide First Nations, Inuit, and Métis (Health Canada, 2010)

### Dietary Reference Intakes

The original dietary reference intakes (DRIs) were developed by the Institute of Medicine (IOM) of the National Academies of Sciences, Engineering, and Medicine in 1997 to reflect the latest understanding about nutrient requirements based on optimizing health in individuals and groups. They are quantitative estimates of nutrient intakes, which can be used to plan and assess the diets of healthy people in Canada, to prevent disease and deficiencies. The recommended dietary allowances (RDAs) form the basis for the DRIs. The adequate intakes are to be used whenever there is not enough evidence to include a nutrient in the RDAs. See Box 21.1, for details on these components and suggested uses.

It is important to note that the DRIs are updated only when deemed necessary. In 2008, the Canadian and US governments decided there were enough new studies as well as concern about vitamin D, in particular, to warrant the development of new DRIs for vitamin D and calcium. The latest updates were published in late 2010. In 2014, the Canadian and US governments formed a working group to assess the need to align the DRIs with levels that not only prevent chronic diseases but also reduce the impact of poor health for those presently living with chronic diseases. The revision of the vitamin D and calcium DRIs as well as changes to align with chronic disease management demonstrates that DRIs continue to be researched and revised as more information and evidence-informed studies become available.

There are some controversies over DRIs because there may be limited data relating to genetic diversity in the population or specific groups such as children, pregnant women, and older persons. However, they are a good starting point based on best available evidence and probability of harm or benefit.

As the DRIs are intended to be applied to healthy people, it is possible that a provider might override the DRI for a specific nutrient on the basis of clinical judgement and recommend more or less for a particular recipient. It is also helpful to remember that whereas DRIs may be used for individuals, ideally, they are guidelines for population groups and apply over time. So, if an individual does not meet the recommendation for a specific nutrient, such as vitamin C, on a certain day, that is not a cause for alarm. It is the trend that matters with respect to food sources as opposed to supplements.

After this discussion of DRIs, the twentieth-century anthropologist Margaret Mead's statement that "people eat food, not nutrition" seems particularly apt. Nutrition recommendations stated in terms of micrograms or milligrams of nutrients are of

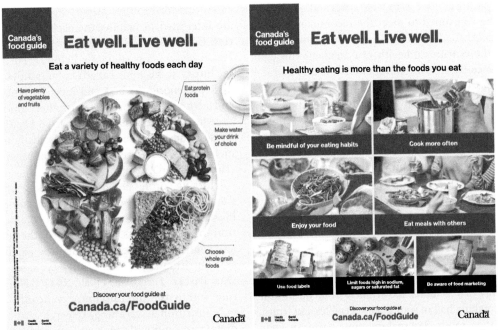

**Fig. 21.3** Canada's Dietary Guidelines: Learn about healthy eating at https://food-guide.canada.ca/en/. ((c) All rights reserved. *Canada's Food Guide: Snapshot.* Health Canada, 2019. Adapted and reproduced with permission from the Minister of Health, 2020.)

---

## BOX 21.1  Dietary Reference Intake Components and Definitions

### Estimated Average Requirement

Estimated average requirement (EAR) is the (median) daily intake that meets the estimated nutrient needs of half of the individuals in a particular life stage and gender group. It is used as a basis for developing the recommended dietary allowance (RDA) and is especially useful for evaluating adequacy of nutrient intake of a group (or groups) and for planning how much the group(s) should consume.

### Recommended Dietary Allowance

RDA is the average dietary intake level that is sufficient to meet the nutrient requirement of nearly all (97–98%) healthy individuals in a particular life stage and gender group. It is computed with use of the EAR. In the past, the RDA of most nutrients represented the levels needed to prevent deficiency diseases. Now an RDA also includes the goal of preventing chronic diseases (e.g., heart disease or osteoporosis, where applicable). As a variety of Institute of Medicine dietary reference intake (DRI) publications note, the RDA should not be used to assess or plan nutrient intake for groups but may be useful in some individual applications (National Academies of Sciences, Engineering and Medicine, 2017).

### Adequate Intake

An adequate intake (AI) is set to fill the gap (e.g., infants) when there is not enough scientific evidence to determine the RDA. The AI is based on estimates of observed or experimentally determined mean nutrient intake of a group (or groups) of healthy people and assumes that the amount consumed is adequate to promote health. The level is set to meet or exceed the needs of almost all people in a particular life stage and gender group. This is the most controversial component in the DRIs.

### Tolerable Upper Intake Level

This is the highest average daily intake that can be safely eaten continuously and still be considered safe for almost all healthy individuals in a specified group. The upper limit (UL) is not intended to be a recommended level of intake. No established benefit exists for individuals to consume nutrients at levels above the RDA or AI. As intake increases above the UL, the potential risk of side effects increases. For most nutrients the UL would include total intakes from any of the following (alone or in combination): food, fortified food, and nutrient supplements. It is important to note that ULs are set only when there is a strong pool of scientific data. In cases where the evidence is limited or inconclusive, a UL will not be established. In that case, eating levels close to the RDA or AI (as applicable) is not advised.

### Acceptable Macronutrient Distribution Range

This is the range of intake for a particular energy source (e.g., carbohydrate, fat, protein) that is associated with reduced risk of chronic disease while providing intakes of essential nutrients for a healthy person within an identified life stage and gender group. An intake outside the acceptable macronutrient distribution range (AMDR) carries the potential of increased risk of chronic diseases and/or insufficient intakes of essential nutrients. For example, the AMDR for carbohydrates for a 19-year-old woman (in the life stage and gender group of female, 19–30 years old) is 45 to 65% of calories.

### Estimated Energy Requirement

This is the average dietary energy intake predicted to maintain energy balance in a healthy adult of a specific life stage and gender group calculated with a reference weight, height, and level of physical activity that is consistent with good health.

Source: National Academies of Sciences, Engineering, and Medicine. (2017). *Guiding principles for developing dietary reference intakes based on chronic disease.* Washington, DC: The National Academies Press. Retrieved from https://www.nap.edu/catalog/24828/guiding-principles-for-developing-dietary-reference-intakes-based-on-chronic-disease.

no use unless people are advised as to what types and quantities of foods should be consumed to meet the recommendations. The intent of *Canada's Food Guide* has been to guide food selection to promote the nutritional health of Canadians through translation of science-based nutrient requirements into a practical pattern of food choices.

The DRIs are also important in the design and implementation of nutrition-related programs, including federal nutrition programs for families, children, and older persons. These guidelines also provide nutrition education initiatives for the general public of adults and children aged 2 years or older.

## Canada's Dietary Guidelines: Healthy Eating Recommendations 2019

Key recommendations from the 2019 *Canada's Dietary Guidelines* (Health Canada, 2019) include suggestions to:

- Make it a habit to eat a variety of healthy foods each day.
  - Include plenty of vegetables and fruits in your meals and snacks. Try making half of your plate vegetables and fruits.
  - Eat whole grain foods. Try making one quarter of your plate whole grain foods such as quinoa, whole grain pasta, whole grain bread, whole grain oats or oatmeal, and whole grain brown or wild rice.
  - Eat protein foods and choose protein food that come from plants more often. Try making one quarter of your plate protein food such as eggs, lean meats and poultry, nuts and seeds, fish and shellfish, lower fat dairy products, beans, peas and lentils, and fortified soy beverages, tofu, soybeans, and other soy products.
  - Make water your drink of choice. Replace sugary drinks with water.
  - Limit your intake of highly processed foods by preparing meals and snacks using ingredients that have little to no added sodium, sugars, or saturated fat, and by choosing healthier meal options when eating out.
- Healthy eating is more than the foods you eat. It is also about where, when, why, and how you eat.
  - Be mindful of your eating habits by taking time to eat and noticing when you are hungry and when you are full.
  - Cook more often by planning what you eat and involving others in planning and preparing meals.
  - Enjoy your food by incorporating culture and food traditions as part of your healthy eating habits.
  - Eat meals with others.

Other topics addressed in detail include guidance for specific life stages: infant feeding and nutrition, teens, parents, adults, and older persons. A discussion of how to build healthy eating patterns through meal planning, healthy grocery shopping, and healthy cooking methods, as well as how to take steps towards being physically active, is also included in *Canada's Dietary Guidelines* (for details, see https://food-guide.canada.

ca/en/tips-for-healthy-eating/). For nursing professionals who are interested in helping themselves or others balance calories, *Canada's Dietary Guidelines for Health Professionals and Policy Makers* is particularly helpful. (For more information, see https://food-guide.canada.ca/en/guidelines/.)

Representing the best and most current scientific evidence and advice from nutrition experts, these guidelines are intended to reduce Canada's major diet-related health problems such as obesity and other chronic diseases including type 2 diabetes mellitus, heart disease, certain types of cancer, and osteoporosis (Health Canada, 2019).

Nursing professionals play a key role in promoting *Canada's Dietary Guidelines* as one component of healthy lifestyles. Nurses play an important role in supporting nutrition in their patients, they often fill the role of assessing for and counselling patients on nutrition challenges as dieticians and nutritionists are not always available to meet this need (Xu, Parker, Ferguson, et al., 2017). Nurses play a crucial role within the interdisciplinary health care team to provide nutritional screening, referral, and implementation of dietary recommendations, and should therefore understand the importance of good nutrition on the overall health and wellness of their patients. *Canada's Dietary Guidelines for Health Professionals and Policy Makers* introduces important healthy eating guidelines and considerations that are relevant to the Canadian context. This includes the following:

1. Nutritious foods are the foundation for healthy eating: vegetables, fruit, whole grains, and protein foods should be consumed regularly. Among protein foods, consume plant-based more often. Foods that contain mostly unsaturated fat should replace foods that contain mostly saturated fat, and water should be the beverage of choice.
2. Processed or prepared foods and beverages that contribute to excess sodium, free sugars, or saturated fats undermine healthy eating and should not be consumed regularly.
3. Food skills are needed to navigate the complex food environment and support healthy eating. Cooking and food preparation using nutritious foods should be promoted as a practical way to support healthy eating. Food labels should be promoted as a tool to help Canadians make informed food choices.

Although *Canada's Dietary Guidelines* reflect general eating patterns of Canadians, they have enough flexibility for different cultural preferences and food traditions, including vegetarians (see Diversity Awareness).

Recognizing that in recent years almost 15 million adults and children have found it difficult to obtain enough food to meet their needs, the Government of Canada's website on *Canada's Food Guide* (https://food-guide.canada.ca/en/) includes an emphasis on resources for healthy eating on a budget. The Government of Canada also has resources available in French. The website continues to be updated, so it is worth checking periodically.

## ⊕ DIVERSITY AWARENESS

### *Food and Culture*

The reasons why people eat the ways they do are numerous. Although it is true that without food people cannot survive, food is much more than a tool of survival. Food is also a source of pleasure ("Let's eat out tonight"), a source of comfort ("Right now, I could use some of my mother's chicken soup"), a symbol of hospitality ("Please come to my house for brunch on Sunday"), and an indicator of social status (consider an expensive T-bone steak versus a hamburger). Food also has ritual significance. Drinking champagne to celebrate an important event, the bride and groom saving the top layer of their wedding cake, and people of the Jewish faith sharing challah (braided bread) at their Sabbath (Friday evening) meal are examples.

To a large extent the environment determines what people typically eat. For example, wheat that is plentiful in Canada is the principal grain in North America, whereas rice enjoys a similar status in Asian countries. Typical wheat-based staples in Canada and the United States include a slice of wheat bread, a bowl of wheat cereal, wheat crackers, pastries made from wheat flour, and pasta made from wheat. Rice-based foods form the backbone of the Chinese diet.

Every culture has its particular food ways, or activities related to food. Food ways include the activities that surround procuring, distributing, storing, consuming, and disposing of food, all of which define what is fit to eat, or what is edible. Factors that affect everyone's food choices and factors that affect food selections of new arrivals to a community should be examined. It is important to remember, however, that just because a person is from a specific culture does not mean the person follows his or her cultural food patterns. These general guidelines are helpful as a starting point, but do not assume—ask questions to clarify specific eating habits with individuals and families.

Among traditional Chinese people, health and disease are believed to relate to the balance between the forces of yin and yang in the body. Diseases that are caused by yang forces may be treated with yin forces to restore balance. Yin foods include low-calorie-density, low-protein foods, such as fresh fruits and vegetables. Yang foods are high in calories, cooked in oil, and irritating to the mouth, or are red, orange, or yellow. Examples include most meats, chili peppers, tomatoes, garlic, ginger, and alcoholic beverages. The hot-cold theory in Puerto Rico follows the same basic principles as do yin and yang, but the food groupings differ somewhat.

Religious beliefs affect the food choices of millions of people worldwide. Many religions, including Buddhism, Hinduism, Islam, Judaism, and Seventh Day Adventism, specify the foods that may be eaten and how they should be prepared. The following is a very basic summary of the principal dietary practices of these five major world religions (adapted from Barer-Stein, 1979, and Kittler & Sucher, 2000).

Many Buddhists practise vegetarianism. Foods of plant origin are viewed as the most appropriate for consumption, except pungent foods (garlic, leeks, scallions, chives, and onions), which are believed to generate lust when eaten cooked and to cause rage when eaten raw. For most Buddhists, however, dietary rules such as these are observed on a voluntary basis. What characterizes all Buddhists is the belief that all forms of life share a common link and are thus sacred. Therefore, rather than the specific type of food eaten, more important is the attitude of the person receiving the food and the person's sincere gratitude for the lives of the plants and animals contained in the meal that have served to sustain and further enhance the life of the individual.

Many Hindus practise vegetarianism, but those who originate from the cold northern areas of India usually eat meat (except for beef, which is considered sacred and prohibited).

Many Muslims follow Islamic food laws, which include foods that are halal (permitted), haram (prohibited), and questionable (*mashbooh*). Foods believed to be unclean, or haram, are animals that are improperly slaughtered or already-dead animals such as carrion, swine/pork and its by-products (bacon, lard, shortening), carnivorous animals with fangs (dogs, cats, and lions), birds of prey, and land animals without ears (frogs and snakes). Alcohol and intoxicants are also prohibited. Halal-certified products are used.

Conservative Jews follow Judaic food laws, which prohibit the consumption of swine/pork, carrion, carrion eaters (scavengers), shellfish, animals with a cloven (split) hoof and that do not chew their cud (horses), and animals not slaughtered by the appropriate ritual method or kosher (fit). According to Jewish kosher dietary laws, meat (beef, lamb, veal, and poultry), fish, and meat products (eggs) cannot be served at the same meal or be cooked or eaten in the same vessels as dairy products. Kosher-certified products are used.

The dietary practices of Seventh Day Adventists focus on health, so many Seventh Day Adventists practise vegetarianism as the foundation of their dietary standard. They also abstain from alcohol, and many do not drink caffeine-containing beverages.

#### Reflective Questions

Health care providers, including registered nurses, must examine their own cultural backgrounds and ask themselves and their patients questions related to values, beliefs, and practices. Examples include the following:

- What are some of your health-related values, beliefs, and practices related to nutrition?
- How might these values, beliefs, and practices affect or influence the way you provide nutritional care and education?

Sources: Barer-Stein, T. (1979). Multiculturalism and nutrition counseling. *Journal of the Canadian Dietetic Association, 40*(2), 112–116; Kittler, P. G., & Sucher, K. P. (2000). *Cultural foods: Traditions and trends.* Belmont, CA: Wadsworth.

## NUTRITIONAL SUPPLEMENTS AND NATURAL AND NONPRESCRIPTION HEALTH PRODUCTS

In recent decades the popularity of supplemental vitamins, minerals, proteins, fibre, and herbs has earned a high profile in the health field. It was the explosion of the use of single-component dietary supplements in the 1980s that helped to spur the change from the old RDAs to the DRIs. New evidence indicated that perhaps ranges of nutrients could be used that were higher than the old "one size fits all" RDAs. At the same time, there appeared to be a point at which a nutrient could pose more of a risk than an advantage. As a result, tolerable upper limit (UL) guidelines were developed for specific life stages, ages, and gender (Taylor, 2008).

According to Statistics Canada (2017b), 45.6% of Canadians aged 1 year and older (approximately 15.7 million people) used at least one nutritional supplement, with women being more likely than men to use supplements. Under the *Natural Health Products Regulations* (Government of Canada, 2015) natural health products include vitamins and minerals, herbal remedies, homeopathic medicines, traditional medicines such as Chinese medicines, probiotics, and other products link amino acids and essential fatty acids. People use supplements as if they were medications. Additionally, they are marketed in the same manner as over-the-counter medications. To distinguish a dietary supplement from an over-the-counter medication, the lot number appearing on the product label will end with DIN-HM for homeopathic medicines and NPN for all other products (Ministry of Justice, 2018). The labels may carry certain types of structure-function claims about certain common conditions associated with aging, pregnancy, menopause, and adolescence that do not relate to disease (i.e., "calcium builds strong bones" or "fibre maintains bowel regularity"). In other words, health claims that refer to diseases or health-related conditions listed in Appendix A of the *Evidence for Safety and Efficacy of Finished Natural Health Products Guidance Document* are not permitted on the label. Claims of traditional use must be prefaced with qualifiers such as "traditionally used." If the claim uses terminology specific to a particular culture or system of medicine, that culture or healing paradigm must be specified in the claim. Furthermore, if a health claim is supported by only scientific evidence, it must not include the words "traditionally used (Health Canada, 2006).

All natural health products (NHPs) sold in Canada are conditional to the licensing provisions of the *Natural Products Regulations*, which came into effect in 2004. The purpose of the Regulations is to help assure the Canadians have access to NHPs that are safe, effective, and meet quality standards (Government of Canada, 2015). In order to be legally sold in Canada, all NHPs must have a product licence, and the Canadian sites which manufacture, package, label and import these products must obtain and hold site licences (Government of Canada, 2015). In addition, there are specific labelling and packaging requirements as well as good manufacturing practice standards and evidence norms that must be met in order to obtain and continue to hold site licences (Government of Canada, 2015). Also important to note are the evidence requirements for safety and efficacy. Any safety and efficacy claims associated with NHPs must be supported by appropriate evidence so that both consumers and Health Canada can be certain that products are safe and effective (Government of Canada, 2015). The type and among of supporting evidence required is dependent on the proposed heath claim of the product and its overall risks (Government of Canada, 2015).

Although the desirable way for the general public to obtain recommended levels of nutrients is by eating a variety of foods, if people take dietary supplements, they should avoid taking them in excess of the UL of the DRI for those nutrients for their age and gender group to preclude possible side effects. An example of this is a recent study of the effects of dietary as well as calcium supplementation in fracture prevention in which it was concluded that there was no such association (Bolland, Leung, Tai, et al., 2015). For other types of supplements, such as herbals or botanicals, caution is also advised. Natural is not always better. For example, the Canadian Medical Association (CMA, 2015) encourages Canadians to become educated about their own heath and health care, and to appraise health information critically.

## Vitamin and Mineral Toxicity

Toxic levels of certain micronutrients can cause a host of health problems. For example, it is important to advise individuals not to overuse the fat-soluble vitamins (vitamins A, D, E, and K). Of particular concern is vitamin A, an excess of which may be teratogenic during pregnancy or may increase the risk of lung cancer for current or former smokers (Dietitians of Canada, 2013). On the other hand, water-soluble vitamins such as vitamin C and the B-complex vitamins may pose less danger because the body is able to excrete them through the urine.

Nutrient imbalances and toxicities are unlikely to occur when nutrients are derived from foods in a normal diet. Most nutrient toxicities occur through supplementation, and in some cases with a combination of supplementation and fortification of foods. The estimated toxic doses for daily oral consumption of vitamins and minerals by adults are as low as five times the recommended intake for selenium, and as high as 25 to 50 times or more the recommended intakes for folic acid and vitamins C and E. The toxicities of high doses of nutrients such as vitamin A, vitamin $B_6$, vitamin D, niacin, iron, and selenium are well established.

Large doses of vitamin A may be teratogenic. Because of this risk, supplementation with preformed vitamin A should be avoided during the first trimester of pregnancy unless there is evidence of deficiency (Quality and Safety Scenario). Excess preformed vitamin A supplements (more than 10,000 international units [IU]) during the first trimester of pregnancy has been linked to birth defects of the eyes, lungs, skull, and heart (Maia et al., 2019). Such a risk in early pregnancy raises the need for caution about general vitamin and mineral supplement use by women of child-bearing age.

### ⚡ QUALITY AND SAFETY SCENARIO
#### *Supplements/Vitamin A*

Adele is a 32-year-old married Black woman with no children and a history of one miscarriage. She and her husband have been trying to conceive for the past 4 years and have recently started talking about going to a fertility clinic. Always one to try the "natural way" first, she read that vitamin A is important for normal fetal development and decides to take a multivitamin supplement with 25,000 IU of preformed vitamin A. Adele knows that she can get vitamin A from food, but she also makes an effort to read nutrition labels and choose fortified foods that have 20% or more vitamin A content. She comes into the health care provider's office for a regular routine visit. It is common knowledge that she and her husband are trying to have a baby.

**Reflective Questions**
- Why is it important to discuss the use and type of supplements (and potentially fortified food use) during preconception/pregnancy?
- What is the vitamin A dietary reference intake recommendation for a woman of her age?
- How can learning about simple changes in her eating habits/supplement use affect her risk of a spontaneous abortion or a birth defect in the event of pregnancy?
- What would your next step be in this situation?

*Note:* One retinol activity equivalent = 1 mcg of all-*trans*-retinol = 3.33 IU from retinol = 2 mcg of supplemental all-*trans*-β-carotene = 12 mcg of dietary all-*trans*-β-carotene = 24 mcg of other dietary provitamin A carotenoids.

Besides problems with direct toxicity of some individual nutrients, there may be problems related to nutrient imbalances or adverse interactions with prescribed medication. Often, high doses of a single nutrient may reflect interactions that result in a relative deficiency of another nutrient (American Dietetic Association, 2009). Some examples follow:

- High doses of vitamin E can interfere with vitamin K action and enhance the effect of warfarin as one of the anticoagulant medications. Examples such as this are one of the reasons that health care providers may ask about supplement use before surgery and recommend discontinuation of use of certain supplements for 1 week before and 1 week after surgery. Large amounts of calcium inhibit absorption of iron and possibly other trace elements.
- Folic acid can mask hematological signs of vitamin $B_{12}$ deficiency, which, if untreated, can result in irreversible neurological damage. Folic acid can also interact adversely with anticonvulsant medications.
- Zinc supplementation can reduce copper levels, impair immune responses, and decrease levels of high-density lipoprotein (HDL) cholesterol ("good" cholesterol).

Nursing professionals can help people who suspect an adverse supplement effect by reporting the event to the Canada Vigilance Program, or by encouraging the individual to file a report. This should be done as soon as possible when there is a suspected problem. Information on how to do this is available at https://www.canada.ca/en/health-canada/services/drugs-health-products/medeffect-canada/adverse-reaction-reporting.html. Another avenue is to alert the product's manufacturer or distributor to any serious side effects through the address or phone number listed on the supplement's label. According to Canada's *Food and Drugs Act*, it is mandatory for manufacturers and distributors to submit side effect reports to Health Canada (Health Canada, 2017b).

## Circumstances When Nutrient Supplementation Is Indicated

Nutrient supplements or fortified foods, or sometimes a combination of both, are sometimes necessary for specific populations to obtain desirable amounts of particular nutrients (Dietitians of Canada, 2019). Some examples follow:

- Folic acid (400 mcg) from fortified enriched grains or supplements in addition to folate-rich foods for women who could become pregnant to help prevent neural tube defects.
- Iron supplements during pregnancy when indicated in laboratory tests.
- Calcium and vitamin D supplements in older postmenopausal women to reduce their risk of osteoporosis (levels should not exceed the UL of 2000 mg for calcium or 100 mcg for vitamin D through either supplements or a combination of foods and supplements).
- Vitamin D for those who do not meet the recommended DRI intake (without exceeding the DRI UL of 4000 IU or 100 mcg by a combination of food, supplement, and fortified food).
- Vitamin $B_{12}$ through food fortified with the crystalline form or $B_{12}$ supplements for individuals older than 50 years (who may often have a reduced ability to absorb naturally occurring

vitamin $B_{12}$). In addition, vegans should ensure they have adequate intake of vitamin $B_{12}$ through fortified foods or supplements.

People can get their nutritional requirements from foods and, when necessary, from supplements. However, the amounts needed are generalized to population studies (e.g., amounts for all women during pregnancy). These requirements do not account for individual genetic variations. In the future, it may be possible for specific nutrients to be prescribed to individuals on the basis of genomic maps. This new and exciting study of nutrigenomics explores the effects of nutrients on gene expression. However, when it comes to nutrients in foods and their effects on gene expression, the science is not ready to create diets specific to an individual's genome makeup. As this is an issue of ethics medicine as well as nutrition, it is a field that will move with caution (Pavlidis, Patrinos, & Katsila, 2015).

## FOOD SAFETY

In 2017, Canadian households averaged more than $8500 on food (Statista, 2017), with nearly 30% of the food budget being spent on meals and snacks purchased outside the home (Health Canada, 2019). The combined efforts of the food industry and the regulatory agencies are often credited with making the Canadian food supply among the safest in the world. Nonetheless, the Public Health Agency of Canada (PHAC) reports that each year an estimated one in eight Canadians—a total of 4 million people—become sick from food-borne illnesses caused by contamination by any of a number of microbial pathogens. Of these, an estimated 11,600 people require hospitalization and over 200 people die (PHAC, 2016a).

Attention to food-borne illnesses is becoming increasingly important with the globalization of the world's food supply. New disease-causing organisms have emerged, and food imports from countries without the same safety standards as Canada are on the rise. Furthermore, more consumers are demanding fresh produce and more seafood to be available throughout the year as well as accessibility to less-processed foods, such as raw milk and fresh juices that are not cooked or pasteurized to kill bacteria. Consumers may also ignore warnings about unsafe food habits because of preferences for foods such as raw oysters, rare hamburgers, fresh juices, unpasteurized cheese, and runny egg yolks, which all carry higher risks of contamination.

To protect the public from numerous sources of food contamination (physical, chemical, biological), private industry and numerous federal agencies share responsibilities for regulating the safety of the Canadian food supply. In January 2019, Canada welcomed new legislation termed the *Safe Food for Canadians Regulations* (SFCR). These regulations simplify and strengthen rules for food in Canada, whether produced here or imported into the country. In addition, for the SFCR, food businesses are also subject to the laws described within the *Food and Drugs Act and Regulations*, which further describes how to legally market, distribute, and sell safe food products to consumers in Canada. Furthermore, the Canadian Food Inspection Agency bases its food safety practice on the Hazard Analysis Critical Control Point (HACCP) approach, which is a globally accepted, standardized method to ensure optimal food safety. This have been used since the 1960s and is recommended by the Codex Alimentarius Commission, which is the United Nations international standards organization for food safety.

When the safeguards built into this system fail, however, consumers themselves must serve as the final, and sometimes most important, guardians against unsafe food. Therefore it is essential to be informed and educated about the potential dangers of food-borne illness and ways to avoid contaminated food products.

## Causes of Food-Borne Illness

A food-borne illness is classified according to the source of its contamination (the unintended presence of harmful substances or microorganisms). Food contaminants may be categorized as biological, chemical, or physical. Biological contaminants include bacteria, viruses, parasites, and fungi (yeasts and molds). Chemical contamination refers to the presence of pesticides, kitchen-cleaning supplies, and toxic chemicals in food that have been leached from worn metal cookware and equipment. Physical contamination includes dirt, glass chips, crockery, wood, splinters, stones, hair, jewellery, and metal shavings from dull can openers. Another unintended physical contaminant may be an unintended allergen added to a food product that typically does not include that ingredient (such as peanuts) during food processing in the same location.

## Examples of Common Food-Borne Pathogens

According to the PHAC (2016a), the five most common culprits that cause food-related illness in Canada are: (1) *Norovirus*, (2) *Listeria*, (3) *Salmonella*, (4) *E. Coli 0157*, and (5) *Campylobacter*. Among these top five illness-causing pathogens, *Listeria* is the most fatal with an almost 20% mortality rate (PHAC, 2016a). *Norovirus, Salmonella,* and *Campylobacter,* however, lead to the majority of all food-borne illnesses in Canada (PHAC, 2016a). Most of these species are associated with foods such as beef, dairy, fruits and nuts, leafy vegetables, and poultry. Two common types are discussed next.

### Salmonellosis

*Salmonella* contributes to one in four hospitalization of all food-borne illness in Canada (PHAC, 2016a). Each year in Canada, approximately 88,000 cases of salmonellosis are reported, with 17 deaths from acute salmonellosis (PHAC, 2016a). The actual number of infections may be much higher because milder cases are often not diagnosed or reported. Although the *Salmonella* family includes more than 2300 serotypes of the bacterium, the most common in Canada are *Salmonella enteritidis* and *Salmonella bongori.*

The typical way humans are exposed to salmonellosis is by consuming foods contaminated with animal feces. Foods of animal origin such as beef, poultry, milk, and eggs are often the source of infection. However, *all* foods, including seafood from polluted water and vegetables, may become contaminated. Contamination may also occur from unsanitary handling of foods and utensils by infected food handlers, and contact with the feces of some pets, especially those with diarrhea. Symptoms

of salmonellosis (PHAC, 2016b) include abdominal cramping, mild to severe diarrhea, nausea, vomiting, sudden headache, and fever within 6 to 72 hours after exposure. Symptoms may resolve within 4 to 7 days without treatment; however, infections can become life threatening for people with weakened immune systems such as infants with an immature immune system, young children, pregnant women, older persons, and people with autoimmune disorders or those being treated for cancer. Antibiotics are usually not necessary unless the infection spreads from the intestines. To prevent salmonellosis, avoid uncooked egg dishes, undercooked meat, shellfish, and unpasteurized milk and juice. Adherence to sanitary regulations, as well as proper food handling, is necessary to control salmonellosis outbreaks.

### *Escherichia coli* O157:H7 Infection

Theodor Escherichia, a German pediatrician, first discovered the *E. coli* bacterium in the human colon in 1885. A particularly virulent strain of *E. coli*, known as *E. coli* O157:H7, was first identified in 1982 as a food-borne pathogen during an investigation of an outbreak of severe bloody diarrhea attributable to ingestion of contaminated hamburgers. As a leading cause of food-borne illness, *E. coli* O157:H7 can produce a powerful toxin causing severe illness and damage to the intestinal lining (PHAC, 2017a). The illness is characterized by severe abdominal cramping, watery to bloody diarrhea, dehydration, nausea, and vomiting with or without low-grade fever. Hemorrhagic colitis is usually self-limited and lasts for 5 to 10 days. Most *E. coli* O157:H7 infections (PHAC, 2017a) are food-borne and associated with undercooked or raw ground beef, unpasteurized milk products, and contaminated raw fruits and vegetables, such as leafy greens or sprouts. Moreover, outbreaks can be caused by secondary person-to-person contamination in homes, day cares, nursing homes, and hospitals. Another mode of transmission of *E. coli* O157:H7 is by hand-to-mouth contact with animals or contaminated surfaces at petting zoos and agricultural fairs. Although all people are included in *E. coli* O157:H7 target populations, children, pregnant women, older persons and those with weakened immune systems are more susceptible. In cases confirmed in children, infection may develop into hemolytic uremic syndrome, leading to permanent loss of kidney function.

## Food Safety Practices

The few examples already cited demonstrate how serious food-borne illness can be. Individuals in their own homes can reduce contaminants and keep food safe to eat by following safe food handling practices. Four basic food safety principles work together to reduce the risk of food-borne illness—clean, separate, cook, and chill. The following are some key aspects of food safety regulation for consumers detailed from *Food Safety and You* (Government of Canada, 2014).

Cleaning:

- Wash anything that comes in contact with food to help eliminate bacteria. This includes your hands, utensils, cutting boards, fruit and vegetables, and reusable grocery bags.

- Wash all parts of the hands thoroughly with running warm water with soap and friction for approximately 20 seconds. Teach children to sing the *Happy Birthday* song twice. If no water is available, use alcohol-based hand sanitizers.
- Clean all surfaces with warm, soapy water often (including all appliances, knobs, and handles) and clean up spills immediately. A kitchen sanitizer or bleach solution (5 mL bleach to 750 mL of water) can be used to sanitize surfaces.
- At least once a week, discard refrigerated foods that should no longer be eaten. Cooked leftovers should be discarded after 4 days; raw meat, poultry, fish, and seafood should be discarded 2 to 3 days after purchasing, or they should be frozen before this time.

Separating:
- Do not cross-contaminate. Keep raw meat and poultry separated from foods that will not be cooked while shopping, preparing, or storing foods.
- Rinse fresh fruits and vegetables thoroughly with potable water before eating, cutting, or cooking them (unless they are prepackaged). Scrub firm surfaces (e.g., cantaloupes and cucumbers) with a produce brush. Commercial cleaners are unnecessary.

Cooking:
- Cook food to the proper temperatures (Table 21.2) and use a food thermometer. The appearance or smell of food does not always indicate its safety.
- Seafood, meat, poultry, and egg dishes should be cooked to the recommended safe minimum internal temperature to destroy harmful microbes. Eggs should be cooked thoroughly, and children should not "lick" the bowls of cake mixes using fresh eggs.
- When food is being cooked in a microwave oven, foods should be stirred, rotated, and/or flipped periodically to help them cook evenly.

Chill:
- Refrigerate food promptly within 2 hours. This includes groceries, food being prepared, and leftovers and takeout foods. Keep the refrigerator at 4°C (40°F) or less and the freezer at −18°C (0°F) or less and monitor temperatures with a thermometer.
- Keep hot food hot (60°C [140°F] or higher) and cold foods cold (0–4°C [32–40°F]). Between these temperatures is the danger zone (between 4°C [40°F] to 60°C [140°F]) in which harmful bacteria can grow rapidly, even exponentially.
- Thaw food properly to avoid any bad bacteria: in the refrigerator; in cold water, such as in a leak-proof bag, changing the water for cold water every 30 minutes; or in the microwave oven, never on the countertop.

These guidelines also apply to takeout meals, restaurant leftovers, and home-packed meals to go. If in doubt, discard it.

Making a food safe after it has been handled improperly may not always be possible. For example, certain bacteria found in food that has been left at room temperature too long may produce a heat-resistant toxin that cannot be

**TABLE 21.2  Safe Internal Cooking Temperatures**

| Category | Temperature |
|---|---|
| **Beef, Veal, and Lamb** | |
| Ground meat (burgers, meatballs, sausages) | 71°C (160°F) |
| Pieces and whole cuts | medium-rare: 63°C (145°F) <br> medium: 71°C (160°F) <br> well done: 77°C (170°F) |
| **Pork (Ham, Pork Loin, Ribs)** | |
| Ground pork (burgers, meatballs, sausages) | 71°C (160°F) |
| Pieces and whole cuts | 71°C (160°F) |
| **Poultry (Chicken, Turkey, Duck)** | |
| Ground poultry (burger, meatballs, sausages) | 74°C (165°F) |
| Frozen raw breaded chicken products (nuggets, fingers, strips, burgers) | 74°C (165°F) |
| Pieces (wings, breasts, legs, thighs) | 74°C (165°F) |
| Stuffing (cooked alone or in bird) | 74°C (165°F) |
| Whole | 82°C (180°F) |
| **Eggs** | |
| Egg dishes | 74°C (165°F) |
| **Seafood** | |
| Fish | 70°C (158°F) |
| Shellfish (shrimp, lobster, crab, scallops, clams, mussels, oysters) | 74°C (165°F) *discard any that do not open when cooked* |

Government of Canada. (2015). *Safe cooking temperatures.* Retrieved from https://www.canada.ca/en/health-canada/services/general-food-safety-tips/safe-internal-cooking-temperatures.html © All rights reserved. *Health Canada.* Adapted and reproduced with permission from the Minister of Health, 2019.

destroyed by cooking. Therefore the principal point is to be careful in preparing food, including cooking foods to the right temperatures, keeping track of the time food is exposed to certain temperatures, and being vigilant when eating out. If there is any doubt about the safety of the food, it is better not to eat it.

Without exception, everyone should exercise their best judgement and care when eating out, when handling their own food, or when handling the food of others. Prevention through education is the key to promoting healthy lives that are unscathed by the potentially severe and life-threatening effects of food-borne illness. On a more positive note, normal healthy adults with healthy immune systems are able to withstand the ill effects of most contaminants from the environment and from food.

## HEALTH, NUTRITION, AND FOOD INSECURITY IN CANADA

Household food insecurity, defined as the inadequate or insecure access to food due to financial constraints, is a significant social and public health issue in Canada, affecting both adults and children (Tarasuk, Mitchell, & Dachner, 2016). It has negative impacts on physical, mental, and social health, and costs the Canadian health care system a considerable amount of money and resources. Food insecurity is firmly established in material deprivation, with low income being the strongest predictor. In 2014, when results for the participating provinces and territories (excluding British Columbia, Manitoba, Newfoundland and Labrador, and Yukon) were considered together, 12% of Canadian households experienced some level of food insecurity during the previous 12 months. This figure represents 1.3 million households, or 3.2 million individuals, including nearly 1 million (one in six) children under the age of 18 years (Tarasuk et al., 2016).

## Monitoring Food Insecurity in Canada

Statistics Canada began monitoring food insecurity in 2005 through the Canadian Community Health Survey (CCHS), a cross-sectional survey administered by Statistics Canada that collects health-related information from approximately 60,000 permanently residing Canadians per year. The sample is designed to be representative of the 10 provinces and three territories, yet it excludes individuals living on reserves or Crown Lands, full time members of the Canadian Forces, persons in prisons or care facilities, and the homeless. Although on-reserve Indigenous people and homeless individuals compose relatively small proportions of the populations in each province, their high levels of vulnerability to food insecurity must mean that the true prevalence of food insecurity is, to some extent, underestimated.

Within the CCHS, the Household Food Security Module is included to monitor households' experiences of food insecurity over a 12-month period. The survey module consists of 18 questions pertaining to the presence of food-insecure situations in the household. The situations outlined range from worrying about running out of food, to going for whole days without eating because of inadequate finances. Depending on the number of positive responses, households are classified as food secure or marginally food insecure (worrying about running out of food); moderately food insecure (compromise in quality/quantity of food due to lack of money or food); or severely food insecure (miss meals, reduce intake, and/or go days without food). It is important to note that the Food Security Module is not always included in the CCHS and during cycles of the CCHS where it has been optional, some provinces and territories have opted out of participation (i.e., 2013–2014 cycle: British Columbia, Manitoba, Newfoundland and Labrador, and Yukon; 2015–2016 cycle: Ontario, Newfoundland and Labrador, and Yukon). As a result, there are no national estimates of food insecurity for those years. The next national estimates will be available when the 2017–2018 CCHS data are released.

## Children in Food Insecure Households

Food insecurity is more prevalent among households with children 18 years of age or younger, particularly those run by single mothers (Tarasuk et al., 2016). Current research shows that exposure to severe food insecurity has a lasting impact of children's well-being, manifesting in higher risks for conditions such as asthma, depression, and suicidal ideation in adolescence and early adulthood (Kirkpatrick, McIntyre, & Potestio, 2010; McIntyre, Williams, Lavorato, et al., 2012; McIntyre, Wu, Kwok, et al., 2017). Taking into consideration the provinces and territories that monitored food insecurity in 2013 and 2014 (Alberta, Saskatchewan, Ontario, Quebec, New Brunswick, Nova Scotia, Prince Edward Island, the Northwest Territories, and Nunavut) the following statistics resulted (Tarasuk et al., 2016):

- 17.2% of children lived in households affected by food insecurity.
- Two-thirds of these children resided in households that were classified as moderately or severely food insecure.
- More than half the children living in Nunavut lived in food insecure households, the highest rate in Canada.
- The Northwest Territories have the second highest prevalence of children living in food insecure households at 29%.
- Prince Edward Island, Nova Scotia, and New Brunswick (the Maritime provinces) had rates greater than 20%, meaning more than one in five children were affected by food insecurity in these provinces.
- Quebec and Alberta were found to have the lowest prevalence of children in food-insecure families, both at 16%, yet even in these cases, almost one in six children were affected.

## Indigenous People and Food Insecurity

Indigenous people are the original inhabitants of Canada and include Inuit, Métis, and First Nations living on- and off-reserve. National data on Indigenous people and household food insecurity in Canada primarily comes from the cycles of the CCHS. However, as previously mentioned, the CCHS excludes individuals living on-reserve in Canada, and thus data from these surveys do not represent the experience of on-reserve Indigenous people. This exclusion represents more than one-third of the Indigenous people in Canada.

Research conducted with Indigenous people in Canada repeatedly demonstrates their remarkable vulnerability to household food insecurity (Huet, Rosol, & Egeland, 2012; Power, 2008; Willows, Veugelers, Raine, et al., 2008). Indigenous households in Canada are more likely than non-Indigenous households to experience the sociodemographic risk factors associated with household food insecurity, such as extreme poverty, single-motherhood, living in a rental property, and reliance on social assistance (Willows et al., 2008). Furthermore, even after these factors are adjusted for, Indigenous households continue to exist at a much higher risk of experiencing household food insecurity and are more likely to be categorized as severely food insecure (Willows et al., 2008).

Researchers and practitioners alike continue to emphasize the distinct food practices among Indigenous groups in Canada. The current measures of household food insecurity used in the CCHS were not developed within Indigenous contexts, and therefore do not probe for information that may be important to Indigenous peoples' household food insecurity. For example, household food insecurity may be related to obtaining food from both market and traditional sources (i.e., fishing,

## TABLE 21.3  Select Nutrition Programs

| Program | Mission | To Find Out More |
|---|---|---|
| Nutrition North Canada (NNC) | NNC is a Government of Canada subsidy program aiming to bring healthy food to isolated northern communities. NNC works with stores across the North and food suppliers in southern Canada to help make perishable, nutritious food more affordable and more accessible. | https://www.nutritionnorthcanada.gc.ca |
| Canada Prenatal Nutrition Program (CPNP) | The CPNP is a community-based program that provides support to improve the health and well-being of pregnant women, new mothers, and babies facing challenging life circumstances. The Public Health Agency of Canada (PHAC) currently funds 276 CPNP projects serving over 51,000 pregnant women and parents/caregivers in over 2000 communities across Canada each year. | https://www.canada.ca/en/public-health/services/health-promotion/childhood-adolescence/programs-initiatives/canada-prenatal-nutrition-program-cpnp.html |

Modified from Government of Canada. (2015). *Nutrition Programs*. Ottawa, ON. Retrieved from https://www.canada.ca/en/services/health/nutrition-programs.html.

hunting, gathering), and broader factors such as climate change and environmental pollution may be important considerations due to their impact on the availability of edible plants and animals. Research in the area of household food insecurity among Indigenous people in Canada that is grounded in the realities of Indigenous peoples' culture, beliefs, and political systems is necessary for developing appropriate interventions to reduce household food insecurity among this vulnerable group.

### Community Nutrition Programs

Federal and provincial initiatives such as those aimed at reducing child poverty, programs to increase work force participation, and funding of community-based food and nutrition programs to assist vulnerable populations, may directly or indirectly impact household food insecurity. However, improving the rates of household food insecurity in Canada is not the main focus of these initiatives and little evaluation has been conducted to measure their impact. As previously mentioned, food insecurity continues to be a prevalent and serious problem in Canada, and community food programs are the primary response to the issue.

Currently, when a household is unable to purchase the food that they need, they may reach out to charitable food assistance in the form of food banks and meal/snack programs. However, these programs are limited in their ability to address food insecurity. Groceries provided by food banks are often limited in quantity as well as quality. In addition, research examining meal/snack programs has found that supplying meals and/or snacks is often a secondary service for an employer, and thus the schedule and timing of the meals are designed to fit within the existing operations and resources, and not the food and nutrition needs of the program users (Pettes, Dachner, Gaetz, et al., 2016).

In addition to charitable food assistance, there are a variety of community-based food and nutrition programs that have broad social goals related to the environment and to community engagement (Table 21.3). However, many also strive to increase access to nutritious foods and local foods among low-income and vulnerable groups and are sometimes viewed as food security initiatives. These programs include community kitchens, community gardens, food buying clubs, farmers' markets, and food boxes. The limited research on these types of initiatives suggests very low participation rates, with little potential to impact food insecure households (Loopstra & Tarasuk, 2013).

## NUTRITION SCREENING

Nutrition screening is the process of discovering characteristics or risk factors that are known to be associated with dietary or nutrition problems. Its primary purpose is to identify individuals who are potentially at high risk of complex and involved problems that relate to nutrition. To serve this purpose, screening criteria must be simple, relatively straightforward, and easy to administer. Screening is also helpful in establishing priorities for the most efficient use of valuable time and money (for more information, refer to the Canadian Malnutrition Task Force at http://nutritioncareincanada.ca).

The single largest demographic group at disproportionate risk of malnutrition is older Canadians. Given that malnutrition is not always an obvious condition, nutrition screening holds a tremendous preventive health potential for older persons. One validated and recommended nutrition screening tool is the Canadian Nutrition Screening Tool (CNST) (Canadian Malnutrition Task Force, 2014). The interprofessional medical team (including the registered nurse) should assess the need for nutritional therapy or a referral to a registered dietitian for an individual who has food-related problems that are impacting eating pleasure, health, and quality of life (Canadian Malnutrition Task Force, 2019). Upon formal screening, individuals should be referred to a dietitian when there has been an involuntary decrease in weight of more than 4.5 kg (10 pounds) during the previous 6 months and if food intake has been lower than usual for more than one week (Canadian Malnutrition Task Force, 2014). The pendulum has shifted to reduce unnecessary therapeutic diets for those at risk of unintentional weight loss and undernutrition. There is also controversy about the benefit of weight loss for obese older Canadians, except if their laboratory test results indicate risk of metabolic syndrome. A dietitian or community nutrition program might be appropriate if any of the following are identified in the individual:

- Inappropriate or inadequate food intake
- Desire by obese older person to lose weight—tailoring to provide adequate calories, protein, and physical activity to preserve lean body mass

- Need for nutrient/disease-specific counselling with specific food needs, preferences, cultural taboos, or environmental constraints
- Serum cholesterol levels of more than 6.2 mmol/L with desire to change eating pattern
- Serum albumin level less than 3.5 g/dL
- Inability to self-feed or to prepare and purchase food, or inability to carry out food-related activities of daily living

Additional measurements and clinical presentations suggesting malnutrition include the following:

- Triceps skin-fold thickness less than the tenth percentile (performed by experienced personnel)
- Mid-arm muscle circumference less than the tenth percentile (performed by experienced personnel)
- Evidence of reduced bone mineral density or osteoporosis (indicated by a history of bone pain or fractures, poor nutritional intake, or family history)
- Evidence of vitamin or mineral deficiency (indicated by long-term inadequate or malabsorption secondary to chronic diseases; alopecia, angular stomatitis, glossitis, spoon-shaped nails, bleeding gums; pressure sores in bedbound individuals or poor wound healing

## NUTRITION RISK FACTORS

This section examines the role of nutrition in the cause and prevention of the leading nutrition-related chronic diseases—heart disease, stroke, some forms of cancer, osteoporosis, obesity, and type 2 diabetes.

## Cardiovascular Diseases

Cardiovascular diseases (CVDs) principally coronary heart disease (CHD) and stroke, are among the leading killers of both men and women among all racial and ethnic groups in Canada. Approximately one in every 12 Canadians (or 2.4 million people) has some form of CVD, including hypertension, CHD, and stroke (PHAC, 2017b). Canada is reported to be a leader in the management and prevention of hypertension and cardiovascular disease, demonstrating the impact of public policy, advocacy, and shifts in treatment and management from specialist care to primary care on reducing incidence of disease (Schiffrin, Campbell, Feldman, et al., 2016).

## Heart Disease

### Diet Intervention

In an attempt to reduce the incidence of CVD, the CPHA recommends that people are physically active for 30 to 60 minutes most days of the week, choose healthy foods, including more fruits and vegetables; low-fat dairy products; foods low in saturated fat, trans fat, and sodium; whole grain foods; and protein foods (Research for Evidence-Informed Practice). They also recommend eating less sodium overall; maintaining a healthy weight; limiting alcohol intake to one to two drinks a day, or less; reducing stress, being smoke free; and knowing and controlling your blood pressure (CPHA, n.d.)

---

### ⚕ RESEARCH FOR EVIDENCE-INFORMED PRACTICE

#### Dietary Risk Factors and Heart Disease

Developing guidelines and recommendations for preventing heart disease is a topic that is routinely reassessed. You may ask, "Why do the recommendations change over time?" As with all things scientific, technology is ever-growing and advancing. Such scientific progress brings new findings, for which guidelines are amended. The gold standard in medicine is to base all medical intervention protocols on evidence-informed practice. Evidence-informed practice is the use of current evidence from available research coupled with clinical expertise to establish high-quality patient care.

Cardiovascular disease is among the leading cause of death in Canada, and suboptimal diet quality is the single largest risk factor contributing to death and disability (Statistics Canada, 2016). The Heart and Stroke Foundation notes that the primary contributors to unhealthy dietary habits are insufficient consumption of fruits, vegetables, nuts/seeds, whole grains, and seafood, and an excessively high intake of sodium and sugar (Heart and Stroke Foundation, 2014a). Although the Heart and Stroke Foundation considers the following dietary changes to be modest, providers should be aware that these recommendations do not take into consideration the complexity of the social determinants of health:

- Eat more fruits and vegetables because they are rich in vitamins, minerals, and fibre, and they are low in calories, fat, and salt.
- Choose food higher in fibre, which include vegetables, fruits, whole grains, and legumes such as lentils.
- Cut the salt. Reducing salt intake can reduce the risk of stroke and heart disease by about one-third.
- Choose healthy fats. Saturated and trans fats raise cholesterol levels while unsaturated fats (such as those found in fish, nuts, and vegetable oils) decrease cholesterol.
- Cut the added sugar, as there is no specific amount of sugar recommended as a part of a healthy diet. Added sugar offers no nutritional value.
- Eat moderate portions.

Considering that up to 80% of early heart disease and stroke can be prevented by adopting a healthy, balanced diet and healthy behaviours, there is plenty of room for improving the overall health of Canadians (Heart and Stroke Foundation, 2014b).

Sources: Heart and Stroke Foundation. (2014a). *Position Statement: Dietary sodium, heart disease and stroke.* Retrieved from https://www.heartandstroke.ca/-/media/pdf-files/canada/2017-position-statements/dietary-sodium-ps-eng.ashx; Heart and Stroke Foundation. (2014b). *Position Statement: Sugar, heart disease and stroke.* Retrieved from https://www.heartandstroke.ca/-/media/pdf-files/canada/2017-position-statements/sugar-ps-eng.ashx?la=en&hash=F53E60FC6C6570BBE76A3B5BF9062D8E7D76DE3B; Mozaffarian, D, Benjamin, E. J., Go, A. S., Arnett, D. K., et al. (2016). Heart disease and stroke statistics—2016 update: A report from the American Heart Association. *Circulation, 133,* e38–e360.

---

Many children, adolescents, and adults who already have unhealthy levels of lipids in their blood should receive nutrition counselling (Heart and Stroke Foundation, 2017). In children aged 2 to 20 years, an acceptable level of total cholesterol is less than 4.4 mmol/L.

Individuals with low-density lipoprotein (LDL) cholesterol levels that are higher than 2.59 mmol/L should be advised to restrict their intake of foods high in dietary cholesterol such as egg yolks, organ meats, full-fat dairy products, and processed meats (Heart and Stoke Foundation, 2017). *Canada's Dietary Guidelines for Health Professionals and Policy Makers* does not set specific

## TABLE 21.4 Cholesterol and Lipoprotein Profile Classification

| Cholesterol Reading | Classification |
|---|---|
| **Total Cholesterol (mmol/L)** | |
| <5.2 | Desirable |
| 5.2–6.2 | Borderline |
| >6.2 | High |
| **Low-Density Lipoprotein Cholesterol (mmol/L)** | |
| <2.59 | Optimal |
| 2.59–3.34 | Near optimal |
| 3.37–4.11 | Borderline high |
| 4.14–4.9 | High |
| ≥4.92 | Very high |
| **High-Density Lipoprotein Cholesterol (mmol/L)** | |
| ≥1.55 | Desirable |
| 1–1.55 | Acceptable |
| <1 | Low |
| **Triglycerides (mmol/L)** | |
| <1.7 | Normal |
| 1.7–2.2 | Borderline high |
| 2.2–5.6 | High |
| ≥5.6 | Very high |

Modified from Van Leeuwen, A.M., Bladh, M.L. (2019). *Davis's comprehensive manual of laboratory and diagnostic tests with nursing implications* (8th ed.). Philadelphia: F.A. Davis Co.

quantitative limits for dietary cholesterol consumption per day. However, the healthy eating patterns that are recommended are naturally low in cholesterol. Individuals at risk of heart disease may be advised to further limit their cholesterol intake, particularly if their LDL cholesterol levels are high. After the dietary intervention has been outlined to the individual, follow-up sessions are scheduled to monitor lipid levels and dietary adherence.

The Canadian Cardiovascular Society develops new guidelines periodically, as warranted by research advances. The most recent set of guidelines are the *2016 Canadian Cardiovascular Society Guidelines for the Management of Dyslipidemia for the Prevention of Cardiovascular Disease in the Adult*. These guidelines now recommend lipid screening for both men and women who are 40 years of age or older, and screening for women with a history of hypertensive disease in pregnancy (HDP) with considerations for earlier screening practices in ethnic groups are increased risk, such as South Asian or Indigenous peoples. In addition, new LDL-cholesterol targets have been established for individuals for whom treatment is initiated (LDL-C <2.0 mmol/L) or for recent acute coronary syndrome (ACS) patients (LDL-C <1.8 mmol/L). Key messages of the guidelines include that LDL-cholesterol levels are directly linked to the development of atherosclerosis and its reduction is directly linked to the reduction in cardiovascular disease events as well as the importance of behaviour modification in risk reduction (Table 21.4).

According to the Canadian Cardiovascular Society's (2016) *Dyslipidemia Guidelines*, all patients with the following conditions regardless of age should undergo lipid screening:

- Clinical evidence of atherosclerosis (peripheral arterial disease, abdominal aortic aneurysm, and symptomatic carotid artery disease)
- Age (≥40 years for men and women or postmenopausal)
- Current cigarette smoking
- Arterial hypertension
- Family history of premature CVD (heart disease in a first-degree relative at age less than 55 years for men or at age less than 65 years for women)
- Family history of dyslipidemia
- Diabetes mellitus
- Chronic kidney disease
- Obesity (body mass index [BMI] ≥30 mg/m²)
- Inflammatory disease
- HIV infection
- Erectile dysfunction
- Chronic obstructive pulmonary disease (COPD)
- Hypertensive diseases in pregnancy
- Metabolic syndrome

### Health Behaviour Interventions

The health behaviour interventions that include healthy eating, physical activity, and smoking cessation are recommended for treatment of people who present with type 2 diabetes, elevated levels of LDL, or metabolic syndrome.

Metabolic syndrome describes the presence of a cluster of risk factors that often occur together, which dramatically increases the risk of coronary events. The syndrome is diagnosed when an individual has three or more of the following factors:

- Excessive abdominal fat, as indicated by too large a waist circumference measurement (88 cm [or >35 inches] in women and 102 cm [or >40 inches] in men)
- Elevated triglyceride level (>1.7 mmol/L), which is significantly linked to the degree of heart disease risk
- Low HDL level (<1.3 mmol/L in women and <1.0 mmol/L in men)
- Elevated blood pressure (higher than 130 mm Hg systolic or 85 mm Hg diastolic)
- Elevated fasting plasma glucose (FPG) (≥5.6 mmol/L)

The dietary component of the health behaviour interventions include the following daily intake:

- Target intake of saturated fats of less than 9% of total energy.
- Avoid the intake of trans fats and decrease the intake of saturated fats.
- Target intake of saturated fats of less than 9% of total energy.
- If saturated fats are replaced with mono-unsaturated fatty acids (MUFAs) and carbohydrates then people should choose plant sources of MUFAs such as olive oil, canola oil, nuts, and seeds, and high-quality sources of carbohydrates including whole grains and low glycemic index carbohydrates.
- All individuals should be encouraged to moderate energy (caloric) intake to achieve and maintain a healthy body weight.

A primary treatment goal of the health behaviour interventions is reduction of an elevated LDL level to:

- Target LDL-C consistently: <2.0 mmol/L or >50% reduction of LDL-C for individuals for whom treatment is initiated to lower the risk of CVD events and mortality.
- A >50% reduction of LDL-C for patients with LDL-C >5.0 mmol/L in individuals for whom treatment is initiated to decrease the risk of CVD events and mortality.

The final goal of the health behaviour interventions includes smoking cessation (to reduce CVD risk) and physical activity that accumulates to at least 150 minutes of moderate-to-vigorous intensity per week in bouts of 10 minutes or more (to reduce CVD risk).

### Removing Barriers to Treatment Goals

To improve an individual's adherence to the recommendations made by the Canadian Cardiovascular Society (2016), treatment barriers can be eliminated by the development of protocols to encourage long-term individual adherence and follow-up, such as establishing clinic policy and developing computerized databases for those seeking care, establishing management algorithms, reinforcing and rewarding adherence. The nurse uses behavioural theories to identify a person's level of readiness to change and focus on counselling strategies to match that level of readiness (Snetselaar, 2004).

## Hypertension

Blood pressure, the force of blood against the walls of arteries, is recorded as the systolic pressure (as the heart beats) over the diastolic pressure (as the heart relaxes between beats). The measurement is written with one number above (or before) the other, with the systolic blood pressure (SBP) listed first and the diastolic blood pressure (DBP) listed second. For example, a blood pressure measurement of 120/80 mm Hg is expressed verbally as "120 over 80." Normal blood pressure is less than 120 mm Hg systolic and less than 80 mm Hg diastolic. *Hypertension Canada's 2018 Guidelines for Diagnosis, Risk Assessment, Prevention, and Treatment of Hypertension in Adults and Children* (Nerenberg, Zarnke, Leung, et al., 2018) introduced five new guidelines and revised one existing guideline (Nerenberg et al., 2018). Hypertension Canada produces annually updated, evidence-informed guidelines for health care providers with the intent to provide a framework for evidence-informed care of hypertension.

### Epidemiology

Hypertension is one of the most common chronic diseases affecting Canadians across their lifespan, with approximately 2% of children and adolescents (Statistics Canada, 2015b), to 7% of pregnant women, to 25% of the adult population being affected (Padwal, Bienek, McAlister, et al., 2016). Furthermore, approximately 20% of Canadian adults are either unaware of their hypertension or are aware but are not being treated with antihypertensive medications and, as a consequence, their disease is uncontrolled (Padwal et al., 2016). Hypertension has extensive effects on the overall health of Canadians due to its association with obesity, chronic kidney disease, cardiovascular disease, and death (Padwal et al., 2016). Untreated or uncontrolled hypertension can damage arteries and increase the risk of stroke and heart failure. High blood pressure is also responsible for many cases of kidney failure, requiring dialysis, and increases the risk of kidney failure in people with diabetes.

Indigenous and Black Canadians and people of Asian descent are at higher risk for developing hypertension. Slightly more men than women (71% and 69%, respectively) aged 70 to 79 years have high blood pressure. It appears that having diabetes is the strongest predictor overall of developing hypertension, as it increases the risk by 68% for men and 125% for women.

### Diet Intervention

The modifiable nutrition-related risk factors for stroke include high blood pressure, obesity, habitual high alcohol intake, and high intake of sodium (Padwal et al., 2016). However there appears to be no need to restrict salt intake to less than the suggested 2000 mg per day currently in the guidelines for the prevention of hypertension and to reduce blood pressure. There appears to be a class of hypertensive individuals who are salt sensitive who benefit from sodium restriction (Sanada, Jones, & Jose, 2011). No certain method exists for identifying susceptible people or ascertaining how many of them become hypertensive as a result of excessive salt intake; therefore, the conservative preventive health approach recommends a daily salt intake limited to 5 g or less for adults. This amount is regarded as mild sodium restriction. Ideally, the recommendations are to reduce sodium intake to approximately 1500 mg per day, but this is very difficult with the current prevalence of sodium in packaged and restaurant foods. In 2012, Health Canada published voluntary targets for reducing sodium in processed food, with an end date of 2016. The targets were designed to encourage gradual reductions, while still maintaining food safety, quality, and consumer acceptance. In 2017, Health Canada began an evaluation process of the food industry's efforts to meet these sodium reduction targets. Only 14% of food categories had met the targeted reduction. In total, 48% of companies did not make any meaningful changes toward sodium reduction; and ironically among the 48%, sodium in several categories had increased. The following are the three major sources of sodium in the Canadian diet, in order of predominance:

- Bakery products, which include: breads, muffins, cookies, desserts, crackers, and granola bars are the top food sources (20%) of sodium.
- Mixed dishes such as pizza, lasagna, refrigerated or frozen entrees and appetizers, frozen potatoes, and prepared salads are the second most important contributors to dietary sodium (19%).
- Processed meat products such as sausages, deli meats, canned meats, chicken wings, burgers, and meatballs (11%).

The following recommended food tips are designed to reduce salt and sodium intake:

- Sodium occurs naturally in many foods and is also added to most processed foods; therefore add salt only sparingly in home cooking and at the table.
- Consume fewer foods that have high sodium levels, such as many cheeses; processed meats; most frozen dinners and entrees; packaged mixes; most canned soups and vegetables; salad dressings; and condiments such as soy sauce, pickles, olives, ketchup, and mustard.
- Rinse canned vegetables before warming them.
- Eat salty, highly processed salty, salt-preserved, and salt-pickled foods infrequently.

- Check labels for the amount of sodium in foods and choose products lower in sodium (less than 360 mg of sodium per serving, or less than 15% daily value of sodium).

## Dietary Approaches to Stop Hypertension Eating Plan

Clinical studies show that following the Dietary Approaches to Stop Hypertension (DASH) eating plan helps to lower blood pressure. The US National Heart, Lung, and Blood Institute, with additional support by the National Institutes of Health (NIH), funded the DASH research, with the final results appearing in 1997. The DASH eating plan makes consuming less salt and sodium easier because the plan includes abundant fruits and vegetables, which are lower in sodium but higher in potassium than other foods. Potassium and sodium play important roles as electrolytes in intracellular and extracellular fluid balance. People at high risk of hypertension may have a high sodium intake that may upset the sodium-to-potassium ratio, and eating more vegetables and fruits may account for the success of the DASH diet. The plan also includes more fat-free or low-fat milk and milk products, whole grains, fish, poultry, beans, seeds, and nuts, but contains less sweets, added sugars and sugar-containing beverages, fats, and red meats than the average typical Canadian diet.

The plan is rich in magnesium, potassium, calcium, protein, and fibre. At approximately 2000 calories a day, the nutrients include 4700 mg of potassium, 500 mg of magnesium, and 1250 mg of calcium. These totals are approximately two to three times the amounts that most Canadians receive.

On the basis of the findings of DASH clinical studies, a combination of the eating plan and reduced sodium intake can reduce elevated blood pressure or prevent it when blood pressure is normal. The plan may even eliminate the need for medication or, in the case of severe high blood pressure, allow a reduction in medication. Other steps to control or prevent hypertension should continue to be encouraged, including exercise and weight loss when necessary, not smoking, and limiting alcohol consumption. DASH may also improve health in other ways. The potassium in fruits and vegetables helps reduce hypertension (AHA, 2016) and may reduce the risk of some cancers; the calcium in dairy products may reduce fat mass and thus hypertension (Zemel, 2001). The diet may help lower the risk of osteoporosis, and a diet low in saturated fat and cholesterol can reduce CVD risk. The complete DASH eating plan entitled *Your Guide to Lowering Your Blood Pressure With DASH* (USDHHS, NIH, National Heart, Lung, and Blood Institute, 2006) can be obtained from http://www.nhlbi.nih.gov/health/resources/heart/hbp-dash-index.

## Cancer
### Epidemiology

The Government of Canada estimates that approximately one in two Canadians (49% of men and 45% of women) will receive a diagnosis of some type of cancer in their lifetime. Cancer remains the leading cause of death in Canada and is responsible for 30% of all deaths (Canadian Cancer Society Advisory Committee, 2018).

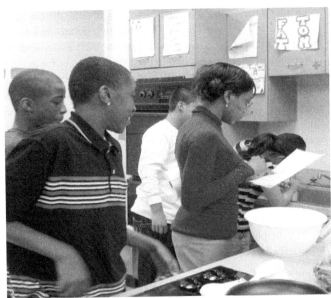

Fig. 21.4 Teenagers who help to prepare safe, nutritious meals become engaged in the healthy eating process. (From Mahan, L. K., & Raymond, J. L. [2017]. *Krause's food & the nutrition care process* [14th ed.]. St Louis: Elsevier.)

The most common cancers in men and women are lung, breast, colorectal, and prostate (excluding nonmelanoma skin cancer); these cancers comprise approximately 50% of new cancer cases. Over 26% of cancer deaths are due to lung cancer. For men in 2017, approximately 50% of new cases will occur at prostate, colorectal, and lung sites; in women the most common sites are breast, lung, and colorectal. Breast cancer alone accounts for 26% of newly diagnosed cancer cases in women (Canadian Cancer Society Advisory Committee, 2018).

Approximately one-third of cancer diagnosed among men and women world-wide can be prevented by eating well, being active, and having a healthy body weight. However, health care providers must be aware that many individuals face barriers to these prevention strategies which are directly associated with the social determinants of health (i.e., income, employment status, education, literacy, etc.) The introduction of a healthy diet (Fig. 21.4) and exercise practices at any time from childhood to old age can promote health and likely reduce cancer risk.

### Diet Intervention for Risk Reduction

Many dietary factors can affect cancer risk: types of foods, food preparation methods, portion sizes, food variety, and overall calorie balance. An overall dietary pattern that balances calorie intake and physical activity for weight management along with inclusion of a high proportion of plant foods (fruits, vegetables, whole grains, and beans) and limited amounts of processed or red meats and whole-fat dairy products, may reduce the risk of cancer. The phytochemicals in fruits and vegetables, in particular, appear to have a protective effect by themselves, but dietary supplements, in particular supplements that exceed DRIs, do not provide the same benefits.

Based on its review of the scientific evidence, the Canadian Cancer Society continually updates its nutrition and physical activity recommendations. The Canadian Cancer Society recommendations are very consistent with the messages of *Canada's Dietary Guidelines for Health Professionals and Policy Makers, Canada's Food Guide* and the Eat Well Plate, and the dietary recommendations of other national agencies for general health promotion and prevention of other diet-related chronic conditions. Although no diet can guarantee full protection against any disease, the Canadian Cancer Society believes that the following recommendations offer the best nutrition information currently available to help Canadians.

For individuals:

- Choose most of the foods you eat from plant sources. Choose fewer and smaller portions of high-fat or calorie-dense foods and beverages. To get the right amount of vegetables and fruit needed each day, make them half your place at every meal and snack. Choose whole-grain breads, cereals, pastas, brown rice, and beans. Limit consumption of processed meat (bacon, sausage, luncheon meats) and red meats such as beef, pork, or lamb. For those who do eat meat, choose leaner cuts and small portions, not more than one-quarter of the plate (similar to the Eat Well Plate recommendation). Many scientific studies show that eating fruits and vegetables (especially green and dark yellow or orange vegetables, foods in the cabbage family, soy products, and legumes) may protect against cancers at many sites, particularly for cancers of the gastrointestinal and respiratory tracts. Grains as well as fruits, vegetables, and dairy products are also an important source of many vitamins and minerals, such as folate, calcium, and selenium, which have been associated with a lower risk of colon cancer in some studies. Beans (legumes) are especially rich in nutrients that may protect against cancer. Consumption of meat, particularly red and processed meats, has been associated with an increased risk of cancer at several sites, most notably the colon, stomach, and prostate.
- Be physically active: achieve and maintain a healthy weight by aiming for 30 minutes of moderate daily activity. Being overweight or obese, by itself or in combination with excess belly fat, increases the risk of cancers at several sites, such as the colon and rectum, prostate, endometrium, breast (among postmenopausal women), and kidney. Both increasing physical activity and balancing food intake to maximize nutrient density within calorie needs are essential. Keeping a healthy BMI without being underweight is ideal. If overweight, avoidance of more weight gain or even losing as little as 5 to 10% of weight can be beneficial.
- For those who drink alcohol, limit consumption. No more than one drink per day for women or two drinks per day for men should be the limit. Alcoholic beverages, along with cigarette smoking and the use of tobacco products, contribute to cancers of the oral cavity, esophagus, and larynx. Studies have also shown drinking about 3.5 drinks a day increases your risk of developing colorectal cancer and breast cancer by 1.5 times (Canadian Cancer Society, 2019). Reducing alcohol consumption is a good way for both men and women who drink regularly to reduce their risk of certain types of cancer.

Nurses may find it is helpful to refer to the sections under the *Prevention and Screening* tab of the Canadian Cancer Society website that refer to other aspects of food intake relating to prevention of cancer. They include more specific suggestions for particular cancers, evidence specific to nutrient supplementation, and answers to other frequently asked questions. It is available at http://www.cancer.ca/en/prevention-and-screening/reduce-cancer-risk/can-cancer-be-prevented/?region=ns.

## Osteoporosis

### Epidemiology

Osteoporosis, is a bone disease characterized by low bone mass leading to fragile bones and an increased risk of hip, spine, and wrist fractures, and is a major public health risk affecting two million Canadians, most commonly those aged 50 years or older (Osteoporosis Canada, n.d.). According to the 2009 CCHS, approximately 19% or women and 3% of men over 50 years of age have been diagnosed with osteoporosis; however, it can occur at any age. Over 80% of all fractures in those 50 years and older are secondary to osteoporosis. Although men and women begin losing bone mass equally in their 30s, women are almost twice as likely to suffer from an osteoporotic fracture compared to men, primarily due to the reduction in bone-protective estrogen after menopause. Direct financial expenditures for management of osteoporotic fracture alone were estimated at $2.3 billion in 2010 and will likely increase given the estimated four-fold increase in prevalence of hip fractures in Canada by 2030 (Papadimitropouos, Coyte, Josse, et al., 1997). These figures underestimate significantly the true costs of osteoporosis because they fail to include the costs of treatment for individuals without a history of fractures or the indirect costs of lost wages or productivity of either the individual or the caregiver.

Osteoporosis Canada (2010) recognizes the following risk factors for osteoporosis that should prompt relevant investigations (i.e., bone mineral density, serological testing).

Younger adults (age <50 years):

- Fragility fracture (breaking a bone as a result of a minor accident)
- Long-term use of glucocorticoids, such as prednisone
- Hypogonadism or premature menopause (age < 45 years)
- Having other disorders strongly associated with rapid bone loss and/or fracture such as rheumatoid arthritis, malabsorption syndrome, and primary hyperparathyroidism.

Older persons (age > 50 years):

- Being 65 years or older
- Clinical risk factors for fracture (menopausal women, men age 50 to 64 years):
  - Fragility fracture (breaking a bone as a result of a minor accident)
  - Long-term use of glucocorticoids, such as prednisone
  - Having a parent who had a hip fracture
  - Having a spine fracture or low bone mass identified on X-ray
  - Being a smoker
  - High alcohol intake (greater than or equal to 3 units per day on a consistent basis)

## TABLE 21.5 Dietary Reference Intakes for Calcium and Vitamin D

| Life Stage Group | CALCIUM | | VITAMIN D | |
| --- | --- | --- | --- | --- |
| | RDA (mg/day) | UL (mg/day) | RDA (IU/day) | UL (IU/day) |
| Infants from birth to 6 months | 200 | 1000 | 400 | 1000 |
| Infants from 7 to 12 months | 260 | 1500 | 400 | 1500 |
| 1–3 years | 700 | 2500 | 600 | 2500 |
| 4–8 years | 1000 | 2500 | 600 | 3000 |
| 9–18 years | 1300 | 3000 | 600 | 4000 |
| 19–50 years | 1000 | 2500 | 600 | 4000 |
| 51–70 years, men | 1000 | 2000 | 600 | 4000 |
| 51–70 years, women | 1200 | 2000 | 600 | 4000 |
| >70 years | 1200 | 2000 | 800 | 4000 |
| 14–18 years, pregnant or lactating | 1300 | 3000 | 600 | 4000 |
| 19–50 years, pregnant or lactating | 1000 | 2500 | 600 | 4000 |

*RDA,* Recommended dietary allowance; *UL,* tolerable upper intake level.
Data from Health Canada. (2019). *Vitamin D and calcium: Updated dietary reference intakes.* Ottawa: Government of Canada.

- Low body weight (less than 60 kg or 132 lbs) or major weight loss (present weight is more than 10% below your weight at age 25)
- Having other disorders strongly associated with rapid bone loss and/or fracture as mentioned above

## Pathophysiology

Osteoporosis develops slowly, resulting in loss of bone mass and fractures, especially in the wrist, hip, and spinal areas. It is defined as a skeletal disorder characterized by compromised bone strength predisposing to an increased risk of fracture. Bone strength reflects the integration of two main features: bone density and bone quality. Bone mineral density is expressed as grams of mineral per area or volume and, in any given individual, is determined by peak bone mass and amount of bone loss. Bone quality refers to architecture, turnover, damage accumulation (microfractures), and mineralization. Osteoporotic bone fractures more easily than healthy bone; as such, osteoporosis is a significant risk factor for fracture.

*Factors involved in building and maintaining skeletal health throughout life.* The bone mass attained early in life, 85 to 90% of which is reached by age 18 years for girls and age 20 years for boys, is perhaps the most important determinant of lifelong skeletal health. Individuals with the highest peak bone mass after adolescence have the greatest protective advantage when there is a decline in bone density with increasing age, illness, and diminished sex steroid production.

Genetic factors exert a strong and perhaps predominant influence on peak bone mass, but physiological, environmental, and modifiable lifestyle factors can also play a significant role. Among these factors are adequate nutrition and body weight, the sex hormones of puberty, and physical activity (particularly weight-bearing activity). Therefore maximizing bone mineral density early in life presents a vital opportunity to reduce the effect of bone loss related to aging. Childhood is a critical time for development of lifestyle habits conducive to maintaining good bone health throughout life. Additionally, cigarette smoking, which may start in adolescence, may have a deleterious effect on bone mass.

## Prevention

Once thought to be a natural part of aging among women, osteoporosis is no longer considered age or sex dependent and is largely preventable, thanks to the recent progress in the understanding of its causes, diagnosis, and treatment. Optimization of bone health is a process that must occur throughout the life span in both men and women so as to prevent osteoporosis. Calcium is often difficult to obtain solely from food sources; therefore supplementation is often recommended. However, studies on the benefits of calcium intake on bone mineral density and on fractures have shown that it may have minimal and no effect, respectively (Bolland et al., 2015; Tai, Leung, Grey, et al., 2015). More well-designed clinical trials are needed to fully comprehend calcium's effects.

A healthy diet, adequate in calories and appropriate nutrients, is essential for normal growth and development of all tissues, including bone. Table 21.5 suggests dietary calcium (and vitamin D) intake recommendations for various stages of life. Factors contributing to low calcium intake include restriction of consumption of dairy/dairy alternative products because of food preferences or lactose intolerance, a generally low level of fruit and vegetable consumption, and a high intake of low-calcium beverages such as soft drinks. Lactose and vitamin D enhance calcium absorption, as does as an acidic environment, seen in superior absorption in calcium-enriched orange juice. Bioavailability is important to consider as well, as different sources of calcium will have differing bioavailability, even if they contain similar amounts of calcium. In addition to calcium and vitamin D, other micronutrients such as vitamin K, magnesium, and zinc are also key contributors to optimal bone health.

Vitamin D is a fat-soluble vitamin encompassing two molecules—vitamin $D_2$ (ergocalciferol) and vitamin $D_3$ (cholecalciferol). Vitamin $D_3$ is the form of vitamin D that best supports bone health. It is synthesized in the body when the skin is exposed to the ultraviolet rays of the sun. This process is complicated by various concerns about sunscreens, clothing, and weather changes. Vitamin D from foods, as well as that from sun exposure, then undergoes a complicated metabolic pathway through the liver and the kidneys, emerging as the hormone 1,25-dehydroxyvitamin $D_3$, the active form. Vitamin D is commonly added to milk, and other food sources of vitamin D include fatty fish (salmon and mackerel); fortified margarine; eggs; and some fortified, ready-to-eat cereals. The percentage of Canadians above the recommended vitamin D blood levels across all age groups resembles a U-shape—it is highest among young children and older persons, and lowest for those aged 20 to 39 (Janz & Pearson, 2013). During adolescence, when consumption of dairy products decreases, vitamin D intake is likely to be inadequate, which may affect calcium absorption adversely. Other nutrients have been evaluated relative to bone health. High dietary protein, caffeine, phosphorus, and sodium intake may adversely affect calcium balance; however, their effects appear to be offset in individuals with adequate calcium intakes.

Food should be selected to provide adequate calcium intake. Women of all ages should make sure they get adequate calcium intake by consuming more calcium-rich foods, including calcium-fortified foods such as orange juice, milk and milk alternatives, and other dairy products as they deliver the most calcium of any food group. Low-fat (1%) and fat-free milk, low-fat yogurt, and low-fat cheeses are the dairy products of choice. Other good sources of calcium include sardines, canned salmon (if the bones are eaten), and some dark green leafy vegetables, especially collard greens. Orange juice, milk and milk alternatives such as soy, almond, and rice milks, and other fortified food products are also good sources of calcium. Supplementation with calcium tablets may be appropriate for high-risk individuals with inadequate calcium intake.

For those who do choose calcium supplements, calcium carbonate (40% elemental calcium), calcium citrate (24%), calcium lactate (14%), and calcium gluconate (9%) are preferred. (Dolomite and bone meal are not recommended because they may be contaminated with lead.) Calcium supplement absorption is most efficient for individuals with adequate gastric acid production at doses no greater than 500 mg at a time when taken with meals.

Anyone younger than 25 years who ingests less than the recommended DRI for calcium should be urged to develop strategies for increasing it. Among Canadian children, girls between the ages of 9 and 18 years show the highest rates of inadequate intakes of calcium (67–70%) (Health Canada, 2019). By modelling appropriate behaviours, health care providers can help prevent or delay the onset of osteoporosis in themselves, their families, and the people in their care.

## Obesity

Overweight (defined in the Body Mass Index Formulas section) can seriously affect health and longevity and is associated with the leading nutrition-related causes of death in Canada: type 2 DM, heart disease, and some cancers. Obesity (defined in the Body Mass Index for Adults section) is also associated with gout and gallbladder disease and may contribute to the development of osteoarthritis in the weight-bearing joints.

### Epidemiology

Overweight and obesity are found worldwide, and the prevalence of these conditions in Canada has approximately doubled since the early 1980s. In 2017, 64% of Canadian adults over the age of 18 were considered to be overweight or obese. In children, 30% of those aged 5 to 17 years were classified as overweight or obese. Lifestyle, genetics, hormonal factors, and social-ecological factors are among the many factors contributing to the problem.

In Canada, obesity is more common in men than in women, and obesity rates have increased more for men than for women since 2003. Furthermore, the highest rates of obesity are found in Atlantic Canada, the Prairie provinces, the Northwest Territories, Nunavut, Yukon, and smaller cities in northern and southwestern Ontario. The lowest rates of people with obesity are found in Toronto, Montreal, Vancouver, and areas of southern British Columbia (Navaneelan & Janz, 2014).

Among Indigenous populations, 26% of off-reserve adults and 36% of on-reserve Indigenous Canadians are considered to be obese (Canadian Institute for Health Information [CIHI] & PHAC, 2011). Although data examining trends in obesity prevalence among Indigenous people are limited, obesity continues to be more evident among adults and children in this population compared to non-Indigenous populations.

### Body Mass Index for Adults

Based on an adult's height and weight, BMI is a helpful indicator of underweight, normal weight, overweight, and obesity (Health Canada, 2011). One can calculate a person's BMI by dividing the person's weight in kilograms by their height in metres squared (https://www.canada.ca/en/health-canada/services/food-nutrition/healthy-eating/healthy-weights/canadian-guidelines-body-weight-classification-adults/body-mass-index-nomogram.html).

*Body mass index formulas.* BMI may be used as an indicator of body fat, but it cannot be interpreted as a specific percentage of body fat. Age and sex influence the relationship between fat and BMI. For example, women are more likely to have a higher percentage of body fat than men have for the same BMI. As weight is part of the BMI calculation, it must be noted that scale weights may be inaccurate if used universally. For example, a well-trained athlete with a higher proportion of muscle to fat will weigh more because muscle weighs more than fat. By the same token, bone weight differs in people with smaller frames compared with those with larger frames and higher bone density. BMI is used to screen and monitor a population to detect the risk of health or nutritional disorders. In an individual, other data must be used to determine whether a high BMI is associated with increased risk of disease and death for that person; use of BMI alone is not diagnostic. Waist circumference is a better indicator of the risk of metabolic syndrome. As mentioned previously, the latter identifies several risk factors associated with morbidity such as elevated level of triglycerides, low HDL level, high LDL level, elevated blood glucose level, and elevated blood pressure. For more details, see Health Canada (2011).

BMI ranges are based on the effect body weight has on disease and death. A BMI from 18.5 to 24.9 kg/m$^2$ is a healthy target range for adults. BMIs higher than 25 kg/m$^2$ are associated with increased risks of developing CVD, gallbladder disease, high blood pressure, and non–insulin-dependent DM (type 2 diabetes).

BMIs for adults are expressed by one number, regardless of age or sex, using the following guidelines established by the WHO (2006):

- Underweight: BMI less than 18.5 kg/m$^2$
- Healthy weight: BMI of 18.5 to 24.9 kg/m$^2$
- Overweight: BMI of 25 to 29.9 kg/m$^2$
- Class 1 obese: BMI of 30 to 34.9 kg/m$^2$
- Class 2 obese: BMI of 35 to 39.9 kg/m$^2$
- Class 3 obese (morbid obesity): BMI of 40 kg/m$^2$ or higher

### Body Mass Index Growth Charts for Children

Pediatric health care providers have used growth charts since 1977, with the newest ones released in 2014 by the WHO to more accurately reflect Canada's diversity. To track growth and development in children and adolescents through age 20 years, pediatricians, nurses, and nutritionists use charts widely to assist in signalling potential developmental and weight problems earlier in childhood/adolescence. They consist of a series of percentile curves that illustrate the distribution in growth of children across Canada.

The BMI is an early warning signal that is helpful as early as age 2 years to help identify children who have the potential to become overweight. Early identification of obesity risk gives parents the opportunity to modify their family eating and activity patterns before their children develop a weight problem.

The WHO's growth charts were first adapted for Canada and put into practice in 2010. The charts were redesigned in March 2014 to address concerns of practitioners who had been using the charts since they were first released. The WHO Growth Charts for Canada are recommended for monitoring and assessment of growth of Canadian infants and Children in primary care and public health by the Canadian Pediatric Society, Canadian Pediatric Endocrine Group, College of Family Physicians of Canada, Community Health Nurses of Canada, and Dietitians of Canada. The charts are available on the Dietitians of Canada website at http://www.whogrowthcharts.ca.

### Diet Intervention in Weight Reduction

With the advances in nutritional genomics it may be possible to individualize dietary recommendations on the basis of a person's genotype, thus having a greater impact on risk reduction in diet-related diseases such as obesity (Genomics). A balanced diet to support weight reduction should include appropriate serving sizes to meet individual nutrient needs. Additionally, exercise is particularly important from the outset, because with exercise there is less need to restrict food intake. Exercise also favours long-term maintenance of body weight (as described in Chapter 22).

## GENOMICS

### Nutritional Genomics[a]

The relatively new field of nutritional genomics is a multidisciplinary field of research that investigates the effects a person's diet has on that person's genes (i.e., nutrigenomics) and how our genetic variations dictate our response to certain nutrients (i.e., nutrigenetics). It has long been accepted that slight variations in our genetic makeup account for the individuality of our physical appearances. Think about how you guess at what your height potential will be. We generally look to our biological parents for answers regarding our physical appearance. Likewise, the study of nutritional genomics is attempting to predict how a specific genetic identity will influence a person's response to food and the nutrients within it.

There are many examples of how such individual genetic variants alter disease treatment in health care. For example, two people with hypertension may need different medications to treat the same condition because of their biological response to certain medications. It stands to reason then that the same two people may also benefit from different dietary interventions. Obesity is one of the primary health concerns in North America and is a significant risk factor for all other major chronic diseases. Nutritional genomics makes possible the use of personalized diet prescription based on an individual's specific genetic profile. Researchers believe that the potential for personalized dietary intervention could drastically change the prevalence of chronic disease, particularly that of obesity (Huang & Hu, 2015). If such diet therapies are more effective in managing or preventing disease, this will allow health care to focus more on health promotion instead of disease management. Such a shift in health care represents a significantly more sustainable and cost-effective strategy to enhance the health of the nation.

For additional information regarding nutritional genomics, refer to the website of the Center of Excellence for Nutritional Genomics at the University of California, Davis. Retrieved from http://nutrigenomics.ucdavis.edu.

[a]With contribution from Staci Nix.
Source: Huang, T., & Hu, F. B. (2015). Gene-environment interactions and obesity: Recent developments and future directions. *BMC Med Genomics, 8*(Suppl 1), S2.

Nurses make referrals to supervised or unsupervised programs as appropriate. People expect this type of advice on maintaining their health. Therefore, nurses can play an important role, although not supervising individuals' weight loss efforts directly. For more information on obesity among children and adults, see the *Towards a Healthier Canada—2017 Progress Report on Advancing the Federal/Provincial/Territorial Framework of Healthy Weights* (Pan-Canadian Public Health Network, 2017).

There are many positive effects of only relatively small amounts of weight loss (5–10% of body weight) for people who are obese, including the following:

- Decreased blood pressure (decreased risk of a heart attack and stroke)
- Reduced abnormally high levels of blood glucose associated with diabetes
- Reduced elevated levels of cholesterol and triglycerides associated with CVD
- Reduced sleep apnea (irregular breathing during sleep)
- Decreased risk of osteoarthritis in the weight-bearing joints
- Decreased depression
- Increased self-esteem

The acronym LEARN has been suggested as a mnemonic device for health professionals. LEARN refers to the steps nurses can take to help the person who needs to improve health-related behaviour (Brownell, 2000). LEARN is particularly useful as a guideline for communicating with the clinically obese individual who has indicated dissatisfaction with his or her current weight:

L—Listen with sympathy and understanding to the person's perception of the problem.

E—Explain personal perceptions of the problem.

A—Acknowledge and discuss differences and similarities.

R—Recommend treatment.

N—Negotiate an agreement.

Fad diets do not provide the best way to lose weight and should be avoided. However, recognizing that people will do almost anything to lose weight when desperate, it is helpful to be able to discuss current fads intelligently and to guide individuals as needed. On an individual basis, for people who cannot or do not choose to maintain a BMI less than 30 kg/m$^2$ as a priority, the paradigm *Health At Every Size [HAES]* (Bacon & Aphramor, 2011) is described in Box 21.2.

Medications have been used to help treat obesity, but only as an accompaniment to nutrition, physical activity, and behaviour-modification therapies. Presently, medications approved for weight loss in Canada are those that decrease nutrient absorption. Medications that decrease food intake by reducing appetite or increasing satiety and medications that increase energy expenditure are not approved for weight loss in Canada.

## Diabetes

### Prevalence and Incidence

Diabetes mellitus (DM) is becoming more prevalent, especially type 2 diabetes, which is associated with obesity. The estimated prevalence of diagnosed DM in Canadian adults is 9.3% (approximately 3.4 million people), and is predicted to rise to 12.1% (5 million people) by 2025 (Diabetes Canada, 2017). DM is the leading cause of blindness, end-stage renal disease, and nontraumatic amputation in Canadian adults. Cardiovascular disease continues to be the leading cause of death in individuals with diabetes and occurs two to four times more often than in people without diabetes. Complications from diabetes are also associated with premature death and it is estimated that one out of every 10 deaths in Canadian adults was attributable to diabetes (PHAC, 2011). In 2015, diabetes-related health expenditure totalled 17 billion US dollars (Diabetes Canada, 2017). In the Indigenous population, diabetes rates are three to five times higher compared to non-Indigenous individuals. In addition, Indigenous people are generally diagnosed at a younger age (Oster, Johnson, Balko, et al., 2012), and Indigenous women experience higher rates of gestational diabetes than non-Indigenous women (Aljohani, Rempel, Ludwig, et al., 2008).

Only about 10% of people with DM have type 1 DM. However, the number of existing cases (prevalence) and new cases (incidence) of individuals with type 2 DM is increasing dramatically due to a number of factors. For example, people are living longer, obesity rates are rising, and lifestyles are becoming increasingly sedentary. In addition, Canada is

---

**BOX 21.2   Health at Every Size (HAES): The Size Acceptance Nondiet Movement**

HAES challenges the value of promoting weight loss and argues for a shift in focus to weight-neutral outcomes such as health behaviours (Bacon & Aphramor, 2011). The following tenets are the foundation of the movement:

- *Respect.* Celebrates body diversity; honours differences in size, age, race, ethnicity, gender, disability, sexual orientation, religion, class, and other human attributes.
- *Critical Awareness.* Challenges scientific and cultural assumptions; values body knowledge and lived experiences.
- *Compassionate self-care.* Finding the joy in moving one's body and being physically active; eating in a flexible and attuned manner that values pleasure and honors internal cues of hunger, satiety, and appetite, while respecting the social conditions that frame eating options

**How to Become a Size-Sensitive Health Professional**

- On the intake form, include a question asking whether the person is satisfied with his or her body size. If the answer is "yes," then try to avoid the issue in the future.
- When the person asks not to be weighed, the request is acknowledged without complaint and automatically taken into account on follow-up office visits. (There are a few cases in which weighing is necessary, such as when certain medications, chemotherapy, or anaesthetics are administered.)
- A size-sensitive health care provider does not necessarily avoid mentioning weight but should avoid making an issue of weight, avoid lectures and humiliation, and respect the individual's wishes with regard to weight discussions.
- When weight contributes to a problem, the professional mentions this situation but also considers other diagnoses and recommends tests to determine the actual diagnosis when appropriate. If weight loss is a recommended treatment for a problem, the compassionate professional may mention this, but at minimum, and recommend and prescribe other treatments. Accept the individual's wish not to use weight loss as a treatment.
- Some health care providers believe that overweight and obesity are not necessarily unhealthy. However, other professionals who believe that fat is unhealthy may acknowledge that weight loss is usually ineffective or that individuals have the right to direct their own treatment.
- Ideally, the waiting area, examining suite, and consultation room are equipped with armless chairs, large blood pressure cuffs, large examination gowns, and other equipment suitable for large people. If this is not the case, then the office staff acknowledges the importance of these items when told.

Sources: Bacon, L., & Aphramor, L. (2011). Weight science: Evaluating the evidence for a paradigm shift. *Nutrition Journal*, 10(1), 9; Spark, A. (2001). Health at any size: The size acceptance nondiet movement. *Journal of the American Medical Women's Association*, 56(2), 69–72.

---

experiencing increased immigration from high-risk populations. These populations include people of Latin American, Asian, South Asian, and African descent (Diabetes Canada, 2017).

### Type 2 Diabetes in Children

Although DM in children and adolescents was believed to be exclusively type 1, type 2 diabetes is now considered a sizeable and growing problem among Indigenous people and an emerging public health problem among other North American ethnic groups. The epidemic of obesity among children and adolescents, the decrease in physical activity, the increase in calorie-dense foods, and the exposure to diabetes in utero are likely contributors to the increase in prevalence of type 2 DM in this population. Young children with type 1 DM or type 2 DM who are either overweight or obese should be observed for metabolic syndrome and CVD risk. The adolescent population is at higher risk because of lifestyle implications, smoking, poor diet adherence, etc., that may put them at risk of chronic disease earlier in life.

Although some children and adolescents are symptomatic, others do not enter the clinical arena until they have severe ketoacidosis and may have a transient insulin requirement. Youth with type 2 diabetes appear to be at a significantly higher risk of developing earlier and severe microvascular and cardiovascular disease compared to youth with type 1 diabetes (Dabelea, Stafford, Mayer-Davis, et al., 2017). In 2018, the Diabetes Canada Clinical Practice Guidelines Expert Committee published clinical practice guidelines for type 2 diabetes in children and adolescents (for more information visit http://guidelines.diabetes.ca/docs/cpg/Ch35-Type-2-Diabetes-in-Children-and-Adolescents.pdf). Generally, children and adolescents with type 2 DM have poor glycemic control. Population mobility, lack of symptoms, denial of illness, absence of family support, and inadequate health care insurance coverage have all been identified as major barriers to adherence to treatment and follow-up and to successful clinical management. Because of a longer duration of disease (from earlier onset), and because glucose control and adherence are challenging during the teenage years, the lifetime complications (microvascular and macrovascular diseases and decreased quality of life) in this population will probably be considerable (Diabetes Canada Clinical Practice Guidelines Expert Committee, 2018).

## Diet Intervention

Medical nutrition therapy (MNT) is the most critical and pivotal component of diabetes care. At the minimum, MNT involves the team efforts of a health care provider, a registered nurse, a registered dietitian, and, in some practice settings, a mental health professional. The purpose of MNT for people with type 2 DM is to delay or prevent the development of complications (blindness, CHD, nephropathy, and neuropathy). No single diabetic diet or Canadian Diabetes Association diet exists. The recommended diet can be defined only as a nutrition prescription based on assessment, treatment goals, and outcomes. Nutrition advice for people with type 2 diabetes is essentially the same as that for the general population: follow Canada's food guide. MNT for people with diabetes should be individualized, with consideration given to usual eating habits, culture, and other lifestyle factors. Nutrition recommendations are then developed and implemented to meet treatment goals and desired outcomes. Monitoring metabolic parameters, including blood glucose levels, glycosylated hemoglobin (HbA1C) levels, lipid values, blood pressure, body weight, renal function (when appropriate), and quality of life, is crucial to ensure successful outcomes. Monitoring HbA1C to less than 6.5% or 7% in most current guidelines is not always the only criterion to use. More importantly the treatment should be started early to prevent further destruction of the beta cells of the pancreas that produce insulin. Studies show that even in people with prediabetes or diabetes there is a loss of 50 to 80% of their beta cells (Aguilar & Zonszein, 2015). The Canadian Diabetes Association further recommends ongoing nutrition self-management education for these individuals.

For people with *hyperglycemia, hyperlipidemia,* obesity, or suboptimal nutrition, start with this nonpharmacological management:

- Determine an appropriate, tailored meal plan based on energy needs for body weight goals (moderate weight loss, weight maintenance, weight gain). With that data, the determination is made with regard to proportions with use of the *Eat Well Plate.* For children and adolescents, their growth needs must be accounted for as well.
- Encourage regular exercise.
- Evaluate the individual with use of the outcome measures listed in Table 21.6. People who have been counselled regarding diet and exercise but who have not responded satisfactorily after 4 to 6 weeks should be referred to a registered dietitian who is a diabetes educator. Those with acute complications, such as hypoglycemia, exercise-related problems, renal disease, autonomic neuropathy, hypertension, or CVD, must first see a health care provider.

A nutrition prescription, which is done after the health care provider has completed a physical and medical assessment, may be general, but it should reflect the individual's therapy goals. The following are some sample orders the nurse might write for the dietitian:

- Individualized diabetic meal plan to achieve clinical goals of diabetes MNT
- MNT to achieve blood glucose levels as near normal as possible
- Individualized meal plan to decrease diabetes control and blood lipid levels
- Diet for improved glycemic control and blood pressure measurements

The registered dietitian with a summary of the planned nutrition intervention may define the prescription further. For example, the dietitian might write:

- Weight-reduction meal plan based on general eating guidelines, 1200 to 1500 calories, three meals, and one snack
- 2300 mg sodium meal plan with weight maintenance
- Carbohydrate-counting meal plan, adjusting carbohydrate and meal timing to achieve target glucose goals

## TABLE 21.6 Goals and Recommendations of Medical Nutrition Therapy for Individuals With Type 2 Diabetes

| Index | Goal | Recommendation |
|---|---|---|
| HbA1c | *For diagnosis must have:* ≥6.5% with a method that is NGSP certified and standardized to DCCT assay | The HbA1c test is the preferred test to diagnose diabetes in nonpregnant adults; other tests listed below may also be used |
| FPG | ≥7.0 mmol/L (126 mg/dL) Fasting is defined as no calorie intake for at least 8 h | The FPG test detects diabetes and prediabetes. It is most reliable when done in the morning |
| 2-h plasma glucose | ≥11.1 mmol/L (200 mg/dL) during OGTT | May also be used with a WHO-approved method and a glucose load of 75 g of anhydrous glucose dissolved in water |
| Random plasma glucose | ≥11.1 mmol/L (200 mg/dL) | In people with classic hyperglycemia or hyperglycemic crisis |
| HbA1c | A reasonable HbA1c goal for many nonpregnant adults is <7%; individualize to ≤6.5% or up to 8% depending on factors such as the level of hypoglycemia, life expectancy, duration of disease, and level of CVD | Perform HbA1c test at least twice a year in individuals who are meeting treatment goals and who have stable glycemic control. Lowering of HbA1c fraction is associated with reduction of microvascular complications of diabetes and possibly macrovascular disease |
| Weight change | For most overweight/obese people (BMI <35 kg/m²) recommend modest weight loss (5–10% of body weight) | Modest weight loss has been shown to reduce insulin sensitivity, glycemic control, and blood pressure |
| MNT | Individuals who have prediabetes or diabetes should receive individualized MNT as needed to achieve treatment goals, preferably provided by a registered dietitian familiar with components of diabetes MNT; meet body's daily nutritional needs and minimized risk of chronic disease | Structure the program to emphasize lifestyle changes, including education and regular physical activity. Modify macronutrient composition to individual and medical condition while meeting DRIs for micronutrients; a variety of meal patterns work (Mediterranean, a lower-fat, lower-carbohydrate pattern, or vegetarian); saturated fat intake should be <7% of total calories; intake of trans fat should be minimized |
| Physical activity | People with diabetes should ideally accumulate a minimum of 150 minutes of moderate-to-vigorous intensity aerobic exercise each week, spread over at least 3 days of the week, with no more than 2 consecutive days without exercise. | Physical activity level gradually increased and sustained at target goal. To improve glycemic control, assist with weight maintenance, and reduce risk of CVD, at least 150 min of moderate-intensity aerobic physical activity per week (64–76% of maximum heart rate) |

*BMI*, Body mass index; *CVD*, cardiovascular disease; *DCCT*, Diabetes Control and Complications Trial; *DRI*, dietary reference intake; *FPG*, fasting plasma glucose; *HbA1c*, glycated hemoglobin; *MNT*, medical nutrition therapy; *NGSP*, National Glycohemoglobin Standardization Program; *OGTT*, oral glucose tolerance test.
Sources: Diabetes Canada Clinical Practice Guidelines Expert Committee. (2018). Definition, classification and diagnosis of diabetes, prediabetes and metabolic syndrome. *Canadian Journal of Diabetes, 42*, S10–S15; Diabetes Canada Clinical Practice Guidelines Expert Committee. (2018). Physical activity and diabetes. *Canadian Journal of Diabetes, 42*, S54–S63; Diabetes Canada Clinical Practice Guidelines Expert Committee. (2018). Nutrition therapy. *Canadian Journal of Diabetes, 42*, S64–S79.

## CASE STUDY

### Obesity/Overweight: Estella

Estella is a 34-year-old single mother of three children sharing a small apartment with her 68-year-old mother in inner-city Toronto. She is a full-time labourer in a local manufacturing facility and attends night classes to obtain her continuing care assistant certification. She is receiving some government assistance but is raising her children, aged 4, 7, and 10 years, on a meager income. Most days she arrives home too tired to prepare a well-balanced meal for her family and admits to eating a lot of fast food. Her mother, despite declining vision, works part-time on evenings at a local fast food restaurant to help with financial difficulties. Her mother is responsible for most of the preparation of meals. Their diet consists mainly of inexpensive carbohydrates: flour tortillas, breads, pasta, cheese, and potatoes. The family budget does not allow for much fresh fruit or vegetables or expensive meats; therefore bologna and hot dogs are frequently served.

Estella has recently been hired at a local hospital as a unregulated care provider (UCP). A required pre-employment physical examination revealed several health risks. At 162.6 cm (5 feet, 4 inches), she weighs 84 kg (185 pounds). Her resting heart rate and blood pressure are also above normal levels. She has a family history of diabetes and heart disease: her father died of a heart attack at age 55 years, and her mother has diabetes that requires daily insulin injections. She was referred to her primary care provider, who recommended immediate lifestyle changes, including walking 30 minutes per day, 4 to 5 days per week, as well as dietary counselling.

#### Reflective Questions

- What social determinants of health may be impacting Estella in being able to feed her family a healthy diet?
- How can learning about simple changes in her eating habits affect Estella's weight and risk of type 2 diabetes?
- What local resources promote inexpensive programs to help Estella lose weight?

## CARE PLAN

### Obesity/Overweight: Estella

**Nursing Issue**

Alteration in current weight related to diet modification and weekly monitoring

**Defining Characteristics**

- Single mother works full-time and attends night school. Is raising three children and supporting her mother on a limited income. Income falls into poverty level for family of five.
- Is a divorced woman with limited support system and resources.
- Current weight is 84.1 kg, at 162.6 cm tall (185 pounds at 5 feet, 4 inches tall). Her body mass index (BMI) is 31.8 kg/m², including her in the obesity category.
- Resting blood pressure is 164/87 mm Hg, and pulse rate is 88 beats/min.
- Father died at age 55 years of a massive heart attack.
- Mother is overweight and has type 1 diabetes and high blood pressure.
- Diet consists of processed foods and a high-fat diet with little fresh fruit or vegetables.
- Recent job change requires her to be on her feet, walking, lifting, and transporting care recipients.
- Inner-city neighbourhood is unsafe to walk in alone or allow her children freedom to play outdoors.
- Single mother of three small boys; she realizes the need to improve her own health to be able to care for and enjoy her children.

**Expected Outcomes**

- Estella's overall health will improve through reduction of all of the following: weight, BMI, resting pulse rate, and blood pressure.
- Establish realistic goals with Estella to improve quality of meals on a limited income.
- Develop a realistic exercise plan that is inexpensive and not time-consuming.

**Interventions**

- Teach meal planning strategy to include *Canada's Dietary Guidelines* basic recommendations for a healthy diet and (as deemed appropriate) refer Estella to a certified diabetes educator or registered dietitian if resources permit.
- Teach Estella easy menus to prepare that use more whole grains, fruits, and vegetables and less processed or fast food. (Resources might include Health Canada's *Healthy Eating on a Budget;* https://food-guide.canada.ca/en/tip-for-healthy-eating/healthy-eating-on-a-budget/).
- Encourage a regular exercise program, beginning with a walking program of 30 minutes per day, four to five times per week. Gradually increase the pace and distance to intensify aerobic benefits.
- Investigate safe options, such as a neighbourhood YMCA or park program, for family activities, or offer other community resources such as cooking and food-preparation courses for low-income adults and children.

## SUMMARY

This chapter has introduced a wide range of subjects, including *Canada's Food Guide* and *Canada's Dietary Guidelines for Health Professionals and Policy Makers*, the most current diet recommendations to reduce the risks of developing nutrition-related diseases, Health Canada regulations for food labelling, government and community nutrition assistance programs, and primary and secondary prevention strategies related to the most common nutrition-related chronic diseases. Many more primary prevention strategies are being discussed as an adjunct to secondary prevention in an effort to make all strategies more successful. Together these topics form the basis of what is known as preventive nutrition, a requisite for the promotion of Canada's public health. All the topics examined in this chapter can be studied further through use of the Internet. High-quality, up-to-date materials and continuing nutrition education literature for professionals are free and online.

**Evolve Chapter Features**

http://evolve.elsevier.com/Canada/Edelman/healthpromotion/

- Review Questions

## REFERENCES

Aguilar, R., & Zonszein, J. (2015). Glycemic control in type 2 diabetes—how low should you go? *Clinical advisor*. Retrieved from http://www.clinicaladvisor.com/cmece-features/glycemic-control-in-type-2-diabeteshow-low-should-you-go/article/441711/.

Aljohani, N., Rempel, B. M., Ludwig, S., et al. (2008). Gestational diabetes in Manitoba during a twenty-year period. *Clinical and Investigative Medicine, 31*(1), 31–37. [Seminal Reference].

American Dietetic Association. (2009). Position of the American dietetic association: Nutrient supplementation. *Journal of the American Dietetic Association, 109*(12), 2073–1085. https://doi.org/10.1016/j.jada.2009.10.020. [Seminal Reference].

American Heart Association (AHA). (2016). *Potassium power: Eating foods rich in this mineral can help reduce the effects of excess sodium*. Retrieved from http://www.heart.org/HEARTORG/Conditions/HighBloodPressure/PreventionTreatmentofHighBloodPressure/How-Potassium-Can-Help-Control-High-Blood-Pressure_UCM_303243_Article.jsp#.WHP-ZXYo7MA.

Bacon, L., & Aphramor, L. (2011). Weight science: Evaluating the evidence for a paradigm shift. *Nutrition Journal, 10*(1), 9. https://doi.org/10.1186/1475-2891-10-9. [Seminal Reference].

Barer-Stein, T. (1979). Multiculturalism and nutrition counseling. *Journal of the Canadian Dietetic Association, 40*(2), 112–116. [Seminal Reference].

Bolland, M. J., Leung, W., Tai, V., et al. (2015). Calcium intake and risk of fracture: Systematic review. *British Medical Journal, 351*, h4580. https://doi.org/10.1136/bmj.h4580. [Seminal Reference].

Brownell, K. (2000). *The LEARN program for weight management 2000*. Dallas: American Health Publishing. [Seminal Reference].

Canadian Cancer Society Advisory Committee. (2018). *Canadian cancer statistics, 2018*. Toronto: Author. Retrieved from http://www.cancer.ca/~/media/cancer.ca/CW/cancer%20information/cancer%20101/Canadian%20cancer%20statistics/Canadian-Cancer-Statistics-2018-EN.pdf?la=en.

Canadian Cancer Society. (2019). *Some sobering facts about alcohol and cancer risk.* Retrieved from http://www.cancer.ca/en/prevention-and-screening/reduce-cancer-risk/make-healthy-choices/limit-alcohol/some-sobering-facts-about-alcohol-and-cancer-risk/?region=ns.

Canadian Cardiovascular Society. (2016). 2016 Canadian cardiovascular society guidelines for the management of dyslipidemia for the prevention of cardiovascular disease in the adult. *Canadian Journal of Cardiology, 32,* 1263–1282.

Canadian Institute for Health Information (CIHI) & Public Health Agency of Canada (PHAC). (2011). *Obesity in Canada, a joint report for the public health agency of Canada and the Canadian Institute of health information.* Retrieved from https://secure.cihi.ca/free_products/Obesity_in_canada_2011_en.pdf. [Seminal Reference].

Canadian Malnutrition Task Force. (2014). *Canadian nutrition screening tool [CNST].* Retrieved from. http://nutritioncareincanada.ca/sites/default/uploads/files/CNST.pdf. [Seminal Reference].

Canadian Malnutrition Task Force. (2019). *Nutrition screening.* Retrieved from http://nutritioncareincanada.ca/tools/screening.

Canadian Medical Association [CMA]. (2015). *Complementary and alternative medicine policy.* Retrieved from https://policybase.cma.ca/documents/policypdf/PD15-09.pdf.

Canadian Obesity Network. (2017). *Report card on access to obesity treatment for adults in Canada 2017.* Edmonton: Canadian Obesity Network.

Canadian Public Health Association (CPHA). (n.d.). *Preventing cardiovascular disease and stroke.* Retrieved from https://www.cpha.ca/preventing-cardiovascular-disease-and-stroke.

Colapinto, C. K., Graham, J., & St-Pierre, S. (2018). Trends and correlates of frequency of fruit and vegetable consumption, 2007 to 2014. *Health Reports, 29*(1), 9–14.

Dabelea, D., Stafford, J. M., Mayer-Davis, E. J., et al. (2017). Association of type 1 diabetes vs type 2 diabetes diagnosed during childhood and adolescence with complications during teenage years and young adulthood. *Journal of the American Medical Association, 317*(8), 825–835. https://doi.org/10.1001/jama.2017.0686.

Dachner, N., & Tarasuk, V. (2018). Tackling household food insecurity: An essential goal of a national food policy. *Canadian Food Studies, 5*(3), 230–247.

Diabetes Canada. (2017). *Diabetes statistics in Canada.* Retrieved from http://guidelines.diabetes.ca/cpg/chapter1#bib0035.

Diabetes Canada Clinical Practice Guidelines Expert Committee. (2018). 2018 clinical practice guidelines: Type 2 diabetes in children and adolescents. *Canadian Journal of Diabetes, 42*(Suppl. 1), S247–S254. https://doi.org/10.1016/j.jcjd.2017.10.037.

Dietitians of Canada. (2013). *Do I need a vitamin or mineral supplement?* Retrieved from https://www.dietitians.ca/Downloads/Factsheets/Do-I-need-a-vitamin-or-mineral-supplement.aspx. [Seminal Reference].

Dietitians of Canada. (2016). *Prevalence, severity and impact of household food insecurity: A serious public health issue.* Retrieved from https://www.dietitians.ca/foodinsecurity.

Dietitians of Canada. (2019). *Vitamins and minerals FAQs.* Retrieved from http://www.unlockfood.ca/en/Articles/Vitamins-and-Minerals/Vitamins-and-Minerals-FAQs.aspx?aliaspath=%2fen%2fArticles%2fNutrients-(vitamins-and-minerals)%2fVitamins-and-Minerals-FAQs.

Food Secure Canada. (2017). *Five big ideas for a better food system: A proposal from food secure Canada for the national food policy.* Retrieved from https://foodsecurecanada.org/policy-advocacy/five-big-ideas-better-food-system.

Gionet, L. (2015). *Breastfeeding trends in Canada.* Ottawa, ON: Report prepared for Statistics Canada. Retrieved from https://www150.statcan.gc.ca/n1/pub/82-624-x/2013001/article/11879-eng.htm.

Government of Canada. (2005). *The integrated pan-Canadian healthy living strategy.* Retrieved from https://www.canada.ca/content/dam/phac-aspc/migration/phac-aspc/hp-ps/hl-mvs/ipchls-spimmvs/pdf/ipchls-spimmvs-eng.pdf. [Seminal Reference].

Government of Canada. (2014). *Food safety and you.* Retrieved from https://www.canada.ca/en/health-canada/services/general-food-safety-tips/food-safety-you.html. [Seminal Reference].

Government of Canada. (2015). *Natural and non-prescription health products.* Retrieved from https://www.canada.ca/en/health-canada/services/drugs-health-products/natural-non-prescription.html.

Government of Canada. (2017). *A food policy for Canada.* Retrieved from https://www.canada.ca/en/campaign/food-policy.html.

Health Canada. (2006). *Labelling guidance document: Natural health products directorate.* Retrieved from https://www.canada.ca/content/dam/hc-sc/migration/hc-sc/dhp-mps/alt_formats/hpfb-dgpsa/pdf/prodnatur/labelling-etiquetage-eng.pdf. [Seminal Reference].

Health Canada. (2010). *Eating well with Canada's food guide First Nations, Inuit and Métis.* Ottawa: Author. Retrieved https://www.health.gov.nl.ca/health/findhealthservices/canada_food_guide_first_nations_inuit_metis.pdf.

Health Canada. (2011). *Canadian guidelines for body weight classification in adults.* Ottawa: Author. Retrieved from https://www.canada.ca/en/health-canada/services/food-nutrition/healthy-eating/healthy-weights/canadian-guidelines-body-weight-classification-adults/questions-answers-public.html. [Seminal Reference].

Health Canada. (2015). *Canadian community health survey—nutrition.* Retrieved from https://www.canada.ca/en/health-canada/services/food-nutrition/food-nutrition-surveillance/health-nutrition-surveys/canadian-community-health-survey-cchs/2015-canadian-community-health-survey-nutrition-food-nutrition-surveillance.html.

Health Canada. (2016). *Healthy eating strategy.* Retrieved from https://www.canada.ca/en/health-canada/services/publications/food-nutrition/healthy-eating-strategy.html.

Health Canada. (2017a). *Sodium intake of Canadians in 2017.* Retrieved from https://www.canada.ca/content/dam/hc-sc/documents/services/publications/food-nutrition/sodium-intake-canadians-2017/2017-sodium-intakes-report-eng.pdf.

Health Canada. (2017b). *Adverse reaction and medical device problem reporting.* Retrieved from https://www.canada.ca/en/health-canada/services/drugs-health-products/medeffect-canada/adverse-reaction-reporting.html.

Health Canada. (2019). *Canada's dietary guidelines for health professionals and policy makers.* Retrieved from https://opha.on.ca/Nutrition-Resource-Centre/NRC-Navigator/Resources/Canada%E2%80%99s-Dietary-Guidelines-for-health-professiona.aspx.

Heart and Stroke Foundation. (2014a). *Position Statement: Dietary sodium, heart disease and stroke.* Retrieved from https://www.heartandstroke.ca/-/media/pdf-files/canada/2017-position-statements/dietary-sodium-ps-eng.ashx. [Seminal Reference].

Heart and Stroke Foundation. (2014b). *Position statement: Sugar, heart disease and stroke.* Retrieved from https://www.heartandstroke.ca/-/media/pdf-files/canada/2017-position-statements/sugar-ps-eng.ashx?la=en&hash=F53E60FC6C6570BBE76A3B5BF9062D8E7D76DE3B. [Seminal Reference].

Heart and Stroke Foundation. (2017). *How to manage your cholesterol*. Retrieved from https://www.heartandstroke.ca/-/media/pdf-files/canada/heart/how-to-manage-your-cholesterol-en.ashx?la=en&hash=BAAD552864358761D53F210A449640100E6B0B53.

Huang, T., & Hu, F. B. (2015). Gene-environment interactions and obesity: Recent developments and future directions. *BMC Med Genomics, 8*(Suppl. 1), S2.

Huet, C., Rosol, R., & Egeland, G. M. (2012). The prevalence of food insecurity is high and the diet quality poor in Inuit communities. *Journal of Nutrition, 142*(3), 541–547. https://doi.org/10.3945/jn.111.149278. [Seminal Reference].

Institute for Health Metrics and Evaluation. (2018). *Global burden of disease (GBD) profile: Canada*. Seattle: Institute for Health Metrics and Evaluation.

Janz, T., & Pearson, C. (2013). *Vitamin D blood levels of Canadians. Statistics Canada*. Retrieved from https://www150.statcan.gc.ca/n1/en/pub/82-624-x/2013001/article/11727-eng.pdf?st=aMS-MU0Ck. [Seminal Reference].

Kirkpatrick, S., McIntyre, L., & Potestio, M. (2010). Child hunger and long-term adverse consequences for health. *Archives of Pediatric & Adolescent Medicine, 164*(8), 754–762. https://doi.org/10.1001/archpediatrics.2010.117. [Seminal Reference].

Kittler, P. G., & Sucher, K. P. (2000). *Cultural foods: Traditions and trends*. Belmont, CA: Wadsworth. [Seminal Reference].

Langlois, K., Garriguet, D., Gonzalez, A., et al. (2019). Changes in total sugars consumption among Canadian children and adults. *Health Reports, 30*(1), 10–19.

Loopstra, R., & Tarasuk, V. (2013). Perspectives on community gardens, community kitchens and the Good Food Box programs in a community-based sample of low-income families. *Canadian Journal of Public Health, 104*(1), 55–59. [Seminal Reference].

Maia, S. B., Souza, A. S., Caminha, M. C., DaSilva, S. L., Cruz, R. D., dos Santos, C. C., et al. (2019). Vitamin A and pregnancy: A narrative review. *Nutrients, 11*(3), 681–699. https://doi.org/10.3390/nu11030681.

McIntyre, L., Williams, J., Lavorato, D., et al. (2012). Depression and suicide ideation in late adolescence and early adulthood are an outcome of child hunger. *Journal of Affective Disorders, 150*(1), 123–129. https://doi.org/10.1016/j.jad.2012.11.029. [Seminal Reference].

McIntyre, L., Wu, X., Kwok, C., et al. (2017). The pervasive effect of youth self-report of hunger on depression over 6 years of follow up. *Social Psychiatry and Psychiatric Epidemiology, 52*(5), 537–547. https://doi.org/10.1007/s00127-017-1361-5.

Ministry of Justice. (2018). *Natural health product regulations*. Retrieved from https://laws-lois.justice.gc.ca/PDF/SOR-2003-196.pdf.

Mozaffarian, D., Rosenberg, I., & Uauy, R. (2018). History of modern nutrition science—Implications for current research, dietary guidelines, and food policy. *BMJ, 361*, k2392. https://doi.org/10.1136/bmj.k2392.

National Academies of Sciences, Engineering, and Medicine. (2017). *Guiding principles for developing dietary reference intakes based on chronic disease*. Washington: The National Academies Press. https://doi.org/10.17226/24828. Retrieved from https://www.nap.edu/catalog/24828/guiding-principles-for-developing-dietary-reference-intakes-based-on-chronic-disease.

National Research Council. (2006). *Dietary reference intakes: The essential guide to nutrient requirements*. Washington: The National Academies Press. Retrieved from http://www.nap.edu/catalog/11537/dietary-reference-intakes-the-essential-guide-to-nutrient-requirements#toc. [Seminal Reference].

National Research Council. (2010). *Dietary reference intakes for calcium and vitamin D*. Washington: The National Academies Press. Retrieved from http://www.nap.edu/catalog/13050/dietary-reference-intakes-for-calcium-and-vitamin-d. [Seminal Reference].

Navaneelan, T., & Janz, T. (2014). *Adjusting the scales: Obesity in the Canadian population after correcting for respondent bias*. Ottawa: Statistics Canada. Retrieved from https://www150.statcan.gc.ca/n1/pub/82-624-x/2014001/article/11922-eng.htm. [Seminal Reference].

Nerenberg, K. A., Zarnke, K. B., Leung, A. A., et al. (2018). Hypertension Canada's 2018 guidelines for diagnosis, risk assessment, prevention, and treatment of hypertension in adults and children. *Canadian Journal of Cardiology, 34*, 506–525. https://doi.org/10.1016/j.cjca.2018.02.022.

Osteoporosis Canada. (2010). *Quick reference guide*. Retrieved from https://osteoporosis.ca/wp-content/uploads/Quick_Reference_Guide_October_2010.pdf. [Seminal Reference].

Osteoporosis Canada. (n.d.). *About the disease*. Retrieved from https://osteoporosis.ca/about-the-disease/.

Oster, R. T., Johnson, J. A., Balko, S. U., et al. (2012). Increasing rates of diabetes amongst status Aboriginal youth in Alberta, Canada. *International Journal of Circumpolar Health, 71*, 1–7. [Seminal Reference].

Padwal, R. S., Bienek, A., McAlister, F. A., & Outcomes Research Task Force of the Canadian Hypertension Education Program., et al. (2016). Epidemiology of hypertension in Canada an update. *Canadian Journal of Cardiology, 32*(5), 687–694. https://doi.org/10.1016/j.cjca.2015.07.734.

Pan-Canadian Public Health Network. (2017). *Towards a healthier Canada—2017 progress report on advancing the federal/provincial/territorial framework of healthy weights*. Retrieved from http://www.phn-rsp.ca/thcpr-vcpsre-2017/index-eng.php.

Papadimitropouos, E. A., Coyte, P. C., Josse, R. G., et al. (1997). Current and projected rates of hip fracture in Canada. *Canadian Medical Association Journal, 158*, 870–871. [Seminal Reference].

Pavlidis, C., Patrinos, G. P., & Katsila, T. (2015). Nutrigenomics: A controversy. *Applied and Translational Genomics, 4*, 50–53. [Seminal Reference].

Pettes, T., Dachner, N., Gaetz, S., et al. (2016). An examination of charitable meal programs in five Canadian cities. *Journal of Health Care for the Poor and Underserved, 27*(3), 1303–1315. https://doi.org/10.1353/hpu.2016.0121.

Power, E. M. (2008). Conceptualizing food security for Aboriginal people in Canada. *Canadian Journal of Public Health, 99*(2), 95–97. [Seminal Reference].

Public Health Agency of Canada (PHAC). (2011). *Diabetes in Canada: Facts and figures from a public health perspective*. Ottawa: Author. Retrieved from https://www.canada.ca/content/dam/phac-aspc/migration/phac-aspc/cd-mc/publications/diabetes-diabete/facts-figures-faits-chiffres-2011/pdf/facts-figures-faits-chiffres-eng.pdf. [Seminal Reference].

Public Health Agency of Canada (PHAC). (2016a). *Food-related illnesses, hospitalization and deaths in Canada*. Retrieved from https://www.canada.ca/en/public-health/services/publications/food-nutrition/infographic-food-related-illnesses-hospitalizations-deaths-in-canada.html.

Public Health Agency of Canada (PHAC). (2016b). *Symptoms of salmonellosis (Salmonella)*. Retrieved from https://www.canada.ca/en/public-health/services/diseases/salmonellosis-salmonella/symptoms.html.

Public Health Agency of Canada (PHAC). (2017a). *E. coli (Escherichia coli) infection*. Retrieved from https://www.canada.ca/en/public-health/services/diseases/e-coli.html.

Public Health Agency of Canada (PHAC). (2017b). *Heart disease in Canada*. Retrieved from https://www.canada.ca/content/dam/phac-aspc/documents/services/publications/diseases-conditions/heart-disease-maladies-coeur-eng.pdf.

Rao, D. P., Kropac, E., Do, M. T., et al. (2016). Childhood overweight and obesity trends in Canada. *Health Promotion and Chronic Disease Prevention in Canada: Research, Policy and Practice, 36*(9), 194–198.

Romieu, I., Dossus, L., Barquera, S., et al. (2017). Energy balance and obesity: What are the main drivers? *Cancer Causes & Control: Cancer Causes & Control, 28*(3), 247–258.

Sanada, H., Jones, J. E., & Jose, P. A. (2011). Genetics of salt-sensitive hypertension. *Current Hypertension Reports, 13*(1), 55–66. [Seminal Reference].

Schiffrin, E. L., Campbell, N., Feldman, R., et al. (2016). Hypertension in Canada: Past, present, and future. *Annals of Global Health, 82*(2), 288–299. https://doi.org/10.1016/j.aogh.2016.02.006.

Singh, R. K., Kumar, P., & Mahalingam, K. (2017). Molecular genetics of human obesity: A comprehensive review. *Comptes Rendus Biologies, 340*(2), 87–108. https://doi.org/10.1016/j.crvi.2016.11.007.

Snetselaar, L. (2004). Counseling for change. In L. K. Mahan, & S. Escott-Stump (Eds.), *Krause's food, nutrition, and diet therapy* (11th ed.) (pp. 519–532). St. Louis: Elsevier. [Seminal Reference].

Statista. (2017). Average annual household expenditure on food in Canada from 2010 to 2017 (*in 1,000 Canadian dollars*). *Statista—The statistics portal.* Retrieved from https://www.statista.com/statistics/436289/average-annual-household-expenditure-on-food-in-canada/.

Statistics Canada. (2015a). *Overweight and obese youth (self-reported), 2013.* Retrieved from https://www150.statcan.gc.ca/n1/pub/82-625-x/2014001/article/14026-eng.htm.

Statistics Canada. (2015b). *Blood pressure of children and youth, 2012 to 2013.* Retrieved from https://www150.statcan.gc.ca/n1/pub/82-625-x/2014001/article/14102-eng.htm.

Statistics Canada. (2016). *Leading causes of death.* Retrieved from https://www150.statcan.gc.ca/t1/tbl1/en/tv.action?pid=1310039401.

Statistics Canada. (2017a). *Canadian community health survey—nutrition: Nutrient intake from food and nutritional supplements.* Retrieved from https://www150.statcan.gc.ca/n1/daily-quotidien/170620/dq170620b-eng.htm.

Statistics Canada. (2017b). *Health fact sheets: Use of nutritional supplements, 2015.* Retrieved from https://www150.statcan.gc.ca/n1/pub/82-625-x/2017001/article/14831-eng.htm.

Tai, V., Leung, W., Grey, A., et al. (2015). Calcium intake and bone mineral density: Systematic review and meta-analysis. *British Medical Journal, 351*, h4183. https://doi.org/10.1136/bmj.h4183.

Tarasuk, V., Mitchell, A., & Dachner, N. (2016). *Household food insecurity in Canada, 2014. Toronto: Research to identify policy options to reduce food insecurity (PROOF).* Retrieved from https://proof.utoronto.ca/resources/proof-annual-reports/annual-report-2014/.

Taylor, C. L. (2008). *Framework for DRI development: Components "known" and components "to be explored".* Background paper. Washington, DC: Institute of Medicine. Retrieved from http://nationalacademies.org/hmd/~/media/Files/Activity%20Files/Nutrition/DRIWS/Background%20Paper%20on%20DRI%20Framework%202008.pdf?la=en. [Seminal Reference].

US Department of Health and Human Services (USDHHS), National Institutes of health (NIH), national heart, lung, and blood Institute. (2006). *Your guide to lowering your blood pressure with DASH.* Retrieved from http://www.nhlbi.nih.gov/health/resources/heart/hbp-dash-index. [Seminal Reference].

Willows, N., Veugelers, P., Raine, K., et al. (2008). Prevalence and sociodemographic risk factors related to household food insecurity in Aboriginal peoples in Canada. *Public Health Nutrition, 12*(8), 1150–1156. https://doi.org/10.1017/S1368980008004345. [Seminal Reference].

World Health Organization (WHO). (2006). *Global database on body mass index.* Retrieved from http://apps.who.int/bmi/index.jsp?introPage=intro_3.html. [Seminal Reference].

Xu, X., Parker, D., Ferguson, C., et al. (2017). Where is the nurse in nutritional care? *Contemporary Nurse, 53*(3), 267–270. https://doi.org/10.1080/10376178.2017.1370782.

Zemel, M. B. (2001). Calcium modulation on hypertension and obesity: Mechanisms and implications. *Journal of the American College of Nutrition, 5*(Suppl. l), 428S–435S. [Seminal Reference].

# 22

# Exercise

Sarah L. West, MSc, PhD

Originating US chapter by *Kevin K. Chui, PT, DPT, DPT, PhD, GCS, OCS, CEAA, FAAOMPT, Frank Tudini, PT, DSc, OCS, COMT, FAAOMPT, Sheng-Che Yen, PT, PhD*

## INTENDED LEARNING OUTCOMES

*After completing this chapter, the reader will be able to:*

- Explain the current national guidelines for physical activity participation, the process involved in creating the guidelines, and the progress made toward meeting these guidelines.
- Describe how physical activity positively influences physical and psychological health.
- Identify the benefits of physical activity throughout the aging process.
- Understand the importance of physical activity within the context of chronic disease.
- Evaluate the prescriptions for and benefits of daily physical activity, aerobic exercise, and resistance training.
- Explain the interventions to promote exercise adherence and compliance.

## KEY TERMS

Aerobic exercise
Anaerobic exercise
Arthritis
Borg scale
Cardiorespiratory fitness
Cool-down period
Exercise
Exercise prescription
Fat mass
Flexibility
High-intensity interval training (HIIT)
Low back pain

Muscular fitness
Obesity
Osteoporosis
Physical activity
Physical fitness
Relaxation response
Resistance training
Rheumatoid arthritis (RA)
Tai chi
Warm-up period
Yoga

## ❓ THINK ABOUT IT

### *Knowing Versus Doing*

Having knowledge of the benefits of exercise does not correlate well with long-term exercise adherence. Confidence in the ability to exercise and a sense of the meaning and purpose (core desire) of exercise ensures better success.

- Why is being active and physically fit important?
- What motivates an individual to put the effort into developing and maintaining an active lifestyle?
- Who or what can help to enable exercise participation in someone's life?
- What does health promotion mean with respect to physical activity participation?

Regular physical activity and exercise are important lifestyle factors that can help improve both physical and psychological health in children and adults. Generally, people who exercise regularly, or those who naturally include physical activity in their daily routine, feel better mentally and physically, improve their health profiles, and safeguard their functional independence as they go through the aging process. A holistic approach to physical activity involves exercise for cardiorespiratory health (endurance), exercise for musculoskeletal health (strength, flexibility, and bone health), and body awareness. Body awareness and mindfulness during exercise facilitate self-inquiry and self-acceptance, helping to relieve psychological stress and preventing physical injury (Box 22.1). Not only is an active lifestyle an important component of primary prevention but regular physical activity is also an essential modality in the treatment of chronic disease (the use of "exercise as medicine"), which establishes the potential for benefit in all aspects of the biopsychosocial and spiritual model of health.

---

## BOX 22.1 Health Impact of Physical Activity

- Improves quality of life
- Improves mood and promotes a sense of well-being
- Increases flexibility
- Builds muscle strength
- Increases endurance
- Increases the efficiency of the heart
- Improves bone health (density and microarchitecture)
- Decreases risk of obesity
- Decreases risk of stroke
- Decreases risk of heart disease
- Decreases risk of diabetes

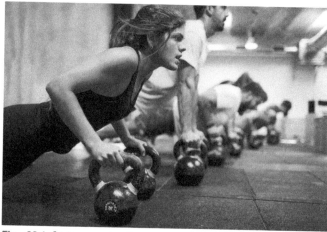

**Fig. 22.1** Some people choose more vigorous types of exercise. (iStockPhoto/Tempura)

## DEFINING PHYSICAL ACTIVITY IN HEALTH

To fully understand the objectives of this chapter, the following definitions will be used:

- Physical activity: body movement that is produced by the contraction of skeletal muscles and that substantially increases energy expenditure; includes transportation and vocational and leisure-time activity. Leisure-time activity can be further categorized into sports, recreational activities, and exercise training (Fig. 22.1).
- Exercise (exercise training): planned, structured, and repetitive body movement performed to improve or maintain one or more components of physical fitness.
- Aerobic exercise: activity that uses large muscle groups in a repetitive, rhythmical fashion over an extended period to increase the efficiency of the oxidative energy-producing system and increase cardiorespiratory endurance; uses stored adipose tissue as a major fuel source.
- Anaerobic exercise: high-intensity, short-duration activity that increases the efficiency of the phosphocreatine and glycolytic energy-producing systems and increases muscle strength, power, and speed of reactivity; uses phosphagens and glucose-glycogen as major fuel sources. High-intensity interval training (HIIT) is an area of anaerobic exercise that includes short bouts of intense aerobic exercise followed by short recovery periods.
- Physical fitness: a set of attributes (cardiorespiratory fitness, muscular fitness, and flexibility) that people have or achieve that relates to the ability to perform physical activity without undue fatigue or risk of injury.
- Muscular fitness: the strength and endurance of muscles that allows participation in daily activities or exercise associated with a lower risk of musculoskeletal injury.
- Flexibility: adequate muscle length and joint mobility to allow free and painless movement through a wide range of motion (ROM).

## PHYSICAL ACTIVITY PARTICIPATION— CURRENT GUIDELINES AND RECOMMENDATIONS

The Canadian Society for Exercise Physiology (CSEP) was founded in 1967, and is an organization of professionals that work to advance the area of exercise and health (CSEP, n.d.). Its mission statement is as follows: "CSEP is the resource for translating advances in exercise science research into the promotion of fitness, performance, and health outcomes for Canadians. CSEP sets the highest standards for qualified exercise professionals through evidence-informed practice and certification" (CSEP, n.d.). CSEP also promotes six goal statements:

- To be the national and international voice for exercise science and prescription in Canada, and to represent and advance CSEP positions.
- To pursue the vision and mission in an ethical, effective, and financially responsible manner.
- To provide members working in exercise physiology and health and fitness with timely, relevant products and services.
- To increase awareness of CSEP in Canada and internationally with funders, within the exercise physiology sector, and among the general public.
- To promote evidence-informed practice through the development of standards, policies, guidelines, and research related to exercise physiology and health and fitness.
- To define, develop, and implement effective knowledge translation activities related to CSEP's evidence-informed body of knowledge and advancing certification in a timely manner. (CSEP, n.d.)

The CSEP organization and community creates an area for excellence in exercise and physical activity knowledge, and therefore is the "go-to" resource for physical activity-related research and guidelines in Canada. Why are physical activity guidelines important? Having well-developed and supported guidelines provides an attainable physical activity goal for the general public, and a goal that promoters of physical activity (such as clinicians, health care providers, or exercise professionals) can use. Guidelines that are well researched provide a reason for being physically active—if you achieve the guidelines for physical activity, it will confer health benefits. Without guidelines, there would be disagreement about how much physical activity to engage in or promote, and people would not know what level of physical activity they should attain.

In 1998, in partnership with Health Canada, CSEP released *Canada's Physical Activity Guide to Healthy Active Living*, which targeted adults between 20 and 55 years of age (Public Health Agency of Canada & Canadian Society for Exercise Physiology [PHAC/CSEP], 1998). This was then followed by updates to include older persons and children and youth, in 1999 and 2002, respectively (PHAC/CSEP, 1999; PHAC/CSEP, 2002). These early iterations of physical activity guidelines were overhauled between 2006 and 2010. With support from the Public Health Agency of Canada (an agency of the Government of Canada that is responsible for public health), CSEP sought to complete an all-encompassing review of physical activity guidelines in Canada. This review would subsequently inform a set of updated, research-based, exercise guidelines. Tremblay, Kho, Tricco, and colleagues (2010) described the review process that was conducted in order to revise the older *Canadian Physical Activity Guidelines*; specifically, the authors discuss the details of the Physical Activity Measurement and Guidelines project (PAMG project). To create supported and informed updated physical activity guidelines, the PAMG project included the following steps (Tremblay, Warburton, Janssen, et al., 2011, pp. 2–4):

- *Phase 1.* Think tank meeting of physical activity experts intended to discuss the current state of the guidelines, expectations, new findings, and initiate a review of the older guidelines. CSEP also convened a Steering Committee on the PAMG project with CSEP and Public Health Agency of Canada representatives; and commissioned 12 papers on various aspects informing physical activity.
- *Phase 2.* There was a meeting of authors to discuss the findings of the commissioned papers, and reach consensus on the evidence to date. Findings of the papers were also presented at research conferences. CSEP submitted a vision document to the Public Health Agency of Canada, with a plan to update the current physical activity guidelines.
- *Phase 3.* CSEP and the Public Health Agency of Canada decided to move forward with developing clinical practice guidelines, with additional reviews being commissioned for further comprehensiveness.

Through this process, CSEP also engaged with international organizations (e.g., in the United Kingdom, United States, Australia, and the World Health Organization [WHO]) to look at making guidelines complementary across countries. Of note, the WHO was also in the process of developing global physical activity guidelines at the time, and thus experts from the PAMG project maintained connection with the WHO during these efforts (Tremblay et al., 2010). Using the highly informed evidence created through the phases above, the committee worked to develop guidelines with a standardized approach. To the knowledge of Tremblay and colleagues, they were the first to use a "methodologically rigorous formal guideline development framework and systematic reviews to inform consensus recommendations in physical activity" (Tremblay et al., 2010, p. 10).

What Tremblay and colleagues, CSEP, and the Public Health Agency of Canada undertook was truly a unique, modern,+4 and comprehensive approach to developing physical activity guidelines. We can appreciate how the creation of the *Canadian Physical Activity Guidelines* was an extensive process that involved a collaborative effort among content experts and the Government of Canada. The long process included a lot of time, research, and effort, leading to physical activity suggestions that were both achievable and associated with the best health effects. The final guidelines were written between 2009 and 2010, and were published in 2011 (Tremblay et al., 2011). A summary of the new *Canadian Physical Activity Guidelines* (Tremblay et al., 2011) follows:

Children (5–11 years old); Youth (12–17 years old)

- The guidelines are intended for all apparently healthy children and youth, irrespective of gender, race, ethnicity, or socioeconomic status.
- Children and youth should participate in activities that support natural development, are part of play, are enjoyable and safe.
- For health benefits, children and youth should engage in at least 60 minutes of moderate- to vigorous-intensity physical activity every day. This should include vigorous activities at least 3 days per week, and activities to strengthen muscle and bone at least 3 days per week. More daily physical activity confers a greater benefit to health.

Adults (18–64 years old)

- The guidelines are intended for all apparently healthy adults, irrespective of gender, race, ethnicity, or socioeconomic status.
- Adults are encouraged to participate in physical activities that are fun and safe, and in a variety of activities.
- The guidelines may be appropriate for adults who are pregnant or have a medical condition, or a disability; however, a medical consultation with a health professional is suggested prior to engaging.
- For health benefits, adults should engage in at least 150 minutes of moderate- to vigorous-intensity physical activity per week, in bouts of 10 minutes or more. It is also of benefit to add muscle and bone strengthening activities at least 2 days per week. More physical activity participation confers a greater benefit to health.

Older Adults (= 65 years old)

- The guidelines are intended for all apparently older persons, irrespective of gender, race, ethnicity, or socioeconomic status.
- Adults are encouraged to participate in physical activities that are fun and safe, and in a variety of activities.
- These guidelines may be appropriate for older persons who are frail, have a medical condition, or a disability; however, a medical consultation with a health professional is suggested prior to engaging.
- For health benefits and to improve functional ability, older persons should engage in at least 150 minutes of moderate- to vigorous-intensity physical activity per week, in bouts of 10 minutes or more. It is also of benefit to add muscle and bone strengthening activities at least 2 days per week. Those with mobility issues should include balance training to prevent falls. More physical activity participation confers a greater benefit to health. (Tremblay et al., 2011)

One major change to the new *Canadian Physical Activity Guidelines* versus the previous version was the removal of specific recommendations for flexibility training. Flexibility was removed because there was limited evidence to support the benefit of flexibility training recommendations; they are not necessarily activities that are discouraged, but they should not be done in place of the recommended activities of the guidelines (Tremblay et al., 2011). The *Canadian Physical Activity*

*Guidelines* are in agreement with international guidelines, such as the current WHO global recommendations for physical activity (WHO, 2010). However, there are still multiple areas of future research needed in the area of physical activity guidelines. As noted earlier, the guidelines were developed for the apparently healthy population; that is, individuals without severe chronic disease. This is because the evidence used to support the creation of the guidelines did not address the individual needs of specific chronic diseases. Later in this chapter, we discuss the role of physical activity in treating some chronic diseases, and towards the end of this chapter we discuss special exercise considerations for two chronic diseases: cardiovascular disease and diabetes. The development of disease-specific guidelines is still an area of research that is needed—this is not to say that the above guidelines will not apply; however, individual considerations for the use of exercise in disease need to be given (Tremblay et al., 2011).

In addition to developing chronic disease specific physical activity guidelines, there is an important consideration in creating 24-hour movement guidelines (Box 22.2). Why would this be necessary? Consider if you have an individual who engages in the recommended 150 minutes of physical activity per week, but spends the remaining time completely sedentary and in front of a screen; while the physical activity guidelines are achieved, this is not a healthy active lifestyle. The amount of sedentary time is extremely high, and research has demonstrated that time spent engaging in sedentary behaviour is independently associated with all-cause mortality (Ku, Steptoe, Liao, et al., 2018), meaning that while participating in physical activity is important, it is also important to consider overall sedentary time as well.

Another area of research that is still lacking is the messaging strategies needed to convey the new guidelines to all Canadians. We understand that it is necessary to have well-supported physical activity guidelines, but how do we make sure that the general public accesses them and uses them? This brings us back to the box at the beginning of the chapter and the concept of knowing versus doing: even if the guidelines are widely read and understood, will people actually do the physical activity?

In 2010, Latimer and colleagues published a systematic review of the effectiveness of three approaches to disseminating physical activity messages. These methods included tailoring messages to best suit individuals who are targeted recipients, framing messages in terms of gains vs. losses, and targeting messages to change self-efficacy. This systematic review found that each type of messaging can lead to increased physical activity participation, but that overall there was not strong evidence to support recommendations for one type of messaging approach over another (Latimer, Brawley, & Bassett, 2010). This presents a health promotion concern—we can promote the guidelines, but how do we promote the physical activity? We will discuss more about health promotion and physical activity later in this chapter.

## BOX 22.2   The Canadian 24-Hour Movement Guidelines

### *Linking Together Physical Activity, Sedentary Time, and Sleep—A Total Day Approach*

At the time the 2010 *Canadian Physical Activity Guidelines* were published, no evidence-informed sedentary behaviour guidelines were available. What does this mean? We have guidelines regarding the amount of physical activity we should be striving to achieve in our daily life (~21 minutes per day for adults), but what about the other 1419 minutes of the day? Are the health benefits the same for someone who meets the physical activity guidelines but spends the rest of the day on the couch versus someone who meets the physical activity guidelines and also engages in an active lifestyle? Studies indicate that yes, time engaging in sedentary behaviour is associated with negative health outcomes independent of physical activity (Ku et al., 2018).

In 2016, the first *Canadian 24-Hour Movement Guidelines* were published. These incorporate not only physical activity but also sedentary time and sleep time. The first set of 24-hour movement guidelines was targeted towards children and youth aged 5–17 years (Tremblay, Chaput, Adamo, et al., 2017). More recently, 24-hour movement guidelines have also been created for children in the Early Years (0–4 years of age). These are highly innovative, as they address a very young age group, with a full-day approach to being healthy. The idea of targeting this age group is to set young children up for a life of healthy active living and the associated benefits. Below is a list of the Canadian 24-Hour Movement Guidelines for the Early Years (0–4), which promote healthy growth and development through recommended physical activity, high quality sedentary time, and sleep:

- Infants (<1 year old): *Move!* Be physically active several times per day (interactive floor-play), at least 30 mins of tummy time if not mobile yet. *Sleep!* 14–17 hours (0–3 months) or 12–16 hours (4–11 months) of good quality sleep including naps per day. *Sit!* Not restrained for more than 1 hour at a time, screen time not recommended.
- Toddlers (1–2 years old): *Move!* Be physically active for at least 180 minutes at any intensity, such as energetic play. *Sleep!* 11–14 hours of good quality sleep including naps per day. Consistent bedtimes and wake-ups. *Sit!* Not restrained for more than 1 hour at a time, screen time not recommended for those <2 years; for those 2 years old, sedentary screen time should be no more than 1 hour.
- Preschoolers (3–4 years old): *Move!* Be physically active for at least 180 minutes every day, with at least 60 minutes of energetic play. *Sleep!* 10–13 hours of good quality sleep which may include a nap. Consistent bedtimes and wake-ups. *Sit!* Not restrained for more than 1 hour at a time, screen time should be no more than 1 hour.

Note that replacing restrained time or sedentary screen time with physical activity can provide health benefits.

Using the above guidelines, how should a day look for a 3-year-old child? The day could include taking a walk to the park, playing at the park and engaging in energetic running and climbing and jumping. It could include walking back home, and then taking a good-quality nap. After nap, the 3-year-old child might be involved in organized play, such as swimming lessons, soccer time, or gymnastics groups. This could be followed up by playing outside on a scooter or a bike. For the after-dinner bedtime routine, the child should be put to bed at an appropriate hour that will allow them to get 11–12 hours of sleep. It is quite easy to promote fun, active play for children at this age, and this is what the 24-hour guidelines promote. Whole-day guidelines offer a change to how we approach daily movement. This is an innovative step forward in guideline work, and allows us to expand our thought from focused exercise sessions to whole day lifestyle adaptations for healthy living.

Source: Tremblay, M.S., Chaput, J.P., Adamo, K.B., Aubert, S., Barnes, J.D. Choquette, L., et al. (2017). Canadian 24-hour movement guidelines for the early years (0–4 years): An integration of physical activity, sedentary behaviour, and sleep. *BMC Public Health, 17*(suppl 5), 874.

## The Current State of Meeting Physical Activity Objectives: Making Progress?

While we have well-defined physical activity guidelines, and also 24-hour movement guidelines for some age groups, unfortunately, and perhaps not surprisingly, both adults and children are not meeting these physical activity guidelines globally (Colley, Garriguet, Janssen, et al., 2011; Ranasinghe, Ranasinghe, Jayawardena, et al., 2013; Marsaux, Celis-Morales, Hoonhout, et al., 2016). The Canadian Health Measures Survey data indicate that only 15% of Canadian adults are accumulating the recommended 150 minutes of moderate-to-vigorous physical activity per week adults; and of this, only 5% of adults accumulate 150 minutes per week in at least 30-minute bouts 5 or more days per week (Colley et al., 2011). According to the Centre for Disease Control and Prevention (CDC) in the United States, only 20.5% of adults in 2015 were participating in the WHO-recommended physical activity guidelines (CDC, 2015). In an international study of 20 countries, the percentage of adults who reported being physically inactive (sedentary) was between 6.9% (China) to 42.3% (Taiwan) (Bauman, Bull, Chey, et al., 2009).

Children are also not achieving the recommended amounts of physical activity: the WHO estimates that globally, 81% of school-aged children are not meeting guidelines of 60 minutes of physical activity per day (WHO, 2017). We know that the new *Canadian 24-Hour Movement Guidelines for the Early Years (0–4 years)* suggest that preschoolers should engage in at least 180 minutes per day of physical activities, 60 minutes of which should be moderate-to-vigorous daily physical activity (Tremblay et al., 2017). However, Chaput et al. (2017) reported that 38.2% of Canadian preschool children (average age ~3.5 years) were not meeting these physical activity recommendations. When the *Canadian 24-Hour Movement Guidelines* were examined in an international sample of over 6000 children, the global prevalence of meeting the recommendations was only 7% (Roman-Vinas, Chaput, Katzmarzyk, et al., 2016)—a number that is staggeringly low. Therefore the problem of physical inactivity is evident across the entire life span, and is a global problem.

### Aging

The biological changes attributed to aging closely resemble the effects of physical inactivity. The list for both aging and inactivity includes an increase in body fat and a decrease in all the following: aerobic capacity, muscle mass (sarcopenia), metabolic rate, strength and flexibility, bone mass, cognitive performance, immune function, and sleep quality.

Among older persons, exercise can improve health, prevent disability, chronic disease and hospitalizations, improve blood lipid profiles, and reduce body fat. We are currently in a phase of accelerated population in Canada (Statistics Canada, 2017a); the number of individuals 85 years of age and older increased by 19.4% between 2011–2016. This is a staggering four times the rate of for the overall Canadian population (Statistics Canada, 2017b). The proportion of aging to young individuals in Canada is changing as well; in 2012 children aged 0–14 years accounted for about 16.2% of the population, with adults aged 65 and older comprised 14.9% of the population (Statistics Canada, 2015). It is expected that the proportions of older persons over 65 will

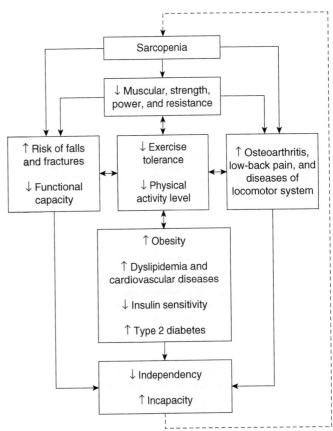

**Fig. 22.2** The interplay of physical activity, disease, physical function, and health in aging. (From Ciolac, E. G. [2013]. Exercise training as a preventive tool for age-related disorders: A brief review. *Clinics [Sao Paulo], 68*[5], 710–717.)

exceed that of children under 15; with older people projected to account for more than one-quarter of the population by 2036 (Statistics Canada, 2015). Trends are similar elsewhere, for example, projected numbers and proportions of the US population of older persons have been reported as follows: 43.1 million or 13.7% in 2012; 56.0 million or 16.8% in 2020; 72.8 million or 20.3% in 2030; 79.7 million or 21.0% in 2040; and 83.7 million or 20.9% in 2050 (Ortman, Velkoff, & Hogan, 2014).

Physical inactivity in the aging population is associated with multiple physiological changes that limit health, well-being, and physical function (Ciolac, 2013) (Fig. 22.2).

Exercise is, therefore, an important lifestyle intervention for the aging population. By exercising, older people can improve levels of cardiovascular, cardiopulmonary, and metabolic functions, including muscle performance and aerobic capacity (Galloza, Castillo, & Micheo, 2017; Turner, Lira, & Brum, 2017). Physical activity also helps to reduce the risk of chronic diseases in a dose-response manner (Warburton, Charlesworth, Ivey, et al., 2010). Several researchers have reported increases in cardiorespiratory fitness, physical performance function such at the 6-minute walk test (Hurst, Weston, McLaren, et al., 2019), significant increases or improvements in strength (Candow, Chilibeck, Abeysekara, et al., 2011), flexibility (Stolee, Zara, & Schuehlein, 2012), self-efficacy (Park, Song, Cho, et al., 2011), quality of life (McGrath, O'Malley, & Hendrix, 2010), balance (Rose & Hernandez, 2010), continence (Shamliyan, Kane, Wyman, & Wilt, 2008), safety (fewer falls and fall-related injuries)

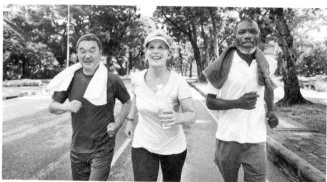

**Fig. 22.3** Older persons and should strive to achieve national physical activity guideline recommendations and maintain an active lifestyle. (iStockPhoto/Rawpixel)

(Caban-Martinez, Courtney, Chang, et al., 2015), and the ability to live independently (Cowan, Radman, Lewis, et al., 2009). Improvements are especially noted in exercise interventions with a combined modality (aerobic and strength training) (Hurst et al., 2019).

Not only can exercise improve psychological and functional health and well-being in aging adults, but it may also help to prevent changes to the brain that happen with aging. Brain atrophy is a consequence of the aging process, specifically, a decrease in grey matter. A recent cross-sectional study examined the impact of tai-chi exercise on slowing the progression of grey matter atrophy in older persons. Compared to controls, those with long-term tai-chi experience had larger grey matter volume in the thalamus and hippocampus, as well as increased emotional stability. Grey matter volume of the thalamus was positively associated with emotional stability (Liu, Li, Liu, et al., 2019). Therefore there might be a protective role of tai-chi exercise on brain matter in aging adults; however, this still needs to be confirmed in larger, longitudinal studies.

Older persons, in particular, need to be concerned about their nutritional status because the potential for malnutrition, a common problem for older persons, is associated with a decline in muscle strength and thus poorer outcomes, such as decreased function and performance (Henwood, Keogh, & Climstein, 2012; Mithal, Bonjour, Boonen, et al., 2013). The way to treat malnutrition in the aging population is still unclear; multiple interventions exist including oral nutritional supplementation with exercise, however there is a lack of high-quality evidence to indicate which interventions are the most effective (Correa-Perez, Abraha, Cherubini, et al., 2019).

Overall, the evidence points to the fact that regular physical activity can help maintain functional independence, health, and improve the quality of life throughout the aging process. Exercise guidelines for older persons (age 65 years and older) were detailed previously in this chapter. Older persons are encouraged to participate in a variety of physical activities, including engaging in planned exercise sessions, and recreational activity in group settings that also offer companionship, thereby conferring increased psychological benefit. But it should be noted that exercise prescription becomes more difficult in the aging population with chronic disease, as extra disease-specific considerations of exercise modality safety and efficacy are necessary.

Unfortunately, according to data from the Government of Canada, most older individuals are not meeting the activity levels recommended by the *Canadian Physical Activity Guidelines*. In 2013, only 13% of men and 11% of women aged 60 to 79 were meeting the guidelines (Government of Canada, 2016; Fig. 22.3). This is a troubling statistic, which indicates there might need to be a bigger focus on how we prescribe and encourage physical activity interventions in older populations. A systematic review found that community-based group exercise programs seem to have long-term adherence (~70%), but that overall, research is still needed that includes the opinions of older people regarding how an exercise program is designed, which may lead to programs with improved adherence (Farrance, Tsofliou, & Clark, 2016).

## CARDIAC RISK FACTORS

The literature strongly demonstrates that the risk of coronary heart disease (CHD) decreases as physical activity increases and that a plausible relationship between the decreased risk and a number of potential physiological and metabolic mechanisms exists (Ghadieh & Saab, 2015; Li, Liu, Tsai, et al., 2015; DeFina, Radford, Barlow, et al., 2019; da Silva, Grande, Roever, et al., 2019; Namgoong, Lee, Hwang, et al., 2018):

- Increasing levels of high-density lipoprotein (HDL) cholesterol
- Decreasing levels of low-density lipoprotein (LDL) cholesterol
- Decreasing total cholesterol levels
- Decreasing serum triglyceride (TRG) levels
- Decreasing high blood pressure
- Improving glucose tolerance and insulin sensitivity
- Decreasing obesity; altering the distribution of body fat
- Reducing the sensitivity of the myocardium to the effects of catecholamines, thereby decreasing the risk of ventricular arrhythmias
- Impacting molecules that promote cardiovascular disease (for example, trimethylamine N-oxide)
- Improved endothelial function

While clearly beneficial, the type of exercise should be carefully considered for CHD. One recent review looked at the time-saving advantages of HIIT compared to more traditional moderate-intensity continuous training in cardiac rehabilitation. Improvement of cardiovascular disease risk factors and measures of cardiac performance indicate that HIIT does not outperform moderate-intensity continuous training, and that adopting only a HIIT approach to cardiac rehabilitation should be done cautiously (Quindry, Franklin, Chapman, et al., 2019). More research is still needed in this area.

### High-Density Lipoprotein and Serum Triglyceride Levels

Exercise has a major influence on lipoprotein metabolism, primarily affecting plasma levels of HDL and TRG. There is a strong negative correlation between CHD and plasma HDL levels. Increases in HDL level reduces the total cholesterol to HDL ratio, thereby reducing CHD risk. Exercise, a common part of treatment of hypertriglyceridemia, has a lowering effect on TRG levels (Vrablík & Češka, 2015; Motallebi, Iranagh, & Mohammadi, 2019). A meta-analysis of randomized controlled trials examined the impact of exercise on cardiorespiratory fitness and cardiometabolic biomarkers in adults, and found that lipid profiles were improved in the exercising groups, including lowered triglyceride levels, higher HDL, and higher apolipoprotein A1 (a protein of HDL) (Lin, Zhang, Guo. et al., 2015). A similar systematic review reported that following exercise, total cholesterol, triglycerides, and LDL decreased, while HDL increased (Glenney, Brockemer, Ng, et al., 2017). In obese children, a systematic review and meta-analysis revealed that the integration of both aerobic and resistance training improves body mass, fat mass and LDL (Garcia-Hermoso, Ramirez-Velez, Ramirez-Campillo, et al., 2018). Combined interventions, such as diet and physical activity, also reduce BMI and triglyceride levels in pediatric obesity (Rajjo, Mohammed, Alsawas, et al., 2017).

The effect of exercise on lipid metabolism may be related more to the volume (duration and frequency) than to the intensity of the exercise. In a systematic review, Tambalis, Panagiotakos, Kavouras, and colleagues (2009) reviewed the literature for responses in the levels of blood lipids to a variety of modes and volumes of exercise. Moderate-intensity aerobic exercise training (less than 60% of maximum heart rate [$\dot{V}o_{2max}$] or six metabolic equivalents) appears to have the greatest effect on HDL levels. However, stronger evidence suggested that high-intensity aerobic training promotes significant increases in HDL levels. This was observed among a wide range of 90 to 200 minutes per week. Resistance training supported a marked reduction in LDL levels, followed by a significant reduction in total cholesterol levels. The review found combining resistance and aerobic exercise can lead to remarkable reductions in LDL levels, significant increases in HDL levels, and significant decreases in total cholesterol levels (Tambalis et al., 2009).

## Hypertension

*Hypertension*, or high blood pressure, is defined as a systolic blood pressure greater than or equal to 140 mm Hg and a diastolic blood pressure greater than or equal to 90 mm Hg. According to Statistics Canada, between 2012 and 2015, the prevalence of hypertension in Canadian adults aged 20 to 79 years was 24%. However, prevalence increased with age, such that 53% of Canadian adults aged 60 to 79 years reported being diagnosed with hypertension (Statistics Canada, 2016). Obesity is an important risk factor for hypertension; according to the Canadian Health Measures Survey, compared to normal-weight adults, adults who were overweight or obese were more than twice as likely to report having hypertension (Statistics Canada, 2016). Heart and Stroke Canada recommends that adults follow national guidelines for exercise participation. This includes participating in 150 minutes of moderate-to-vigorous physical activity per week, in bouts of 10 minutes or more. Examples of aerobic activity could include going for a walk, recreational sports, or even gardening. Heart and Stroke Canada guidelines also align with the national guidelines in suggesting that older persons engage in muscle and bone strengthening activity (resistance training [Box 22.3]) at least 2 days per week (Heart

and Stroke Foundation of Canada, 2019). Note that resistance training can involve the use of handheld weights, but strength training can also include using your own body weight (such as doing push-ups), resistance bands (such as TheraBand®), or even using everyday items (such as filled grocery bags or cans of food). Aerobic exercise, resistance training, and concurrent exercise (i.e., aerobic and resistance) have been all been demonstrated to reduce blood pressure in individuals who are hypertensive (Lopes, Mesquita-Bastos, Alves, et al., 2018). HIIT has also been demonstrated to reduce blood pressure in those who are hypertensive (Boutcher & Boutcher, 2017), which suggests that interval training is a useful exercise modality for hypertension, as well.

The mechanisms underlying the exercise-training effect on lowering blood pressure are not completely clear, but may involve attenuation of sympathetic nervous system activity. This attenuation results in the dilation of peripheral blood vessels, which decreases systemic vascular resistance. Decreasing sympathetic nervous system activity may have a beneficial effect on the insulin resistance that is often observed in hypertensive people. Small improvements of endothelial function confer large benefits in cardiovascular risks; a systematic review and meta-analysis revealed that aerobic exercise leads to improved endothelial function in adults with hypertension (Pedralli, Eibel, Waclawovsky, et al., 2018). The literature has also uncovered significant effects of isometric exercise (i.e., exercise that involves little change in joint angle or muscle length, static exercise) on hypertension. For example, simple isometric handgrip exercise (hand grip strength) is associated with blood pressure reduction in older (50+ years) individuals (Bentley, Nguyen, & Thomas, 2018; Nascimento, Tibana, Benik, et al., 2014). The mechanisms by which this happens are not yet well defined, but improved endothelium-dependent dilation, decreased oxidative stress, and improved autonomic regulation of blood pressure have been suggested (Millar, McGowan, Cornelissen, et al., 2014).

## Hyperinsulinemia and Glucose Intolerance

Diabetes mellitus encompasses a group of metabolic disorders that have in common an increase in blood glucose levels and associated metabolic dysfunction. Type 1 diabetes involves elevated blood glucose levels that are a result of a deficiency of circulating insulin caused by destruction of the pancreatic β cells, and type 2 diabetes involves elevated blood glucose levels from insulin resistance (decreased insulin sensitivity)—largely in skeletal muscles—or impaired insulin secretion (Nathan, 2015). Approximately ~90% of those with diabetes have type 2 diabetes. According to the Government of Canada, about 3 million Canadians were living with diabetes in 2013 and 2014. Approximately one in 300 youth and one in 10 adults (age 20 years and older) have diabetes (Government of Canada, 2017). In addition, adiposity and poor fitness are linked with insulin resistance (Larson-Meyer, Redman, Heilbronn, et al., 2010). Complications of diabetes include heart disease and stroke, peripheral arterial disease, retinopathy, nephropathy, peripheral neuropathy, and lower-extremity amputation (Deshpande, Harris-Hayes, & Schootman, 2008).

## BOX 22.3    Resistive Training Exercises

### Chest Press

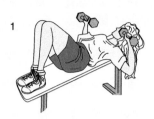

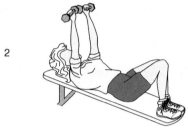

Lie on a bench with feet flat on the bench, or lie on the floor with knees bent and feet flat, whichever is more comfortable.

- Hold weights near shoulders with elbows out and palms facing away from the body.
- Exhale while extending arms straight up, following an "A" pattern with the weights touching at the peak.
- Slowly lower the weights back to original position while inhaling.
- Repeat 8 to 12 times.
- Note: weights can be replaced with canned goods (i.e., soup cans), or for beginners, use no weights at all.

### Chest Fly

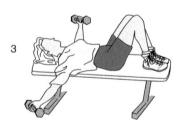

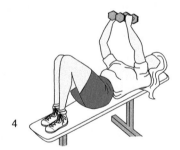

- Lie on a bench with feet flat on the bench, or lie on the floor with knees bent and feet flat, whichever is more comfortable.
- With palms facing each other, extend arms above chest, keeping elbows slightly bent at all times.
- Inhale and lower arms perpendicularly away from the body until arms are out of peripheral vision.
- Exhale while returning to starting position by visualizing arms hugging a barrel that is lying on the chest.

- Repeat 8 to 12 times.
- Note: weights can be replaced with canned goods (i.e., soup cans), or for beginners, use no weights at all.

### Bent Over Row

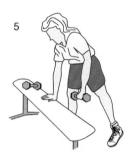

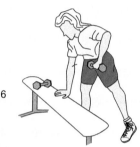

- Bend at waist while supporting the body with one hand (on table, bench, etc.) and holding a weight with the other hand in an overhand grip.
- Keep knees bent while the weight is hanging perpendicular to the torso.
- Slowly pull the weight up to the chest as if starting a lawn mower, exhaling and keeping the elbow away from the body.
- Slowly lower weight back to starting position while inhaling.
- Repeat 8 to 12 times on each side.
- Note: weights can be replaced with canned goods (i.e., soup cans), or for beginners, use no weights at all.

### Dumbbell Curl

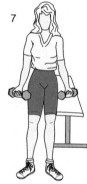
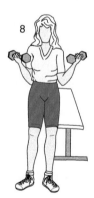

- Stand or sit with weights held at sides in an underhand grip, keeping elbows close to the body, and upper arms stationary.
- Curl weights to the chin or upper chest while exhaling.
- Inhale while slowly lowering weights.
- Keep back straight throughout the duration of motion.
- Repeat 8 to 12 times.
- Note: weights can be replaced with canned goods (i.e., soup cans), or for beginners, use no weights at all.

## BOX 22.3    Resistive Training Exercises—cont'd

**Triceps Extension**

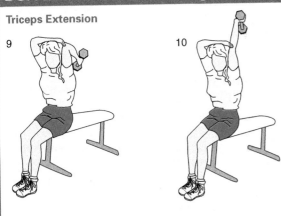

9    10

- While seated or standing in the neutral back position, lift the hand holding the weight straight above the head in alignment with the ear.
- Keeping the upper arm tight, slowly bend the elbow to lower the weight between the shoulder blades.
- Use the free hand to support the elbow and to prevent movement in the upper arm.
- Raise the weight back to its original position by straightening the arm and exhaling.
- Repeat 8 to 12 times on each side.
- Note: weights can be replaced with canned goods (i.e., soup cans), or for beginners, use no weights at all.

Exercise, in addition to diet, is a first-line intervention for diabetes (Gulve, 2008). In a recent meta-analysis of randomized controlled trials, both diet and lifestyle interventions including exercise and physical activity decreased 2-hour plasma glucose and fasting plasma glucose levels in individuals with impaired glucose tolerance (Gong, Kang, Ying, et al., 2015). In a similar meta-analysis of randomized controlled trials, researchers examined the effects of lifestyle interventions including exercise and physical activity on risk factors in individuals with type 2 diabetes and found a significant reduction in the level of hemoglobin A1c (HbA$_{1c}$), among other risk factors (Chen, Pei, Kuang, et al., 2015).

A randomized control trial by Belli, Ribeiro, Ackermann, and colleagues (2011) examined the effects of 12-week overground walking training in individuals with type 2 diabetes. The exercise group performed walking at the ventilatory threshold velocity. When compared with the control group, the exercise group had significant reductions in HbA$_{1c}$ levels (glycemic control) and body composition (body mass and body mass index [BMI]) and a significant increase in exercise capacity (peak oxygen uptake and exercise duration). Several meta-analyses examined the effects of different modes of exercise on glycemic control. Strasser, Siebert, and Schobersberger (2010) examined the effect of resistance training with individuals with abnormal glucose metabolism and found significant improvements in glycemic control, with a mean HbA$_{1c}$ level reduction of 0.48%. Chudyk and Patrella (2011) reported that aerobic exercise alone or combined with resistance training significantly reduced HbA$_{1c}$ levels, systolic blood pressure, and triglyceride levels in individuals with type 2 diabetes. Furthermore, waist circumference was significantly reduced only when aerobic exercise and resistance training were combined. da Silva and colleagues (2019) conducted a systematic review on the impact of HIIT (vs. moderate-intensity interval training) on multiple outcomes in patients with type 2 diabetes. Although only five randomized controlled trials (RCTs) were included, they found that most studies saw significantly improved weight

and BMI with HIIT, but similar improvements to glucose levels with both methods of exercise. More studies are needed to determine the efficacy of HIIT in patients with type 2 diabetes, especially with regard to important outcomes such as HbA$_{1c}$ levels. In addition, technology-based approaches are becoming increasingly popular tools to help increase exercise participation and adherence in type 2 diabetes (Diversity Awareness).

Insulin resistance impedes glucose mobilization into cells, increasing plasma glucose levels and setting the potential for development of type 2 diabetes. Although insulin resistance in skeletal muscles may be the primary defect, the development of disease appears to be related to elevated insulin levels, a result of the body's response to the need to mobilize glucose into the cells. Additionally, this syndrome also often involves elevated TRG levels and hypertension, which contribute to the potential for disease. Exercise increases insulin sensitivity, enhances glucose uptake into the cells via contracting skeletal muscles, improves the inherent effect of endogenous insulin, decreases obesity, and plays a role in lowering TRG levels and blood pressure; therefore, it is recommended in the management of type 2 diabetes (Chen et al., 2015; Gong et al., 2015; Gulve, 2008; Nathan, 2015; Polikandrioti & Dokoutsidou, 2009; Waryasz & McDermott, 2010; Weltman, Saliba, Barrett, et al., 2009; Stanford & Goodyear, 2014). Long-term exercise participation can improve mitochondrial function, increase expression of glucose transporter proteins, and has a favourable effect on a number of metabolic genes (Stanford & Goodyear, 2014). With diet, weight control, and exercise, preventing or decreasing the need for oral antiglycolytic agents and insulin is possible while maintaining normal blood glucose levels. Physical activity may be most beneficial in preventing the progression of type 2 diabetes during the earlier stages of the disease process, before insulin therapy is required. Overall, physical activity has a significant positive effect on a chronic disease that is associated with a high risk of developing CHD.

*The Age of Technology: Using Smartphones and Technology to Encourage Exercise in People With Type 2 Diabetes*

We live in a time when technology has woven its way into many aspects of our lives. With social media platforms, advances in world-wide communication, and the use of technology to play games, it is clear that technology is a prominent component of our lives. Because of the prominence of technology in our daily lives, perhaps it can also be used from a health care perspective, to help advance the health and well-being of populations? This thought has been a focus of researchers in recent years, as they work with smartphones and wearable technology (e.g., wrist-worn smartwatches) to develop applications that can support everything from healthy heart rate mapping to keeping track of exercise and daily activity levels.

The use of technology to help promote physical activity in individuals with type 2 diabetes has been explored by multiple researchers. Since we know that exercise is a potent way to help treat type 2 diabetes, using technology to increased exercise behaviour is a logical step. One recent study developed a smart-phone based, game-like software to promote a healthier, more active lifestyle in middle-aged patients with type 2 diabetes; 36 inactive and overweight patients with type 2 diabetes were randomized to the intervention or control group. The control group received a one-time lifestyle counselling session, while the intervention group was instructed to play the smartphone game and to self-implement recommendations over 24 weeks. Intrinsic motivation to engage in physical activity increased significantly in the intervention group, while it decreased in the control group. The researchers found that the amount of time (minutes) of in-game training was positively associated with intrinsic motivation score, and was accompanied by increased physical activity participation such as walking and strength training. Overall, the integration of technological advancements and exercise prescription to improve chronic disease outcomes is a promising intervention for the future.

**Reflective Questions**

1. Can you think of other examples of different/new technology that can be used to improve health and physical activity?
2. Can you apply the use of technology to increase physical activity to a clinical setting? How might health care providers integrate the use of technology to improve the health of their patients?

Source: Höchsmann, C., Infanger, D., Klenk, C., et al. (2019). Effectiveness of a behavior change technique-based smartphone game to improve intrinsic motivation and physical activity adherence in patients with type 2 diabetes: Randomized controlled trial. *JMIR Serious Games, 7*(1), e11444.

## OBESITY

Overweight and obesity are conditions of excess body fat (adipose tissue). The *Canadian Guidelines for Body Weight Classification in Adults* are a body weight classification system that help to identify weight ranges and health problems associated with these. They are aligned with the WHO recommendations, and thus are internationally similar. The classification uses body BMI and waist circumference as an indicator of abdominal obesity (Government of Canada, 2015). The classification's target use is in adults ≥18 years of age, not including women who are pregnant or lactating. BMI is defined as (body weight in kg) / (height in metres)$^2$.

Health risk classification according to BMI is as follows (Health Canada, 2003):

- Underweight = <18.5 kg/m$^2$
- Normal weight = 18.5–24.9 kg/m$^2$
- Overweight = 25–29.9 kg/m$^2$
- Obese Class I = 30–34.9 kg/m$^2$
- Obese Class II = 35–39.9 kg/m$^2$
- Obese Class III = ≥40 kg/m$^2$

The second component of the *Canadian Guidelines for Body Weight Classification in Adults* is waist circumference. Waist circumference is calculated by measuring the midbody (torso), between the lowest rib and the top of the hip bone (iliac crest). Health risk classification according to waist circumference is:

- Men: ≥102 cm (40 inches)
- Women: ≥88 cm (40 inches)

When both BMI and waist circumference are combined, health classification can be estimated as well. When men have a waist circumference of <102 cm, and women <88 cm, if they have a normal BMI they are at the least risk for adverse health, if they have a BMI in the overweight range they are at increased health risk, and if they have a BMI in the obese range they have a high health risk. When men have a waist circumference of ≥102 cm and women ≥88 cm, if they have a normal BMI they are at an increased risk for adverse health, if they have a BMI in the overweight range they are at high health risk, and if they have a BMI in the obese range they are at very high health risk. This health risk includes risk for diseases such as type 2 diabetes, coronary heart disease, and hypertension (Health Canada, 2003).

It should be noted that there are limitations to the body weight classification system, for example, it can over- or underestimate health risk in certain groups such as in young adults who are not yet fully grown, athletes with a high muscle content, and older persons. However, it does provide an overall indication of whether someone is at risk for metabolic associated health problems.

The prevalence of obesity, as well as overweight and extreme obesity, is typically reported on the basis of BMI values, as is what is reported by Statistics Canada. Unfortunately, the prevalence of obesity in Canada remains high and has been increasing. According to the Statistics Canada data for 2014, 20.2% of Canadians over the age of 18 years were reported as being obese. When you combine those who are overweight with those who are obese, 61.8% of men and 46.2% of women fall within this group. When looking at the numbers provincially, in 2014, the proportion of people who were obese was lower than then national average (20.2%) in both Quebec (18.2%) and British Columbia (16%). However, Newfoundland and Labrador (30.4%), Nova Scotia (27.8%), New Brunswick (26.4%), Manitoba (24.5%), Saskatchewan (25.1%), and Northwest Territories (33.7%) all have rates that are higher than the national average (Statistics Canada, 2014). Obesity prevalence and trends are not only important to assess on a national level, but are of international concern as well. A commissioned report called *The Global Syndemic of Obesity, Undernutrition, and*

*Climate Change: The Lancet Commission Report* was published in 2019. This report details that each of the pandemics of obesity, undernutrition, and climate change are so prevalent globally, that they represent some of the biggest threats to human health and survival. Obesity is now one of the largest factors that contributes to poor health in most countries world-wide. We have known about the epidemic of obesity for decades, however, we still have not seen a reduction in obesity and associated conditions on a global scale—in fact, numbers still continue to rise. The report states that *no country* has decreased the obesity epidemic within its population (Swinburn, Kraak, Allender, et al., 2019). It is clear that obesity remains an important issue, both nationally and internationally; not only is obesity associated with health conditions, it is independently associated with increased mortality (West, Banks, & Wells, 2018).

An increase in fat mass and the development of obesity occur when energy intake exceeds total daily energy expenditure for a prolonged period. Decreased physical activity may be both a cause and a consequence of weight gain over a lifetime. Thus exercise is a modifiable factor that we can use to help decrease obesity. Physical activity:

- Promotes a negative energy balance (burns calories)
- Increases metabolic rate for an extended period after the activity
- Increases metabolic efficiency for burning calories by increasing lean body mass
- Helps counteract the decrease in metabolic rate associated with low-calorie diets by preserving lean body mass
- Is a good alternative to eating when eating is a response to stress rather than to hunger

Research supports the above statements and exercise also reduces BMI and obesity; physical activity also improves physical fitness. Unfortunately, as outlined earlier in this chapter, adults are not meeting recommended physical activity guidelines. Management of obesity needs to involve a comprehensive program of nutrition management, behaviour modification, and physical activity or exercise. The key to normalizing body fatness is long-term adherence and permanent lifestyle changes, not dieting or short-term exercise trials. Individuals who are overweight or obese should strive to achieve the CSEP national guidelines for physical activity, but should consult with a medical professional (doctor, combined with exercise expert) to develop an appropriate exercise program for them. Screening may be required prior to beginning an exercise program, and an individualized program that builds towards guideline achievement is ideal.

The ultimate goal is to have individuals engage in a multicomponent program that aims to decrease the energy intake and increase the energy expenditure, thereby changing the net energy balance to negative, leading to weight loss. There are multiple components to energy expenditure, with daily activity, exercise, and metabolic rate being some of the primary contributors. *Metabolic rate* is how many calories you burn at rest (i.e., how many calories are required

for you to sit awake). Women tend to have a 5 to 10% lower resting metabolic rate than men and a higher percentage of body fat than men of similar weight. Consequently, women have a lower percentage of lean body mass and may not be as metabolically active as are men during exercise. Women may expend up to 40% fewer calories than do men during the same exercise protocol at the same relative intensity (Tremblay, Despres, & Bouchard, 1985). That being said, when fat mass is replaced by lean mass, metabolic rate increases. Therefore, both women and men experience a double benefit with exercise—the energy burned by the exercise itself and the increase in muscle mass that increases energy expenditure at rest.

Unfortunately, the obesity trends are not limited only to adults. There is also a high national and international prevalence of pediatric obesity. In the last 30 years in Canada, obesity rates among children and youth have nearly tripled (Government of Canada, 2019). Pediatric obesity is especially concerning because not only can it impact health and well-being during childhood, but it can also and often does extend into adulthood; those who are obese as a child are more likely to be obese as an adult (Whitaker, Wright, Pepe et al., 1997). For example, in a study by Ortiz-Marrón, Ortiz-Pinto, Cuadrado-Gamarra, and colleagues (2018), researchers from Spain followed more than 2000 4-year-old children and recorded that the prevalence of obesity increased from 5.4 to 10.1% over a two-year follow-up. As well, children who have obese parents have a much higher risk of being obese as adults (Whitaker et al., 1997). In children, obesity-related health concerns include high blood pressure, type 2 diabetes, and fatty liver disease (Güngör, 2014). There can also be emotional and cognitive concerns (Chojnacki, Raine, Drollette et al., 2018; Sagar & Gupta, 2018). The importance of exercise to help reduce obesity in the pediatric population is underscored, but like adults, unfortunately the global prevalence of children meeting the recommendations of the *Canadian 24-Hour Movement Guidelines* was reported as being only 7% (Roman-Vinas et al., 2016).

## OSTEOPOROSIS

Osteoporosis is the most common bone disease and a major global health threat. It is characterized by low bone mineral density (BMD; quantity of bone) and structural weakness of bone tissue, leading to fragility and increased risk of fractures (National Institutes of Health, Osteoporosis and Related Bone Diseases National Resource Center, 2011). In Canada, an estimated 2 million people have osteoporosis (Osteoporosis Canada, 2019). Furthermore, over 80% of fractures in adults over 50 years of age are caused by osteoporosis. The disease affects both men and women, with one in three women and one in five men experiencing an osteoporosis-related fracture in their life (Osteoporosis Canada, 2019). Unfortunately, the incidence of osteoporosis in women is greater than heart attack, stroke, and cancer combined (National Osteoporosis Foundation, 2016).

*Peak bone mass* is defined as the greatest amount of bone that one will have, and is usually reached by the third decade of life (Gordon, Zemel, Wren, et al., 2017). Thereafter, bone loss naturally occurs with aging; thus a higher peak bone mass confers greater protection from future osteoporosis. This age-related bone loss occurs throughout the skeletal system, in all races and in both sexes. However, there are significant differences in bone loss patterns between the sexes, with female sex being a risk factor for osteoporosis. Women tend to achieve a lower peak bone mass than men; and overall, they have less bone mass than men at all ages. An additional factor that impacts BMD in women is menopause; the rate of bone loss accelerates rapidly during the first 5 years after menopause, with annual losses of 3 to 5% being common. By the fifth decade, or during their 40s, women can anticipate a 10% loss of vertebral bone mass. Cumulative bone loss can approach 40% of peak bone mass over a woman's lifetime. Unfortunately, a loss of at least 30% of bone mass is required for detection on plain film radiographs (McKinnis, 2014). Therefore, it is important to detect women who are at risk early in the natural course of the disease, and to target interventions toward maintaining bone heath over the lifespan.

There are many nonmodifiable risk factors that contribute to developing osteoporosis, including being of White/Asian race, a family history, and premature menopause. However, there are also modifiable risk-factors that influence bone health, including long-term smoking, excessive alcohol consumption, nutrition, and physical activity (Mirza & Canalis, 2015; Smith, Wang, & Bloomfield, 2009; Stagi, Cavalli, Seminara, et al., 2014; Behringer, Gruetzner, McCourt, et al., 2014; Julián-Almárcegui, Gomez-Cabello, Huybrechts, et al., 2015; Nakamura, Saito, Kobayashi, et al., 2019). Physical activity is a potent stimulator of bone accrual. Physical activity works by increasing mechanical stresses on the skeleton, which challenges the skeleton to adapt and grow stronger. Bone is a dynamic tissue, constantly changing and adapting to the stresses to which it is subjected. Bone strength depends on stresses applied by muscular and weight-bearing activity (mechanical stress during active movement). Specifically, physical activity that involves weight-bearing activity (such as running and jumping) has a great impact on bone health. Exercise is, therefore, quite important during childhood and adolescence (Gomez-Bruton, Matute-Llorente, Gonzalez-Aguero, et al., 2017), when bone growth is at its greatest, as it provides support for a stronger skeletal foundation throughout aging. Combined exercise (i.e., doing different types of exercise such as aerobic and resistance training) is important in maintaining and preventing bone loss in aging women; a recent systematic review and meta-analysis determined that combined exercise interventions preserve postmenopausal women's BMD at the lumbar spine, hip, and total body (Zhao, Zhang, & Zhang, 2017).

The emphasis on a multimodal approach to exercise in osteoporosis is supported by published recommendations. The American College of Sports Medicine (ACSM) recommends that people with osteoporosis engage in weight-bearing and impact exercises to promote strengthening and cardiovascular conditioning, as well as flexibility, coordination, and balance training to improve quality of life, maintain an active lifestyle, and decrease the risk of falls (Kohrt, Bloomfield, Little, et al., 2004). These recommendations are echoed by Canadian data as well. Giangregorio, Papaioannou, Macintyre, and colleagues (2014) led a consensus process to develop exercise recommendations for men and women with osteoporosis, with and without vertebral fractures. They brought together experts from Canada, Australia, Finland, and the United States, and paired with Osteoporosis Canada to develop appropriate, research-informed exercise guidelines using a rigorous Grading of Recommendation Assessment, Development, and Evaluation (GRADE) approach. The recommendations that resulted from the work of the committee are divided into two categories: (1) for individuals with osteoporosis, and (2) for individuals with osteoporotic vertebral fractures:

For individuals with osteoporosis:

- Engage in a multicomponent exercise program including resistance training and balance training.
- Individuals do not engage in aerobic exercise *to the exclusion* of resistance or balance training.

For individuals with osteoporotic vertebral facture:

- Consult a physiotherapist to ensure safe appropriate exercise. Engage in a multicomponent exercise program including resistance training and balance training.
- Individuals do not engage in aerobic exercise *to the exclusion* of resistance or balance training. (Giangregorio et al., 2014)

These guidelines clearly emphasize that exercise should not be limited to one type (i.e., aerobic), and should include resistance training and balance training (Box 22.4). Resistance and balance training can also help reduce fall risk by strengthening important muscles. Some further special considerations for exercise programs in those with osteoporosis include ensuring that programs are designed to limit the risk of falls or fractures, and learn how to safely move (i.e., proper twisting and bending).

Another important initiative to help inform proper exercise in osteoporosis was led by Osteoporosis Canada, with the help of an advisory team of expert clinicians and academics. They developed courses called Bone Fit™, which are aimed to help train both fitness and rehab professionals working with both uncomplicated and complicated cases of individuals with osteoporosis (Osteoporosis Canada, 2017). These workshops are designed to provide instruction for how to provide the safest, most effective exercises for those with bone loss and complement the guidelines discussed above.

### BOX 22.4 Balance Training for Osteoporosis

- Should accumulate 2 hours of balance training per week (15–20 minutes per day)
  - Can be done in short bouts throughout the day
  - Great to incorporate into daily activities
- Balance exercise examples include:
  - Standing on one leg
  - Standing on heels or toes only
  - Sit-to-stand
  - Tai chi

Source: Giangregorio, L. M., Papaioannou, A., Macintyre, N. J., et al. (2014). Too fit to fracture: Exercise recommendations for individuals with osteoporosis or osteoporotic vertebral fracture. *Osteoporosis International, 25*(3), 821–835.

An important goal of exercise training in osteoporosis is to decrease the risk of fractures through fall prevention. One type of exercise, tai chi, involves a lot of balance and coordinated muscle movements. It is a low-impact exercise, and thus may not improve BMD, but might be important to help reduce falls. A meta-analysis summarized research on the ability of tai chi to prevent falls in older persons. Research indicates that tai chi may reduce the risk of falls and injury related falls over the short term, by between 43 and 50% (Lomas-Vega, Obrero-Gaitan, Molina-Ortega, et al., 2017). More research is still needed to continue to improve our understanding how the interplay between exercise, muscle, falls, bone health, and fractures work. See the Research for Evidence-Informed Practice box, which presents a research spotlight on a recent pilot study that investigated the feasibility of an at home exercise program in reducing the risk of falls and fractures for older women with a history of vertebral fracture.

## RESEARCH FOR EVIDENCE-INFORMED PRACTICE

### The Feasibility of an At-Home Exercise Program for Reducing the Risk of Falls and Fractures for Older Women With a History of Vertebral Fracture

Giangregorio, Gibbs, Templeton, and colleagues (2018) conducted a pilot study to examine the feasibility of a 12-month, at home, exercise protocol in older women with vertebral fracture.

*Objectives.* To examine the feasibility of an exercise randomized controlled trial (RCT), looking at the efficacy and safety of exercise for reducing fractures in people who already have vertebral fractures. This pilot study was important for determining if a larger, more resources-dependent trial is warranted.

*Design.* This was a multicentre study with 7 sites (in Australia and Canada) participating.

*Participants.* Women ≥65 years old with a confirmed vertebral fracture were included. Intervention: Participants were randomly assigned to one of two groups: (1) exercise (12-month home exercise program, including resistance, balance, and posture exercises, as well as aerobic activity for a min of 30 min) ($n = 71$), and (2) equal attention control group ($n = 70$). Both groups received six home visits from a physiotherapist over the 12 months. The exercise group was given instruction on exercise, and the control group received a discussion about health-related topics (excluding exercise).

*Measurements.* The primary outcome measures included retention and adherence measurements, number of falls, and fractures.

*Results.* Overall retention and adherence were good; 92% completed the study, and adherence was on average 66%. The exercise group did not differ in the number of falls, or fractures compared to the control group.

*Conclusion.* An at-home RCT of home exercise in women with vertebral fractures was feasible, but there were issues with achieving initial recruitment. The pilot trail was not designed with statistical power to detect differences in falls or fractures. Future trials should consider an active control group, a larger number of recruitment sites, recruitment integrated with clinical visits as well as other methods of increasing recruitment potential. This type of protocol is promising; but overall researchers are encouraged to work together to develop large multicentre trials.

Source: Giangregorio, L. M., Gibbs, J. C., Templeton, J. A., et al. (2018). Build better bones with exercise (B3E pilot trial): Results of a feasibility study of a multicenter randomized controlled trial of 12 months of home exercise in older women with vertebral fracture. *Osteoporosis International, 29,* 2545–2556.

## ARTHRITIS

Arthritis is associated with a deterioration in joint health. Although rheumatoid arthritis and osteoarthritis have different causes and attack different parts of the joint, impaired joint function is the result. Cartilage is destroyed, and irregularities occur in the bone ends. As proper joint alignment changes, normal ROM is decreased, normal muscle balance and activity are altered, and disfigurement and dysfunction occur; and ultimately normal movement patterns are altered. Although there is an ongoing progression in arthritis that cannot be reversed by exercise, physical activity helps to restore health to synovium and cartilage, increase strength and flexibility, decrease joint vulnerability, and delay the onset of dysfunction. Most importantly, exercise has been shown to reduce pain and joint stiffness, reduce fatigue, and improve function and psychological well-being in adults with arthritis (Cooney, Law, Matschke, et al., 2010; Kelley, Kelley, & Hootman, 2015; Kujala, 2009; Nelson, Allen, Golightly, et al., 2014).

Using exercise to counteract the effects of inactivity associated with arthritis is certainly a component to effective management (American College of Sports Medicine [ACSM], 2009b). Although researchers have concluded that regular exercise cannot cure arthritis, exercise has the following quality-of-life benefits for people with arthritis (ACSM, 2009b; Cooney et al., 2010; Metsios, Stavropoulos-Kalinoglou, & Kitas, 2015):

- Improvement in joint function and increase of ROM
- Increase in muscle strength and aerobic fitness that enhance daily activities of living
- Improvement in psychological state
- Decrease in loss of bone mass, and may promote increased BMD
- Decrease in the risk of chronic disease, including cardiovascular risk in rheumatoid arthritis

Consequently, exercise programs based on individual needs and interests should emphasize exercises to increase joint ROM and flexibility (performed before aerobic or strength activities) and should also include muscle-strengthening (two to three times per week) and aerobic exercises (5–10 minutes with progression to a 30-minute session 3–5 days per week) and be functionally based (ACSM, 2009a).

The collective evidence strongly and consistently suggests that exercise is beneficial for individuals with *osteoarthritis (OA)*. The specific aspects of exercise prescription for individuals with OA have been studied to differing extents. In terms of the different modes of exercise, various forms of exercise have been shown to be effective for OA. For example, aquatic exercise has been demonstrated to have a beneficial effect on pain, disability, and quality of life in individuals with knee or hip OA (Franco, Morelhao, de Carvalho, et al., 2017). A systematic review examined the effects of aquatic exercise on symptoms and function associated with lower extremity OA and reported significant effects for pain, self-reported function, physical functioning, stiffness, and quality of life (Waller, Ogonowska-Slodownik, Vitor, et al., 2014). With respect to fall risk, the available evidence produces mixed results with use of aquatic exercise to reduce fall risk in individuals with hip and/or knee OA, supporting the use of aquatic exercise in conjunction with fall risk education to effectively reduce fall risk, but not the use of aquatic exercise alone (Arnold & Faulkner, 2010; Hale, Waters, & Herbison, 2012). Long-term effects have not been shown to date, and determining the intensity, frequency, and duration (i.e., optimal protocol) has not been established (Franco et al., 2017); thus, we suggest aquatic exercise either be incorporated into a broader exercise program or be modified and exercise increase regularly to promote adaptation to and avoid accommodation to the training stimulus.

With respect to non–aquatic-based exercise, an umbrella review found high-quality evidence supporting the beneficial effects of exercise on pain and function in individuals with OA of the knee (Jamtvedt, Dahm, Christie, et al., 2008). Similarly, a systematic review of the effects of strength training alone, exercise therapy alone, and a combination of exercise and manual therapy in individuals with OA of the knee concluded that these modes of treatment improved function and reduced pain to a small degree, with the addition of manual therapy to treatment producing a moderate effect on pain (Jansen, Viechtbauer, Lenssen, et al., 2011). Another systematic review incorporating adults and older persons with knee OA supported progressive resistance exercise and aerobic exercise as having a modest beneficial effect on strength, pain, and function (Keysor & Brembs, 2011). Physical therapies including strength training, tai chi, and aerobic exercises have also been demonstrated to lead to improved balance outcomes and decreased fall risk in older individuals with knee OA (Mat, Tan, Kamaruzzaman, & Ng, 2015). Overall, there is no firm evidence that any specific type of exercise (aerobic, resistance, etc.) is more effective than another for reducing OA pain and disability; what is evident is that patients should engage in a lifestyle that encourages long-term exercise participation multiple days per week (Knapik, Pope, Orr, et al., 2018).

Furthermore, additional evidence suggests that increased belief that physical activity can be beneficial to manage arthritis leads to higher levels of participation in physical activity (Ehrlich-Jones, Lee, Semanik, et al., 2011) and is significantly associated with decreased pain and fatigue, increased function, and a self-perceived positive effect (Bezalel, Carmeli, & Katz-Leurer, 2010; Hewlett, Ambler, Almeida, et al., 2011; Pisters, Veenhof, Schelleves, et al., 2010). Exercise intensity is another important consideration for exercise prescription in individuals with OA; however, unlike the mode of exercise, intensity has received little attention. There is limited research available that compares the outcomes in individuals with OA with the intensity of training. More research is needed to determine the optimal parameters for exercise in individuals with OA, and an impairment-based, person-centred approach with consideration of comorbidities and accessibility is required (Regnaux, Lefevre-Colau, Trinquart, et al., 2015).

Rheumatoid arthritis (RA), unlike OA, is an autoimmune disease. This results in chronic inflammation of the joints (similar to OA) as well as other complications (such as cardiovascular involvement; different from OA). Exercise has been demonstrated to improve functional ability and reduce cardiovascular manifestations in RA (Metsios et al., 2015). Evidence supports the use of a combination of aerobic and strength exercises to improve outcomes in those with RA (Cooney et al., 2010). The use of tai chi as a form of activity in individuals with RA has also been considered. A case series study of the use of tai chi in individuals with RA

supported significant reduction in swelling of joints and increase in strength and endurance as measured by the "timed sit to stand test," and suggests practicing tai chi may help individuals with RA increase their level of physical activity (Uhlig, Fongen, Steen, et al., 2010). More intense exercise has also been investigated in RA. In a recent pilot study, Bartlett, Willis, Slentz, and colleagues (2018) examined the impact of HIIT on rheumatoid arthritis disease activity and aerobic fitness. They recruited 12 inactive older persons with rheumatoid arthritis and had them complete 10 weeks of high-intensity interval walking (3 × 30-minute sessions per week, that included 10 ≥60-second intervals of high-intensity activity with low intensity bouts in between). Following the intervention, cardiorespiratory fitness improved, as did resting blood pressure and heart rate. Importantly, disease activity (as determined by joint swelling and blood indices) was reduced by 38% post-intervention. The exercise program was also well tolerated by participants (Bartlett et al., 2018). HIIT is a promising area of exercise research in rheumatoid arthritis, but it needs further investigation before formal recommendations can be made.

Motivation to engage in exercise remains an important factor for participation in individuals with RA. A systematic review examined the correlates in four categories (sociodemographic, physical, psychological, and social variables) with levels of physical activity in individuals with RA (Larkin & Kennedy, 2014). Positive correlations with physical activity were found for motivation, self-efficacy, health perception, and previous physical activity levels, whereas negative correlations were found for fatigue, a coerced regulation style (i.e., the extent to which the person believes the physical activity goal was set not by himself or herself but by others), and certain physiological variables. Further to this, a more recent narrative review suggested that exercise should enhance self-efficacy in order to achieve long-term adherence in those with RA; and that proper support from health professionals, as well as friends and family, is important in encouraging physical activity for those with RA. There remains a need for interventions that target improving physical activity participation in patients with RA through overcoming barriers to exercise to sustain behaviour (Veldhuijzen van Zanten, Rouse, Hale, et al., 2015).

## LOW BACK PAIN

Low back pain is a problem frequently associated with disability and absence from work. The spinal column is composed of 24 vertebrae that are stacked vertically, forming natural curves that allow the bony column to function with the resiliency of a spring. The intervertebral disks help with mobility and shock absorption. The health of the bony vertebrae and the cartilaginous disks depends on movement. The cartilage receives its nutrients from cyclical compression and decompression as a function of weight-bearing and non–weight-bearing movement. Similarly, repeated weight-bearing and non–weight-bearing activity stimulates vertebral bone integrity.

Muscles are intimately involved in the support and function of the spinal column. Maintaining the proper curves (anterior and posterior convexities) of lordosis in the cervical and lumbar vertebrae and kyphosis in the thoracic vertebrae is vital for sustaining the spring and shock-absorption qualities of the spine. The lumbar curve is especially influenced by three sets of muscles that are attached to the pelvis and the lumbar vertebrae. By altering the tilt of the pelvis, these muscles can increase (iliopsoas muscle) or decrease (abdominal and hamstring muscles) the lumbar curve. In addition, the deep muscles of the back (paraspinal muscles) work in controlled synergistic and antagonistic fashions to control spinal planes of motion; they are also influential in supporting the spinal curves in posture. Weakness or shortening of any of these muscles can adversely impact posture and increase stress on the back. The result can be back pain from muscle strain, altered joint function (facet joints), and abnormal force on the intervertebral disks.

Low back pain is a multifactorial disorder that is unlikely to be caused by a single factor. Obesity is associated with an increased risk of low back pain, as well as an increased likelihood of seeking care for subacute and chronic low back pain (Shiri, Karppinen, Leino-Arjas, et al., 2010). The risk of low back pain increases as BMI increases: 2.9% when BMI is 20 to 25 kg/m$^2$, 5.2% when BMI is 26 to 30 kg/m$^2$, 7.7% when BMI is 31 to 35 kg/m$^2$, and 11.6% when BMI is 36 kg/m$^2$ or greater (Smuck, Kao, Brar, et al., 2014). Higher levels of muscular and aerobic fitness are also associated with a decreased risk of low back pain (Heneweer, Picaret, Staes, et al., 2012).

Exercise has a positive influence on low back pain. A 2015 meta-analysis concluded that aerobic exercise can reduce pain and improve the physical and psychological functioning of individuals with chronic low back pain (Meng & Yue, 2015). Another study found a positive synergistic effect of a rehabilitation program consisting of 14 exercises and treadmill exercises on the low back extensor strength in individuals with chronic low back pain (Cho, Kim, Jung, et al., 2015). Olaya-Contreras, Styf, Arvidsson, and colleagues (2015) examined the effects of advising a group of people with acute severe low back pain to "stay active in spite of the pain," and they found no difference in pain intensity trajectory and a significantly higher level of physical activity when this group was compared with a group that was instructed to "adjust activity to the pain." Given the acknowledged detriments of bed rest, staying active is good advice for individuals with low back pain.

Chronic back pain can affect many populations, from athletes to aging adults, and exercise appears to be beneficial for all groups with low back pain. Recreational runners often report chronic lower back pain, which can contribute to reduced ability to train and engage in continued running. One study examined the effect of 8 weeks of lower limb exercises compared to lumbar extensor or stabilization exercises (which are more traditionally used to help low back pain) in 84 recreational runners who reported low back pain. Self-rated running capability and knee extension strength improved to a greater extent in the lower limb exercise group (vs. the extensor and stabilization groups). All exercise types improved pain and back muscle function. The authors concluded that for runners with lower back pain, lower limb exercises may be a newer exercise therapy to help reduce low back pain while simultaneously improving running outcomes (Cai, Yang, & Kong, 2017). In ballet dancers, an exercise program that targeted trunk muscles decreased low back pain, which might translate to a decrease in the incidence of injuries (Kovácsné Bobály, Szilagyi, Makai, et al., 2017).

A recent systematic review and meta-analysis examined the impact of various interventions on low back pain in aging adults.

Interestingly, they reported that interventions (including exercise), did not produce a clinically significant reduction of pain or disability due to low back pain. The authors importantly noted that evidence on interventions to manage low back pain in older persons is weak; and suggested that higher quality RCTs are needed in this area in the future (Nascimento et al., 2014). Another study examined the impact of 12 weeks of tai chi or core stabilization exercises on pain and functional disability in older persons with low back pain. Both the core stabilization and the tai chi exercise groups experienced improved pain intensity following the intervention. Overall, exercises improved pain but not lower limb proprioception (as hypothesized) in older persons (Liu et al., 2019). Aquatic therapy may be beneficial in adults with low back pain; indeed, a 4-week aquatic physiotherapy program led to improved disability scores, and core muscle endurance in adults with low back pain (So, Ng, & Au, 2019). A hybrid approach (that is highly individualized), which includes both motor-control and/or psychological approaches to treating low back pain may also be a model to benefit those who are suffering (Hodges, 2019), but research is still needed in this area.

The goal of exercise programs for individuals with low back pain is to prevent debilitation as a result of inactivity and to increase endurance, strength, and flexibility, allowing a return to usual functional activities. Exercise recommendations and progression of activity are highly individualized on the basis of the origin, duration, and severity of pain. A referral to a physiotherapist is warranted in most, if not all, cases of low back pain to allow there to be proper comprehensive management, which may include exercise as well as other safe and effective interventions.

## IMMUNE FUNCTION

Exercise can have both a positive effect and a negative effect on immune function (Gleeson, 2007). Exercise and immune response have a somewhat complex and conflicting relationship in the literature. The relationship between exercise and immune function has a fairly long history of study, and the interest that grew out of the human immunodeficiency virus (HIV) epidemic continues to stimulate investigations in this area. Several studies demonstrate that people with impaired immune function can exercise safely without risk to their health status and can enhance their physiological and psychological well-being with regular exercise (Fillipas, Oldmeadow, Bailey, et al., 2006; Galantino, Shepard, Krafft, et al., 2005; Gomes-Neto, Conceiçao, Carvalho, et al., 2013; Sax, 2006; Terry, Sprinz, Stein, et al., 2006). A systematic review concluded that progressive resistive exercise may increase body weight and limb girth and aerobic exercise may improve adipose levels and lipid profiles by decreasing fat in tissues and blood in individuals with HIV (Fillipas et al., 2010). Another systematic review concluded that resistance exercise may improve body composition by decreasing body fat and increasing muscle strength, aerobic exercise may also improve body composition and increase aerobic capacity, and concurrent training may improve all outcomes evaluated in individuals with HIV (Gomes-Neto et al., 2013).

Furthermore, two recently updated meta-analyses suggest that aerobic exercise, either alone or in conjunction with progressive resistance exercise, can be safely performed by adults with HIV/acquired immunodeficiency syndrome (AIDS) and may increase fitness and improve body composition and well-being (O'Brien, Nixon, Tynan, et al., 2009, 2010). Recommended parameters include exercising at least three times per week for 20 minutes over a period of 5 weeks or more (O'Brien, Nixon, Tynan, et al., 2010).

The effect of exercise on immune system markers (e.g., CD4 levels, CD4/CD8 ratio, or viral load) in people with HIV/AIDS is unclear. Reviews discuss the effects of exercise on immune function in individuals with HIV/AIDS and report conflicting findings (Anderson, 2006; Dudgeon, Phillips, Bopp, et al., 2004). A meta-analysis compared aerobic exercise groups with nonexercising groups and found no significant differences in CD4 count, CD4 percentage, or viral load (Nixon, O'Brien, Glazier, et al., 2005). Similarly, meta-analytic data compared the combination of aerobic and progressive resistance exercise with no exercise and found no significant differences in CD4 count (O'Brien, Nixon, Glazier, et al., 2004). Despite the fact that the CD4 count did not differ between exercising and non-exercising groups, there were significant beneficial changes in depressive symptoms, mean body weight, mean arm and thigh girth, and maximum heart rate for those in the exercising groups (Nixon et al., 2005; O'Brien, Nixon, Glazier, et al., 2004). In another study, Jaggers, Hand, Dudgeon, and colleagues (2015) examined the effects of combined aerobic and resistance training on the psychological well-being of adults with HIV and found significant decreases in depression and mood states (Profile of Mood States) for the exercise group. The control group, the members of which were allowed to engage in sedentary activities, showed a significant increase in the perception of stress (Perceived Stress Scale). Evidence suggests that regular exercisers and athletes are less likely to become ill than sedentary women (Nieman, 1994) and middle-aged men and women (Matthews, Ockene, Freedson, et al., 2002). In direct contrast, evidence also suggests that athletes are also at increased risk of infection during increased periods of training or after competition (Nieman, 1994; Nieman, Johanssen, Lee, et al., 1990; Pedersen & Bruunsgaard, 1995; Peters-Futre, 1997). Another reported finding is that after exercise, sedentary individuals have a higher risk of infection than active individuals (Kiwata, Anouseyan, Desharnais, et al., 2014). A recent review concluded that immune function, both innate and acquired, of athletes under heavy training is often observed to decrease by approximately 15% to 25%, but studies on whether this change increases infection risk remain inconclusive (Walsh, Manor, Hausdorff, et al., 2015).

Classic epidemiological studies indicate that a J-curve relationship may exist between the intensity of exercise and the risk of upper respiratory tract infection (URTI) (Nieman, 1994; Pedersen, Rohde, & Ostrowski, 1998). That is, in theory, moderate exercise may decrease the risk of URTI below that of a sedentary individual, but high-intensity exercise may raise the risk above average. In direct contrast, Lee, Meehan, Robinson, and colleagues (1992) concluded that immune function was not linked to the risk of URTI in a group of cadets during basic training, and Pyne, Baker, Fricker, and colleagues (1995) reported similar rates of URTI between elite swimmers under intense training and age- and gender-matched sedentary controls. Similarly, Gleeson, Bishop, Oliveira, and colleagues (2013) reported that high-exercising (≥11 hrs/wk) and medium-exercising (7–10 hrs/wk) groups had more URTI episodes than the low-exercising (3–6 hrs/wk) group. Factors that confound studies on the relationship between exercise and URTI

include failure to distinguish between new infection and the clinical manifestations of a dormant infection (Gleeson, Pyne, Austin, et al., 2002) and failure to distinguish between airway hyperresponsiveness and URTI (Langdeau & Boulet, 2001). In a recent study in nonelite marathon runners, 17% of participants presented with a lower respiratory tract infection following the marathon race. Changes in salivary immunity were present as well in these individuals, and the findings of this study suggests that salivary immunity might have an important role in the immunity of long-distance runners (Cantó, Roca, Perea, et al., 2018). Another study also supports this idea that salivary immunity can predict the risk upper respiratory tract symptoms in endurance athletes. It was also suggested by these authors that it is a combination of various stressors that may increase infection susceptibility—exercise immune depression post competition, but that also environmental conditions, psychological stress, lack of sleep etc. may all work together to impact immune response in athletes (Keaney, Kilding, Merien, et al., 2018). This phenomenon still needs to be examined in more detail.

Immune system changes that are apparently related to the intensity of exercise have been identified. Moderate-endurance exercise stimulates the neuroendocrine system, which causes changes in the function and numbers of various immune system cells, such as the natural killer, CD4, and CD8 cells. Evidence also indicates that moderate exercise is associated with a prolonged improvement in the killing capacity of neutrophils (one of the most efficient phagocytes). Several immune marker changes suggest increased risk of illness in those who engage in high-intensity exercise, including a low level of salivary immunoglobulin (antibodies), low serum complement levels, low lymphocyte count, depressed natural killer cell activity, low helper and suppressor T cell ratio, and decreased neutrophil phagocytic capacity (Mackinnon, 1992; Nieman, 1994; Pedersen & Ullum, 1994). Most aspects of immunity in male and female athletes are not significantly different (Gleeson, Bishop, Oliveira, et al., 2011).

Changes in immune cell counts and activity may be related to hormonal immunoregulation. Moderate exercise increases the release of immunostimulatory hormones, such as growth hormone and endogenous opiates (β-endorphin and methionine enkephalin). The increase in the levels of β-endorphins with exercise seems to have a positive effect on natural killer cell activity. Conversely, intense exercise is associated with increases in the levels of catecholamine and corticosteroid (cortisol), which have immunosuppressive characteristics (Mackinnon, 1992). High-intensity exercise is also associated with muscle cell damage and inflammation. The immune system is involved in tissue repair. It is theorized that while immune cells are busy with the repair process, host protection may suffer. A window of opportunity for infection during recovery from high-intensity exercise appears to exist. Accordingly, rest is recommended after vigorous exercise to allow the body to recover, and moderate exercise may be the better choice for enhancement of health and well-being. However, recent findings have challenged this early exercise immunity information, suggesting that athletes with high-volume training actually suffer fewer URTI episodes, and URTI incidence decreases around competition time (Walsh & Oliver, 2016). Therefore, the precise effect of exercise on immune function is still conflicting.

If immunity level does decrease in response to high-intensity training, is there a way to protect the athletes from getting sick? This is important, since infection and sickness can impact training, and potentially even performance (Gleeson, 2007). Some studies have investigated the impact of supplementing athletes with antioxidants, and there has been some support of attenuated immune blunting with vitamin C and E use (Gleeson, 2007). Other approaches include carbohydrate ingestion during exercise, as this might reduce cortisol levels and other negative immune responses (Gleeson, 2007). One recent study examined salivary immunity and lower respiratory tract infections in nonelite marathon runners; more specifically, the impact of a standardized polysaccharide-based multi-ingredient supplement on salivary secretory factors before and after a marathon. The authors found that compared to athletes who did not take the supplement ($n = 21$), athletes who took the supplement for 15 days prior to the marathon ($n = 20$) had lower levels of anti-inflammatory chemokines, which overall suggested that there was a positive effect on immune response after strenuous exercise with supplementation (Roca, Canto, Nescolarde, et al., 2019).

Evidence that exercise, while negatively temporarily impacting virus protection, leads to reduced inflammation, may be important with regard to chronic disease prevention. Inflammation has been implicated in many chronic diseases such as CVD and cancer. There is convincing evidence that exercise has a significant protective effect against colon cancer (Martin, 2011). A recent meta-analysis concluded that physical activity may reduce all-cause breast cancer–related deaths and breast cancer events in breast cancer survivors (Lahart, Metsios, Nevill, et al., 2015). Another meta-analysis concluded that physical activity may decrease the risk of prostate cancer, and encouraged men to engage in regular physical activity (Liu, Hu, Li, et al., 2011). A synthesis of clinical practice guidelines, systematic reviews, meta-analyses, and individual studies suggests that exercise may minimize or prevent adverse physiological effects of cancer and its treatment (Ingram & Visovsky, 2007). A position statement on immune function and exercise (Walsh, Gleeson, Shephard, et al., 2011) offered the following conclusion: "There is consensus that exercise training protects against some types of cancers. Training also enhances aspects of anti-tumour immunity and reduces inflammatory mediators. However, the data linking immunological and inflammatory mechanisms, physical activity, and cancer risk reduction remains tentative (p. 39)".

## MENTAL HEALTH

People who exercise regularly generally state that they feel better, have increased self-esteem, and have a more positive outlook on life. Not only do they feel better physically, they also they feel better mentally. The mental health benefits of physical activity as an intervention have been summarized elsewhere, and include promoting mental health and well-being in healthy adults, preventing and treating mental health disorders, and supporting psychosocial rehabilitation (Nyström, Neely, Hassmen, et al., 2015; Wang, Chan, Ho, et al., 2014; Wang, Lee, Wu, et al., 2014). Epidemiological research with both men and women suggests that physical activity may be associated with improvements in positive affect and general sense of well-being (USDHHS, 2015).

Much of the work has focused on depression and stress (Stanton & Reaburn, 2014), anxiety (Stubbs, Vancampfort, Rosenbaum, et al., 2017), and schizophrenia (Firth, Stubbs, Rosenbaum, et al., 2017).

Evidence from a review of the literature (prospective studies, randomized controlled trials, and meta-analyses) found that exercise protects against and is an intervention for mild to major depression (Graven, Brock, Hill, et al., 2011; Nahas & Sheikh, 2011). A large meta-analysis found that exercise has an overall moderate effect on depression (effect size = 0.56) (Wegner, Helmich, Machado, et al., 2014). Exercise is suggested as a first-line treatment for mild/moderate depression, and can be used in combination with medication to alleviate symptoms (Carek, Laibstain, & Carek, 2011). Exercise also alleviates anxiety; in another meta-analysis, exercise decreased anxiety more than control conditions (Stubbs et al., 2017). Exercise can also help alleviate depression in those with chronic disease; exercise reduces depressive symptoms in individuals with arthritis and other rheumatic conditions (Kelley et al., 2015), and in individuals with type 2 diabetes (de Groot et al., 2019).

Investigations have also focused on populations across the life span, including children, young adults, and older persons. Based on a limited number of small trials, a Cochrane Review concluded that, when compared with no intervention, exercise reduces anxiety and depression in children and young adults (Larun, Nordheim, Ekeland, et al., 2009). Research suggests that hippocampal volume (an area of the brain associated with lower depression) may be modified by exercise. A recent study found that in over 4000 children 9 to 11 years of age, sport involvement was positively correlated with hippocampal volume. Hippocampal volume also helped to predict depressive symptoms, and thus may be one mechanism by which exercise helps to alleviate depression in children (Gorham, Jernigan, Hudziak, et al., 2019). Muscle strength, cardiovascular function, and speed are associated with executive function in children who are overweight and obese, suggesting that exercise interventions could benefit this outcome as well in children (Mora-Gonzalez, Esteban-Cornejo, Cadenas-Sanchez, et al., 2019). Another Cochrane Review suggests that long-term exercise, of various types, is most likely to have a beneficial effect on mood in adults; however, the magnitude of the effect is indeterminate at this point (Mead, Morley, Campbell, et al., 2009). Researchers examining major depressive disorder recommended an exercise prescription that is supervised, individually customized, at least 30 minutes, and at least three times per week (Nyström et al., 2015). Yoga has also been shown to be effective in treating depression (Cramer, Lauche, Langhorst, et al., 2013; de Manicor, Bensoussan, Smith, et al., 2016).

In a recent systematic review and meta-analysis of the effect of exercise on cognitive function in older persons, Northey, Cherbuin, Pumpa, and colleagues (2018) found that exercise improved cognitive function in adults over the age of 50 years. They reported that many types of exercise, including aerobic, resistance training, tai chi all benefited cognition. For benefit, the authors suggest that exercise should be at least 45 to 60 minutes in duration, and of moderate intensity to see cognitive benefits (Northey et al., 2018). Exercise may also help to maintain and improve cognitive function in individuals who have chronic disease associated with cognitive decline, such as in end-stage kidney disease (Chu & McAdams-DeMarco, 2019).

Furthermore, the effect of exercise on individuals with various disorders or diseases, such as schizophrenia, cancer, or other chronic diseases has been studied. In a systematic review, Herring, O'Connor, & Dishman (2010) concluded that although exercise in sedentary persons with a chronic illness reduces anxiety, training programs lasting as few as 12 weeks and consisting of sessions of at least 30 minutes resulted in the largest reductions in anxiety. A Cochrane Review of the psychological and physical effects of dance and movement therapy on persons with cancer was unable to arrive at a conclusion because of a dearth of high-quality studies in this area, although there may be a positive effect on quality of life in persons with breast cancer (Bradt, Goodill, & Dileo, 2011). A more recent study found that yoga may improve quality of life, fatigue, and depression in patients with breast cancer, but acknowledged that more research is still needed (McCall, 2018). Exercise had been shown in two meta-analyses to improve health-related quality of life in those scheduled to receive, actively undergoing, or having completed cancer treatment (Mishra, Scherer, Snyder, et al., 2014, 2015). Clinical practice guidelines have been developed with exercise recommendations for people living with cancer that also address safety concerns for this population (Segal, Zwaal, Green, et al., 2017).

Various types and modalities of exercise have been used in studies; an example of one such intervention is tai chi. In a systematic review and meta-analysis of the effect of tai chi on psychological well-being, Wang, Bannru, Ramel, and colleagues (2010) demonstrated an apparent association with reductions in anxiety, depression, mood disturbance, and stress, as well as improvements in self-esteem. Another review examining various populations again supported the benefits of tai chi for treatment of depression, treatment of anxiety, general stress management, and exercise self-efficacy (Wang et al., 2014). In a more recent review that qualitatively assessed tai chi's effect on mental health, it was found that there is poor evidence to support the role of tai chi in improving mental health, even though tai chi has been found to improve mood and anxiety in many studies (Jiang, Kong, & Jiang, 2016). However, tai chi continues to be associated with improved quality of life, including in a recent study of older men (Tajik, Rejeh, Heravi-Karimooi, et al., 2018). Yoga has also been shown to decrease depression and anxiety in a variety of conditions (Pascoe & Bauer, 2015). Yoga may also be of benefit for adolescent mental health; we are currently experiencing an observed increase in mental health challenges in teenagers, and a recent case study suggested that yoga might be a safe and effective intervention for the growing number of adolescents/teens who are experiencing mental health challenges (Stephens, 2019).

## EXERCISE PRESCRIPTION

The literature certainly reflects both the physiological and the psychological benefits that can be experienced with commitment to an active lifestyle. In short, regular physical activity or exercise can help people feel better, perform better, and be healthier. Unfortunately, as discussed, Canadians, and individuals around the world, have failed to embrace the concept and health value of an active lifestyle. Perhaps they are overwhelmed by the misperception that to gain health benefits they must perform vigorous, continual exercise.

People need to be reminded that many of their activities of daily living are actually important and add up; they may also contribute to increased exercise levels. This approach to physical activity serves as a good foundation to a healthy lifestyle. However, when possible, individuals should also be encouraged to include more formal exercise training in their overall activities to promote optimal cardiorespiratory fitness and significantly increase muscle strength and endurance. The amount of exercise required to achieve these goals is determined by the parameters of an exercise prescription:

| **F** (frequency) | Aerobic exercise three to five times a week |
| | Resistance training two to three times a week |
| **I** (intensity) | Moderate to vigorous, by heart rate and perceived exertion |
| | Able to complete each resistance exercise, 8 to 12 repetitions, without strain |
| **T** (time) | 20 to 60 minutes, plus warm-up and cool-down periods |
| | 15 to 30 minutes to complete a series of 8 to 10 resistance exercises |
| **T** (type) | Aerobic (walking, jogging, biking, swimming, rowing, cross-country skiing, elliptical trainer, NordicTrack, StairMaster, aerobics, dancing, skating, or rollerblading) |
| | Resistance training (weight machines, free weights, and calisthenics such as push-ups, sit-ups, or pull-ups) (ACSM, 2013) |

*Exercise is Medicine ® Canada* (EIMC) encourages a healthy lifestyle that incorporates physical activity and exercise into daily routines (EIMC, 2019). The EIMC Professional Network recommends assessment of the Exercise Vital Sign (EVS) with all patients and use of counselling strategies to promote behaviour change. EIMC Recognized exercise professionals have the ability to work with individuals at risk of, or with existing chronic disease who are medically cleared for independent or supervised exercise prescription (CSEP, 2019).

### Aerobic Exercise

The benefits of aerobic exercise are cumulative; therefore a frequency of three to five times a week is recommended. Every other day is a good frame of reference and allows recovery between training sessions, potentially decreasing the chance of overuse injuries. Physical activity guidelines indicate a

## TABLE 22.1 Rating of Perceived Exertion, From the Borg Scale of Perceived Exertion

| Borg Rating | How Exertion Might be Described | Examples (For Most Adults <65 Years Old) |
|---|---|---|
| 6 | None | Reading a book, watching television |
| 7 to 8 | Very, very light | Tying shoes |
| 9 to 10 | Very light | Chores like folding clothes that seem to take little effort |
| 11 to 12 | Fairly light | Walking through the grocery store or other activities that require some effort but not enough to speed up your breathing |
| 13 to 14 | Somewhat hard | Brisk walking or other activities that require moderate effort and speed our heart rate and breathing but don't make you out of breath |
| 15 to 16 | Hard | Bicycling, swimming, or other activities that take vigorous effort and get the heart pounding and make breathing very fast |
| 17 to 18 | Very hard | The highest level of activity you can sustain |
| 19 to 20 | Very, very hard | A finish kick in a race or other burst of activity that you can't maintain for long |

Source: Borg G.A. (1982). Psychophysical bases of perceived exertion. *Medicine and Science in Sports and Exercise, 14,* 377–381. Retrieved from https://www.hsph.harvard.edu/nutritionsource/borg-scale/.

dose-response relationship with exercise; more exercise can confer greater health benefits. However, the benefits of exercising more than five times a week need to be considered, and weighed against the risk of injury, especially with higher-impact activities. When more frequent exercising is a goal, cross-training is recommended. *Cross-training* means performing different types of exercise on different days of the week or performing different types of exercise within one session. The benefits of cross-training include a decreased risk of musculoskeletal injury, an increased potential for total body conditioning, and improved long-term compliance because variety decreases boredom and eliminates the exercise barrier of limited choices.

The intensity of exercise that results in health and fitness benefits ranges from moderate to vigorous and is comfortable, but challenging (brisk). Intensity is defined by the objective measure of heart rate (HR) and the subjective measure of perceived exertion. The increase in HR during exercise has a strong linear relationship with exercise intensity and aerobic capacity. Resting heart rate is the HR measured at rest. Maximum heart rate is the rate measured at the highest workload tolerated during exercise. Maximum heart rate also decreases with age; a generic formula for determining maximum heart rate is 220 minus age. Formulas for determining appropriate exercise HRs have been developed that take resting heart rate and maximum heart rate into consideration.

The Borg scale for rating perceived exertion is a psychophysical category scale for the subjective rating of sensations associated with the intensity of physical work (Borg, 1973, 1982) (Table 22.1). The scale uses ratings based on the individual's overall feeling of exertion and physical fatigue. These ratings correspond well with metabolic responses to exercise, such as HR and oxygen consumption. The strong linear relationship between HR and the rating of perceived exertion (RPE) was originally suggested by Borg and has been verified by subsequent studies. Correlation coefficients from 80 to 90% have been reported consistently with use of a variety of work tasks and exercise conditions (Borg, 1973, 1982; Skinner, Hutsler, Bergsteinova, et al., 1973). A meta-analysis has shown the Borg scale to be a valid measure of exercise intensity with a strong link between RPE and HR (Chen, Fan, & Moe, 2002). In addition, recent studies support use of the Borg scale for various populations, including individuals with stroke (Sage, Middleton, Tang, et al., 2013), obesity (Coquart, Tourny-Chollet, Lemaitre, et al., 2012), and fibromyalgia (Soriano-Maldonado, Ruiz, Alvarez-Gallardo, et al., 2015), and have quantified its ability to predict $Vo_{2max}$ (or $Vo_2$ peak) (Coquart, Garcin, Parfitt, et al., 2014). However, perceptions of exertion and the relationship with HR are influenced by both physiological and psychological factors (aches, cramps, pain, fatigue, shortness of breath, anxiety, depression, and introversion or extroversion). Smutok, Skrinar, & Pandolf (1980) noted that some individuals are more accurate in regulating exercise intensity by RPE than are others and that this variability may be more the result of psychological than physiological factors. Other factors that may alter the strong relationship between HR and RPE are drug-related situations (β-blockers), age, and disease states (Hautala, Kiviniemi, Karjalainen, et al., 2013; Mampuya, 2012).

Despite this potential for variability in perception, RPE correlates well with HR clinically, and together they form a complementary means of helping individuals determine a comfortable, beneficial level of exercise intensity. An RPE of 11 to 14 corresponds well with 50% to 85% of maximum heart rate (see Table 22.1). Subjective parameters include being slightly short of breath, but not out of breath; being able to talk without difficulty, but unable to sing a song easily; being pleasantly fatigued, but not exhausted; and having mild musculoskeletal discomfort, but no pain.

Attention to RPE helps a person develop a sense of body awareness and an appreciation for the body's response to the stress of activity. Awareness of RPE helps people listen to their bodies and become aware of how it feels to move, where they carry tension, and where they have discomfort. With this increased awareness, individuals can choose how they want to respond, adjusting their exercise practice on a daily basis, making the activity more enjoyable, decreasing the risk of injury, and improving long-term exercise adherence.

The recommended duration of aerobic conditioning exercise is generally 20 to 60 minutes. Less than 20 minutes usually provides minimal benefit—this is why the *Canadian Physical Activity Guidelines* note that exercise should be done in bouts of

10 minutes or greater. Increases in cardiorespiratory fitness can also be accrued from intermittent bouts of moderate-to-vigorous exercise (10-minute segments) on a workout day. However, for people who are unaccustomed to exercising or for those who are greatly deconditioned, short durations are permissible, gradually increasing to a beneficial, comfortable level as tolerance and confidence increase. Everyone has to start somewhere, and doing a little is much better than doing nothing at all. The range of acceptable duration allows greater flexibility, giving reassurance of benefit to the individual who varies exercise choices daily on the basis of capability, interests, and life demands.

As mentioned, many different choices for the mode of aerobic exercise are available. A question that is often asked is "What is the best type of aerobic exercise?" The answer is "The one that the individual is willing to do on a regular basis." Different aerobic exercises have different benefits; they all have their advantages and disadvantages. From a cardiovascular point of view, with relative intensity, frequency, and duration being equal, the benefit is about the same for all modes. Probably the best scenario is cross-training, which results in the greatest number of optimal all-around benefits. However, the most important recommendation is that the person starts moving—choosing the person's favourite exercise will increase the likelihood of adhering to an exercise program.

Walking is probably the most accessible and popular form of aerobic exercise. Done briskly, walking provides a good cardiorespiratory challenge in 60 to 80% of the adult population. Walking is also an activity that nearly everyone can do, requires little equipment or cost, can be done almost anywhere, and can be a social or a solitary activity, depending on individual needs. Walking is often the recommended exercise of choice for people who are greatly deconditioned or for those who have physical limitations. Considered a low-impact activity, walking can be easily regulated to accommodate a wide range of fitness levels and motor abilities. Cycling, rowing, and swimming (or water walking or other water aerobics) are non–weight-bearing to low–weight-bearing activities that may be good choices for individuals with physical limitations. Aquatic exercise is a good alternative for individuals with musculoskeletal limitations who need some weight relief with exercise, such as individuals with advanced osteoarthritis. Although the buoyancy of the water provides this weight relief, the water also provides resistance to the limbs as they move, encouraging an increase in intensity and conditioning. Individuals should be encouraged to do the types of aerobic exercise that best fit their needs, interests, and lifestyles while providing reasonable benefits.

## Warm-Up and Cool-Down Periods

In addition to the endurance phase of exercise, warm-up and cool-down periods should be a regular part of the exercise session. The warm-up period usually lasts 5 to 10 minutes and may include light stretching or performance of the chosen aerobic activity at a low intensity. This approach prepares both the musculoskeletal system and the cardiorespiratory system for the transition from rest to exercise by increasing blood flow, respiration, body temperature, and muscle flexibility.

The cool-down period follows the endurance phase and usually lasts 5 to 10 minutes. This phase allows the body to readjust gradually from the demands of exercise back to the baseline. Stretching and slow, rhythmical movement help to increase muscle elasticity, prevent blood pooling and hypotension, and facilitate dissipation of body heat and removal of lactic acid. The result is the prevention of injury, light-headedness, fatigue, and muscle soreness.

Yoga is an excellent example of one form of exercise to use during warm-up and cool-down periods. The word yoga means union or "established in being," which implies a mind-body connection. Simply defined, yoga is mindful stretching. The mind is quiet, and awareness is focused on feeling the body as it moves. Movement into and out of yoga postures (called asanas) provides the necessary stimulation of weight-bearing activity to help keep bones strong, provides the movement to increase joint ROM, and stretches and tones muscles. The sun salute (*surya namaskar*), a series of 12 flexion-extension yoga postures linked together as one fluid movement by the breath rhythm, is a wonderful practice to include in the warm-up and cool-down phases of exercise, providing both physiological and mind-body benefits.

Yoga also helps develop an appreciation for the experience of the basic resting state, a mindfulness of how it feels to be relaxed physically and mentally during the activity. In this form, exercise becomes an inner experience: that is, quiet and settled on the inside, dynamic and lively on the outside. The yoga philosophy encourages an appreciation of body sensations, slow stretching, and maintenance of proper posture, all of which help to prevent injury and promote health. There is a growing body of evidence to support the use of yoga to increase ROM, reduce pain, improve posture, function, mental health, and sleep patterns, reduce disability, and improve quality of life in select populations (Alfonso, Hachul, Kozasa, et al., 2012; Büssing, Osterman, Lüdtke, et al., 2012; Ebnezar, Nagarathna, Yogitha, et al., 2012; Holtzman & Beggs, 2013; Visceglia & Lewis, 2011). Yoga should not only be considered as a useful warm-up and cool-down tool; it has also been linked with improved health and well-being (including quality of life, stress, anxiety, mind-body connection biomarkers, inflammation, immunity, neuromuscular function, and/or reducing blood pressure) in a variety of populations such as those with cancer, Alzheimer's disease, multiple sclerosis, hypertension, HIV, and stroke (Danhauer, Addington, Cohen, et al., 2019; Dunne, Balletto, Donahue, et al., 2019; Green, Huynh, Broussard, et al., 2019; Harris, Austin, Blake, et al., 2019; Wu, Johnson, Acabchuk, et al., 2019).

## Flexibility

Flexibility is a basic component of physical fitness. Although not formally part of the *Canadian Physical Activity Guidelines*, warm-up and cool-down periods provide the opportunity to work on stretching muscles and increasing joint ROM. A safe stretch is one that is gentle and relaxing; a little discomfort may be felt as the muscle stretches, but the discomfort should never reach the point of pain. Stretching mindfully, as in yoga, will ensure a safe stretch. Holding the position for 10 to 20 seconds and repeating the stretch three to five times will encourage optimal flexibility (ACSM, 2013).

## Resistance Training

Studies suggest that people who maintain or increase their flexibility and strength are better able to perform daily activities and avoid injury and disability (Pate, Pratt, Blair, et al., 1995). Resistance training increases muscle strength and endurance, increases muscle mass, increases metabolic efficiency, maintains or increases bone quantity and quality, prevents limitations in performance of everyday tasks, decreases the effort required to perform these tasks, and decreases the potential for injury during physical activity.

On average, after their early 20s people lose approximately half a pound of muscle every year through lack of use. This reduction in muscle mass is largely responsible for a decrease in resting metabolic rate, which may translate into weight gain. Resistance training is recommended for the general population because it has a positive effect on many of the degenerative problems associated with the aging process.

Every individual should try to perform activities throughout the day that stimulate muscle strength and endurance. Activities that involve lifting, carrying, or performing repetitive movement against a resistance (vacuuming, raking, or shoveling) help preserve lean body mass. If these types of activities are not performed on a regular basis, then the guidelines for resistance training provided in Box 22.3 are suggested. These guidelines are not meant to represent workouts performed by bodybuilders and competitive weight lifters; they are not meant to result in significant muscular hypertrophy. The purpose of weight training from a health perspective is to develop healthy muscles that provide the strength to do daily activities without risk of injury and to stimulate bone health.

The figures in Box 22.3 demonstrate several suggested resistance exercises for upper body strengthening. Resistance training for all major muscle groups is appropriate, but individuals often choose to concentrate on the upper body because these muscles tend to be neglected in daily activity and other exercise regimens. The ACSM (2013) recommends the incorporation of bilateral and unilateral, and single- and multijoint exercises, including total body exercises. Although many people believe that they need to do three sets of each exercise, excellent results can be attained by doing one set (Hass, Garzarella, de Hoyos, et al., 2000). A meta-analysis of the effect of single versus multiple sets on muscle hypertrophy showed multiple sets yielded a 40% greater increase in muscle hypertrophy (Krieger, 2010). The ACSM recommends three to five sets of 8 to 12 repetitions (ACSM, 2013). The weight that is lifted should result in near muscle fatigue at the end of each set (this differs substantially depending on the muscle being trained, the amount of resistance, and the fitness level of the individual) and should be performed without strain and while maintaining proper form. Once 12 to 15 repetitions can be completed without fatigue, the resistance can be increased (by 5% or less), or the same weight can be used to do an additional set to fatigue. The movements should be performed slowly, preferably coordinated with the breath. Rest intervals differ substantially in the literature; however, a review suggested that 3 to 5 minutes allows hypertrophy and power development and 1 to 3 minutes allows endurance gains (de Salles, Simao, Miranda, et al., 2009). The ACSM suggests 1 to 3 minutes of rest between sets to develop endurance and 3 to 5 minutes to develop strength and power. Slow, controlled movements result in greater benefits, lower risk of injury,

and more appreciation of how the body feels as its muscles are challenged. The recommended frequency, as per the CSEP guidelines, for adults is at least 2 days per week. The exercise variables that constitute the exercise prescription must always be chosen to meet the specific needs and limitations of each individual.

## EXERCISE AND RELAXATION RESPONSE

Exercise should not be considered merely a physical regimen with objective outcomes (calories burned and repetitions completed). Exercise is also a process of challenging the body and the mind to gain a sense of well-being and a feeling of accomplishment, an opportunity to learn about who we really are.

Most people understand the physical benefits of exercise, and some people enjoy the challenge of being physically active, but few realize the learning potential inherent in physical activity. Success in embracing a physically active lifestyle may involve a change in focus from the mechanics of exercise to an appreciation for how it feels and what it means to move. Physical activity can be time spent in meditation that fuels both the body and the spirit.

The relaxation response (RR) is an inborn set of physiological changes that offset those of the fight-or-flight (stress) response. When elicited, the RR results in a "letting go" of physical, emotional, and mental tension. It is a physiological response inborn in everyone and, although it can sometimes occur without the individual being aware of it, people generally need to develop techniques that help them let go on a more regular basis. Some techniques that are used commonly to elicit the RR include diaphragmatic breathing, meditation, imagery, mindfulness, yoga stretching, and repetitive exercise.

The RR can be combined with exercise to facilitate the release of tension and improve self-awareness and the feeling of well-being. However, a shift in attitude about exercise is also involved, with the focus becoming the process and awareness of movement. Successful elicitation of the RR involves two basic components: a repetitive focus (the breath, a mantra, and the cadence or rhythm of physical activity) and a nonjudgmental attitude (about everyday thoughts and the quality of performance) (Benson & Stuart, 1992). Berger and Owen (1988) have developed exercise characteristics that facilitate stress reduction and support an exercise environment that allows the successful elicitation of the RR. Activities must:

- Be pleasant and enjoyable.
- Be noncompetitive (competition implies judgement about the self and others).
- Be predictable (elicitation of the RR involves a shift in awareness from the external to the internal environment that will happen only with a sense of safety and reliability).
- Be repetitive and rhythmical (the cadence of activity provides a focus for awareness).
- Facilitate abdominal breathing (watching the breath serves to anchor thoughts in the moment; in combination with cadence, it provides a focused awareness).
- Continue for 20 to 30 minutes at a comfortable intensity on most days of the week (continuity restores a sense of serenity).

All forms of exercise can be used to gain this experience. As discussed, yoga involves mindful stretching with a breathing focus, providing an environment for successful elicitation of the RR. Tai chi is another exercise practice with relaxation potential. Known as moving meditation, tai chi combines movement with focused awareness, involving a physical and cognitive focus for moving in choreographed forms that become a meditation.

The quality of body awareness can also be brought into a more traditional exercise practice. Aerobic exercise lends itself well to the elicitation of the RR, because it has rhythmical and repetitive form and because it facilitates abdominal breathing. The practitioner can focus on the breath rhythm, the step cadence of walking or jogging, the pedaling cadence of bicycling, or the stroke cadence of swimming. Mantras can be used to create a positive mindset and to focus the mind in the present moment as the experience unfolds. Resistance training takes on new meaning when coordinated with the breath. Focusing on the muscles and how it feels to move through the ROM enhances the knowledge of what feels good and what does not, providing feedback on accepting physical challenge.

Exercise focus can and should vary on a daily basis depending on need, mood, and intent. Some days it feels right to focus on the more physical aspects of the activity, appreciating the challenge of working harder or longer. Other exercise sessions may be more contemplative, letting creativity run, working through the tension of a lingering stressor, quieting the mind for relaxation, listening to music, or appreciating nature. Focusing on the process rather than the outcomes brings meaning and purpose to the activity and helps achieve something more valuable than mere physical outcomes.

When exercise integrates mind and body, it stops being something that has to be done and instead becomes something desired. Being mindful during physical activity and exercising in the moment increase awareness. With awareness comes choices in the possibilities of self-care. Exercise for fitness of the spirit, walk for the soul, and just let the body do the work. There is a growing body of evidence to support the use of tai chi to improve balance in confidence, decrease pain, improve cognitive function, mental health, and functional mobility, decrease disability, increase self-efficacy and quality of life, and reduce fall risk in select populations (Hall, Maher, Lam, et al., 2011; Huang, Yang, & Liu, 2011; Leung, Chan, Tsang, et al., 2011; Rand, Miller, Yiu, et al., 2011; Wayne, Walsh, Taylor-Piliae, et al., 2014).

## SPECIAL CONSIDERATIONS

Many adults do not need to consult a physician before starting a moderate-intensity physical activity program. However, older individuals who plan a vigorous program (intensity more than 60% of maximum heart rate or $Vo_{2max}$), those who have never been active or have not been active for a long time, or those who have either chronic disease or risk factors for chronic disease should consult an appropriate health care provider before starting exercise.

The use of prescreening tools for participation in exercise may be appropriate for assessing someone's readiness for exercise participation. For example, the Physical Activity Readiness Questionnaire (PAR-Q) and the Physical Activity Readiness Medical Evaluation (PARmed-X) are two internationally used screening tools that were developed and based on experts' opinion in the field. The PAR-Q/

PARmed-X are surveys to assess your readiness to engage in an exercise program and to help you determine if you should consult with a medical professional prior to physical activity participation. Use of an approved preparticipation tool is a requirement for CSEP-qualified exercise professionals (CSEP, 2019).

In 2011, CSEP supported an evidence-informed consensus process (with funding from the Public Health Agency of Canada) to revise the document to improve and address some limitations of the PAR-Q and PARmed-X. They conducted a systematic review process and found that the benefits of physical activity participation outweighed the risks in the majority of asymptomatic and symptomatic individuals. A new risk continuum and decision tree process was created (Warburton, Jamnik, Bredin, et al., 2011). The PAR-Q+ and ePARmed-X+ (http://eparmedx.com/) are currently available for use. For example, the PAR-Q+ asks questions about ones blood pressure, chest pain during activity, dizziness or loss of consciousness symptoms, diagnosis with medical conditions, medication use, bone or joint problems, if you have ever been told by a doctor you should engage in medically supervised physical activity (PAR-Q+ Collaboration, 2018). Using the answers to the survey, it determines if you are able to begin an exercise program on your own, or if you need to seek medical evaluation or assistance from exercise professionals first. The PAR-Q+/ PARmed-X+ is free, and easily accessible (PAR-Q+ Collaboration, 2018).

Despite the PAR-Q+/PARmed-X+ questionnaire improvements, more recently (in 2017), CSEP commissioned a panel of experts to address remaining barriers associated with screening tools. One of the most predominant issues associated with existing tools was the high rate of false-positive tests; in other words, test results that indicated individuals should seek medical advice prior to exercise participation when this was not necessary. This is problematic because it might discourage people from getting physically active if they have to take another step (seeking medical clearance) before they can engage in exercise. Therefore, they created a new tool that is currently endorsed by CSEP, the *Get Active Questionnaire* (CSEP, 2017). Similar to the questionnaires previously described, the *Get Active Questionnaire* helps someone determine if they should seek advice from health care or exercise professionals before becoming physically active (CSEP, 2017) (Box 22.5), with the idea that this updated questionnaire is more inclusive and permissive for participation.

It should be noted that while the Get Active Questionnaire is the current CSEP-endorsed prescreening tool, a recent paper found that in older persons (~75 years old), when compared to an actual exercise stress test, the Get Active Questionnaire did a good job of screening in individuals (i.e., saying that they were able to participate in exercise), but was not as precise when needing to screen out individuals (i.e., saying that they needed to seek medical advice prior to participation). Thus the *Get Active Questionnaire* may not appropriately tell older individuals if they should be seeking exercise clearance (Petrella, Gill, & Petrella, 2018). This area still needs more research. As well, it is important to note that prescreening questionnaires, while valid and useful in most populations, cannot catch every physiological problem prior to exercise, such as in the case with sudden cardiac death (Quality and Safety Scenario).

## BOX 22.5  Symptoms and Signs Suggestive of Cardiopulmonary Disease

- Pain, discomfort (or other anginal equivalent) in the chest, neck, jaw, arm, or other areas that may be ischaemic in nature
- Shortness of breath at rest or with mild exertion
- Dizziness or syncope
- Orthopnea or paroxysmal nocturnal dyspnea
- Ankle edema
- Palpitations or tachycardia
- Intermittent claudication
- Known heart murmur
- Unusual fatigue or shortness of breath with usual activities

These symptoms must be interpreted in the clinical context in which they appear because they are not all specific to cardiopulmonary or metabolic disease. The *Get Active Questionnaire* helps screen for the presence of some of these symptoms prior to engaging in a physical activity program.

Source: Johri, A.M., Poirier, P., Dorian, P., et al. (2019). Society position statement. Canadian Cardiovascular Society/Canadian Heart Rhythm Society joint position statement on the cardiovascular screening of competitive athletes. *Canadian Journal of Cardiology, 35*(1), 1–11. https://doi.org/10.1016/j.cjca.2018.10.016.

## ⚡ QUALITY AND SAFETY SCENARIO

### Sudden Cardiac Death—Canadian Position

Sudden cardiac death (SCD) is a tragic situation and is a rare outcome in young, seemingly healthy athletes. Cases of SCD are often published in the news; they receive a lot of public attention and there is a strong reaction from the communities the individual is from. SCD is often unexpected, and in young athletes has often been associated with a pre-existing (but unknown) congenital cardiac condition. So what can we do? Should all young competitive athletes, who train a lot, be getting tested to rule out any cardiac abnormality?

The Canadian Cardiovascular Society and the Canadian Hearth Rhythm Society issued a joint position statement on the cardiovascular screening of competitive athletes. Specifically, they addressed whether or not routine electrocardiogram (ECG) was something that should be performed in athletes. The position stand recommended the following:

- That the cardiac screening of athletes in Canada be composed of a tiered approach to identify cardiac risk, emphasizing the limitations of screening tools such as ECG.
- That 12-lead ECG should not be used for mass screening of competitive athletes
- Rather, screening should be more of a systematic approach that includes assessments, appropriate investigations, interpretation of findings, and management of these findings. As well, counselling and follow-up should be included.

This holistic approach includes treating and creating policy and procedures for the management of these types of incidents in sport. It is a more comprehensive approach, with an end goal of keeping athletes safe and healthy.

Prescribing exercise programs to individuals with chronic disease requires additional considerations. For example, people with CHD or diabetes have special exercise needs. Earlier in this chapter the ways in which exercise and physical activity positively affect primary and secondary prevention in both disease processes were discussed. Limitations in the ability to exercise are related to the severity of the disease and the signs and symptoms of intolerance. For people with CHD and diabetes mellitus, safety

with starting a new exercise program requires supervision and guidance from knowledgeable health care providers and exercise professionals. Before starting the program, these individuals should have a medical evaluation, including an exercise tolerance test, to determine functional capacity and the severity of disease.

## Coronary Heart Disease

Exercise plays a strong role in rehabilitation after a cardiac event such as myocardial infarction (MI), coronary artery bypass surgery, percutaneous transluminal coronary angioplasty or stent placement, and angina. Symptoms suggestive of cardiopulmonary disease are presented in Box 22.5 (earlier). Increased physical activity appears to benefit individuals from all these groups. The benefits include the following (Cornelissen, Fagard, Coeckelberghs, et al., 2011; Heran, Chen, Ebrahim, et al., 2011; Lavie & Milani, 2011; Menezes, Lavie, Milani, et al., 2012; Milani, Lavie, Mehra, et al., 2011; Oerkild, Frederiksen, Hansen, et al., 2011):

- Reduction in blood pressure (systolic and diastolic)
- Reduction in total and cardiovascular mortality
- Reduction in hospital admissions
- Reduction of symptoms
- Reduction in obesity
- Increase in exercise tolerance and functional capacity
- Increase in the confidence and ability to carry out usual activities of daily living
- Improvement in psychological well-being and quality of life

Despite the numerous benefits noted previously, cardiac rehabilitation and exercise training is underused by older persons (Menezes et al., 2012).

Generally, people with CHD demonstrate a reduction in $Vo_{2max}$ and the ability to do submaximal levels of work. With exercise training, the increase in $Vo_{2max}$ in persons with CHD averages approximately 20% after 3 months. This improvement in conditioning is the result of both central (cardiac) and peripheral (muscular) changes (ACSM, 2009b). Some of the most significant increases in exercise tolerance have been noted in individuals with angina. With a decrease in submaximal HR or a decrease in systolic blood pressure resulting from conditioning, myocardial oxygen demand is decreased and individuals are able to do a greater amount of work before reaching the anginal threshold. This boost is reflected in an observed increase in the heart rate–pressure product (RPP: HR × SBP) at the anginal threshold (ACSM/AHA, 2007). An increase in functional capacity allows progression of exercise tolerance and progression with daily activities and leisure or vocational activities.

Appropriately prescribed and conducted exercise training programs increase exercise tolerance and physical fitness in individuals with CHD. Moderate and vigorous regimens are of value, but care must be taken to determine safe exercise parameters for each individual. The parameters of the exercise prescriptions are the same as those for the general population, including frequency, intensity, duration, and mode of exercise.

Aerobic exercise increases cardiorespiratory fitness and functional capacity. Any of the aforementioned aerobic exercises are acceptable for this population, depending on the level of fitness and musculoskeletal limitations. Traditionally, resistance training was not commonly recommended for individuals with CHD.

The belief was that lifting weights resulted in a disproportionate rise in blood pressure, increased the myocardial oxygen demand, and increased the risk of angina and MI. However, data from several studies indicate that moderate, supervised weight training is feasible, tolerable, and beneficial for individuals with hypertension and CHD. Strength training can keep the heart healthy by helping to control body weight, reduce cholesterol levels, and regulate blood glucose levels. Guidelines for determination of appropriate individual training include an aerobic capacity of at least four to five metabolic equivalents, an ejection fraction of greater than 30%, and the absence of severe, symptomatic aortic stenosis. However, clinical experience demonstrates that people with severe disease can use small hand weights to increase muscle tone without risk of cardiovascular compromise.

The exercise intensity for persons who have had a cardiac event but who have not had a symptom-limited exercise tolerance test should be kept at a low level based on an elevated heart rate of 20 to 30 beats per minute above the resting heart rate and an RPE of less than 12. After an exercise tolerance test has been performed, intensity should then be prescribed on the basis of 50 to 85% of maximum heart rate and an RPE of 11 to 14, or below the ischaemic, anginal, or arrhythmic threshold. The duration and frequency recommendations are similar to those for the general population. People who are the most deconditioned may need to exercise at lower intensities, for short durations, and more frequently throughout the day. Generally, a reasonable goal is three to five times per week for 20 to 40 minutes, plus 5 to 10 minutes for each warm-up and cool-down period (ACSM/AHA, 2007). The Canadian Cardiovascular Society provides a link of a variety of guidelines and position statements related to cardiovascular disease; and embedded in some of these are exercise recommendations (http://www.ccs.ca/index.php/en/guidelines/guidelines-library.).

## Diabetes

Exercise has long been regarded as part of the triad in the management of diabetes in conjunction with diet and medication (insulin or oral medication). In the early 1900s it was determined that exercise lowers the blood glucose concentration of people with diabetes. After the introduction of insulin, studies revealed that exercise can potentiate the hypoglycemic effect of injected insulin. More recently, findings suggest that in individuals who have poor control (i.e., excessive blood glucose levels), exercise may induce a further increase in blood glucose levels, resulting in ketosis. On average, people with diabetes have a lower maximum heart rate, achieve a lower cardiac output at maximal exercise, and have a higher blood pressure during exercise, resulting in lower maximal oxygen consumption. However, these individuals can increase their exercise capacity with training and can experience the benefits related to overall fitness and cardiorespiratory training similar to the benefits gained by people without diabetes.

Apparently, both benefits and risks from exercise exist for people with diabetes. The overall goals regarding physical activity should be to teach individuals to incorporate activity into their daily life, pursue an exercise program if they wish, and develop strategies to avoid the complications of exercise. A combined approach to improving health and well-being, including nutrition, is an ideal intervention in those with type 2 diabetes. The largest randomized control trial to date that evaluated a physical activity and dietary intervention was The Look AHEAD (Action for Health in Diabetes) trial. This trial of older persons with type 2 diabetes had an intense lifestyle intervention group that needed to obtain at least 175 min/week of exercise, and a control group that received standard of care. Compared to controls, the intense lifestyle intervention group reported a greater weight loss, better glycemic control, improved cardiorespiratory fitness, improved blood pressure better lipid profile, among many other findings (Look, Wing, Bolin, et al., 2013).

In 2018, Diabetes Canada (via the Diabetes Canada Clinical Practice Guidelines Expert Committee) published exercise guidelines for those with diabetes (Sigal, Armstrong, Bacon, et al., 2018). They reported that most individuals with diabetes who do not have coronary problems are able to begin an exercise program without medical clearance before starting a low- or moderate-intensity exercise program. If individuals are planning to begin a high-intensity program, they should speak with a medical professional before beginning. An important consideration that was outlined was that specific side-effects associated with diabetes need to be assessed before an exercise program begins. For example, retinopathy should be treated and should be stable before an exercise program is undertaken. Those who have peripheral neuropathy need to keep an eye on their feet, and wear appropriate footwear when exercising. The guidelines indicate that those who have peripheral neuropathy can safely engage in exercise as long as they do not have active foot ulcers. Those who have cardiac involvement, or angina, shortness of breath, etc. should have an ECG (rest) and an ECG exercise stress test performed before beginning exercise (Sigal et al., 2018). Other special considerations include that those with diabetes have an increased risk of heat-related injury. Due to the reduced ability to properly dissipate heat, individuals who are exercising should make note of their heat-related symptoms and should avoid exercising in excessive heat conditions (like outside in the sun on a hot summer day; or participating in hot yoga). It is also important to maintain hydration with exercise (Sigal et al., 2018).

People with type 2 diabetes should monitor their blood glucose levels and determine their responses to exercise. Although the same exercise benefits can be achieved by people with type 1 diabetes, the inherent behaviour and function of endogenous insulin makes exercising a more difficult proposition for these individuals (see Genomics box). The major functions of insulin are to promote glucose uptake into the cells and to control metabolic homeostasis during exercise, working in synergy with the counterregulatory hormones. With exercise, insulin secretion decreases slightly and the concentrations of counterregulatory hormones increase. This increase stimulates hepatic glucose production, which balances the increased use of glucose by the working muscles, maintaining normoglycemia. However, with injected insulin the plasma insulin concentration does not decrease with exercise, hepatic glucose is not produced as quickly as it is used, and a decrease in blood glucose concentration results. In contrast, people who have poorly controlled diabetes with decreased plasma insulin concentrations already have elevated blood glucose levels because there is insufficient insulin to assist glucose transport into cells. During exercise the liver is stimulated to produce more glucose, which causes a further elevation in blood glucose levels, worsening the hyperglycemic condition. Ketosis may also result from increased mobilization and incomplete combustion of free fatty acids in muscle cells and accelerated ketone body formation in the liver (Federici & Benedetti, 2006).

Individuals with diabetes who take insulin can help reduce exercise-associated hypoglycemia by reducing basal insulin by 20% for the days when they are engaging in exercise. Intermittent exercise (with rest), or engaging in resistance training before aerobic exercise might also be strategies to reduce the likelihood of exercise induced hypoglycemia. Timing of exercise might also be important, since exercise performed in the evening could increase the chance of overnight hypoglycemia.

### BOX 22.6  How to Reduce the Risk of Hypoglycemia in Type 1 Diabetes

Consider use of the following strategies, either alone or in combination:
- Reduce the bolus dose of the insulin that is most active at the time of exercise.
- Significantly reduce, or suspend (only if the activity is ≤45 minutes), basal insulin for the exercise duration, and lower the basal rate overnight after exercise by ~20%.
- Increase carbohydrate consumption prior to, during, and after exercise, as necessary.
- Perform brief (10 seconds), maximal-intensity sprints at the start of exercise, periodically during the activity, or at the end of exercise.
- Perform resistance exercise before aerobic exercise.

Source: Sigal, R.J., Armstrong, M.J., Bacon, S.L., Boulé, N.G., Dasgupta, K., Kenney, G.P., & Riddell, M.C. (2018). Physical activity and diabetes. *Canadian Journal of Diabetes, 42*(Suppl 1), S59–60.

Changing exercise time or altering insulin injections at bedtime might be ways to manage this (Sigal et al., 2018).

Although each person with diabetes should be evaluated and given individual exercise recommendations, the *2018 Clinical Practice Guidelines* from Diabetes Canada offer the following key messages for people with diabetes:
- Physical activity often improves glucose control and facilitates weight loss, but has multiple other health benefits even if weight and glucose control do not change.
- It is best to avoid prolonged sitting. Try to interrupt sitting time by getting up briefly every 20 to 30 minutes.
- Try to get at least 150 minutes per week of aerobic exercise (like walking, bicycling, or jogging).
- Using a step monitor (pedometer or accelerometer) can be helpful in tracking your activity.
- In addition to aerobic exercise, try to do at least two sessions per week of strength training (like exercises with weights or weight machines).
- If you decide to begin strength training, you should ideally get some instruction from a qualified exercise specialist.
- If you cannot reach these recommended levels of activity, doing smaller amounts of activity still has some health benefits. (Sigal et al., 2018)

Innovative Practice presents exercise prescription examples from Diabetes Canada. Box 22.6 describes how to reduce risk of hypoglycemia in type 1 diabetes. The Genomics box presents findings from a meta-analysis that examines the association between genetics and the odds/risk of type 2 diabetes.

## INNOVATIVE PRACTICE

### Exercise Prescription Examples From Diabetes Canada

**Aerobic Exercise**
- Start by walking at a comfortable pace for as little as 5 to 15 minutes at one time.
- Gradually progress over 12 weeks to up to 50 minutes per session (including warm-up and cool down) of brisk walking.
- Alternatively, shorter exercise sessions in the course of a day, for example, 10 minutes three times a day after meals, can replace a single longer session of equivalent length and intensity.

**Resistance Exercise**
- Choose approximately six to eight exercises that target the major muscle groups in the body.
- Gradually increase the resistance until you can perform three sets of 8 to 12 repetitions for each exercise, with 1 to 2 minutes of rest between sets.
- The best evidence supports strength training with weight machines or free weights. Resistance bands may not be as effective to improve glycemic control, but they can help increase strength and can be a starting point to progress to other forms of resistance training.
- If you wish to begin resistance exercise, you should receive initial instruction and periodic supervision by a qualified exercise specialist to maximize benefits, while minimizing risk of injury, at least for the initial sessions.

**Interval Exercise**
- Exercise performed in intervals, alternating between higher intensity and lower intensity, can be used by participants who have trouble sustaining continuous aerobic exercise, or can be used to shorten total exercise duration or

increase variety. Try alternating between 3 minutes of faster walking and 3 minutes of slower walking.
- Another form of interval training, high-intensity interval training (HIIT), can be performed through shorter intervals of higher-intensity exercise (e.g., 30 seconds to 1 minute at near maximal intensity alternating with 1–3 minutes of lower-intensity activity), and can be performed with walking/running or other modalities, such as stationary cycling.
- Start with just a few intervals and progress to longer durations by adding additional intervals.

**Other Types of Exercise**
- Aquatic exercise can have similar benefits as other forms of exercise and help minimize barriers from conditions, such as osteoarthritis. Aquatic exercise can include walking briskly in the water, swimming or classes that include a variety of exercises.
- Other types of exercise or exercise classes, such as yoga, may be appealing for reasons, such as stress management.

**Using Pedometers or Accelerometers**
- Encourage people with diabetes to self-monitor physical activity with a pedometer or accelerometer. Ask them to record values, review at visits, set step count targets and formalize recommendations with a written prescription

**Breaking up Sedentary Time**
- It is best to avoid prolonged sitting. Try to interrupt sitting time by getting up briefly every 20 to 30 minutes.

Source: Sigal, R.J., Armstrong, M.J., Bacon, S.L., et al. (2018). Physical activity and diabetes. *Canadian Journal of Diabetes, 42*(Suppl 1), S58–59.

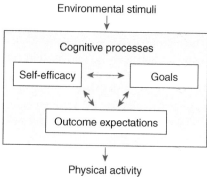

**Fig. 22.4** Three interacting cognitive processes of Bandura's social-cognitive theory. (Modified from Dzewaltowski, D. A. [1995]. Physical activity determinants: A social-cognitive approach. *Medicine and Science in Sports and Exercise, 26,* 1395–1399.)

## BUILDING A RHYTHM OF PHYSICAL ACTIVITY

We know from our discussion earlier that although exercise and physical activity are clearly beneficial for health and well-being, there is a great disconnect and many people are not achieving the recommended physical activity guidelines.

### Adherence and Compliance

Physiological, behavioural, and psychological variables all influence the decision to adhere to diabetes treatment, including physical activity and medications. Each person is unique, and success with exercise over the long term comes from recognition of personal motivation or core desire and support from the social environment. Core desire defines the purpose behind putting the effort into developing and maintaining an active lifestyle; it is what motivates the individual to exercise. Consider the Ottawa Charter for Health Promotion, which supports the process of enabling individuals to not only improve, but also control, their health and well-being (Dugani, Bhutta, & Kisson, 2017; WHO, 1986). An individual needs to be empowered to be able to make appropriate choices for their health, and having support systems in place can help this to occur. As outlined in the Ottawa Charter, this includes building public policy, supporting creative environments, strengthening community action, and reorienting health care services towards disease prevention (Dugani et al., 2017; WHO, 1986). At the level of the individual, people need to be able to access affordable means to be able to increase the physical activity appropriately—if someone is empowered and decides they desire to be active, they need the support in place to effectively do so. This remains an issue that we currently battle with; ensuring equitable access to proper physical activity training and resources for all.

Finding meaning and purpose in an active lifestyle can enhance behaviour. Biopsychosocial and spiritual variables need to be considered in promoting physical activity. An individual's biopsychosocial factors and spiritual beliefs affect the behavioural and attitudinal factors that influence the motivation

and ability to adhere to an active lifestyle. Generally, however, physical activity is more likely to be initiated and maintained if the individual (Pentecost & Taket, 2011):

- Perceives a net benefit
- Chooses an enjoyable activity
- Feels competent doing the activity
- Feels confident in overcoming barriers that may interfere with the activity
- Feels safe doing the activity
- Can access the activity easily on a regular basis
- Perceives no significant negative financial or social cost
- Experiences minimal musculoskeletal discomfort
- Is able to address competing time demands
- Is readily able to fit the activity into the daily schedule
- Balances the use of labor-saving devices with activities that involve physical exertion

In addition, measures to increase satisfaction and increase adherence to medication use have been explored and include (García-Pérez, Alvarez, Dilla, et al., 2013):

- Complexity of dosing regimens: reducing the complexity of therapy by fixed-dose combination pills and less frequent dosing regimens
- Safety and tolerability: using medications that are associated with fewer adverse events (e.g., hypoglycemia or weight gain)
- Perceptions of medication: educational initiatives
- Care recipient-provider interaction: improved care recipient–health care provider communication
- Economic considerations: social support to help reduce costs

Educating the public about physical activity helps to provide guidelines for safe and effective exercise, to reinforce potential benefits, and to alleviate misperceptions that may interfere with the decision to change behaviour. However, knowledge of exercise and the intent to exercise do not correlate well with an individual's uptake of physical activity behaviour. Confidence in the ability to be physically active—and the confidence that overcoming barriers produces positive benefits that are related to personal goals (self-efficacy)—is strongly related to participation (Fig. 22.4). Exercise self-efficacy is increased when people perform exercise successfully, receive positive feedback about success, view exercise role models, and learn more about the relationships among exercise, health, and body awareness (see the Case Study and Care Plan at the end of this chapter).

## Creating a Climate That Supports Exercise

Clearly exercise and fitness need to be social norms. A climate that supports and encourages physical activity should be fostered. Other people and organizations in the individual's social environment can influence the adoption and maintenance of physical activity.

### Health Care Providers

People are more likely to increase their physical activity if counseled to do so by clinicians or other health care providers, such as nurses (Bakhshi, Sun, & Murrells, 2015). Primary health care workers who interact with patients on a daily basis have an integral role in managing the burden of obesity and associated secondary diseases by counselling patients towards healthier living. They can inquire about exercise habits, communicate the benefits of increased activity, assist the person in initiating activity, and provide adequate follow-up. Challenging perceived individual barriers to exercise and offering alternative viewpoints can help create new exercise paradigms (Lascar, Kennedy, Hancock, et al., 2014; Leone & Ward, 2013; Veldhuijzen van Zanten et al., 2015). Teixeira, Carraça, Markland, and colleagues (2012) published an informative systematic review that summarizes the evidence for self-determination theory, which can be used to improve our understanding of exercise motivation and the importance of autonomous regulations in promoting physical activity. Health care providers also serve as role models by demonstrating enthusiasm for and the health benefits of being physically active.

However, we do still face challenges regarding health care provider-based exercise prescription. Let's use nursing as an example. Unfortunately, despite nurses' important role as health advocates for their patients, research suggests that individuals in the nursing profession have a high level of obesity. One study reported that almost 55% of ~5000 nurses surveyed were overweight or obese (Miller, Alpert, & Cross, 2008). Although nurses acknowledge that obesity is an important health concern that requires immediate attention and action, over three-quarters of nurses do not pursue this topic with their overweight and obese patients (Miller et al., 2008). In 2018, Reed, Prince, Pipe, and colleagues provided the first objective measure of exercise in a cohort of Canadian nurses ($n = 410$), and reported that only 23% of nurses met Canadian exercise guidelines of 150 minutes of moderate/vigorous physical activity per week. Furthermore, nurses who worked longer shifts, rotating shifts, or were casually employed participated in less exercise. Additionally, nurses reported having negative perceptions of obesity and had poor professional attitudes towards these individuals (Brown, 2006; Poon & Tarrant, 2009). There is a large disconnect between the problem of obesity, exercise counselling, and nursing practise, and this disconnect is not only present among nurses; health care practitioners, in general, are unsure of how to prescribe exercise to their patients.

One recent study by Brannan, Bernardotto, Clarke, and colleagues (2019) attempted to narrow this knowledge gap regarding exercise prescription in health care practitioners. The Moving Healthcare Professional Project (MHPP) was developed as an overarching model capturing all stages of medical education at all levels (undergraduate to continuing medical education), and embedding prevention and physical activity promotion into clinical practice. This study looked at the early implementation of the MHPP in the England and its ongoing development. There are multiple phases of this project, but an overall important takeaway is that through their model, they have trained just over 17,000 GP trainees, other doctors, nurses, and other health care practitioners (Brannan et al., 2019). Evaluation of the model is still underway; however, it might be that full-system knowledge-based interventions like this are needed in order to inform and train our health care providers about the importance of physical activity for themselves, and for their patients.

### Family and Friends

Social support can be a valuable resource for behavioural change. Significant others or friends can serve as buddies, providing a source of companionship and motivation. These people can offer to share daily responsibilities to make time for exercise (e.g., provide child care). Parents can support their children's activity by having family outings and providing transportation, praise, and encouragement. Joining a fitness club or an exercise group at work provides various forms of stimulation and socialization, which increases the potential for new friendships grounded in an appreciation of the rewards of exercise.

### Schools

Schools are one of the most important resources for increasing physical activity. Strategies must be developed to facilitate increased activity in children because it is clear that children are becoming less active and more obese. Schools are providing less opportunity and poorer quality time for physical activity during school hours. All schools should provide opportunities for physical activity that:

- Are appropriate and enjoyable for children of all skill levels and are not limited to competitive sports or physical education classes
- Appeal to girls and boys and to children from diverse backgrounds
- Are offered daily
- Can serve as a foundation for activities throughout life

Schools can also serve as a resource for the community. Expanding operating hours at either end of the school day creates a safe, indoor environment for hall walking. In fact, Ontario saw the integration of more physical activity within the school system as being important. In 2005, the Ontario Government (Ministry of Education) created the Daily Physical Activity Policy (DPA). This mandated that school boards need to ensure that all elementary school students have a minimum of 20 minutes of moderate-to-vigorous physical activity each day during instructional time. There was the unique piece with this policy—the activity did not include activity during lunch break, recess, or after school. The intention was to help fill in activity gaps on days when physical education was not offered (Public Health Ontario, 2019). Like many policies, there have been challenges in adopting this program (Allison, Vu-Nguyen, Ng, et al., 2016). An evaluation of policy implementation revealed that while administrators and teachers both perceived the DPA as being beneficial, there was a sense that both administrators and teachers did not think it was realistic and achievable, and that there were many barriers, including competing curriculum priorities, lack of time, lack of teacher readiness, and lack of space (Allison et al., 2016).

## Communities

Participation in regular physical activity at the community level depends in large part on the availability and proximity of facilities and safe environments. For example, encouraging active transportation to and from school (i.e., walking and not driving to school). Community government agencies, local health agencies, schools, and places of worship have the potential to provide activity resources to the population at large. Churches seem to be particularly successful in reaching ethnic minorities and older persons. Making neighbourhoods safe for outdoor activities can have a major effect on improving activity habits, especially among low socioeconomic and disadvantaged populations, who report lower levels of daily physical activity.

Recognizing that many of the previous recommendations require a financial commitment, government agencies must respond to reports by health agencies and establish public policies that support the importance of physical activity for the general population. Individuals should make a personal commitment to be physically active, but that commitment needs to be supported by a social and political environment that values this type of lifestyle choice.

## CASE STUDY

### Exercise Self-Efficacy: Sharon G.

Sharon G. is a 53-year-old account executive who is 2 years after menopause, has insomnia, and has chronic low back pain and knee pain.

#### History

Motor vehicle accident (2014), resulting in bone graft to left leg (her left leg is shorter than her right leg). As part of rehabilitation, Sharon started jogging, which was more comfortable than walking with chronic right-sided sacroiliac joint pain. She started running marathons in 2016 and continued until 2017. In 2018 she began to add more variety to exercise and decreased her running, but she still identified herself as being an athlete.

In 2019 Sharon had a fall that resulted in chronic low back pain, and she was unable to continue aerobic exercise. She began to experience depression and insomnia; exercise had been a significant coping mechanism in the past, and now her whole sense of well-being was being affected. As Sharon attempted to rebuild her exercise practice, she would alternate between over-exercising, exacerbating symptoms, and then having to stop and recuperate, reinforcing her negative self-image.

#### Reflective Questions

- What are some of her barriers to exercise?
- How will a regular practice of mindfulness and the relaxation response benefit Sharon's exercise practice?
- How might exercise in Sharon's case be both a positive and negative component in her life?
- What would your suggestion for physical activity (exercise prescription) be for Sharon, moving forward?

## CARE PLAN

### Exercise Self-Efficacy: Sharon G.

#### Nursing Issue
Altered sleep pattern related to low back pain, depression, and recent weight gain

#### Medications
- Oxazepam (Serax) 30 mg, four to six times a week
- Ginkgo biloba

#### Defining Characteristics
- Insomnia
- Chronic low back and knee pain
- Depression
- Upset about recent weight gain of 4.53 kg (10 lb) (156 cm [61.5 inches], 53.52 kg [118 lb]); sees her ideal body weight as 49 kg (108 lb)

#### Expected Outcomes
- Walking, treadmill, bicycling, and low-impact aerobics (30 minutes, three to four times per week)
- Weights three to four times per week
- Stretching three to four times per week
- Daily relaxation response
- Build mindfulness into exercise practice

#### Interventions
- Treadmill and walking daily for 30 minutes
- Weights two to three times per week
- Yoga and stretching daily

# SUMMARY

It is important that people incorporate physical activity into their lifestyles on a long-term basis; exercise in the short term is of little overall benefit. Helping individuals gain the knowledge (benefits of exercise and recommended parameters for exercise), skills (self-monitoring), and attitude (core desire) increases the likelihood of incorporating daily physical activity. Behavioural change is cyclical rather than linear; success often comes with repeated movement through stages of change, and it helps to explore the reasons for a change in physical activity, and to view the change as a learning experience rather than a failure. The goal is to ensure an overall healthy lifestyle approach.

The benefits and enjoyment derived from a physically active lifestyle have a significant effect on the quality of life. However, this lifestyle is successful only when it is supported by a degree of self-awareness and self-care. People must realize that they are worth the effort of doing something good for themselves, that they have the right to be happy and healthy, and that exercise can help them achieve that end. By adding a mind-body component to physical activity and not regarding it solely as a physical regimen, people can experience true health rather than mere fitness. A great deal of body exercise is not required; 30 minutes a day can make a significant difference. Success comes with building a rhythm of physical activity into everyday life. The following are some suggestions for a lifestyle approach to exercise:

- Something is better than nothing.
- Attempt small changes over time (gradualism).
- Emphasize moderate intensity.
- Make activity an integral part of life.
- Focus on the process rather than the outcome.
- Clinicians can provide a knowledgeable, supportive, and enthusiastic environment to encourage the change to a healthier, more active way of life.

## Evolve Chapter Features

http://evolve.elsevier.com/Canada/Edelman/healthpromotion/
- Review Questions

# REFERENCES

Alfonso, R. F., Hachul, H., Kozasa, E. H., et al. (2012). Yoga decreases insomnia in postmenopausal women: A randomized clinical trial. *Menopause*, *19*(2), 186–193. https://doi.org/10.1097/gme.0b013e318228225f.

Allison, K. R., Vu-Nguyen, K., Ng, B., et al. (2016). Evaluation of daily physical activity (DPA) policy implementation in Ontario: Surveys of elementary school administrators and teachers. *BMC Public Health*, *16*, 746. https://doi.org/10.1186/s12889-016-3423-0.

American College of Sports Medicine (ACSM). (2009a). American College of Sports Medicine position stand. Progression models in resistance training for healthy adults. *Medicine & Science in Sports & Exercise*, *41*(3), 687–708. [Seminal Reference].

American College of Sports Medicine (ACSM). (2009b). *ACSM's exercise management for persons with chronic diseases and disabilities* (3rd ed.). Champaign, IL: Human Kinetics. [Seminal Reference].

American College of Sports Medicine (ACSM). (2013). *ACSM's guidelines for exercise testing and prescription* (9th ed.). Philadelphia: Lippincott Williams & Wilkins.

American College of Sports Medicine & American Heart Association (ASCM/AHA). (2007). Exercise and acute cardiovascular events: Placing the risks into perspective. *Medicine & Science in Sports & Exercise*, *39*(5), 886–897. [Seminal Reference].

Anderson, S. L. (2006). Physical therapy for patients with HIV/AIDS. *Cardiopulmonary Physical Therapy Journal*, *17*(3), 103–109. [Seminal Reference].

Arnold, C. M., & Faulkner, R. A. (2010). The effect of aquatic exercise and education on lowering fall risk in older adults with hip osteoarthritis. *Journal of Aging and Physical Activity*, *18*(3), 245–260. [Seminal Reference].

Bakhshi, S., Sun, F., Murrells, T., et al. (2015). Nurses' health behaviours and physical activity-related health promotion practices. *British Journal of Community News*, *20*(6), 289–296. doi:10:12968/bjcn.2015.20.6.289.

Bartlett, D. B., Willis, L. H., Slentz, C. A., et al. (2018). Ten weeks of high-intensity interval walk training is associated with reduced disease activity and improved innate immune function in older adults with rheumatoid arthritis: A pilot study. *Arthritis Research & Therapy*, *20*, 127. https://doi.org/10.1186/s13075-018-1624-x.

Bauman, A., Bull, F., Chey, T., et al. (2009). The international prevalence study on physical activity: Results from 20 countries. *International Journal of Behavioral Nutrition and Physical Activity*, *6*, 21. https://doi.org/10.1186/1479-5868-6-21. [Seminal Reference].

Behringer, M., Gruetzner, S., McCourt, M., et al. (2014). Effects of weight-bearing activities on bone mineral content and density in children and adolescents: A meta-analysis. *Journal of Bone and Mineral Research: The Official Journal of the American Society for Bone and Mineral Research*, *29*(2), 467–478.

Belli, T., Ribeiro, L. F. P., Ackermann, M. A., et al. (2011). Effects of 12-week overground training at ventilatory threshold velocity in type 2 diabetic women. *Diabetes Research and Clinical Practice*, *93*(3), 337–343. https://doi.org/10.1016/j.diabres.2011.05.007. [Seminal Reference].

Benson, H., & Stuart, E. (1992). *The wellness book: The comprehensive guide to maintaining health and treating stress-related illness*. New York: Simon & Schuster. [Seminal Reference].

Bentley, D. C., Nguyen, C. H. P., & Thomas, S. G. (2018). High-intensity handgrip training lowers blood pressure and increases heart rate complexity among postmenopausal women: A pilot study. *Blood Pressure Monitoring*, *23*(2), 71–78. https://doi.org/10.1097/mbp.0000000000000313.

Berger, B., & Owen, D. (1988). Stress reduction and mood enhancement in four exercise modes: Swimming, body conditioning, hatha yoga, and fencing. *Research Quarterly for Exercise and Sport*, *59*(2), 148–159. https://doi.org/10.1080/02701367.1988.10605493. [Seminal Reference].

Bezalel, T., Carmeli, E., & Katz-Leurer, M. (2010). The effect of a group education programme on pain and function through knowledge acquisition and home-based exercise among patients with knee osteoarthritis: A parallel randomised single-blind clinical trial. *Physiotherapy*, *96*(2), 137–143. https://doi.org/10.1016/j.physio.2009.09.009. [Seminal Reference].

Borg, G. A. (1973). Perceived exertion: A note on "history" and methods. *Medicine & Science in Sports & Exercise*, *5*(2), 90–93. [Seminal Reference].

Borg, G. A. (1982). Psychophysical bases of perceived exertion. *Medicine & Science in Sports & Exercise, 14*(5), 377–381. [Seminal Reference].

Boutcher, Y. N., & Boutcher, S. H. (2017). Exercise intensity and hypertension: What's new? *Journal of Human Hypertension, 31*(3), 157–164. https://doi.org/10.1038/jhh.2016.62.

Bradt, J., Goodwill, S. W., & Dileo, C. (2011). Dance/movement therapy for improving psychological and physical outcomes in cancer patients. *The Cochrane Database of Systematic Reviews, 1*, CD007103.

Brannan, M., Bernardotto, M., Clarke, N., et al. (2019). Moving healthcare professionals—a whole system approach to embed physical activity in clinical practice. *BMC Medical Education, 19*, 84. https://doi.org/10.1186/s12909-019-1517-y.

Brown, I. (2006). Nurses' attitudes towards adult patients who are obese: Literature review. *Journal of Advanced Nursing, 53*(2), 221–232. [Seminal Reference].

Büssing, A., Ostermann, T., Lüdtke, R., et al. (2012). Effects of yoga intervention on pain and pain-associated disability: A meta-analysis. *Journal of Pain, 13*(1), 1–9. https://doi.org/10.1016/j.jpain.2011.10.001.

Caban-Martinez, A. J., Courtney, T. K., Chang, W. R., et al. (2015). Leisure-time physical activity, falls, and fall injuries in middle-aged adults. *American Journal of Preventive Medicine, 49*(6), 888–901. https://doi.org/10.1016/j.amepre.2015.05.022.

Cai, C., Yang, Y., & Kong, P. W. (2017). Comparison of lower limb and back exercises for runners with chronic low back pain. *Medicine & Science in Sports & Exercise, 49*(12), 2374–2384. https://doi.org/10.1249/MSS.0000000000001396.

Canadian Society for Exercise Physiology (CSEP). (2017). *Get active questionnaire*. Ottawa: Author. Retrieved from http://www.csep.ca/home.

Canadian Society for Exercise Physiology CSEP. (2019). *Pre-screening for physical activity preparation*. Ottawa: Author. Retrieved from https://www.csep.ca/view.asp?ccid=517.

Canadian Society for Exercise Physiology (CSEP). (n.d.). *About the Canadian Society for Exercise Physiology*. Ottawa: Author. Retrieved from https://www.csep.ca/en/about-csep/about-the-canadian-society-for-exercise-physiology.

Candow, D. G., Chilibeck, P. D., Abeysekara, S., et al. (2011). Short-term heavy resistance training eliminates age-related deficits in muscle mass and strength in healthy older males. *Journal of Strength and Conditioning Research, 25*(2), 326–333. doi:10.1519/JSC.0b013e3181bf43c8. [Seminal Reference].

Cantó, E., Roca, E., Perea, L., et al. (2018). Salivary immunity and lower respiratory tract infections in non-elite marathon runners. *PLoS One, 13*(11), e0206059. https://doi.org/10.1371/journal.pone.0206059.

Carek, P. J., Laibstain, S. E., & Carek, S. M. (2011). Exercise for the treatment of depression and anxiety. *International Journal of Psychiatry In Medicine, 41*(1), 15–28. https://doi.org/10.2190/PM.41.1.c.

Centers for Disease Control and Prevention (CDC). (2015). *Nutrition, physical activity, and obesity: Data, trends and maps*. Retrieved from https://nccd.cdc.gov/dnpao_dtm/rdPage.aspx?rdReport=DNPAO_DTM.ExploreByLocation&rdRequestForwarding=Form.

Chaput, J. P., Colley, R. C., Aubert, S., et al. (2017). Proportion of preschool-aged children meeting the Canadian 24-hour movement guidelines and associations with adiposity: Results from the Canadian Health Measures Survey. *BMC Public Health, 17*(Suppl. 5), 829. doi:10:1186/s12889-017-4844-y.

Chen, L., Pei, J. H., Kuang, J., et al. (2015). Effect of lifestyle intervention in patients with type 2 diabetes: A meta-analysis. *Metabolism: Clinical and Experimental, 64*(2), 338–347. https://doi.org/10.1016/j.metabol.2014.10.018.

Chen, M. J., Fan, X., & Moe, S. T. (2002). Criterion-related validity of the Borg Kratings of perceived exertion scale in healthy individuals: A meta-analysis. *Journal of Sports Sciences, 20*(11), 873–899. [Seminal Reference].

Cho, Y. K., Kim, D. Y., Jung, S. Y., et al. (2015). Synergistic effect of a rehabilitation program and treadmill exercise on pain and dysfunction in patients with chronic low back pain. *Journal of Physical Therapy Science, 27*(4), 1187–1190. https://doi.org/10.1589/jpts.27.1187.

Chojnacki, M. R., Raine, L. B., Drollette, E. S., et al. (2018). The negative influence of adiposity extends to intraindividual variability in cognitive control among preadolescent children. *Obesity (Silver Spring), 26*(2), 405–411. https://doi.org/10.1002/oby.22053.

Chu, N. M., & McAdams-DeMarco, M. A. (2019). Exercise and cognitive function in patients with end-stage kidney disease. *Seminars in Dialysis*. https://doi.org/10.1111/sdi.12804.

Chudyk, A., & Patrella, R. J. (2011). Effects of exercise on cardiovascular risk factors in type 2 diabetes. A meta-analysis. *Diabetes Care, 34*(5), 1228–1237.

Ciolac, E. G. (2013). Exercise training as a preventive tool for age-related disorders: A brief review. *Clinics (Sao Paulo), 68*(5), 710–717. https://doi.org/10.6061/clinics/2013(05)20.

Colley, R. C., Garriguet, D., Janssen, I., et al. (2011). Physical activity of Canadian children and youth: Accelerometer results from the 2007 to 2009 Canadian Health Measures Survey. *Health Reports, 22*(1), 7–14. [Seminal Reference].

Cooney, J. K., Law, R., Matschke, V., et al. (2010). Benefits of exercise in rheumatoid arthritis. *Journal of Aging Research, 13*, 1–14. https://doi.org/10.4061/2011/681640. [Seminal Reference].

Coquart, J. B., Garcin, M., Parfitt, G., et al. (2014). Prediction of maximal or peak oxygen uptake from ratings of perceived exertion. *Sports Medicine, 44*(5), 563–578.

Coquart, J. B., Tourny-Chollet, C., Lemaitre, F., et al. (2012). Relevance of the measure of perceived exertion for the rehabilitation of obese patients. *Annals of Physical and Rehabilitation Medicine, 55*(9-10), 623–640. https://doi.org/10.1016/j.rehab.2012.07.003.

Cornelissen, V. A., Fagard, R. H., Coeckelberghs, E., et al. (2011). Impact of resistance training on blood pressure and other cardiovascular risk factors: A meta-analysis of randomized, controlled trials. *Hypertension, 58*(5), 950–958.

Correa-Perez, A., Abraha, I., Cherubini, A., et al. (2019). Efficacy of non-pharmacological interventions to treat malnutrition in older persons: A systematic review and meta-analysis. The SENATOR project ONTOP series and MaNuEL knowledge hub project. *Ageing Research Reviews, 49*, 27–48. https://doi.org/10.1016/j.arr.2018.10.011.

Cowan, D., Radman, H., Lewis, D., & Turpie, I. (2009). A community-based physical maintenance program for frail older adults: The Stay Well program. *Topics in Geriatric Rehabilitation, 25*(4), 355–364. [Seminal Reference].

Cramer, H., Lauche, R., Langhorst, J., et al. (2013). Yoga for depression: A systematic review and meta-analysis. *Journal of Depression and Anxiety, 30*(1), 1068–1083.

da Silva, D. E., Grande, A. J., Roever, L., et al. (2019). High-intensity interval training in patients with type 2 diabetes mellitus: A systematic review. *Current Atherosclerosis Reports, 21*(2), 8. https://doi.org/10.1007/s11883-019-0767-9.

Danhauer, S. C., Addington, E. L., Cohen, L., et al. (2019). Yoga for symptom management in oncology: A review of the evidence base and future directions for research. *Cancer*. https://doi.org/10.1002/cncr.31979.

de Groot, M., Shubrook, J. H., Hornsby, W. G., Jr., et al. (2019). Program ACTIVE II: Outcomes from a randomized, multistate community-based depression treatment for rural and urban adults with type 2 diabetes. *Diabetes Care, 42*(7), 1185–1193. https://doi.org/10.2337/dc18-2400.

de Manincor, M., Bensoussan, A., Smith, C. A., et al. (2016). Individualized yoga for reducing depression and anxiety, and improving well-being: A randomized controlled trial. *Depress Anxiety*, 33(9), 816–828. https://doi.org/10.1002/da.22502.

de Salles, B. F., Simao, R., Miranda, F., et al. (2009). Rest interval between sets in strength training. *Sports Medicine*, 39(9), 765–777. [Seminal Reference].

DeFina, L. F., Radford, N. B., Barlow, C. E., et al. (2019). Association of all-cause and cardiovascular mortality with high levels of physical activity and concurrent coronary artery calcification. *JAMA Cardiology*, 4(2), 174–181. https://doi.org/10.1001/jamacardio.2018.4628.

Deshpande, A. D., Harris-Hayes, M., & Schootman, M. (2008). Epidemiology of diabetes and diabetes-related complications. *Physical Therapy*, 88(11), 1254–1264. [Seminal Reference].

Dudgeon, W. D., Phillips, K. D., Bopp, C. M., et al. (2004). Physiological and psychological effects of exercise interventions in HIV disease. *AIDS Patient Care and STDs*, 18(2), 81–98. https://doi.org/10.1089/108729104322802515. [Seminal Reference].

Dugani, S., Bhutta, Z. A., & Kissoon, N. (2017). Empowering people for sustainable development: The Ottawa Charter and beyond. *Journal of Global Health*, 7(1), 010308. https://doi.org/10.7189/jogh.07.010308.

Dunne, E. M., Balletto, B. L., Donahue, M. L., et al. (2019). The benefits of yoga for people living with HIV/AIDS: A systematic review and meta-analysis. *Complementary Therapies in Clinical Practice*, 34, 157–164. https://doi.org/10.1016/j.ctcp.2018.11.009.

Ebnezar, J., Nagarathna, R., Yogitha, B., et al. (2012). Effects of integrated approach of Hatha yoga therapy on functional disability, pain, and flexibility in osteoarthritis of the knee joint: A randomized controlled study. *Journal of Alternative and Complementary Medicine*, 18(5), 463–472.

Ehrlich-Jones, L., Lee, J., Semanik, P., Cox, C., et al. (2011). Relationship between beliefs, motivation, and worries about physical activity and physical activity participation in persons with rheumatoid arthritis. *Arthritis Care & Research*, 63(12), 1700–1705.

Exercise is Medicine Canada (EIMC). (2019). *Exercise is Medicine® Canada*. Retrieved from https://exerciseismedicine.org/canada/.

Farrance, C., Tsofliou, F., & Clark, C. (2016). Adherence to community based group exercise interventions for older people: A mixed-methods systematic review. *Preventive Medicine*, 87, 155–166. https://doi.org/10.1016/j.ypmed.2016.02.037.

Federici, M. O., & Benedetti, M. M. (2006). Ketone bodies monitoring. *Diabetes Research & Clinical Practice*, 74(2), S77–S81. https://doi.org/10.1016/S0168-8227(06)70004-3. [Seminal Reference].

Fillipas, S., Cherry, C. L., Cicuttini, F., et al. (2010). The effects of exercise training on metabolic and morphological outcomes for people living with HIV: A systematic review of randomised controlled trials. *HIV Clinical Trials*, 11(5), 270–282. https://doi.org/10.1310/hct1105-270.

Fillipas, S., Oldmeadow, L. B., Bailey, M. J., et al. (2006). A six-month, supervised, aerobic and resistance exercise program improves self-efficacy in people with human immunodeficiency virus: A randomized controlled trial. *Australian Journal of Physiotherapy*, 52(3), 185–190. [Seminal Reference].

Firth, J., Stubbs, B., Rosenbaum, S., et al. (2017). Aerobic exercise improves cognitive functioning in people with schizophrenia: A systematic review and meta-analysis. *Schizophrenia Bulletin*, 43(3), 546–556. https://doi.org/10.1093/schbul/sbw115.

Franco, M. R., Morelhao, P. K., de Carvalho, A., et al. (2017). Aquatic exercise for the treatment of hip and knee osteoarthritis. *Physical Therapy*, 97(7), 693–697. https://doi.org/10.1093/ptj/pzx043.

Galantino, M. L., Shepard, K., Krafft, L., et al. (2005). The effect of group aerobic exercise and t'ai chi on functional outcomes and quality of life for persons living with acquired immunodeficiency syndrome. *Journal of Alternative and Complementary Medicine*, 11(6), 1085–1092. [Seminal Reference].

Galloza, J., Castillo, B., & Micheo, W. (2017). Benefits of exercise in the older population. *Physical Medicine and Rehabilitation Clinics of North America*, 28(4), 659–669. https://doi.org/10.1016/j.pmr.2017.06.001.

Garcia-Hermoso, A., Ramirez-Velez, R., Ramirez-Campillo, R., et al. (2018). Concurrent aerobic plus resistance exercise versus aerobic exercise alone to improve health outcomes in paediatric obesity: A systematic review and meta-analysis. *British Journal of Sports Medicine*, 52(3), 161–166. https://doi.org/10.1136/bjsports-2016-096605.

García-Pérez, L. E., Alvarez, M., Dilla, T., Gil-Guillen, V., et al. (2013). Adherence to therapies in patients with type 2 diabetes. *Diabetes Therapy*, 4(2), 175–194. https://doi.org/10.1007/s13300-013-0034-y. [Seminal Reference].

Ghadieh, A. S., & Saab, B. (2015). Evidence for exercise training in the management of hypertension in adults. *Canadian Family Physician Médecine De Famille Canadienne*, 61(3), 233–239.

Giangregorio, L. M., Papaioannou, A., Macintyre, N. J., et al. (2014). Too fit to fracture: Exercise recommendations for individuals with osteoporosis or osteoporotic vertebral fracture. *Osteoporosis International*, 25(3), 821–835. https://doi.org/10.1007/s00198-013-2523-2.

Giangregorio, L. M., Gibbs, J. C., Templeton, J. A., et al. (2018). Build better bones with exercise (B3E pilot trial): Results of a feasibility study of a multicenter randomized controlled trial of 12 months of home exercise in older women with vertebral fracture. *Osteoporosis International*, 29(11), 2545–2556. https://doi.org/10.1007/s00198-018-4652-0.

Gleeson, M. (2007). Immune function in sport and exercise. *Journal of Applied Physiology (1985)*, 103(2), 693–699. https://doi.org/10.1152/japplphysiol.00008.2007. [Seminal Reference].

Gleeson, M., Bishop, N., Oliveira, M., et al. (2013). Influence of training load on upper respiratory tract infection incidence and antigen-stimulated cytokine production. *Scandinavian Journal of Medicine & Science in Sports*, 23(4), 451–457.

Gleeson, M., Bishop, N., Oliveira, M., et al. (2011). Sex differences in immune variables and respiratory infection incidence in an athletic population. *Exercise Immunology Review*, 17, 122–135.

Gleeson, M., Pyne, D. B., Austin, J. P., et al. (2002). Epstein-Barr virus reactivation and upper-respiratory illness in elite swimmers. *Medicine & Science in Sports & Exercise*, 34(3), 411–417. https://doi.org/10.1097/00005768-200203000-00005. [Seminal Reference].

Glenney, S. S., Brockemer, D. P., Ng, A. C., et al. (2017). Effect of Exercise training on cardiac biomarkers in at-risk populations: A systematic review. *Journal of Physical Activity and Health*, 14(12), 968–989. https://doi.org/10.1123/jpah.2016-0631.

Gomes-Neto, M., Conceiçao, C. S., Carvalho, V. O., et al. (2013). A systematic review of the effects of different types of therapeutic exercise on physiologic and functional measurements in patients with HIV/AIDS. *Clinics (São Paulo, Brazil)*, 68(8), 1157–1167. https://doi.org/10.6061/clinics/2013(08)16.

Gomez-Bruton, A., Matute-Llorente, A., Gonzalez-Aguero, A., et al. (2017). Plyometric exercise and bone health in children and adolescents: A systematic review. *World J Pediatr*, 13(2), 112–121. https://doi.org/10.1007/s12519-016-0076-0.

Gong, Q. H., Kang, J. F., Ying, Y. Y., et al. (2015). Lifestyle interventions for adults with impaired glucose tolerance: A systematic review and meta-analysis of the effects on glycemic control. *Internal Medicine (Tokyo, Japan)*, 54(3), 303–310.

Gordon, C. M., Zemel, B. S., Wren, T. A., et al. (2017). The determinants of peak bone mass. *Journal of Pediatrics, 180*, 261–269. https://doi.org/10.1016/j.jpeds.2016.09.056.

Gorham, L. S., Jernigan, T., Hudziak, J., et al. (2019). Involvement in sports, hippocampal volume, and depressive symptoms in children. *Biological Psychiatry Cognitive Neuroscience and Neuroimaging, 4*(5), 484–492. https://doi.org/10.1016/j.bpsc.2019.01.011.

Government of Canada. (2015). *Canadian guidelines for body weight classification in adults.* Ottawa: Author. Retrieved from https://www.canada.ca/en/health-canada/services/food-nutrition/healthy-eating/healthy-weights/canadian-guidelines-body-weight-classification-adults.html.

Government of Canada. (2016). *Health status of Canadians 2016: Report of the chief public health officer—What is influencing our health? Physical activity.* Retrieved from https://www.canada.ca/en/public-health/corporate/publications/chief-public-health-officer-reports-state-public-health-canada/2016-health-status-canadians/page-13-what-influencing-health-physical-activity.html.

Government of Canada. (2017). *Diabetes in Canada: Highlights from the Canadian chronic disease surveillance system.* Retrieved from https://www.canada.ca/en/public-health/services/publications/diseases-conditions/diabetes-canada-highlights-chronic-disease-surveillance-system.html.

Government of Canada. (2019). *Childhood obesity.* Retrieved from https://www.canada.ca/en/public-health/services/childhood-obesity/childhood-obesity.html.

Graven, C., Brock, K., Hill, K., et al. (2011). Are rehabilitation and/or care co-coordination interventions delivered in the community effective in reducing depression, facilitating participation and improving quality of life after stroke? *Disability and Rehabilitation, 33*(17/18), 1501–1520.

Green, E., Huynh, A., Broussard, L., et al. (2019). Systematic review of yoga and balance: Effect on adults with neuromuscular impairment. *American Journal of Occupational Therapy, 73*(1). https://doi.org/10.5014/ajot.2019.028944. 7301205150p1–7301205150p11.

Gulve, E. A. (2008). Exercise and glycemic control in diabetes: Benefits, challenges, and adjustments to pharmacotherapy. *Physical Therapy, 88*(11), 1297–1321. [Seminal Reference].

Güngör, N. K. (2014). Overweight and obesity in children and adolescents. *Journal of Clinical Research in Pediatric Endocrinology, 6*(3), 129–143. https://doi.org/10.4274/Jcrpe.1471.

Hale, L. A., Waters, D., & Herbison, P. (2012). A randomized controlled trial to investigate the effects of water-based exercise to improve falls risk and physical function in older adults with lower-extremity osteoarthritis. *Archives of Physical Medicine and Rehabilitation, 93*(1), 27–34. https://doi.org/10.1016/j.apmr.2011.08.004. [Seminal Reference].

Hall, A. M., Maher, C. G., Lam, P., et al. (2011). Tai chi exercise for treatment of pain and disability in people with persistent low back pain: A randomized controlled trial. *Arthritis Care & Research, 63*(11), 1576–1583. [Seminal Reference].

Harris, A., Austin, M., Blake, T. M., et al. (2019). Perceived benefits and barriers to yoga participation after stroke: A focus group approach. *Complementary Therapy in Clinical Practice, 34*, 153–156. https://doi.org/10.1016/j.ctcp.2018.11.015.

Hass, C. J., Garzarella, L., de Hoyos, D., et al. (2000). Single versus multiple sets in long-term recreational weightlifters. *Medicine & Science in Sports & Exercise, 32*(1), 235–242. [Seminal Reference].

Hautala, A. J., Kiviniemi, A. M., Karjalainen, J. J., et al. (2013). Peak exercise capacity prediction from a submaximal exercise test in coronary artery disease patients. *Frontiers in Physiology, 4*, 1–6. https://doi.org/10.3389/fphys.2013.00243. [Seminal Reference].

Health Canada. (2003). *Canadian guidelines for body weight classification in adults—quick reference. (Catalogue no. H49-179/2003-1E).* Ottawa: Author. Retrieved from L. [Seminal Reference].

Heart, & Stroke Foundation of Canada. (2019). *How much physical activity do you need?* Retrieved from https://www.heartandstroke.ca/get-healthy/stay-active/how-much-physical-activity-do-you-need.

Heneweer, H., Picavet, H. S., Staes, F., et al. (2012). Physical fitness, rather than self-reported physical activities, is more strongly associated with low back pain: Evidence from a working population. *European Spine Journal, 21*(7), 1265–1272. https://doi.org/10.1007/s00586-011-2097-7.

Henwood, T., Keogh, J., & Climstein, M. (2012). Sarcopenia in older adults. *Australian Nursing Journal, 19*(9), 39–40. https://doi.org/10.1097/BOR.0b013e328358d59b.

Heran, B. S., Chen, J. M., Ebrahim, S., et al. (2011). Exercise-based cardiac rehabilitation for coronary heart disease. *The Cochrane Database of Systematic Reviews, 7*, CD001800. https://doi.org/10.1002/14651858.CD001800.pub2.

Herring, M. P., O'Connor, P. J., & Dishman, R. K. (2010). The effect of exercise training on anxiety symptoms among patients: A systematic review. *Archives of Internal Medicine, 170*(4), 321–331. https://doi.org/10.1001/archinternmed.2009.530. [Seminal Reference].

Hewlett, S., Ambler, N., Almeida, et al. (2011). Self-management of fatigue in rheumatoid arthritis: A randomised controlled trial of group cognitive-behavioural therapy. *Annals of the Rheumatic Diseases, 70*(6), 1060–1067.

Hodges, P. W. (2019). Hybrid approach to treatment tailoring for low back pain: A proposed model of care. *Journal of Orthopedic Sports Physical Therapy, 49*(6), 1–37. https://doi.org/10.2519/jospt.2019.8774.

Holtzman, S., & Beggs, R. T. (2013). Yoga for chronic low back pain: A meta-analysis of randomized controlled trials. *Pain Research & Management, 18*(5), 267–272. https://doi.org/10.1155/2013/105919.

Huang, T. T., Yang, L. H., & Liu, C. Y. (2011). Reducing the fear of falling among community-dwelling elderly adults through cognitive-behavioural strategies and intense tai chi exercise: A randomized controlled trial. *Journal of Advanced Nursing, 67*(5), 961–971.

Hurst, C., Weston, K. L., McLaren, S. J., et al. (2019). The effects of same-session combined exercise training on cardiorespiratory and functional fitness in older adults: A systematic review and meta-analysis. *Aging Clinical and Experimental Research.* https://doi.org/10.1007/s40520-019-01124-7.

Ingram, C., & Visovsky, C. (2007). Exercise intervention to modify physiologic risk factors in cancer survivors. *Seminars in Oncology Nursing, 23*(4), 275–284. https://doi.org/10.1016/j.soncn.2007.08.005. [Seminal Reference].

Jaggers, J., Hand, G. A., Dudgeon, W. D., et al. (2015). Aerobic and resistance training improves mood state among adults living with HIV. *International Journal of Sports Medicine, 36*(2), 175–181.

Jamtvedt, G., Dahm, K. T., Christie, A., et al. (2008). Physical therapy interventions for patients with osteoarthritis of the knee: An overview of systematic reviews. *Physical Therapy, 88*(1), 123–136. [Seminal Reference].

Jansen, M. J., Viechtbauer, W., Lenssen, A. F., et al. (2011). Strength training alone, exercise therapy alone, and exercise therapy with passive manual mobilisation each reduce pain and disability in people with knee osteoarthritis: A systematic review. *Journal of Physiotherapy, 57*(1), 11–20. https://doi.org/10.1016/S1836-9553(11)70002-9.

Jiang, D., Kong, W., & Jiang, J. J. (2016). The role of tai chi in mental health management: Lessons learned from clinical trials. *Reviews on Recent Clinical Trials, 11*(4), 324–332.

Julián-Almárcegui, C., Gomez-Cabello, A., Huybrechts, I., et al. (2015). Combined effects of interaction between physical activity and nutrition on bone health in children and adolescents: A systematic review. *Nutrition Reviews, 73*(3), 127–139.

Keaney, L. C., Kilding, A. E., Merien, F., et al. (2018). The impact of sport related stressors on immunity and illness risk in team-sport athletes. *Journal of Science & Medicine in Sport, 21*(12), 1192–1199. https://doi.org/10.1016/j.jsams.2018.05.014.

Kelley, G. A., Kelley, K. S., & Hootman, J. M. (2015). Effects of exercise on depression in adults with arthritis: A systematic review with meta-analysis of randomized controlled trials. *Arthritis Research & Therapy, 17*(21). https://doi.org/10.1186/s13075-015-0533-5.

Keysor, J. J., & Brembs, A. (2011). Exercise: Necessary but not sufficient for improving function and preventing disability? *Current Opinion in Rheumatology, 23*(2), 211–218. https://doi.org/10.1097/BOR.0b013e3283432c41.

Kiwata, J., Anouseyan, R., Desharnais, R., et al. (2014). Effects of aerobic exercise on lipid-effector molecules of the innate immune response. *Medicine and Science in Sports and Exercise, 46*(3), 506–512. https://doi.org/10.1249/MSS.0000000000000137.

Knapik, J. J., Pope, R., Orr, R., et al. (2018). Osteoarthritis: Pathophysiology, prevalence, risk factors, and exercise for reducing pain and disability. *Journal of Special Operations Medicine: A Peer Reviewed Journal for SOF Medical Professionals, 18*(3), 94–102.

Kohrt, W. M., Bloomfield, S. A., Little, K. D., et al. (2004). American College of Sports Medicine Position stand: Physical activity and bone health. *Medicine & Science in Sports & Exercise, 36*(11), 1985–1996. [Seminal Reference].

Kovácsné Bobály, V., Szilagyi, B., Makai, A., et al. (2017). Improvement of lumbal motor control and trunk muscle conditions with a novel low back pain prevention exercise program. *Orv Hetil, 158*(2), 58–66. https://doi.org/10.1556/650.2017.30640. [Article in Hungarian].

Krieger, J. W. (2010). Single vs. multiple sets of resistance exercise for muscle hypertrophy: A meta-analysis. *Journal of Strength & Conditioning Research, 24,* 1150–1159. https://doi.org/10.1519/JSC.0b013e3181d4d436. [Seminal Reference].

Ku, P. W., Steptoe, A., Liao, Y., et al. (2018). A cut-off of daily sedentary time and all-cause mortality in adults: A meta-regression analysis involving more than 1 million participants. *BMC Medicine, 16,* 74.

Kujala, U. M. (2009). Evidence on the effects of exercise therapy in the treatment of chronic disease. *British Journal of Sports Medicine, 43*(8), 550–555. https://doi.org/10.1136/bjsm.2009.059808. [Seminal Reference].

Lahart, I. M., Metsios, G. S., Nevill, A. M., et al. (2015). Physical activity, risk of death and recurrence in breast cancer survivors: A systematic review and meta-analysis of epidemiological studies. *Acta Oncologica, 54*(5), 635–654. https://doi.org/10.3109/0284186X.2014.998275.

Langdeau, J. B., & Boulet, L. P. (2001). Prevalence and mechanisms of development of asthma and airway hyperresponsiveness in athletes. *Journal of Sports Medicine, 31*(8), 601–616. [Seminal Reference].

Larkin, L., & Kennedy, N. (2014). Correlates of physical activity in adults with rheumatoid arthritis: A systematic review. *Journal of Physical Activity and Health, 11*(6), 1248–1261. https://doi.org/10.1123/jpah.2012-0194.

Larson-Meyer, D. E., Redman, L., Heilbronn, L. K., et al. (2010). Caloric restriction with or without exercise: The fitness versus fatness debate. *Medicine & Science in Sports & Exercise, 42*(1), 152–159. https://doi.org/10.1249/MSS.0b013e3181ad7f17. [Seminal Reference].

Larun, L., Nordheim, L. V., Ekeland, E., et al. (2009). Exercise in prevention and treatment of anxiety and depression among children and young people. *The Cochrane Database of Systematic Reviews* (3), CD004691. [Seminal Reference].

Lascar, N., Kennedy, A., Hancock, B., et al. (2014). Attitudes and barriers to exercise in adults with type 1 diabetes (T1DM) and how best to address them: A qualitative study. *PLoS ONE, 9*(9), e108019. https://doi.org/10.1371/journal.pone.0108019.

Latimer, A. E., Brawley, L. R., & Bassett, R. L. (2010). A systematic review of three approaches for constructing physical activity messages: What messages work and what improvements are needed? *International Journal of Behavioral Nutrition and Physical Activity, 7,* 36. https://doi.org/10.1186/1479-5868-7-36.

Lavie, C. J., & Milani, R. V. (2011). Cardiac rehabilitation and exercise training in secondary coronary heart disease prevention. *Progress in Cardiovascular Diseases, 53*(6), 397–403. https://doi.org/10.1016/j.pcad.2011.02.008. [Seminal Reference].

Lee, D. J., Meehan, R. T., Robinson, C., et al. (1992). Immune responsiveness and risk of illness in US Air Force Academy cadets during basic cadet training. *Aviation, Space, and Environmental Medicine, 63*(6), 517–523. [Seminal Reference].

Leone, L. A., & Ward, D. S. (2013). A mixed methods comparison of perceived benefits and barriers to exercise between obese and non-obese women. *Journal of Physical Activity & Health, 10*(4), 461–469. https://doi.org/10.1123/jpah.10.4.461.

Leung, D. P., Chan, C. K., Tsang, H. W., et al. (2011). Tai chi as an intervention to improve balance and reduce falls in older adults: A systematic and meta-analytical review. *Alternative Therapies in Health and Medicine, 17*(1), 40–48.

Li, C. S., Liu, C. C., Tsai, M. K., et al. (2015). Motivating patients to exercise: Translating high blood pressure into equivalent risk of inactivity. *Journal of Hypertension, 33*(2), 287–293. https://doi.org/10.1097/HJH.0000000000000392.

Lin, X., Zhang, X., Guo, J., et al. (2015). Effects of exercise training on cardiorespiratory fitness and biomarkers of cardiometabolic health: A Systematic review and meta-analysis of randomized controlled trials. *Journal of the American Heart Association, 4*(7), e002014. https://doi.org/10.1161/jaha.115.002014.

Liu, S., Li, L., Liu, Z., et al. (2019). Long-term tai chi experience promotes emotional stability and slows gray matter atrophy for elders. *Frontiers in Psychology, 10,* 91. https://doi.org/10.3389/fpsyg.2019.00091.

Liu, Y., Hu, F., Li, D., et al. (2011). Does physical activity reduce the risk of prostate cancer? A systematic review and meta-analysis. *European Urology, 60*(5), 1029–1044. https://doi.org/10.1016/j.eururo.2011.07.007.

Lomas-Vega, R., Obrero-Gaitan, E., Molina-Ortega, F. J., et al. (2017). Tai chi for risk of falls: A meta-analysis. *Journal of the American Geriatric Society, 65*(9), 2037–2043. https://doi.org/10.1111/jgs.15008.

Look, A. R. G., Wing, R. R., Bolin, P., et al. (2013). Cardiovascular effects of intensive lifestyle intervention in type 2 diabetes. *New England Journal of Medicine, 369*(2), 145–154. https://doi.org/10.1056/NEJMoa1212914.

Lopes, S., Mesquita-Bastos, J., Alves, A. J., et al. (2018). Exercise as a tool for hypertension and resistant hypertension management: Current insights. *Integrated Blood Pressure Control, 11,* 65–71. https://doi.org/10.2147/ibpc.S136028.

Mackinnon, L. T. (1992). *Exercise and immunology.* Champaign, IL: Human Kinetics. [Seminal Reference].

Mampuya, W. M. (2012). Cardiac rehabilitation past, present and future: An overview. *Cardiovascular Diagnosis and Therapy, 2*(1), 38–49.

Marsaux, C. F., Celis-Morales, C., Hoonhout, J., et al. (2016). Objectively measured physical activity in European adults: Cross-sectional findings from the Food4Me study. *PLoS One, 11*(3), e0150902. https://doi.org/10.1371/journal.pone.0150902.

Martin, D. (2011). Physical activity benefits and risks on the gastrointestinal system. *Southern Medical Journal, 104*(12), 831–837. https://doi.org/10.1097/SMJ.0b013e318236c263. [Seminal Reference].

Mat, S., Tan, M. P., Kamaruzzaman, S. B., et al. (2015). Physical therapies for improving balance and reducing falls risk in osteoarthritis of the knee: A systematic review. *Age and Ageing, 44*(1), 16–24. https://doi.org/10.1093/ageing/afu112.

Matthews, C. E., Ockene, I. S., Freedson, P. S., et al. (2002). Moderate to vigorous physical activity and risk of upper-respiratory tract infection. *Medicine & Science in Sports & Exercise, 34*(8), 1242–1248. https://doi.org/10.1097/00005768-200208000-00003. [Seminal Reference].

McCall, M. (2018). Yoga intervention may improve health-related quality of life (HRQL), fatigue, depression, anxiety and sleep in patients with breast cancer. *Evidence-Based Nursing, 21*(1), 9. https://doi.org/10.1136/eb-2017-102673.

McGrath, J. A., O'Malley, M., & Hendrix, T. J. (2010). Group exercise mode and health-related quality of life among healthy adults. *Journal of Advanced Nursing, 67*(3), 491–500. https://doi.org/10.1111/j.1365-2648.2010.05456.x. [Seminal Reference].

McKinnis, L. N. (2014). *Fundamentals of orthopedic radiology* (4th ed.). Philadelphia: F.A. Davis.

Mead, G. E., Morley, W., Campbell, P., et al. (2009). Exercise for depression. *The Cochrane Database of Systematic Reviews* (3), CD004366. [Seminal Reference].

Menezes, A. R., Lavie, C. J., Milani, R. V., et al. (2012). Cardiac rehabilitation and exercise therapy in the elderly: Should we invest in the aged? *Journal of Geriatric Cardiology, 9*(1), 68–75. https://doi.org/10.3724/SP.J.1263.2012.00068.

Meng, X. G., & Yue, S. W. (2015). Efficacy of aerobic exercise for treatment of chronic low back pain: A meta-analysis. *American Journal of Physical Medicine & Rehabilitation/Association of Academic Physiatrists, 94*(5), 358–365. https://doi.org/10.1097/PHM.0000000000000188.

Metsios, G. S., Stavropoulos-Kalinoglou, A., & Kitas, G. D. (2015). The role of exercise in the management of rheumatoid arthritis. *Expert Review of Clinical Immunology, 11*(10), 1121–1130. https://doi.org/10.1586/1744666x.2015.1067606.

Milani, R. V., Lavie, C. J., Mehra, M. R., et al. (2011). Impact of exercise training and depression on survival in heart failure due to coronary heart disease. *American Journal of Cardiology, 107*(1), 64–68. https://doi.org/10.1016/j.amjcard.2010.08.047. [Seminal Reference].

Millar, P. J., McGowan, C. L., Cornelissen, V. A., et al. (2014). Evidence for the role of isometric exercise training in reducing blood pressure: Potential mechanisms and future directions. *Sports Medicine, 44*(3), 345–356. https://doi.org/10.1007/s40279-013-0118-x.

Miller, S. K., Alpert, P. T., & Cross, C. L. (2008). Overweight and obesity in nurses, advanced practice nurses, and nurse educators. *Journal of the American Academy of Nurse Practitioners, 20*(5), 259–265. https://doi.org/10.1111/j.1745-7599.2008.00319.x. [Seminal Reference].

Mirza, F., & Canalis, E. (2015). Management of endocrine disease: Secondary osteoporosis: Pathophysiology and management. *European Journal of Endocrinology/European Federation of Endocrine Societies, 173*(3), R131–R151. https://doi.org/10.1530/EJE-15-0118.

Mishra, S. I., Scherer, R. W., Snyder, C., et al. (2014). Are exercise programs effective for improving health-related quality of life among cancer survivors? A systematic review and meta-analysis. *Oncology Nursing Forum, 41*(6), 326–342. https://doi.org/10.1188/14.ONF.E326-E342. [Seminal Reference].

Mishra, S. I., Scherer, R. W., Snyder, C., et al. (2015). The effectiveness of exercise interventions for improving health-related quality of life from diagnosis through active cancer treatment. *Oncology Nursing Forum, 42*(1), E33–E53.

Mithal, A., Bonjour, J. P., Boonen, S., et al. (2013). Impact of nutrition on muscle mass, strength, and performance in older adults. *Osteoporosis International, 24*(5), 1555–1566. https://doi.org/10.1007/s00198-012-2236-y.

Mora-Gonzalez, J., Esteban-Cornejo, I., Cadenas-Sanchez, C., et al. (2019). Physical fitness, physical activity, and the executive function in children with overweight and obesity. *Journal of Pediatrics, 208*, 50–56. https://doi.org/10.1016/j.jpeds.2018.12.028.

Motallebi, S. A., Iranagh, J. A., & Mohammadi, F. (2019). Effect of a physical activity program on serum biochemical parameters among elderly women. *Reviews on Recent Clinical Trials, 14*(3), 209–216. https://doi.org/10.2174/1574887114666190201113809.

Nahas, R., & Sheikh, O. (2011). Complementary and alternative medicine for the treatment of major depressive disorder. *Canadian Family Physician, 57*(6), 659–663.

Nakamura, K., Saito, T., Kobayashi, R., et al. (2019). Physical activity modifies the effect of calcium supplements on bone loss in perimenopausal and postmenopausal women: Subgroup analysis of a randomized controlled trial. *Archives of Osteoporosis, 14*(1), 17. https://doi.org/10.1007/s11657-019-0575-4.

Namgoong, H., Lee, D., Hwang, M. H., et al. (2018). The relationship between arterial stiffness and maximal oxygen consumption in healthy young adults. *Journal of Exercise Science & Fitness, 16*(3), 73–77. https://doi.org/10.1016/j.jesf.2018.07.003.

Nascimento, D. C., Tibana, R. A., Benik, F. M., et al. (2014). Sustained effect of resistance training on blood pressure and hand grip strength following a detraining period in elderly hypertensive women: A pilot study. *Clinical Interventions In Aging, 9*, 219–225. https://doi.org/10.2147/cia.S56058.

Nathan, D. M. (2015). Diabetes: Advances in diagnosis and treatment. *JAMA: The Journal of the American Medical Association, 314*(10), 1052–1062. https://doi.org/10.1001/jama.2015.9536.

National Institutes of Health, Osteoporosis and Related Bone Diseases National Resource Center. (2011). *Osteoporosis*. Retrieved from http://www.niams.nih.gov/Health_Info/Bone/Osteoporosis.

National Osteoporosis Foundation. (2016). *Fast facts about osteoporosis*. Retrieved from https://cdn.nof.org/wp-content/uploads/2016/04/Fast-Facts-About-Osteoporosis.pdf.

Nelson, A. E., Allen, K. D., Golightly, Y. M., Goode, A. P., & Jordan, J. M. (2014). A systematic review of recommendations and guidelines for the management of osteoarthritis: The chronic osteoarthritis management initiative of the U.S. bone and joint initiative. *Seminars in Arthritis and Rheumatism, 43*(6), 701–712. https://doi.org/10.1016/j.semarthrit.2013.11.012.

Nieman, D. (1994). Exercise, upper respiratory tract infection, and the immune system. *Medicine & Science in Sports & Exercise, 26*(2), 128–139. https://doi.org/10.1249/00005768-199402000-00002. [Seminal Reference].

Nieman, D. C., Johanssen, L. M., Lee, J. W., et al. (1990). Infectious episodes in runners before and after the Los Angeles Marathon. *Journal of Sports Medicine and Physical Fitness, 30*(3), 316–328. [Seminal Reference].

Nixon, S., O'Brien, K., Glazier, R. H., et al. (2005). Aerobic exercise interventions for adults living with HIV/AIDS. *The Cochrane Database of Systematic Reviews* (2), CD001796. [Seminal Reference].

Northey, J. M., Cherbuin, N., Pumpa, K. L., et al. (2018). Exercise interventions for cognitive function in adults older than 50: A systematic review with meta-analysis. *British Journal of Sports Medicine, 52*(3), 154–160. https://doi.org/10.1136/bjsports-2016-096587.

Nyström, M. B., Neely, G., Hassmen, P., et al. (2015). Treating major depression with physical activity: A systematic overview with recommendations. *Cognitive Behaviour Therapy*, 44(4), 341–352. https://doi.org/10.1080/16506073.2015.1015440.

O'Brien, K., et al. (2009). Progressive resistive exercise interventions for adults living with HIV/AIDS. *The Cochrane Database of Systematic Reviews* (4), CD004248,. pub2. [Seminal Reference].

O'Brien, K., Nixon, S., Glazier, R. H., et al. (2004). Progressive resistive exercise interventions for adults living with HIV/AIDS. *The Cochrane Database of Systematic Reviews* (4), CD004248. [Seminal Reference].

O'Brien, K., Nixon, S., Tynan, A. M., et al. (2010). Aerobic exercise interventions for adults living with HIV/AIDS. *The Cochrane Database of Systematic Reviews* (8), CD001796. [Seminal Reference].

Oerkild, B., Frederiksen, M., Hansen, J. J., et al. (2011). Home-based cardiac rehabilitation is as effective as centre-based cardiac rehabilitation among elderly with coronary heart disease: Results from a randomised clinical trial. *Age and Ageing*, 40(1), 78–85. https://doi.org/10.1093/ageing/afq122. [Seminal Reference].

Olaya-Contreras, P., Styf, J., Arvidsson, D., et al. (2015). The effect of the stay active advice on physical activity and on the course of acute severe low back pain. *BMC Sports Science, Medicine and Rehabilitation*, 7, 19. https://doi.org/10.1186/s13102-015-0013-x.

Ortiz-Marrón, H., Ortiz-Pinto, M. A., Cuadrado-Gamarra, J. I., et al. (2018). Persistence and variation in overweight and obesity among the pre-school population of the community of Madrid after 2 years of follow-up: The ELOIN Cohort. *Revista Española De Cardiología (English Edition)*, 71(11), 902–909. https://doi.org/10.1016/j.rec.2017.12.024.

Ortman, J. M., Velkoff, V. A., & Hogan, H. (2014). *An aging nation: The older population in the United States*. US Department of Commerce.

Osteoporosis Canada. (2017). *Bone Fit*™. Toronto: Author. Retrieved from https://bonefit.ca/.

Osteoporosis Canada. (2019). *Fast facts*. Retrieved from https://osteoporosis.ca/about-the-disease/fast-facts.

Park, Y. H., Song, M., Cho, B. L., et al. (2011). The effects of an integrated health education and exercise program in community-dwelling older adults with hypertension: A randomized controlled trial. *Patient Education and Counseling*, 82(1), 133–137.

PAR-Q+ Collaboration. (2018). *Home page*. Retrieved from http://eparmedx.com/.

Pascoe, M. C., & Bauer, I. E. (2015). A systemic review of randomized control trials on the effects of yoga on stress measures and mood. *Journal of Psychiatric Research*, 68, 270–282. https://doi.org/10.1016/j.jpsychires.2015.07.013.

Pate, R. R., Pratt, M., Blair, S. N., et al. (1995). Physical activity and public health. A recommendation for the Centers for Disease Control and Prevention and the American College of Sports Medicine. *Journal of the American Medical Association*, 273(5), 402–407. https://doi.org/10.1001/jama.1995.03520290054029. [Seminal Reference].

Pedersen, B. K., & Bruunsgaard, H. (1995). How physical exercise influences the establishment of infections. *Sports Medicine*, 19(6), 393–400. https://doi.org/10.2165/00007256-199519060-00003. [Seminal Reference].

Pedersen, B., & Ullum, H. (1994). NK cell response to physical activity: Possible mechanisms of action. *Medicine & Science in Sports & Exercise*, 26(2), 140–146. https://doi.org/10.1249/00005768-199402000-00003. [Seminal Reference].

Pedersen, B., Rohde, T., & Ostrowski, K. (1998). Recovery of the immune system after exercise. *Acta Physiologica Scandinavica*, 162(3), 325–332. https://doi.org/10.1046/j.1365-201X.1998.0325ex. [Seminal Reference].

Pedralli, M. L., Eibel, B., Waclawovsky, G., et al. (2018). Effects of exercise training on endothelial function in individuals with hypertension: A systematic review with meta-analysis. *Journal of the American Society of Hypertenion*, 12(12), e65–e75. https://doi.org/10.1016/j.jash.2018.09.009.

Pentecost, C., & Taket, A. (2011). Understanding exercise uptake and adherence for people with chronic conditions: A new model demonstrating the importance of exercise identity, benefits of attending and support. *Health Education Research*, 26(5), 908–922. https://doi.org/10.1093/her/cyr052. [Seminal Reference].

Peters-Futre, E. M. (1997). Vitamin C, neutrophil function, and upper respiratory tract infection risk in distance runners: The missing link. *Exercise Immunology Review*, 3, 32–52. [Seminal Reference].

Petrella, A. G., Gill, D. P., & Petrella, R. J. (2018). Evaluation of the Get Active Questionnaire in community-dwelling older adults. *Applied Physiology, Nutrition, and Metabolism*, 43(6), 587–594. https://doi.org/10.1139/apnm-2017-0489.

Pisters, M. F., Veenhof, C., Schelleves, F. G., et al. (2010). Exercise adherence improving long-term patient outcome in patients with osteoarthritis of the hip and/or knee. *Arthritis Care & Research*, 62(8), 1087–1094. https://doi.org/10.1002/acr.20182. [Seminal Reference].

Polikandrioti, M., & Dokoutsidou, H. (2009). The role of exercise and nutrition in type II diabetes mellitus management. *Health Science Journal*, 3(4), 216–221 [Seminal Reference].

Poon, M. Y., & Tarrant, M. (2009). Obesity: Attitudes of undergraduate student nurses and registered nurses. *Journal of Clinical Nursing*, 18(16), 2355–2365. https://doi.org/10.1111/j.1365-2702.2008.02709.x. [Seminal Reference].

Public Health Agency of Canada & Canadian Society for Exercise Physiology (PHAC/CSEP). (1998). *Canada's physical activity guide to healthy active living*. Ottawa: Author. [Seminal Reference].

Public Health Agency of Canada & Canadian Society for Exercise Physiology (PHAC/CSEP). (1999). *Physiology: Canada's physical activity guide to healthy active living for older adults*. Ottawa: Author. [Seminal Reference].

Public Health Agency of Canada & Canadian Society for Exercise Physiology (PHAC/CSEP). (2002). *Physiology: Canada's physical activity guide for children and youth*. Ottawa: Author. [Seminal Reference].

Public Health Ontario. (2019). *Daily physical activity in Ontario*. Toronto: Ontario Agency for Health Protection and Promotion. Retrieved from https://www.publichealthontario.ca/en/health-topics/health-promotion/physical-activity/dpa.

Pyne, D. B., Baker, M. S., Fricker, P. A., et al. (1995). Effects of an intensive 12-wk training program by elite swimmers on neutrophil oxidative activity. *Medicine & Science in Sports & Exercise*, 27(4), 536–542. [Seminal Reference].

Quindry, J. C., Franklin, B. A., Chapman, M., et al. (2019). Benefits and risks of high-intensity interval training in patients with coronary artery disease. *American Journal of Cardiology*, 123(8), 1370–1377. https://doi.org/10.1016/j.amjcard.2019.01.008.

Rajjo, T., Mohammed, K., Alsawas, M., et al. (2017). Treatment of pediatric obesity: An umbrella systematic review. *Journal of Clinical Endocrinology & Metabolism*, 102(3), 763–775. https://doi.org/10.1210/jc.2016-2574.

Ranasinghe, C. D., Ranasinghe, P., Jayawardena, R., et al. (2013). Physical activity patterns among South-Asian adults: A systematic review. *The International Journal of Behavioral Nutrition and Physical Activity*, 10(1), 116. https://doi.org/10.1186/1479-5868-10-116.

Rand, D., Miller, W. C., Yiu, J., et al. (2011). Interventions for addressing low balance confidence in older adults: A systematic review and meta-analysis. *Age & Aging*, 40(3), 297–306. https://doi.org/10.1093/ageing/afr037.

Reed, J. L., Prince, S. A., Pipe, A. L., et al. (2018). Influence of the workplace on physical activity and cardiometabolic health: Results of the multi-centre cross-sectional Champlain Nurses' study. *International Journal of Nursing Studies, 81*, 49–60. https://doi.org/10.1016/j.ijnurstu.2018.02.001.

Regnaux, J. P., Lefevre-Colau, M. M., Trinquart, L., et al. (2015). High-intensity versus low-intensity physical activity or exercise in people with hip or knee osteoarthritis. *Cochrane Database Systematic Reviews, 10*, Cd010203. https://doi.org/10.1002/14651858.CD010203.pub2.

Roca, E., Canto, E., Nescolarde, L., et al. (2019). Effects of a polysaccharide-based multi-ingredient supplement on salivary immunity in non-elite marathon runners. *Journal of the International Society of Sports Nutrition, 16*(1), 14. https://doi.org/10.1186/s12970-019-0281-z.

Roman-Vinas, B., Chaput, J. P., Katzmarzyk, P. T., et al. (2016). Proportion of children meeting recommendations for 24-hour movement guidelines and associations with adiposity in a 12-country study. *International Journal of Behavioral Nutrition and Physical Activity, 13*(1), 123–133. https://doi.org/10.1186/s12966-016-0449-8.

Rose, D. J., & Hernandez, D. (2010). The role of exercise in fall prevention for older adults. *Clinics in Geriatric Medicine, 26*(4), 607–631. https://doi.org/10.1016/j.cger.2010.07.003. [Seminal Reference].

Sagar, R., & Gupta, T. (2018). Psychological aspects of obesity in children and adolescents. *The Indian Journal of Pediatrics, 85*(7), 554–559. https://doi.org/10.1007/s12098-017-2539-2.

Sage, M., Middleton, L. E., Tang, A., Sibley, K. M., Brooks, D., & McIlroy, W. (2013). Validity of rating of perceived exertion ranges in individuals in the subacute stage of stroke recovery. *Topics in Stroke Rehabilitation, 20*(6), 519–527. https://doi.org/10.1310/tsr2006-519. [Seminal Reference].

Sax, P. E. (2006). Strategies for management and treatment of dyslipidemia in HIV/AIDS. *AIDS Care, 18*(2), 149–157. [Seminal Reference].

Segal, R., Zwaal, C., Green, E., et al. (2017). Exercise for people with cancer: A clinical practice guideline. *Current Oncology, 24*(1), 40–46. https://doi.org/10.3747/co.24.3376.

Shamliyan, T. A., Kane, R. L., Wyman, J., et al. (2008). Systematic review: Randomized, controlled trials of nonsurgical treatments for urinary incontinence in women. *Annals of Internal Medicine, 148*(6), 459–473. [Seminal Reference].

Shiri, R., Karppinen, J., Leino-Arjas, P., et al. (2010). The association between obesity and low back pain: A meta-analysis. *American Journal of Epidemiology, 171*(2), 135–154. https://doi.org/10.1093/aje/kwp356. [Seminal Reference].

Sigal, R. J., Armstrong, M. J., Bacon, S. L., et al. (2018). Physical activity and diabetes. *Canadian Journal of Diabetes, 42*(Suppl.1), S54–S63. https://doi.org/10.1016/j.jcjd.2017.10.008.

Skinner, J. S., Hutsler, R., Bergsteinova, V., et al. (1973). The validity and reliability of a rating scale of perceived exertion. *Medicine & Science in Sports & Exercise, 5*(2), 94–96. [Seminal Reference].

Smith, S. S., Wang, C. H., & Bloomfield, S. A. (2009). *Osteoporosis. ACSM's exercise management for persons with chronic diseases and disabilities* (3rd ed.). Champaign, IL: Human Kinetics, 270–279. [Seminal Reference].

Smuck, M., Kao, M. C., Brar, N., et al. (2014). Does physical activity influence the relationship between low back pain and obesity? *The Spine Journal: Official Journal of the North American Spine Society, 14*(2), 209–216. https://doi.org/10.1016/j.spinee.2013.11.010.

Smutok, M., Skrinar, G., & Pandolf, K. (1980). Exercise intensity: Subjective regulation by perceived exertion. *Archives of Physical Medicine & Rehabilitation, 61*(12), 569–574. [Seminal Reference].

So, B. C. L., Ng, J. K., & Au, K. C. K. (2019). A 4-week community aquatic physiotherapy program with Ai Chi or Bad Ragaz Ring Method improves disability and trunk muscle endurance in adults with chronic low back pain: A pilot study. *Journal of Back and Musculoskeletal Rehabilitation*, 1–13. https://doi.org/10.3233/bmr-171059.

Soriano-Maldonado, A., Ruiz, J. R., Alvarez-Gallardo, I. C., et al. (2015). Validity and reliability of rating perceived exertion in women with fibromyalgia: Exertion-pain discrimination. *Journal of Sports Sciences, 33*(14), 1515–1522. https://doi.org/10.1080/02640414.2014.994661.

Stagi, S., Cavalli, L., Seminara, S., et al. (2014). The ever-expanding conundrum of primary osteoporosis: Aetiopathogenesis, diagnosis, and treatment. *Italian Journal of Pediatrics, 40*(55), 1–18. https://doi.org/10.1186/1824-7288-40-55.

Stanford, K. I., & Goodyear, L. J. (2014). Exercise and type 2 diabetes: Molecular mechanisms regulating glucose uptake in skeletal muscle. *Advances in Physiology Education, 38*(4), 308–314. https://doi.org/10.1152/advan.00080.2014. [Seminal Reference].

Stanton, R., & Reaburn, P. (2014). Exercise and the treatment of depression: A review of the exercise program variables. *Journal of Science and Medicine in Sport, 17*(2), 177–182. https://doi.org/10.1016/j.jsams.2013.03.010. [Seminal Reference].

Statistics Canada. (2014). *Overweight and obese adults (self-reported), 2014. Health fact sheets (Catalogue no. 82-625-X)*. Ottawa: Author. Retrieved from https://www150.statcan.gc.ca/n1/pub/82-625-x/2015001/article/14185-eng.htm.

Statistics Canada. (2015). *Section 2: Population by age and sex. Annual demographic estimates: Canada, provinces, and territories (Catalogue no. 91-215-X)*. Ottawa: Author. Retrieved from https://www150.statcan.gc.ca/n1/pub/91-215-x/2012000/part-partie2-eng.htm.

Statistics Canada. (2016). *Blood pressure of adults, 2012 to 2015. Health fact sheets (Catalogue no. 82-625-X)*. Ottawa: Author. Retrieved from https://www150.statcan.gc.ca/n1/pub/82-625-x/2016001/article/14657-eng.htm.

Statistics Canada. (2017a). *Age and sex, and type of dwelling data: Key results from the 2016 Census. The daily, may 3*. Ottawa: Author. Retrieved from https://www150.statcan.gc.ca/n1/daily-quotidien/170503/dq170503a-eng.htm.

Statistics Canada. (2017b). *Census in brief: A portrait of the population aged 85 and older in 2016 in Canada*. Ottawa: Author. Retrieved from. https://www12.statcan.gc.ca/census-recensement/2016/as-sa/98-200-x/2016004/98-200-x2016004-eng.cfm.

Stephens, I. (2019). Case report: The use of medical yoga for adolescent mental health. *Complementary Therapies in Medicine, 43*, 60–65. https://doi.org/10.1016/j.ctim.2019.01.006.

Stolee, P., Zara, C., & Schuehlein, S. (2012). Evaluation of a volunteer-led in-home program for home-bound older adults. *Work (Reading, Mass.), 41*(3), 339–354. https://doi.org/10.3233/WOR-2012-1304.

Strasser, B., Siebert, U., & Schobersberger, W. (2010). Resistance training in the treatment of the metabolic syndrome. *Sports Medicine, 40*(5), 397–415. [Seminal Reference].

Stubbs, B., Vancampfort, D., Rosenbaum, S., et al. (2017). An examination of the anxiolytic effects of exercise for people with anxiety and stress-related disorders: A meta-analysis. *Psychiatry Research, 249*, 102–108. https://doi.org/10.1016/j.psychres.2016.12.020.

Swinburn, B. A., Kraak, V. I., Allender, S., et al. (2019). The global syndemic of obesity, undernutrition, and climate change: The Lancet Commission report. *The Lancet, 393*(10173), 791–846. https://doi.org/10.1016/S0140-6736(18)32822-8.

Tajik, A., Rejeh, N., Heravi-Karimooi, M., et al. (2018). The effect of Tai Chi on quality of life in male older people: A randomized controlled clinical trial. *Complementary Therapies in Clinical Practice, 33*, 191–196. https://doi.org/10.1016/j.ctcp.2018.10.009.

Tambalis, K., Panagiotakis, D. B., Kavouras, S. A., et al. (2009). Responses of blood lipids to aerobic, resistance, and combined aerobic with resistance exercise training: A systematic review of current evidence. *Angiology, 60*(5), 614–832. https://doi.org/10.1177/0003319708324927. [Seminal Reference].

Teixeira, P. J., Carraça, E. V., Markland, D., et al. (2012). Exercise, physical activity, and self-determination theory: A systematic review. *Inter-*

national Journal of Behavioral Nutrition and Physical Activity, 9(78), 1–30. https://doi.org/10.1186/1479-5868-9-78. [Seminal Reference].

Terry, L., Sprinz, E., Stein, R., et al. (2006). Exercise training in HIV-1-infected individuals with dyslipidemia and lipodystrophy. Medicine & Science in Sports & Exercise, 38(3), 411–417. https://doi.org/10.1249/01.mss.0000191347.73848.80. [Seminal Reference].

Tremblay, A., Despres, J. P., & Bouchard, C. (1985). The effects of exercise-training on energy balance and adipose tissue morphology and metabolism. Sports Medicine, 2(3), 223–233. https://doi.org/10.2165/00007256-198502030-00005. [Seminal Reference].

Tremblay, M. S., Chaput, J. P., Adamo, K. B., et al. (2017). Canadian 24-hour movement guidelines for the early years (0–4 years): An integration of physical activity, sedentary behaviour, and sleep. BMC Public Health, 17(Suppl. 5), 874. https://doi.org/10.1186/s12889-017-4859-6.

Tremblay, M. S., Kho, M. E., Tricco, A. C., et al. (2010). Process description and evaluation of Canadian Physical Activity Guidelines development. International Journal of Behavioral Nutrition and Physical Activity, 7, 42. https://doi.org/10.1186/1479-5868-7-42. [Seminal Reference].

Tremblay, M. S., Warburton, D. E., Janssen, I., et al. (2011). New Canadian physical activity guidelines. Applied Physiology, Nutrition, and Metabolism, 36(1), 36–46, 47–58. https://doi.org/10.1139/H11-009.

Turner, J. E., Lira, V. A., & Brum, P. C. (2017). New insights into the benefits of physical activity and exercise for aging and chronic disease. Oxidative Medicine and Cellular Longevity, 2017, 2503767. https://doi.org/10.1155/2017/2503767. [Seminal Reference].

Uhlig, T., Fongen, C., Steen, E., et al. (2010). Exploring tai chi in rheumatoid arthritis: A quantitative and qualitative study. BMC Musculoskeletal Disorders, 11(43), 1–7. https://doi.org/10.1186/1471-2474-11-43. [Seminal Reference].

U.S. Department of Health and Human Services (USDHHS). (2015). Prevention and wellness. Retrieved from https://www.hhs.gov/programs/prevention-and-wellness/index.html.

Veldhuijzen van Zanten, J. J., Rouse, P. C., Hale, E. D., et al. (2015). Perceived barriers, facilitators and benefits for regular physical activity and exercise in patients with rheumatoid arthritis: A review of the literature. Sports Medicine (Auckland, N.Z.), 45(10), 1401–1412. https://doi.org/10.1007/s40279-015-0363-2.

Visceglia, E., & Lewis, S. (2011). Yoga as an adjunctive treatment for schizophrenia: A randomized, controlled pilot study. Journal of Alternative & Complementary Medicine, 17(7), 601–607. https://doi.org/10.1089/acm.2010.0075. [Seminal Reference].

Vrablík, M., & Češka, R. (2015). Treatment of hypertriglyceridemia: A review of current options. Physiological Research/Academia Scientiarum Bohemoslovaca, 64(Suppl. 3), S331–S340.

Waller, B., Ogonowska-Slodownik, A., Vitor, M., et al. (2014). Effect of therapeutic aquatic exercise on symptoms and function associated with lower limb osteoarthritis: Systematic review with meta-analysis. Physical Therapy, 94(10), 1383–1395. [Seminal Reference].

Walsh, J. N., Manor, B., Hausdorff, J., et al. (2015). Impact of short- and long-term tai chi mind-body exercise training on cognitive function in healthy adults: Results from a hybrid observational study and randomized trial. Global Advances in Health and Medicine, 4(4), 38–48. https://doi.org/10.7453/gahmj.2015.058.

Walsh, N. P., & Oliver, S. J. (2016). Exercise, immune function and respiratory infection: An update on the influence of training and environmental stress. Immunology and Cell Biology, 94(2), 132–139. https://doi.org/10.1038/icb.2015.99.

Walsh, N. P., Gleeson, M., Shephard, R. J., et al. (2011). Position statement. Part one: Immune function and exercise. Exercise Immunology Review, 17, 6–63. [Seminal Reference].

Wang, C. W., Chan, C. H., Ho, R. T., et al. (2014). Managing stress and anxiety through qigong exercise in healthy adults: A systematic review and meta-analysis of randomized controlled trials. BMC Complementary and Alternative Medicine, 14(8). https://doi.org/10.1186/1472-6882-14-8.

Wang, C., Bannru, R., Ramel, J., et al. (2010). Tai chi on psychological well-being: Systematic review and meta-analysis. BMC Complementary and Alternative Medicine, 10, 23. https://doi.org/10.1186/1472-6882-10-23. [Seminal Reference].

Wang, F., Lee, E. K., Wu, T., et al. (2014). The effects of tai chi on depression, anxiety, and psychological well-being: A systematic review and meta-analysis. International Journal of Behavioral Medicine, 21(4), 605–617. https://doi.org/10.1007/s12529-013-9351-9.

Warburton, D. E., Charlesworth, S., Ivey, A., et al. (2010). A systematic review of the evidence for Canada's Physical Activity Guidelines for Adults. International Journal of Behavioral Nutritional and Physical Activity, 7, 39. https://doi.org/10.1186/1479-5868-7-39.

Warburton, D. E., Jamnik, V. K., Bredin, S. S., et al. (2011). Evidence-based risk assessment and recommendations for physical activity clearance: An introduction. Applied Physiology, Nutrition and Metabolism, 36(Suppl. 1), S1–S2. https://doi.org/10.1139/h11-060. [Seminal Reference].

Waryasz, G. R., & McDermott, A. Y. (2010). Exercise prescription and the patient with type 2 diabetes: A clinical approach to optimizing patient outcomes. Journal of American Academy of Nurse Practitioners, 22, 217–227. https://doi.org/10.1111/j.1745-7599.2010.00490.x. [Seminal Reference].

Wayne, P. M., Walsh, J. N., Taylor-Piliae, R. E., et al. (2014). The impact of tai chi on cognitive performance in older adults: A systematic review and meta-analysis. Journal of the American Geriatrics Society, 62(1), 25–39. https://doi.org/10.1111/jgs.12611.

Wegner, M., Helmich, I., Machado, S., et al. (2014). Effects of exercise on anxiety and depression disorders: Review of meta analyses and neurobiological mechanisms. CNS and Neurological Disorders Drug Targets, 13(6), 1002–1014. https://doi.org/10.1139/h11-060.

Weltman, N. Y., Saliba, S. A., Barrett, E. J., et al. (2009). The use of exercise in the management of type 1 and type 2 diabetes. Clinics in Sports Medicine, 28(3), 423–439. https://doi.org/10.1016/j.csm.2009.02.006. [Seminal Reference].

West, S. L. C., Caterini, J., Banks, L., et al. (2018). The epidemic of obesity and poor physical activity participation: Will we ever see a change? Journal of Functional Morphometry and Kinesiology, 3(2), 34. https://doi.org/10.3390/jfmk3020034.

Whitaker, R. C., Wright, J. A., Pepe, M. S., et al. (1997). Predicting obesity in young adulthood from childhood and parental obesity. New England Journal of Medicine, 337(13), 869–b873. https://doi.org/10.1056/nejm199709253371301. [Seminal Reference].

World Health Organization (WHO). (2017). 10 facts on physical activity. Retrieved from http://www.who.int/features/factfiles/physical_activity/en/.

World Health Organization (WHO). (2010). Global recommendations on physical activity for health. Geneva: Author. Retrieved from https://www.who.int/dietphysicalactivity/global-PA-recs-2010.pdf. [Seminal Reference].

World Health Organization (WHO). (1986). The Ottawa charter for health promotion: 1st international conference on health promotion. Ottawa, ON, 17–21. [Seminal Reference]

Wu, Y., Johnson, B. T., Acabchuk, R. L., et al. (2019). Yoga as antihypertensive lifestyle therapy: A systematic review and meta-analysis. Mayo Clinic Proceedings, 94(3), 432–446. https://doi.org/10.1016/j.mayocp.2018.09.023.

Zhao, R., Zhang, M., & Zhang, Q. (2017). The effectiveness of combined exercise interventions for preventing postmenopausal bone loss: A systematic review and meta-analysis. Journal of Orthopedic Sports Physical Therapy, 47(4), 241–251. https://doi.org/10.2519/jospt.2017.6969.

# 23

# Stress Management

*Shannon Dames, MPH, EdD*

Originating US chapter by *June Andrews Horowitz, FAAN, CNS-BC, PMH, RN, PhD*

## INTENDED LEARNING OUTCOMES

*After completing this chapter, the reader will be able to:*

- Analyze concepts of stress, stressor, eustress, and distress.
- Evaluate physical, psychological, social, spiritual, and behavioural stressors that are potential contributors to physical and mental health disorders.
- Analyze the pathophysiology of the stress response and effects on health and illness.
- Examine primary and secondary cognitive appraisals of stress.
- Develop evidence-informed stress-management interventions that can be used in clinical practice.
- Explain the nurse's role in stress management and crisis intervention.

## KEY TERMS

Active listening
Acupuncture
Affirmation
Anxiety sensitivity
Aromatherapy
Assertive communication
Burnout
Caregiver stress/burden
Cognitive restructuring
Coping
Distress
Empathy
Eustress
Exercise
Expressive writing
Fight-or-flight response

Goal setting
Healthy diet
Healthy pleasures
Homeostasis
Homeodynamics
Humour
Hypnosis
Interplay
Journal writing
Meridian
Mindfulness
Mini relaxations
Presence
Primary appraisal
Reiki
Relaxation response

Sandwich generation
Secondary appraisal
Self-awareness
Self-care
Sleep hygiene
Social support
Sociophysiology
Spillover stress
Spiritual practice
Stress
Stress management
Stress response
Stress warning signs
Stressor
Values clarification
Yoga

## ❓ THINK ABOUT IT

### *Do We Live to Work or Work to Live?*

When asked about yourself, what is your first response? Do you say what you do for work, or do you describe your characteristics? For most of us, our work roles, including being students, define us to a great extent. For most adults who live in industrialized countries and many other societies, employment is a primary source of income and social connection; working also contributes to a personal sense of accomplishment. However, how much work is too much? Canadians take fewer yearly vacation days than most of their counterparts in other industrialized countries, and workplace pressures can increase the risk of a variety of disorders. Work-related stress can be a significant problem.

- What aspects of work typically create stress?
- How do people manage work-related stress? Which strategies are effective and which strategies increase health risks?
- How do people manage the work–home life balance (spillover stress)?
- What health-promotion strategies could you implement to reduce your own work-related stress?
- What could you do to promote workplace health in your own practice?

Stress is an excellent paradigm for understanding the relationships among the determinants of health, the leading health indicators, and health outcomes. Stress has been shown to cause or exacerbate many of the leading health problems in the Canada today, such as those related to obesity, alcohol, and drug abuse, poverty, and sexually transmitted infections (Government of Canada, 2018; Sampasa-Kanyinga & Chaput, 2017). In 2014, 23% of Canadians over the age of 15 years reported that most days were highly stressful (Statistics Canada, 2014). Consequently, helping individuals, families, and communities to find more effective ways to respond to stress is an important health-promotion goal. The Public Health Agency of Canada works to support Canadian people in making healthy choices where they live and work.

Stress management has been an effective intervention framework for health promotion, disease prevention, and symptom management. Stress-management strategies such as relaxation and imagery, self-monitoring, goal setting, cognitive restructuring, mindfulness, and problem-solving have long been staples of community health-promotion programs, including Alcoholics Anonymous, Smoke Enders, and Weight Watchers. These strategies help people to modify health risk behaviours and thereby improve quality of life. However, national health trends indicate the need for continued and expanded use of these modalities across the life span. Although the Canada's health care system provides excellent care, it fails to address many preventable conditions, including those related to stress. Moreover, to ameliorate many harmful effects of stress, community-level health promotion is essential. Continuing to shift focus from providing acute care for individuals to enhancing the health of communities by successful community health-promotion initiatives holds promise for the future.

The goal of stress management is to improve quality of life by increasing healthy, effective coping and self-care, thereby reducing unhealthy consequences of distress. This process produces a dynamic interaction of mind, body, and spirit, which influences physical health and well-being. Self-care describes our ability to consciously take a nurturing action that promotes our mental, emotional, physical, and/or spiritual health. Stress management is thus an essential tool for expert nursing practice, which recognizes the interface of knowledge on behaviour change. The use of critical reasoning to examine multiple factors contributing to symptom development provides a valuable contribution to improving the health of Canadians. While stress begins in the mind as a result of threatening thoughts, it has profound effects on our mental and physical health. In addition to the mental health impacts, stress contributes to high blood pressure, stroke, heart disease, immunity, and circulatory consequences (Statistics Canada, 2014). This chapter outlines the multifaceted psychophysiological aspects of stress, examines strategies shown to mediate its harmful effects, reviews examples of clinical situations in which stress management has been effective, and explores the unique perspective nurses bring that helps individuals identify healthy stress-management strategies.

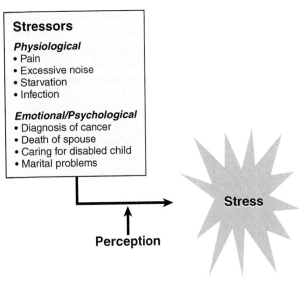

**Fig. 23.1** Stressors can be physiological or emotional/psychological. Perception of the stressors will determine whether they cause stress. (From Lewis, S. L., Dirksen, S. R., Heitkemper, M. M., et al. [2014]. *Medical-surgical nursing: Assessment and management of clinical problems* [9th ed.]. St Louis: Mosby.)

## SOURCES OF STRESS

A stressor is any psychological, social, environmental, physiological, or spiritual stimulus that disrupts the tendency of a system, especially the physiological system of higher animals, to maintain internal stability, owing to the coordinated response of its parts to any situation or stimulus that would tend to disturb its normal condition or function. Although in use for more than 100 years, the term has suggested balance and stability but has also denoted interchange and continuous regulated or balanced change (Bortz, 2015). In other words, homeostasis has connoted a state of balance thereby requiring change or adaptation—not a static state (Fig. 23.1). To reflect advances in science that underscore the continuously changing nature of and interaction among life processes in all of its manifestations, the term homeodynamics has emerged in the past decade (Bortz, 2015) as a better descriptor:

*Homeodynamics extends homeostasis into a more inclusive term. It is evident that there is no stasis in life. All of life is dynamic. 98% of a body's atoms are replaced each year. The Krebs cycle turns over 2.66 × 10²¹ times per minute. The half-life of an intestinal cell is measured in days. Stasis is nowhere to be found. Life is a verb rather than a noun.*

Stress is understood as a state of threatened homeostasis/homeodynamics that triggers an array of adaptive physiological, behavioural, and even social responses in an effort to re-establish homeostasis or relative balance to avoid chaos. These descriptions of stress underscore important ideas: even welcome events, such as a child's wedding, are stressors because they precipitate change. Nonetheless, stress is not intrinsically bad or unhealthy, and stress is experienced psychophysiologically and socially (i.e., as an *interplay* across all domains of individual and communal living). Stress is an essential component of being alive. Stress can be situational or maturational. One's coping strategies and resources will determine the outcomes of each stressful experience. Moreover, family and communal/social response will also affect many responses to shared stress. In this age of instant messaging and 24/7 news cycles, the communal shared nature of stress is intensified.

Individuals encounter a variety of physical, psychological, social, spiritual, and environmental stressors. These stressors are not simply an additive but rather have an interactive effect within a homeodynamic human–ecological system. Stressors range from health and illness experiences, such as childbirth, physical illness, trauma, or blood loss, to activities of daily living, such as caring for children, meeting work deadlines, and cleaning or repairing the house, to less common events, such as taking a critical examination, experiencing the death of a relative, losing possessions in a fire, losing a job, getting a divorce, or getting married, and environmental contexts. As a useful rubric, stressors can be organized into three categories: stressors over which people have no control (extrinsic factors), such as the weather, a traffic jam, or the death of a spouse; stressors that individuals can modify by changing their environment, social interactions, or behaviours; and stressors created or exacerbated (intrinsic factors) by poor time management, procrastination, poor communication, catastrophic negative thinking (expecting the worst), or struggling with self-defeating behaviours. However, stressors can never be neatly boxed into simple categories; stress is a person–environment process. The person–environment fit model indicates that the person appraises a situation as taxing or as exceeding his or her resources and endangering well-being. Moreover, links between biological pathways and social adversity to subsequent adverse health outcomes underscore the importance of stress as a health determinant (Berger, Juster, & Sarnyai, 2015; Lazarus & Folkman, 1984; Weber, 2011).

Workplace stress is another major source of stress for many. For example, in caregiving professions, the research shows that workplace stress has alarming physical and mental consequences (Leiter, Price, & Spence Laschinger, 2010). In 2017, the Canadian Medical Association's National Physician Health Survey found that 49% of residents and 33% of physicians screened positive for depression, and 38% of residents and 29% of physicians screened positive for burnout (Simon & McFadden, 2017). In 2015, the Manitoba Nurses Union launched a formal strategy to address the 64% of caregivers suffering from emotional exhaustion and the 52% suffering from critical incident stress and post-traumatic stress disorder (Manitoba Nurses Union, 2015).

When basic human needs go unmet, we experience chronic stress (emerging as anxiety and/or depression) until they are satisfied (Dames, 2018; Maslow, 1943). As caregivers, we don't get to thrive while under the cloud of chronic stress that rises up when our basic human needs go unsatisfied. If unchecked, chronic stress leads to emotional exhaustion and eventual burnout. Prolonged levels of stress, fuelled

by feelings of insecurity, is a normal part of the work for many caregivers.

Burnout affects every care provider, if not directly then indirectly, as they feel the ripple effects from struggling coworkers. Burnout is comprised of three components: (1) emotional exhaustion, (2) depersonalization (detachment from the "real" self), and (3) diminished sense of accomplishment (Maslach & Jackson, 1986). Work environments that fail to meet basic human requirements drive the ubiquity and severity of this caregiver stress. In turn, caregiver stress is fuels addiction, anxiety, depression, suicide, and attrition rates among caregivers.

Stress appraisal is an important concept that helps to explain why two people react in different ways to the same situation. In addition, models of stress have evolved from an individualistic perspective to consideration of family-level and community-level stress and coping (Weber, 2011).

The shared situation of Ms. Khan (86 years old) and Ms. Goldman (86 years old), both in good health, provides a case in point. Both individuals are about to become new residents at an assisted living retirement community in their hometown. Ms. Khan perceives this move as an opportunity to increase the ease of her socializations and activities of daily living, and is looking forward to making new friends and participating in new recreational activities. In contrast, Ms. Goldman views this move as abandonment by her family and fears that the available resources will be inadequate. Although the event is virtually the same for both Ms. Khan and Ms. Goldman, the homeodynamic consequences are personalized because each woman perceives her situation differently. Even though the move to the new environment is the same, each woman has different coping styles and each has different support systems, so the experience will differ in its perception and thereby its level of stress.

Stress is the physical, psychological, social, or spiritual effect of life's pressures and events. Stress is an interactive hemodynamic process that involves appraisal and response to loss or the threat of loss of well-being at individual, family, and community levels (Weber, 2011). Canadian physiologist Hans Selye (1950, 1974, 1982) first introduced the general adaptation syndrome, which led the way to continual interest in stress and the effect on the body. Selye reported that, to a certain extent, stress can be challenging and useful, which he identified as eustress. Selye also observed that when stress becomes chronic or excessive, the body is unable to adapt and maintain homeostasis, and thus the process becomes distress. Stress can be both useful and harmful. As stress increases, efficiency and performance also increase, but not endlessly. At a certain point performance and efficiency start to decrease significantly if stress continues unabated. It is important to understand the many causes of stress and the negative physical, psychosocial, and spiritual consequences of distress. Understanding the many-sided sources of stress provides the rationale for a multifaceted approach to its management. It is noteworthy that even in its early understanding, scientists and clinicians recognized the dynamic

As an example of how stress can contribute to disease, researchers exploring the relationship between stress and breast cancer have demonstrated a relationship among stress (personality traits, stressful life events, and responses to stress), the immune system, genetics, and environmental factors. The physiological influences of stress on breast cancer may be mediated by the immune system. Although women may be unable to prevent stress in their lives, learning stress management strategies may improve the quality of life for individuals and their families with or at risk of breast cancer.

Growing research evidence supports this understanding of the complex interactions between life stress and breast cancer risk. For example, Kruk (2012) examined the relationship between severe life events and breast cancer risk. Kruk used case-control examination of 858 Polish patients with invasive breast cancer and 1095 controls matched for age and place of residence. Data on life events, sociodemographic characteristics, reproductive factors, family history of breast cancer, current weight and height, and lifestyle habits were collected via a self-administered questionnaire. Unconditional logistic regression analyses with odds ratios with 95% confidence intervals were estimated. After adjustment for potential breast cancer risk factors, women with four to six individual major life events had 5.33 times higher risk of breast cancer compared with those in the lowest quartile. Similarly, women with a high lifetime life change score had approximately five times higher risk compared to women with corresponding scores in the lowest range. Several life events (death of a close family member, personal injury or illness, imprisonment/trouble with the law, retirement) were significantly associated with breast cancer risk. Those findings suggest that major life events may have an important etiological role in the development of breast cancer. Surviving breast cancer also poses ongoing challenges to women who experienced breast cancer and their partners (Gregorio et al., 2012).

Sources: Gregorio, S. W., Carpenter, K. M., Dorfman, C. S., Yang, I. L. C., Simonelli, L. F., & Carson III, W. E. (2012). Impact of breast cancer recurrence and cancer-specific stress on spouse health and immune function. *Brain, Behavior, & Immunity, 26*(2), 228–233; Kruk, J. (2012). Self-reported psychological stress and the risk of breast cancer: A case-control study. *Stress, 15*(2), 162–171; National Cancer Institute. (n.d.). *Psychological stress and cancer: Questions and answers.* Retrieved from http://www.cancer.gov/cancertopics/factsheet/Risk/stress.

changing nature of stress and its many human system responses (Box 23.1).

In nursing, we have operated within multiple frameworks to understand stress and its outcomes. Historically nursing has been grounded in the biological and medical sciences because of our long-standing roles in health promotion and caring for people experiencing illness. Yet over many decades nursing frameworks have also embraced concepts of continuous change and interaction in human-environmental fields. Most notably Martha Rogers's science of unitary human beings (Phillips, 2015; Willis, DeSanto-Madeya, Ross, et al., 2015), Neuman's systems model, and Roy's adaptation model (Willis et al., 2015) have stressed the dynamic, interactive nature of human life. As a result, nurses have learned to balance and integrate the worldviews of traditional medical and bench science with the evolving and sometimes rather heretical nursing frameworks that focused more on continual change and interaction within and among human-environmental systems. Thus in this chapter, examining stress,

its manifestations, and approaches to ameliorate distress and associated health problems involves weaving knowledge and understanding generated from diverse and sometimes conflicting perspectives.

The models for understanding human stress are multifaceted and complex. In the past, scientists and clinicians tended to examine and understand stress from their own disciplinary or scientific silos. In other words, understanding stress was typically split into neurobiological and psychosocial camps. However, in recent decades sociophysiology has emerged as a multidisciplinary perspective to integrate the "social" and "biological" worlds to answer the following question (Barchas & Barchas, 2011): "How do social processes impact the physiology of the organism and how does that altered physiology affect future social behaviour?"

Nursing science has long held an interest in the dynamic interaction among human systems. Outstanding among nurses' voices calling for innovative perspectives to topple the traditional and accepted mechanistic, medical worldview was Martha Rogers's theory of unitary human beings (Phillips, 2015). Phillips, a valued colleague of Rogers, described her as a heretic and heroine because of her then revolutionary view about nursing and health and illness. Today her ideas resonate well with contemporary understandings of the rapidly evolving interplay across all spheres of human life.

Thus understanding stress and its management involves attention to the *interactions* of social and biological life at individual and family/communal levels. It follows that stress-management strategies/interventions need to be multifaceted and could be aimed at neurophysiological and interpersonal/social stressors and/or interactions and responses. Establishing empathy by the nurse in understanding stress is beneficial in designing interventions aimed at primary, secondary, and tertiary levels of prevention.

## PHYSICAL, PSYCHOLOGICAL, SOCIOBEHAVIOURAL, AND SPIRITUAL/ HOMEODYNAMIC CONSEQUENCES OF STRESS

To begin, it is necessary to set the groundwork for understanding stress and its multifaceted/interactive consequences. In the discussion that follows, facets of human responses are artificially categorized and discussed to help the learner to discern the many aspects of stress responses. In no way should this content be interpreted as meaning that stress responses are isolated to specific human systems or simply additive. Growing understanding of the homeodynamic interplay, including epigenetics, within individuals and across human and ecological systems, forces us to examine the ever-changing nature of our knowledge of our world. As a startling example, in 2016 the Zika virus emerged on the global stage to pose multiple human health risks, with a specific threat to pregnant women and their fetuses for microcephaly, a devastating birth anomaly: the effects reverberated across continents with lightning speed and had global effects on health, travel, and prevention efforts (Sifferlin, 2016). Thus we all must remain cognizant of the ongoing interplay within and among human, social, and ecological systems, even as we examine knowledge focused predominantly at specific response areas (i.e., human systems). Nevertheless, understanding stress effects at a variety of micro to macro levels is needed to comprehend a holistic picture. The future challenges to do so are indeed exciting!

## Physiological Effects of Stress

An individual's homeodynamic response to stress provides a model to examine changes across biopsychosocial–spiritual domains. In response to a perceived threat (i.e., stressor), the body prepares to meet the challenge. Perception of threat stimulates a physiological pattern of neuroendocrine activation and behavioural changes mediated by the central nervous system. Moreover, chronic stressful life circumstances likely exacerbate conditions favourable to adverse health outcomes (Fig. 23.2) (Berger et al., 2015). Nonetheless, in most cases, this reaction is an adaptive, short-term, acute response to a stressor. First termed the fight-or-flight response (Cannon, 1914) and later called the stress response (Selye, 1950, 1974, 1982), the individual's reaction to a real or imagined threat prepares the body for emergency reaction and fosters survival in circumstances of immediate, time-limited threat. The hypothalamus signals the sympathetic nervous system to release epinephrine and norepinephrine, along with other related hormones. A resultant state of arousal is characterized by increased metabolism, pulse rate, blood pressure, respiration rate, and muscle tension. This physiological arousal proceeds along three main pathways: the musculoskeletal system, the autonomic nervous system, and the psychoneuroendocrine system.

The musculoskeletal system responds by increasing tension and tone. At the same time, the autonomic nervous system, via the sympathetic branch, orchestrates a generalized arousal that includes increases in heart rate, blood pressure, and respiration rate. In addition, a heightened awareness of the environment is triggered, and blood shifts from the visceral organs to the large muscle groups. Concurrently the psychoneuroendocrine system stimulates the hypothalamic-pituitary-adrenal axis and the secretion of corticosteroids (primarily cortisol) and other neuroendocrine substances into the systemic circulation, increasing blood glucose levels, influencing sodium retention, and, in the acute phase, increasing the anti-inflammatory response.

Chronic stress exposure increases the risk of poor health outcomes for a host of health conditions (Slavich, 2016). Pro-inflammation associated with stress is emerging as a common pathway in a variety of diseases, such as asthma, angina, cardiac arrhythmias, pain, tension headaches, insomnia, depression, and gastrointestinal disorders. Additionally, stress can produce hyperreactivity or hyporeactivity of hormones regulated by the psychoneuroendocrine system (Ebner & Singewald, 2017).

As mentioned previously, in most cases the stress response is a beneficial adaptive pattern that increases the efficiency and quality of performance, but it can prove maladaptive when a stressor continues indefinitely. Maladaptive stress (distress) is an enduring and sometimes self-sustaining cascade of responses that degenerate physical, psychosocial, and spiritual well-being. Not surprisingly, stress and specifically depression have been associated with increased susceptibility to cardiovascular disease, as well as poor response to its treatment. Inflammation has been suggested as one of the processes underlying the association between cardiovascular disease and depression, two debilitating conditions (Nikkheslat, Zunszin, Horowitz, et al., 2015). Nonetheless, indirect influences of stress and depression on self-caring health behaviours also help to explain associations between these diseases. Needless to say, further investigation is needed to demonstrate direct causal links, as well as effectiveness of psychological intervention for people with cardiovascular disease (Richards, Anderson, Jenkinson, et al., 2017).

## Psychological Effects of Stress

The psychological effects of stress are best illustrated by its contributory role in negative mood states, including anxiety, depression, hostility, and anger. Exposure to stressful stimuli is associated with elevated cortisol levels and resultant effects on the immune system. The duration, intensity, and timing of a stressor have been shown to affect immune responses in animals. Although systematic studies to explain different patterns of immune response with humans are not yet adequate, the interactive nature of the mind and immune system is an exciting area of investigation that may contribute to future evidence-informed practice (Louveau, Harris, & Kipnis, 2015).

A growing body of clinical research outcomes illustrates the interplay of stress and various health outcomes. For example, research evidence is convincing that individuals with post-traumatic stress disorder (PTSD) are at higher risk for eating disorders (Trottier & MacDonald, 2017). The relationship between stress and cardiac symptoms also is well documented. Stress is more about one's interpretation of the event rather than about the event itself. Clinical implications include reducing perceived stress and ruminative, angry coping styles by encouraging reappraisal and support seeking. In conclusion, the evidence to date demonstrates a strong association between chronic stress and negative health effects for individuals and their family members.

## Sociobehavioural Effects of Stress

In response to stress, individuals often revert to or increase their reliance on less healthy behaviours, such as over-eating, excessive use of alcohol or drugs, and smoking. Recognizing that such behaviours are inconsistent with the healthy behaviours needed to cope with stress is easy; however, stopping these behaviours and using health-promoting strategies instead is not. For example, stress promotes addictive behaviours such as smoking, substance abuse, and overeating, leading to increased morbidity and mortality (Canadian Centre on Substance Use and Addiction & University of Victoria, 2018; Sinha & Jastreboff, 2013). Conversely, exercise, healthy diet, smoking cessation, healthy weight maintenance, and social interaction are

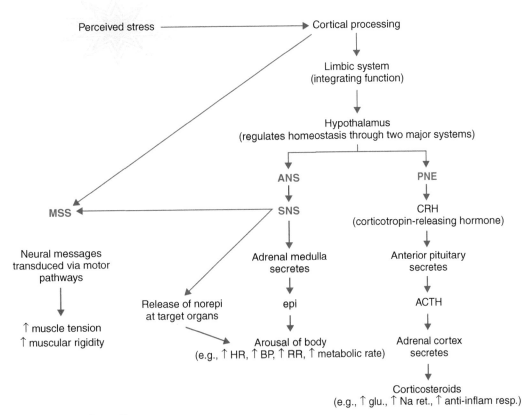

**Fig. 23.2 The Stress Response**
*ACTH,* Adrenocorticotropic hormone; *ANS,* autonomic nervous system; *anti-inflam resp.,* anti-inflammatory response; *BP,* blood pressure; *CRH,* corticotropin-releasing hormone; *epi,* epinephrine; *glu.,* blood glucose level; *HR,* heart rate; *MSS,* musculoskeletal system; *Na ret.,* sodium retention; *norepi,* norepinephrine; *PNE,* pituitary-neuroendocrine system; *RR,* respiration rate; *SNS,* sympathetic nervous system. (From Wells-Federman, C., Stuart-Shor, E., Deckro, J., Mandle, C. L., Baim, M., & Medich, C. [1995]. The mind/body connection: The psychophysiology of many traditional nursing interventions. *Clinical Nurse Specialist, 9,* 60.)

leading indicators of health (World Health Organization [WHO], 2018). Encouraging these health behaviours supports the goals of the Public Health Agency of Canada to support Canada's public health priorities (PHAC, 2017). However, unless we understand how psychosocial factors affect health behaviours, promotion of effective self-care is an unrealistic goal (Box 23.2).

## Spiritual Effects of Stress

Interest in the connection between spirituality and health is significant. Spirituality is defined in many ways, but key components are typically that spirituality comprises feelings, thoughts, experiences, and behaviours that arise from a search for meaning and may include interconnectedness with self, others, nature, and a higher force called God, a life-force/higher power, nature, or the transcendent. Spirituality and religion intersect for many, yet they are not synonymous. Many individuals feel spiritual without a formal religious affiliation or practice. In response to stress, people often feel disconnected from life's meaning and purpose; harmful effects on their health and well-being can result. Stressful events can shatter individuals' spiritual centre or conversely can move individuals to seek comfort in spirituality or religious practice, beliefs, or community. Encouraging

involvement with one's religious/spiritual practices is recommended as a helpful intervention for stress-related problems (Weber, 2011).

Examination of spiritual healing in the aftermath of men's childhood mistreatment through nursing research unearthed the following themes (Willis et al., 2015):

- Exploring spiritual faith traditions as a foundation for spiritual healing
- Being in spiritual community serves as a foundation for spiritual healing
- Being in spiritual community facilities healing connections with other human beings and the transcendent
- Cultivating spiritual consciousness through prayer, music, yoga, nature, and reading spiritual material expands awareness of one's spiritual being
- Loving and letting go reflects one's spirituality and humanity
- Believing in a cosmic energy, divine purpose, or higher power can bring a sense of healing

These themes provide foundations for nursing interventions to be tested (Willis et al., 2015). Engaging a pastoral counsellor of the individual's choice in the treatment team can be an effective strategy to promote spiritual healing. However, the source of mistreatment must be carefully explored sensitively with the

## BOX 23.2   Health-Related Quality of Life and Well-Being

Health-related quality of life (HRQoL) is multi-faceted, including factors related to physical, mental, emotional, and social functioning; it goes beyond independent measures of health, to focus on the link between health status and quality of life. A related concept of HRQoL is well-being, which reflects the positive aspects of life, such as pleasant emotions and satisfaction with life. As explained in this chapter, stress is a challenge to HRQoL; therefore, stress management promotes HRQoL.

Source: US Department of Health and Human Services. (2014). *Health-related quality of life & well-being.* Retrieved from http://healthypeople.gov/2020/topicsobjectives2020/overview.aspx?topicid=19.

individual in advance to determine the acceptability of engaging a member of the clergy.

The previous section discussed how stress can adversely affect biological, cognitive, emotional, behavioural, and spiritual well-being. This understanding of the psychophysiology of the mind-body-spirit connection is fundamental to the application of stress management in nursing and provides an obvious rationale for a multifaceted approach. Further support is provided from research endorsing the health-promoting effects of managing stress (Gregorio, Carpenter, Dorfman, et al., 2012) (Research for Evidence-Informed Practice).

## RESEARCH FOR EVIDENCE-INFORMED PRACTICE

### Impact of Breast Cancer Recurrence and Cancer-Specific Stress on Spouse Health and Immune Function

Spouses of people with cancer are often primary informal caregivers for their partners. As a group, they experience a variety of poor health outcomes. This study examined the relative contributions of cancer recurrence—a cancer-specific stressful event—and the subjective experience of cancer-specific stress in a sample of male spouses of breast cancer survivors. The investigators hypothesized that stress would contribute to poorer physical health and compromised immune function.

Given the difficulty of random assignment for this type of study, the researchers used a matched-control design, comparing spouses of women with recurrence to a cohort of spouses whose wives were disease-free but had a history of breast cancer. Spouses of women experiencing a first recurrence were matched to spouses of women with no evidence of disease. The results showed that cancer recurrence status was not a significant predictor of spouses' physical health or immune function; however, among all spouses, cancer-specific stress symptoms were associated with increased physical symptoms and altered T-cell blastogenesis. These findings suggest that health effects for these caregiving spouses were more strongly connected to their subjective experience of cancer as stressful, rather than their partners' current disease status. A practice implication is that exploring spouses' appraisals of the experience should be an essential component of family care when one partner has breast cancer.

Source: Gregorio, S. W., Carpenter, K. M., Dorfman, C. S., et al. (2012). Impact of breast cancer recurrence and cancer-specific stress on spouse health and immune function. *Brain, Behavior, & Immunity, 26,* 228–233.

## HEALTH BENEFITS OF MANAGING STRESS

A growing body of evidence underscores the importance of controlling stress to promote health and quality of life for people with a variety of health problems. "The association between stressors and biomarkers specific to physiological systems (i.e., cardiovascular, neuroendocrine, immune, etc.) is an emerging area of interest in biomedical research … with evidence that specific stressors may differentially affect various physiological systems" (Paradies, 2011). Thus interventions that reduce the stress response are an important component of comprehensive disease prevention and management. Psychotherapeutic approaches, such as interpersonal and cognitive–behavioural psychotherapies that focus on self-care and perception and management of life stressors, are effective treatments for depression and related mental health disorders (Sadock & Sadock, 2015). These psychotherapies have been incorporated into a range of treatment and secondary prevention programs, such as cardiac rehabilitation, with great potential for wider adapted use (Menezes, Milani, O'Keefe, et al., 2011). Targeting primary prevention programs is the aim of nurses in assisting individuals with stress reduction before becoming symptomatic.

Promoting a positive attitude and development of skills to cope with stress is foundational to many stress-management interventions. As early as 1982, Kobasa, Maddi, and Kahn (1982) made a groundbreaking contribution to our understanding of the stress-illness relationship when they identified characteristics of hardiness. They described individuals with stress-hardy characteristics who, when exercising and accessing social support, were less vulnerable to stress-related symptoms and diseases. The characteristics of stress hardiness are control, challenge, and commitment. For stress-hardy individuals, stress is viewed as a challenge rather than a threat; they feel in control of situations in their lives, and they are committed to rather than alienated from work, home, and family. Hardiness continues to be assessed (recognized) by nurses in assisting individuals and families dealing with a crisis and promoting the strengths of survivorship in dealing with new stressors. Another term that is used is *resiliency*.

Stress management is especially important in situations such as caregiving that extend over long periods. Caregiver stress/burden can be described as the appraisal of the experience of caregiving including the taxing nature of behaviours of the recipient of care, role conflict or strain, and physical and mental health effects on the caregiver (McLennon, Habermann, & Rice, 2011). As the setting for care increasingly is the home and family members take on mounting responsibility for care of loved ones (i.e., children, spouses, or aging parents with chronic conditions), the importance of caring for the caregiver to prevent significant burnout grows. As a result of current trends of delayed parenting and increased life span, the "sandwich generation" of middle-aged adults who have concurrent responsibility for their children and aging parents is at particular risk of severe caregiver burden. Research evidence supports the usefulness of interventions aimed at helping caregivers to find meaning in their activities and role for buffering caregiver stress (McLennon et al., 2011; Quinn, Clare, & Woods, 2011;

Wood, Gonzalez, & Barden, 2015). Moreover, the quality of the caregiver–care recipient relationship can affect the caregiver's well-being (Quinn et al., 2011).

In summary, the evidence is conclusive that thoughts, feelings, behaviours, beliefs, and biological activity are interrelated. Perceptions, or the way individuals view situations, can lead to stress, and, in turn, adversely affect biological activity, emotions, behaviour, and the connection with life meaning and purpose. This interaction among perceptions, stress, and multifaceted effects, in turn, can increase stress and foster a negative stress cycle. The remainder of this chapter presents assessment of stress relating to the homeodynamic framework, including the facets of physical, psychosocial, and spiritual health and well-being of individuals, and describes the application of a variety of strategies shown to help break the negative stress cycle and mitigate its harmful effects across the biological, psychosocial, and spiritual domains.

## ASSESSMENT OF STRESS

Assessment of the stress-coping abilities of an individual, family, or community is part of a comprehensive health assessment that includes past and present subjective and objective data. Collection of these data enables the individual and the nurse to determine the status of the person's stress-coping pattern, and actual and potential strengths and weaknesses.

The nurse thoroughly collects data during the history, physical examination, and health patterns assessment (see Chapters 7–8 and 19). Identifying the stress-coping pattern is especially important. Asking for specific examples of events with probes to elicit the person's thoughts, feelings, and actions leads to discussion of appraisal and ideas for alternative actions in the future. Each individual is the primary data source; no other person can explain accurately the individual's perceptions of the stressors, stress responses, and resources to prevent or alleviate the stress.

Stress is experienced across biological, psychosocial, and spiritual domains; therefore, all perceptions are important for the assessment. Throughout the assessment process, individuals may become aware of information of which they were previously unaware, or they may identify information related to their perceived problems. For example, a man may be aware of the stress of his job but may be unaware that his high blood pressure was caused at least in part by this stress.

Lazarus and Folkman (1984) proposed a theory comprising primary and secondary appraisals of stressful events, situations, or demands and the effectiveness of an individual's coping skills. Primary appraisal of coping includes descriptions of perceived actual and potential positive and negative outcomes. Negative outcomes refer to harm, whereas positive outcomes refer to the challenges resulting from stressors that an individual perceives can be overcome. Examples of negative outcomes include physical injury; disease; loss of a cherished relationship, position, or possession; and death. Positive outcomes include graduation, promotion, and development of important relationships (see the Case Study and Care Plan at the end of this chapter).

Secondary appraisal follows primary appraisal. Secondary appraisal consists of the individual's identification of choices to cope with the actual or potential harm, threat, or challenge. The choices may be internal or external resources and responses. For example, a social resource in coping with the needs of a toddler might be learning strategies in a parent-effectiveness training course. A coping response to the challenges of parenting a toddler might be restructuring the toddler's and parent's schedules to allow for more frequent cycles of activities and rest.

The individual's primary and secondary appraisals of stress provide opportunities to consider the stress experiences in different ways. Resources that had been forgotten may be remembered, or a threat may be newly viewed as a challenge and an opportunity for enhanced development and status. The appraisal process mediates stress responses. This understanding supports use of cognitive–behavioural therapy (CBT) as an effective intervention approach for stress-related problems (Wood et al., 2015). Nurses appropriately may refer individuals for CBT and are also encouraged to obtain advanced training in CBT to integrate this evidence-informed intervention into their practice. Use of good-quality health texts aimed at the general population is also an effective psychoeducational approach. For example, Marchant's (2016) highly readable book *Cure: A Journey Into the Science of Mind Over Body* and Kaku's (2014) interesting text *The Future of the Mind* are examples of materials that can serve as springboards for discussion of ways to adjust the meaning of life stressors, responses, and ways to cope.

Measuring stress and related symptoms/responses is important in assessment and evaluation of treatment outcomes. By using measurement instruments with established reliability and validity, nurses can improve assessment of an individual's stress and coping. Tools can help nurses distinguish between diagnoses that have many signs and symptoms in common. For example, disturbances in thinking and feeling processes can be difficult to distinguish and may have confounding clinical pictures. These disturbances can occur separately or simultaneously in the same person. An example of this complexity is the overlapping symptoms of depression and dementia. The nurse determines whether one health problem is actually the cause of the other so as to develop an effective plan of care (see the Case Study and Care Plan at the end of this chapter).

A wide variety of instruments are available to help nurses assess orientation, attention, cognitive skills and patterns, traits and states of emotions, symptoms of mental health distress and disorders, and overall quality of life. For example, the Schedule of Recent Experiences (Holmes, 1981) and the Impact of Event Scale (Horowitz, Wilner, & Alvarez, 1979) are two well-established instruments used widely in clinical assessment and research to measure stress associated with life changes and events. Burnout, be it work-related or personal, is understood as emotional exhaustion, depersonalization, and a sense of reduced personal accomplishment. The Maslach Burnout Inventory (Maslach & Jackson, 1986) is a psychometrically robust instrument to assess perceptions about work–life balance. Before using any instrument, clinicians and researchers need to check information about its reliability and validity, updates/revisions, training requirements, and copyright restrictions (e.g., purchase requirements) that can affect access to its use. Older instruments typically have a long-established record of demonstrated reliability and validity; however, phenomena may evolve with time, and revised versions may have been developed and tested for specific populations. Therefore exploration of the literature to seek updated information to inform use is always wise. In addition, the seeking of consultation from clinical experts/researchers regarding instrument selection is recommended.

Use of standardized instruments promotes accuracy in developing diagnoses and care plans and assists in evaluating the effectiveness of care. For example, a nurse may compare an individual's self-evaluation and/or symptom preintervention scores with postintervention scores and revise the care plan accordingly. Additionally, nurses may analyze population baseline scores for relevant characteristics and develop programs of research and quality improvements aimed at improving outcomes.

Assessment at the family and community levels is also recommended. Family assessment consists of three major categories: structural, developmental, and functional components of the family (Wright & Leahey, 2019). Environmental factors also contribute to the determinants of health and, thus, to stress, so a thorough nursing assessment requires consideration of the community. For example, examination of community-level data for unemployment, population density, housing, school quality, crime, suicide incidence, and disease occurrence patterns (i.e., health profiles of the community), as well as availability of various amenities such as green space and access to transportation and healthy foods, provides a more complete stress assessment than does individual assessment alone (DeMarco & Segraves, 2011). Moreover, family and community assessment can point to possible stress-reduction interventions, such as marshalling available social support or engaging in outdoor activities and exercise.

## STRESS-MANAGEMENT INTERVENTIONS

Stress-management strategies are beneficial to people across a broad spectrum of chronological, gender, cultural, and ethnic characteristics. Men and women, young and old, from divergent socioeconomic, cultural, and ethnic backgrounds can benefit from stress-management interventions. Sensitivity to the needs and values of individuals and communities, particularly for high-risk groups (i.e., vulnerable populations), guides assessment, and intervention techniques. The language, belief system, and cultural distinctions of individuals and families in the community guide the choice and adoption of stress-management strategies. Understanding stress and its management involves attention to the *interactions* of social and biological life at individual and family/communal levels (Barchas & Barchas, 2011); therefore, interventions may need to encompass a variety and combination of psychosocial and biological approaches at the primary, secondary, and tertiary levels of prevention. Additionally, many individual stress management recommendations are also applicable for population-based interventions, expanding from the individual to the community and to a system- or population-focused practice (Harkness & DeMarco, 2012). For example, mindfulness and exercise may start as an individual strategy to manage stress, but can be expanded to apply to systems and workplace cultures by encouraging walking

meetings and providing quiet spaces for people to step away from the environmental stimuli and/or engage in meditation.

### Developing Self-Awareness

Self-awareness is one of the most effective stress-management tools. Self-awareness helps people learn about interactions among mind, body, and spirit; increases a sense of control; and counters self-defeating perceptions. Interventions that promote self-awareness help people make sense of life events and circumstances that may be bewildering or discomforting. Many experiences in life lead to feelings of emptiness and disharmony because people are unable to connect the experience with thoughts, feelings, actions, and physiological responses. Self-awareness helps individuals recognize stress that they create through negative, exaggerated, unrealistic thinking. This recognition affords an opportunity to change these negative thought patterns, thereby decreasing stress and increasing control. Strategies that increase self-awareness can empower individuals to make new connections and to reframe and reinterpret their experiences in light of their own inner strengths and wisdom.

A closely related concept is mindfulness, nonjudgemental self-awareness characterized by intentional acceptance of the unfolding of experience in the moment. Mindfulness can be understood as having two components: "the intentional self-regulation of attention so that it remains focused on present-moment experiences (i.e., thoughts and feelings) as they arise" (Baer, 2014) and "an attitude of openness, acceptance, and curiosity toward whatever arises" (Baer, 2014). Mindfulness requires dedicated practice both to achieve and to use to reduce negative stress effects. While a variety of mindfulness approaches have been proposed and tested, those with the best empirical support are mindfulness-based stress reduction, dialectical behaviour therapy, and acceptance and commitment therapy (Baer, 2014). Mindfulness interventions can be combined with other efficacious treatments or can serve as primary interventions for stress management. Mindfulness as both a state and an intervention is not simple although it may appear so at first. Therefore nurses are urged to obtain specialized training in mindfulness approaches so they can use them in their practice. Mindfulness interventions have shown promise to improve quality of life in coping with various health conditions. For example, Lengacher, Reich, Craig, and colleagues (2015) demonstrated the cost effectiveness and efficacy of a mindfulness stress-reduction program in improving quality of life for breast cancer survivors.

The neuroscience basis of mindfulness remains a fruitful field of investigation. As is common to new areas of research, the studies to date generally lack robust methods and offer only speculative conclusions (Tang, Holzel, & Posner, 2015). Nonetheless, there is developing evidence that mindfulness meditation may precipitate neuroplastic changes "in the structure, and function of brain regions involved in regulation of attention, emotion and self-awareness" (Tang et al., 2015). The horizons are vast and exciting for future nurse scientists to engage in team science to explore the underpinnings of interventions such as mindfulness.

## Techniques for Developing Self-Awareness

*Monitoring stress warning signs.* The negative stress cycle can be difficult to interrupt. Recognizing warning signs of stress is a necessary first step. Often individuals have long ignored physical, emotional, or behavioural cues or reactions to a stressor that are stress warning signs. A man who has chronic, intermittent backaches and ignores the daily muscle tension caused by poor posture that precedes the backaches provides an example. If he had attended to his early stress warning signs of poor posture and muscle tension, he might have avoided the backache that kept him from exercising and socializing. Becoming aware of these stress warning signs is the first step. Attending to these cues is the next step. After this connection has been made, the development of skills to reduce negative mood states, unhealthy behaviours, and physical symptoms becomes much easier. Furthermore, some people misinterpret physiological signs of anxiety (e.g., shortness of breath, racing heartbeat) as indicative of serious physical danger (e.g., suffocation, myocardial infarction). This tendency to misinterpret physical anxiety cues is referred to as anxiety sensitivity, a belief that body sensations associated with anxiety indicate imminent and dangerous outcomes, and is associated with various anxiety disorders and health anxiety. In a study of gender differences in anxiety sensitivity, Thompson, Keogh, and French (2011) found that distraction worked better than sensation focusing in reducing stress for males. By assisting individuals who are prone to anxiety sensitivity to interpret body sensations accurately or to distract from the sensation, nurses can help reduce individuals' misinterpretations, as well as the likelihood of escalation of anxiety symptoms and possibly even development of anxiety disorders.

Nurses teach people to identify their warning signals of stress and to stop, take a few breaths, and break the cycle. Fig. 23.3 shows a sample form for identifying and recording this information. These signals or cues differ among individuals and can be physical, emotional, behavioural, cognitive, relational, or spiritual. When asked to monitor their responses to a particular event, individuals become more consciously aware of these cues. Although this heightened awareness initially may increase an individual's consciousness of physical pain or emotional discomfort, awareness is a necessary first step in recognizing the negative effects of stress and the relationship of thoughts, feelings, behaviour, and biological processes. In addition, nurses and other clinicians have a responsibility to screen individuals for emotional distress to help them recognize and monitor their own physical and mood states. For individuals with health conditions such as coronary artery disease, which is known to have high comorbidity with emotional distress and specifically depression, routine screening should be the standard of care (Menezes et al., 2011).

Try this: ask an individual to identify a stressful experience and the physical or emotional reactions (stress warning signals) to that particular experience. For example, after being instructed to stop, take a breath, and notice the physical and emotional response to a stressful situation, one woman related the following:

*On my way to work yesterday, I sat in a huge traffic jam. I noticed that my heart was racing, my breathing had changed, and my hands were gripping the steering wheel. I felt angry and frustrated because I was going to be late for work.*

Although these responses seem quite obvious, most people are unaware of the effects of stress on their minds and bodies. In the preceding example, the building of the woman's stress may continue to escalate at work, influencing her interactions with coworkers. Once individuals become aware of these effects, they may be able to release tension more easily, countering the negative effects of stress and increasing a sense of control. Techniques that help to reduce negative effects of stress include use of distraction by purposefully shifting focus to pleasant thoughts or engaging in a diversion activity, and use of a relaxation response technique, as described in the following section.

*Learning and practising a relaxation response technique.* Eliciting the relaxation response is another technique to help people develop awareness and counter the negative effects of stress. Relaxation response techniques oppose the stress response by reducing sympathetic arousal (Benson, 1975). The immediate physiological effects of relaxation are decreases in heart rate, blood pressure, respiration rate, and muscle tension. The long-term physiological effect is a decrease in central nervous system arousal with a concomitant decrease in musculoskeletal system, autonomic nervous system, and psychoneuroendocrine system arousal. To the extent that stress causes or exacerbates a symptom, elicitation of the relaxation response can break this stress–symptom cycle. In addition to these physiological changes, psychological changes such as improved mood and behavioural changes, including a reduction in risky behaviours, can occur. Finally, using biofeedback tools—which provide instant biological feedback—as a mechanism to maximize effectiveness of relaxation exercises can counteract stress, buffering individuals from a host of stress-related disease processes (Tonhajzerova & Mestanik, 2017).

The relaxation response is an innate physiological response (Benson, 1975); therefore a number of techniques that involve mental focusing can be used. All of these techniques have two basic components:

- The repetition of a word, sound, phrase, prayer, image, or physical activity
- The passive disregard of everyday thoughts when they occur

Electronic recordings (e.g., DVDs, CDs, MP3/MP4 files, and mobile apps/downloads) can be used to help guide this process of focusing, especially during the initial learning phase.

Nurses can often introduce individuals to the immediate calming effects of the relaxation response in less than 5 minutes. One effective way is to have the person make a fist and notice what happens to the breathing pattern. Most people have a tendency to hold their breath while tensing a body part. Now ask the person to take a few deep diaphragmatic breaths while making a fist. Most people will notice that the tension is much harder to maintain while taking a deep breath. This awareness helps to recognize the relationship between breath and tension. Lamaze techniques for helping women manage pain during labour and delivery are based on this connection between breathing and relaxation. Most people hold their breath when they perceive a threat (stress), feel anxious, or become angry. By stopping and taking a few deep breaths when they become aware of physical changes (holding the breath or clenching the jaw) or emotional changes (feeling anxious or angry), individuals can elicit the relaxation response,

## Physical Symptoms

—— Headaches
—— Indigestion
—— Stomachaches
—— Sweaty palms
—— Sleep difficulties
—— Dizziness

—— Back pain
—— Tight neck and shoulders
—— Racing heart
—— Restlessness
—— Tiredness
—— Ringing in ears

## Behavioural Symptoms

—— Excess smoking
—— Bossiness
—— Compulsive gum chewing
—— Attitude critical of others

—— Grinding of teeth at night
—— Overuse of alcohol
—— Compulsive eating
—— Inability to get things done

## Emotional Symptoms

—— Crying
—— Nervousness and anxiety
—— Boredom (no meaning to things)
—— Edginess (ready to explode)
—— Feeling powerless to change things

—— Overwhelming sense of pressure
—— Anger
—— Loneliness
—— Unhappiness for no reason
—— Easily upset

## Cognitive Symptoms

—— Trouble thinking clearly
—— Lack of creativity
—— Memory loss
—— Forgetfulness

—— Inability to make decisions
—— Thoughts of running away
—— Constant worry
—— Loss of sense of humour

## Spiritual Symptoms

—— Emptiness
—— Loss of meaning
—— Doubt
—— Unforgiving
—— Martyrdom
—— Looking for magic
—— Loss of direction
—— Cynicism
—— Apathy
—— Needing to "prove" self

## Relational Symptoms

—— Isolation
—— Intolerance
—— Resentment
—— Loneliness
—— Lashing out
—— Hiding
—— Clamming up
—— Lowered sex drive
—— Nagging
—— Distrust
—— Lack of intimacy
—— Using people

**Fig. 23.3 Stress Warning Signals** (From *Medical symptom reduction clinic patient notebook*. [n.d.]. Boston: The Benson-Henry Institute for Mind Body Medicine of Massachusetts General Hospital, Harvard Medical School.)

reduce sympathetic arousal, calm negative mood states, and gain a sense of control. Yoga and deep breathing can assist with *mindfulness* (i.e., awareness of perception) and promote relaxation.

***Using mini relaxations.*** Mini relaxations can be taught quickly and used throughout the day to help develop awareness and to counter the negative effects of stress on the mind, body, and spirit. Individuals can be taught to monitor minor stress warning signs (jaw and shoulder tension) and to use a mini-relaxation exercise to keep these initial symptoms of stress from developing into an incapacitating tension headache. A mini-relaxation exercise can be anything from a few conscious, deep diaphragmatic breaths to several minutes of sitting quietly (Quality and Safety Scenario). Practice is needed to elicit the response quickly when stress, pain, or tension is recognized. The power of using relaxation, including visualization, and breathing techniques is illustrated by the personal experience of a nurse who had coached pregnant women and partners in Lamaze preparation for childbirth for 10 years before having her third baby. During pitocin induction due to a postdate determination, the woman was experiencing significant contractions. Her very experienced labour nurse commented that she was an advertisement for childbirth preparation. The woman managed a smile in response. The woman reflected:

*The contractions were tough. I think that the pitocin escalated the process so that contractions increased quickly from mild to intense. Did my Lamaze relaxation techniques help? Oh yes. Was it still painful—oh yes. However, I was able to make it through this and two previous labours and deliveries without an epidural by using relaxation techniques that I had taught and practised. I cannot emphasize enough that relaxation techniques including breathing, visualization, distraction, and partner/nurse coaching support are powerful tools. These techniques require practice to be called upon in an instant of pain or stress. Medication and/or anaesthesia remain as helpful tools in situations of acute pain such as labour, surgery, injury, or ongoing stress, but the power of our capacities to harness our own abilities are powerful and should not be overlooked. Let's empower ourselves so that pharmacotherapeutics is not the immediate go-to solution for stress and pain!*

### ⚡ QUALITY AND SAFETY SCENARIO

#### A Stress-Management Strategy for Nurses

Develop the skill of personal presence. Presence is the gift of self through availability and attention to needs. Presence means "being there" for another person. To be available to others in this way, first practise the skill of being present with yourself. One effective way of developing this skill is through mindfulness, which is the ability to focus attention on what you are experiencing from moment to moment. Mindfulness encompasses the abilities of slowing down and bringing your full attention (thoughts, feelings, and body sensations) to the action in which you are engaged at the moment. The practice can be particularly useful in allowing yourself to extend the benefits of eliciting the relaxation response in more areas of your daily life.

The following are some ideas for practising personal presence (mindfulness):

- When you awaken each morning, bring your full attention to your breathing. Allow your awareness to expand gradually into the room and then slowly begin to listen to the sounds of the outdoors.
- On your way to work, focus on how you walk, drive, or ride the transit. Take some deep diaphragmatic breaths and relax your body as you travel.
- Take a moment to attend to your breath, relax your body, and focus your mind before entering a care recipient's room.
- As you eat a meal, carefully examine it through all of your senses—the sight, smell, touch, taste, and the sound of each bite. Mindfully enjoy this new experience.
- Recurring events of the day can become cues for a mini relaxation (the ringing telephone; auscultating a heartbeat; answering a call light, before, during, and after rounds or report).
- Make the transition home from work mindful. Leave thoughts and worries of work at work and be conscious of your home environment each day.

Once again, focus on your breathing and become completely aware of your surroundings as you go to sleep. Practise mindfully letting go of today and tomorrow as you allow your mind and body to get some much-needed rest.

Source: Modified from Benson-Henry Institute for Mind Body Medicine of Massachusetts General Hospital. (n.d.). *Stress*. Retrieved from https://www.bensonhenryinstitute.org/.

***Alternative and complementary therapies.*** Most Canadians use alternative and complementary therapies such as vitamins, herbs, acupuncture, hypnosis, aromatherapy, naturopathy, Indigenous healing, reflexology, and reiki (Government of Canada, 2015). A variety of alternative and complementary therapies can prevent and reduce harmful effects of stress. These approaches have developed outside the mainstream of traditional Western medicine; however, developing evidence of efficacy has promoted growing acceptance of some of these approaches. People are increasingly using alternative and complementary practices as self-help measures, and research to study their effects has exploded in recent years. Nurses can help individuals evaluate the safety and efficacy of various alternative and complementary therapies.

Acupuncture is an ancient Chinese technique used to reduce pain and to prevent and manage various disorders by placement of fine needles at specific meridian points on the body. Acupuncture is not a self-help approach, so seeking treatment from an experienced acupuncturist is required. The Western scientific community cannot explain why acupuncture works but acknowledges its effectiveness. Even the WHO has listed illnesses that can be managed with acupuncture (Stuart, 2013), and some health insurance plans provide reimbursement for acupuncture treatments.

*Hypnosis* comes from a Greek word meaning sleep. Hypnosis narrows consciousness and elicits relaxation, inertia, and passivity, like sleep, yet awareness is never lost completely and the hypnotized person can respond (Brann, Owens, & Williamson, 2011). The exact mechanisms through which hypnosis works are not known, although perhaps its ability to induce deep relaxation and its possible action in shifting brain activity from the "analytical" left side to the "nonanalytical" right side might be explanatory. Nevertheless, its effectiveness in managing a variety of conditions, notably smoking and anxiety-related problems, and managing pain is well recognized. Trained therapists provide hypnotherapy to manage stress and various mental health problems, including phobias, addictions, and posttraumatic stress disorder. Self-hypnosis, a form of deep relaxation similar to the relaxation techniques described in this chapter, can be a useful stress-reduction tool.

Reiki (pronounced ray-kee) is made up of two Japanese words: *rei*, or universal spirit (sometimes thought of as a supreme being), and *ki*. Thus the word reiki means universal life energy. Reiki is a therapy that uses energy fields with the intent to affect health. To transmit ki, believed to be a life-force energy, the reiki practitioner places hands on or near the person receiving treatment. Some studies show that self-Reiki may be an effective stress management tool (Helali, 2016).

***Expressive writing.*** Transforming thoughts and emotions related to stressful experiences into written language has demonstrated positive effects on health (North, Pai, Hixon, et al., 2011). In its therapeutic meaning, expressive writing involves telling a "story" about traumatic, emotionally charged, or stressful events and personal reactions. Journal writing—more specifically, self-confessional writing—is a form of expressive writing that is typically done via entries in a journal over time that describe unfolding personal responses to life events. Expressive writing is useful in disclosing and processing emotions, and in measurably improving physical and mental health.

Expressive writing, including journalling, can help people reflect on stressful events and their reactions to these events. Such reflection is an opportunity to reform perceptions and to consider alternative ways to manage stress. Individuals may find resolutions to conflicts that work uniquely for them. These resolutions may then increase a sense of control and mediate negative consequences of stress. This self-reflective process shares elements of CBT—an intervention effective in reducing harmful effects of stress.

Nurses can advise people to get a special notebook or a journal (or use an electronic tablet or computer) and write about a stressful event for 15 minutes a day in a setting in which they will not be interrupted. From a health perspective, people will be more effective when they make themselves the only audience. The nurse should warn the individual that he or she may feel sad or depressed immediately after the writing session, but these feelings usually dissipate within an hour. Nonetheless, exploring deep thoughts and feelings on paper is not a panacea. When an individual is coping with death, divorce, or some other major stressor, feeling better instantly after writing cannot be expected. A person can, however, develop a clearer understanding of feelings and of the situation through journal writing. In other words, journal writing helps people objectify experiences, identify the influence of stress on symptoms, and develop insights into more effective problem solving. Some individuals may recognize the need for psychotherapeutic support through journal writing, and an appropriate referral can then be made. Nurses can use the same approaches to examine their own stressful work-related situations to reflect, analyze their responses/reactions, and generate effective responses to similar experiences in the future.

## Nutrition: Healthy Diet

Countering negative effects of stress requires caring for physical health and well-being. The mind and body are connected; therefore paying attention to one while ignoring the other does not promote overall health. The body requires rest, a healthy diet of balanced food choices, and exercise. In the last few decades, nutrition has moved to the forefront as a major component of health promotion, disease prevention, and symptom management. Food is now viewed as a positive influence on health, physical performance, and state of mind rather than simply a fuel needed to prevent disease and sustain life. Adaptive eating is characterized by balanced eating patterns and calorie intake as well as appropriate body weight for height. Nutrition is an important component of early intervention strategies to improve physical, cognitive, emotional, social, and spiritual functioning. However, the North American lifestyle has made practising healthy eating habits increasingly difficult. Many Canadians have difficulty finding affordable foods that are low in salt and sugar and contain adequate vitamins and minerals (Schermel, Mendoza, Henson, et al., 2014).

One of the frustrations that nurses experience is trying to help children and adults develop healthy eating habits. This effort requires planning and correctly choosing a variety of foods and eating a diet low in fat, saturated fat, and cholesterol, with plenty of vegetables, fruits, and grain products. *Canada's Dietary Guidelines* aim to maximize health and vitality by educating Canadians about how much food they need, what types of food provide adequate nutrition, and the importance of regular physical activity (Health Canada, 2019). Daily food choices should be made from a variety of food groups. Key recommendations also highlight the importance of calorie control and physical activity. Guidelines continue to undergo evaluation and revision; for example, guidelines about "healthy foods" are under ongoing review, so nurses are urged to check for updated guidelines. A detailed discussion of the health benefits of balanced nutrition and guidelines throughout the life span can be found in Chapter 21.

Encouraging healthier dietary choices helps people to recognize that control over their health and well-being is possible. This knowledge, in turn, helps counter the negative effects of stress and lower the stress-disinhibition effect that can influence poor dietary choices. Nurses encourage people to monitor their daily dietary patterns to gain awareness of how they use food in times of stress. Tools such as food diaries (24-hour recall) help people to monitor the amount and quality of what they eat and drink and to set realistic goals. A variety of free online resources provide nutrition tips and ways to monitor portions and exercise.

## Physical Activity

Combining a healthy diet with a regular exercise routine has many health benefits and can positively affect quality of life. For example, one of the most effective ways to lose weight and improve self-esteem is to combine exercise with nutritious eating. Exercise (physical activity that increases strength and flexibility and improves conditioning) and balanced nutrition serve as protective factors against several major chronic diseases. Regular physical activity reduces the risk of breast cancer, colon cancer, diabetes, ischemic heart disease, and strokes (Kyu, Bachman, Alexander, et al., 2016). Exercise helps prevent high blood pressure and helps lower blood pressure in people with elevated levels. Regular physical activity, even at moderate levels, is associated with lower death rates for adults of any age. Psychological well-being is enhanced, and the risk of developing depression can be reduced; regular physical activity appears to reduce symptoms of depression and anxiety and to improve mood.

Additionally, children and adolescents need weight-bearing exercise for normal skeletal development, and young adults need this type of exercise to achieve and maintain peak bone mass (Gunter, Almstedt, & Janz, 2012). Regular physical activity also reduces cognitive impairments and increases the ability of older persons, and those with certain chronic and disabling conditions, to perform activities of daily living (McPhee, French, Jackson, et al., 2016). Nevertheless, high stress could increase injury risk for athletes, and injured athletes may experience greater stress than noninjured peers when they are sidelined from competition. Chapter 22 provides a comprehensive discussion of the benefits of exercise and its clinical application throughout the life span.

Regular physical activity helps people adopt a more active lifestyle as they begin to feel better physically and emotionally, thereby breaking the negative stress cycle (Fig. 23.4). Positive effects can be obtained with exercise of only moderate intensity. For example, a brisk walk of 30 to 60 minutes, three to five times a week, promotes fitness and decreases the risk of disease. Being physically active on a daily basis is extremely important; therefore nurses can help individuals increase their physical activity by suggesting a variety of activities in which they might engage each day (Box 23.3). An exercise diary can generate a baseline for usual activity to set realistic goals and monitor progress. By simply changing a few daily routines, individuals can gain enormous physical, psychosocial, and spiritual rewards that promote health and break the negative stress cycle.

### Sleep Hygiene

Health and the ability to meet life's many demands and manage stress effectively require proper rest. Many people experience sleep deprivation and sleep disorders (e.g., sleep apnea) that can cause or exacerbate conditions such as depression and fatigue and contribute to poor concentration and ineffective problem-solving. Insomnia can be induced by stress or other cognitive–behavioural factors, such as unrealistic expectations, inappropriate scheduling of sleep, trying too hard to sleep, consuming caffeine, getting inadequate exercise, and a number of other factors, including illness, alcohol use, or drug use (Stuart, 2013). Determining the extent to which sleep disturbance is the result of behaviour or stress-related issues is a necessary assessment. Overcoming sleep disturbances cannot be done quickly. Changing these behaviours requires patience and persistence. Once the factors associated with sleep disturbance have been identified, nurses can help individuals improve their sleep patterns by counselling them to follow several sleep hygiene or behaviour guidelines (keeping a sleep diary, having a regular sleep-wake cycle, and making prudent dietary changes). Referral for appropriate evaluation of possible disorders such as sleep apnea is also a necessary nursing intervention. Assisting people to make healthy behaviour changes in their sleep habits provides another opportunity for people to increase self-regulation, confidence, and control, thereby reducing stress and improving quality of life. Box 23.4 presents several sleep hygiene strategies.

### Cognitive–Behavioural Restructuring

Many stressful situations can be created or exacerbated by negative, exaggerated, catastrophic thinking. CBT is a conceptually based short-term intervention to modify this thinking and related behaviours, and thereby reduce stress. In the

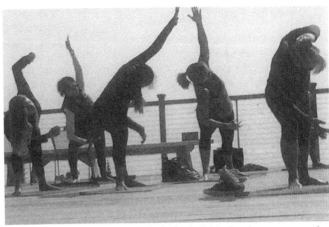

**Fig. 23.4** Regular physical activity helps individuals adopt a more active lifestyle.

---

#### BOX 23.3  Helping Individuals Increase Physical Activity

Nurses can suggest ways for individuals to increase physical activity throughout the day, including:

- Have fun and play active games with children.
- Engage in a sport.
- Find a friend with whom to walk or jog.
- Take a class in yoga or tai chi.
- Get and walk a dog.
- Garden on the weekends.
- Walk or bicycle to school or work.
- Take the stairs, never the elevator.
- Park the car at the farthest point in the parking lot at work, at school, or when shopping.

By simply changing a few daily routines, a person can gain enormous physical, psychosocial, and spiritual rewards that promote health and break the negative stress cycle.

---

context of therapy, cognitive–behavioural restructuring is a technique or a series of strategies that help people evaluate their thoughts, challenge them, and replace them with more rational cognitive and behavioural responses (Beck, 1976, 1979; Clark & Beck, 2012; Dowd, Hogan, McGuire, et al., 2015). Although advanced training is needed to provide CBT and nurses are encouraged to do so, nurses can safely and effectively use basic strategies. A helpful resource for nurses is the Beck Institute for Cognitive Behavior Therapy (2012).

Appraisal, or the way in which a situation is viewed, can be a major cause of stress, making CBT especially suited for stress management. When situations are viewed in a negative, distorted, or illogical manner, such perceptions can adversely affect emotions, behaviours, beliefs, and physiological parameters. Cognitive–behavioural restructuring teaches people to recognize that negative thinking often causes emotional distress and associated behaviours. This recognition, in turn, alters problematic thinking and behaviour, reduces the negative consequences of stress, and enhances health (Stuart, 2013).

## BOX 23.4 Sleep Hygiene Strategies

Nurses find the following suggestions to be helpful for individuals with sleep disturbance resulting from behavioural or stress-related issues:

- Keep a sleep diary, which helps determine sleep patterns more accurately, assess progress, and reinforce behaviour change.
- Challenge irrational beliefs.
- Reduce consumption of alcohol and caffeine. (Chapter 21 gives some tips.)
- Avoid use of sleeping pills.
- Have a regular sleep-wake schedule, even on the weekends.
- If you are unable to fall asleep within 20 to 30 minutes, or if you wake up and are unable to fall back to sleep within that time, get out of bed and do something until you are groggy and sleepy again.
- Focus on relaxation, not sleep. Use a relaxation tape, and practise diaphragmatic breathing. Limit naps during the day to less than 45 minutes. Longer naps reset the biological clock and disturb nighttime sleep.
- Exercise within 3 to 6 hours of bedtime. Exercise improves sleep by producing a significant rise in body temperature, followed by a compensatory drop a few hours later, making it easier to fall asleep and stay asleep. Furthermore, because exercise is a physical stressor, the brain compensates for this by increasing the amount of deep sleep.
- Take a hot bath 2 hours before bedtime. The temperature drop after the bath helps to induce sleep.
- Sleep in a cool room. Individuals become sleepier and less active when body temperature falls.

Source: Stuart, G. W. (2013). *Principles and practice of psychiatric nursing* (10th ed.). St. Louis: Mosby.

### INNOVATIVE PRACTICE

#### The Four-Step Approach to Cognitive Restructuring Enhanced With Technology

To help individuals develop the skill of cognitive restructuring, nurses can teach them to examine a stressful situation using the following four-step approach:

- *Stop* (break the cycle of escalating, negative thoughts).
- *Breathe deeply* (elicit the relaxation response and release tension).
- *Reflect* (ask "What is going on here? What am I thinking? Is the thought true? Is the thought helpful? Am I jumping to conclusions or magnifying the situation?").
- *Choose* a more realistic, rational response. Try out the alternative response in a future situation.

#### Alternative Approach

Teaching/coaching can be done face-to-face or can be provided via technology (e.g., a website and/or smartphone application that shows the previous steps with a feedback interface). Via technology, feedback can be given via text or e-mail messages to correct negative thoughts and to provide suggestions and positive reinforcement for steps two to four when success is reported. Phone and/or face-to-face interaction can augment contact via technology when possible. Tracking successful cognitive restructuring via online entry can provide useful outcome data. As Internet and smartphone penetration increase and costs decrease, use of such technological interventions will increasingly be cost-effective ways to reach more individuals and can be applied across a range of technological platforms (e.g., computers, smartphones, and tablets). Reminder generic affirmations also can be added via text messaging at very low cost to encourage practice of the steps.

Source: Modified from Clark, D. A., & Beck, A. T. (2012). *The anxiety and worry workbook: The cognitive behavioral solution.* New York: Guilford Press; Stuart, G. W. (2009). Psychophysiological responses and somatoform and sleep disorders. In G. W. Stuart & M. T. Laraia (Eds.), *Principles and practice of psychiatric nursing* (9th ed., p. 241). St Louis: Mosby; Stuart, G. W. (Ed.) (2013). *Principles and practice of psychiatric nursing* (10th ed.). St. Louis: Mosby.

Cognitive–behavioural restructuring does not gloss over or deny misfortune, suffering, or negative feelings. Many circumstances exist in peoples' lives for which it is appropriate to feel sad, anxious, angry, or depressed. More accurately, cognitive–behavioural restructuring is a technique that helps some people become unstuck from these moods so that they can experience a broader range of feelings and try out new behaviours (Stuart, 2013). In this structured method, individuals are asked to consider their cognitive appraisal of a situation and how this assessment affects feelings, behaviours, and physiological processes. Reframing, or cognitive reappraisal, educates individuals in monitoring thoughts and replacing those that are negative and irrational with those that are more realistic and helpful. Adding behaviours that are consistent with reframed thinking follows.

For example, a woman may have had plans to meet a friend for lunch on a day she woke up with a migraine headache. She might begin to think such thoughts as "This always happens to me when I have plans," "This headache will never go away," "I shouldn't have to deal with this," or "My day is ruined." The result of this negative, irrational self-talk is disappointment, frustration, and anger. This emotional arousal will, in turn, increase muscle tension and a variety of other stress-related symptoms, which may exacerbate the headache. To help individuals develop the skill of cognitive–behavioural restructuring, nurses can teach them to examine a stressful situation using the four-step innovative practice CBT approach highlighted in the Innovative Practice box.

In the previous example, the woman may reflect that "I am having a migraine headache, and I hate that it is on a day that I had made plans, but I will take my medication, listen to my relaxation tapes, and rest. I'll call my friend and see if we can change our plans. Perhaps she can come over to visit me for tea this afternoon if I feel better." Although it is understandable that anyone would be disappointed and upset over this situation, application of the four-step cognitive restructuring technique can help individuals identify healthy choices and gain a sense of control.

Based on the work of pioneers such as Beck (1976, 1979) and Albert Ellis (Ellis, 1962; Ellis & Dryden, 1987), cognitive therapy has emerged during the past several decades as a treatment designed to alter dysfunctional beliefs and thoughts associated with depression, anxiety disorders, and other emotional problems (Clark & Beck, 2012). Over time, theorists, clinical researchers, and clinicians recognized the effectiveness of this approach for many people, as well as the value of linking helpful alterations in thinking to complementary behavioural changes. As a result, CBT emerged. CBT is an efficacious treatment approach for many stress-related and mental health disorders. For example, researchers have shown that CBT is effective, alone or with other therapies or medication, in alleviating post-partum depression (Bobo & Yawn, 2014). Evidence provides strong support for use of cognitive–behavioural restructuring as a stress-management approach. A comparison of an online mindfulness-based cognitive therapy intervention (Mindfulness in Action) with online pain management psychoeducation showed positive outcomes in self well-being from both approaches, yet Mindfulness in Action was associated with more pronounced positive outcomes (Dowd et al., 2015). Although the results were promising, more research is needed to demonstrate efficacy. Sensitivity to stress appraisals is also situated within a person's culture and experience. Cultural safety to such influences is critical to providing quality care. The Diversity Awareness box presents relevant information related to the effects of racial/ethnic discrimination on cognitive appraisals of interactions as threatening and harmful, resulting in increased overall stress burden.

---

### 🌐 DIVERSITY AWARENESS

#### Social Stressors Can Lead to Discrimination for Vulnerable Populations

Health is perceived through one's spiritual beliefs, holistic practice, and bio-medical perspectives. Nurses understand cultural safety when providing care and the importance of clear communication in multicultural care. Greater concern for health literacy and improved coordination with support organizations are needed. Barriers such as discrimination and geopolitical tension may affect the ability to cope through frustration and may influence health care outcomes. In order to close the gap and support health equity, we must by address issues such as chronic disease and infant mortality rates, which are compounded by inequities. For example, social stressors have been linked to increased depressive symptoms among antepartum black American women (Dailey et al., 2011). Thus in addition to the need for universal symptom screening, it is essential that nurses develop and test interventions to ameliorate effects of social stressors such as discrimination for vulnerable populations.

**Reflective Question**
- What examples can you identify in your local health care culture that demonstrate how social inequities lead to an increased risk for chronic stressors and/or physical health problems

Source: Dailey, D. E., Dawn, E., & Humphreys, J. C. (2011). Social stressors associated with antepartum depressive symptoms in low-income African American women. *Public Health Nursing, 28*, 203–212.

---

## Affirmations

Affirmations can be an effective stress-management and cognitive–behavioural restructuring skill because they are a method of countering self-defeating negative thoughts and attitudes in addition to being helpful in addressing spiritual needs. An affirmation is a positive thought, in the form of a short phrase or saying, which has meaning for the individual. By reinforcing new ways of thinking or behaving in the present moment, affirmations are statements that people can use to reaffirm new intentions and to clarify goals.

Nurses coach individuals to create an affirmation as a way of developing a more helpful, realistic belief system. For example, thoughts such as "I can't handle this" and "My day is ruined"

can be countered with "I can handle this" and "I know ways to increase my comfort." Repeating an affirmation often throughout the day, perhaps after elicitation of the relaxation response or as part of a breathing exercise, can become second nature and can help to enhance self-esteem and reduce stress.

## Social Support

Having supportive family, friends, and coworkers is for many individuals an important contributor to effective coping and stress hardiness (Kobasa et al., 1982). Many people believe that confiding in others and talking out problems can be a helpful way to get good advice or uncritical support. Social support comprises a network of close family, friends, coworkers, and professionals. The social support literature notes that both the number of supports and the quality of the relationships are important (van Woerden, Poortinga, Bronstering, et al., 2011). Research outcomes demonstrate the protective health effects of social support. However, influences may differ by type or source of support. For example, van Woerden and colleagues (2011) examined the effects of social support from personal, professional, and community networks and other factors in relation to self-rated health using a cross-sectional postal and Web-based survey with a random sample of 10,000 households in Wandsworth, London. The results demonstrated that social support from family or friends, at work, and by civic participation was associated with a lower likelihood of poor self-rated health, but that social support from neighbours was associated with a higher likelihood of reporting poor health. The outcomes suggest that most of the health effects of social support are complementary. Nonetheless, the finding that the health effects of family social support were insignificant after the other social support variables had been controlled for suggests that it can be compensated by support from other sources. Sociodemographic variables (e.g., sex, age, being married, being employed, owning a home) were also associated with better self-rated health. The principal message is that a variety of sources of social support may promote health and that nurses should ask individuals about all types of social support so as to help them cultivate and use support from many sources. In addition, substituting support from a different source when it is lacking from one usual source such as the family can be a helpful strategy.

Nursing interventions are aimed at facilitating social support to promote effective coping and reduce stress. Nurses can promote information available in their local communities or through national organizations, support groups, website chat rooms, social networking sites, educational classes, and exercise facilities. Individuals and their families are often referred to volunteer organizations such as the Lung Association, the Heart and Stroke Foundation of Canada, the Canadian Cancer Society, and the Arthritis Society for resources related to specific health-promotion/maintenance needs that also may provide social support opportunities.

## Assertive Communication

Effective communication is an important stress-management skill. An important coping and problem-solving skill, communication can be adversely affected by exaggerated negative thoughts and deeply held negative beliefs and assumptions (Stuart, 2013). People who have difficulty with communication usually have one or all of the following problems:

- Incongruence between what they say (statement) and what they want (intent)
- Confusion about or resistance to stating clearly how they feel, what they want, or what they need (lack of assertiveness), with either a tendency to deny their own feelings (passiveness) or indifference toward the feelings of others (aggressiveness)
- Difficulty listening to others

The importance of matching the statement with intention is illustrated by the following example:

> As Timothy is leaving for his basketball game on a Saturday afternoon, his mother tells him, "Remember to be home early tonight." When Timothy arrives home at 9:00 pm, his mother, who is waiting at the front door, yells, "Where were you? Is this your idea of early? You know your father and I had plans tonight. We were counting on you. You think only of yourself. This always happens. You'll never change. You'll always be irresponsible and selfish."

The first guideline for effective communication is that people need to be clear about what they want and what they need (intent) in statements to others. Although it would be wonderful if a son or daughter, spouse, friend, or others were great mind readers, assuming that people automatically know what is meant does little to help with communication. Nurses help individuals match statements with intentions. This process requires that individuals recognize distorted, exaggerated thoughts and emotions and take responsibility for their part of the conversation. Communicating effectively is a learned art and skill.

In our reviewing the previous example, it is helpful to note that if the mother's intention was to have her son home before 8:00 p.m., then her statement needed to indicate this. She could have said "I hope you enjoy the game, but remember your father and I are going out tonight. We need to have you home before 8:00 p.m. to take care of your sister." It is important that the person understands that the other person in the conversation is not obligated to respond as one would wish. However, a request can be much clearer when the statement reflects the intent.

The next guideline for effective communication is to be assertive. Assertive communication, in most cases, is the most effective way to communicate. An assertive statement is non-judgemental, expresses feelings and opinions, and reaffirms perceived rights. The general format of an assertive statement is: *I feel* [emotion], *when you* [the behaviour], *because* [explanation].

The formula requires that all three elements be included. Cognitive restructuring, as described earlier, facilitates assertive communication because it requires individuals to identify their thoughts and feelings. In the previous example, Timothy's mother could:

- *Stop* (breaking the cycle of escalating, negative thoughts)
- *Breathe deeply* (releasing physical tension; promoting relaxation)
- *Reflect*:
  - How do I feel emotionally? (e.g., frustrated)
  - What are my automatic thoughts? ("If he cared about us, then he would have been home on time. He's always selfish and irresponsible. He's never going to change.")
- *Choose*:
  - A more realistic, helpful way of thinking ("He's not always selfish and irresponsible. Even though it feels like he doesn't care about us when he does this, I know he cares.")

Becoming aware of her automatic thoughts and feelings would help Timothy's mother plan an assertive statement when Timothy comes home. She could then say "I feel frustrated [emotion] when you are late [behaviour] because I expected you would be home in time to care for your sister while your father and I went out, or that you would have called if you were going to be late [explanation]." This statement both makes her feelings clear and explains why she feels this way, which in turn provides a better opportunity to work on problem solving. When people cannot verbalize both their feelings and their needs, others are forced to figure out what they are. When others fail to do so correctly, individuals may feel victimized and blame the others for not understanding. Nurses help people recognize that they have a right and a responsibility to speak up and to do so in an assertive manner. The nurse helps individuals in matching their emotions with the explanation (frustration equals unmet expectation). It is important to remind them that this way of communicating may feel awkward and uncomfortable at first. Practising this technique many times will be required before communication improves. Role play can be a useful technique to practise. Other people need time to become accustomed to the changes. Effective communication takes both practice and patience with everyone involved.

## Empathy

Empathy is an effective stress-management intervention because it assists with communication. Empathy is the ability to consider another person's perspective and to communicate this understanding back to that person. Empathy guides individuals to become better listeners.

Empathy can be facilitated through the technique of active listening. Active listening requires conscious, empathic, non-judgemental awareness. Listening also helps clarify the issues involved and can de-escalate many emotional exchanges. The use of focus groups can assist the nurse in understanding concerns, such as a parent group concerned about nutrition choices in the lunch room. For example, during a situation in which a parent announces, "I'm fed up with the food selection in the cafeteria," the response may be important to resolving the issues without promoting further miscommunications and increasing problems. Rather than being caught by a defensive, emotional reaction, individuals can learn to communicate empathetically using the four-step approach:

- *Stop* (breaking the cycle of escalating, negative thoughts)
- *Breathe deeply* (releasing physical tension; promoting relaxation)
- *Reflect*:
  - How do I feel emotionally? (hurt, angry)

- What are my automatic thoughts? ("How could [person] say that? It's not my fault. I have things to do. [Person] always accuses me. This is never going to change.")
- What are the thoughts and emotions being expressed by the other person?
- *Choose:*
  - "My feelings are hurt, but I don't have to react defensively."
  - "I'm going to try to understand [person's] perspective using this phrase: 'You sound ____about____' and listen to [person's] response."

By using this phrase ("You sound ____about____"), an individual can gain awareness from another person's perspective (Rogers, 1951). If we continue with the scenario, the response might be "You sound upset about the choice of food available … ." Possible responses to this empathetic statement might include "It's not just about that. Everything went wrong today, and this was just one more thing when my child complains about lunch," and "You're right. I hate having to pay for food that my child will not eat."

When one uses active listening, the other person often feels heard. An opportunity to clarify any misunderstanding becomes available. This exercise may help reduce emotional arousal, defensive behaviour, and conflict. Active listening allows the individual to buy time and to get a better perspective on what the other person is thinking and feeling. Individuals can then make a choice as to how they want to respond. They may choose to use assertive communication or to step away from the interaction. Active listening promotes empathic, objective, and nonjudgemental communication. Nurses recommend use of stress-management skills that include active listening techniques to facilitate effective communication, which, in turn, reduces conflict and stress.

## Healthy Pleasures

Engaging in healthy pleasures (activities that bring feelings of peace, joy, and happiness), is, for most individuals, an important part of life. However, for individuals who are feeling overwhelmed with daily hassles of work–life balance, illness, or loss, this practice may have been lost. Individuals may feel that they do not deserve to have pleasure or that they are waiting for happiness until they feel better, until the stressors are resolved, or until they go away. This belief makes breaking the stress cycle even more challenging; however, rewards motivate behaviour (Stuart, 2013). By nurses asking people to pursue a healthy and pleasurable activity every week, motivating them to become more involved in their lives and break this cycle is often easier. The activity can be simple, and it need not cost money. For example, people often find pleasure in enjoying nature, spending time with a friend, reading a book, or watching a movie. Hobbies are purposeful leisure-time activities that can balance hectic, stressful lives. A hobby should be chosen from interest and/or talent. Many hobbies have added benefits of increasing activity (e.g., gardening) or promoting social engagement (e.g., a book club or chorus). Nurses advise individuals to make leisure-time activities a regular part of the week as a purposeful and conscious plan to break the stress cycle.

## Spiritual Practice

In response to stress, people can feel disconnected from life's meaning and purpose, which in turn affects spiritual health and well-being. Meeting spiritual needs may be facilitated by spiritual practice or activities that help people find meaning, purpose, and connection. For example, individuals may choose to elicit the relaxation response through prayer. This focused, relaxed state of mind might help them develop a spiritual perspective that can engender a shift in values and beliefs to help them cope with a stressor they cannot change, such as chronic illness or loss of a loved one. Expression of anger or confusion in the face of difficulties, trauma, or tragedy also can provide a therapeutic outlet, but conversely may engender spiritual or religious doubt, or a sense of alienation from one's beliefs. Nurses suggest a referral to a chaplain or clergy member, provide spiritual music or art work, recommend spiritual reading material, and provide personal presence (see Quality and Safety Scenario box, earlier). Willis and colleagues (2015) explicated how spiritual healing manifested itself in the aftermath of childhood maltreatment and point out the potential helpfulness of "constructing caring-healing interventions aimed at both cultivating spiritual consciousness and facilitating loving-kindness and acts of letting go in the healing process."

Nurses propose activities that provide a sense of meaning and purpose. Keeping a journal can be an important strategy to help individuals focus on aspects of life that are more positive and that become clouded from view when a person is feeling overwhelmed by stress. Finding ways of helping others (e.g., tutoring children, reading to the blind, or visiting an older person) can have a positive influence on spiritual health and well-being. Altruism, generosity, kindness, and service to others are more than moral virtues. These attributes not only help to make the world a better place but also help people find meaning and purpose in life. Religious and existential well-being has provided some defense against depression for people with chronic and life-threatening conditions. Older, chronically ill, and homebound people can be encouraged to produce written or oral histories that can be a legacy or, when able, to contact others needing care or to make telephone calls to raise funds for a favourite charity. In addition, nurses and other health care professionals can assist individuals and families to describe and clarify their personal religious and spiritual perspectives, especially in light of evolving practices/meaning structures and high rates of interfaith marriages/partnerships (Walsh, 2011). Spirituality and religious affiliation cannot be equated. Additionally, being part of a "faith community" may provide an important source of social support for many people. Within faith communities, nurses (also known as "parish" nurses) act as facilitators, educators, and referrers to individuals and families in promoting holistic care. Nurses can encourage individuals to search for a community that is comfortable, accepting, and supportive.

## Clarifying Values and Beliefs

To manage stress and develop a balanced lifestyle, people must recognize the things and values that are important to them, reflect on where they are in life, evaluate what needs to be changed, and generate an action plan for that change. This process is known as values clarification. The first step is to identify what is important, meaningful, and valuable so as to assess whether actions are consistent with beliefs. What people believe and value guides their actions by endorsing certain behaviours and changing others.

When people assess their values and beliefs, they use the ability to make their own choices rather than relying on beliefs and values dictated to them by others.

One method nurses use to help people identify what they value and, ultimately, to help them clarify the relationship between their beliefs and actions is to ask them to identify what is important or meaningful to them. The form in Fig. 23.5 is an example of questions used in the Medical Symptom Reduction Program at the Benson-Henry Institute for Mind Body Medicine of Massachusetts General Hospital in Boston. Individuals are asked to identify what is important and meaningful to them in eight domains. Nurses change the domains to reflect more accurately the values and beliefs of the individuals they are counseling. After reviewing the results, individuals may find that they have not been doing certain things that are important to them (becoming more physically active, eating a healthier diet, volunteering, or spending time with their children). When people detect inconsistencies between their values and their actual living habits, they can begin to develop a working plan for correcting these inconsistencies. This process enables them to make conscious choices and to have more control (see Fig. 23.5).

## Setting Realistic Goals

Developing an action plan for change to work toward a more balanced health-promoting lifestyle that is consistent with a person's values and beliefs is an important stress-management strategy. Setting realistic, attainable goals facilitates this exercise. Goal setting is a dynamic process that involves both the individual and the nurse. Goals should be specific, concrete, measurable, and achievable. Nurses facilitate this process by respecting the individual's input and using a values clarification exercise (such as the one mentioned) to facilitate a more complete database to guide individuals to identify and prioritize problems to be addressed, and set mutually agreed on long-term and short-term goals. Nurses encourage individuals to challenge themselves when their behaviours are not consistent with what they identified as important and meaningful to them. For example, when an overweight man with hypertension and high cholesterol levels continues to smoke and eat high-fat foods, nurses help him to look at these behaviours relative to what is meaningful to him, such as his family. The cost and benefit are usually clear, and the responsibility for the change is with the individual, not the nurse. Nurses ask the following questions to help individuals clarify long-term goals:

- What is important to you?
- What would you like to change about your life?
- What can you do to start that change?
- When will you take that action?
- How will you measure success?
- How will you maintain the desired change?
- How can I help you to reach your goal?

Setting realistic, attainable goals helps to create a sense of confidence and achievement and to build enthusiasm to set future goals. This process, in turn, increases a sense of control and mitigates the negative effects of stress.

## Humour

Humour is an enjoyable and effective antidote to stress for many people. Humour can have health-promoting properties (Konradt, Hirsch, Jonitz, et al., 2013; Stuart, 2013). When acting as a stress reducer, humour produces laughter. Laughter creates predictable physiological changes in the body. Human emotions associated with humour, such as joy, and the act of laughing do not only have significant psychophysiological impacts, but they also improve social connections and one's ability to manage emotions and to focus (Savage, Lujan, Thipparthi, et al., 2017).

Humour can open different perspectives on problems and facilitate objectivity, which increases a sense of self-protection and control. Finding humour in a stressful situation can help people to reframe perceptions of the event. Some hospital staffs are using laughter libraries, humour rooms, and comedy carts that can be wheeled into an individual's hospital room, and clowns to bring laughter and joy to the bedside. Humour has potential as an accessible, enjoyable, and inexpensive stress-reduction strategy that can offer people new perspectives on their world and themselves. Nevertheless, recognizing that humour can mask conflict or be hurtful is critically important in judging when and how to use it in clinical and work setting encounters (Box 23.5).

## Engaging in Pleasurable Activities

A variety of activities can promote the relaxation response. Finding activities that are enjoyable to the person can be a key strategy to reduce stress and promote healthy behaviours. For example, Wong in her engaging book *Scales to Scalpels* (Wong & Viagas, 2012) described how the Longwood Symphony Orchestra in Boston, a talented group of medical professionals who practise at an elite centre of health care and research, helps them to thrive as artists. Carving out the time to create music within this ensemble in the midst of demanding clinical and academic lives allows these musician/clinicians to practise the healing art of music for themselves and in turn to be better healers. Wong's engaging narrative underscores the value of integrating various art therapies into our care plans as a valuable strategy for health promotion and stress reduction. Additionally, it points to the importance of self-care for clinicians.

## EFFECTIVE COPING

When people believe that they can cope effectively, the harmful effects of stress can be minimized. The stressful situation is perceived as a challenge rather than a threat. This often-elusive difference has vital mind, body, and spirit effects. When people believe that their lives are more balanced and under control, they are productive, but not driven; are aroused, but not anxious; and they may even be physically or mentally tired, but not exhausted.

Effective coping helps people face great adversity (such as illness) and recognize the opportunity that the situation often presents. First and foremost, individuals must recognize that coping is the ability to find a balance between

*"What Is Important and Meaningful to You in Life?"*

In each of the following areas, what do you want for yourself, today, next week, a year from now?

Under each of the following categories, please ask yourself these important questions.

*Professional, educational, and intellectual*
Today _____
Next week _____
A year from now _____

*Relationships*
Today _____
Next week _____
A year from now _____

*Creative things*
Today _____
Next week _____
A year from now _____

*Spiritual*
Today _____
Next week _____
A year from now _____

*Volunteer and altruistic*
Today _____
Next week _____
A year from now _____

*Health*
Today _____
Next week _____
A year from now _____

*Fun and play*
Today _____
Next week _____
A year from now _____

*Material objects*
Today _____
Next week _____
A year from now _____

**Fig. 23.5** What Is Important and Meaningful to You in Life? (From *Medical symptom reduction program patient notebook*. [n.d.]. Boston: The Benson-Henry Institute for Mind Body Medicine of Massachusetts General Hospital, Harvard Medical School.)

acceptance and action, between letting go and taking control. Many stress-management strategies help individuals distinguish these differences by providing a format for observing or objectifying their experiences. Other strategies such as exercise and balanced nutrition help individuals promote physical health and well-being to counter the harmful effects of stress. In addition, epigenetics (i.e., how environmental factors such as nutrition and stress trigger or mute the expression of genetic traits) is a vast canvas for the exploration of causes and intervention across a variety of physical and mental health disorders for individuals and populations (Dauncey, 2014) (Genomics).

Nurses help individuals improve effective coping by guiding them in the art of choosing the right strategy at the right time. In doing so, people gain a sense of control that minimizes or buffers harmful effects of stress. Nurses use the interventions described in this chapter to assist individuals to manage extrinsic and intrinsic stressors.

## GENOMICS

Epigenetic regulators modify gene expression without changes in DNA sequence. Nutrition is such a regulator that affects the brain throughout life, with profound implications for cognitive decline and dementia. Effects are mediated by changes in expression of multiple genes, and responses to nutrition are in turn affected by individual genetic variability. Epigenetic mechanisms are central to brain development, structure, and function. Epigenetics promote cell-specific and age-related gene expression that can be highly stable but also reversible in response to factors such as nutrition. Health and brain function, in particular, result from highly complex interactions between numerous genetic and environmental factors, including nutrition, physical activity, age, and stress. The interplay of genetic and environmental factors, including nutrition and stress, is critical to our understanding the causes of many health disorders and developing effective interventions.

Source: Modified from Dauncey, M. J. (2014). Nutrition, the brain and cognitive decline: Insights from epigenetics. *European Journal of Clinical Nutrition, 68*(11), 1179–1185.

### BOX 23.5  Humour Strategies for Stress Reduction

Nurses help individuals use humour for health promotion and stress reduction in a variety of ways, including:
- Keeping a humour journal: looking for the unintentional amusing remark, watching for funny things young children say or do, and looking in the newspaper for humorous grammatical errors or an inappropriate choice of words and writing them in a journal
- Looking on the Internet for humorous resources
- Creating a scrapbook of humorous cartoons, pictures, stickers, poems, and songs
- Reading a cartoon or joke in the newspaper every day and sharing it with a friend
- Watching funny movies or reruns of old television programs
- Finding and spending time with funny, light-hearted people

When individuals cannot control or influence the situation (extrinsic stressors), nurses advise them to do the following:
- Take care of physical health and well-being: exercise; eat healthy, balanced meals; and practise sleep hygiene.

- *Accept:* learn to accept that some situations or people cannot be changed or avoided. Forgiveness and letting go of resentment are often a part of acceptance.
- *Use distraction:* distraction involves putting a worry aside, when necessary, until the situation can be dealt with directly. This prioritizing is quite different from procrastinating or denial, because it is a necessary delay rather than avoidance.
- *Reduce emotional arousal:* practise mini relaxations, listen to a relaxation recording, use the four-step cognitive–behavioural restructuring technique, exercise, seek social support, pray, meditate, use humour and affirmations, write in a journal, or engage in a healthy pleasure.

When individuals can alter or influence the situation, or when they are contributing to or creating the stress (intrinsic stressors), nurses advise them to do the following:
- Take care of physical health and well-being: exercise; eat healthy, balanced meals; and practise sleep hygiene.
- Reduce emotional arousal: practise mini relaxations, listen to music or a relaxation DVD or CD, engage in exercise, seek social support, pray, meditate, use humour and affirmations, write in a journal, engage in a healthy pleasure, and/or use the four-step cognitive–behavioural restructuring strategy:
  - *Stop* (breaking the cycle of escalating, negative thoughts)
  - *Breathe deeply* (eliciting the relaxation response and releasing tension)
  - *Reflect* (asking "What is going on here? What am I thinking? Is the thought true? Is the thought helpful? Am I jumping to conclusions or magnifying the situation?")
  - *Choose* a more realistic, rational response and related behavioural reaction.
- Problem solve:
  - Clarify values, beliefs, and expectations.
  - Gather information.
  - Seek advice, support, assistance, or information.
  - Use assertive communication and empathy.
  - Set realistic goals, design action strategies, and determine the best steps to handle the problem.
  - Take action.
See the Care Plan for John DeMarco for an example of a plan for effective coping.

## CASE STUDY

### Health Assessment: John DeMarco

John DeMarco, a 29-year-old man separated from his wife, walked into the health clinic stating he had a severe sore throat, could not eat, had not worked for a day, and was feeling "awful." He wanted to see the physician and get a prescription for an antibiotic. The medical record revealed two episodes within the last 9 months of reports of a sore throat, culture of organism, and antibiotic treatment. The separation from his wife occurred 1 year ago. He had not had a physical examination in 2 years. During the assessment interview, the nurse gathered the following information: John DeMarco appeared tired; he presented his problem in short, terse statements; he was irritable about the clinic's slow service; and he expressed a need to get back to work. Within the last 3 weeks he had been required to work overtime because he faced deadline penalties, and his boss said that Mr. DeMarco's promotion, due in 2 months, depended on his performance now. The company is struggling, and layoffs may be pending. Mr. DeMarco said that, in general, things were fine. His wife was

apparently happy without him, and he was too busy to care or to think about that relationship. He made one remark about his boss: "What do you do with a nervous boss?" He described his diet as fast food "taken on the run." He said he gets about 6 hours of sleep per night and awakens one to two times near morning. He has infrequent contact with family members, who live in the area. In accordance with the clinical protocol for the health centre, the nurse collects a throat culture.

**Reflective Questions**
- As Mr. DeMarco's nurse, how would you comprehensively assess his health?
- What are several different diagnoses and possible individual, family, and etiological factors to consider?
- What work-related health issues may be a concern?
- What other issues may impact the community where Mr. DeMarco is employed?

## CARE PLAN

**Plan for Effective Coping: John DeMarco**

**Nursing Issue**
Inadequate coping related to increased stress at work and limited coping strategies

**Defining Characteristics to Assess**
- Physiological disturbances
- Abuse of alcohol or drugs
- Participation in potentially dangerous activities
- Engaging in lifestyle with risk to health
- Impairment of social role functioning:
  - Nonproductive lifestyle
  - Failure to function in usual social roles
  - Nonperformance of activities of daily living
  - Inappropriate behaviours in social situations
  - Self-absorption
  - Lack of concern for or detachment from usual social supports
- Poor morale:
  - Unhappiness
  - Lack of future orientation
  - Hopelessness
  - Unacceptable quality of life
  - Pessimism
- Defensive patterns:
  - Inflexibility
  - Hypervigilance
  - Avoidance
  - Inertia
  - Refusal or rejection of help

**Expectations**
Mr. DeMarco will:
- Report increased information on and consequences to himself of stressors experienced.
- Practise the relaxation response for 20 to 30 minutes every day through prayer or contemplation; use multiple mini relaxations throughout each day.
- Report increasing weekly exercise or activity and healthy changes in nutrition and sleep or rest patterns.
- Develop effective coping and problem-solving abilities to manage stress, beginning with the stress at work.
- Evaluate the result of throat culture and consult with his primary care provider if the result is positive and an antibiotic is indicated.

**Interventions**
- Promote an attitude of openness to new information.
- Enroll him in a cognitive–behavioural group program to learn stress-management strategies and health promotion.
- Monitor his daily practice of relaxation response.
- Monitor his changes in exercise or activity, nutrition, sleep or rest patterns, and mood.
- Guide him to develop two coping strategies through cognitive–behavioural restructuring.
- Schedule a follow-up appointment or telephone check-in to monitor his well-being.

## SUMMARY

Health and the ability to cope effectively with the many demands of work–life balance require management of stress. Combining careful assessment and choice of strategies, thoughtful and honest feedback, and continued support, nurses assist people to cope more effectively with the innumerable actual and potential stressors they may encounter. Research to discern the interplay of homeodynamic physiological, psychological, social, and spiritual responses to stress has yielded important knowledge for practice. However, uncovering the intricate workings of the brain within the context of human stress and coping experiences is a daunting and critical challenge for today's health researchers.

Stress-management strategies provide an opportunity for individuals to acquire the necessary skills to cope more successfully and become confident in self-management. Such awareness enables the individual to challenge and change perceptions, decrease stress reactivity, improve self-management skills, and minimize the harmful consequences of stress. This process positively influences health promotion, disease prevention, and symptom management. Challenges remain to expand intervention testing to families and communities. Understanding the influences of stress on health and illness is essential to all nursing practice.

**Evolve Chapter Features**
http://evolve.elsevier.com/Canada/Edelman/healthpromotion/
- Review Questions

## REFERENCES

Baer, R. A. (2014). *Mindfulness-based treatment approaches: Clinician's guide to evidence base and applications.* Cambridge, MA: Academic Press.

Barchas, P. R., & Barchas, J. D. (2011). Sociophysiology 25 years ago: Early perspectives of an emerging discipline now as part of neuroscience. *Annals of the New York Academy of Sciences, 1231,* 1–16.

Beck, A. T. (1976). *Cognitive therapy and the emotional disorders.* New York: International Universities Press. [Seminal Reference].

Beck, A. T. (1979). *Cognitive therapy of depression.* New York: Guilford Press. [Seminal Reference].

Beck Institute for Cognitive Behaviour Therapy. (2012). *Beck Institute for cognitive behaviour therapy.* Retrieved from https://beckinstitute.org/.

Benson, H. (1975). *The relaxation response.* New York: William Morrow & Co. [Seminal Reference].

Benson-Henry Institute for Mind Body Medicine of Massachusetts General Hospital. (n.d.). Stress. Retrieved from https://www.bensonhenryinstitute.org/.

Berger, M., Juster, R. P., & Sarnyai, Z. (2015). A mental health consequences of stress and trauma: Allostatic load markers for practice and policy with a focus on indigenous health. *Australasian Psychiatry, 23*(6), 644–649. https://doi.org/10.1177/1039856215608281.

Bobo, W. V., & Yawn, B. (2014). Concise review for physicians and other clinicians: Postpartum depression. *Mayo Clinic Proceedings, 89*(6), 835–844.

Bortz, W. M. (2015). Updating homeostasis. *Biological Systems: Open Access, 4*, 138.

Brann, L., Owens, J., & Williamson, A. (2011). *The handbook of contemporary clinical hypnosis: Theory and practice.* Chichester, England: John Wiley & Sons.

Canadian Centre on Substance Use and Addiction & University of Victoria Canadian Institute for Substance Use Research. (2018). *Canadian substance use costs and harms (CSUCH) 2007–2014.* Retrieved from http://www.ccsa.ca/Resource Library/CSUCH-Canadian-Substance-Use-Costs-Harms-Report-2018-en.pdf.

Cannon, W. (1914). The emergency function of the adrenal medulla in pain and the major emotions. *American Journal of Physiology, 33*(2), 356–372. [Seminal Reference].

Clark, D. A., & Beck, A. T. (2012). *The anxiety and worry workbook: The cognitive behavioral solution.* New York: Guilford Press.

Dailey, D. E., Dawn, E., & Humphreys, J. C. (2011). Social stressors associated with antepartum depressive symptoms in low-income African American women. *Public Health Nursing, 28*(3), 203–212.

Dames, S. (2018). THRIVEable work environments: A study of interplaying factors that enable novice nurses to thrive. *Journal of Nursing Management, 26*, 6. https://doi.org/10.1111/jonm.12712.

Dauncey, M. J. (2014). Nutrition, the brain and cognitive decline: Insights from epigenetics. *European Journal of Clinical Nutrition, 68*(11), 1179–1185.

DeMarco, R., & Segraves, M. M. (2011). Community assessment. In G. Harkness, & R. DeMarco (Eds.), *Community and public health nursing: Evidence for practice* (pp. 175–191). Philadelphia: Lippincott Williams & Wilkins.

Dowd, H., Hogan, M. J., McGuire, B. E., et al. (2015). Comparison of an online mindfulness-based cognitive therapy intervention with online pain management psychoeducation: A randomized controlled study. *The Clinical Journal of Pain, 31*(6), 517–527. https://doi.org/10.1097/AJP.0000000000000201.

Ebner, K., & Singewald, N. (2017). Individual differences in stress susceptibility and stress inhibitory mechanisms. *Current Opinion in Behavioral Sciences, 14*, 54–64. https://doi.org/10.1016/j.cobeha.2016.11.016.

Ellis, A. (1962). *Reason and emotion in psychotherapy.* New York: L. Stuart. [Seminal Reference].

Ellis, A., & Dryden, W. (1987). *The practice of rational emotive therapy (RET).* New York: Springer. [Seminal Reference].

Government of Canada. (2015). *Natural and non-prescription health products.* Retrieved from https://www.canada.ca/en/health-canada/services/drugs-health-products/natural-non-prescription.html.

Government of Canada. (2018). *Mental health: Coping with stress.* Retrieved from https://www.canada.ca/en/health-canada/services/healthy-living/your-health/lifestyles/your-health-mental-health-coping-stress-health-canada-2008.html.

Gregorio, S. W., Carpenter, K. M., Dorfman, C. S., et al. (2012). Impact of breast cancer recurrence and cancer-specific stress on spouse health and immune function. *Brain, Behavior, and Immunity, 26*(2), 228–233.

Gunter, K. B., Almstedt, H. C., & Janz, K. F. (2012). Physical activity in childhood may be the key to optimizing lifespan skeletal health. *Exercise and Sport Sciences Reviews, 40*(1), 13–21.

Harkness, G., & DeMarco, R. (Eds.). (2012). *Community and public health nursing: Evidence for practice.* Philadelphia: Lippincott Williams & Wilkins.

Health Canada. (2019). *Canada's dietary guidelines (Catalogue No. H164-231/2019E-PDF).* Ottawa: Author. Retrieved from https://food-guide.canada.ca/static/assets/pdf/CDG-EN-2018.pdf.

Helali, A. (2016). *The effects of daily self-reiki practice on nurses' level of burnout.* ProQuest Dissertation Publishing.

Holmes, T. H. (1981). *The schedule of recent experiences.* Seattle: University of Washington Press. [Seminal Reference].

Horowitz, M., Wilner, N., & Alvarez, W. (1979). Impact of event scale: A measure of subjective stress. *Psychosomatic Medicine, 41*(3), 209–218. [Seminal Reference].

Kaku, M. (2014). *The future of the mind.* New York: Doubleday.

Kobasa, S. C., Maddi, S. R., & Kahn, S. (1982). Hardiness and health: A prospective study. *Journal of Personality and Social Psychology, 42*, 391–404. [Seminal Reference].

Konradt, B., Hirsch, R. D., Jonitz, M. F., et al. (2013). Evaluation of a standardized humor group in a clinical setting: A feasibility study for older patients with depression. *International Journal of Geriatric Psychiatry, 28*(8), 850–857.

Kruk, J. (2012). Self-reported psychological stress and the risk of breast cancer: A case-control study. *Stress: The International Journal on the Biology of Stress, 15*(2), 162–171.

Kyu, H. H., Bachman, V. F., Alexander, L. T., et al. (2016). Physical activity and risk of breast cancer, colon cancer, diabetes, ischemic heart disease, and ischemic stroke events: Systematic review and dose-response meta-analysis for the global burden of disease study. *BMJ, 354.* https://doi.org/10.1136/bmj.i3857.

Lazarus, R., & Folkman, S. (1984). *Stress, appraisal, and coping.* New York: Springer. [Seminal Reference].

Leiter, M. P., Price, S. L., & Spence Laschinger, H. K. (2010). Generational differences in distress, attitudes and incivility among nurses: Generational differences among nurses. *Journal of Nursing Management, 18*(8), 970–980. https://doi.org/10.1111/j.1365-2834.2010.01168.x.

Lengacher, C. A., Kip, K. E., Reich, R. R., et al. (2015). A cost-effective mindfulness stress reduction program: A randomized control trial for breast cancer survivors. *Nursing Economics, 33*(4), 210–232.

Louveau, A., Harris, T. H., & Kipnis, J. (2015). Revisiting the mechanisms of CNS immune privilege. *Trends in Immunology, 36*(10), 569–577. https://doi.org/10.1016/j.it.2015.08.006.

Manitoba Nurses Union. (2015). *Helping manitoba's wounded healers: Post-traumatic stress disorder in the nursing profession.* Retrieved from http://traumadoesntend.ca/wp-content/uploads/2015/04/75005-MNU-PTSD-BOOKLET-SCREEN.pdf.

Marchant, J. (2016). *Cure: A journey into the science of mind over body.* New York: Crown Publishers.

Maslach, C., & Jackson, S. E. (1986). *Maslach burnout inventory manual* (2nd ed.). Palo Alto, CA: Consulting Psychologists Press. [Seminal Reference].

Maslow, A. H. (1943). A theory of human motivation. *Psychological Review, 50*(4), 370–396. https://doi.org/10.1037/h0054346. [Seminal Reference].

McLennon, S. M., Habermann, B., & Rice, M. (2011). Finding meaning as a mediator of burden on the health of caregivers of spouses with dementia. *Aging & Mental Health, 15*, 522–530.

McPhee, J. S., French, D. P., Jackson, D., et al. (2016). Physical activity in older age: Perspectives for healthy ageing and frailty. *Biogerontology, 17*(3), 567–580. https://doi.org/10.1007/s10522-016-9641-0.

Menezes, A. R., Lavie, C. J., Milani, R. V., O'Keefe, J., & Lavie, T. J. (2011). Psychological risk factors and cardiovascular disease: Is it all in your head? *Postgraduate Medicine, 123*(5), 165–176. https://doi.org/10.3810/pgm.2011.09.2472.

Nikkheslat, N., Zunszain, P. A., Horowitz, M. A., et al. (2015). Insufficient glucocorticoid signaling and elevated inflammation in coronary heart disease patients with comorbid depression. *Brain, Behavior, and Immunity, 48*, 8–18. https://doi.org/10.1016/j.bbi.2015.02.002.

North, R. J., Pai, A. V., Hixon, G., et al. (2011). Finding happiness in negative emotions: An experimental test of a novel expressive writing paradigm. *The Journal of Positive Psychology, 6*(3), 192–203. https://doi.org/10.1080/17439760.2011.570365.

Paradies, Y. (2011). A theoretical review of psychosocial stress and health. In A. B. Barnes, & J. E. Montefuscio (Eds.), *Role of stress in psychological disorders* (pp. 1–19). New York: Nova Science Publishers.

Phillips, J. R. (2015). Martha E. Rogers: Heretic and heroine. *Nursing Science Quarterly, 28*, 42–48.

Public Health Agency of Canada (PHAC). (2017). *Departmental results report 2016–2017.* Retrieved from https://www.canada.ca/en/public-health/corporate/transparency/corporate-management-reporting/departmental-performance-reports/2017-2018-departmental-results-report.html.

Quinn, C., Clare, V., & Woods, R. T. (2011). The impact of motivation and meanings on the wellbeing of caregivers of people with dementia. *International Psychogeriatrics, 22*, 43–55.

Richards, S. H., Anderson, L., Jenkinson, C. E., Whalley, B., Rees, K., Davies, P., et al. (2017). Psychological interventions for coronary heart disease. *Cochrane Database of Systematic Reviews, 4*, CD002902.

Rogers, C. (1951). *Client-centered therapy.* Boston: Houghton Mifflin. [Seminal Reference].

Sadock, B. S., & Sadock, V. A. (2015). *Kaplan & Sadock's synopsis of clinical psychiatry* (11th ed.). Philadelphia: Wolters Kluwer.

Sampasa-Kanyinga, H., & Chaput, J. (2017). Associations among self-perceived work and life stress, trouble sleeping, physical activity, and body weight among Canadian adults. *Preventive Medicine, 96*, 16–20. https://doi.org/10.1016/j.ypmed.2016.12.013.

Savage, B. M., Lujan, H. L., Thipparthi, R. R., et al. (2017). Humor, laughter, learning, and health! A brief review. *Advances in Physiology Education, 41*(3), 341–347. https://doi.org/10.1152/advan.00030.2017.

Schermel, A., Mendoza, J., Henson, S., et al. (2014). Canadians' perceptions of food, diet, and health—a national survey. *PloS One, 9*(1), e86000. https://doi.org/10.1371/journal.pone.0086000.

Selye, H. (1950). *Stress.* Montreal: Acta Inc. [Seminal Reference].

Selye, H. (1974). *Stress without distress.* Philadelphia: J. B. Lippincott & Co. [Seminal Reference].

Selye, H. (1982). History and present status of the stress concept. In L. Goldberger, & S. Breznitz (Eds.), *Handbook of stress: Theoretical and clinical aspects* (pp. 7–17). New York: Free Press. [Seminal Reference].

Sifferlin, A. (2016). What you need to know about Zika: How to beat the virus and the mosquitoes that carry it. *Time, 187*(18), 32–41.

Simon, C., & McFadden, T. (2017). *National physician health survey: The process, preliminary data, and future directions Canadian Medical Association (CMA). Canadian conference on physician health.* 2017 Sep 7–9; Ottawa.

Sinha, R., & Jastreboff, A. M. (2013). Stress as a common risk factor for obesity and addiction. *Biological Psychiatry, 73*(9), 827–835.

Slavich, G. M. (2016). Life stress and health: A review of conceptual issues and recent findings. *Teaching of Psychology, 43*(4), 346–355. https://doi.org/10.1177/0098628316662768.

Statistics Canada. (2014). *Perceived live stress. National physician health survey.* Retrieved from https://www150.statcan.gc.ca/n1/pub/82-625-x/2015001/article/14188-eng.htm.

Stuart, G. W. (Ed.). (2013). *Principles and practice of psychiatric nursing* (10th ed.). St. Louis: Mosby.

Tang, Y. Y., Holzel, B. K., & Posner, M. I. (2015). The neuroscience of mindfulness meditation. *Nature Reviews Neuroscience, 16*(4), 213–225. https://doi.org/10.1038/nrn3916.

Thompson, T., Keogh, E., & French, C. C. (2011). Sensory focusing versus distraction and pain: Moderating effects of anxiety sensitivity in males and females. *The Journal of Pain, 12*, 849–858.

Tonhajzerova, I., & Mestanik, M. (2017). New perspectives in the model of stress response. *Physiological Research, 66*, S173.

Trottier, K., & MacDonald, D. E. (2017). Update on psychological trauma, other severe adverse experiences and eating disorders: State of the research and future research directions. *Current Psychiatry Reports, 19*(8), 1–9. https://doi.org/10.1007/s11920-017-0806-6.

van Woerden, H. C., Poortinga, W., Bronstering, K., et al. (2011). The relationship of different sources of social support and civic participation with self-rated health. *Journal of Public Mental Health, 10*(3), 126–139. https://doi.org/10.1108/17465721111175010.

Walsh, A. (2011). The relaxation response: A strategy to address stress. *International Journal of Athletic Therapy & Training, 16*(2), 20–23.

Weber, J. G. (2011). *Individual and family stress and crises.* Thousand Oaks, CA: Sage Publications. [Seminal Reference].

Willis, D. G., DeSanto-Madeya, S., Ross, R., et al. (2015). Spiritual healing in the aftermath of childhood maltreatment: Translating men's lived experiences utilizing conceptual models and theory. *Advances in Nursing Science, 38*(3), 162–174. https://doi.org/10.1097/ANS.0000000000000075.

Wong, L., & Viagas, R. (2012). *Scales to scalpels.* New York: Pegasus Books.

Wood, A. W., Gonzales, J., & Barden, S. M. (2015). Mindful caring: Using mindfulness-based cognitive therapy with caregivers of cancer survivors. *Journal of Psychosocial Oncology, 33*(1), 66–84. https://doi.org/10.1080/07347332.2014.977418.

World Health Organization (WHO). (2018). *2018 global reference list of 100 core health indicators (plus health-related SDGs).* Geneva: WHO. 2018. Licence: CC BY-NC-SA 3.0 IGO. Retrieved from http://apps.who.int/iris/bitstream/handle/10665/259951/WHO-HIS-IER-GPM-2018.1-eng.pdf;jsessionid=B5C58F65276B-62C00DDD5A7B9E2D65BC?sequence=1.

Wright, L. M., & Leahey, M. (2019). *Nurses and families: A guide to family assessment and intervention* (7th ed.). Philadelphia: F. A. Davis.

# 24

# Complementary and Alternative Strategies

*Bernie Garrett, RN, PGCE, PhD*

## INTENDED LEARNING OUTCOMES

*After completing this chapter, the reader will be able to:*

- Compare and contrast alternative and biomedical health modalities.
- Explore the nature of commonly encountered alternative, complementary, and salutogenic approaches to health.
- Discuss tensions and issues with the use of alternative health care in respect to health promotion.

- Discuss the safety and effectiveness of complementary and alternative medicine.
- Describe the nursing role in supporting patients who engage with alternative health care.
- Identify alternative medicine resources.

## KEY TERMS

Alternative medicine
Allopathic medicine
Biomedicine

Complementary and alternative medicine (CAM)
Integrative medicine/health care
Salutogenic medicine

## ? THINK ABOUT IT

Ms. Sun is a 45-year-old in a state of good health who works as a part-time receptionist for a car dealer. She has a 92-year-old mother and was advised by her physician to get an influenza vaccination for the coming winter flu season. Ms. Sun is a keen believer in natural health and, at a recent consultation with her naturopath, was advised by the naturopath that "from strictly a health perspective, the flu vaccine is not necessarily in your mother's very best long-term interest." The naturopath also talked of other natural benefits from getting the flu, such as reducing the risk of brain tumours, and suggested that rather than getting the vaccination, her mother could come to her clinic for an intravenous (IV) vitamin supplement to boost her immune system. She provided Ms. Sun with a leaflet telling her how if her mother does get influenza, she could easily treat the fever by wearing ice-cold wet socks overnight. After looking at sites on the Internet that advocate against vaccination, Ms. Sun believes that these therapies recommended by the naturopath might be better than getting an influenza vaccination for her mother. She also feels somewhat overwhelmed and confused regarding what is best for her mother, because her physician and friends suggest she should get the flu shot, but her naturopath is advising alternative strategies instead.

- What is the difference between a naturopath and a physician?
- What does best evidence and Health Canada policy suggest regarding health-promotional strategies for influenza?
- What is the best understanding of the biomedical mechanisms for these therapies?
- What is the best understanding of the safety of these therapies?
- Which therapies are available for free or covered by her health insurance?
- Would the therapies suggested by the naturopath be considered complementary, alternative, or integrative?

## BACKGROUND

Most human societies are now reliant on science and the technologies that it has provided, and we now live in a highly technological world. Yet many people crave explanations for things which hold more personal meaning to them and hold strong faith-based beliefs, which often influence their health behaviours. In a liberal and diverse society this is to be expected, and there has been a growth of alternative health care along with ongoing research into the motivations of people using it (Nahin, Barnes, & Stussman, 2016; Sirois, 2008; Thorne, Paterson, Russell, et al., 2002). Interestingly, if one raises the subject of alternative health care, you are likely to find a range of opinions, and it is often a very polarizing issue. However, as with most health-related concerns, things are rarely black and white, and the use of alternative health strategies in health promotion is no exception.

A practical description of complementary and alternative health care is that it represents therapeutic modalities that originate from alternative cultural traditions that are distinct from biomedical science. Alternative health care is focused on personal physical, emotional, and mental well-being and predominantly exists outside of public health care provision (Ernst & Cassileth, 1998; Garrett, 2018; Offit, 2012; Thorne et al., 2002). Some therapies are used to supplement biomedical health care, such as meditation or acupuncture for anxiety and pain management. A key feature is that a scientific consensus on the efficacy of these therapies has yet to be established. Overall, evidence supporting these practices is generally weak or even, in some cases, indicates that they do not work. Some alternative health practitioners will argue that their practices are science based (when they may not be); also, many are often argued to be beyond scientific analysis by their supporters, and many of them (such as faith-healing) are difficult to validate in empirical terms.

While alternative health care practices are widely used by Canadians, nurses and physicians may have a limited knowledge about their use, in many cases because of a lack of perceived scientific research to evaluate effectiveness (Gaboury, April, & Verhoef, 2012; Gaboury, Johnson, Robin, et al., 2016). Thus complementary therapies are typically not a part of public health care provision. For example, the Canadian Medical Association policy on complementary and alternative medicine (CAM) advises caution regarding the use of CAMs by physicians because indiscriminate use and unrestricted acceptance could result in adverse health effects or failure by patients to access more appropriate care (Canadian Medical Association, 2015). Nevertheless, use of alternative medicine in North America is increasing and, far from being a homespun activity, it now represents a major economic sector. Many of these practices are based upon ancient and traditional health systems, such as Ayurvedic medicine, that people in India have used for more than 5000 years. Other practices arose from more modern roots such as the Western counter-culture movements of the 1960s promoting natural health and holistic well-being, whole foods, and mindfulness. Many of these strategies have now become a part of more mainstream health-promotional practice today.

Overall, more than 70% of Canadians regularly use some form of complementary and alternative health care therapies today such as vitamins and minerals, herbal products, homeopathic medicines, and other alternative health products to stay healthy and improve their quality of life (Public Health Agency of Canada, 2019). In 2016, the Fraser Institute conducted a national survey to determine Canadians' use of and attitude toward complementary and alternative therapies. They found increased use over the past decade: approximately 80% of Canadians had used at least one form of complementary therapy, in total spending more than $8 billion on alternative therapies. This included $6.5 billion spent on provider treatment such as homeopathy, chiropractic, reiki, and acupuncture, and another $2.3 billion spent on herbs, vitamins, special diet programs, equipment, and literature (Esmail, 2017). A 2019 industry report suggested that the global market will be worth $210 billion by 2026 (Grand View Research, 2019).

The rapid growth and commercialization of alternative health care has instigated much research into the factors associated with its use. Psychological theory has suggested several personality traits that correlate with its uptake. Research suggests that strong predictors of complementary and alternative therapies include chronological age (35–44 years), chronic health conditions, and pain (Canizares, Hogg-Johnson, Gignac, et al., 2017; Esmail, 2017). The increasing trend toward consumer use is suggestive of a proactive self-care approach to health care and health promotion. Overall, rather than people who live alternative lifestyles, research suggests that alternative health care users are more likely to be women, well-educated, who do not have a regular care provider, and often have chronic health issues (Bromfield & McGwin, 2013; Canizares et al., 2017; Sirois, Salamonsen, & Kristoffersen, 2016). People who have chronic illnesses that conventional medicine cannot cure are often challenged with the ongoing process of self-care management, and so they seek options. The supplementary use of alternative medicine is well-documented here. People who have inflammatory bowel disease (IBD), multiple sclerosis (MS), arthritis, and cancer are all significant users of alternative medicine (Buckner, Lafrenie, Dénommée, et al., 2018; Gilmour, Ramage-Morin, & Wong., 2018; Luctkar-Flude, Groll, & Tyerman, 2017; Opheim, Lie Høivik, Bernklev, et al., 2016; Zhang, Dennis, Bishop, et al., 2019).

Generally, alternative health care advocates will argue this growth in use is because it focuses on prevention of illness rather than on cure, and on forms of holistic medicine that are wholesome, natural, and harmless. This is not necessarily true, however, and unfortunately the less well-regulated alternative health care sector has also been taken advantage of by some deceptive practitioners (Garrett, Murphy, Jamal, et al., 2019), so care is needed when examining the use of such strategies.

## TERMINOLOGY

Alternative health care has multiple confusing names and definitions, so before investigating further, exploring this terminology is useful. However, this presents challenges in itself, as there is actually no consensus on the terms used, and multiple synonyms are in use. CAM is probably the most widely used term, representing the diverse set of health practices that typically lie outside of mainstream medicine and those used in a complementary fashion to it. Although the acronym CAM has become well established, there is ongoing disagreement as to what it means, even amongst its advocates. If people call themselves CAM practitioners, it may be assumed that they practice health care techniques that are outside of the scope of physicians and allied health professionals, and use them in combination with conventional medical treatments. In essence, *complementary* refers to additional health-promoting activities. The term "complementary" infers that the intervention is somehow adjunctive to a medical focus on treating disease. Nevertheless, in modern health care, multiple therapeutic modalities are employed. Modern health care is an interdisciplinary approach, focused on the maintenance and promotion of good health and the prevention, alleviation, or cure of disease. It is delivered at individual, community, and population levels by a wide range of health professionals. What seems to differentiate conventional public health care from CAM practices is an established scientific foundation for practice, not whether the therapies are used alone or in combination with others.

Other than CAM, common terms used in the field include alternative medicine, alternative health, traditional complementary and alternative medicine (TCAM), integrative/integrated medicine, holistic medicine, traditional medicine, salutogenic, and non-allopathic medicine, to name but a few.

This multiplicity gives rise to other issues. The terms *allopathic* and *salutogenic* tend to be used as antonyms. The term allopathic medicine is the conventional practice of science-based curative biomedicine in which medical doctors and other health care providers, such as nurses, pharmacists, and physiotherapists, treat the symptoms and diseases using medications and other biomedical therapeutics.

Salutogenic medicine describes a new paradigm in health care that incorporates positive psychology, employing positive organizational behaviours. Rather than focusing on biomedicine and pathogenesis, the focus of salutogenesis was described as the "birth of health," helping the individual pursue wellness, both mentally and physically, with the goal of preventive health and overall well-being. These terms are frequently espoused by alternative health practitioners to help explain their approach.

There is not a clear consensus regarding the meaning of alternative medicine in any significant sense (Micozzi, 2018). However, many provincial regulatory bodies, such as the British Columbia College of Nursing Professionals (BCCNP), recognize and use the term "alternative medicine." For example, "complementary" practices are used *alongside* mainstream health care, while "alternative" practices are used *in place of* mainstream health care practices (BCCNP, 2018). These arguments serve to illustrate the ongoing complexity in using these terms, and the adversarial stance that alternative health practices often provoke.

## Integrative Medicine and Health Care

Problems inherent to our current public health care systems, along with arguments for more compassionate care, have given rise to attempts to integrate alternative medicine into medicine and public health care, usually referred to as integrative or integrated medicine. The University of Toronto, McGill University, University of Alberta, Mount Royal University, Harvard University, the Mayo Clinic, and the University of Texas offer various programs to health care providers. Leading US cancer centres increasingly present integrative medicine content on their websites, and the majority of them provide these services to patients (Yun, Sun, & Mao, 2017). There is also an *Integrative Medicine Research* journal published by Elsevier. The aims of these approaches sound highly laudable in terms of health promotion, in that they argue that integrative health emphasizes therapeutic relationships and makes use of all appropriate therapies—conventional, complementary, and alternative—to provide a holistic approach. They also promote the goals of examining alternative therapies through scientific research.

Nonetheless, a significant criticism of this approach remains. One problem with the notion of integrative medicine is that it neglects the existing interdisciplinary nature of public health care, and particularly the role of nursing within it. Nursing has been critiqued as being difficult to understand in terms of its focus, but the whole nature of nursing practice is focused upon the holistic integrated person and community-centred care. It will be the nurse who, in addition to providing medical care, also asks patients how they are feeling overall, what else helps them relieve their symptoms, what supplements are they taking,

> ### BOX 24.1   Hot Topics
>
> Key issues in the field of alternative health care include the following:
> - Should we treat the evidence base for alternative health practices differently from that for biomedicine?
> - How do we best differentiate and classify alternative health care practices?
> - How should alternative health care providers be regulated?
> - Should marketing claims for alternative therapeutics be more rigorously controlled than they are currently?
> - Should qualified nurses provide faith-based alternative therapies?
> - Does integrative health care offer a rational way to meet public health needs? What are the potential issues in adopting this approach?
> - Should scientific medicine be regulated as one option in a publicly funded health care system that incorporates diverse approaches in more of a *laissez-faire* system?

how is this illness affecting their lifestyle/employment, how is the family coping, are their religious/spiritual needs being catered for, and who is looking after their pets. In the community, nurse-led clinics support a wide range of health-promotion initiatives, from quitting smoking to breastfeeding programs. In addition to doctors and nurses providing treatment, other science-based professionals in the system support people's specialist health care needs, such as dentists, physiotherapists, psychologists, and social workers. Therefore it is something of a misrepresentation to suggest that the current system is solely disease focused and unholistic in its approach to health, unless one adopts "holism" as an exclusively spiritual term.

Another problem is that this concept of integration involves bringing together different things to improve practice as a whole. In the public view, integrative centres appear to equate the value of conventional and alternative treatments. However, combining faith-based and empirical therapies together with the notion of inclusivity may well result in a mélange of practices that is difficult to defend. Health care is only science based and ethical if its practitioners are science-based and ethical, and integrative medicine supports the potential for serious quality and ethical issues to arise. Some proponents of integrative health care have also acknowledged this. Minimal research is being undertaken to demonstrate the theoretical basis for the alternative therapies that are being applied in these centres.

In reviewing research output from integrative health centres, independent researchers found that only a small number of randomized controlled trials (RCTs) were undertaken and these used small numbers of patients and lacked adequate control groups (Khorsan, Coulter, Crawford, et al., 2011). A recent review of integrative medicine clinical guidelines in China in 2017 also found that the quality was poor (Yao, Wei, Chen, et al., 2017).

The use of any therapeutics also has associated costs, so the argument to adopt alternative therapies in publicly funded integrative health facilities without existing quality evidence of efficacy also raises ethical concerns. The use of public funding for therapeutics that have poor evidence (or even suggesting that the patient pays for these therapies) is questionable. These concerns mean the role of integrative health care in health promotion remains to be demonstrated (Box 24.1).

## TABLE 24.1 Categories and Examples of Complementary and Alternative Therapies

| | |
|---|---|
| Alternative Health Belief Systems | Chinese traditional medicine (including acupuncture), homeopathy, naturopathy, Ayurvedic medicine, Indigenous, and traditional medicine systems |
| Physical Manipulative Interventions | Massage, chiropractic, reflexology, hydrotherapy, craniosacral therapy |
| Herbal and Nutritional Interventions | Herbal remedies, vitamins, dietary supplements, diets, aromatherapy, detoxification therapies |
| Mind–Body Interventions | Meditation, guided imagery, hypnotherapy, music therapy, neurofeedback, biofeedback, yoga, tai chi, qigong, dance |
| Energy Interventions | Reiki, therapeutic touch, magnetic field therapy, faith-healing |

## ALTERNATIVE HEALTH CARE THERAPIES AND PRACTICES

In order to adequately classify and explore alternative practices, it is necessary to define conventional biomedical practice. Biomedicine can be regarded as those health care practices derived from scientific methods, which have evolved under the influences of biomedical and evidence–based approaches, and which currently receive broad international acceptance as a primary mode of health care in the majority of the economically developed world. In contrast, alternative health care is marked by a wide diversity and lack of standardization. A popular approach to the classification of these practices, based on that originally suggested by the National Centre for Complementary and Integrative Health (NCCIH), organizes alternative approaches into five broad systems of practice, which for clarity are presented here as follows: (1) Alternative Health Belief Systems, (2) Physical Manipulative Interventions, (3) Herbal and Nutritional Interventions, (4) Mind–Body Interventions, and (5) Energy Interventions (Table 24.1). However, there are hundreds of alternative therapies, from homeopathy to beer spas, many of which have practices that overlap. For example, homeopathy is usually described as an alternative health belief system, and yet characterizes illness as disturbances in the body's vital energy or life force; thus it is also an energy-based approach. Yoga is often regarded as a mind–body intervention, but it is also a part of Ayurvedic medicine.

It is beyond the scope of this book to explore every type of alternative health practice, and new ones frequently arise. Nonetheless, it is useful to explore the most common ones that nurses are likely to encounter in their practice from each of these categories.

### Alternative Health Belief Systems

These alternative strategies are characterized by complete systems of beliefs about health that do not employ biomedical explanations as their rationale. There are many, including traditional Indigenous belief systems, although in North America, the main ones that nurses will most likely encounter are traditional Chinese medicine (TCM), homeopathy, naturopathy, and Ayurvedic medicine.

### Traditional Chinese Medicine and Acupuncture

Aspects of TCM have been around for several thousand years, but it was first advanced as a national approach to Chinese health by Chairman Mao Zedong as a part of the communist cultural revolution in China during the 1960 and 1970s, and continues to be promoted by the Chinese government today (Dashtdar, Dashtdar, Dashtdar, et al., 2016; Dong, 2013; Li, Dai, Thurston, et al., 1994; Lu & Lu, 2013). TCM is based on a wide-ranging collection of different philosophies and therapeutics, from acupuncture to demonology. The theoretical framework includes the notion of complementary yet opposing *yin* and *yang* life forces, and the balance and harmony of a vital energy or life force that flows through the body known as *qi*. Other theoretical aspects from Chinese traditions include the concept of wind and its direction (one of the six excesses in TCM, which comprise wind, cold, heat, dryness, moisture, and the heat of summer), which is also believed to affect health (Dashtdar et al., 2016). In TCM, multiple herbs and medicines are prescribed together by the practitioner, and a formula may contain up to 20 herbs that each have different actions, organ focus, and functions. Many herbal TCM remedies do in fact work and, therefore, TCM should not be regarded as a completely supernatural framework. However, the acceptance of TCM does risk conflating the possible effectiveness of many traditional remedies with the other metaphysical beliefs attached to it.

Acupuncture represents one of the most successful components of TCM, and is often argued to be an exemplar of an alternative therapy adopted by conventional medicine that has been shown to work. It is said to have been developed in ancient China, and acupuncture points mapped across the body are theorized to correspond to flows of *qi* energy of these pathways of energy flow, and are known as *meridians* in the body. Acupuncture involves stimulating these energy points on the body by using needles that penetrate the skin to alleviate pain or to treat various health conditions. There are various forms of this needling, including electro-acupuncture, which uses electrical stimulation.

Studies conducted by scientists across Europe and North America have demonstrated that acupuncture can be useful in helping treat pain and nausea, and it is available in many Canadian pain clinics. However, outside of China and North Korea there is, as yet, no scientific evidence that the meridians or acupuncture points exist, or that acupuncture can effectively treat any other condition. Although the practice is reported to be over 2000 years old, only relatively recently have high-quality studies been undertaken, using mock acupuncture devices (e.g., using false non-penetrating needles, or needling at non-acupuncture points) as a placebo (Brinkhaus, Witt, Jena, et al., 2007; Haake, Müller, Schade-Brittinger, et al., 2007; Han, 2015; Kluger, Rakowski, Christian, et al., 2016; Paley & Johnson, 2015; Vas, Aranda, Modesto, et al., 2015). The results of a study of acupuncture for the treatment of fibromyalgia-related pain in 2017 found that both acupuncture and sham acupuncture appeared to work better than conventional medications, and exercise alone (Lin, 2017). Clearly there was some effect, but the researchers were unable to demonstrate that it was more than a placebo effect. Following further studies, the

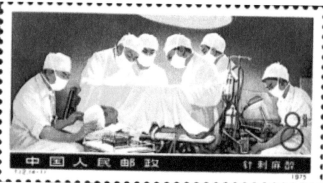

**Fig. 24.1** Chinese stamp depicting use of acupuncture for general anaesthesia during open-heart surgery, 1975. (From Cheng, T. O. [2000]. Stamps in cardiology: Acupuncture anaesthesia for open heart surgery. *Heart [British Cardiac Society]*, *83*[3], 256. Retrieved from https://doi.org/10.1136/heart.83.3.256.)

National Institute for Clinical Excellence (NICE) in the UK withdrew its support for the use of acupuncture for low back pain. Evidence now suggests that acupuncture may actually work more as a powerful distraction for pain (Colquhoun & Novella, 2013). It is well established that pain perception is hugely impacted by psychological factors, so this may explain the effects observed in other studies. Researchers are also now suggesting that neurochemistry may better explain the effects of acupuncture on pain and nausea, and that the proposed pathways (or meridians) of *qi* generally follow the routes of the peripheral nervous system (Li, Yang, Sun, et al., 2013; Moffet, 2006; Yu, Liu, Gao, et al., 2011). However, the neurochemical explanation is not a popular view in the public domain, or a view that is currently promoted by the Chinese authorities. For example, Chinese acupuncturists report how an open-heart surgery operation was performed using acupuncture for anaesthesia in 1975 (Lu & Lu, 2013). This was even commemorated on a Chinese postage stamp at the time (Fig. 24.1).

Acupuncture remains a popular therapy and the evidence base is large but generally of low quality. Chinese medical studies make up the majority of the research work in this area, as well as numerous studies of acupuncture that have problematic study designs with multiple confounding variables. Although acupuncture has observable physical and psychological effects, the current underdetermined mode of action, poor quality of clinical studies, and findings that mock acupuncture also has similar effects, means that the real value of acupuncture as a therapeutic tool remains unclear. For efficacy in pain, there is some data, and many people report benefits, but there remains little quality evidence that acupuncture works better than other interventions. For conditions such as infertility, heart disease, or other significant diseases where efficacy is claimed, no evidence of clinical value has been established.

## Homeopathy and Naturopathy

Two well-established alternative health belief systems are those of homeopathy and naturopathy. Although separate disciplines, they may be considered together here as they have distinct similarities. Both involve the belief of vitalism, and both also have shared a substantial growth in popularity over the last few decades.

Homeopathy is based upon the philosophy of vitalism that interprets diseases and sickness as caused by disturbances in the body's vital energy or life force. It represents a form of alternative medicine where practitioners treat patients using highly diluted preparations of substances believed to cause their symptoms. The German physician Samuel Hahnemann (1755–1843) first elaborated the basic principles of homeopathy in 1796, invoking ideas of curing "like with like" (Canadian Society of Homeopathy, 2019). The theoretical basis is that a substance that in large doses produces symptoms of a specific disease will, in extremely small doses, cure it. Hahnemann originally experimented with cinchona tree bark that is used as a traditional remedy for malaria; it contains large amounts of quinine. He found that he experienced symptoms similar to malaria when he ingested it, and so concluded that he could treat diseases by using small amounts of substances that caused similar symptoms. This thinking also reflects earlier medieval beliefs in metaphysical rather than physical links between cause and the cure (Garrett, 2018).

Homeopathic remedies are prepared from plants, animals, and minerals and known as either *sarcodes* (from healthy organisms) or *nosodes* (from pathological substances). They are listed in a professional *Homeopathic Materia Medica,* and include substances like belladonna, wolfsbane *(Aconitum)*, lithium, silver, tree cancers, and even the livers of rabbit with anthrax. There appears to be no global standard because the contents of this database change around the world.

Despite its popularity, there remains conflicting evidence regarding the effectiveness of homeopathy (Hawke, van Driel, Buffington, et al., 2018; Mathie, Frye, & Fisher, 2015; Mathie, Ramparsad, Legg, et al., 2017; Mathie, Ulbrich-Zürni, Viksveen, et al., 2018). Homeopathy, therefore, is often considered a faith-based practice that many people continue to believe in. Even in the absence of strong scientific evidence of efficacy, homeopathy is generally harmless if used as an adjunctive therapy, because the preparations do not typically contain active ingredients.

Naturopathy is a related and somewhat confusing field, as definitions of it and levels of education vary considerably. Naturopaths are now recognized as doctorly prepared practitioners (naturopathic doctors; NDs) and regulated as a legal health profession in much of North America, including Alberta, British Columbia, Nova Scotia, and Ontario in Canada. There are around 2400 registered naturopaths in Canada, and the profession has gained some popularity, with some strong advocates. Overall, it may be considered a form of alternative medicine based on a belief in natural health with a basis in vitalism. Their vitalist beliefs suggest that disease results from an imbalance in the vital energies that distinguish living from nonliving matter, and this vital force is seen to guide the bodily processes such as metabolism, reproduction, growth, and adaptation. Like TCM practitioners, they use arguments of holistic medicine to explain their approach to health care (Canadian Association of Naturopathic Doctors [CAND], 2019).

Naturopathy has its roots in the nineteenth-century natural health movement of Europe, which arose in part as a reaction to the ineffectiveness and harsh nature of medical treatments of the time. The term *naturopathy* was coined in 1895 by the

German homeopath John Scheel, and adopted by Benedict Lust, a German hydrotherapist (water therapist) and osteopath (therapist that externally manipulates tissues), whom naturopaths consider to be the father of modern naturopathy in North America.

Modern naturopathy supports prevention of disease through healthy living, positive mind–body–spirit strength, and therapeutics to enhance the body's innate healing processes. Naturopathy attributes illness to the violation of natural laws, suggesting that standard medical practices merely treat or suppress symptoms (described as allopathic or salutogenic). The CAND states:

> Naturopathic medicine is a distinct primary health care system that blends modern scientific knowledge with traditional and natural forms of medicine. The naturopathic philosophy is to stimulate the healing power of the body and treat the underlying cause of disease. Symptoms of disease are seen as warning signals of improper functioning of the body, and unfavourable lifestyle habits. Naturopathic Medicine emphasizes disease as a process rather than as an entity.
>
> (CAND, 2019)

On the surface, this definition seems not so very different from the approach of modern medicine, other than the limitation of focus to primary and natural health care. However, many of the natural/traditional interventions that naturopaths support are based on a number of unsubstantiated theories and a collection of faith-based practices, including homeopathy, herbalism, nutritional supplements, detoxification, the use of essential oils, and even faith-healing.

In British Columbia, naturopathic medicine has been legally regulated since 1936 and naturopathy is recognized as doctorly prepared and a self-regulated health profession. It is also one of the few health professions, along with physicians and midwives, that is explicitly identified as being able to give orders to nurses under our professional health laws. British Columbia, Ontario, and Alberta are the only Canadian provinces that allow certified NDs to prescribe pharmaceuticals and perform minor surgeries, but there are only two naturopathic colleges in Canada; neither is currently affiliated with any Canadian public university, and the curricular emphasis is upon homeopathic practice rather than pharmacological science.

Today, naturopaths treat with a range of therapeutics, although chief amongst them are homeopathic remedies. Other therapeutics range from infrared saunas, detox baths, tonics for autism, colonic irrigation, nutritional supplements, and intravenous megadose vitamins to coffee enemas. The claims of effectiveness used in the marketing of these various treatments are often based on very poor-quality, or unscientific evidence (such as testimonials). Many represent boutique therapies that are marketed to people who want to try experimental things that aren't available in mainstream medicine. However, most naturopathic therapies remain faith-based endeavours, and the current state of scientific knowledge offers no support for these beliefs, or treatments based upon them (Garrett, 2018; Murdoch, Carr, & Caulfield, 2016).

In 2011, the Canadian Association of Naturopathic Doctors suggested that a strong healthy immune system will provide adequate protection against illness and that vaccinations actually prevent the body from naturally responding to external pathogens (CAND, 2011). Following significant criticism, CAND has now withdrawn from promoting any advice against vaccination. As a result of the 2019 anti-vaccination crisis, some naturopathic regulators in Canada have started reminding their members that they should not advise clients on vaccination (College of Naturopathic Physicians of BC [CNPBC], 2019; World Health Organization, 2019). However, recent activity by naturopaths offering counter-vaccination advice indicates that this is still a widely held belief. Although many have removed explicit references against immunization from their websites under direction from their regulatory colleges, many continue to support and practice against Health Canada policy on immunization (Young, 2018).

Although naturopaths may offer some good advice on healthy lifestyles and nutrition, the majority of naturopathic therapeutics remain faith-based interventions that are currently unsupported by high-quality scientific evidence. Many of their health-promotion practices also run counter to Health Canada recommendations, and so nurses advising clients who are consulting naturopaths should be aware of these issues.

## Ayurvedic Medicine

Ayurveda evolved in India several thousand years ago. Two ancient Sanskrit texts are considered to be the basis of the practice and identify eight branches of Ayurvedic medicine: internal medicine; surgery; treatment of head and neck disease; gynecology/obstetrics; pediatrics; toxicology; care of older persons and rejuvenation; and sexual vitality. Ayerveda utilizes herbs, massage, and diets, based upon the "seasons of life" (stages of the life span) and treatment of three mind–body (Prakriti) types: *vata* (governs all movement in the mind and body, blood flow, elimination, breathing, and the movement of thoughts); *pitta* (governs heat, metabolism, digestion, transformation in the mind and body, sensory perceptions, and morality); and *kapha* (governs all structure and lubrication in the mind and body, weight, growth, joints and lungs, and formation of all tissues). These are called the *doshas* and their balance is seen to result in health, while imbalance is seen to result in disease (Jaiswal & Williams, 2017).

The goals of Ayurveda are seen as the treatment of disease, prevention of disease, and improving a person's quality of life, by balancing the body, mind, and spirit. Basic premises include the beliefs that all living and nonliving things in the universe are joined together and good health is achieved when one's mind and body are in harmony. Ayurvedic supplements can be made either of herbs only or a combination of herbs, metals, and minerals. Treatment practices include eliminating impurities, decreasing symptoms, increasing resistance to disease, reducing worry, and increasing harmony. Although widely used in India and popularized by the celebrity author Deepak Chopra in North America, currently no provinces or states license Ayurvedic practitioners. According to the Canadian Cancer Society, no significant scientific evidence has demonstrated the effectiveness of Ayurveda for the treatment of cancer. Some research demonstrates that certain approaches used in Ayurveda are helpful as complementary therapies (e.g., yoga and meditation can relieve stress and anxiety in people living with cancer [Canadian Cancer Society, 2019]). Similarly, reviews of Ayurveda (such as for diabetes mellitus) by the Cochrane Library have found that no firm conclusions can be drawn about its efficacy, due to weak methods and small number of participants in the evaluated studies (Sridharan, Mohan, Ramaratnam, et al., 2011).

## Physical Manipulative Interventions

Physical manipulative interventions involve manual treatments that are designed to resolve health issues. There are a number of them, including reflexology (which uses massage to treat illness, based on the theory that there are reflex points on the feet, hands, and head that are linked to every part of the body) and craniosacral therapy (which uses manipulations of the skull), believed to harmonize a natural rhythm in the central nervous system. Hydrotherapy, or water therapy, is a more common form, where water at various temperatures or ice or steam is used to relieve discomfort and promote physical well-being and is very commonly used as a relaxation therapy throughout North America. However, the most commonly consulted alternative practitioners in this category in North America are chiropractors and massage therapists.

## Chiropractic

The most popular form of alternative health care practice in this category is chiropractic, which is well established in North America and Europe. The American Chiropractic Association estimates that there are roughly 77,000 chiropractors in the United States, while the Canadian Chiropractic Association identifies 9000 in Canada. It represents a system of medicine that is based on the diagnosis and manipulative treatment of the spinal vertebrae, which are believed to cause disorders by affecting the nerves, muscles, and organs. The theory of chiropractic rests on three theoretical assumptions, in that (1) spinal vertebrae become misplaced, (2) displacement of these vertebrae interferes with nerve action, and (3) manipulating the spine to realign the vertebrae removes the nerve interference, improving the flow of nervous stimulation (or for straight chiropractors, also the flow of vitalistic life force) to restore health. Chiropractors gain a Doctor of Chiropractic (DC) qualification from private chiropractic colleges, with the exception of the Université du Québec à Trois-Rivières.

Chiropractors maintain they are diagnostic practitioners and can help treat a variety of musculoskeletal conditions, including whiplash injuries, sciatica, herniated discs, persistent pain, and sports performance (but also migraines). There is some evidence that when people have back pain or a crick in their neck, manipulating or exercising it may help relieve the pain and discomfort. Similar to acupuncture, there is a significant body of literature and studies that support the use of chiropractic spinal manipulative therapy (SMT) for pain-related issues (notably low back pain), but little quality research exploring the nature of the mechanism. Whether chiropractic works more effectively than other techniques such as exercise and physiotherapy is currently also unknown.

A number of *Cochrane Systematic Reviews* of the published research focusing on chiropractic interventions for conditions such as asthma, infantile colic, neck pain, bed-wetting, period pain, and carpal tunnel syndrome have identified either no effect or cite insufficient evidence to support its effectiveness.

In Canada, there has been significant criticism for chiropractic over the last few years regarding two specific issues. First, the growth of pediatric chiropractic and, secondly, the role of chiropractors in the ongoing anti-vaccination crisis. Infant chiropractic has developed as a trend that involves chiropractors advertising to treat newborn babies and children on the basis that they are correcting misalignments of the spine caused during childbirth or normal growth. Another example of this is chiropractic research suggesting that chiropractic helped improve cognitive function in children (Cuthbert & Barras, 2009). None of these claims are currently supported by independent scientific evidence. With infants and children under 18 years old, bones are still in a phase of growth, development, and remodeling, and the vertebral end-plate growth is incomplete. In younger children, the cartilaginous growth areas in the bones are immature and potentially vulnerable to injury if subjected to manipulation. Additionally, back pain in children is rare and, when it does occur, it is potentially a more serious problem and should always be brought to the attention of a pediatrician rather than a chiropractor. A 2002 paper from the Canadian Paediatric Society reported that there were no satisfactory studies of chiropractic treatments for back pain in children. Some studies had suggested that chiropractic manipulation of the neck could provide short-term relief of neck pain in children, but its efficacy hadn't been compared with other therapies (Spigelblatt, 2002). In 2008, two chiropractors published a review of chiropractic manipulation in pediatric health conditions, indicating that chiropractic as a health care intervention for children's medical conditions continued to be supported by poor scientific evidence (Gotlib & Rupert, 2008; Homola, 2010). Criticism of infant chiropractic has met significant resistance from the profession, and yet the practice has expanded (Armstrong, Gavin, & Kruse Michael, 2019; Barrett & Homola, 2019; Colquhoun, 2008; Gorski, Novella, Atwood, et al., 2019). In March 2019, the regulatory body for chiropractors in British Columbia (The College of Chiropractors of British Columbia [CCBC]) confirmed that they would undertake a thorough review of the scientific evidence about chiropractic treatments for children following a number of complaints. In a bid to move toward better standards for a scientific basis for chiropractic, the CCBC has also banned chiropractors from claiming to effectively treat various childhood conditions where evidence of efficacy was not available, including autism, ear infections, and cancer.

Although, many people report success with back pain treatment by chiropractors, additional research is needed to confirm if it is an effective therapy compared with other approaches, or even how or if it works. Nevertheless, the profession has established a popular appeal and is a commonly used alternative therapy.

## Massage Therapy

Massage therapy is generally used for the treatment of body stress or pain and involves the physical manipulation of soft tissues by touch. The title 'massage therapist' has been recognized as a professional title for those who have been professionally trained to give therapeutic massage (Registered Massage Therapists in Canada). It is an increasingly popular health care option across Canada (Esmail, 2017). It remains one of the less controversial alternative health strategies and there is some evidence that it can help with relaxation, relieve stress and anxiety, and help support rehabilitation and mild pain reduction in some circumstances, mainly through muscle relaxation, increasing perfusion to tissues, and possibly helping endorphin release (Furlan, Giraldo, Baskwill, et al., 2015). Due to its widespread acceptance, it is regarded less as an alternative therapeutic, and simply a useful adjunctive therapy. However, like other alternative strategies, it has a weak theoretical base, and some claims of the efficacy of massage for specific conditions (such as for lymphedema or tendonitis) remain unevidenced (Pichonnaz, Bassin, Lécureux, et al., 2016). As such, its role as an adjunctive health promotion therapy may be useful to help reduce stress, depression, and anxiety in clients, but other than that, there is no significant evidence that supports its use for other conditions.

## Herbal and Nutritional Interventions

Herbal remedies, vitamins, dietary supplements, and specialist diets are some of the oldest forms of alternative health strategies, and also represent a major sector of modern health care business. This category includes the use of natural herbs, vitamins, minerals, probiotics, and also aromatherapy and detoxification therapies and nutritional counselling. The principle of these approaches is either that the particular herb or substance has curative properties (such as garlic for asthma), that there is a dietary deficit of the substance (such as vitamins), or that there is an overabundance of a substance which is toxic (e.g., mercury or polychlorinated biphenyls).

### Botanical and Herbal Remedies

Botanical remedies were inventoried in great detail in ancient Egyptian, Chinese, and Indian cultures and in the Middle Ages in Europe. Herbal therapy is the use of herbs to treat specific conditions or to enhance the function of various body systems, such as claims of boosting the immune system, treating allergies, or preventing a cold. Herbal medicines may act on the body like prescription medications (and most medications are simply attenuated forms of plant-based substances, such as aspirin being derived from willow bark). The efficacy of various herbal and botanical remedies varies. There are hundreds of these remedies, and because such herbal supplements may interact with prescription medication, it is important for health care providers to elicit what clients are taking and in what doses as part their care management.

### Dietary Interventions

Multiple studies have demonstrated the efficacy of nutritional interventions, vitamins, and therapeutic diets (such as low-potassium and protein diets in renal failure) to help stabilize inter-dialysis biochemistry (Garagarza, Valente, Oliveira, et al., 2015), and nutritional interventions for those undergoing chemotherapy to help maintain weight and muscle mass and improve survival (De Waele, Mattens, Honoré, et al., 2015). However, those are accepted medical interventions, and most hospitals have highly qualified Registered Dietitians on staff to provide dietary advice for a range of conditions.

Probiotic supplements—live microorganisms found in the human digestive tract, and often called "friendly bacteria"—are another example here. They are ingested to enhance the digestive system either as a supplement or in natural forms, such as in yogurt or other fermented foods.

The singling out of an individual problem nutrient, superfood, or specialist diet is not necessarily a good indicator of the complexity of nutrition and other lifestyle factors that may affect personal health. Nevertheless, diet fads identifying the latest supernutrient come and go very frequently. Antioxidants are a key example, and nutritional advice focused on antioxidant intake, aging, and cancer health continues to be popular in the media, despite a lack of evidence for their effectiveness.

Much of the uptake of dietary health-promotional advice is from alternative nutritionists, many who claim that specific foods or specific supplements can improve general health and well-being or, in the most extreme examples, can cure serious diseases such as cancer (Jarry, 2018). Many of these promote fashionable diets such as alkaline water, juice diets, or the paleo or keto diet, and they have become remarkably prevalent in popular culture despite a lack of good scientific foundation.

### Aromatherapy

Aromatherapy, also known as essential oil therapy, is the use of extracted oils from plants that are claimed to balance, harmonize, and promote the health of body, mind, and spirit via inhalation, external application, or, sometimes, ingestion. Like many alternative therapists, the levels and training of aromatherapists is not standardized and the discipline is unregulated. There is currently no quality evidence that aromatherapy can either prevent, treat, or cure any disease, and RCTs are difficult to design because the point of most aromatherapy is the smell of the agent (Lee, Choi, Posadzki, et al., 2012). There is some evidence that it may be effective in combating postoperative nausea and vomiting, and it remains popular, but like many of the therapies discussed here, its use is mainly based upon faith rather than scientific evidence (Hines, Steels, Chang, et al., 2018).

### Mind–Body Interventions

Mind and body interventions are rather a wide categorization based on alternative therapies that are focused on the body and mind. One such intervention that is showing promising results is the use of neurofeedback or biofeedback, in which individuals receive feedback on the electrical activity occurring in the brain. Neurofeedback operates in a manner similar to biofeedback (e.g., heart rate monitoring) because it monitors brainwave activity, then provides audio or visual feedback to the user. Certain levels of electrical activity are associated with sleep, mental stimulation, and mood. Neurofeedback provides feedback to the brain related to maladaptive patterns of electrical activity to help train the user to voluntarily increase or decrease electrical activity in order to help the brain to operate more effectively (Harris, Hundley, & Lambie, 2019). There is promising research that supports the effectiveness of neurofeedback for treating post-traumatic stress disorder (PTSD), attention-deficit/hyperactivity disorder (ADHD), stress and anxiety, pain, and post-chemotherapy cognitive impairment (PCCI) (Emmert, Breimhorst, Bauermann, et al., 2017; Harris et al., 2019; Luctkar-Flude et al., 2017; Reiter, Andersen, & Carlsson, 2016; Van Doren, Arns, Heinrich, et al., 2019).

Other mind–body therapies include various methods of body movement, meditation, and mindfulness. Movement-based therapies (such as yoga and tai chi), meditation (or mindfulness) for progressive relaxation, guided imagery, and hypnotherapy are the most popular alternative health-promotional therapies in this category (Clarke, Black, Stussman, et al., 2015; Esmail, 2017).

### Movement-Based Therapies

Movement therapies use movement and body work to promote physical, mental, emotional, and spiritual well-being. Practices such as yoga, tai chi, and qigong involve gentle exercise and are helpful as health-promotional activities where they have some well-evidenced benefits, and for improving general health, pain management, psychological state (reducing depression, stress, and anxiety) and for improving mobility. Physical benefits observed also include increasing flexibility, function, and strength (Büssing, Michalsen, Khalsa, et al., 2012; Clarke et al., 2015; Kim, Pascual-Leone, Johnson, et al., 2016; Prathikanti, Rivera, Cochran, et al., 2017; Qaseem, Wilt, McLean, et al., 2017). Outside of health-promotional benefits, there is less quality evidence of specific efficacy of movement-based therapies for other common medical conditions such as diabetes or renal failure, and positive effects are probably due to demonstrated health benefits of engaging in social exercise and relaxation activities (Cramer, Lauche, Klose, et al., 2017; Marks, 2017; Yang, Wang, Ren, et al., 2015).

Yoga is a meditative movement practice that originated in India as a form of spiritual practice and that aids in flexibility, agility, balance, and relaxation. Qigong is part of TCM, combining relaxed movements with a meditative aspect and controlled breathing. Tai chi began as a Chinese martial art and combines physical movement, breath control, and meditation in a dance-like sequence of poses based on the movements of animals. All these movement therapies involve moment-to-moment–based sequences of physical activity that are designed to produce a positive, relaxed, and meditative state.

Dance therapy is another movement-based mind–body modality that uses dance to allow the body and mind to move freely in response to music. This, too, has some evidence of effectiveness as a health-promotional activity (McNeely, Duncan, & Earhart, 2015; Tortora, 2019).

### Meditation and Mindfulness

Meditation is a method of focused attention to increase relaxation, quiet the mind, and reduce stress. It is a part of several religious cultures (such as Zen Buddhism) and can be practised while one is still or active, such as during walking. Like massage, different types of meditation have a variety of purposes and techniques. Breath meditation is a simple example that involves the person emptying their mind and focusing all of their attention on their breathing. Centring is another technique that involves focusing on a chosen word. Mindfulness meditation is a way of paying attention to or being mindful of a variety of topics, such as thoughts, actions, or the environment. Walking meditation is another form of mindfulness, because the individual is mindful of the interaction of the inner body, the external body, and the environment with each step. There is some compelling evidence that such activities can change brain activity and have some health-promotional benefits, such as helping people to quit smoking, and helping people maintain a more positive mental state for dealing with stress, anxiety, and depression (Kocovski, Fleming, Blackie, et al., 2019; Ma & Fang, 2019; Spears, Abroms, Glass, et al., 2019). Currently, however, the mechanisms involved and the scale of benefits remain unclear.

### Guided Imagery

Similar to mindfulness, visual or guided imagery is another approach that encourages individuals to relax by focusing on calming thoughts or experiences. Imagery is a gentle technique that uses the use of the imagination to promote a sense of well-being and to help relaxation. Its reported benefits are similar to those of mindfulness (Charalambous, Giannakopoulou, Bozas, et al., 2015; Zehetmair, Tegeler, Kaufmann, et al., 2019).

### Hypnotherapy

Hypnotherapy is a form of guided deep relaxation that focuses attention of the unconscious mind. It has been used with some reported success as a health-promotion activity for such things as behavioural change (e.g., quitting smoking or dealing with phobias), memory recall of suppressed events, and improving positive self-esteem (Badaoui, Kassm, & Naja, 2019; Birnie, Noel, Chambers, et al., 2018; Hirsch, 2018). Currently, the mechanisms involved and the benefits compared with other approaches remain unclear. For example, a recent Cochrane review found insufficient evidence to determine whether hypnotherapy was more effective for smoking cessation than other forms of behavioural support (Barnes, McRobbie, Dong, et al., 2019).

## Human Energy Field Therapies

In North American nursing, there has been a significant interest in proposed human energy field (HEF)-based alternative health practices over the last 40 years, such as therapeutic touch (TT) or reiki. They represent modern interpretations of a number of Indigenous faith-based therapeutic interventions and beliefs.

### Therapeutic Touch

Dora Kunz (a psychic) and Dolores Krieger (a nurse educator at New York University) developed TT in the 1980s. Kunz suggested that it had origins in ancient Sanskrit Yogic texts, described as a *pranic* healing method (another belief in a vital, life-sustaining force in living beings). The technique is now taught in approximately 80 colleges and universities in the United States, and in many other countries, including Langara College in British Columbia, Canada. Many nurses support this idea of mystical therapeutic energies (Dossey, Keegan, Barrere, et al., 2018; Koerner, 2007).

TT practitioners claim to be able to detect and manipulate a proposed HEF by passing their hands over the patient and smoothing out their HEF. It does not normally involve any physical contact. There have been several attempts to establish scientific evidence for TT over the years (Hanley, Coppa, & Shields, 2017; Shields, Fuller, Resnicoff, et al., 2017).

Some scientific suggestions have been made to indicate that physical energies could be occurring and taking place with TT practitioners (Jhaveri, Walsh, Wang, et al., 2008). However, empirical methods for measuring them have not been taken up by the community of practitioners, and none of the work has been independently validated. Hence, despite numerous low-quality and small-scale studies exploring TT, there is currently no quality scientific evidence that HEFs exist, or that TT interventions work any better than placebo. Therefore, as an alternative therapeutic strategy, TT currently remains a faith-based approach that is indistinguishable from faith healing.

### Reiki

Reiki is an Asian form of this therapeutic approach and identifies the channelling of divine universal energy *(ki)* as its focus. It was developed in 1922 by the Japanese Buddhist Mikao Usui (1865–1926) and has been adapted by various teachers in varying traditions. Japanese practitioners purport to manipulate *ki* by the intuitive skill of knowing where to place the hands to provide therapeutic health benefits (known as *Reiji-hō*). The Western tradition uses a similar process on specific points *(chakras)* on the body where the *ki* is said to conjoin. Nurses have also been advocates for reiki (Bossi, Ott, & DeCristofaro, 2008; Burke, 2010; Kryak & Vitale, 2011; Toms, 2011). Nevertheless, no empirical evidence for its efficacy currently exists, and a 2008 systematic review of the research concluded: "The evidence is insufficient to suggest that reiki is an effective treatment for any condition. Therefore, the value of reiki remains unproven" (Lee, Pittler, & Ernst, 2008, p. 593). A 2015 high-quality systematic review of reiki research for depression and anxiety found "insufficient evidence to say whether or not reiki is useful for people over 16 years of age with anxiety or depression or both" and that the quality of the evidence was moderate, "which, on top of a dearth of evidence, weakens the findings further" (Joyce & Herbison, 2015, p. 2).

## SAFETY AND EFFECTIVENESS

Although much alternative medicine is mainly harmless, the implications of using it are not always clear and serious injuries and deaths have occurred, just as they have with conventional medicine.

Using alternative medicine in place of conventional medicine and putting off seeing a doctor or nurse may have serious health implications. One recent case involved an Alberta couple whose son died of meningitis after being treated with natural remedies from a naturopath, and who had delayed seeking medical advice from a physician (Aldach, 2016). Another Calgary couple was jailed for 32 months for criminal negligence after their 14-month-old son died of a treatable staphylococcus bacterial infection because his parents searched online for natural remedies and he was not taken to a physician until it was too late. (Krugel, 2019). Some alternative therapeutics present significant risks of harm if used instead of conventional medicines (Caulfield, 2015; Johnson, Park, Gross, et al., 2018).

A common issue is people not informing their physician that they are taking supplemental alternative remedies that could interact with their medical prescription medications. This has led to serious health issues due to combined effects. A 2002 systematic review identified that older patients frequently suffered harm from alternative therapies, and herbal treatments have been associated with adverse events through unwanted medication interactions as well as direct toxicity (Ernst, 2002; Temple, 2012). Because supplemental alternative remedies are used but not necessarily professionally guided, concerns remain regarding their use. Health care providers must complete comprehensive health histories which include the identification of both prescribed and non-medically supervised interventions.

## EVIDENCE-INFORMED PRACTICE

A significant problem with much of the alternative medicine sector is that most of the practices are not well substantiated in terms of good-quality scientific evidence. In its most fundamental form, EIP involves the practitioner asking: "What is the best solution to this particular health issue?" Then looking at the alternative therapeutic interventions available using the best evidence of effectiveness (does it work), pragmatic issues (is it readily available, legally approved, affordable, and usable in this context), and patient preference (what does the patient want). Then the health professional can select and advise the patient on the most appropriate therapeutic intervention. Overall, these elements can be summarized as:

- Scientific evidence of a demonstrated positive (or negative) effect of a specific action/intervention
- Social and personal acceptability of the intervention
- Clinical expert judgement as to the efficacy of the intervention in the specific case considered, or any adaptations required in its implementation
- Economic viability of the intervention (Garrett, 2018)

This process involves consideration of the level of evidence to support a practice, which requires significant scientific expertise. Much of the evidence in the alternative sector relies on testimonials; personal reports; small-scale studies; in vitro, animal, or unreplicated studies lacking independently verified experiments; and studies published in self-interest disciplinary journals. This makes it difficult to justify these practices in empirical

## ⚡ QUALITY AND SAFETY SCENARIO

### How Should Complementary and Alternative Medicine (CAM) Be Evaluated?

- What standards of evidence should the nurse require before adopting an alternative therapy in clinical practice?
- How do the standards of evidence used in medicine and nursing today compare with those used in the alternative/complementary sector?
- Government and consumer advocates are beginning to require the same oversight, regulation, and monitoring of CAM practices as for other forms of professional health care. How can this best be achieved?

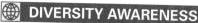

## 🌐 DIVERSITY AWARENESS

### Respecting Patient Choices

In respecting alternative belief systems, it is important to respect the patient's choice and desires to select unorthodox therapies, just as the nurse should respect differing sociocultural and religious beliefs. However, such therapies may run counter to evidence-informed therapies. For example, an Indigenous patient may express a wish to pursue natural traditional cultural health practices rather than scientific biomedical ones.

**Reflective Questions**
- What is the role of the nurse in advising and helping such patients meet their health goals?
- What strategies can help patients with unorthodox health beliefs meet their health needs while respecting diversity?
- If a patient wishes to use a cultural health practice that is not legally permitted in Canada (such as female genital cutting for young girls after puberty), how should the nurse best help the patient meet health goals, and support cultural diversity?

terms. Some researchers have even suggested that a new set of research methods is needed to study CAM, to bypass demonstrating scientific efficacy, and simply focus on patient preference and economic viability (Herman, D'Huyvetter, & Mohler, 2006). Nevertheless, bypassing scientific proof of effectiveness does not help resolve the issue of justifying public health care expenditure on therapeutics that have not been demonstrated to work.

Of course, this does not mean we should ignore these disciplines or clients' wishes to engage with them. It is important for nurses to support clients in their personal health promotion choices as much as we support clients in meeting their diverse spiritual needs. However, the adoption of alternative strategies within public health care settings presents a complex set of issues. Integrating faith-based health-promotion strategies requires careful consideration by the nurse, because advocating for the best evidence-informed health practices is also an important aspect of person-centred nursing care (Quality and Safety Scenario). Nevertheless, of primary importance is respect for the client's personal health choices (Diversity Awareness).

## HEALTH POLICY AND ALTERNATIVE MEDICINE

The health care system is responding to the increase in CAM use and new models of integrative health care that combine CAM and conventional medicine. However, much of this is piecemeal rather than the result of systematic planning, and it remains unclear whether these changes are safe and effective and how they will affect Canadian health care. Alternative health care is also marked by a lack of standardization of qualifications and accreditation.

There is also a significant issue with deceptive practices in this sector (Garrett et al., 2019). The lack of nationally and internationally recognized accreditation standards and effective control of qualifications and practices makes policy initiatives to regulate them and protect the public extremely difficult. Issues with CAM practices in children are particularly complex because the well-being of the child has to be considered alongside the wishes of the parents. The ongoing debates regarding the provision and regulation of CAM are likely best understood in the context of wider policies and sociopolitical changes in society (Saks, 2015).

## ▎SUMMARY

Alternative health strategies continue to be popular with the public and represent a growing sector of health care provision in North America. However, as they remain predominantly faith-based therapies, they persist outside of orthodoxy, and governments seek to put positive regulatory frameworks in place to maintain and control them while also protecting the public. Many have been practiced in other cultures for thousands of years, some as religious practices. However, good-quality scientific evidence to support these alternative health strategies remains lacking, creating ongoing tensions between the evidence-informed practice movement and CAM advocates. Additionally, some alternative products and services are not well regulated, and deceptive practices frequently occur. Many consumers remain convinced that these practices help promote and maintain health or cure a variety of health conditions, and the placebo effect (although well understood) may have a strong influence on the results of much research in the field. Nurses need to understand alternative health strategies and remain aware of them in order to best support a client's personal health choices as a fundamental part of evidence-informed care, offering them current advice and to make informed decisions in terms of their health-promotional choices, while respecting and supporting them.

**Evolve Chapter Features**

http://evolve.elsevier.com/Canada/Edelman/healthpromotion/
- Review Questions

## CASE STUDY

### Chiropractic as a Complementary Treatment for Back Pain: David

David, a 62-year-old man, was referred to the hospital pain clinic by his doctor reporting low back pain of 4 months' duration following a skiing injury. He was previously treated with ibuprofen, acetaminophen, and oxycodone, as well as physiotherapy. At the time of his clinic visit, he was still taking ibuprofen but had stopped taking oxycodone because his pain "wasn't bad enough." He rated his daily, back pain as 4–6 on the Visual Analogue Scale (VAS) for pain (from 0 to 10). He also confirmed that the pain was worse when driving and that this prevented him going too far. To help, he said had now booked a series of chiropractic appointments.

The primary goal of treatment for David is pain relief and return of normal function in his daily activities. David is seen at the pain clinic weekly for a total of six times for further review of his medication and work with a physiotherapist, who has advocated yoga stretches for the back, neck, and shoulders daily (five gentle repetitions each time) and other physical exercises. David also received chiropractic spinal manipulation weekly for 6 weeks, was given some simple exercises for his back by the chiropractor, and was advised to perform the exercises daily. His pain rating at the end of his treatment was averaging at 2–3 daily on the VAS, and he had stopped taking ibuprofen and oxycodone completely. He was also driving further and working in his garden again. He continued his yoga stretches and has started performing daily physical exercises to maintain his functionality.

#### Reflective Questions

- David reports that he felt the chiropractic treatment seemed to have helped him the most. How would it be possible to determine the respective effects of the different therapies?
- What other health strategies might be used to relieve David's pain and to help him increase his range of motion?
- After the treatment goals have been reached, what health strategies would you recommend to assist David in maintaining and promoting health?

## CARE PLAN

### Use of Therapeutic Touch: David P.

**Nursing Issue**
Disrupted energy field due to the slowed or blocked energy field

**Defining Characteristics**
- Perceptions of changes in patterns of energy flow, such as:
- Temperature changes: warmth, coolness
- Visual changes: image, color Resting blood pressure is 164/87 mm Hg, and pulse rate is 88 beats/min.
- Disruption of the field: vacant, hole, spike, bulge
- Movement: wave, spike, tingling, dense, flowing
- Sounds: tone, words

**Related Factors**
- Pathophysiological: illness, injury
- Treatment-related: immobility, perioperative experience, labor and delivery.
- Situational: pain, fear, anxiety, grieving
- Maturational: age-related developmental difficulties or crises

**Expected Outcomes**
- The person will report increased sense of relaxation
- The person will report decreased anxiety and tension
- The person will demonstrate evidence of physical relaxation (e.g., decreased blood pressure, pulse, respiratory rate, and muscle tension).
- The person will report an increased sense of well-being

**Interventions**
- Provide privacy if possible.
- Explain energy therapy (therapeutic touch, reiki, healing touch), and obtain permission to treat the person.
- Position the person comfortably.
- Become quiet and still (centered) and bring the focus to the person.
- Assess (scan) the energy field for openness and flow.
- Clear the exterior energy field by combing through the field from head to toe (unruffling).
- Move the palms of the hands toward the person, 2 to 4 inches over the person's body, from head to feet in a smooth, light movement.
- Sense the cues to energy imbalance (i.e., warmth, coolness, tightness, heaviness, tingling, emptiness).
- Focus on perceived areas of imbalance to repattern the energy flow.
- Reassess and smooth the exterior energy field, ensuring that the energy flow is open in the feet.
- Gently stop the treatment and allow the person time to rest.
- Encourage the person to discuss the experience.

## REFERENCES

Aldach, K. (2016). *Alberta parents whose toddler died of meningitis were told to visit doctor, trial hears.* CBC News Calgary. March 8. Retrieved from http://www.cbc.ca/news/canada/calgary/raymond-toddler-death-trial-stephan-1.3481958.

Armstrong, R., Gavin, A., & Kruse, M. (2019). *Bad science watch—important issues, sound science, real change.* Retrieved from https://www.badsciencewatch.ca/.

Badaoui, A., Kassm, S. A., & Naja, W. (2019). Fear and anxiety disorders related to childbirth: Epidemiological and therapeutic issues. *Current Psychiatry Reports, 21*(4), 27.

Barnes, J., McRobbie, H., Dong, C. Y., et al. (2019). Hypnotherapy for smoking cessation. *Cochrane Database of Systematic Reviews*, CD001008. https://doi.org/10.1002/14651858.CD001008.pub3.

Barrett, S., & Homola, S. (2019). *Chirobase: A guide to chiropractic history, theories, and practices.* Retrieved from https://www.chirobase.org/.

Birnie, K. A., Noel, M., Chambers, C. T., et al. (2018). Psychological interventions for needle-related procedural pain and distress in children and adolescents. *Cochrane Database of Systematic Reviews*, CD005179. https://doi.org/10.1002/14651858.CD005179.pub4.

Bossi, L. M., Ott, M. J., & DeCristofaro, S. (2008). Reiki as a clinical intervention in oncology nursing practice. *Clinical Journal of Oncology Nursing*, 12(3), 489–494. [Seminal Reference].

Brinkhaus, B., Witt, C. M., Jena, S., et al. (2007). Physician and treatment characteristics in a randomised multicentre trial of acupuncture in patients with osteoarthritis of the knee. *Complementary Therapies in Medicine*, 15(3), 180–189. [Seminal Reference].

British Columbia College of Nursing Professionals (BCCNP). (2018). *Complementary and alternative healthcare fact sheet for RNs and NPs*. Vancouver, BC. Retrieved from https://www.bccnp.ca/Standards/RN_NP/StandardResources/437CompandAlternativeHealthCare.pdf.

Bromfield, S. G., & McGwin, G. (2013). Use of complementary and alternative medicine for eye-related diseases and conditions. *Current Eye Research*, 38(12), 1283–1287. [Seminal Reference].

Buckner, C. A., Lafrenie, R. M., Dénommée, J. A., et al. (2018). Complementary and alternative medicine use in patients before and after a cancer diagnosis. *Current Oncology*, 25(4), e275. https://doi.org/10.3747/co.25.3884.

Burke, S. (2010). Reiki: Ancient healing art for today's new healthcare vision. *American Nurse Today*, 5(3), 43–56. [Seminal Reference].

Büssing, A., Michalsen, A., Khalsa, S. B. S., et al. (2012). Effects of yoga on mental and physical health: A short summary of reviews. *Evidence-based Complementary and Alternative Medicine*, 2012, 165410. https://doi.org/10.1155/2012/165410. [Seminal Reference].

Canadian Association of Naturopathic Doctors (CAND). (2011). *Position paper on flu vaccines*. Ottawa: Author. Retrieved from https://web.archive.org/web/20131005225723/http://www.cand.ca/Position_Papers.papers.0.html. [Seminal Reference].

Canadian Association of Naturopathic Doctors (CAND). (2019). *About naturopathic medicine*. Retrieved from https://www.cand.ca/about-naturopathic-medicine/.

Canadian Cancer Society. (2019). *Ayurveda*. Retrieved from https://www.cancer.ca/en/cancer-information/diagnosis-and-treatment/complementary-therapies/ayurveda/?region=on.

Canadian Medical Association. (2015). *CMA policy: Complementary and alternative medicine*. Retrieved from https://policybase.cma.ca/documents/policypdf/PD15-09.pdf.

Canadian Society of Homeopathy. (2019). *What is homeopathy?* Retrieved from http://www.csoh.ca/Homeopathy_What_Is_Hx.htm.

Canizares, M., Hogg-Johnson, S., Gignac, M. A., et al. (2017). Changes in the use practitioner-based complementary and alternative medicine over time in Canada: Cohort and period effects. *PloS One*, 12(5), e0177307. https://doi.org/10.1371/journal.pone.0177307.

Caulfield, T. A. (2015). *Is Gwyneth Paltrow wrong about everything? When celebrity culture and science clash*. Boston: Beacon Press.

Charalambous, A., Giannakopoulou, M., Bozas, E., et al. (2015). A randomized controlled trial for the effectiveness of progressive muscle relaxation and guided imagery as anxiety reducing interventions in breast and prostate cancer patients undergoing chemotherapy. *Evidence-based Complementary and Alternative Medicine*, 2015, 270876. https://doi.org/10.1155/2015/270876.

Clarke, T. C., Black, L. I., Stussman, B. J., et al. (2015). Trends in the use of complementary health approaches among adults: United States, 2002–2012. *National Health Statistics Reports*, 79, 1–16. Retrieved from http://www.ncbi.nlm.nih.gov/pubmed/25671660.

College of Naturopathic Physicians of BC (CNPBC). (2019). *Media release*. Retrieved from http://www.cnpbc.bc.ca/media-release/.

Colquhoun, D. (2008). *An ex-chiropractor speaks out: Again*. Retrieved from http://www.dcscience.net/2008/12/07/an-ex-chiropractor-speaks-out-again/. [Seminal Reference].

Colquhoun, D., & Novella, S. P. (2013). Acupuncture is theatrical placebo. *Anesthesia & Analgesia*, 116(6), 1360–1363. [Seminal Reference].

Cramer, H., Lauche, R., Klose, P., et al. (2017). Yoga for improving health-related quality of life, mental health and cancer-related symptoms in women diagnosed with breast cancer. *Cochrane Database of Systematic Reviews*, CD010802. https://doi.org/10.1002/14651858.CD010802.pub2.

Cuthbert, S. C., & Barras, M. (2009). Developmental delay syndromes: Psychometric testing before and after chiropractic treatment of 157 children. *Journal of Manipulative and Physiological Therapeutics*, 32(8), 660–669. [Seminal Reference].

Dashtdar, M., Dashtdar, M. R., Dashtdar, B., et al. (2016). The concept of wind in traditional Chinese medicine. *Journal of Pharmacopuncture*, 19(4), 293–302.

De Waele, E., Mattens, S., Honoré, P. M., et al. (2015). Nutrition therapy in cachectic cancer patients. The tight caloric control (TiCaCo) pilot trial. *Appetite*, 91, 298–301.

Dong, J. (2013). The relationship between traditional Chinese medicine and modern medicine. *Evidence-based Complementary and Alternative Medicine*, 2013, 153148. https://doi.org/10.1155/2013/153148. [Seminal Reference].

Dossey, B. M., Keegan, L., Barrere, C. C., et al. (2018). *Holistic nursing: A handbook for practice* (7th ed.). Burlington, MA: Jones & Bartlett Learning.

Emmert, K., Breimhorst, M., Bauermann, T., et al. (2017). Active pain coping is associated with the response in real-time fMRI neurofeedback during pain. *Brain Imaging and Behavior*, 11(3), 712–721. https://doi.org/10.1007/s11682-016-9547-0.

Ernst, E. (2002). Adverse effects of unconventional therapies in the elderly: A systematic review of the recent literature. *Journal of the American Aging Association*, 25(1), 11–20. [Seminal Reference].

Ernst, E., & Cassileth, B. R. (1998). The prevalence of complementary/alternative medicine in cancer: A systematic review. *Cancer*, 83(4), 777–782. [Seminal Reference].

Esmail, N. (2017). *Complementary and alternative medicine: Use and public attitudes 1997, 2006, 2016*. Vancouver: Fraser Institute. Retrieved from https://www.fraserinstitute.org/studies/complementary-and-alternative-medicine-use-and-public-attitudes-1997-2006-and-2016.

Furlan, A. D., Giraldo, M., Baskwill, A., et al. (2015). Massage for low-back pain. *Cochrane Database of Systematic Reviews*, 9.

Gaboury, I., April, K. T., & Verhoef, M. (2012). A qualitative study on the term CAM: Is there a need to reinvent the wheel? *BMC Complementary and Alternative Medicine*, 12(1), 131.

Gaboury, I., Johnson, N., Robin, C., et al. (2016). Complementary and alternative medicine: Do physicians believe they can meet the requirements of the Collège des Médecins du Québec? *Canadian Family Physician*, 62(12), e772–e775.

Garagarza, C. A., Valente, A. T., Oliveira, T. S., et al. (2015). Effect of personalized nutritional counseling in maintenance hemodialysis patients. *Hemodialysis International*, 19(3), 412–418.

Garrett, B. (2018). *Empirical nursing: The art of evidence-based care*. Bingley, UK: Emerald Publishing Limited.

Garrett, B., Murphy, S., Jamal, S., et al. (2019). Internet health scams—Developing a taxonomy and risk of deception assessment tool. *Health and Social Care in the Community*, 27(1), 226–240.

Gilmour, H., Ramage-Morin, P. L., & Wong, S. L. (2018). Multiple sclerosis: Prevalence and impact. *Health Reports*, 29(1), 3–8.

Gorski, D., Novella, S., Atwood, K. C., et al. (2019). *Science-based medicine—chiropractic*. Retrieved from https://sciencebasedmedicine.org/reference/chiropractic/.

Gotlib, A., & Rupert, R. (2008). Chiropractic manipulation in pediatric health conditions—an updated systematic review. *Chiropractic and Osteopathy, 16*(1), 11. [Seminal Reference].

Grand View Research. (2019). *Complementary and alternative medicine market size, share & trends analysis report by intervention (botanical, acupuncture, mind, body, yoga), by distribution (direct contact, e-training), and segment forecasts, 2019–2026.* San Francisco, CA. Retrieved from https://www.grandviewresearch.com/industry-analysis/aternative-medicine-therapies-market.

Haake, M., Müller, H.-H., Schade-Brittinger, C., et al. (2007). German acupuncture trials (gerac) for chronic low back pain: Randomized, multicenter, blinded, parallel-group trial with 3 groups. *Archives of Internal Medicine, 167*(17), 1892–1898. [Seminal Reference].

Han, J. S. (2015). *Acupuncture. Treatment of chronic pain by integrative approaches.* New York: Springer, 123–136.

Hanley, M. A., Coppa, D., & Shields, D. (2017). A practice-based theory of healing through therapeutic touch: Advancing holistic nursing practice. *Journal of Holistic Nursing, 35*(4), 369–381.

Harris, S., Hundley, G., & Lambie, G. (2019). The effects of neurofeedback on depression, anxiety, and academic self-efficacy. *Journal of College Student Psychotherapy.* https://doi.org/10.1080/87568225.2019.1606689.

Hawke, K., van Driel, M. L., Buffington, B. J., et al. (2018). Homeopathic medicinal products for preventing and treating acute respiratory tract infections in children. *Cochrane Database of Systematic Reviews,* CD005974. https://doi.org/10.1002/14651858.CD005974.pub5.

Herman, P. M., D'Huyvetter, K., & Mohler, M. J. (2006). Are health services research methods a match for CAM? *Alternative Therapies in Health & Medicine, 12*(3), 78–83. [Seminal Reference].

Hines, S., Steels, E., Chang, A., et al. (2018). Aromatherapy for treatment of postoperative nausea and vomiting. *Cochrane Database of Systematic Reviews,* CD007598. https://doi.org/10.1002/14651858.CD007598.pub2.

Hirsch, J. A. (2018). Integrating hypnosis with other therapies for treating specific phobias: A case series. *American Journal of Clinical Hypnosis, 60*(4), 367–377.

Homola, S. (2010). *Pediatric chiropractic care: Scientifically indefensible?* Retrieved from https://sciencebasedmedicine.org/pediatric-chiropractic-care-scientifically-indefensible/. [Seminal Reference].

Jaiswal, Y. S., & Williams, L. L. (2017). A glimpse of Ayurveda—the forgotten history and principles of Indian traditional medicine. *Journal of Traditional and Complementary Medicine, 7*(1), 50–53.

Jarry, J. (2018). *"Cancer is a good thing!!!"; Says Montreal's own food babe.* Montreal: Office for Science and Society, McGill University. Retrieved from https://www.mcgill.ca/oss/article/quackery/cancer-good-thing-says-montreals-own-food-babe.

Jhaveri, A., Walsh, S. J., Wang, Y., et al. (2008). Therapeutic touch affects DNA synthesis and mineralization of human osteoblasts in culture. *Journal of Orthopaedic Research, 26*(11), 1541–1546. [Seminal Reference].

Johnson, S. B., Park, H. S., Gross, C. P., et al. (2018). Use of alternative medicine for cancer and its impact on survival. *Journal of the National Cancer Institute, 110*(1), 121–124.

Joyce, J., & Herbison, G. P. (2015). Reiki for depression and anxiety. *Cochrane Database of Systematic Reviews,* CD006833. https://doi.org/10.1002/14651858.CD006833.pub2.

Khorsan, R., Coulter, I. D., Crawford, C., et al. (2011). Systematic review of integrative healthcare research: Randomized control trials, clinical controlled trials, and meta-analysis. *Evidence-Based Complementary and Alternative Medicine (ECAM), 2011.* https://doi.org/10.1155/2011/636134. [Seminal Reference].

Kim, T. H. M., Pascual-Leone, J., Johnson, J., et al. (2016). The mental-attention tai chi effect with older adults. *BMC Psychology, 4*(1), 29.

Kluger, B. M., Rakowski, D., Christian, M., et al. (2016). Randomized, controlled trial of acupuncture for fatigue in Parkinson's disease. *Movement Disorders, 3*(7), 1027–1032.

Kocovski, N. L., Fleming, J. E., Blackie, R. A., et al. (2019). Self-help for social anxiety: Randomized controlled trial comparing a mindfulness and acceptance-based approach with a control group. *Behavior Therapy, 50*(4), 696–709.

Koerner, J. G. (2007). *Healing presence: The essence of nursing.* New York: Springer.

Krugel, L. (2019). *Sentencing decision for Calgary couple convicted in toddler's infection death.* CTV News. June 5. Retrieved from https://www.ctvnews.ca/canada/sentencing-decision-for-calgary-couple-convicted-in-toddler-s-infection-death-1.4452332.

Kryak, E., & Vitale, A. (2011). Reiki and its journey into a hospital setting. *Holistic Nursing Practice, 25*(5), 238–245.

Lee, M. S., Choi, J., Posadzki, P., & Ernst, E. (2012). Aromatherapy for healthcare: An overview of systematic reviews. *Maturitas, 71*(3), 257–260.

Lee, M. S., Pittler, M. H., & Ernst, E. (2008). Effects of reiki in clinical practice: A systematic review of randomised clinical trials. *International Journal of Clinical Practice, 62*(6), 947–954.

Li, Z., Dai, H., Thurston, A. F., et al. (1994). *The private life of Chairman Mao: The memoirs of Mao's personal physician.* New York: Random House. [Seminal Reference].

Lin, K. (2017). *Effectiveness of acupuncture treating fibromyalgia. (Unpublished doctoral dissertation).* Anaheim, CA: South Baylo University.

Li, C., Yang, J., Sun, J., et al. (2013). Brain responses to acupuncture are probably dependent on the brain functional status. *Evidence-based Complementary and Alternative Medicine, 2013,* 175278. https://doi.org/10.1155/2013/175278. [Seminal Reference].

Luctkar-Flude, M., Groll, D., & Tyerman, J. (2017). Using neurofeedback to manage long-term symptoms in cancer survivors: Results of a survey of neurofeedback providers. *European Journal of Integrative Medicine, 12,* 172–176.

Lu, D. P., & Lu, G. P. (2013). An historical review and perspective on the impact of acupuncture on U.S. medicine and society. *Medical Acupuncture, 25*(5), 311–316. [Seminal Reference].

Ma, Y., & Fang, S. (2019). Adolescents' mindfulness and psychological distress: The mediating role of emotion regulation. *Frontiers in Psychology, 10,* 1358.

Marks, R. (2017). Qigong exercise and arthritis. *Medicines (Basel, Switzerland), 4*(4).

Mathie, R. T., Frye, J., & Fisher, P. (2015). Homeopathic oscillococcinum for preventing and treating influenza and influenza-like illness. *Cochrane Database of Systematic Reviews,* CD001957. https://doi.org/10.1002/14651858.CD001957.pub6.

Mathie, R. T., Ramparsad, N., Legg, L. A., et al. (2017). Randomised, double-blind, placebo-controlled trials of non-individualised homeopathic treatment: Systematic review and meta-analysis. *Systematic Reviews, 6*(1), 63.

Mathie, R., Ulbrich-Zürni, S., Viksveen, P., et al. (2018). Systematic review and meta-analysis of randomised, other-than-placebo controlled, trials of individualised homeopathic treatment. *Homeopathy, 107*(04), 229–243.

McNeely, M. E., Duncan, R. P., & Earhart, G. M. (2015). A comparison of dance interventions in people with Parkinson disease and older adults. *Maturitas, 81*(1), 10–16. [Seminal Reference].

Micozzi, M. S. (2018). *Fundamentals of complementary, alternative, and integrative medicine* (6th ed.). St. Louis: Elsevier.

Moffet, H. H. (2006). How might acupuncture work? A systematic review of physiologic rationales from clinical trials. *BMC Complementary and Alternative Medicine, 6*(1), 25.

Murdoch, B., Carr, S., & Caulfield, T. (2016). Selling falsehoods? A cross-sectional study of Canadian naturopathy, homeopathy, chiropractic and acupuncture clinic website claims relating to allergy and asthma. *BMJ Open, 6*(12), e014028.

Nahin, R. L., Barnes, P. M., & Stussman, B. J. (2016). Expenditures on complementary health approaches: United States, 2012. *National Health Statistics Reports, 95*, 1–11.

Offit, P. A. (2012). Studying complementary and alternative therapies. *Journal of the American Medical Association, 307*(17), 1803–1804. [Seminal Reference].

Opheim, R., Lie Høivik, M., Bernklev, T., et al. (2016). The use of complementary and alternative medicine among patients with inflammatory bowel disease is associated with reduced health-related quality of life. *Gastroenterology Research and Practice, 2016*, 6453657. https://doi.org/10.1155/2016/6453657.

Paley, C. A., & Johnson, M. I. (2015). Investigation into the effects of using two or four acupuncture needles with bidirectional rotation on experimentally-induced contact heat pain in healthy subjects. *Acupuncture in Medicine, 33*(1), 23–29.

Pichonnaz, C., Bassin, J.-P., Lécureux, E., et al. (2016). Effect of manual lymphatic drainage after total knee arthroplasty: A randomized controlled trial. *Archives of Physical Medicine and Rehabilitation, 97*(5), 674–682.

Prathikanti, S., Rivera, R., Cochran, A., et al. (2017). Treating major depression with yoga: A prospective, randomized, controlled pilot trial. *PloS One, 12*(3), e0173869.

Public Health Agency of Canada. (2019). *Complementary and alternative health—Canadian Health Network*. Retrieved from http://www.phac-aspc.gc.ca/chn-rcs/cah-acps-eng.php.

Qaseem, A., Wilt, T. J., McLean, R. M., et al. (2017). Noninvasive treatments for acute, subacute, and chronic low back pain: A clinical practice guideline from the American college of physicians. *Annals of Internal Medicine, 166*(7), 514–530.

Reiter, K., Andersen, S. B., & Carlsson, J. (2016). Neurofeedback treatment and posttraumatic stress disorder: Effectiveness of neurofeedback on posttraumatic stress disorder and the optimal choice of protocol. *The Journal of Nervous and Mental Disease, 204*(2), 69–77. https://doi.org/10.1097/NMD.0000000000000418.

Saks, M. (2015). *Health policy and complementary and alternative medicine. The Palgrave international handbook of healthcare policy and governance*. London: Palgrave Macmillan UK, 494–509. https://doi.org/10.1057/9781137384935_30.

Shields, D., Fuller, A., Resnicoff, M., et al. (2017). Human energy field: A concept analysis. *Journal of Holistic Nursing, 35*(4), 352–368.

Sirois, F. M. (2008). Provider-based complementary and alternative medicine use among three chronic illness groups: Associations with psychosocial factors and concurrent use of conventional health-care services. *Complementary Therapies in Medicine, 16*(2), 73–80. [Seminal Reference].

Sirois, F. M., Salamonsen, A., & Kristoffersen, A. E. (2016). Reasons for continuing use of complementary and alternative medicine (CAM) in students: A consumer commitment model. *BMC Complementary and Alternative Medicine, 16*(1), 75.

Spears, C. A., Abroms, L. C., Glass, C. R., et al. (2019). Mindfulness-based smoking cessation enhanced with mobile technology (iQuit Mindfully): Pilot randomized controlled trial. *JMIR MHealth and UHealth, 7*(6), e13059.

Spigelblatt, L., & Canadian Paediatric Society, & Community Paediatrics Committee (2002). Chiropractic care for children: Controversies and issues. *Paediatrics and Child Health, 7*(2), 85–89. [Seminal Reference].

Sridharan, K., Mohan, R., Ramaratnam, S., et al. (2011). Ayurvedic treatments for diabetes mellitus. *Cochrane Database of Systematic Reviews*, CD008288. https://doi.org/10.1002/14651858.CD008288.pub2. [Seminal Reference].

Temple, N. J. (2012). The marketing of dietary supplements: Profit before health. In N. Temple, T. Wilson, & D. Jacobs, Jr. (Eds.), *Nutritional health: Nutrition and health*. Totowa, NJ: Humana Press. [Seminal Reference].

Thorne, S., Paterson, B., Russell, C., et al. (2002). Complementary/alternative medicine in chronic illness as informed self-care decision making. *International Journal of Nursing Studies, 39*(7), 671–683. https://doi.org/10.1016/S0020-7489(02)00005-6. [Seminal Reference].

Toms, R. (2011). Reiki therapy. *Critical Care Nursing Quarterly, 34*(3), 213–217. [Seminal Reference].

Tortora, S. (2019). Children are born to dance! Pediatric medical dance/movement therapy: The view from integrative pediatric oncology. *Children, 6*(1), 14–15.

Van Doren, J., Arns, M., Heinrich, H., et al. (2019). Sustained effects of neurofeedback in ADHD: A systematic review and meta-analysis. *European Child & Adolescent Psychiatry, 28*(3), 293–305. https://doi.org/10.1007/s00787-018-1121-4.

Vas, J., Aranda, J., Modesto, M., et al. (2015). *True acupuncture for back pain no better than sham or placebo*. PainScience.com. Retrieved from https://www.painscience.com/biblio/true-acupuncture-for-back-pain-no-better-than-sham-or-placebo.html.

World Health Organization. (2019). *Ten threats to global health in 2019*. Retrieved rom https://www.who.int/emergencies/ten-threats-to-global-health-in-2019.

Yang, G. Y., Wang, L. Q., Ren, J., et al. (2015). Evidence base of clinical studies on tai chi: A bibliometric analysis. *PloS One, 10*(3), e0120655.

Yao, S., Wei, D., Chen, Y., et al. (2017). Quality assessment of clinical practice guidelines for integrative medicine in China: A systematic review. *Chinese Journal of Integrative Medicine, 23*(5), 381–385.

Young, L. (2018). *Here's what naturopaths and chiropractors shouldn't be advising you about. Global News,* May 2. Retrieved from https://globalnews.ca/news/4248401/naturopath-chiropractor-advice-vaccination/.

Yu, L., Liu, R., Gao, X., et al. (2011). Development of studies on neurochemical mechanism of acupuncture underlying improvement of depression. *Zhen Ci Yan Jiu (Acupuncture Research), 36*(5), 383–387. [Seminal Reference].

Yun, H., Sun, L., & Mao, J. J. (2017). Growth of integrative medicine at leading cancer centers between 2009 and 2016: A systematic analysis of NCI-designated comprehensive cancer center websites. *JNCI Monographs, 2017*(52). https://doi.org/10.1093/jncimonographs/lgx004.

Zehetmair, C., Tegeler, I., Kaufmann, C., et al. (2019). Stabilizing techniques and guided imagery for traumatized male refugees in a German state registration and reception center: A qualitative study on a psychotherapeutic group intervention. *Journal of Clinical Medicine, 8*(6), 894.

Zhang, Y., Dennis, J. A., Bishop, F. L., et al. (2019). Complementary and alternative medicine use by U.S. adults with self–reported doctor–diagnosed arthritis: Results from the 2012 National Health Interview Survey. *Physical Medicine and Rehabilitation*, 1–11. https://doi.org/10.1002/pmrj.12124.

# 25

# Health Promotion for the Twenty-First Century: Throughout the Life Span and Throughout the World

*Robin Humble, MPH*

Originating US chapter by *Ratchneewan Ross, FAAN, RN, PhD, Rosanna F. Hess, MA, MSN, DNP, RN*

## INTENDED LEARNING OUTCOMES

*After completing this chapter, the reader will be able to:*

- Identify global trends and directions for health promotion and disease prevention, including the sustainable development goals and immunization programs.
- Discuss recent and emerging infectious disease, including Ebola virus disease, Zika virus disease, human papilloma virus and cervical cancer, and methicillin-resistant *Staphylococcus aureus* infection.
- Describe problems and implications related to HIV/AIDS.
- Discuss problems and implications related to violence.
- Discuss problems and implications related to bioterrorism and terrorism.

## KEY TERMS

Anthrax (*Bacillus anthracis*)
Bioterrorism
Botulism
Ebola virus disease (EVD)
Essential public health services
Human immunodeficiency virus (HIV)
Human papilloma virus (HPV)
Malnutrition
Methicillin-resistant *Staphylococcus aureus* (MRSA)
Plague

Self-abuse
Social determinants of health
Smallpox (variola major)
Suicide
Sustainable development goals (SDG)
Terrorism
Violence
World Health Organization
Zika virus disease (ZVD)

## ? THINK ABOUT IT

### Human Papilloma Virus Infection and Cultural Practices

Adila lives in Ghana, West Africa, with her husband and her two daughters, aged 13 and 10 years. Adila learned 6 weeks ago that she has cervical cancer. When Adila told her husband that she had cervical cancer and needed treatment, he accused her of having sexual relations with another man and refused to give her money. He also refused to have his daughters vaccinated against human papilloma virus (HPV), which would prevent them from contracting cervical cancer. He said that this immunization would make them more sexually promiscuous as teenagers.

- What kind of problems would you anticipate that Adila will encounter if she does not have treatment for her cervical cancer?
- How could Adila's husband be encouraged and educated to change his mind about his wife and daughters?
- What do you think could be done in this Ghanaian village to prevent further HPV infections *in addition* to an immunization campaign?

Visit the World Health Organization website (https://www.who.int/) to identify the incidence and prevalence of HPV and cervical cancer in West African countries.

## BOX 25.1    A Social Gradient Approach to Addressing Health Inequities: Norway's Social Gradient Approach to the Social Determinants of Health

A social gradient approach to addressing health inequities has emerged in Norway, with universal policies and programs aimed at the whole spectrum of the socioeconomic gradient, and additional measures directed at the most disadvantaged in the population (Whitehead & Popay, 2010). Norway's social gradient initiative includes upstream social reform, midstream risk reduction, and downstream effect reduction (Fosse & Helgesen, 2017). Norway's public health action plan recognizes the social structure of the whole population and that behaviours are related to social conditions; and that, therefore, empowering individuals to change behaviours is not possible unless there is success in improving their entire life situation in relation to the social determinants of health (Vallgarda, 2008). The social gradient approach also includes non-stigmatizing measures to serve those who are entrenched in absolute poverty through measures of taxation, access to health care, behaviour health promotion, and prevention of social exclusion (Vallgarda, 2008). This universal approach is described as upstream or "farsighted," preventing health and socioeconomic inequities from developing in the first place rather than attempting to address issues after poverty arises (Vallgarda, 2008). Adopted in 2012, the Norwegian Public Health Act uses health promotion as the guiding principles in all public health policies and reduces social inequalities in health by taking direct action to change the social gradient (Fosse & Helgesen, 2017).

Norway remains a world leader in developing active labour market policies, safe working conditions, action plans to prevent social exclusion, universal health care, high-quality and low-cost child care, social security safety nets, supportive affordable housing, unemployment and child benefits, improved living conditions for those disadvantaged, free education up to 19 years of age, and universal eligibility for subsidized loans and grants for higher education (Grimm, Helgesen, & Fosse, 2013).

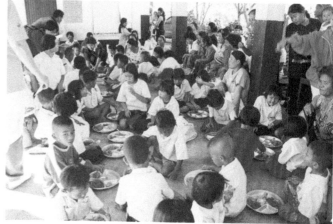

**Fig. 25.1** Lunchtime for schoolchildren in a remote area of Thailand. The food was made possible through donations from health care providers.

In the current millennium, the gap in life expectancies between people in high-, middle-, and low-income countries has been widening. In many developed nations, such as Japan, France, Monaco, and Canada, people have a life expectancy at birth ranging from 81 to 89 years, whereas residents of some countries, such as Chad, Guinea-Bissau, and Afghanistan, can have a life expectancy as low as 50 years (Central Intelligence Agency [CIA], 2017), attributable primarily to political instability and a high level of poverty, inadequate nutrition, lack of clean water and sanitation, high rates of human immunodeficiency virus (HIV) infections, limited access to health resources and interventions, and low quality of life (CIA, 2016, 2017; Joint United Nations Programme on HIV/AIDS [UNAIDS], 2017a).

In 2016 there were 56.9 million deaths worldwide: 71% were due to noncommunicable diseases (cardiovascular diseases, cancer, chronic lung diseases, and diabetes); more than 75% occurred in low- to middle-income countries, with a disproportionate rise in low-income countries. Over 5 million children younger than 5 years died in 2017, a steady decline since 2000, but still a rate equivalent to one in 26 children dying in 2017 per day (World Health Organization [WHO], 2019b). The mortality rate of children younger than 5 years remains high, with an average of 69 deaths per 1000 live births of children under 5 years, compared with 5.4 deaths per 1000 live births in high-income countries. Sub-Saharan Africa continues to have

the highest under-five mortality rate, with 76 deaths per 1000 live births in 2017 (United Nations Children's Fund [UNICEF], 2018). On the basis of WHO's 2016 statistics, lower respiratory tract infections, HIV/AIDS (acquired immunodeficiency syndrome), diarrheal diseases, and stroke were the leading causes of death for people in low-income countries, whereas ischemic heart disease and stroke were the leading causes of deaths in lower-middle-income, upper-middle-income, and high-income countries (WHO, 2017) (Box 25.1).

Since 2016, the number of undernourished people has increased globally with 11%, or 815 million people being undernourished. All but 10% of them live in developing countries with food insecurities that are attributable to violent conflict, economic slowdowns, and climate-related shocks. Sub-Saharan Africa experiences the highest prevalence of undernourished people, at 22.7% of the population (Food and Agriculture Organization of the United Nations, International Fund for Agricultural Development, UNICEF, et al., 2017). Annually, more than 3.1 million children die of starvation, and one out of four children under the age of 5 years is affected by growth stunting (Food and Agriculture Organization of the United Nations et al., 2017). Undernutrition heightens the effect of every disease (Fig. 25.1). At the other end of the spectrum, obesity is a rising cause of health problems in both medium- and high-income countries. The number of the world population with obesity more than doubled from 1980 to 2008, and almost 41 million children 5 years or younger were obese in 2016 (WHO, 2018f). Whereas urgent interventions to combat hunger and infectious diseases (such as HIV infection and diarrheal diseases) are needed in many developing countries, broad societal public health education, initiatives, and interventions to fight cardiovascular disorders and obesity are crucial in medium-income and high-income countries.

To address global health trends, the sustainable development goals (SDG) were developed in 2016 by the United Nations Development Programme (UNDP) as a universal call to action "… to end poverty, protect the planet and ensure that all people enjoy peace and prosperity" (UNDP, 2016, p. 1). The SDGs act as a blueprint for addressing global challenges, with a purpose of achieving an improved and more sustainable future for all (United Nations, n.d). The 17 SDGs are as follows: eradicate poverty; end hunger and malnutrition; good health and well-being; quality education; gender equality; clean water and sanitation; affordable and clean energy; decent work and economic growth; industry, innovation, and infrastructure; reduced inequalities; sustainable cities and communities; responsible consumption and production; climate action; life below water; life on land; peace, justice, and strong institutions; and partnerships for the goals (UNDP, 2016). Achieving the SDG targets by 2030 requires mutual partnerships and commitments from governments, the private sector, citizens, and civil society around the world. More information on the United Nations SDGs can be found at https://www.un.org/sustainabledevelopment/sustainable-development-goals/.

## THE SOCIAL DETERMINANTS OF HEALTH

The term "social determinants of health" first appeared in the Canadian literature in 1996 to describe social and economic factors that influence people's health (Rootman, Dupere, Pederson, et al., 2012). Since then, the social determinants of health have gained international recognition and application: for example, with the creation of the WHO Commission of the Social Determinants of Health (Rootman et al., 2012). The social determinants of health are defined as the living environments, conditions, or contexts that an individual experiences on a daily basis and are thus directly correlated with the health and well-being of that individual (Jones, Jones, Perry, et al., 2009; Mikkonen & Raphael, 2010). The WHO describes the social determinants of health as being "the circumstances in which people are born, grow up, live, work and age, and the systems put in place to deal with illness" (WHO, 2019d, p. 1).

The Canadian social determinants of health are as follows: income and social status, employment and working conditions, education and literacy, childhood experiences, physical environments, social supports and coping skills, healthy behaviours, access to health services, biology and genetic endowment, gender, culture, and race/racism (Government of Canada, 2019). The Canadian government, in conjunction with the Public Health Agency of Canada (PHAC) and public health practitioners, actively focus on upstream health-promotion and disease-prevention initiatives through community, governmental, and structural policies to address underlying health inequities resulting from the social determinants of health. Although behavioural components that determine health are important, Canadian public health moves away from historical behavioural strategies that focus solely on lifestyle choices as the primary cause of poor health (Sieppert, Te Linde, & Rutherford, 2004). The Canadian social determinants of health shift health promotion away from a biomedical deficit model and focus, instead, on assets and resilience for health potential (Mikkonen & Raphael, 2010).

Intrinsic to SDG outcomes and the social determinants of health, emerging infections, various forms of intercultural and interpersonal violence, terrorism, and bioterrorism also pose public health threats and risks to populations around the world.

This chapter presents information on malnutrition, Ebola virus disease (EVD), Zika virus disease (ZVD), methicillin-resistant *Staphylococcus aureus* (MRSA), HIV, and HPV infections, violence, bioterrorism, and terrorism, followed by a discussion of their important implications for the future.

## MALNUTRITION

The WHO defines malnutrition as "deficiencies, excesses, or imbalances in a person's intake of energy and/or nutrients" and includes three broad groups of conditions: undernutrition (wasting, stunting, and underweight); micronutrient-related malnutrition (lack of important vitamins and minerals); and overweight, obesity, and diet-related noncommunicable diseases (such as stroke, heart disease, and diabetes) (WHO 2018b). This chapter addresses only undernutrition (protein–energy malnutrition resulting in wasting, stunting, and underweight), because it is the most serious among the three types (WHO, 2000, 2018b).

### Undernutrition

Undernutrition due to protein–energy malnutrition, a lack of calories and protein, is widespread in low-income countries and is the most lethal form of malnutrition/hunger (World Hunger Education Service, 2018). Humans convert food into energy, and the energy contained in food is measured in calories. Protein is necessary for key body functions, including provision of essential amino acids and development and maintenance of muscles (WHO & United Nations Children's Fund [UNICEF], 2009). Protein–energy malnutrition can be severely harmful to the mental and physical development of individuals, especially children younger than 5 years (WHO, 2016d). Worldwide, one in two deaths among children younger than 5 years old stem from protein–energy malnutrition (WHO, 2016d). One in four children are underweight, and one in three children are stunted (WHO, 2016d).

### Severe Acute Malnutrition

WHO defines severe acute malnutrition as the presence of serious wasting and/or edema (WHO & UNICEF, 2009). Severe wasting is defined as the weight of a child being less than 70% (or less than three standard deviations [3 SD]) of the median weight for height (WHO, 2011) and/or having a mid-upper arm circumference less than 115 mm—a new cut-off (WHO & UNICEF, 2009). Children with severe acute malnutrition require immediate treatment because they have a higher risk of death than children without severe acute malnutrition (WHO & UNICEF, 2009). Severe wasting is caused by loss of subcutaneous fat and skeletal muscle and is highly noticeable because of underdeveloped buttocks, thighs, and upper arms. It is also characterized by sunken eyes, visible ribs, and protruding shoulder blades (WHO, 2013). Children with severe wasting usually have a distended abdomen and a general overall appearance in some way similar to that of an older person. In general, these children are irritable, anxious, and cry easily; yet they will often have an absence of tears while crying because of lacrimal gland atrophy (WHO, 2013).

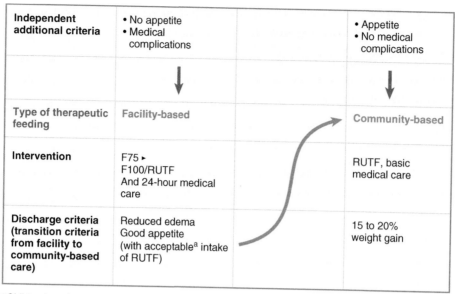

| Independent additional criteria | • No appetite<br>• Medical complications | | • Appetite<br>• No medical complications |
|---|---|---|---|
| Type of therapeutic feeding | Facility-based | | Community-based |
| Intervention | F75 ►<br>F100/RUTF<br>And 24-hour medical care | | RUTF, basic medical care |
| Discharge criteria (transition criteria from facility to community-based care) | Reduced edema<br>Good appetite<br>(with acceptable[a] intake of RUTF) | | 15 to 20% weight gain |

[a]Child eats at least 75% of their calculated RUTF ration for the day

**Fig. 25.2** Severe acute malnutrition management. *RUTF*, Ready-to-use therapeutic food. (Reprinted with permission from World Health Organization. [2011]. *The WHO child growth standards.* Retrieved from https://www.who.int/childgrowth/en/.)

Treating children with severe acute malnutrition involves providing special therapeutic, milk-based foods called ready-to-use therapeutic foods (RUTFs), which are soft, crushable, and tasty, nutrient- and energy-rich foods that can be consumed by children 6 months of age or older (WHO & UNICEF, 2009). When a child has a good appetite with no medical conditions (e.g., hypoglycemia, hypothermia, dehydration, electrolyte imbalance, and/or infections), use of RUTFs under community-based care is appropriate. However, when a child does not have an appetite and/or medical conditions are present, the child needs to receive facility-based care (WHO & UNICEF, 2009). The child may be transferred from a facility-based care setting to a community-based setting when the following conditions are met: the child does not have bilateral edema, regains a good appetite, and eats at least 75% of the calculated RUTF ration for the day (WHO & UNICEF, 2009). Children can be discharged from a community-based care setting when they have a weight gain of 15% since admission (WHO & UNICEF, 2009) (Fig. 25.2).

### Addressing Malnutrition at the Global Level

The US Centers for Disease Control and Prevention (CDC), the World Health Organization (WHO), and UNICEF have worked collaboratively to create several initiatives to address the malnutrition issue. These include the Baby Friendly Hospital Initiative programs to manage nutrition needs during emergencies, global nutrition data banks, a global network of collaborating centres in nutrition (UNICEF, 2018), and the International Micronutrient Malnutrition Prevention and Control (IMMPaCt) program (CDC, 2015a).

The Baby Friendly Hospital Initiative, launched in 1991 by UNICEF and WHO, has as its goal to promote exclusive breastfeeding during the first 4 months of life when it is most required by the infant (UNICEF & WHO, 2018). The program involves at least 170 countries and more than 16,000 hospitals (UNICEF & WHO, 2018). Through the initiative a mother starts breastfeeding as soon

as her child is born and continues to breastfeed her child exclusively, unless medically otherwise indicated or until the child is 4 months old. This includes avoiding supplemental food and drink until the older child is ready for such intake (UNICEF & WHO, 2018).

The IMMPaCt program, established in 2000 by the CDC, works with global partners such as WHO, UNICEF, and the US Agency for International Development to provide its skills and resources to eradicate vitamin and mineral deficiencies around the globe (CDC, 2015a). The IMMPaCt program's activities include conducting surveys; providing micronutrients to infants, young children, and women of child-bearing age; and monitoring and evaluating intervention systems (CDC, 2015a). Since its establishment, the IMMPaCt program has provided assistance and/or training in more than 70 countries around the world.

## EMERGING INFECTIONS

### Severe Acute Respiratory Syndrome (SARS)

In 2002 to 2004, the rapidly spreading severe acute respiratory syndrome (SARS) coronavirus drew global attention, with 8500 probable cases and over 900 deaths globally. Outside of Asia, Canada was the hardest-hit country, documenting 438 probable SARS cases and 44 deaths (The Canadian Encyclopedia, 2015). Due to its sudden, widespread emergence and high virulence through exhaled droplets and body secretions, SARS became a global health care crisis in an era of globalization and international tourism and migration (For more information on the SARS virus see the Government of Canada information page: https://www.canada.ca/en/health-canada/services/healthy-living/your-health/diseases/severe-acute-respiratory-syndrome-sars.html.)

As a result of the SARS crisis, Canada's vulnerability and lack of organizational resources to protect Canadians from an infectious disease outbreak became apparent, with the Government of Canada appointing the National Advisory Committee on SARS and Public Health to investigate Canada's response to the SARS outbreak. The committee's historic report, *Learning from SARS: Renewal of Public Health in Canada* (Health Canada, 2003), otherwise known as the Naylor Report for its author, Dr David Naylor, has since shaped the Canadian public health system.

The goal of the report was to evaluate the epidemiology, management, communication, and international coordination of the SARS outbreak, identify systemic deficiencies, and make recommendations regarding future emerging infectious diseases and public health services within Canada. The report called for a "comprehensive renewal of both the public health system in general, and the nation's capacity to detect, prevent, understand, and manage outbreaks of significant infectious diseases" (Health Canada, 2003, p. iii).

Since 2003, the 75 recommendations from the Naylor Report remain a catalyst for public health reform in Canada, including calls for a $1.3 billion increase in federal spending, coordination between funding agencies, the creation of a national public health–monitoring body, a "CDC North," and appointment of a chief public health officer, among others (Canadian Broadcasting Corporation, 2003).

The Public Health Agency of Canada (PHAC) and the Chief Public Health Officer position were created in 2004, in direct response to recommendations from the Naylor Report and growing concerns of Canada's public health system capacity to anticipate, identify, and effectively respond to public health threats. Activities of the PHAC include disease and injury prevention, supporting evidence-informed decision making with regard to infectious diseases, chronic diseases, travel health, food safety, biosafety and biosecurity, immunization and vaccines, health promotion, and emergency preparedness and response. For more information on the PHAC, see the Government of Canada information page: https://www.canada.ca/en/public-health.html.

## Coronavirus Disease 2019 (COVID-19)

The 2002-2004 SARS coronavirus outbreak pales in comparison to the 2019-2020 COVID-19 coronavirus pandemic. Originating in China COVID-19 quickly developed into a global pandemic with infections and fatalities reported in almost every country around the world. Learnings from the SARS outbreak positioned the Canadian government, the national British Columbia Center for Disease Control (BCCDC), and the PHAC to implement a timely and effective response to COVID-19 with a primary goal of protecting the health and safety of Canadians. Information on the PHAC and BCCDC's response to COVID-19 can be found at the following links https://www.canada.ca/en/public-health/services/diseases/coronavirus-disease-covid-19.html; https://www.bccdc.ca/health-info/diseases-conditions/covid-19.

## Ebola Virus Disease

Ebola virus disease (EVD), originally known as Ebola hemorrhagic fever, emerged on to the world scene of deadly infections in the mid-1970s in the African countries of the Democratic Republic of Congo and what is now known as South Sudan. The most recent major outbreak occurred in three countries in West Africa: Guinea, Sierra Leone, and Liberia. Case-fatality rates for EVD average approximately 50%, with deaths in some outbreaks as high as 90%. The virus spreads by human-to-human contact from an index case infected by contaminated blood,

secretions, or bodily organs of a wild animal such as a fruit bat or monkey. Humans can be infected by contact with bedding and clothing of an infected person (CDC, 2018a; WHO, 2018a). The risk of transmission by sexual contact is an important concern, and research is ongoing (Fischer & Wohl, 2016). Current recommendations include abstinence from sexual intercourse for 3 months after development of symptoms or use of condoms if abstinence is not feasible (Rogstad & Tunbridge, 2015).

Although an experimental Ebola vaccine has shown strong promise in protection when trialled during a 2015 outbreak in Guinea, community involvement is vital for the prevention and control of an outbreak. Control measures include careful case management, contact tracing, a viable laboratory service, safe internment of deceased persons, and risk reduction for spread of the virus. See the section entitled "Prevention and control" in WHO (2018a) for details on these measures. Cultural practices differ greatly from country to country, region to region, and even village to village. The diversity of cultures must be taken into consideration when one is expecting a public health response (Alexander, Sanderson, Marathe, et al., 2015). Burial practices, bushmeat consumption, use of traditional medicines, beliefs about modern medicine and health care interventions, and stigmatization of Ebola survivors are topics to include (Alexander et al., 2015). Ways to modify practices particularly related to the preparation of a dead body for burial must be found to curtail the spread of Ebola virus. This must be done in conjunction with an understanding of other nonpharmaceutical interventions (Shuaib, Musa, Muhammad, et al., 2017).

The prevention of the spread of infection in the health care setting must start with standard precautions when any patient is being cared for: basic hand hygiene, personal protective equipment, and respiratory hygiene. If EVD is suspected, health care workers must add extra protective measures to avoid contact with all bodily fluids and contaminated surfaces during direct patient care (Lupton, 2015; Marion, Charlebois, & Kao, 2016). Protective clothing must include a face shield of some type, a long-sleeved gown, and gloves. Laboratory workers must follow strict protection protocols. In the community, safe burial practices using the same techniques health care workers have instituted are essential.

Follow-up of EVD survivors is important for surveillance and treatment of long-term complications. Tiffany, Vetter, Mattia, and colleagues (2016) found that 57% of EVD survivors followed up in Sierra Leone developed ocular complications. Others complications included arthralgia, fatigue, headaches, abdominal pains, and anemia. Even more difficult for survivors is the stigmatization they experience when discharged from the hospital. In a study of 81 EVD survivors in Sierra Leone (Nanyonga, Saidu, Ramsay, et al., 2016), 96% reported being rejected by their communities, leading to fear and anxiety about returning home. Economic hardships accompanied the physical and psychosocial sequelae. A full range of services are needed to care for these survivors.

## Zika Virus Disease

ZVD burst onto the global scene in 2015, with reports of hundreds of children in Brazil born with microcephaly to mothers who had been ill because of this virus. Zika virus was actually identified in the 1940s. The main vector is *Aedes* mosquitos known to live in Africa, the Americas, Asia, and the Pacific. Classic transmission is from the bite of an infected mosquito to a human. It is also now known that Zika virus can be transmitted from men who are infected with the virus during sexual contact. As the virus can stay in semen longer than it can in blood, the virus can be transmitted before a man develops symptoms, during the symptom phase, and even after symptoms have disappeared. Although transmission of Zika virus from male to female sexual partners is more likely (Coelho, Durovni, Saraceni, et al., 2016), reports confirm that female-to-male transmission is also possible (CDC, 2018f; PHAC, 2019). For couples in which the woman could get pregnant, a condom should be used during every sexual contact or the couple should abstain from sexual relations to prevent infection with Zika virus for at least 6 months after symptoms appeared. If there were no symptoms but the man has travelled to a Zika virus–infested region, the couple should use a condom or abstain from sex for 8 weeks after the man returns (CDC, 2018f, CDC, 2018h; PHAC, 2019).

Most people infected with Zika virus will not exhibit symptoms. If symptoms appear, they are usually mild and can last up to 1 week. The symptoms include fever, joint and muscle pain, headache, and a rash. The virus can be detected by a laboratory test confirming its presence in blood, urine, and/or saliva. The incubation period is not yet well established but is believed to be a few days from bite to symptoms.

In 2015, public health officials in Brazil observed an increase in the number of patients with Guillain–Barré syndrome and an increase in the number of babies born with microcephaly at the same time as there was an increase in the number of cases of ZVD. Research has attributed the Zika virus as being the cause of these apparent complications. In 2016, the WHO Director-General declared the Zika virus and its associated health complications an international public health concern (WHO, 2018g).

Prevention of ZVD requires elimination of mosquitos' breeding sources and reduction in opportunities for mosquitos to bite people. Any objects that can contain and hold water should be removed or cleaned: pots, tires, buckets, gutters, etc. People should cover their skin as much as possible, screen windows and doors, sleep under mosquito nets, and use insect repellant (WHO, 2018g). A number of promising Zika virus vaccines have moved into clinical trials, and are expected to be widely available in the coming years (Wilder-Smith, Vannice, Durbin, et al., 2018).

The PHAC provides numerous tools, in pdf documents, on its website for health care providers to use when they are caring for patients who may have or who have contracted Zika virus. These tools include testing algorithms for pregnant women who have travelled to regions of the world known to have Zika virus, for pregnant women who live in these same regions, and for infants whose mothers reside in or travelled to Zika virus–infested areas of the world. Other tools include one to measure an infant's head circumference, fact sheets on testing for the virus, and preconception counselling (PHAC, 2019). There is also a page on the CDC website with details about a US Zika Pregnancy Registry. This page includes links to fact sheets for health care providers in general, one specific to pediatric health care providers, and one for pregnant women (CDC, 2018e).

## Human Papilloma Virus Infection

Human papilloma virus (HPV) is a group of approximately 150 related viruses, each with an assigned number. HPV is named for the warts it causes called papillomas. An estimated 70% of sexually active Canadian women and men will have an HPV infection over the course of their lives, making it the most common sexually transmitted infection (PHAC, 2017). HPV is transmitted by intimate vaginal, anal, or oral contacts, even if the person is asymptomatic. Most HPV infections are asymptomatic and disappear without causing any problems; persistent ones, however, may lead to precancerous lesions, progressing years later to cervical cancer. HPV infections occur in men and women. Most HPV infections are acquired shortly after a person becomes sexually active with a person or persons infected with the virus. Abstinence, delay in becoming sexually active, use of condoms, limits on the number of sexual partners, and vaccination against HPV should slow down the increase in the number of people who carry and propagate HPV (WHO, 2019c).

### Vaccination

WHO (2014b) guidelines include the following elements: vaccinate all girls aged 9 to 13 years with two doses of the HPV vaccine; screen women with HPV tests; and promote screening to a larger audience. Men should be included in any screening awareness efforts because, without their support, women in many cultures will not participate in screening practices (Learmonth, van Vuuren, & De Abreu, 2015; Lim & Ojo, 2016; Modibbo, Bamisaye, Dareng, et al., 2016; Tsu, Njama-Meya, Lim, et al., 2018).

The HPV vaccine was introduced in 2006. The current Health Canada–approved vaccines against HPV are Gardasil, Cervarix, and Gardasil 9 (White, Waldrop, & Waldrop, 2016). National vaccination programs have been conducted in Rwanda, Uganda, and Uzbekistan, to name a few countries (GAVI Alliance, 2016). The prevalence of vaccine-type HPV infections is decreasing in vaccinated Canadian girls (Steben, Thompson, Rodier, et al., 2018). The PHAC recommends that sexually active young men be vaccinated against HPV, starting at the age of 11 years (PHAC, 2015). Barriers to HPV vaccination include social norms related to sexual activity, financial constraints, vulnerable populations (immigrants, those with disability, and visible minority groups) and levels of trust or distrust in vaccination programs (Vahabi & Lofters, 2018). An increase in high-risk sexual behaviour has not been associated with HPV vaccination in young females (Donken, Ogilvie, Bettinger, et al., 2018).

### Human Papilloma Virus and Cervical Cancer

HPV triggers a sexually acquired infection that may lead to cervical cancer. Cervical cancer is the world's fourth deadliest, but preventable, forms of cancer. There are more than 570,000 new cases each year (International Agency for Research on Cancer, 2018; WHO, 2019c). Approximately 85% of the approximately 311,000 annual deaths occur in the developing world. Cervical cancer incidence rates in sub-Saharan Africa are the highest in the world (Bouassa, Prazuck, Lethu, et al., 2017). The risk factors for persistent HPV infection and progression to cervical cancer include early first sexual intercourse, multiple sexual partners, and a compromised immune system (WHO, 2019c). Lack of access to effective screening and to services that promote early detection and treatment may explain the dramatic differences in prevalence.

## Screening and Testing

Screening recommendations in Canada are set by the PHAC and the Society of Obstetricians and Gynaecologists of Canada. The current recommendations for routine cervical screening are as follows (Canadian Partnership Against Cancer, 2016): start at age 25 years and continue through to age 65 to 70 years; conventional or liquid-based cytological tests (Papanicolaou test) for women every 3 years; the testing recommendations are the same for women, regardless of whether they have been vaccinated against HPV or not; refer women with abnormal test results to an appropriate provider for follow-up. Barriers to cervical screening include fear of diagnosis, lack of access, lack of partner support, lack of finances, cultural modesty (only wanting a female provider), not knowing about cervical cancer, and not seeing self as having risk factors (Compaore, Ouedraogo, Koanda, et al., 2015; Lim & Ojo, 2016). A promising WHO prequalified global screening test is careHPV (Lorenzi, Fregnani, Possati-Resende, et al., 2016; Jeronimo, Bansil, Lim, et al., 2014).

Health care providers have an important role to play in the promotion of vaccinations against HPV and screening for HPV and cervical cancer. Studies have noted that when health care providers, particularly nurses, educate women and recommend the vaccine, immunization rates increase (Walling, Benzoni, Dornfeld, et al., 2016). Fact sheets, continuing education courses, and vaccination schedules and recommendations for use by health care providers in combating HPV infections and subsequent cancer risks can be found on the PHAC website (PHAC, 2015).

## Methicillin-Resistant *Staphylococcus aureus* Infection

Colonization of *S. aureus* in the nasal area is common and asymptomatic in one in three healthy individuals (CDC, 2015b; PHAC, 2008). On the other hand, MRSA, a form of staphylococcus bacteria that causes skin/soft-tissue infections, is estimated to be colonized in only 1% of healthy individuals (CDC, 2015b). It is resistant to β-lactams (e.g., methicillin, oxacillin, penicillin, amoxicillin) (CDC, 2016b).

Health care–associated MRSA (HA-MRSA) infection may occur in hospitalized individuals who undergo medical or surgical procedures, such as administration of ventilation apparatus or introduction of a nasogastric tube or catheter (particularly in those with minimized immune functions), and can lead to life-threatening infections, such as pneumonia and bacteremia. MRSA infections in Canada continued to rise from 1995 until 2008; however, recent research has shown a 25% decrease in MRSA infection rates since 2008 (PHAC, 2016).

In the community setting, community-associated MRSA (CA-MRSA) strains have emerged as serious threats in the past two decades and can cause dermatitis and soft tissue infections (British Columbia Centre for Disease Control [BCCDC], 2014; BCCDC, n.d), with the ability to also cause fatal infections in the lungs (e.g., necrotizing pneumonia, purpura fulminans, and postviral toxic shock syndrome) (BCCDC, n.d; Schlievert, Nemeth, Davis, et al., 2010). Most CA-MRSA cases are mild and include a skin or soft-tissue infection (i.e., a boil or abscess).

Usually, the infected area resembles a red, swollen, and painful "spider bite" (BCCDC, 2014). Pus or other drainage may be present. If the infection is limited to the skin, it can be difficult to distinguish CA-MRSA from HA-MRSA (BCCDC, 2014; BCCDC, n.d.).

Among severely CA-MRSA-infected people, complications may include serious necrotizing infection, septicemia, pneumonia, and death (BCCDC, 2014; BCCDC, n.d.).

CA-MRSA cases have been reported by emergency departments, day care centres, schools, correctional facilities, sports facilities, dormitories, and military stations (CDC, 2015b; Sedighi, Moez, & Alikhani, 2011). People who are generally healthy can contract the bacteria through close skin-to-skin contact, cuts in or abrasions of the skin, crowded conditions, shared utilities (e.g., clothing items and towels), and poor hygiene (CDC, 2015b; Kirkland & Adams, 2008). In addition, those who are taking or have previously received antibiotic therapy have a greater risk of infections than those who do not have a history of antibiotic intake (Fekete, 2007).

The most up-to-date Canadian clinical guidelines for CA-MRSA management were published in 2014 by the BCCDC. The guidelines suggest that CA-MRSA skin infections, such as boils or abscesses, may be treated by incision and drainage. Antibiotic regimens guided by sensitivity test results should be administered to infected individuals. Intravenous antibiotic treatment should be considered among hospitalized individuals who show signs of oral therapy nonadherence. Oral antibiotics may include sulfamethoxazole-trimethoprim, clindamycin, doxycycline, minocycline, and linezolid.

Knowledge of this disease is essential to enable health care providers to initiate appropriate infection control. In general, CA-MRSA spreads more easily, has higher recurrence rates, and causes more skin problems and serious damage than the traditional HA-MRSA found in hospital settings (BCCDC, 2014; BCCDC, n.d.). Standard precautions—a combination and expansion of universal precautions and body substance isolation—are required among health care providers to prevent cross-contamination Meticulous handwashing has been found to be important and is recommended as a cost-effective everyday practice: see BCCDC (2014) for more details. Current recommendations by the BCCDC for various sectors of the community are on the BCCDC website: http://www.bccdc.ca/health-professionals/clinical-resources/mrsa.

## Human Immunodeficiency Virus/Acquired Immunodeficiency Syndrome

In 2017, approximately 37 million people worldwide were infected with HIV, with 25.7 million in sub-Saharan Africa, 5.3 million in Asia and the Pacific, 1.8 million in Latin America, 1.4 million in eastern Europe and Central Asia, 2.2 million in western/central Europe and North America, 220,000 in the Middle East/North Africa, and 310,000 in the Caribbean (UNAIDS, 2018).

The number of newly infected people continues to decline each year (2.9 million new HIV infections in 2000, and 1.8 million new HIV infections in 2017), with 940,000 AIDS-related deaths and 21.7 million people accessing antiretroviral therapy in 2017 (UNAIDS, 2018). Overall, the number of people living with HIV reflects the fact that people receiving antiretroviral therapies are living longer (UNAIDS, 2018).

In some low-income countries, HIV prevalence rates in the adult population are higher than those in high-income countries. For instance, the 2016 rate was 27.2% in Swaziland and 21.9% in Botswana (CIA, 2016). The rate is approximately 0.2% in Sweden and the Netherlands (CIA, 2016). Although economic level is sometimes negatively associated with HIV rates, evidence also shows that cultural beliefs and practices are significant factors contributing to HIV infections.

The modes of HIV transmission include sexual contact with persons of the opposite sex, sexual contact with persons of the same sex, from mother to baby at birth or through breast milk, contact with objects contaminated with HIV such as needles, syringes, and knives, and through blood transfusions of HIV-infected blood. In east and southern Africa, 60% to 95% of the new infections are occurring among the heterosexual population, people with multiple sex partners, their usual partners, and couples in a mutually faithful discordant relationship (*discordant relationship* in this context is defined as one partner infected with HIV and the other partner HIV-negative) (AVERT, 2019). In Caribbean and Latin American countries, the largest group of new infections is in men who have sex with men, although there are sizeable new infections also among sex workers and their clientele, and in the general heterosexual population. In Eastern Europe, newly infected individuals are mostly those who are intravenous drug users and their sexual partners. In Asia, male risk behaviours dominate the transmission methods (Gouws & Guchi, 2015).

Clearly, the challenges of reducing HIV/AIDS rates are complex and the solutions require multidisciplinary and multidimensional approaches. Ordinary people, community leaders, health care providers, and organizations at all levels must work collaboratively. Together, we can consider gender/social inequalities and cultural/religious beliefs and practices as we work to identify barriers to understanding and facilitate the reduction of HIV infections (Box 25.2). Support from all parties will enable us to set priorities and fight HIV/AIDS more effectively at the global level. UNAIDS (2017a) is working collaboratively with its partner organizations, such as UNICEF, UNESCO (United Nations Educational, Scientific, and Cultural Organization), WHO, and the World Bank. In meeting the ambitious visions of the SDG, the ultimate goal of UNAIDS is to end the AIDS epidemic by 2030, with zero new HIV infections, zero AIDS-related deaths, and zero discrimination; the commitment is that everyone globally should have universal access to HIV prevention, treatment, care, and support (UNAIDS, 2018). To reach this ultimate goal, UNAIDS has outlined three strategic directions: by 2020, 90% of all people living with HIV will know their status, will have received sustained antiretroviral therapy, and will have viral suppression as a result of antiretroviral therapy (UNAIDS, 2017b).

*Revolutionizing HIV prevention* means that the focus is shifted from HIV rates of "prevalence" to "incidence" (UNAIDS, 2017b). "Incidence" deals with the number of new HIV infections in a particular population during a certain period, whereas HIV "prevalence" is the percentage of all cases (new and old) of HIV infections at a certain time point (AVERT, 2012). In this focus, hot spot transmissions need to be identified, and empowerment (especially among young people) needs to be encouraged so that all people involved will adopt more proactive behaviours to decrease the number of new HIV infections. UNAIDS (2015) has announced its support of political change in terms of HIV, new approaches to technology, the reduction of stigma and discrimination associated with HIV, and comprehensive sex education for HIV-positive individuals, networks, and related key populations.

*Catalyzing the next generation of treatment, care, and support* involves universal access to antiretroviral treatment for all HIV-positive individuals who need medication (Research for Evidence-Informed Practice). UNAIDS (2015) expects that all HIV-positive individuals and their families will have access to essential care and support. UNAIDS (2015) will act with each nation to make it possible that simpler, more effective, and more affordable therapy will be universally accessible so that HIV deaths related to tuberculosis infection will be minimized.

## RESEARCH FOR EVIDENCE-INFORMED PRACTICE

### Prophylactic Use of Antiretrovirals to Assist in the Prevention of HIV Infection Among High-Risk Groups in Namibia

With a prevalence rate of 12.1% in populations aged 15 to 49, Namibia has one of the highest prevalence and incidence rates of sexually transmitted HIV, with 75% of new sexually transmitted HIV infections in Namibia occurring among girls and women aged 15 to 24 (CDC, 2019b). The Namibian Medicines Regulatory Council has approved the prophylactic use of antiretrovirals emtricitabine/tenofovir disoproxil fumarate (TDF/FTC) to assist in the prevention of HIV infection among high-risk groups (Management Sciences for Health, 2017). This daily administration of antiretrovirals to HIV-uninfected people is known as pre-exposure prophylaxis (PrEP), reducing the risk of sexually transmitted HIV by over 90% in high-risk populations (Telesur, 2018). As a part of their *National Strategic Framework for HIV and AIDS Response*, Namibia has expanded PrEP to include antiretroviral-based injectables, impregnated vaginal rings for at-risk women, patches, and oral/anal gels (Republic of Namibia, 2017).

Advancing human rights and gender equality for the HIV response means working toward the day when gender inequality, violence against women and girls, and stigmatization and discrimination related to HIV will be eradicated (UNAIDS, 2015). Punitive laws and practices against HIV-positive individuals need to be eliminated. UNAIDS (2015) will work with each government to reinforce the rights of HIV-positive individuals and to better educate infected individuals about their rights. UNAIDS proposes to accelerate the full implementation of these goals within countries by building synergies with communities and other organizations.

## Nongovernmental Organizations

UNAIDS has recognized the importance of the inclusion of nongovernmental organizations (NGOs) in the worldwide fight against the spread of HIV/AIDS. The UNAIDS Programme Coordinating Board (PCB) has as its nonvoting members representatives, two NGOs from each of the following regions: Africa; Asia and the Pacific; Europe; Latin America and the Caribbean; and North America. The mission of the NGO delegation is to

*bring to the PCB the perspectives and expertise of people living with, most affected by, and most at risk of, vulnerable to, marginalized by, and affected by HIV and AIDS…to ensure that their human rights and equitable, gender-sensitive access to comprehensive HIV prevention, treatment, care and support are reinforced by the policies, programs, strategies and actions of the PCB and UNAIDS (UNAIDS, 2012)*

# VIOLENCE

Violence can happen to individuals anywhere, regardless of gender, age, or nationality, and is among the leading causes of physical, sexual, reproductive, and mental health problems worldwide. Each year, violence has been estimated to cause the loss of 1.6 million lives globally. In addition, violence costs nations immeasurable amounts of money in terms of health care, law enforcement, and loss of productivity (WHO, 2019a). The cost of violence containment to the world economy was approximately US $9.8 trillion in 2014 (Morgan, 2015).

## Definition of Violence

Violence is defined differently in different parts of the world, depending on people's beliefs and cultures. The definition proposed by WHO is used in this chapter. According to WHO (2014a), violence is defined as

*intentional use of physical force or power, threatened or actual, against oneself, another person, or against a group or community, that either results in or has a high likelihood of resulting in injury, death, psychological harm, maldevelopment or deprivation.*

In response to violence, WHO has proposed a four-step public health approach that includes the following steps: defining the problem; identifying risks and protective factors; devising and testing means of dealing with violence; and applying successful

means on a large scale (WHO, 2019e). Successful response prevention of violence should be based on rigorous research and collaboration among health care providers and other experts in areas such as epidemiology, criminology, education, and economics. The CDC is an example of an organization in the United States that is applying the preceding four-step public health model. Activities, projects, and funding supported by the CDC are outlined in the following sections as an exemplar.

### Defining the Problem

To understand the magnitude of violence in Canada, different data sources are needed. Such sources may include police reports, medical examiner files, vital records, medical records, population-based surveys, and research results. Extrapolation of the data from these sources can help us to learn about violence frequencies, places, trends, and perpetrators. The CDC has provided funding to studies deemed to be helpful in defining violence problems. The National Violent Death Reporting System is an example of a project funded by the CDC to ensure that timely, complete, and accurate data are collected about violent deaths for different states in the United States. It is hoped that the data will enable each state to gain a clearer picture of violence so as to respond more effectively (CDC, 2018c).

### Identifying Risk and Protective Factors

A "risk factor" is defined as "a characteristic that increases the likelihood of a person becoming a victim or perpetrator of violence," and a "protective factor" is defined as "a characteristic that decreases the likelihood of a person becoming a victim or perpetrator of violence" (CDC, 2018c). Knowing risk and protective factors can help responsible organizations and personnel to estimate violence magnitudes and devise appropriate prevention measures. It is important to note that the identification of risk factors should be used not to blame victims of violence but rather as a focus for intervention.

### Devising and Testing Means for Dealing With Violence

In this step, data on violence from all available sources are extrapolated and assessed. On the basis of the evidence, programs and interventions are planned. Such programs and interventions are then implemented, tested, and rigorously evaluated to determine their effectiveness. An example of step 3 activities is the Choose Respect project—a communication initiative for Grade 6 to 8 students to guide adolescents in forming healthy relationships so as to prevent dating violence (CDC, 2018c). Technology also plays a role in protecting violence victims. The MyPlan app is a web-based safety planning tool that helps violence victims to respond to dating violence. It enhances victims' decisional conflict and safety behaviour (Glass, Clough, Hanson, et al., 2015).

### Applying Successful Means on a Large Scale

After a program has been tested successfully for its effectiveness, large-scale dissemination should occur. At this stage, communities are encouraged to adopt a program tailored to their own problems and needs. The program should be evaluated in each community. Training, networking, technical assistance, and process evaluations are to be supported by all parties involved. An example of step 4 activities initiated by the CDC is the National Youth Violence Prevention Resource Center with its goal to prevent youth violence and suicide. In this project, a website, toll-free hotline, and fax-on-demand service were created as helpful resources for youth. Any interested community can request more information from the CDC.

## Forms and Context of Violence

WHO (2019d) classifies violence into three major categories: interpersonal, self-directed, and collective.

### Interpersonal Violence

Interpersonal violence (IPV) is violence committed by an individual or a small group of people in a wide range of acts and behaviours (emotional, physical, sexual, and psychological). The violence could happen to people of any age (adolescents, children, and older persons). It could also occur anywhere, including the home, workplace, neighbourhood, and unfamiliar places.

Whereas violence in the community (e.g., youth violence or crimes) is highly visible, violence in the home is usually hidden. The impact of such hidden violence is complicated by the fact that authorities or health personnel are less willing or prepared to deal with it (Koistinen & Holma, 2015).

The risk factors for IPV include a victim's low self-esteem, low self-control, and personality/conduct disorders (CDC, 2018c). Other risk factors are reported to be lack of social support, dysfunctional family structure, family history of violence, and drug and alcohol abuse (Canadian Domestic Homicide Prevention Initiative, 2016; Ross, Saenyakul, Stidham, et al., 2015). Alcohol intoxication may increase violent actions by impairing the drinker's cognitive functions and processes through alterations of social cue perceptions and inhibitions (Bernardin, Maheut-Bosser, & Paille, 2014; PHAC, 2012). According to the Canadian Centre on Substance Use and Addiction (CCSA, 2018), between 40% and 50% of convicted crimes in Canada occurred while the offender was under in the influence of illicit drugs or alcohol.

In addition, four subtypes of male perpetrators are reported as the mentally ill, under-controlled/dysregulated, chronic batterer, and over-controlled/catathymic subtypes (Koistinen & Holma, 2015). Shared characteristics were found among the four subtypes of male perpetrators. For example, most of them were abused as children, tend to be in their mid-30s to late 30s, and tend to show pathology (Koistinen & Holma, 2015).

Mothers who are victims of violence, along with their children who witness such violence, are at risk of physical, emotional, psychological, and developmental damage, requiring trauma- and violence-informed approaches to decrease the risk for harm, retraumatization, enhance safety, and resilience (McFarlane, Symes, Binder, et al., 2014; PHAC, 2018c). In Canada, IPV accounts for 30% of all police-reported violent crimes, 79% of these being against women (Government of Canada, 2017a).

Culture and gender inequality are also significant factors in IPV. Evidence shows that women in countries where gender equality is emphasized experience violence less than those in countries with gender inequality (Fulu, Jewkes, Roselli, et al., 2013). Fulu and colleagues (2013) reported that that the highest rate of physical and/or sexual violence among women was in Papua New Guinea (80.0%), whereas a rate of 25% was reported in Indonesia.

A study among 245 women in Thailand revealed that the rate of emotional abuse was 88.2%, that of physical abuse was 59.2%, and that of sexual abuse was 23.9% (Ross et al., 2015). Predictors of emotional abuse included partner's drug use and gambling behaviour. The predictor of physical abuse was drug abuse. No predictor was found for sexual abuse. Violence in this study was found to be associated with depression and physical problems (Ross et al., 2015). This result aligns with a study that summarizes the literature concerning history of childhood sexual abuse and depression or depressive symptoms among pregnant and postpartum women, which revealed that women who were abused reported higher rates of postpartum depression than those who did not experience abuse (Wosu, Gelaye, & Williams, 2015). Social support was found to mediate the effects of IPV on depression and physical health in the Thai study (Ross et al., 2015).

It is important for health care providers to understand the seriously negative impact that IPV can have on individuals. They should be able to identify such violence and be aware of helpful resources for people affected by violence, as well as their children. Local domestic violence crisis contact information (i.e., phone numbers and counselling services) should be readily provided to these people. A domestic violence assessment and care guide provided by the Canadian Department of Justice is a helpful resource for health care providers who work with females, families, and at-risk populations who seek care related to violence (Millar, Code, & Ha, 2013). A review and recommendation of risk assessment tools is also available for multidisciplinary care providers who work with care recipients who may have experienced intimate partner violence, including physical, sexual, verbal, social, financial, and emotional violence (Knox, 2018; Millar, Code, & Ha, 2013).

### Self-Directed Violence

Self-directed violence is defined by WHO (2018e) as "violence in which the perpetrator and the victim are the same individual and is subdivided into self-abuse and suicide." It is estimated that 800,000 individuals die by suicide annually (a person commits suicide every 40 seconds) (WHO, 2018c). Previously, suicide rates had been highest among the older male. However, the rates among young people aged 15 to 29 years have been increasing to such an extent that suicide is the second leading cause of death in this age group in some developed and developing countries (WHO, 2018c). Although the major factors contributing to suicide in Europe and North America include mental health disorders, especially depression, and alcohol use disorders, impulsiveness and high pressure to be successful is found to be a major factor in Asian countries (WHO, 2018e).

In 2019, the WHO (2018e) published their National Suicide Prevention Strategies, which recommend that effective suicide prevention interventions should include restriction of access to common methods of suicide where possible, or when prudent,

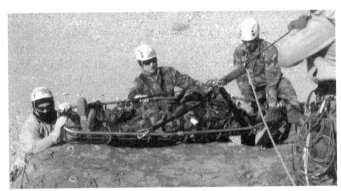

Fig. 25.3 Armed conflicts can be within or between states and nations.

along with effective prevention and treatment of depression and alcohol and substance abuse. However, there are clearly challenges to such interventions. In many countries, for example, a lack of awareness about suicide and the taboo to discuss suicide openly exist. Many countries will need to initiate training for prevention of suicide, including appropriate certification for health care personnel, and to seek the involvement of individuals from sectors other than health care, including education, labour, law, politics, police, justice, religion, and the media.

## Collective Violence

Collective violence is defined as the instrumental use of violence by a particular group of people for specific political, economic, or social objectives. Such violence may include armed conflicts within or between states or nations, genocide, terrorism, repression, and other abuses of human rights (WHO, 2018c) (Fig. 25.3).

In the twentieth century, it is estimated that 191 million people lost their lives as a result of armed conflict. More than half of these people were civilians. In 2011, 86,307 people died because of collective violence. Most victims lived in the poorer regions of the world (WHO, 2018c). Besides death, the aftermath of collective violence includes physical and psychological disabilities that exert burdens on families, communities, and nations. Young children and refugees are usually among the most vulnerable to the aftermaths of disease and post-traumatic stress disorders (PTSDs) related to violence (WHO, 2014a).

The WHO is committed to working with its partners at the regional, national, and international levels to prevent collective violence. Its goal is to identify and implement preventive strategies. Data collection systems are used to support and evaluate the success of the strategies. In this effort, political commitment and momentum are required from a wide variety of concerned parties to strengthen and increase violence prevention endeavours in the next 5 years (WHO, 2014a).

## TERRORISM

The threat of terrorism—whether homegrown or international—creates a unique brand of fear among individuals and communities within our increasingly interconnected global cultures (Santoro, 2018). Moreover, the need to be able to respond to terrorism—potential or actual—poses important challenges

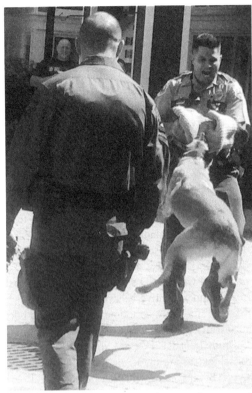

Fig. 25.4 The need to be able to respond to terrorism poses important challenges to all.

to health care providers and community planners at all levels of our society (Fig. 25.4). The International Council for Nurses describes its position on the role of nursing concerning disaster preparedness to include risk assessment as well as management strategies bridging multiple disciplines and system levels.

Nursing plays a key role in responding to the short-, medium-, and long-term requirements of populations stricken by disaster. The establishment of a set of tailor-made disaster nursing core competencies for the community and the development of a comprehensive curriculum for public health will help nurses plan for and streamline health care responses to such mass events internationally (Loke & Fung, 2014; Veenema, Griffin, Gable, et al., 2016). Much work in laying the foundations for such a broader, more global preparedness has already been started.

Research on the surgical responses to the 2008 terrorist attacks in Mumbai, India, reveals the importance of an initial disaster management plan to treat casualties. The earliest victims of firearm and blast trauma were received in a primary triage zone and then sent to different stations for further treatment. The study concluded that onsite triage—established as soon as a site is found to be safe—optimizes the treatment of bullet and blast injuries (Bhandarwar, Bakhshi, Tayade, et al., 2012). Another study examined the effectiveness of including a pediatric trauma centre (PTC) in responding to victims of a disaster surge. This study added a hypothetical PTC to the response of the Israel Defense Forces field hospital to the Haiti earthquake in 2010 and measured its effectiveness mathematically, concluding that "aggressive inclusion of PTCs in planning for disasters by public health agencies" (Barthel,

Pierce, Goodhue, et al., 2011) can significantly increase overall rates of admission and greatly reduce treatment times (Barthel et al., 2011). Regarding the responses of health care providers to the repercussions of mass disasters, the results from the literature are sometimes conflicting. In the United Sates, studies among victims of the World Trade Center (WTC) disaster in terms of PTSD suggest that early and brief interventions at the work site were most effective in responding to PTSD, and that informal support from family, friends, and spiritual communities was also beneficial. Conversely, more extensive post-disaster psychotherapy was not found to be beneficial and sometimes led to worse outcomes (Boscarino & Adams, 2008). Mental resilience following the WTC disaster tended to be linked with victims having Hispanic ethnicity, pre-9/11 psychiatric history, degree of exposure to the WTC, life stressors, and/or maladaptive coping (Feder, Mota, Salim, et al., 2016). A "greater sense of purpose in life," a "higher perceived preparedness," and "positive emotion-focused coping" were negatively associated with PTSD symptom trajectories (Feder et al., 2016). In Thailand, cognitive-behavioural therapy as a means to treat PTSD was studied in a randomized controlled effectiveness trial. The researchers found that cognitive-behavioural therapy can successfully treat PTSD, even "in settings where very regular [terrorist] attacks are made upon communities in which the patient lives" (Bryant, Ekasawin, Chakrabhand, et al., 2011).

Among its overarching influences, one must also weigh terrorism's negative consequences for economies around the world. These include direct and indirect repercussions affecting human life, physical damage, lost growth of gross domestic product (GDP), human relocation, tourism, transportation, and the cost of attending to victims (Buesa & Baumert, 2018). Such economic changes affect the lives of everyday people and, in turn, their health. The threat of terrorism is thus real, and its actual and potential negative effects are pervasive and far-reaching, spanning cultures and ranging from the concrete and immediate to the psychosocial and lasting. Nurses and health care providers must be among the front lines of response.

## Bioterrorism

Bioterrorism is the deliberate terrorist release of a biological agent such as a virus, bacteria, or germ with the intention of causing death or illness. Biological agents are found in nature, but can be modified to amplify the symptoms of a disease, improve resistance to medicine, or increase transmission. Biological agents can be released through the air, water, or food. Some biological agents, such as smallpox, can be spread from person to person, while others, such as anthrax, cannot (BCCDC, n.d).

The preceding definition reflects what many people in different nations may feel or know about bioterrorism. As health care providers, we are required to be knowledgeable about possible diseases/agents that could be used for bioterrorism and the proper responses we should make to an act of bioterrorism.

Bioterrorism is classified by the CDC (2017a) into three different categories: A, B, and C. These categories are based on the ease with which the disease or agent might be spread; the potential negative impact it could have on public health; the extent to which it could cause public panic or social disruption; and the degree to which it would require the public to prepare for an attack.

### Category A Diseases/Agents

Category A diseases/agents include various biological agents and pathogens that are not usually seen in the United States and pose the highest risks and have the highest priority. They include anthrax, botulism, plague, smallpox, tularemia, and viral hemorrhagic fevers.

*Anthrax (Bacillus anthracis).* Since the anthrax (*Bacillus anthracis*) mailing attacks on a few recipients in the United States in 2001, no other attacks have been reported (CDC, 2016a). These unfortunate mail recipients contracted the bacillus either cutaneously or inhalationally. Cutaneous anthrax contractors developed erythema (red, inflamed area similar to cellulitis) on exposed areas of the hands, arms, or face that later transformed into painful vesicles and then necrotic painless, depressed, black eschar. Inhalation anthrax contractors had fever, dyspnea, cough, and chest discomfort (CDC, 2016c). Usually, respiratory failure and hemodynamic collapse will follow. Other symptoms may include lymphangitis and painful lymphadenopathy. It is recommended that individuals receive a complete treatment of ciprofloxacin, levofloxacin, doxycycline, or penicillin for 60 days (Heine, Shadomy, Boyer, et al., 2017). Vaccines against anthrax have been developed, and evidence shows that they can be effective in preventing the disease (Hendricks, 2017). The CDC (2018d) and its partners are working collaboratively to develop more effective anthrax vaccines. Questions and answers about anthrax vaccines can be found at https://www.cdc.gov/vaccines/vpd/anthrax/public/index.html.

*Smallpox (variola major).* It is believed that smallpox (variola major) was eradicated in 1977. However, there are fears that a strain kept in a laboratory could be used as a bioweapon. According to Health Canada (2019), the PHAC has three types of smallpox vaccine stockpiled in the event of a smallpox outbreak. The side effects from smallpox vaccination mostly involve a mild fever, soreness in the injection area, and enlarged glands in the armpit (Health Canada, 2019). (In rare circumstances, severe side effects may occur and need medical attention.) To learn more about potentially serious and life-threatening side effects, visit https://www.canada.ca/en/public-health/services/publications/healthy-living/canadian-immunization-guide-part-4-active-vaccines/page-21-smallpox-vaccine.html.

Smallpox symptoms usually resemble influenza symptoms, which include fever and myalgia, followed by a rash. Rashes in smallpox can be differentiated from those of chickenpox (varicella). A rash from smallpox is most prominent on the face and extremities, with the same stage of lesion development. A rash from chickenpox is more prominent on the trunk, with different stages of lesion development and resolution. Health Canada (2019) provides an acute, generalized vesicular or pustular rash illness testing protocol in Canada.

### Category B Diseases/Agents

Category B diseases/agents are those that pose the second highest risks for world and national security. They include brucellosis; food safety threats (e.g., *Salmonella* sp., *Escherichia coli* O157:H7, *Shigella*); glanders; melioidosis; psittacosis; Q fever; ricin toxin; staphylococcal enterotoxin B; typhus fever; viral encephalitis; and water safety threats (e.g., *Vibrio cholerae, Cryptosporidium parvum*).

## Category C Diseases/Agents

Category C diseases/agents are emerging pathogens that could be reproduced for mass dissemination. They include emerging infectious diseases such as Nipah virus and hantavirus.

## Epidemic and Pandemic Alert and Response

The Government of Canada has created a public health emergency response guide to help public health professionals at the federal, provincial, territorial, and municipal levels respond to an emergency in the first 24 hours (Government of Canada, 2017b). Health care providers should be alerted to any unusual symptoms indicative of an infectious outbreak related to bioterrorism. In turn, if a bioterrorist action is suspected, health care providers should report it to their provincial/territorial health department. According to the CDC (2017b), indications of bioterrorism include

> an unusual temporal or geographic clustering of illness (e.g., persons who attended the same public event or gathering) or individuals presenting with clinical signs and symptoms that suggest an infectious disease outbreak (e.g., more than two persons presenting with an unexplained febrile illness associated with sepsis, pneumonia, respiratory failure, or rash or a botulism-like syndrome with flaccid muscle paralysis, especially if occurring in otherwise healthy persons); an unusual age distribution for common diseases (e.g., an increase in what appears to be a chickenpox-like illness among adult persons, but which might be smallpox); and a large number of cases of acute flaccid paralysis with prominent bulbar palsies, suggestive of a release of botulinum toxin.

To learn more about clinical diagnosis, management, and responses to bioterrorism, refer to the Infection Prevention and Control Canada (IPAC) website at https://ipac-canada.org/bioterrorism-resources.php.

At the international level, responses to bioterrorism have also been prepared. WHO is a core organization responding to the needs for such preparation at this level. WHO works collaboratively with agencies in many countries to gather reports of suspected outbreaks and rumors regarding bioterrorism through advanced technologies from all sources available, both formally and informally.

The Global Public Health Intelligence Network, a significant source of informal information related to outbreaks, was also collaboratively established by Health Canada and WHO. Its multilingual capabilities are Internet based, and are constantly searching data worldwide to identify information regarding disease outbreaks that can place international public health sectors at risk (WHO, 2016b).

The 2005 International Health Regulations (IHR)—legally binding regulations across countries led by WHO—are embraced by most nations throughout the world. Their mission is to provide legal frameworks to ensure health security among nations without unnecessary international traffic and trade interference (WHO, 2016a). To learn more about the IHR, see WHO (2016a).

## NATURAL DISASTERS

Natural disasters have existed since Earth was formed. They are phenomena that occur through natural forces involving land, air, or water, and they often have large-scale negative impacts on humans who live in the affected areas. Examples of natural disasters include tsunamis, earthquakes, floods, landslides, mudslides, tornadoes, hurricanes, cyclones, typhoons, wildfires, volcano eruptions, extreme heat, and winter weather (CDC, 2019a). Natural disasters in recent decades have been reported to cause more harm in developing countries than developed countries, attributable in part to deforestation and inadequate warning and emergency management systems (Cameron & Shah, 2015). Health care providers should be aware of recent large-scale natural disasters and be familiar with their negative impact on human well-being. Critically, lessons learned from the successful or unsuccessful management of these disasters should be shared among health care providers so as to appropriately address and minimize the effects of future disasters.

### Effects of Natural Disasters on Human Well-Being

All humans are affected by natural disasters economically, physically, and psychologically. In the past 10 years, 2 billion people were affected by a reported 3751 natural disasters in 141 countries, costing an estimated $1658 billion globally (International Federation of Red Cross and Red Crescent Societies [IFRC & RCS], 2018). Earthquakes remain the largest killer, causing 351,968 deaths, 49% of all natural disaster–related deaths (IFRC & RCS, 2018).

Concerning the physical effects of natural disasters, victims tend to have limited access to essential infrastructures for survival related to food, water, shelter, and sanitation. These deficiencies can lead to infectious disease outbreaks, infections, and undernutrition (Hattori, Chagan-Yasutan, Shiratori, et al., 2016; Phalkey & Louis, 2016). Undernutrition, in turn, can lead to malnutrition and starvation—especially among infants and children in low-resource countries (Food & Agriculture Organization et al., 2017). Infection outbreaks commonly diagnosed after a typhoon, earthquake, and flood in the Philippines in 2013 included diarrhea, acute respiratory tract infections, open wounds, bruises and burns, high blood pressure, skin disease, and fever (Salazar, Pesigan, Law, et al., 2016).

In terms of the psychological impact of natural disasters, PTSD is a classic negative effect that occurs among victims of all ages. Natural disasters can cause a significant amount of stress, especially from the loss of loved ones (Bromet, Atwoli, Kawakami, et al., 2017). A survey of flood victims in 2000 in Hunan province, China, showed that PTSD among the victims still existed 13 years later. No relationship was found between demographic characteristics and the recovery from PTSD (Hu, Cofie, Tan, et al., 2015). A follow-up study in China among 1573 adolescent survivors at 6, 12, 18, and 24 months after an earthquake found that negative life events, less social support, and less positive coping were common predictors of poor recovery (Fan, Zhou, Long, et al., 2015). A cross-sectional study of 350 survivors from the Mount Merapi volcanic eruption in Indonesia reported that female adults aged between 18 and 59 years, and individuals who owned their own home, experienced the highest levels of negative psychosocial impact (Warsini, Mills, Buettner, et al., 2015). In conclusion, psychological trauma has been reported as a result of natural disasters regardless of age or country of residence.

## Natural Disaster Responses and Preparedness

In general, immediate medical care and rapid emergency response are important to address natural disasters, especially among children and women. Unfortunately, such care and response are reported to be inadequate, regardless of the country type. However, the inadequacy of emergency care is heightened in developing nations (Van Berlaer, Staes, Danschutter, et al., 2017). For example, with the 2010 earthquake in Haiti, more than 220,000 people lost their lives, with 1.5 million people losing shelter (Oxfam International, 2015). As the poorest country in the Western world, Haiti already had limited resources before the earthquake. As many as 40% of rural Haitians did not have access to primary health care before the disaster, and 70% of health provisions in Haiti overall before the disaster were offered by NGOs (Gelting, Bliss, Patrick, et al., 2013). Although psychiatric mental health needs surged after the earthquake, existing mental health services in Haiti were damaged by the two crumpled, understaffed psychiatric hospitals as a consequence of the earthquake.

The psychiatrist-to-person ratio was 0.2 to 100,000 before the earthquake, and this ratio became worse when some health care workers were among the injured (WHO, 2018d). Vodou, a common belief about magic and illness in Haiti, is deemed by some to function as the main Haitian health care system (McAlister, 2016). Vodou beliefs might be considered by some professionals as a hindrance to modern mental health acquisition. Yet evidence shows that if a strong collaboration is established between traditional healers and health care providers, mental health services can be enhanced in the process (Khoury, Kaiser, Keys, et al., 2012).

### International Standard Guidelines for Emergency Mental Health Response

Before 2007, there was a lack of consensual international guidelines for emergency mental health response (WHO, 2016c). However, after the Asian tsunami in 2004, a taskforce was established composed of both governmental and nongovernmental experts from more than 100 various organizations and 27 different countries (WHO, 2016c). This taskforce, the Inter-Agency Standing Committee (IASC), developed the 2007 "IASC Guidelines on Mental Health and Psychosocial Support in Emergency Settings," reflecting standards for appropriate emergency mental health care for victims around the world (WHO, 2016c). The IASC guidelines are consistent with WHOs recommendations for emergencies among developing nations in that all victims and affected families should have access to emergency assistance with equality and dignity, and that helping people to remain resilient after a disaster is important. Besides these general principles, the minimum response for primary care clinics to help victims with severe psychological needs is outlined by the IASC and includes 10 major tenets (WHO, 2016c):

- Each victim is assessed holistically.
- Each victim will have access to essential psychiatric medications.
- At least one emergency primary health care (PHC) provider is available to tend to victims' mental health in the affected area.
- The care provided by the PHC provider is adequately supervised.
- PHC providers will be assigned to specific trainings and will not be overwhelmed by unnecessary training sessions.

- Additional mental health service points will be established for victims' accessibility.
- Unnecessary duplicating services should be avoided.
- All people affected by a disaster are informed about available mental health services.
- Primary care clinics should work collaboratively with local community agencies to discover, visit, and help the target population.
- Primary care clinics should have a major role in collaboration with other mental health agencies.

To learn more about the IASC's guidelines and related work, see WHO (2016c).

### Emergency Management for Infants in Developed Countries

Most infants in developing countries are breastfed. Thus, when natural disasters occur, they tend to do better than infants in developed countries, because their mothers have mobile fresh milk supplies for them as long as they are with their mothers during the disaster (Gribble, 2018; Gribble & Berry, 2011). Infants in developed countries whose primary food is based on formula feeding can be vulnerable, because of a lack of supplies during a disaster (Gribble, 2018; Gribble & Berry, 2011). Therefore, emergency preparedness for these infants should be in place. In general, it is recommended that a week's supply of necessary items is available for infants. For exclusively breastfed infants, 100 diapers and 200 wipes are the only items needed. For bottle-fed infants, more items are recommended for their survival (Gribble & Berry, 2011). Mothers of infants with ready-to-use formula require: 56 single servings of the formula, 84 L of drinking water, 56 feeding bottles, 56 zip-lock plastic bags, 120 antiseptic wipes, detergent, 100 diapers, and 200 wipes (Gribble & Berry, 2011). Mothers of infants with powdered infant formula will need the following items: 2 cans of infant formula, 170 L of drinking water, a feeding cup, a large storage container, a measuring cup, a large cooking pot with a lid, a kettle, a gas stove, a box of matches/lighters, 14 kg of liquid cooking gas, a metal knife, a pair of metal tongs, 120 antiseptic wipes, detergent, 300 sheets of paper towels, 100 diapers, and 200 wipes (Gribble & Berry, 2011). Health care providers who care for mothers with their infants should be trained to provide appropriate information to the mothers based on their feeding strategy. The PHAC (2018a) offers information on emergency preparedness and response to many potential public health emergencies. Information can be found on their website: https://www.canada.ca/en/public-health/services/emergency-preparedness-response.html. Similarly, the Office of Public Health Preparedness and Response provides very helpful information about the steps and types of emergency responses on the US CDC website (CDC, 2018b).

## IMPLICATIONS

The health-promotion and disease-prevention priorities that have been outlined in this chapter present challenges and opportunities for health care providers—as individuals and as a collective profession—to play key roles in emerging systems emphasizing health promotion and disease prevention. The goals for optimal health of individuals include greater longevity and quality of life, while decreasing sex, racial, and ethnic disparities through the development of cultural safety (Purnell, 2008). The principles of primary prevention, health care policies, cultural diversity, cultural safety, and multidisciplinary teamwork in health promotion are critical to a new era that strives to achieve dramatic changes in health care delivery (Purnell, 2008). Through a perspective on the development of community-based, health-promotion programs, health care providers can bring a balance to decisions that will be made about the appropriate use of traditional and newer health care resources.

In 2007, the PHAC, in collaboration with public health practitioners across Canada, developed the *Core Competencies for Public Health in Canada,* which includes 36 competency statements within the following seven categories: public health science, assessment and analysis; policy and program planning; implementation and evaluation; partnerships; collaboration; advocacy; and, diversity, communication and leadership (PHAC, 2007).

Core competencies are the essential knowledge, skills, and attitudes necessary for the practice of public health. They transcend the boundaries of specific disciplines and are independent of program and topic. They provide the building blocks for effective public health practice, and the use of an overall public health approach. Generic core competencies provide a baseline for what is required to fulfill public health system core functions (PHAC, 2007, p. 1).

The development of *Core Functions* for public health in Canada, arose after the SARS public health emergency in 2003, and subsequent Canadian reports (*Learning from SARS, The Future of Public Health in Canada* [CIHR report], and the *Naylor Report on Public Health*) that outlined the need to bring structure and organization to public health in order to prevent injury, disability, and disease, improving the health of Canadians (Public Health Association of British Columbia [PHABC], 2006). Although development of national public health services remains a work in progress, the Government of Canada recognizes six public health functions in the legislation for the PHAC. These comprise:

- *Health protection.* Actions to ensure water, air, and food are safe; a regulatory framework to control infectious diseases; protection from environmental threats; and expert advice to food and drug safety regulators.
- *Health surveillance.* The ongoing, systematic use of routinely collected health data for the purpose of tracking and forecasting health events or health determinants. Surveillance includes: collection and storage of relevant data; integration, analysis, and interpretation of this data; production of tracking and forecasting products with the interpreted data, and publication/dissemination of those products; and provision of expertise to those developing and/or contributing to surveillance systems, including risk surveillance.
- *Disease and injury prevention.* Investigation, contact tracing, preventive measures to reduce the risk of infectious disease emergence and outbreaks, and activities to promote safe, healthy lifestyles to reduce preventable illness and injuries.
- *Population health assessment.* Understanding the health of communities or specific populations, as well as the factors that underlie good health or pose potential risks, to produce better policies and services.

- *Health promotion.* Preventing disease, encouraging safe behaviours, and improving health through public policy, community-based interventions, active public participation, and advocacy or action on environmental and socioeconomic determinants of health.
- *Emergency preparedness and response.* Planning for both natural disasters (e.g., floods, earthquakes, fires, dangerous infectious diseases) and man-made disasters (e.g., those involving explosives, chemicals, radioactive substances or biological threats) to minimize serious illness, overall deaths, and social disruption. (PHAC, 2008)

Although great strides in public health initiatives have improved the health of Canadians, considerable challenges remain. These include motor vehicle accidents, changes in the environment such as rising temperatures and extreme weather events, air quality, water contaminants, mental illnesses, chronic illness and obesity, and, significantly, poverty, which is linked to low employment and education levels, and subsequent lower levels of health on average (PHAC, 2008). Migrant, First Nations, Inuit, and Métis, and other minority groups within Canada have the highest risk of being impacted by adverse public health challenges (PHAC, 2018b).

An increasing demand for PHC providers will continue to spur the need for more advanced practice nurses, including nurses with degrees of doctor of nursing practice and doctor of philosophy. This demand can be met if undergraduate students are introduced early to concepts of health promotion and disease prevention, with an emphasis on evidence-informed practice, human rights, cultural diversity, cultural safety, and with a global perspective (Purnell, 2008). Undergraduate and graduate programs in public health, social dimensions of health, and global health are becoming increasingly popular at universities across Canada. As this global consciousness trend grows, a focus on health promotion, quality of life, and socioeconomic justice might become increasingly valued in cultures throughout the world.

In addition, health care educational programs in culturally diverse global frameworks that teach about malnutrition, emerging diseases, HIV/AIDS, bioterrorism, violence, and other contemporary challenges will help nurses and other professionals play innovative roles in health care and maximize the quality of life around the world. Faculty and students will ideally increase their work together in interdisciplinary teams, using an expanding variety of health-promotion services and guided by national and international standards. Given the increasing focus on cultural diversity and self-care in disease prevention and health promotion, nurses can respond directly to the health needs of individuals, families, communities, and groups by focusing on health promotion and disease prevention tailored to particular cultures and spiritual beliefs and by supporting new ways to work and live.

In the area of research, understanding health care practices and the impact of culture on people from different nations will enable health care providers to create appropriate health-promotion and disease-prevention interventions. Thus, international collaborative research is important. The United Nations Declaration on the Rights of Indigenous Peoples was adopted in 2007. With an estimated 370 million Indigenous peoples globally, representing a rich diversity of cultures, religions, traditions, languages, and histories,

Indigenous peoples continue to be among the world's most marginalized population groups (WHO, 2007). From a global perspective, Indigenous peoples suffer higher rates of ill health and have dramatically shorter life expectancy than other groups living in the same countries. This inequity results in Indigenous peoples suffering unacceptable health problems and they are more likely to experience disabilities and dying at a younger age than their non-Indigenous counterparts (United Nations, 2015, p. IV).

Other social determinants impacting Indigenous peoples' health status include living conditions; income levels; employment rates; access to safe water; sanitation; health services; food availability; loss of traditional lands, territories and resources; climate change and environmental contamination; and barriers in accessing health care, further compounded by discrimination and racism (UN General Assembly, 2015). The UN 2030 Sustainable Development Goals continue to engage a global partnership with nations, recognizing that strategies for the improvement of health and reduction of inequality for all peoples, must go hand-in-hand with ending poverty and other deprivations (UN General Assembly, 2015).

To be advocates for newly emerging priorities for disease prevention and health promotion, nurses in the twenty-first century need to engage in the following:

- Participate in policy development for health promotion, as the health care of individuals in acute settings shifts from hospitals to home and community settings. Thus, the attention to health-promoting behaviours in home and community environments provides an entry point for the development of models of primary care that emphasize both health promotion and disease prevention in communities.
- Influence public expectations about health promotion. Presentations and other forms of public dialogue and education will help raise awareness of the value of individual and community health promotion. Nurses have the collective

capacity to change the philosophy of the system, from selling health care in the marketplace to creating a milieu for changing health behaviours. Encouraging meaningful community participation in addressing health issues provides a significant opportunity to narrow the gap between what is possible in terms of health promotion in each country and what is reality. As mentioned earlier, violence and emerging diseases are among the challenges today that require heightened public awareness.

- Promote equitable access to preventive health care. Given the higher rates of preventable conditions among populations in resource-poor countries and in vulnerable sub-populations within high-resource countries, the need to promote the justified distribution and utilization of preventive health services is apparent. Community-based efforts that combine public and private resources should be targeted to those most in need of health care. Delivery models that focus on integrating preventive and primary care should be expanded.

Preventive health care delivery should be based on broad research agendas that encompass multiple health and social science perspectives. Health care providers should participate in areas of research that will cost-effectively influence both personal and community health. Service delivery can also benefit from expanded health service research agendas that foster collaboration among disciplines and countries. Most important, preventive health care should be adapted to the health and social problems of specific groups and cultures. Alternative approaches to health-promotion and preventive service delivery should be used where they are most effective to meet new international health challenges, including mobile vans, school and work-site clinics, and other community-based, collaborative actions (Innovative Practice).

---

### INNOVATIVE PRACTICE

#### Haitian Health Foundation: A Charitable Outreach to Neighbours in Need

A volunteer effort of health professionals initiated in Haiti in 1982 by Dr Jeremiah Lowney and his wife Virginia has grown into an outpatient health care facility supported by a nondenominational foundation called the Haitian Health Foundation (HHF). In 1985, after working for 4 years in Port-au-Prince, HHF moved its outreach to Jeremie, Haiti, at the suggestion of Mother Teresa of Calcutta, to bring health care, hope, and opportunity to this especially poor and remote area. The clinic at Jeremie employs 105 people, including 2 full-time physicians, 1 full-time dentist, 10 registered nurses, 2 licensed practical nurses, a medical technician, a dental assistant, and 70 to 80 auxiliary personnel (all Haitians). The clinic provides health care to more than 120,000 Haitians yearly (Lowney, 2016).

The Haitian agents de santé program currently employs villagers in 936 villages surrounding Jeremie. This program was initiated by a nurse who enlisted an individual who had a seventh- grade education in each village. After being educated in health promotion, the person became the health agent of that village. These health agents are trained by HHF to provide preventive and basic health care and education. Many villages have also begun mothers' groups, by which women can share experiences and knowledge relating to nutrition, health care, and other topics that have an effect on their quality of life. Breastfeeding classes and immunization programs are available.

Another program was begun by the building of a food distribution pavilion. This building will be used to store and distribute food to more than 1000 children and pregnant women three times a week. The pavilion will also be used to educate participants in nutrition and preventive health care. Much of the education in these programs is accomplished through song, primarily because this approach appears to enable the Haitians to remember what is being taught.

For more than 8 years, another education program has provided access to schools for poor children in a country in which education is neither free nor mandatory. In 2016, almost 3300 students attended school through this program. Tuition, uniforms, books, and shoes are provided by HHF funds or through the Save-a-Family Plan.

HHF relies heavily on the generosity of donors and the many volunteers who donate their time and talents to supplement the staff in Haiti. Volunteers travel to Jeremie at their own expense from Canada, the United States, and Europe to share their skills and resources with the poor. These volunteers include health care providers, electricians, plumbers, teachers, clergy, and students.

These programs are only a few examples of the health-promotion programs sponsored by HHF. These efforts show how dedicated professionals can make a difference, even in developing countries in which health care resources are rare.

Source: Courtesy of Jeremiah Lowney. (2016). *Our impact.* Haitian Health Foundation. Retrieved from http://www.haitianhealthfoundation.org/our-impact/.

## CASE STUDY

### Nutrition: Don

Don is a 4-year-old boy who is brought to a rural health department clinic by his grandmother. Don and his family are recent immigrants from Laos and have lived in this area for less than 1 year. This is Don's first visit to the clinic. Don looks weak, with sunken eyes and a dry mouth. His weight is less than 70% (or less than 3 SD) of the median weight for height, and he has underdeveloped buttocks, thighs, and upper arms. Through a translator, Don's grandmother tells the community health nurse that Don has had diarrhea for more than 2 days and that the family can barely "make ends meet." Don's parents are seasonal farmworkers and are at work today.

**Reflective Questions**

- Who is Don's caretaker during the day?
- How can the nurse help Don's family learn about the resources available in their community?
- Where does the nurse direct Don's family for immediate help?
- How would the nurse follow up with the family to prevent further problems with this child?

## CARE PLAN

### Nutrition: Don

**Nursing Issue**

Inadequate nutrition—lower than body requirement related to inadequate food intake and diarrhea, as evidenced by a weight of less than 70% (or less than 3 SD) of the median weight for height; underdeveloped buttocks, thighs, and upper arms; and sunken eyes and dry mouth

**Defining Characteristics**

- A weight of less than 70% (or less than 3 SD) of the median weight for height
- Underdeveloped buttocks, thighs, and upper arms
- Sunken eyes, dry mouth, and a history of diarrhea

**Related Factors**

- Poverty, lack of knowledge about available resources

**Short-Term Expected Outcomes**

The grandmother will:
- Increase health-promotion and health-maintenance knowledge regarding Don's nutrition.
- Increase health-promotion and health-maintenance practices regarding Don's nutrition.

- Gain access to available resources, such as food vouchers and Canadian Food Bank programs for families, women, infants, and children.

**Long-Term Expected Outcome**

- Don will show no signs of malnutrition.

**Interventions**

- Give Don fluids/food per protocol.
- Observe Don's fluid/food intake and monitor his signs and symptoms.
- If necessary, refer Don to an appropriate health care setting.
- Assess the grandmother's knowledge and practices regarding Don's nutrition.
- Educate the grandmother about the negative effects of malnutrition on Don's growth and development.
- Educate the grandmother about appropriate food choices for Don.
- Assist the family to access and connect with available nutrition community resources.
- Assist Don's parents to access the community career centre.
- Provide follow-ups to monitor Don's physical progress (body weight for age and height) and the family's access to available resources.

## SUMMARY

This chapter has presented priority issues and future directions for health professions in the areas of health promotion and disease prevention from a world perspective. Current emerging health care reform efforts pose significant challenges and opportunities for health care providers, educators, and researchers, with the emphasis on human rights, cultural diversity, and cultural sensitivity; health promotion and disease prevention; evidence-informed practice and advanced technology; and global perspectives. Nurses today are required to have sufficient vision, expertise, and the ability to truly make a difference in the health of the people for whom they care at individual, local community, national, and international levels. Through leadership, creativity, and determination, nurses and other health care providers can establish a healthier future for people around the globe with a respect for human needs, cultural diversity, and human rights.

**Evolve Chapter Features**

http://evolve.elsevier.com/Canada/Edelman/healthpromotion/

- Review Questions

## REFERENCES

Alexander, K. A., Sanderson, C. E., Marathe, M., et al. (2015). What factors might have led to the emergence of Ebola in West Africa? *PLoS Neglected Tropical Diseases, 9*(6), e0003652. https://doi.org/10.1371/journal.pntd.0003652.

AVERT. (2012). *Understanding HIV and AIDS statistics.* Retrieved from http://www.avert.org/statistics.htm.

AVERT. (2019). *HIV and AIDS in east and southern Africa.* Retrieved from https://www.avert.org/professionals/hiv-around-world/sub-saharan-africa/overview. [Seminal Reference].

Barthel, E. R., Pierce, J. R., Goodhue, C. J., et al. (2011). Availability of a pediatric trauma center in a disaster surge decreases triage time of the pediatric surge population: A population kinetics model. *Theoretical Biology and Medical Modeling, 8*(38), 1–32.

Bernardin, F., Maheut-Bosser, A., & Paille, F. (2014). Cognitive impairments in alcohol dependent subjects. *Frontiers in Psychiatry, 5*(78), 1–6.

Bhandarwar, A. H., Bakhshi, G. D., Tayade, M. B., et al. (2012). Surgical response to the 2008 Mumbai terror attack. *British Journal of Surgery, 99*(3), 368–372. https://doi.org/10.1002/bjs.7738.

Boscarino, J. A., & Adams, R. E. (2008). Overview of findings from the World Trade Center disaster outcome study: Recommendations for future research after exposure to psychological trauma. *International Journal of Emergency Mental Health, 10*(4), 275–290.

Bouassa, M., Prazuck, T., Lethu, T., et al. (2017). Cervical cancer in sub-saharan Africa: An emerging and preventable disease associated with oncogenic human papillomavirus. *Médecine et Santé Tropicales, 27*(1), 16–22. https://doi.org/10.1684/mst.2017.0648.

British Columbia Centre for Disease Control (BCCDC). (n.d.). *MRSA guidelines.* Retrieved from http://www.bccdc.ca/health-professionals/clinical-resources/mrsa#References.

British Columbia Centre for Disease Control (BCCDC). (2014). *Guidelines for the management of community-associated methicillin-resistant* Staphylococcus aureus *(CA-MRSA)–related skin and soft tissue infections in primary care.* Retrieved from http://www.bccdc.ca/resource-gallery/Documents/Statistics%20and%20Research/Statistics%20and%20Reports/Epid/Antibiotics/MRSAguidelineFINALJuly7.pdf.

British Columbia Centre for Disease Control (BCCDC). (n.d). A National Centre for Disease Control British Columbia. Retrieved from www.health.gov.bc.ca/library/publications/year/misc/diseasecontrol.pdf.

Bromet, E. J., Atwoli, L., Kawakami, N., et al. (2017). Post-traumatic stress disorder associated with natural and human-made disasters in the World Mental Health Surveys. *Psychological Medicine, 47*(2), 227–241. https://doi.org/10.1017/S0033291716002026.

Bryant, R. A., Ekasawin, S., Chakrabhand, S., et al. (2011). A randomized controlled effectiveness trial of cognitive behavior therapy for post-traumatic stress disorder in terrorist-affected people in Thailand. *World Psychiatry, 10*, 205–209.

Buesa, M., & Baumert, T. (2018). The economic impact of terrorism. In *Routledge handbook of terrorism and counterterrorism* (pp. 211–220). London: Routledge.

Cameron, L., & Shah, M. (2015). Risk-taking behavior in the wake of natural disasters. *Journal of Human Resources, 50*(2), 484–515.

Canadian Broadcasting Corporation (CBC). (2003). *Federal report: Learning from SARS renewal of public health in Canada.* Retrieved from https://www.cbc.ca/news2/background/sars/sars_report.html.

Canadian Centre on Substance Use and Addiction (CCSA). (2018). *Canada's national alcohol strategy.* Retrieved from http://www.ccsa.ca/national-alcohol-strategy-monitoring-project-status-report.

Canadian Domestic Homicide Prevention Initiative. (2016). *Domestic violence risk assessment: Informing safety planning and risk management.* Retrieved from http://endingviolence.org/wp-content/uploads/2016/12/Risk-Assessment-Brief.pdf.

Canadian Partnership Against Cancer. (2016). *New cervical cancer screening guidelines.* Retrieved from https://www.partnershipagainstcancer.ca/news-events/news/article/cervical-cancer-new-guidelines-shifting-overscreening-young-women/.

Centers for Disease Control and Prevention (CDC). (2015a). *Global health programs: International Micronutrient Malnutrition Prevention and Control Program (IMMPaCT).* Retrieved from https://www.cdc.gov/nutrition/micronutrient-malnutrition/index.html?CDC_AA_refVal=https%3A%2F%2Fwww.cdc.gov%2Fimmpact%2Findex.html.

Centers for Disease Control and Prevention (CDC). (2015b). *MRSA and the workplace.* Retrieved from http://www.cdc.gov/niosh/topics/mrsa/.

Centers for Disease Control and Prevention (CDC). (2016a). *A history of anthrax.* Retrieved from https://www.cdc.gov/anthrax/resources/history/index.html.

Centers for Disease Control and Prevention (CDC). (2016b). *Precautions to prevent spread of MRSA.* Retrieved from https://www.cdc.gov/mrsa/healthcare/clinicians/precautions.html.

Centers for Disease Control and Prevention (CDC). (2016c). *Symptoms.* Retrieved from https://www.cdc.gov/anthrax/basics/symptoms.html.

Centers for Disease Control and Prevention (CDC). (2017a). *Bioterrorism agents/diseases.* Retrieved from https://emergency.cdc.gov/agent/agentlist-category.asp.

Centers for Disease Control and Prevention (CDC). (2017b). *Syndrome definitions for diseases associated with critical bioterrorism-associated agents.* Retrieved from http://emergency.cdc.gov/bioterrorism/surveillance.asp.

Centers for Disease Control and Prevention (CDC). (2018a). *Ebola (Ebola virus disease).* Retrieved from http://www.cdc.gov/vhf/ebola.

Centers for Disease Control and Prevention (CDC). (2018b). *Emergency preparedness and response.* Retrieved from https://emergency.cdc.gov/.

Centers for Disease Control and Prevention (CDC). (2018c). *Intimate partner violence: Risk and protective factors.* Retrieved from http://www.cdc.gov/violenceprevention/intimatepartnerviolence/riskprotectivefactors.html.

Centers for Disease Control and Prevention (CDC). (2018d). *Prevention.* Retrieved from http://www.cdc.gov/anthrax/medical-care/prevention.html.

Centers for Disease Control and Prevention (CDC). (2018e). *US Zika pregnancy registry.* Retrieved from https://www.cdc.gov/pregnancy/zika/research/registry.html.

Centers for Disease Control and Prevention (CDC). (2018f). *Zika virus and sexual transmission.* Retrieved from https://www.cdc.gov/zika/prevention/sexual-transmission-prevention.html.

Centers for Disease Control and Prevention (CDC). (2018h). *Zika virus. Tools for health care providers.* Retrieved from https://www.cdc.gov/zika/hc-providers/.

Centers for Disease Control and Prevention (CDC). (2019a). *Emergency preparedness and response.* Retrieved from https://emergency.cdc.gov/disasters/.

Centers for Disease Control and Prevention (CDC). (2019b). *Namibia country profile.* Retrieved from https://www.cdc.gov/globalhivtb/where-we-work/namibia/namibia.html.

Central Intelligence Agency (CIA). (2016). *HIV/AIDS adult prevalence rates.* Retrieved from https://www.cia.gov/library/publications/the-world-factbook/rankorder/2155rank.html.

Central Intelligence Agency (CIA). (2017). *Life expectancy at birth.* Retrieved from https://www.cia.gov/library/publications/the-world-factbook/rankorder/2102rank.html.

Coelho, F. C., Durovni, B., Saraceni, V., et al. (2016). Higher incidence of Zika in adult women than adult men in Rio de Janeiro suggests a significant contribution of sexual transmission from men to women. *International Journal of Infectious Diseases, 51*, 128–132. https://doi.org/10.1016/j.ijid.2016.08.023.

Compaore, S., Ouedraogo, C. M. R., Koanda, S., et al. (2015). Barriers to cervical cancer screening in Burkina Faso: Needs for patient and professional education. *Journal of Cancer Education*, 1–7. https://doi.org/10.1007/s13187-015-0898-9.

Donken, R., Ogilvie, G. S., Bettinger, J. A., et al. (2018). Effect of human papillomavirus vaccination on sexual behaviour among young females. *Canadian Family Physician/Medecin de Famille Canadien, 64*(7), 509–513.

Fan, F., Zhou, Y., Long, K., et al. (2015). Longitudinal trajectories of post-traumatic stress disorder symptoms among adolescents after the Wenchuan earthquake in China. *Psychological Medicine, 45*(13), 2885–2896. https://doi.org/10.1017/S0033291715000884.

Feder, A., Mota, N., Salim, R., et al. (2016). Risk, coping and PTSD symptom trajectories in World Trade Center responders. *Journal of Psychiatric Research, 82*, 68–79. https://doi.org/10.1016/j.jpsychires.2016.07.003.

Fekete, T. (2007). Emerging infections: What you need to know, part 1. *Consultant, 47*(12), 1013–1016. [Seminal Reference].

Fischer, W. A., & Wohl, D. A. (2016). *Confronting Ebola as a sexually transmitted infection. Clinical infectious diseases.* An Official Publication of the Infectious Diseases Society of America. https://doi.org/10.1093/cid/ciw123.

Food and Agriculture Organization of the United Nations, International Fund for Agricultural Development, UNICEF, World Food Program, & World Health Organization. (2017). *The state of food insecurity in the world 2017. Building resilience for peace and food security.* Rome: Author. Retrieved from http://www.fao.org/3/a-I7695e.pdf.

Fosse, E., & Helgesen, M. (2017). Advocating for health promotion policy in Norway: The role of the county municipalities. *Societies, 7*(5), 1–10. https://doi:10.3390/soc7020005. Retrieved from file:///C:/Users/rhumb/Downloads/societies-07-00005-v2%20(1).pdf.

Fulu, E., Jewkes, R., Roselli, T., et al. (2013). Prevalence of and factors associated with male perpetration of intimate partner violence: Findings from the UN multi-country cross-sectional study on men and violence in Asia and the Pacific. *The Lancet Global Health, 1*(4), e187–e207. https://doi.org/10.1016/S2214-109X(13)70074-3.

GAVI Alliance. (2016). *Review of GAVI support for HPV vaccine.* Retrieved from https://www.gavi.org/search/?SearchText=HPV.

Gelting, R., Bliss, K., Patrick, M., Lockhard, G., & Handzel, T. (2013). Water, sanitation and hygiene in Haiti: Past, present, and future. *The American Journal of Tropical Medicine and Hygiene, 89*(4), 665–670.

Glass, N., Clough, A., Hanson, G., et al. (2015). A safety app to respond to dating violence for college women and their friends: The MyPlan study randomized controlled trial protocol. *BMC Public Health, 15*(1), 871. https://doi.org/10.1186/s12889-015-2191-6.

Gouws, E., & Guchi, P. (2015). Focusing on HIV response through estimating the major modes of HIV transmission: A multi-country analysis. *Sexually Transmitted Infections, 88*(Suppl. 2), i76–i85. https://doi.org/10.1136/sextrans-2012-050719.

Government of Canada. (2017a). *Section 2: Police-reported intimate partner violence in Canada, 2017.* Retrieved from https://www150.statcan.gc.ca/n1/pub/85-002-x/2018001/article/54978/02-eng.htm.

Government of Canada. (2017b). *Federal/provincial/territorial public health response plan for biological events.* Retrieved from https://www.canada.ca/en/public-health/services/emergency-preparedness/public-health-response-plan-biological-events.html.

Government of Canada. (2019). *Social determinants of health and health inequalities.* Retrieved from https://www.canada.ca/en/public-health/services/health-promotion/population-health/what-determines-health.html.

Gribble, K. (2018). Supporting the most vulnerable through appropriate infant and young child feeding in emergencies. *Journal of Human Lactation, 34*(1), 40–46. Retrieved from https://journals.sagepub.com/doi/pdf/10.1177/0890334417741469.

Gribble, K. D., & Berry, N. (2011). Emergency preparedness for those who care for infants in developed country contexts. *International Breastfeeding Journal, 6*(16). Retrieved from http://www.internationalbreastfeedingjournal.com/content/pdf/1746-4358-6-16.pdf.

Grimm, M. J., Helgesen, M. K., & Fosse, E. (2013). Reducing social inequities in health in Norway: Concerted action at state and local levels? *Health Policy, 113*(3), 228–235. https://doi.org/10.1016/j.healthpol.2013.09.019.

Hattori, T., Chagan-Yasutan, H., Shiratori, B., et al. (2016). Development of point-of-care testing for disaster-related infectious diseases. *Tohoku Journal of Experimental Medicine, 238*(4), 287–293. https://doi.org/10.1620/tjem.238.287.

Health Canada. (2003). *Learning from SARS: Renewal of public health in Canada.* A report of the National Advisory Committee on SARS and public health. Retrieved from http://www.phac-aspc.gc.ca/publicat/sars-sras/pdf/sars-e.pdf.

Health Canada. (2019). *Canadian immunization guide: Smallpox vaccine.* Ottawa: Government of Canada. Retrieved from https://www.canada.ca/en/public-health/services/publications/healthy-living/canadian-immunization-guide-part-4-active-vaccines/page-21-smallpox-vaccine.html.

Heine, H. S., Shadomy, S. V., Boyer, A. E., et al. (2017). Evaluation of combination drug therapy for treatment of antibiotic-resistant inhalation anthrax in a murine model. *Antimicrobial Agents and Chemotherapy, 61*(9), e00788 -17. https://doi.org/10.1128/AAC.00788-17.

Hendricks, K. A. (2017). *Centers for Disease Control and Prevention Anthrax Vaccine Workgroup.* Updating recommendations for use of anthrax vaccine in the United States. Retrieved from https://stacks.cdc.gov/view/cdc/58929.

Hu, S. H., Cofie, R., Tan, H., et al. (2015). Recovery from post-traumatic stress disorder after a flood in China: A 13-year follow-up and its prediction by degree of collective action. *BMC Public Health, 15*(615), 2–7. https://doi.org/10.1186/s12889-015-2009-6.

International Agency for Research on Cancer. (2018). *Latest world cancer statistics. Global cancer burden rises to 18.1 million new cases and 9.6 million cancer deaths in 2018*, Press release no. 263. Retrieved from https://www.iarc.fr/wp-content/uploads/2018/09/pr263_E.pdf.

International Federation of Red Cross (IFRC) and Red Crescent Societies (RCS). (2018). *World disaster report 2018.* Retrieved from https://media.ifrc.org/ifrc/world-disaster-report-2018/.

Jeronimo, J., Bansil, P., Lim, J., et al. (2014). A multicountry evaluation of care: HPV testing, visual inspection with acetic acid, and Papanicolaou testing for the detection of cervical cancer. *International Journal of Gynecological Cancer, 24*(3), 576–585.

Joint United Nations Programme on HIV/AIDS (UNAIDS). (2015). *90-90-90: Treatment for all.* Retrieved from http://www.unaids.org/en/resources/909090.

Joint United Nations Programme on HIV/AIDS. (UNAIDS). (2017b). *State of the AIDS epidemic.* Retrieved from http://www.unaids.org/sites/default/files/media_asset/2017_data-book_en.pdf.

Joint United Nations Programme on HIV/AIDS (UNAIDS). (2012). *Independent review: NGO/Civil society participation in the UNAIDS Programme Coordinating Board.* Retrieved from http://files.unaids.org/en/media/unaids/contentassets/documents/pcb/2012/20121116_PCB31_CRP3_Review_Civil_Society_Participation_in_UNAIDS_Final_en.pdf.

Joint United Nations Programme on HIV/AIDS (UNAIDS). (2017a). *Getting to zero: How will we fast track the aids response?* Discussion paper for consultations on UNAIDS strategy 2016–2021. Retrieved from http://www.icad-cisd.com/pdf/UNAIDS/Strategy-Consultations/1-UNAIDS-Discussion-Paper_2016-2021-Strategy-Consultations.

Joint United Nations Programme on HIV/AIDS (UNAIDS). (2018). *Fact sheet—world AIDS day 2018. Commemorating 30 years.* Retrieved from http://www.unaids.org/sites/default/files/media_asset/UNAIDS_FactSheet_en.pdf.

Jones, C. P., Jones, C. Y., Perry, G. S., et al. (2009). Addressing the social determinants of children's health: A cliff analogy. *Journal of Health Care for the Poor and Underserved, 20*(4A), 1–12.

Khoury, N. M., Kaiser, B. N., Keys, H. M., et al. (2012). Explanatory models and mental health treatment: Is vodou an obstacle to psychiatric treatment in rural Haiti? *Culture, Medicine and Psychiatry, 36*(3), 514–534.

Kirkland, E. B., & Adams, B. B. (2008). Methicillin-resistant *Staphylococcus aureus* and athletes. *Journal of the American Academy of Dermatology, 59*(3), 494–502.

Knox, B. (2018). Screening women for intimate partner violence: Creating proper practice habits. *The Nurse Practitioner, 43*(5), 14–20. https://doi.org/10.1097/01.NPR.0000531918.92139. ca Retrieved from https://journals.lww.com/tnpj/Fulltext/2018/05000/Screening_women_for_intimate_partner_violence_.3.aspx.

Koistinen, I., & Holma, J. (2015). Finnish health care professionals' views of patients who experience family violence. *Sage Open, 5*(1). https://doi.org/10.1177/2158244015570392.

Learmonth, D., van Vuuren, A. J., & De Abreu, C. (2015). The influence of gender roles and traditional healing on cervical screening adherence amongst women in a Cape Town peri-urban settlement. *South African Family Practice, 57*(2), 62–63. https://doi.org/10.1080/20786190.2014.978096.

Lim, J. N. W., & Ojo, A. A. (2016). Barriers to utilisation of cervical cancer screening in sub-saharan Africa: A systematic review. *European Journal of Cancer Care, 26*(1). https://doi.org/10.1111/ecc.12444.

Loke, A. Y., & Fung, O. W. M. (2014). Nurses' competencies in disaster nursing: Implications for curriculum development and public health. *International Journal of Environmental Research and Public Health, 11*(3), 3289–3303.

Lorenzi, A. T., Fregnani, J. H. T., Possati-Resende, J. C., et al. (2016). Can the careHPV test performed in mobile units replace cytology for screening in rural and remote areas? *Cancer Cytopathology, 124*(8), 581–588. https://doi.org/10.1002/cncy.21718.

Lowney, J. (2016). *Our impact.* Haitian Health Foundation. Retrieved from http://www.haitianhealthfoundation.org/our-impact/.

Lupton, K. (2015). Preparing nurses to work in Ebola treatment centres in Sierra Leone. *British Journal of Nursing, 24*(3), 168–172. https://doi.org/10.12968/bjon.2015.24.3.168.

Management Sciences for Health. (2017). *A powerful new ally in the effort to prevent HIV in Namibia.* Retrieved from https://www.msh.org/news-events/stories/a-powerful-new-ally-in-the-effort-to-prevent-hiv-in-namibia.

Marion, D., Charlebois, P. B., & Kao, R. (2016). The healthcare workers' clinical skill set requirements for a uniformed international response to the Ebola virus disease outbreak in West Africa: The Canadian perspective. *Journal of the Royal Army Medical Corps, 162*(3), 207–211.

McAlister, E. A. (2016). *Vodou: Haitian religion.* Retrieved from http://www.britannica.com/topic/Vodou.

McFarlane, J., Symes, L., Binder, B. K., et al. (2014). Maternal-child dyads of functioning: The intergenerational impact of violence against women on children. *Maternal and Child Health Journal, 18*(9), 2236–2243. https://doi.org/10.1007/s10995-014-1473-4.

Mikkonen, J., & Raphael, D. (2010). *Social determinants of health: The Canadian facts.* Toronto: York University, School of Health Policy and Management.

Millar, A., Code, R., & Ha, L. (2013). *Inventory of spousal violence risk assessment tools used in Canada.* Ottawa: Research and Statistics Division, Department of Justice Canada. Retrieved from https://www.justice.gc.ca/eng/rp-pr/cj-jp/fv-vf/rr09_7/rr09_7.pdf.

Modibbo, F. I., Bamisaye, P., Dareng, E., et al. (2016). Qualitative study of barriers to cervical cancer screening among Nigerian women. *BMJ Open, 6*(1):e008533. https://doi.org/10.1136/bmjopen-2015-008533.

Morgan, T. (2015). Putting a price on peace: The total cost of violence to the global economy. In L. Bouckaert, & M. Chatterji (Eds.), *Business, ethics and peace (contributions to conflict management, peace economics and development)* (Vol. 24) (pp. 247–264). Bingley, UK: Emerald Group Publishing Limited.

Nanyonga, M., Saidu, J., Ramsay, A., et al. (2016). Sequelae of Ebola virus disease, kenema district, Sierra Leone. *Clinical Infectious Diseases, 62*(1), 125–126. https://doi.org/10.1093/cid/civ795.

Oxfam International. (2015). *Haiti earthquake, our response.* Retrieved from https://www.oxfam.org/en/haiti-earthquake-our-response.

Phalkey, R. K., & Louis, V. R. (2016). Two hot to handle: How do we manage the simultaneous impacts of climate change and natural disasters on human health? *The European Physical Journal—Special Topics, 225*(3), 443–457. https://doi.org/10.1140/epjst/e2016-60071-y.

Public Health Agency of Canada (PHAC). (2007). *Core competencies for public health in Canada.* Ottawa: Author. Retrieved from http://www.phac-aspc.gc.ca/php-psp/ccph-cesp/pdfs/cc-manual-eng090407.pdf.

Public Health Agency of Canada (PHAC). (2008). *Chief Public Health Officer's reports on the state of public health in Canada 2008: Addressing health inequalities.* Retrieved from https://www.canada.ca/en/public-health/corporate/publications/chief-public-health-officer-reports-state-public-health-canada/report-on-state-public-health-canada-2008/chapter-2a.html.

Public Health Agency of Canada (PHAC). (2012). *WHO facts on alcohol and violence: Intimate partner violence and alcohol.* Retrieved from https://www.canada.ca/en/public-health/services/health-promotion/stop-family-violence/prevention-resource-centre/women/who-facts-on-alcohol-violence-intimate-partner-violence-alcohol.html.

Public Health Agency of Canada (PHAC). (2015). *Update on the recommended Human Papillomavirus vaccine immunization schedule.* Ottawa: Author. Retrieved from https://www.canada.ca/en/public-health/services/publications/healthy-living/update-recommended-human-papillomavirus-vaccine-immunization-schedule.html.

Public Health Agency of Canada (PHAC). (2016). *MRSA in Canada.* Ottawa: Author. Retrieved from https://www.canada.ca/en/public-health/services/publications/drugs-health-products/canadian-antimicrobial-resistance-surveillance-system-report-2016.html#a4-2-3.

Public Health Agency of Canada (PHAC). (2017). *Human papillomavirus (HPV).* Ottawa: Author. Retrieved from https://www.canada.ca/en/public-health/services/infectious-diseases/sexual-health-sexually-transmitted-infections/human-papillomavirus-hpv.html#sm.

Public Health Agency of Canada (PHAC). (2018a). *Emergency preparedness and response.* Ottawa: Author. Retrieved from https://www.canada.ca/en/public-health/services/emergency-preparedness-response.html.

Public Health Agency of Canada (PHAC). (2018b). *First nations and Inuit health.* Ottawa: Author. Retrieved from https://www.canada.ca/en/indigenous-services-canada/services/first-nations-inuit-health.html.

Public Health Agency of Canada (PHAC). (2018c). *Trauma and violence-informed approaches to policy and practice*. Ottawa: Author. Retrieved from https://www.canada.ca/en/public-health/services/publications/health-risks-safety/trauma-violence-informed-approaches-policy-practice.html.

Public Health Agency of Canada (PHAC). (2019). *Zika virus: Symptoms and treatment*. Ottawa: Author. Retrieved from https://www.canada.ca/en/public-health/services/diseases/zika-virus/health-professionals.html.

Public Health Association of British Columbia (PHABC). (2006). *Public health core functions implementation*. Retrieved from https://phabc.org/presentation/public-health-core-functions-implementation/.

Purnell, L. D. (2008). Transcultural diversity and health care. In L. D. Purnell, & B. J. Paulanka (Eds.), *Transcultural health care: A culturally competent approach* (pp. 1–18). Philadelphia: F.A. Davis.

Republic of Namibia. (2017). *National strategic framework for HIV and AIDS response in Namibia 2017/18 to 2021/22*. Ministry of health and social services directorate of special programmes. Retrieved from https://www.unaids.org/sites/default/files/country/documents/NAM_2018_countryreport.pdf.

Rogstad, K. E., & Tunbridge, A. (2015). Ebola virus as a sexually transmitted infection. *Current Opinion in Infectious Diseases, 28*(1), 83–85. https://doi.org/10.1097/QCO.0000000000000135.

Rootman, I., Dupere, S., Pederson, A., et al. (2012). *Health promotion in Canada* (3rd ed.). Toronto: Canadian Scholars Press.

Ross, R., Saenyakul, P., Stidham, A. W., et al. (2015). Intimate partner violence, emotional support, and health outcomes among Thai women: A mixed methods study. *Journal of the Royal Thai Army Nurses, 16*(1), 14–24.

Salazar, M. A., Pesigan, A., Law, R., et al. (2016). Post-disaster health impact of natural hazards in the Philippines in 2013. *Global Health Action, 9*(1), 31320. https://doi.org/10.3402/gha.v9.31320.

Santoro, D. (2018). A cosmopolitanism of fear: The global significance of terrorism after the 9/11. *Knowledge Cultures, 6*(3), 28. https://doi.org/10.22381/KC6320182.

Schlievert, P. M., Nemeth, K. A., Davis, C. C., et al. (2010). *Staphylococcus aureus* exotoxins are present *in vivo* in tampons. *Clinical and Vaccine Immunology: CVI, 17*(5), 722–727. https://doi.org/10.1128/CVI.00483-09.

Sedighi, I., Moez, H. J., & Alikhani, M. Y. (2011). Nasal carriage of methicillin resistant staphylococcus aureus and their antibiotic susceptibility patterns in children attending day-care centers. Acta Microbiologica Et Immunologica Hungarica, 58(3), 227.

Shuaib, F. M., Musa, P. F., Muhammad, A., et al. (2017). Containment of Ebola and polio in low-resource settings using principles and practices of emergency operations centers in public health. *Journal of Public Health Management and Practice: JPHMP, 23*(1), 3–10. https://doi.org/10.1097/PHH.0000000000000447.

Sieppert, J., Te Linde, J., & Rutherford, G. (2004). Addressing poverty as a determinant of health: Capturing the voices of low income calgarians. *Canadian Review of Social Policy/Revue canadienne de politique sociale, 53*, 122–139.

Steben, M., Thompson, M. T., Rodier, C., et al. (2018). A review of the impact and effectiveness of the quadrivalent human papillomavirus vaccine: 10 years of clinical experience in Canada. *JOGC, 40*(12), 1635–1645. https://doi.org/10.1016/j.jogc.2018.05.024.

Telesur. (2018). *Namibia: HIV fight is gaining ground*. Retrieved from https://www.telesurenglish.net/news/Namibia-HIV-Fight-is-Gaining-Ground-20181202-0005.html.

The Canadian Encyclopedia. (2015). *Severe acute respiratory syndrome*. Retrieved from https://www.thecanadianencyclopedia.ca/en/article/sars-severe-acute-respiratory-syndrome.

Tiffany, A., Vetter, P., Mattia, J., et al. (2016). Ebola virus disease complications as experienced by survivors in Sierra Leone. *Clinical Infectious Diseases, 62*(11), 1360–1366. https://doi.org/10.1093/cid/ciw158.

Tsu, V. D., Njama-Meya, D., Lim, J., et al. (2018). Opportunities and challenges for introducing HPV testing for cervical cancer screening in sub-Saharan Africa. *Preventive Medicine, 114*, 205–208. https://doi.org/10.1016/j.ypmed.2018.07.012.

United Nations. (2015). *State of the world's Indigenous peoples: Indigenous peoples' access to health services*. Geneva: United Nations, Department of Economic and Social Affairs. Retrieved from https://www.un.org/development/desa/indigenouspeoples/wp-content/uploads/sites/19/2018/03/The-State-of-The-Worlds-Indigenous-Peoples-WEB.pdf.

United Nations Children's Fund (UNICEF) & WHO. (2018). *The baby friendly hospital initiative*. Retrieved from https://www.who.int/nutrition/bfhi/en/.

United Nations Children's Fund (UNICEF). (2018). *Levels & trends in child mortality*. Retrieved from http://www.childmortality.org/files_v22/download/UN%20IGME%20Child%20Mortality%20Report%202018.pdf.

United Nations Development Programme. (2016). *Sustainable development goals*. Retrieved from https://www.undp.org/content/undp/en/home/sustainable-development-goals.html.

United Nations General Assembly. (2015). *Transforming our world: The 2030 agenda for sustainable development*. Retrieved from https://www.un.org/sustainabledevelopment/sustainable-development-goals/.

United Nations (n.d.). *Sustainable development goals: About the sustainable development goals*. Retrieved from https://www.un.org/sustainabledevelopment/sustainable-development-goals/.

Vahabi, M., & Lofters, A. (2018). HPV self-sampling: A promising approach to reduce cervical cancer screening disparities in Canada. *Current Oncology, 25*(1), 13. https://doi.org/10.3747/co.25.3845.

Vallgarda, S. (2008). Social inequality in health: Dichotomy or gradient? *Health Policy, 85*(1), 71–82.

Van Berlaer, G., Staes, T., Danschutter, D., et al. (2017). Disaster preparedness and response improvement: Comparison of the 2010 Haiti earthquake-related diagnoses with baseline medical data. *European Journal of Emergency Medicine, 24*(5), 382. https://doi.org/10.1097/MEJ.0000000000000387.

Veenema, T. G., Griffin, A., Gable, A. R., et al. (2016). Nurses as leaders in disaster preparedness and response—a call to action. *Journal of Nursing Scholarship, 48*(2), 187–200. https://doi.org/10.1111/jnu.12198.

Walling, E. B., Benzoni, N., Dornfeld, J., et al. (2016). Interventions to improve HPV vaccine uptake: A systematic review. *Pediatrics, 138*(1):e20153863. https://doi.org/10.1542/peds.2015-3863. Retrieved from http://pediatrics.aappublications.org/content/pediatrics/138/1/e20153863.full.pdf.

Warsini, S., Mills, J. E., Buettner, P., et al. (2015). Post-traumatic stress disorder among survivors two years after the 2010 Mount Merapi volcano eruption: A survey study. *Nursing and Health Sciences, 17*(2), 173–180. https://doi.org/10.1111/nhs.12152.

Whitehead, M., & Popay, J. (2010). Swimming upstream? Taking action on the social determinants of health inequalities. *Social Science & Medicine, 71*(7), 1234–1236.

White, L., Waldrop, J., & Waldrop, C. (2016). Human papillomavirus and vaccination of males: Knowledge and attitudes of registered nurses. *Pediatric Nursing, 42*(1), 21–35.

Wilder-Smith, A., Vannice, K., Durbin, A., et al. (2018). Zika vaccines and therapeutics: Landscape analysis and challenges ahead. *BMC Medicine, 16*(1), 84. https://doi.org/10.1186/s12916-018-1067-x.

World Health Organization (WHO) & United Nations Children's Fund (UNICEF). (2009). *Child growth standards and the identification of severe acute malnutrition in infants and children.* Retrieved from http://www.who.int/nutrition/publications/severemalnutrition/9789241598163_eng.pdf.

World Health Organization (WHO). (2000). *Turning the tide of malnutrition: Responding to the challenge of the 21st century.* WHO/NHD/00.7. Geneva: Author. Retrieved from https://apps.who.int/iris/bitstream/handle/10665/66505/WHO_NHD_00.7.pdf?sequence=1&isAllowed=y.

World Health Organization (WHO). (2007). *Health of indigenous peoples.* Retrieved from https://www.who.int/mediacentre/factsheets/fs326/en/.

World Health Organization (WHO). (2011). *The WHO child growth standards.* Retrieved from http://www.who.int/childgrowth/standards/en/.

World Health Organization (WHO). (2013). *Guideline: Updates on the management of severe acute malnutrition in infants and children.* Geneva: Author. Retrieved from http://www.kznhealth.gov.za/family/MCWH/Servere-acute-malnutrition-infants-and-children.pdf.

World Health Organization (WHO). (2014a). *Global status report on violence prevention 2014.* Retrieved from https://www.who.int/violence_injury_prevention/publications/violence/en/.

World Health Organization (WHO). (2014b). *New WHO guide to prevent and control cervical cancer.* Retrieved from http://www.who.int/mediacentre/news/releases/2014/preventing-cervical-cancer/en/.

World Health Organization (WHO). (2016a). *Alert, response, and capacity building under the international health regulations (IHR).* Retrieved from http://www.who.int/features/qa/39/en/index.html.

World Health Organization (WHO). (2016b). *Epidemic intelligence—systematic event detection.* Retrieved from http://www.who.int/csr/alertresponse/epidemicintelligence/en/.

World Health Organization (WHO). (2016c). *IASC guidelines on mental health and psychosocial support in emergency settings.* Retrieved from http://www.who.int/mental_health/emergencies/IASC_guidelines.pdf.

World Health Organization (WHO). (2016d). *What is malnutrition?.* Retrieved from http://www.who.int/features/qa/malnutrition/en/.

World Health Organization (WHO). (2017). *The top 10 causes of death.* Retrieved from https://www.who.int/en/news-room/fact-sheets/detail/the-top-10-causes-of-death.

World Health Organization (WHO). (2018a). *Ebola virus disease.* Retrieved from https://www.who.int/en/news-room/fact-sheets/detail/ebola-virus-disease.

World Health Organization (WHO). (2018b). *Malnutrition: Key facts.* Retrieved from https://www.who.int/news-room/fact-sheets/detail/malnutrition.

World Health Organization (WHO). (2018c). *Mental health.* Retrieved from https://www.who.int/en/news-room/fact-sheets/detail/suicide.

World Health Organization (WHO). (2018d). *Mental health atlas 2017: Haiti.* Retrieved from https://www.who.int/mental_health/evidence/atlas/profiles-2017/HTI.pdf.

World Health Organization (WHO). (2018e). *National suicide prevention strategies: Progress, examples and indicators.* Retrieved from https://apps.who.int/iris/bitstream/handle/10665/279765/9789241515016-eng.pdf?ua=1.

World Health Organization (WHO). (2018f). *Obesity and overweight.* Retrieved from https://www.who.int/en/news-room/fact-sheets/detail/obesity-and-overweight.

World Health Organization (WHO). (2018g). *Zika virus.* Retrieved from http://www.who.int/topics/zika/en/.

World Health Organization (WHO). (2019a). *Definition and typology of violence.* Retrieved from http://www.who.int/violenceprevention/approach/definition/en/.

World Health Organization (WHO). (2019b). *Global health observatory data.* Retrieved from http://www.who.int/gho/ncd/mortality_morbidity/en/.

World Health Organization (WHO). (2019c). *Human papillomavirus (HPV) and cervical cancer.* Retrieved from https://www.who.int/en/news-room/fact-sheets/detail/human-papillomavirus-(hpv)-and-cervical-cancer.

World Health Organization (WHO). (2019d). *Social determinants of health.* Retrieved from https://www.who.int/social_determinants/thecommission/finalreport/key_concepts/en/.

World Health Organization (WHO). (2019e). *Violence and injury prevention.* Retrieved from https://www.who.int/violence_injury_prevention/violence/en/.

World Hunger Education Service. (2018). 2018 *World hunger and poverty facts and statistics.* Retrieved from https://www.worldhunger.org/world-hunger-and-poverty-facts-and-statistics/.

Wosu, A. C., Gelaye, B., & Williams, M. A. (2015). History of childhood sexual abuse and risk of prenatal and postpartum depression or depressive symptoms: An epidemiologic review. *Archives of Women's Mental Health, 18*(5), 659–671. https://doi.org/10.1007/s00737-015-0533-0.

# INDEX

Page numbers followed by '*f*' indicate figures, '*t*' indicate tables, and '*b*' indicate boxes.